AIDS and Other Manifestations of HIV Infection

Second Edition

AIDS and Other Manifestations of HIV Infection

Second Edition

Editor

Gary P. Wormser, M.D.

Chief, Division of Infectious Diseases
Professor of Medicine and Pharmacology
New York Medical College
Westchester County Medical Center
Valhalla, New York

Raven Press · New York

Raven Press, Ltd., 1185 Avenue of the Americas, New York, New York 10036

Made in the United States of America

Library of Congress Cataloging-in-Publication Data

AIDS and other manifestations of HIV infection/edited by Gary P. Wormser.—2nd ed.
   p. cm.
  Rev. ed. of: AIDS acquired immune deficiency syndrome, and other manifestations of HIV infection. ©1987.
  Includes bibliographical references and index.
  ISBN 0-88167-881-3
  1. AIDS (Disease) 2. HIV infections. I. Wormser, Gary P.
II. AIDS, acquired immune deficiency syndrome, and other manifestations of HIV infection.
  [DNLM: 1. Acquired Immunodeficiency Syndrome. 2. HIV. 3. HIV Infections. WD 308 A28762]
RC607.A26A3455535 1992
616.97′92—dc20
DNLM/DLC
for Library of Congress   92-3572
                                              CIP

9 8 7 6 5 4 3 2 1

To
John I. Wormser, Ronald P. Wormser,
and to the
memory of Ruth S. Wormser

Contents

Contributing Authors

G. L. Ada, D.Sc. *Department of Immunology and Infectious Diseases, Johns Hopkins University School of Hygiene and Public Health, 615 North Wolfe Street, Baltimore, Maryland 21205; Present Address: Division of Cell Biology, John Curtin School of Medical Research, Australian National University, Canberra, ACT 2601, Australia*

Ronald Bayer, Ph.D. *Columbia University, School of Public Health, 600 West 168th Street, New York, New York 10032*

Anita L. Belman, M.D. *Department of Neurology, State University of New York at Stony Brook, Stony Brook, New York 11794*

Robert C. Bollinger, M.D., M.P.H. *Department of Medicine, Johns Hopkins University School of Medicine, Baltimore, Maryland 21205*

Edward J. Bottone, Ph.D. *Departments of Microbiology and Pathology, Mount Sinai Medical Center, 1 Gustave L. Levy Place, New York, New York 10029-6574*

Dania Caron, M.D. *Department of Medicine, New York University Medical Center, 426 First Avenue, New York, New York 10016; Present Address: Department of Clinical Affairs, Immunex Corporation, Seattle, Washington 98101*

Clay J. Cockerell, M.D. *Departments of Dermatology and Pathology, Division of Dermatopathology, University of Texas Southwestern Medical Center, 5323 Harry Hines Boulevard, Dallas, Texas 75235-9072*

John M. Coffin, Ph.D. *Department of Molecular Biology and Microbiology, Tufts University School of Medicine, 136 Harrison Avenue, Boston, Massachusetts 02111*

Mary Ann Adler Cohen, M.D., F.A.C.P. *Department of Psychiatry, New York Medical College, Metropolitan Hospital Center, 1900 Second Avenue, New York, New York 10029*

Richard Conviser, Ph.D. *New Jersey Medical and Dental School; and Children's Hospital, Newark, New Jersey 07103*

Don C. Des Jarlais, Ph.D. *Chemical Dependency Institute, Beth Israel Medical Center, First Avenue and 16th Street, New York, New York 10013*

D. Peter Drotman, M.D., M.P.H., F.A.C.P.M. *Division of HIV/AIDS, National Center for Infectious Diseases, Centers for Disease Control, 1600 Clifton Road, Atlanta, Georgia 30333*

Brad M. Dworkin, M.D., F.A.C.G., F.A.C.N. *Department of Gastroenterology, Westchester County Medical Center, New York Medical College, Valhalla, New York 10595*

Debra Fertel, M.D. *Pulmonary Division, University of Miami School of Medicine, 1201 Northwest 16th Street, Miami, Florida 33125*

James L. Finley, M.D. *Department of Pathology and Laboratory Medicine, East Carolina University School of Medicine, Moye Boulevard, Greenville, North Carolina 27858-4354*

Donald P. Francis, M.D., D.Sc.
Department of Health Services, Berkeley, California 94704

Samuel R. Friedman, Ph.D. *Narcotic and Drug Research, Inc., 11 Beach Street, New York, New York 10013*

Patricia N. Fultz, Ph.D. *Department of Microbiology, University of Alabama at Birmingham, School of Medicine, 1918 University Avenue, Birmingham, Alabama 35294*

Murray B. Gardner, M.D. *Department of Medical Pathology, California Primate Research Center, University of California, Davis, California 95616*

Helene D. Gayle, M.D., M.P.H. *International Activity, Division of HIV/AIDS, National Center for Infectious Diseases, Centers for Disease Control, 1600 Clifton Road, Atlanta, Georgia 30333*

Howard E. Gendelman, M.D. *Department of Cellular Immunology, Walter Reed Army Institute of Research, 9620 Medical Center Drive, Suite 200, Rockville, Maryland 20850; and the Henry M. Jackson Foundation for the Advancement of Military Medicine, Washington, D.C. 20037*

Parkash S. Gill, M.D. *Division of Hematology, Department of Internal Medicine, University of Southern California School of Medicine, Los Angeles, California 90033*

Deborah Greenspan, B.D.S., D.Sc. *Department of Stomatology, University of California at San Francisco, San Francisco, California 94143-0512*

John S. Greenspan, B.D.S., Ph.D., F.R.C.Path *Department of Stomatology, University of California at San Francisco, Box 0512, San Francisco, California 94143-0512*

Samuel Grubman, M.D. *University of Medicine and Dentistry of New Jersey/New Jersey Medical School; and Children's Hospital, 15 South Ninth Street, Newark, New Jersey 07107*

John W. Hadden, M.D. *Department of Medicine, University of South Florida Medical College, 12901 North 30th Street, Tampa, Florida 33612*

William L. Heyward, M.D., M.P.H. *International Activity, Division of HIV/AIDS, National Center for Infectious Diseases, Centers for Disease Control, 1600 Clifton Road, Atlanta, Georgia 30333*

Scott D. Holmberg, M.D., M.P.H. *Division of HIV/AIDS, National Center for Infectious Diseases, Centers for Disease Control, Public Health Service, U.S. Department of Health and Human Services, 1600 Clifton Road, Atlanta, Georgia 30333*

Harold Horowitz, M.D. *Division of Infectious Diseases, Department of Medicine, New York Medical College, Westchester County Medical Center, Valhalla, New York 10595*

Douglas A. Jabs, M.D. *Departments of Ophthalmology and Medicine, Johns Hopkins University School of Medicine, 550 North Broadway, Suite 700, Baltimore, Maryland 21205*

Daniel Jacobson, M.D. *Division of Oncology, New York University Medical Center, New York, New York 10016; and Research Service, New York VA Medical Center, 423 East 23rd Street, New York, New York 10010*

Carol Joline, R.N., B.A. *AIDS Management Program, Westchester County Medical Center, Valhalla, New York 10595*

Vijay V. Joshi, M.D., Ph.D. *Department of Pathology and Laboratory Medicine, East Carolina University School of Medicine, Pitt County Memorial Hospital, Brody Boulevard, Greenville, North Carolina 27858*

D. Chester Kalter, M.D. *Department of Cellular Immunology, Walter Reed Army Institute of Research, 9620 Medical Center Drive, Rockville, Maryland 20850; and the Henry M. Jackson Foundation for the Advancement of Military Medicine, Washington, D.C. 20037*

Phyllis J. Kanki, D.V.M., S.D.
Department of Cancer Biology, Harvard School of Public Health, 677 Huntington Avenue, Building 1, Room 909, Boston, Massachusetts 02115

Barbara W. Kilbourne, R.N., M.P.H.
Division of HIV/AIDS, Center for Infectious Diseases, Centers for Disease Control, Public Health Service, U.S. Department of Health and Human Services, 1600 Clifton Road, Atlanta, Georgia 30333

Barbara S. Koppel, M.D. *Department of Neurology, New York Medical College, Valhalla, New York 10595; and Metropolitan Hospital, 1901 First Avenue, New York, New York 10029*

Lauren B. Krupp, M.D. *Department of Neurology, State University of New York at Stony Brook, Stony Brook, New York 11794*

Jeffrey Laurence, M.D. *Department of Medicine, Division of Hematology-Oncology, Cornell University Medical College, 411 East 69th Street, New York, New York 10021*

Howard L. Leaf, M.D. *Infectious Diseases Section, New York Veterans Administration Medical Center; and New York University School of Medicine, 423 East 23rd Street, New York, New York 10016*

Alexandra M. Levine, M.D. *Division of Hematology, University of Southern California School of Medicine, Norris Comprehensive Cancer Center, 1441 Eastlake Avenue, Los Angeles, California 90033*

Paul A. Luciw, Ph.D. *Department of Medical Pathology, California Primate Research Center, University of California, Davis, California 95616*

Benjamin J. Luft, M.D. *Health Sciences Center, State University of New York at Stony Brook, Stony Brook, New York 11794*

Peter Mariuz, M.D. *Health Sciences Center, State University of New York at Stony Brook, Stony Brook, New York 11794*

Lauri E. Markowitz, M.D. *Division of Immunizations, Center for Prevention Services, Centers for Disease Control, 1600 Clifton Road, Atlanta, Georgia 30333*

Anthony Martinez, M.D. *Critical Care Medicine, National Institutes of Health, Bethesda, Maryland 20892*

William J. Martone, M.D. *Hospital Infections Program, Center for Infectious Diseases, Centers for Disease Control, 1600 Clifton Road, Atlanta, Georgia 30333*

Joseph R. Masci, M.D. *Division of Infectious Diseases, Department of Medicine, City Hospital Center at Elmhurst, Elmhurst, New York 11373*

Timothy D. Mastro, M.D., D.T.M.H.
International Activity, Division of HIV/AIDS, National Center for Infectious Diseases, Centers for Disease Control, 1600 Clifton Road, Atlanta, Georgia 30333

Henry Masur, M.D. *Clinical Center, National Institutes of Health, 9000 Rockville Pike, Bethesda, Maryland 20892*

Pratik Multani, B.S. *Department of Pathology, Beth Israel Hospital, 330 Brookline Avenue, Boston, Massachusetts 02215*

Abdollah Bijan Naficy, M.D. *Department of Medicine, Elmhurst Hospital, 79-01 Broadway, Elmhurst, New York 11373*

James S. A. Neill, M.D. *Department of Pathology and Laboratory Medicine, East Carolina University School of Medicine, Greenville, North Carolina 27858-4354*

Thomas R. O'Brien, M.D., M.P.H.
Division of HIV/AIDS, National Center for Infectious Diseases, Centers for Disease Control, Public Health Service, U.S. Department of Health and Human Services, 1600 Clifton Road, Atlanta, Georgia 30333

James Oleske, M.D., M.P.H. *University of Medicine and Dentistry of New Jersey; and Children's Hospital, Newark, New Jersey 07103*

Ida M. Onorato, M.D. *Division of HIV/AIDS, National Center for Infectious Diseases, Centers for Disease Control, 1600 Clifton Road, Atlanta, Georgia 30333*

Jan M. Orenstein, M.D. *Department of Pathology, George Washington University Medical Center, Washington, D.C. 20037*

Arthur E. Pitchenik, M.D. *Department of Medicine, University of Miami, Veterans Administration Medical Center, 1201 Northwest 16th Street, Miami, Florida 33125*

Michael Poon, M.D. *Clinical Microbiology Laboratories, The Mount Sinai Hospital, New York, New York 10029-6574; Present Address: Division of Cardiology, Department of Medicine, The Mount Sinai Hospital, New York, New York 10029*

Richard W. Price, M.D. *Department of Neurology, University of Minnesota Medical School, 420 Delaware Street Southeast, Minneapolis, Minnesota 55455*

Chester Roberts, Ph.D. *Department of Diagnostic Retrovirology, Water Reed Army Institute of Research, 9620 Medical Center Drive, Rockville, Maryland 20850*

Martha F. Rogers, M.D. *Epidemiology Branch, Division of HIV/AIDS, Center for Infectious Diseases, Centers for Disease Control, Public Health Service, U.S. Department of Health and Human Services, 1600 Clifton Road, Atlanta, Georgia 30333*

Syed Zaki Salahuddin, M.S. *Division of Hematology, Department of Internal Medicine University of Southern California, Los Angeles, California 90033*

Robert T. Schooley, M.D. *Infectious Diseases Division, University of Colorado Health Sciences Center, 4200 East Ninth Avenue, Denver, Colorado 80134*

Paul S. Shneidman, M.D. *Department of Neuropathology, University of Pennsylvania School of Medicine, Philadelphia, Pennsylvania 10904*

John J. Sidtis, Ph.D. *Department of Neurology, University of Minnesota Health Science Center, 420 Delaware Street, Southeast, Minneapolis, Minnesota 55455*

Robert F. Siliciano, M.D., Ph.D. *Department of Medicine, Johns Hopkins University School of Medicine, 1721 East Madison Street, Baltimore, Maryland 21205*

Michael S. Simberkoff, M.D. *Infectious Diseases Section, New York Veterans Administration Medical Center, New York University School of Medicine, 423 East 23rd Street, New York, New York 10016*

Rosemary Soave, M.D. *Division of Infectious Diseases, New York Hospital-Cornell Medical Center, 525 East 68th Street, New York, New York 10021*

Ana Sotrel, M.D. *Department of Pathology, Beth Israel Hospital, Harvard Medical School, 330 Brookline Avenue, Boston, Massachusetts 02115*

Steven Specter, Ph.D. *Departments of Medicine, Microbiology, and Immunology, University of South Florida College of Medicine, Tampa, Florida 33612*

Anthony F. Suffredini, M.D. *Critical Care Medicine, National Institutes of Health, Bethesda, Maryland 20892*

Jerome I. Tokars, M.D., M.P.H. *Hospital Infections Program, Center for Infectious Diseases, Centers for Disease Control, 1600 Clifton Road, Atlanta, Georgia 30333*

Russell H. Tomar, M.D. *Department of Pathology and Laboratory Medicine, University of Wisconsin Hospitals and Clinics, 600 Highland Avenue, Madison, Wisconsin 53792*

Christina Walsh, M.D. *Department of Medicine, New York University Medical Center, 462 First Avenue, New York, New York 10016*

John W. Ward, M.D. *Division of HIV/ AIDS, National Center for Infectious Diseases, Centers for Disease Control, Atlanta, Georgia 30333*

Stanley H. Weiss, M.D. *Division of Infectious Diseases Epidemiology, Department of Preventive Medicine and Community Health, University of Medicine and Dentistry of New Jersey, 30 Bergen Street, Newark, New Jersey 07107*

Gary P. Wormser, M.D. *Division of Infectious Diseases, Department of Medicine, Westchester County Medical Center, New York Medical College, Valhalla, New York 10595*

Robert L. Yarrish, M.D. *Infectious Diseases Section, St. Vincent's Hospital and Medical Center of New York, 153 West 11th Street, New York, New York 10011*

Foreword

For many readers of this book, it will be difficult to imagine that the first cases of AIDS in the world were reported as recently as 1981. We now know that there was a rapid spread of HIV infection in many countries during the 1970s; sporadic AIDS cases are reported to have occurred even as early as the 1950s. Nonetheless, for all practical purposes, the HIV epidemic is a "new" scourge upon humankind.

In the 1980s and early 1990s there has been considerable progress in the scientific recognition and understanding of the virus itself, diagnosis of clinical conditions associated with HIV infection, and methods of clinical management and therapy. Even more rapid than the scientific progress, however, has been the spread of the virus throughout the world. The World Health Organization (WHO) estimated that 9 to 11 million persons were infected with HIV by 1991 and that this number will grow to 30 to 40 million by the turn of the century.

The epidemic in the United States is coming into clear focus. HIV/AIDS has become endemic and is being recognized as a leading cause of death among young adults. When final mortality statistics are reported for 1991, HIV infection will be the second leading cause of death in men age 25–44, with black men suffering a death rate three times greater than white men. Similarly, HIV infection will be one of the five leading causes of death for women age 15–44, with black women having nine times the mortality rate of white women. It is also becoming clear that many aspects of the HIV/AIDS epidemic will require commitments beyond the control of scientists and clinicians. The public health problem of HIV/AIDS has exposed many societal problems that have resisted public prioritization and easy solution. Examples include injection drug abuse, inadequate preparation of youths for sexual maturity, inadequacies in health care distribution and financing, and erosion of the family public health infrastructure. Even more general problems (such as poverty and urban crowding) or attitudes (such as racism or homophobia) form barriers to addressing the HIV/AIDS problem.

In many other parts of the world, however, the dimensions of the HIV/AIDS epidemic remain uncertain. In Asia and in parts of South and Central America, the rapid rise of HIV infection dwarfs current clinical cases of AIDS, preceding the true public awareness that an AIDS epidemic will bring. In these areas of the world, the virus is winning the battle against us. When confronted with the WHO projections and the potential for human misery they imply, we see that the need for a vaccine is urgent.

HIV/AIDS challenges us not only to perform our medical, public health, and scientific roles with competence but also to provide leadership for our respective communities in the worldwide struggle. Meeting both of these challenges requires that we have up-to-date and accurate information on the full spectrum of clinical, laboratory, public health, and social aspects of HIV infection.

The Second Edition of *AIDS and Other Manifestations of HIV Infection* provides us with important information needed to help us meet those challenges.

James W. Curran, M.D., M.P.H.
Associate Director for HIV/AIDS Programs
Centers for Disease Control
Atlanta, Georgia

Preface

AIDS has now been with us for more than a decade and is widely appreciated as a worldwide problem of immense and growing proportions. Well over 200,000 cases have been diagnosed and over 130,000 deaths reported in the United States alone. The first edition of *AIDS and Other Manifestations of HIV Infection* was published in 1987. It was written to provide a comprehensive overview of the biologic properties of the etiologic viral agent, its clinico-pathological manifestations, the epidemiology of its infection, and present and future therapeutic and preventive options. The goals for this second edition are unchanged. Every chapter has been extensively revised in accordance with a vast amount of new knowledge. New chapters on "Viral Cofactors in the Pathogenesis of HIV Disease"; "Virologic and Biologic Features of HIV-2"; "Simian Retroviruses"; "Care of the Adult Patient with HIV Infection"; "Gastrointestinal Manifestations of AIDS"; "Oral Lesions Associated with HIV Infection"; "Ophthalmologic Aspects of HIV Infection"; "Occupational Issues Related to the HIV Epidemic"; "Immunizations, Vaccine-Preventable Diseases, and HIV Infection"; and "AIDS and the Ethics of Prevention, Research, and Care", have been added. Readers may also refer to the extensive bibliographical material provided throughout the book. The interested reader is referred to the first edition for more extensive coverage of topics such as "The Discovery of AIDS"; "AIDS in Prisons"; "HIV Infection in the Military"; "Feline Leukemia Virus"; "Ultrastructural Changes in AIDS"; and the "Pathology of AIDS in Children", which (among others) are not included as separate chapters in this volume.

It is our hope and intention that this second edition will provide a reference source for essential information needed by most practitioners and specialists and will contribute not only to a better understanding of HIV infection, but also to assisting health care workers render the highest level of care possible to their patients.

Gary P. Wormser, M.D.

Acknowledgments

Special thanks go to Mrs. Shirley Gamble for her assistance with this project; to my Infectious Diseases colleagues, research team, office staff, and Fellows for their understanding; to Richard D. Levere, Edward Stolzenberg, Jack McGiff, Kerry Willis, Zalman Arlin, Soldano Ferrone, Richard Gorlin, and Glen Braunstein for their general support; and to my special friends Edward Bottone, Rosalyn Stahl, and Joni Laden, who have helped in so many ways.

AIDS and Other Manifestations of HIV Infection

Second Edition

AIDS and Other Manifestations of HIV Infection,
Second Edition, Edited by Gary P. Wormser.
Published by Raven Press, Ltd., New York 1992.

CHAPTER 1

Epidemiology of HIV and AIDS

John W. Ward and D. Peter Drotman

Historically, public responses to epidemics have been characterized all too often by panic and overreaction. Among the advances in societal response to epidemics are not only medical interventions on behalf of those afflicted, but also public health systems. The scientific response to epidemics can be traced back to Dr. John Snow's analysis of neighborhood clusters of cholera deaths during the 1850s in London. Since then, surveillance, epidemiologic investigation, and prevention methods have been developed for a wide spectrum of infectious and noninfectious diseases and health conditions.

Public health surveillance in the United States is inextricably tied to the medical care system. Physicians or other clinicians diagnose cases and report unusual cases or clusters to public health departments. Epidemiologists analyze the reported data, provide information to clinicians, and make recommendations for prevention or control. This system proved its utility in the initial recognition of the AIDS epidemic.

RECOGNITION OF THE EPIDEMIC

In the spring of 1981, the Centers for Disease Control (CDC) received reports of the unexpected occurrence of *Pneumocystis carinii* pneumonia (PCP) and Kaposi's sarcoma (KS) among young gay men in California and New York City (1,2). These illnesses were associated with an acquired cellular immunodeficiency of a type not previously described. Subsequent reports in 1981 and 1982 identified persons with hemophilia, recipients of blood and blood components, intravenous drug users, and their heterosexual partners and children who had similar opportunistic conditions associated with unex-

plained immunodeficiency (3–7). The occurrence of these conditions in epidemiologically distinct populations suggested the immunosuppression was caused by an infectious agent transmitted sexually, through exposure to blood, and perinatally from mother to fetus or infant, but all findings were consistent with other etiologic hypotheses as well. In late 1981, CDC established a surveillance case definition that formally listed the opportunistic illnesses indicative of underlying immunosuppression (8). Beginning in 1982, this immune disorder and the accompanying illnesses became known as the acquired immunodeficiency syndrome, or AIDS. The cases reported through that system formed the initial database upon which the case-control and other studies would be established that would ultimately point the way for the laboratory investigators who isolated a unique retrovirus from persons with AIDS or at risk for it (9).

Their findings supported the conclusion that AIDS was caused by an infectious agent (10,11). Various terminology was initially used to label this virus but it has been known as the human immunodeficiency virus (HIV) since 1986 (12). The subsequent development of antibody tests to detect evidence of infection with HIV led to the finding that the number of persons infected with HIV was much larger than the number with AIDS (13–15). The so-called iceberg model was strongly supported and proved useful for several years. However, as incidence of HIV infections eventually comes under control (an admittedly optimistic view), the base of the iceberg will not grow in proportion to the tip, which represents AIDS cases. Cases are projected to increase, as many persons with HIV develop AIDS.

Since the initial case reports of AIDS, the number of persons with HIV infection and AIDS has grown rapidly in the United States and around the world. HIV infection has become a leading cause of morbidity and mortality. Although no curative therapies or effective vaccines

J. W. Ward and D. P. Drotman: Division of HIV/AIDS, National Center for Infectious Diseases, Centers for Disease Control, Atlanta, Georgia 30333.

have become available, a growing number of drugs or specific interventions serve to delay the natural history of HIV infection and prevent related illnesses (16–19). Of course, these too play a role in shaping the iceberg of the future. Understanding the epidemiology of HIV infection in the United States is important to maximize the effectiveness of national prevention and education efforts, as well as to provide appropriate and thorough patient management services.

NATIONAL AIDS SURVEILLANCE SYSTEM

All 50 States, the District of Columbia, and all territories of the United States require AIDS cases to be reported to local health authorities. The diagnosis of AIDS is based on uniform case definitions for adults and children developed by CDC in collaboration with others. Reports of all cases that meet these definitions are forwarded to CDC with standard information. No patients' names (only code numbers) are reported to CDC or the U.S. Public Health Service, so as to preclude the same case being reported multiple times from hospitals or clinicians in different counties or states. Public health departments have established an excellent record of confidentiality of the names of patients reported to them with AIDS.

The initial AIDS case definition was developed to be highly specific for use in an acute outbreak of a then-rare condition. It included opportunistic infections and neoplasms indicative of underlying immunosuppression (8). In the absence of previously described causes of immunosuppression, a diagnosis of one of these conditions was defined as AIDS. Using this case definition, clinicians nationwide began to report cases to CDC. By June 20, 1983, 2 years after the first recognized cases, 1,641 cases of AIDS had been reported from 38 states (20).

CDC and others retrospectively investigated physician and hospital records and death certificates to identify earlier cases of AIDS that had gone unrecognized or unreported. Investigators eventually located 125 cases diagnosed from 1977 to 1981. These data provided evidence that AIDS was a relatively new disease in the country. Although a few cases compatible with AIDS were retrospectively diagnosed in the 1950s and 1960s, the AIDS epidemic in the United States clearly started in the mid- to late 1970s (21–23).

The original AIDS case definition was modified in 1985 and 1987 (24,25), and another modification to include all persons with severe HIV-related immunosuppression (CD4+ lymphocyte count of less than 200/mm^3) was planned for 1992. As knowledge of the clinical spectrum of AIDS grew, a broader range of indicator diseases and conditions was incorporated into the definition, and use of HIV antibody tests improved both the sensitivity and specificity of the definition. Two major issues come under scrutiny in any alteration of criteria

for diagnosing an illness of public health importance such as AIDS: epidemiologic uses of surveillance data and clinical practice in applying diagnostic techniques. For the first issue, public health authorities must weigh the disadvantages of possibly losing track of trend data when clinical criteria are altered against the advantage of making the criteria more sensitive, i.e., counting more of the affected patients. In 1985 and 1987, the deliberations were strongly swayed by progress in understanding the natural history of HIV infection, such as the recognition of HIV wasting syndrome and encephalopathy, conditions that were not known in 1981. For the second issue, presumptive diagnoses appeared to become of major importance in providing care to large numbers of severely ill HIV-infected persons, mainly women, children, the poor, intravenous drug users, and those without adequate access to health care services. Thus, revisions to the case definition have all resulted in more patients being defined as having AIDS.

The 1985 revision added disseminated histoplasmosis, chronic isosporiasis, and certain non-Hodgkin's lymphomas. As a result, the reported number of AIDS cases increased by an estimated 3–4% (26).

The 1987 revision had a much larger impact on AIDS case surveillance. For patients with laboratory evidence of HIV infection, this revision incorporated HIV encephalopathy, wasting syndrome, and other indicator diseases that are diagnosed presumptively (i.e., without definitive laboratory evidence of the opportunistic disease) and allowed them to be reported as AIDS patients. Compared with patients who met the pre-1987 case definition, a higher proportion of patients who met only the 1987 case definition were female, black or Hispanic, or intravenous drug users (27). The number of cases reported may have increased by as much as 28% in some areas (27).

An increasing proportion of cases began to be diagnosed presumptively, rather than definitively. Of nearly 40,000 cases diagnosed prior to 1987, 7% met only the criteria of the 1987 case definition. (These cases were reported months or years after diagnosis.) The proportion increased to 19% for cases diagnosed in 1987, to 28% in 1988, to 31% in 1989, and to 34% in 1990. By 1992, the understanding of HIV immunopathogenesis had progressed to the point at which early clinical intervention had become the standard of medical care. The CD4+ lymphocyte is the primary target for HIV infection because of the affinity of the virus for the CD4 surface marker (28). As the number of CD4+ lymphocytes decreases, the risk and severity of opportunistic illnesses increases (29,30). Measures of CD4+ lymphocytes are currently used to guide clinical and/or therapeutic actions for HIV-infected persons. As a result, antiretroviral therapy is recommended for all persons with a CD4+ lymphocyte count of less than 500/mm^3, and prophylaxis against PCP, the most common serious opportunistic infection diagnosed in AIDS patients, is recommended for all persons with CD4+ lymphocyte counts of less than 200/mm³ (31,32). In fact, earlier diagnosis of HIV infection and specific antiretroviral therapy and PCP prophylaxis has influenced the epidemiologic pattern of AIDS by delaying the onset of opportunistic illnesses included in the 1987 surveillance case definition. In acknowledgment of this clinical trend, the expanded case definition for 1992 includes all persons with a CD4+ lymphocyte count of less than 200/mm³ regardless of symptomatology.

COMPLETENESS OF AIDS REPORTING

AIDS case surveillance aims to provide a consistent database that can guide public health officials, biomedical scientists, clinicians, public policy formulators, legislators, and others. The goals of any surveillance system are to yield accurate information on disease or death trends, health care use, prevention efforts, and other parameters. These goals can be achieved with less than 100% complete reporting. Indeed, tracking every diagnosed AIDS case would probably be an imprudent expenditure of public health resources and effort when equally useful conclusions can be reached with a dataset of documented consistency. By observing what determines why cases do or do not get reported, public health officials can assess the extent of case reporting and become sensitive to changes in patterns of reporting. As long as the goals of reporting continue to be met, the absolute level of completeness of reporting is of lesser importance.

Clinicians should not be lulled into complacency about their duty to report cases because of the statistical capabilities of public health departments. Reporting is a legal requirement in all states, and the more complete the case count, the more accurate the data tend to be. Furthermore, social expenditures and services often depend on officially reported case counts in cities, counties, or states. Therefore, the more cases clinicians report, the more resources tend to be allocated to provide social services for their patients.

The completeness of reporting of diagnosed cases of AIDS varies according to many factors including number of previously reported cases, geography, staffing of health departments, facility of diagnosis, specialty of diagnostician, the patient's wish, age, sex, race, and vital status of patient, and many others. A good public health surveillance system can employ either a passive or an augmented-active case-finding method or both. A passive system receives reports of diagnosed cases from physicians, hospitals, and laboratories. In a study of three areas that relied on passive surveillance, 55–70% of AIDS cases were reported (33).

The reporting of AIDS cases tends to be more complete when local or state health departments augment passive surveillance with solicitations to physicians and infection control practitioners as well as reviews of hospital records, death certificates, and a variety of disease registries. Studies of cases reported from 1985 through 1988 in seven states using active surveillance methods indicated that 90–99% of persons with AIDS were reported (33). Studies in South Carolina and Oregon found that only 60% and 64%, respectively, of the cases identified by active surveillance were reported via the passive surveillance system (34,35). As a result, beginning in 1988, CDC provided funds to all states to carry out active surveillance (and had done so earlier in many states). The AIDS surveillance system receives reports for an estimated 85% of all AIDS cases diagnosed and 70–90% of HIV-related deaths among men 25–44 years of age (36,37). This rate of reporting is as good as or better than surveillance for other reportable illnesses (38,39).

TRENDS IN AIDS CASE SURVEILLANCE

As of December 31, 1990, 161,073 cases of AIDS were reported to CDC (40). Since 1981, the number of reported cases has increased annually. However, the rate of increase (slope of the epidemic curve) has varied. From January 1982 to December 1984, the number of cases increased by 150–200% annually and this steep increase can be seen in Figure 1. In 1987, the curve appeared to become more linear and less steep. This "bend" was perceived as a true change by participants in a late 1989 Public Health Service workshop to evaluate projection estimates for HIV infection and AIDS (41). The slowing of case reporting for homosexual/bisexual men was most dramatic for New York, Los Angeles, and San Francisco (42). Possible reasons include the effect of antiviral treatments, which slowed the natural history of HIV infection. By 1987, thousands of homosexual/bisexual men with severe immunodeficiency had received zidovudine from its manufacturer even before its full licensure, which could have contributed to the slowing of the increase in the epidemic curve (43). The slowing may also have been due to a decreased incidence of new HIV infections dating from the early 1980s in gay communities. Cohort studies have demonstrated this decreased incidence, and the rate of other sexually transmitted diseases has also fallen sharply among white homosexual/bisexual men (44,45). As the diagnosis of AIDS becomes more of an outpatient procedure performed in physicians' offices and clinics, the lag time between diagnosis and case reporting may increase (46). Despite progress, or at least hopeful developments in some populations, the number of new AIDS cases was projected to increase through at least 1993 (41). Between 52,000 and 57,000 cases of AIDS were projected to have been diagnosed during 1990 and the annual count was expected to increase to 61,000–98,000 diagnosed during 1993. Thus, by the end of 1993, an estimated 390,000–480,000 Amer-

TABLE 1. AIDS cases by age group, exposure category, and sex, reported in 1989 and 1990 and cumulative totals, by age group and exposure category, through December 1990, United States

Adult/adolescent exposure category	Males		Females		Totals		
	1989 No. (%)	1990 No. (%)	1989 No. (%)	1990 No. (%)	1989 No. (%)	1990 No. (%)	Cumulative total[a] No. (%)
Male homosexual/bisexual contact	19,891 (64)	23,738 (63)	—	—	19,891 (58)	23,738 (56)	94,126 (59)
Intravenous (IV) drug use (female and heterosexual male)	6,218 (20)	7,689 (20)	1,871 (51)	2,329 (48)	8,089 (23)	10,018 (24)	34,398 (22)
Male homosexual/bisexual contact and IV drug use	2,214 (7)	2,295 (6)	—	—	2,214 (6)	2,295 (5)	10,557 (7)
Hemophilia/coagulation disorder	283 (1)	329 (1)	6 (0)	11 (0)	289 (1)	340 (1)	1,386 (1)
Heterosexual contact	778 (3)	1,054 (3)	1,232 (34)	1,657 (34)	2,010 (6)	2,711 (6)	8,440 (5)
Sex with IV drug user	390	469	770	1,062	1,160	1,531	4,470
Sex with bisexual male	—	—	109	129	109	129	498
Sex with person with hemophilia	1	2	20	26	21	28	79
Born in pattern-II country[b]	247	305	132	117	379	422	2,036
Sex with person born in pattern-II country	19	22	12	22	31	44	130
Sex with transfusion recipient with HIV infection	13	24	22	40	35	64	151
Sex with HIV-infected person, risk not specified	108	232	167	261	275	493	1,076
Receipt of blood transfusion, blood components or tissue[c]	469 (2)	501 (1)	308 (8)	365 (7)	777 (2)	866 (2)	3,684 (2)
Other/undetermined[d]	1,093 (4)	2,061 (5)	222 (6)	528 (11)	1,315 (4)	2,589 (6)	5,696 (4)
Adult/adolescent subtotal	30,946 (100)	37,667 (100)	3,639 (100)	4,890 (100)	34,585 (100)	42,557 (100)	158,287 (100)

4

Pediatric (<13 years old) exposure category

Category							
Hemophilia/coagulation disorder	24 (7)	31 (7)	1 (0)	—	25 (4)	31 (4)	139 (5)
Mother with/at risk for HIV infection	282 (84)	342 (82)	283 (92)	339 (92)	565 (88)	681 (87)	2,327 (84)
IV drug use	139	167	123	147	262	314	1,163
Sex with IV drug user	67	75	61	75	128	150	487
Sex with bisexual male	8	3	7	5	15	8	48
Sex with person with hemophilia	—	1	—	1	—	2	9
Born in pattern-II country	27	20	28	20	55	40	213
Sex with person born in pattern-II country	1	2	2	4	3	6	12
Sex with transfusion recipient with HIV infection	1	1	5	—	6	1	12
Sex with HIV-infected person, risk not specified	10	15	16	21	26	36	98
Receipt of blood transfusion, blood components, or tissue	4	5	6	7	10	12	47
Has HIV infection, risk not specified	25	53	35	59	60	112	238
Receipt of blood transfusion, blood components, or tissue	25 (7)	26 (6)	15 (5)	13 (4)	40 (6)	39 (5)	252 (9)
Undetermined	5 (1)	16 (4)	10 (3)	15 (4)	15 (2)	31 (4)	68 (2)
Pediatric subtotal	336 (100)	415 (100)	309 (100)	367 (100)	645 (100)	782 (100)	2,786 (100)
Total	**31,282**	**38,082**	**3,948**	**5,257**	**35,230**	**43,339**	**161,073**

[a] Includes three patients known to be infected with human immunodeficiency virus type 2 (HIV-2).

[b] Countries where heterosexual transmission predominates including sub-Saharan African and Caribbean countries.

[c] Includes 14 transfusion recipients who received blood screened for HIV antibody, and 1 tissue recipient.

[d] "Other" refers to three health care workers who seroconverted to HIV and developed AIDS after occupational exposure to HIV-infected blood. "Undetermined" refers to patients whose mode of exposure to HIV is unknown. This includes patients under investigation; patients who died, were lost to follow-up, or refused interview; and patients whose mode of exposure to HIV remains undetermined after investigation.

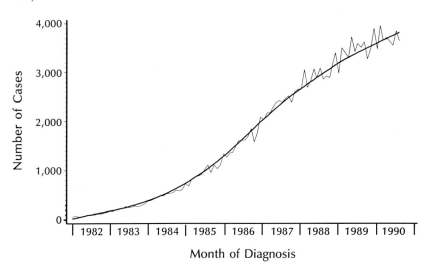

FIG. 1. AIDS cases by month of diagnosis, adjusted for reporting delays, January 1982 through September 1990, United States. From CDC (40).

icans will have developed AIDS. Of these, between 285,000 and 340,000 persons with AIDS were projected to die by the end of 1993.

The distribution of HIV transmission risks has evolved. This evolution will continue. About 56% of the AIDS cases reported in 1990 occurred in homosexual/bisexual men compared with 70% of cases reported in 1987 (26,40). Over this same interval, the proportion of AIDS patients who reported a history of intravenous drug use increased from 14% to 24%. The most rapidly growing population of AIDS patients in 1990 was heterosexually infected adults whose yearly total increased by more than one-third over the total reported in 1989 (see Table 1). Many increases were magnified by the greatly increased number of cases reported annually.

The incidence of AIDS began to plateau for some other persons at risk. The number of AIDS cases among adult transfusion recipients increased by only 89 (11%) in 1990 and the number of newly reported cases actually decreased by one for pediatric transfusion recipients (40). Most persons with hemophilia- and transfusion-associated AIDS were infected with HIV prior to 1985. In 1985, measures were adopted to protect the blood supply by instituting HIV antibody screening of blood and plasma donations and heat treatment to inactivate HIV in pooled plasma from which clotting factor concentrates are derived (14,47). Since the adoption of these measures, transmission of HIV through blood transfusion has become rare (48). As of the end of 1990, only 14 of the 3,935 transfusion-associated AIDS cases were infected by blood that screened negative for HIV antibody.

AIDS IN MEN

Nearly 90% (144,295) of patients reported with AIDS by the end of 1990 have been males. The median age at diagnosis has been 36 years. Of men with AIDS, 94,126 (66%) were homosexual/bisexual in orientation, 26,540

(19%) were intravenous drug users, and 10,557 (7%) reported both of these exposure categories. Another 1,352 (1%) had hemophilia A or B or some other coagulation disorder, 2,252 (2%) had only a history of a blood transfusion, and 3,367 (2%) had heterosexual contact with persons at risk for AIDS. This latter category included 1,483 men (44%) who were born in countries where heterosexual transmission of HIV predominated. The proportion of all men with AIDS born in these countries has decreased from 4% of cases before 1984 to 1% of cases in 1990.

AIDS IN WOMEN

As of December 31, 1990, 16,778 women were reported with AIDS, constituting more than 10% of all reported adult and adolescent cases. The 4,890 women reported with AIDS in 1990 accounted for 11.5% of adult and adolescent cases reported that year and was an increase from the 8% of reported cases in 1987. Women with AIDS have a mean age of about 36 years. Of women with AIDS, 7,858 (51%) have a history of intravenous drug use, 1,432 (9%) have received blood transfusions or tissue transplants, and 5,073 (33%) reported heterosexual contact with persons with or at risk for HIV infection. From 1984 through 1990, the proportion of women with AIDS who had sex partners at risk for HIV infection increased from 15% to 33%. Of women with AIDS whose HIV infections were ascribed to heterosexual contact, 3,183 (63%) were sex partners of intravenous drug users and 553 (11%) were born in countries with predominantly heterosexual transmission of HIV.

AIDS CASES WITH NO IDENTIFIED RISK

Of the 158,287 AIDS cases reported in adults or adolescents (>13 years) by the end of 1990, 5,696 (3.6%) were in persons who did not have a risk of HIV infection identified (40). When additional investigation is carried out, the risks for HIV infection will be identified for most of these persons (49). Of 10,224 adult and adolescent AIDS patients initially reported with an undetermined risk for infection through 1990, 4,979 have had additional investigation and 4,528 (91%) had a risk for HIV infection identified and were reclassified into the appropriate transmission category.

Of the 451 persons who remained with "no identified risk," three were health care workers who seroconverted to HIV and developed AIDS after occupational exposure to blood of HIV-infected patients. For the remaining 448, 69 are also health care workers. Of 63 who responded to a questionnaire, 36 (57%) reported needle-stick and/or mucous membrane exposures. However, none of the source patients was known to be infected with HIV at the time of exposure. Of these 448 cases, 393 responded to an additional interview; 126 (35%) respondents gave a history of another sexually transmitted disease, and 84 (34%) of 247 men interviewed reported having had sexual contact with a prostitute. Clearly, some AIDS patients classified as not having risk represent unreported or unrecognized heterosexual transmission or other risk behavior for HIV and a few may have incurred infection in health care settings.

AIDS AMONG RACIAL AND ETHNIC MINORITY POPULATIONS

Of the 161,073 AIDS cases reported through 1990, 55% were in whites, 28% in blacks, and 16% in Hispanics (Table 2). African Americans and Hispanics have had the highest annual incidence rates for AIDS (34.9 and 28.9 cases per 100,000 population, respectively, in 1988) followed by whites (9.6), Asians/Pacific Islanders (5.4), and American Indians/Alaskan Natives (2.2) (26). The numbers of new cases reported among minority populations are increasing faster than among whites. From 1988 to the end of 1989, the number of blacks and Hispanics with AIDS increased by 22% and 14%, respectively, in comparison to an increase of 10% in whites (50). The largest increase was among American Indians/Alaska Natives, with the number of reported cases having increased by 91% in 1989 (50).

From 1981 through 1988, the cumulative incidence of AIDS was 3.0 times higher among black men and 2.8 times higher among Hispanic men than among white men (26). A much larger proportion of black (39%) and Hispanic (40%) adult/adolescent AIDS patients reported a history of intravenous drug use than did whites (8%) with AIDS, and 70% of AIDS patients who reported intravenous drug use were black or Hispanic (Table 2).

Of the 15,493 women reported with AIDS through 1990, 11,221 (72%) were black or Hispanic. More than

78% of the 7,858 women with AIDS associated with intravenous drug use were black or Hispanic. Sexual contact with male intravenous drug users was the most frequently reported risk factor for women who did not report use of such drugs. This has been true for black and Hispanic women as well as for white women.

AIDS-RELATED MORTALITY

Of 158,287 adults and adolescents reported with AIDS through 1990, 99,372 (63%) are known to have died. The crude mortality rate among AIDS patients increases sharply over time. Of the 8,136 persons diagnosed with AIDS from January to June 1986, 86% were known to have died by the end of 1990. Earlier diagnosis dates tend to have even higher fatality rates, but no cohort had recorded a 100% death rate by 1991. This may be artifactual, as the mortality rate of reported AIDS cases underestimates the true rate due to incomplete reporting of death information to the AIDS surveillance system.

Because HIV infection and AIDS is most common among young adults, the increase in mortality is most profound for this age group. As a result, the AIDS epidemic has had a profound impact on mortality when measured by the years of potential life lost (YPLL). From 1987 to 1988, YPLL before the age of 65 attributed to AIDS and HIV infection increased by 30% and became the sixth leading cause of YPLL before the age of 65 (51).

After a number of years of declining mortality rates, death rates in men 25–44 years of age increased from 212 deaths/100,000 population in 1983 to 236/100,000 in 1987. Most of this increase was due to HIV infection and AIDS. By the end of 1987, mortality related to AIDS and other HIV-associated illnesses accounted for 10% of all deaths in men in this age group (32). A review of mortality data for 1987 found that death due to HIV infection and AIDS was the fourth leading cause of death among black males and females and the fifth leading cause of death for the 20–24-year age group (52).

HIV infection and AIDS has emerged as an important cause of mortality in U.S. women aged 15–44 years. Deaths attributable to HIV infection and AIDS increased from 18 (0.03/100,000 in women aged 25–44 years) in 1980 to 1,430 (2.24/100,000) in 1988. AIDS represented 3% of all deaths of women in this age group (53). In 1988, HIV infection and AIDS-related death rates among black women (10.3/100,000) was nine times greater than the rate among white women (1.2/100,000). In New York and New Jersey in 1987, HIV infection and AIDS was the third leading cause of death in all women 15–44 years of age and the leading cause of death among black women in this age group. AIDS was expected to become one of the five leading causes of

TABLE 2. *AIDS cases by age group, exposure category, and race/ethnicity, reported through December 1990, United States*

	White, not Hispanic	Black, not Hispanic	Hispanic	Asian/ Pacific Islander	American Indian/ Alaskan Native	Total[a]
	No. (%)	No. (%)	No. (%)	No. (%)	No. (%)	No. (%)
Adult/adolescent exposure category						
Male homosexual/bisexual contact	67,049 (76)	15,966 (36)	10,051 (40)	733 (74)	123 (54)	94,126 (59)
Intravenous (IV) drug use (female and heterosexual male)	6,954 (8)	17,232 (39)	10,050 (40)	44 (4)	38 (17)	34,398 (22)
Male homosexual/bisexual contact and IV drug use	6,112 (7)	2,852 (6)	1,526 (6)	21 (2)	30 (13)	10,557 (7)
Hemophilia/coagulation disorder	1,153 (1)	95 (0)	110 (0)	16 (2)	8 (4)	1,386 (1)
Heterosexual contact	1,799 (2)	5,039 (11)	1,535 (6)	37 (4)	10 (4)	8,440 (5)
Sex with IV drug user	*980*	*2,264*	*1,191*	*16*	*7*	*4,470*
Sex with bisexual male	*274*	*155*	*58*	*9*	*1*	*498*
Sex with person with hemophilia	*68*	*7*	*3*	*1*	*—*	*79*
Born in pattern-II country[b]	*8*	*2,004*	*16*	*4*	*—*	*2,036*
Sex with person born in pattern-II country	*41*	*80*	*8*	*—*	*—*	*130*
Sex with transfusion recipient with HIV infection	*96*	*26*	*26*	*1*	*—*	*151*
Sex with HIV-infected person, risk not specified	*332*	*503*	*233*	*6*	*2*	*1,076*
Receipt of blood transfusion, blood components, or tissue[c]	2,580 (3)	638 (1)	380 (2)	70 (7)	6 (3)	3,684 (2)
Other/undetermined[d]	2,093 (2)	2,205 (5)	1,278 (5)	64 (6)	12 (5)	5,696 (4)
Adult/adolescent subtotal	87,740 (100)	44,027 (100)	24,930 (100)	985 (100)	227 (100)	158,287 (100)
Pediatric (<13 years old) exposure category						
Hemophilia/coagulation disorder	95 (16)	18 (1)	23 (3)	3 (25)	—	139 (5)
Mother with/at risk for HIV infection	366 (61)	1,326 (92)	617 (86)	4 (33)	6 (100)	2,327 (84)
IV drug use	*181*	*657*	*318*	*1*	*2*	*1,163*
Sex with IV drug user	*77*	*211*	*196*	*1*	*1*	*487*
Sex with bisexual male	*18*	*21*	*9*	*—*	*—*	*48*
Sex with person with hemophilia	*6*	*2*	*1*	*—*	*—*	*9*
Born in pattern-II country	*2*	*209*	*2*	*—*	*—*	*213*
Sex with person born in pattern-II country	*—*	*11*	*—*	*—*	*—*	*12*
Sex with transfusion recipient with HIV infection	*5*	*3*	*3*	*—*	*—*	*12*
Sex with HIV-infected person, risk not specified	*20*	*46*	*29*	*1*	*1*	*98*
Receipt of blood transfusion, blood components, or tissue	*16*	*19*	*12*	*—*	*—*	*47*
Has HIV infection, risk not specified	*41*	*147*	*47*	*1*	*2*	*238*
Receipt of blood transfusion, blood components, or tissue	133 (22)	56 (4)	58 (8)	5 (42)	—	252 (9)
Undetermined	8 (1)	39 (3)	21 (3)	—	—	68 (2)
Pediatric subtotal	602 (100)	1,439 (100)	719 (100)	12 (100)	6 (100)	2,786 (100)
Total	**88,342**	**45,466**	**25,649**	**997**	**233**	**161,073**

[a] Includes 386 persons whose race/ethnicity is unknown.
[b] Countries where heterosexual transmission predominates including sub-Saharan African and Caribbean countries.
[c] Includes 14 transfusion recipients who received blood screened for HIV antibody, and 1 tissue recipient.
[d] "Other" refers to three health care workers who seroconverted to HIV and developed AIDS after occupational exposure to HIV-infected blood. "Undetermined" refers to patients whose mode of exposure to HIV is unknown. This includes patients under investigation; patients who died, were lost to follow-up, or refused interview; and patients whose mode of exposure to HIV remains undetermined after investigation.

death among women of reproductive age by the early 1990s (53).

GEOGRAPHIC DISTRIBUTION OF AIDS CASES

AIDS cases have been reported from all 50 states, the District of Columbia, and all U.S. territories, but the geographic distribution of these cases is uneven. In 1990, the annual incidence rates by geographic areas varied from 0.3 cases/100,000 persons in North Dakota to 121.1 in the District of Columbia (Fig. 2).

The geographic distribution has changed with time. Before 1983, New York, New Jersey, and Pennsylvania reported 63% (541 of 856) of all AIDS cases in the United States. This proportion has gradually decreased to 32% (10,279 of 32,311) in 1988 and 28% (12,060 of 43,339) of cases reported in 1990. Cases reported from the Northeastern United States have increased by diminishing increments yearly, while reporting in small cities and rural areas, particularly in the South and in the Midwest increased sharply in the late 1980s. In 1989, the number of reported cases increased by 32% for cities with populations of 500,000 or less compared to only a 5% increase for metropolitan areas of 1,000,000 popula-

tion or more (50). The rate of reported cases actually decreased by 7% in the more populous Northeastern part of the country versus 18% and 22% increases, respectively, in the number of cases reported from the South and Midwest (50). In New York City, from July 1988 through June 1989, the number of reported cases among intravenous drug users decreased by 22% compared with the previous 12 months. Accordingly, a greater proportion of cases associated with intravenous drug use was reported from the rest of the country. From 1984 through 1986, the Southeastern United States reported only 9.2% (551 of 5,978) of AIDS cases among intravenous drug users, and 15.5% (88 of 568) of AIDS cases among sex partners of intravenous drug users. For the years 1987–1989, the Southeast reported 13.8% of the AIDS cases among intravenous drug users (2,836 of 20,513) and 27.9% of the AIDS cases in sex partners of intravenous drug users (854 of 3,066) (54).

Reported cases of AIDS among homosexual and bisexual males has decreased in some of the major metropolitan areas of the country. Compared with 1986, the rate of increase in reporting of AIDS cases among homosexual and bisexual males slowed in 1988 in New York (26% to 11%), San Francisco (28% to 8%), and Los An-

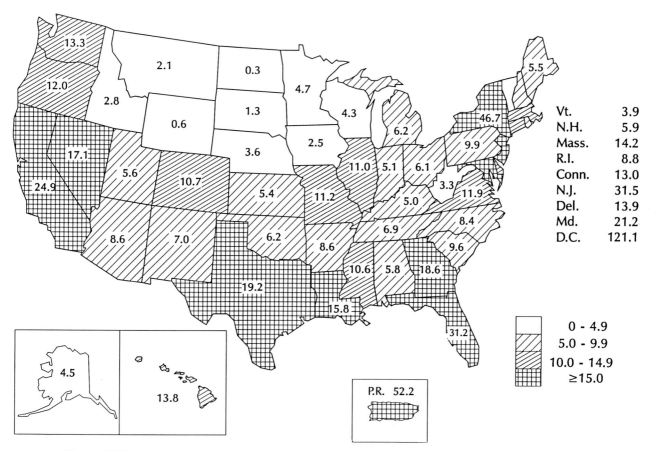

FIG. 2. AIDS annual rates per 100,000 population, for cases reported to CDC in 1990, United States. From CDC (40).

geles (32% to negative 6%) (55). The reasons for this apparent trend may include early saturation of the at-risk population with HIV infection, underreporting of cases, delays in reporting, differences in medical practices, and behavior changes that served to interrupt HIV transmission.

SURVEILLANCE OF HIV INFECTION

HIV seroprevalence studies are the best means to address such key questions as "what is the magnitude of the problem?" and "How successful are our prevention efforts?" They also are useful to identify trends in HIV transmission, risk factors for infection and vulnerable populations, and communities in need of HIV-related prevention and health care services. Some HIV seroprevalence surveys have been performed on specimens not linked to the individual so as to reduce the likelihood of self-selection bias, which may result in an underestimate of the HIV seroprevalence rate. Other surveys collect only specimens linked to specific patients so that information on HIV-associated risk factors can be correlated with HIV seroprevalence. CDC has conducted national HIV seroprevalence studies in populations at risk for HIV infection, women of reproductive age, persons in various clinical settings, and certain large groups that are subject to mandatory or routine testing such as blood donors or military recruits. The methods for these studies and surveys were published in 1990 in a special issue of *Public Health Reports* (Volume 105).

HOMOSEXUAL/BISEXUAL MEN

HIV-seroprevalence studies from 1984, when HIV antibody was first detected, to 1987 demonstrated that a large proportion of homosexual and bisexual men already had been infected with HIV. In the mid-1980s, the HIV seroprevalence among these men ranged from 36% (24/74) in New York City and 42% (38/90) in Los Angeles to 70% (4,676/6,680) in San Francisco (56). In other cities, where studies were primarily conducted in sexually transmitted disease (STD) clinics, HIV seroprevalence ranged from 12% in Arizona and New Mexico to 48% in Denver and 58% in Seattle (56). Later studies of HIV infection among homosexual/bisexual men in areas not initially impacted by the AIDS epidemic found that 25% (12/48) of homosexual/bisexual men in North Carolina, and 28% (45/159) in Oregon were infected with HIV (57,58). Because many such studies of homosexual/bisexual men were conducted in STD clinics, they may have been biased toward identifying men with high risk sexual behavior. Beginning in 1988, CDC conducted HIV-seroprevalence surveys of anonymously obtained specimens from patients of 85 STD clinics in 31 metropolitan areas (59). Of the homosexual/bisexual men with a newly diagnosed STD in these clinics, 38% were HIV antibody positive.

The incidence of HIV infection in homosexual/bisexual men dropped during the late 1980s (56). However, new HIV infections continued to occur. Young homosexual men appeared to be at particular risk of new HIV infections. A group of over 3,000 homosexual men followed for a 6-year period in four U.S. cities initially demonstrated a decrease in the rate of new HIV infections. The rate of new infections increased in some study sites, and younger men (less than 29 years) had higher rates of HIV seroconversion (60). In addition, studies in San Francisco STD clinics in 1989 revealed a 41% HIV seroprevalence rate among men 20 to 24 years of age (61). This high rate of HIV infection suggests that these persons became infected after AIDS was recognized and prevention programs established for homosexual/bisexual men.

INTRAVENOUS DRUG USERS

The initial HIV-seroprevalence studies demonstrated very high rates of HIV infection among intravenous drug users in the northeastern United States. Of drug users recruited primarily in drug treatment centers, 34–61% of drug users in New York City and New Jersey were HIV infected (56). However, the prevalence of HIV infection varies strikingly by geographic region. In contrast to the epidemic among homosexual and bisexual men, in which seroprevalence is substantial in all geographic areas, only 3% of intravenous drug users tested in drug treatment centers in Los Angeles, 5% in San Francisco, and 1% in San Antonio, Texas were HIV seropositive (56). Although the highest rates of HIV infection were seen in the Northeast, the rates of HIV infection among drug users in many areas of the country have increased. Studies in Chicago and Boston drug treatment centers conducted in the late 1980s revealed seroprevalence rates of 23% and 21%, respectively (62,63). Studies conducted in 1987–1989 in Atlanta and San Francisco drug treatment centers found 19% of intravenous drug users infected with HIV (64). CDC conducted HIV-seroprevalence studies in drug treatment centers in 27 metropolitan areas. Of the 15,000 intravenous drug users tested, 5.0% were HIV seropositive (range 0–47.7%) (65). The rate of HIV infection was higher in the Northeast (median, 18.2%) than in the rest of U.S. (median, 2.5%).

The rate of HIV infection is related to the frequency of sharing injection equipment with other persons, the use of "shooting galleries" where the sharing of equipment is common, and other factors (66). Black and Hispanic intravenous drug users tend to have higher seroprevalence rates than do white intravenous drug users. It is not known if this finding is due to less safe injection practices or the additional risk of heterosexual HIV transmission in these populations (65).

Public health prevention programs have encouraged intravenous drug users to stop using drugs, to seek treatment, not to share injection equipment, and to clean injection equipment with bleach if needles and syringes are not new or sterile. Studies in San Francisco, Chicago, and New Jersey have shown that after implementation of education programs, the use of bleach for cleaning equipment increases and the frequency of sharing equipment decreases. Efforts to increase the use of condoms to reduce sexual transmission among drug users have been less successful (67). HIV-infected drug users in San Francisco were shown to have high rates of gonorrhea and syphilis, suggesting transmission related to unsafe sexual practices (68).

PERSONS WITH HEMOPHILIA

Many persons with coagulation abnormalities, primarily hemophilia, require clotting factor replacement derived from plasma pools donated by hundreds or even thousands of different individuals. Because clotting factor concentrate users were exposed to plasma of so many donors, the chance of having one or more exposures to HIV was enormous until 1985 when HIV antibody screening of donors and heat treatment of the lyophilized factor concentrate began. As a result, many of the estimated 15,500 persons with hemophilia A or B were infected with HIV. A study conducted by the National Hemophilia Foundation tested 7,214 patients between 1985 and 1989; 50% (3,633 of 7,214) were HIV seropositive (69). Persons with hemophilia A, which is far more common than hemophilia B (also called Christmas disease), tend to require more clotting factor therapy than do persons with hemophilia B, and thus have higher rates of HIV infection; in the National Hemophilia Foundation study, 56% of patients who received factor VIII concentrate (hemophilia A) and 31% of patients who received factor IX concentrate (hemophilia B) were HIV infected (69). Because clotting factor concentrates are manufactured by a small number of suppliers for use throughout the country and internationally, HIV-infected persons with hemophilia are found in all geographic areas (69). The classic epidemiologic paradigm that applies to this aspect of the HIV epidemic is that of a point-source contamination with widespread distribution of a tragically tainted product. Although the HIV epidemic in persons with hemophilia essentially ended with the eradication of the contamination at its source, the AIDS epidemic that followed will be with us for years, and sexual and perinatal transmission prevention have become important priorities for persons with hemophilia and their loved ones.

HETEROSEXUAL TRANSMISSION

Studies of heterosexual partners of HIV-infected persons have shown varied but appreciable rates of transmission. What may be surprising to some is that the observed risk is below 100%. Prevalence of HIV infection in heterosexual partners has ranged from 0 to 58% with a median of 24% (56). The risk of male to female transmission appears to be greater than that for female to male. Severity of the HIV illness in the index partner, cooccurrence of other sexually transmitted diseases, and possibly the lack of circumcision of the male partner may be factors that increase the likelihood of HIV transmission (70). Many potential host, agent, and environmental factors may play roles in as yet undetermined ways to influence risk of sexual transmission of HIV.

HIV INFECTION IN WOMEN OF REPRODUCTIVE AGE

The rate of HIV infection among young women has increased since the onset of the AIDS epidemic. Women have been infected with HIV primarily through intravenous drug use or sexual contact with intravenous drug users. Surveys of women in clinical settings in the late 1980s revealed HIV seroprevalence rates ranging from less than 1% to approximately 4% (71). Most of the rates above 1% were from inner-city hospitals in the Northeast, the region that has had the country's highest incidence of AIDS in women.

In a CDC survey of 100,000 women aged 15–44 years in 32 metropolitan areas, the median rate of HIV infection was 0.2% (range 0–2.3%), with the median seroprevalence rate among black women (0.5%; range, 0–3.5%) greater than that for white (0%; range, 0–4.3%) and Hispanic women (0%; range, 0–2.5%) (72).

Prevalence of HIV infection in childbearing women can be determined by testing blood samples that are routinely collected from all newborn infants for early diagnosis of hereditary metabolic disorders. These samples are suitable for detection of HIV antibody that is passively transferred to all infants of seropositive mothers. Thus newborn screening yields direct information about maternal infection but indirect information about the infants because less than half of such children acquire HIV infection. This technique was applied anonymously and in an unlinked fashion in many states and cities across the country in 1989. The initial results proved compelling and very useful to public health leaders.

CDC coordinated surveys in 24 states by testing anonymous specimens collected from newborns for maternal HIV antibody (73). The HIV seroprevalence rate was 0.15% in the childbearing women tested; if this rate were projected nationally, an estimated 1,500–2,000 children born in 1989 would have been infected with HIV perinatally.

HOSPITAL ADMISSIONS

HIV seroprevalence rates among persons admitted to hospitals varies greatly (74–78). A CDC sentinel hospital survey of 26 acute-care hospitals in 21 cities during January 1988 through June 1989 showed some rather high rates in specific subpopulations and regions (79). Specimens from a sample of patients were stripped of personal identifiers and *excluded* if the patient had an admitting diagnosis of AIDS or any other medical condition likely to be associated with HIV. Of 89,547 blood specimens tested, 1,201 (1.3%) were found to contain HIV antibody. The seroprevalence rates among the participating hospitals ranged from 0.1% to 7.8%. Hospitals with high rates of HIV infection tended to be in areas of the country with high rates of HIV infection and AIDS, mainly urban centers in the northeast and along the Atlantic coast. Higher rates were found in men, blacks, and Hispanics, and in patients aged 25 to 44 years.

PERSONS WITH TUBERCULOSIS

All persons with tuberculous infection or tuberculosis need to be assessed for HIV infection (19). *Mycobacterium tuberculosis* infection is frequently found among HIV-infected persons. Of 79,329 cases of AIDS reported to CDC through 1988, 3,301 (4%) patients had tuberculosis (80). Although AIDS cases with TB have been reported from 44 states, 70% of these cases were reported from New York, New Jersey, Florida, and Texas. In 1989, CDC conducted HIV-seroprevalence studies among patients at 20 tuberculosis clinics in 14 metropolitan areas (81). The HIV-seroprevalence rates in TB patients had a median of 3% (range, 0–46%); the median rate of HIV infection was higher among male patients (75%). HIV-infected persons with tuberculosis tend to be located in the northeastern United States and along the Atlantic coast, where rates were extremely high, approaching 50% in some clinics, and the HIV-seroprevalence rate was highest for persons 30–34 years of age (15%) (81).

POPULATION-BASED SURVEYS

Large groups of persons who are tested on a routine basis provide unique opportunities for researchers and public health scientists. These include blood donors, civilian applicants for military service, and applicants to the Job Corps Residential Training Program conducted by the U.S. Department of Labor. These sources are valuable, but they are biased to the degree to which persons at high risk for HIV infection are restricted from these populations. Homosexual and bisexual men or those who have used intravenous drugs are actively discouraged from applying for military service or from donating blood. The HIV seroprevalence among voluntary blood donors in the United States is low: 0.020% of approximately 12.6 million blood donations collected from April 1985 through May 1987 (56). The overall level of HIV infection among blood donors declined from 0.035% in mid-1985 to 0.01% in early to mid-1988 (82). This was accomplished by permanently deferring previously identified HIV-seropositive donors.

Among civilian applicants for military service, the crude prevalence of HIV infection was 0.12% of 2.5 million applicants screened from October 1985 through 1989 (82). Rates were higher in male (0.14%) than in female applicants (0.06%) and higher in blacks (0.35%) than Hispanics (0.20%), American Indians/Alaskan Natives (0.10%), whites (0.06%), or Asians/Pacific Islanders (0.05%) (82). The rates have tended to decline over time, but this trend has not been readily interpretable due to active discouragement of at-risk applicants.

From March 1987 through March 1988, antibody screening was implemented for Job Corps entrants; of the first 84,089 residential Job Corps entrants tested, 0.4% were positive for HIV antibody (82). Entrants into this program tend to be disadvantaged youths 16–21 years of age who are drawn heavily from racial and ethnic minorities and include both inner-city and rural poor.

THE CHALLENGE OF PROJECTING AIDS/HIV TRENDS

In 1989, the Public Health Service convened a working group of epidemiologists, statisticians, and mathematical modelers to derive estimates of trends for AIDS cases and HIV infection prevalence and incidence (36). Based on analysis presented at the workshop, it was estimated that 750,000 persons in the United States were infected with HIV at the beginning of 1986. The estimate of HIV prevalence in 1989 was derived from various statistical models and ranged from 650,000 to 1.4 million; this estimate was derived after adjustments for deaths due to AIDS, underreporting of AIDS cases, and nonascertainment of HIV disease outside the AIDS surveillance definition.

The incidence, or rate of new HIV infections, is an indicator of the growth of the epidemic. Incidence can be observed directly from cohorts that are repeatedly screened for HIV infection, such as blood donors, or estimated from serial seroprevalence measurements carried out in similar populations, such as young gay men attending the same STD clinic over a number of years. The screening of active duty military personnel from 1987 to 1989 yielded a rate of approximately 0.6 to 0.8 seroconversions/1,000 military personnel per year. If the lower estimate of 0.6/1,000 is extrapolated to be the rate for the U.S. population of young adults, then at least 40,000 new HIV infections occurred in adults and adolescents in the United States during 1989 (36). This is probably an underestimate. Simply dividing the difference between the workshop participants' estimates of 750,000 prevalent infections in 1986 and about 1,000,000 in 1989 by the 3-year difference in time would suggest an incidence of at least 80,000 infections per year, even before considering deaths. Thus, 40,000–80,000 infections per year probably represents the minimum reasonable estimate of HIV incidence in the United States in the late 1980s.

HIV-RELATED ILLNESSES AND NATURAL HISTORY

Patients may develop clinical illnesses soon after infection with HIV. The acute retroviral syndrome typically occurs within 2–6 weeks after HIV infection and may include fever, myalgia, arthralgia, photophobia, sore throat, lymphadenopathy, and maculopapular rash (83). Evidence from several studies suggests that between 37% and 53% of adults may develop these symptoms following HIV infection (83).

Prospectively followed cohorts of HIV-infected persons have shed considerable light on the risk of developing AIDS or other clinical conditions in HIV-infected persons. In general, these studies have shown that the risk of AIDS increases over time. It is unusual for HIV-related illness to develop in the first few years after acquisition of HIV infection (84,85). Only 1–2% of HIV-infected adults have been shown to develop AIDS within 2 years of infection. The proportion who have developed AIDS rises steadily over time to at least 33–49% of adults who have been shown to develop AIDS within 7 years of infection (84,85).

Persons infected with HIV through different routes may have different risks of developing AIDS. Persons with transfusion-associated HIV infection have been shown to develop AIDS more quickly than homosexual/bisexual men (84). In addition, older adults with hemophilia have been shown to develop AIDS faster than HIV-infected homosexual/bisexual men (86). This may reflect differences in viral strains, the inoculum of virus received, and the immune function status and older age of persons with hemophilia and transfusion recipients, or other factors.

Reasonable estimates of the average incubation time between HIV infection and AIDS have been approximately 8–11 years. Analysis using different methods for adults with HIV infection gave similar results of 8.2 and 9.8 years (87,88).

What proportion of HIV-infected persons will ultimately develop AIDS is not known. Possibly all HIV-infected persons eventually may develop signs and symptoms of illness. One analysis based on 114 homosexual men concluded that between 65% and 100% of infected men would develop AIDS within 16 years (89). However, some men have remained immunologically and clinically healthy despite 8 or more years of infection. Thus, to define the full scope of HIV-related illnesses, longitudinal study of HIV-infected persons is necessary.

FUTURE DIRECTIONS

Surveillance systems for HIV infection and AIDS must evolve in accordance with clinical and public health needs for information. The reporting of AIDS cases will continue to be the best indicator of severe HIV-related immunosuppression and morbidity. However, as more therapeutic progress is achieved, either by restoring immune function to immunodeficient patients or in delaying the development of opportunistic illnesses, the current AIDS case definitions may need to evolve. Additional illnesses indicative of HIV-related immunosuppression may be recognized as the natural history of HIV infection is more completely described in women, children, and racial and ethnic minorities. To continue as an effective clinical and public health tool, the definition of AIDS may need to include more laboratory (both virologic and immunologic) parameters and become less dependent on long lists of HIV-related clinical illnesses.

AIDS case reporting will continue to serve as a basis to track the scope of the epidemic, to make projections about trends, and to help plan the allotment of health care resources. The scope of information collected about AIDS cases and HIV infections will need to be expanded beyond demographic and risk factor characteristics to include access to health care and family planning services, drug use rehabilitation, and HIV and other sexually transmitted disease prevention programs. These data will help to identify gaps in these services and help to evaluate prevention efforts.

The systematic reporting of all HIV infections may be an effective way to augment AIDS case surveillance efforts. Because lymphocyte subpopulation enumerations play a large role in determining diagnostic and therapeutic strategies, information on such key laboratory results will be increasingly valuable. Information regarding all diagnosed HIV infections and the clinical status of the patients would allow for a better understanding of the full burden of HIV-related illnesses in a given area, and could result in better allocation of resources for health services and HIV prevention programs.

The collaborative surveillance system supported by CDC and operated by all state and local health departments is clearly dependent on the work of thousands of dedicated clinicians, infection control practitioners, public health and laboratory workers, and others. Keeping all participants in this system trained, informed, and motivated will require continued commitment and will be well worth the effort.

REFERENCES

1. CDC. *Pneumocystis* pneumonia—Los Angeles. *MMWR* 1981;30:250-2.
2. CDC. Kaposi's sarcoma and *Pneumocystis* pneumonia among homosexual men—New York City and California. *MMWR* 1981;30:305-8.
3. CDC. Update on Kaposi's sarcoma and opportunistic infections in previously healthy persons—United States. *MMWR* 1982;31:294-301.
4. CDC. *Pneumocystis carinii* pneumonia among persons with hemophilia A. *MMWR* 1982;31:365-7.
5. CDC. Possible transfusion-associated acquired immune deficiency syndrome (AIDS)—California. *MMWR* 1982;31:652-4.
6. CDC. Unexplained immunodeficiency and opportunistic infections in infants—New York, New Jersey, California. *MMWR* 1982;31:665-7.
7. CDC. Immunodeficiency among female sexual partners of males with acquired immune deficiency syndrome (AIDS)—New York. *MMWR* 1983;31:697-8.
8. CDC. Update on the acquired immune deficiency syndrome (AIDS)—United States. *MMWR* 1982;31:507-8, 513-4.
9. Jaffe HW, Choi K, Thomas PA, et al. National case-control study of Kaposi's sarcoma and *Pneumocystis carinii* pneumonia in homosexual men: Part 1, Epidemiologic results. *Ann Intern Med* 1983;99:145-51.
10. Klatzmann D, Barre-Sinoussi F, Nugeyre MT, et al. Selective tropism of lymphadenopathy associated virus (LAV) for helper-inducer T lymphocytes. *Science* 1984;225:59-63.
11. Gallo RC, Salahuddin SZ, Popovic M, et al. Frequent detection and isolation of cytopathic retroviruses (HTLV-III) from patients with AIDS and at risk for AIDS. *Science* 1984;224:500-3.
12. Coffin J, Haase A, Levy J, et al. Human immunodeficiency viruses [Letter]. *Science* 1986;232:697.
13. CDC. Antibodies to a retrovirus etiologically associated with acquired immunodeficiency syndrome (AIDS) in populations with increased incidences of the syndrome. *MMWR* 1984;33:377-9.
14. CDC. Provisional Public Health Service inter-agency recommendations for screening donated blood and plasma for antibody to the virus causing acquired immunodeficiency syndrome. *MMWR* 1985;34:1-5.
15. CDC. Update: Acquired immunodeficiency syndrome in the San Francisco cohort study, 1978-85. *MMWR* 1985;34:573-5.
16. Volberding PA, Lagakos SW, Koch MA, et al. Zidovudine in asymptomatic human immunodeficiency virus infection. *N Engl J Med* 1990;322:941-9.
17. CDC. Guidelines for prophylaxis against *Pneumocystis carinii* pneumonia for persons infected with human immunodeficiency virus disease. *MMWR* 1989;38 [Suppl. S5].
18. CDC. General recommendations on immunization. *MMWR* 1989;38:207-27.
19. CDC. Screening for tuberculosis and tuberculous infection in high-risk populations and the use of preventive therapy for tuberculous infection in the United States. Recommendations of The Advisory Committee for Elimination of Tuberculosis. *MMWR* 1990;39:RR-8.
20. CDC. Acquired immunodeficiency syndrome (AIDS) update—United States. *MMWR* 1983;32:309-11.
21. Garry RF, Witte MH, Gottlieb AA, et al. Documentation of an AIDS virus infection in the United States in 1968. *JAMA* 1988;260:2085-7.
22. Corbitt G, Bailey AS, Williams G. HIV infection in Manchester, 1959. *Lancet* 1989;336:51.
23. Huminer D, Rosenfeld JB, Pitlik SD. AIDS in the pre-AIDS era. *Rev Infect Dis* 1987;9:1102-8.
24. CDC. Revision of the case definition of acquired immunodeficiency syndrome for national reporting—United States. *MMWR* 1985;34:373-5.
25. CDC. Revision of the CDC surveillance case definition for acquired immunodeficiency syndrome. *MMWR* 1987;36:1-15S.
26. CDC. Update: Acquired immunodeficiency syndrome—United States, 1981-1988. *MMWR* 1989;38:229-36.
27. Selik RM, Buehler JW, Karon JM, et al. Impact of the 1987 revision of the case definition of the acquired immunodeficiency syndrome in the United States. *J AIDS* 1990;3:73-82.
28. McDougal JS, Kennedy MS, Sligh JM, et al. Binding of the HTLV-III/LAV to T4+ T cells by a complex of the 110K molecule and the T4 molecule. *Science* 1985;231:382-5.
29. Goedert JJ, Biggar RJ, Melbye M, et al. Effect of T4 count and cofactors on the incidence of AIDS in homosexual men infected with human immunodeficiency virus. *JAMA* 1987;257:331-4.
30. Nicholson JKA, Spira TJ, Aloisio CH, et al. Serial determinations of HIV-1 titers in HIV-infected homosexual men: association of rising titers with CD4 T cell depletion and progression to AIDS. *AIDS Res Hum Retroviruses* 1989;5:205-15.
31. NIH. State-of-the-art conference on azidothymidine therapy for early HIV infection. *Am J Med* 1990;89:335-44.
32. CDC. Guidelines for prophylaxis against *Pneumocystis carinii* pneumonia for persons infected with human immunodeficiency virus. *MMWR* 1989;38:1-9.
33. Buehler J, Berkelman R, Stehr-Green J, Leary L. Completeness of AIDS surveillance, United States. 6th International Conference on AIDS, San Francisco, June, 1990;Th.C.698 (abst).
34. Conway GA, Colley-Niemeyer B, Pursley C, et al. Underreporting of AIDS cases in South Carolina, 1986 and 1987. *JAMA* 1989;262:2859-63.
35. Modesitt SK, Hulman S, Fleming D. Evaluation of active versus passive AIDS surveillance in Oregon. *Am J Public Health* 1990;80:463-4.
36. CDC. Estimates of HIV prevalence and projected AIDS cases: Summary of a workshop, October 31–November 1, 1989. *MMWR* 1990;39:110-2, 117-9.
37. Buehler JW, Devine OJ, Berkelman RL, Chevarley FM. Impact of the human immunodeficiency virus epidemic on mortality trends in young men, United States. *Am J Public Health* 1990;80:1080-6.
38. Thacker SB, Choi K, Brachman PS. The surveillance of infectious disease. *JAMA* 1983;249:1181-5.
39. Vogt RL, Clark SW, Kappel S. Evaluation of the state surveillance system using hospital discharge diagnoses, 1982-83. *Am J Epidemiol* 1986;123:197-8.
40. CDC. HIV/AIDS surveillance report, January 1991;1-22.
41. CDC. HIV prevalence estimates and AIDS projections for the United States: report based on a workshop. *MMWR* 1990;39:1-31.
42. Thomas PA, Hindin R, Greenberg A, Lopez E, Bernard G, Weisfuse I. Decreased incidence of reported AIDS cases, New York City. 6th International Conference on AIDS, San Francisco, June 1990;Th(abst).
43. Gail MH, Rosenberg PS, Goedert JJ. Therapy may explain recent deficits in AIDS incidence. *J Acquired Immune Deficiency Syndrome* 1990;3:296-306.
44. Winklestein W, Wiley JA, Padian NS, et al. The San Francisco Men's Health Study: continued decline in HIV seroconversion rates among homosexual/bisexual men. *Am J Public Health* 1988;78:1472-4.
45. CDC. Declining rates of rectal and pharyngeal gonorrhea among males–New York City. *MMWR* 1984;33:295-7.
46. Lieb L, Nahlen B, Wakamatsu P. Increasing AIDS case reporting delay in Los Angeles County, 1984-1989. 6th International Conference on AIDS, San Francisco, June, 1990;Th.C.704 (abst).
47. CDC. Safety of therapeutic products used for hemophilia patients. *MMWR* 1988;37:441-4,449-50.
48. Ward JW, Holmberg SD, Allen JR, et al. Human immunodeficiency virus (HIV) transmission by blood transfusions screened negative for HIV antibody. *N Engl J Med* 1988;318:473-8.
49. Castro KG, Lifson AR, White CR, et al. Investigations of AIDS patients with no previously identified risk factors. *JAMA* 1988;259:1338-42.
50. CDC. Acquired immunodeficiency syndrome. United States, 1989. *MMWR* 1990;39:81-6.
51. CDC. Years of potential life lost before ages 65 and 85—United States, 1987 and 1988. *MMWR* 1990;39:20-2.

52. Kilbourne BW, Chu SY, Oxtoby MJ, Rogers MF. Mortality due to HIV infection in adolescents and young adults. 6th International Conference on AIDS, San Francisco, June, 1990;Th.C.743 (abst).

53. Chu SY, Buehler JW, Berkelman RL. Impact of the human immunodeficiency virus epidemic on mortality in women of reproductive age, United States. *JAMA* 1190;264:225–9.

54. Berkelman R, Fleming P, Green T, Gwinn M, Stehr-Green J, Curran J. The epidemic of AIDS in intravenous drug users (IVDUs) and their heterosexual partners in the southeastern United States. 6th International Conference on AIDS, San Francisco, June, 1990;Th(abst).

55. Berkelman R, Karon J, Thomas P, Kerndt P, Rutherford G, Stehr-Green J. Are AIDS cases among homosexual males leveling? 5th International Conference on AIDS, Montreal, Canada, June, 1989;W.A.O.13 (abst).

56. CDC. Human immunodeficiency virus infection in the United States: a review of current knowledge. *MMWR* 1987;36 [Suppl S-6]:1–48.

57. Fleming D, Bennett D, Klockner R, Gould J, Cassidy D, Foster L. HIV infected STD clients who decline HIV counseling and testing. 5th International Conference on AIDS, Montreal, Canada, June, 1989;M.A.O.22 (abst).

58. Landis S, Schoenbach V, Weber D, Mittal M, Koch G, Levine P. HIV-1 seroprevalence in sexually transmitted disease (STD) clinic patients in central North Carolina. 5th International Conference on AIDS, Montreal, Canada, June, 1989;M.A.O.23 (abst).

59. McCray E, Onorato IM, and State and Local Health Departments. HIV seroprevalence in clients attending sexually transmitted disease (STD) clinics in the United States, 1988–90. 6th International Conference on AIDS, San Francisco, June, 1990;F.C.44 (abst).

60. Kingsley LA, Bacellar H, Zhou S, et al. Temporal trends in HIV seroconversion: a report from the multicenter AIDS cohort study (MACS). 6th International Conference on AIDS, San Francisco, June, 1990;F.C.550 (abst).

61. Kellogg TA, Marelich WD, Wilson MJ, Lemp GF, Bolan G, Rutherford GW. HIV prevalence among homosexual and bisexual men in the San Francisco Bay area: evidence of infection among young gay men. 6th International Conference on AIDS, San Francisco, June, 1990;F.C.556 (abst).

62. Weibel W, Lampinen T, Chene D, Stevko B. HIV-1 seroconversion in a cohort of street intravenous drug users in Chicago. 6th International Conference on AIDS. San Francisco, June, 1990;F.C.556 (abst).

63. Steger KA, Zawacki A, Allen D, Werner BG, Coppola D, Craven DE. Antibody to HIV-1 in intravenous drug users (IVDU) entering methadone treatment programs (MTP) in Boston. 6th International Conference on AIDS. San Francisco, June, 1990;F.C.558 (abst).

64. Hahn RA, Onorato IM, Jones TS, Dougherty J. Prevalence of HIV infection among intravenous drug users in the United States. *JAMA* 1989;261:2677–84.

65. Allen DM, Onorato IM, Sweeney PA, State and Local Health Departments. Seroprevalence of HIV infection in intravenous drug users (IVDUs) in the United States (U.S.). 6th International Conference on AIDS, San Francisco, June, 1990;F.C.551 (abst).

66. Des Jarlais DC, Friedman SR, Novick DM, et al. HIV-1 infection among intravenous drug users in Manhattan, New York City, from 1977 through 1987. *JAMA* 1989;261:1008–12.

67. van den Hoek A JAR, van Haastrecht HJA, Coutinho RA. Heterosexual behaviour of intravenous drug users in Amsterdam: implications for the AIDS epidemic. *AIDS* 1990;4:449–53.

68. Chaisson RE, Bacchetti P, Osmond D, et al. Cocaine use and HIV infection in intravenous drug users in San Francisco. *JAMA* 1989;261:561–5.

69. Augustyniak L, Kramer AS, Fricke W, Brownstein A, Evatt B. U.S. HIV seroprevalence surveillance project: regional seropositivity rates for HIV infection in patients with hemophilia. 6th International Conference on AIDS. San Francisco, June, 1990;F.C.565 (abst).

70. Holmberg SC, Horsburgh CR, Ward JW, Jaffe HW. Biologic factors in the sexual transmission of human immunodeficiency virus. *J Infect Dis* 1989;160:116–25.

71. Sweeney PA, Allen D, Onorato I, et al. HIV seroprevalence among women of reproductive age seeking clinic services, United States, 1988–1990. 6th International Conference on AIDS, San Francisco, June, 1990;F.C.568 (abst).

72. Gwinn M, George JR, Hannon WH, et al. Estimates of HIV seroprevalence in childbearing women and incidence of HIV infection in infants, United States. *Abstract* 6th International Conference on AIDS, San Francisco, June, 1990;F.C.43 (abst).

73. Gwinn M, Pappaioanou M, George JR, et al. Prevalence of HIV infection in childbearing women in the United States. *JAMA* 1991;265:1704–8.

74. Kelen GD, DiGiovanna T, Bisson L, Kalainov D, Sivertson KT, Quinn TC. Human immunodeficiency virus infection in emergency department patients: epidemiology, clinical presentations, and risk to health care workers: The Johns Hopkins experience. *JAMA* 1989;262:516–22.

75. Soderstrom CA, Furth PA, Glasser D, Dunning RW, Groseclose SL, Cowley RA. HIV infection rates in a trauma center treating predominantly rural blunt trauma victims. *J Trauma* 1989;29: 1526–30.

76. Lewandowski C, Ognjan A, Rivers E, Pohlod D, Belian B, Saravolatz LD. HIV-1 and HTLV-I seroprevalence in critically ill resuscitated emergency department patients. 5th International Conference on AIDS, Montreal, Canada, June, 1989;Th.A.P.9 (abst).

77. Gordin FM, Gibert C, Hawley HP, Willoughby A. Prevalence of human immunodeficiency virus and hepatitis B virus in unselected hospital admissions: implications for mandatory testing and universal precautions. *J Infect Dis* 1990;161:14–17.

78. Risi GF, Gaumer RH, Weeks S, Leete JK, Sanders CV. Human immunodeficiency virus: risk of exposure among health care workers at a southern urban hospital. *South Med J* 1989;82:1079–82.

79. St. Louis ME, Rauch KJ, Petersen LR, et al. Seroprevalence rates of human immunodeficiency virus infection at sentinel hospitals in the United States. *N Engl J Med* 1990;323:213–8.

80. Cauthen GM, Bloch AB, Snider DE. Reported AIDS patients with tuberculosis in the United States. 6th International Conference on AIDS, San Francisco, June, 1990;Th(abst).

81. Hnath R, McCray E, Onorato IM, and State and Local Health Departments. HIV seroprevalence in patients attending tuberculosis clinics in the United States, 1989–90. 6th International Conference on AIDS, San Francisco, June, 1990;Th.C.726 (abst).

82. CDC. *National HIV seroprevalence surveys: summary of results,* 2nd ed. Washington: U.S. Department of Health and Human Services. 1990;1–26.

83. Tindall B, Barker S, Donovan JB, et al. Characterization of the acute clinical illness associated with human immunodeficiency virus infection. *Arch Intern Med* 1988;148:945–9.

84. Ward JW, Bush TJ, Perkins HA, et al. The natural history of HIV infection: factors influencing progression to disease. *N Engl J Med* 1989;321:947–52.

85. Hessol NA, Rutherford GW, Lifson AR, et al. The natural history of HIV infection in a cohort of homosexual and bisexual men: a decade of follow-up. 4th International Conference on AIDS, Stockholm, June, 1988;4096 (abst).

86. Goedart JJ, Kesler CM, Aledort LM, et al. A prospective study of human immunodeficiency virus type 1 infection and the development of AIDS in subjects with hemophilia. *N Engl J Med* 1989;321:1141–8.

87. Longini IM, Clark WS, Horsburgh CR, et al. Statistical analysis of the stages of HIV infection using a Markov model. 5th International Conference on AIDS, Montreal, Canada, June 1988; T.A.O.36 (abst).

88. Lui KJ, Darrow WW, Rutherford GW. A model-based estimate of the mean incubation period for AIDS in homosexual men. *Science* 1988;240:1333–5.

89. Lemp GF, Hessol NA, Rutherford GW, et al. Projections of AIDS morbidity and mortality in San Francisco using epidemic models. 4th International Conference on AIDS, Stockholm, Sweden, June, 1988;4682 (abst).

AIDS and Other Manifestations of HIV Infection,
Second Edition, Edited by Gary P. Wormser.
Published by Raven Press, Ltd., New York 1992.

CHAPTER 2

Epidemiology of Pediatric HIV Infection

Martha F. Rogers and Barbara W. Kilbourne

The first cases of the acquired immunodeficiency syndrome (AIDS) in children were reported to the Centers for Disease Control (CDC) in 1982. Since that time over 3,000 cases of AIDS in children under 13 years of age have been reported, half in the past 2 years. AIDS is now among the top ten leading causes of death in children over 1 year of age (1). Over the next decade, many more pediatric cases are likely to occur as the number of human immunodeficiency virus (HIV)-infected women of childbearing age increases because of intravenous drug and heterosexual transmission. Over the past 2 years, greater percentage increases have occurred in women compared with men, in children compared with other age groups, and in persons infected via heterosexual and perinatal transmission compared with other transmission groups (2). Based on data from the National Survey of Childbearing Women, CDC estimates that approximately 6,000 infants are born each year to HIV-infected women in the United States (3).

Although HIV infection in women and children has been concentrated in large urban areas along the east coast, the epidemic is spreading rapidly to smaller urban and even rural areas and other regions of the country (2). Pediatric HIV infection and AIDS is becoming an increasingly common disease. Understanding the epidemiology, transmission, and occurrence of HIV infection in the pediatric population is important for early recognition and diagnosis of this infection in children. This chapter reviews these topics.

EPIDEMIOLOGY IN CHILDREN

Cases of AIDS and HIV infection among children in the United States represent a relatively small but increasingly important proportion of total cases. In the United States, 2,786 (2%) of the 161,073 cases of AIDS reported to CDC as of December 31, 1990, occurred in children under the age of 13 years (pediatric cases) and another 629 cases occurred in adolescents, ages 13–19 years (Fig. 1). The number of cases reported each year continues to increase, with 782 pediatric cases reported in 1990, a 21% increase over 1989.

Children in the United States have acquired HIV infection primarily through two routes: perinatally (mother to infant) and transfusion of blood or blood products. In the United States, most pediatric AIDS cases are attributable to perinatal transmission (Table 1), and this distribution has not changed remarkably over time. However, HIV transmission patterns have changed, but these changes are not yet apparent among AIDS cases due to the relatively long incubation period for the disease (4). In most developed countries, transmission of HIV through blood products virtually ended in 1985 when donor screening for HIV antibody began (5). Both donor screening and heat treatment of blood clotting factor products have virtually stopped most new infections in persons with hemophilia (6). In the United States, only two children with AIDS following HIV infection acquired from screened blood have been reported to CDC. In these cases, the donors were seronegative at the time of donation, but later seroconverted. Only 18 cases in persons with hemophilia receiving heat-treated factor products have been published (6). In contrast, perinatal transmission of HIV continues to rise as more women become infected and bear children.

The demographic characteristics of children acquiring HIV through these various routes differ markedly. Characteristics of children with perinatally acquired AIDS parallel those of women with AIDS. In the United States, most of these children are from large urban areas in the East (Table 2), and they are largely of minority race and ethnicity (Table 3). The male:female ratio in these children is 1:1, indicating that mothers probably transmit

M. F. Rogers and B. W. Kilbourne: Division of HIV/AIDS, Center for Infectious Diseases, Centers for Disease Control, Public Health Service, U.S. Department of Health and Human Services, Atlanta, Georgia 30333.

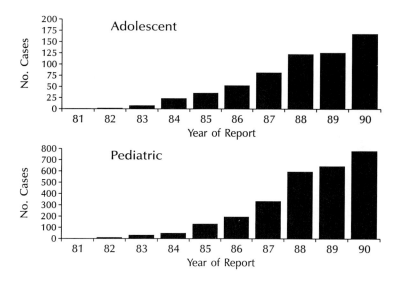

FIG. 1. Pediatric (<13 years of age) and adolescent (13–19 years of age) AIDS cases by year of report to CDC, United States.

equally to male and female infants. The majority of the mothers of these children acquired HIV infection through intravenous drug use (50%) or heterosexual transmission (38%) (Table 1).

The demographic characteristics of children with transfusion-acquired AIDS reflect the characteristics of children receiving transfusions (Table 3). In the United States, most children with transfusion-acquired AIDS were transfused in infancy as a result of perinatal problems such as prematurity or congenital abnormalities. There is a slight male predominance (Table 3). In a study of blood transfusion practices, male infants were more likely to receive transfusions than female infants (7). In contrast to children with perinatally acquired AIDS, most children with transfusion-acquired AIDS are white; however, compared with the U.S. population, blacks and Hispanics are also overrepresented among children with transfusion-acquired AIDS. Although little information exists on the race distribution of persons receiving transfusions, minority children are more likely to suffer from perinatal morbidity (8) and may be more likely to receive transfusions in infancy.

Children with clotting factor disorders have also been at increased risk for HIV infection and account for 5% of pediatric AIDS cases and 31% of cases in adolescents in

the United States. Since most cases occur in persons with sex-linked genetic disorders, 98% of these cases occur in males. Racially, they are more reflective of the U.S. population: 68% are white, 13% are black, 17% are Hispanic, and 2% are of other race/ethnicity.

TABLE 2. *Geographic distribution of children (less than 13 years of age) with AIDS reported to CDC as of December 31, 1990, United States*

Metropolitan areas with populations of 500,000 or more	No. (%)
New York City, NY	728 (26)
Miami, FL	163 (6)
Newark, NJ	126 (5)
San Juan, PR	106 (4)
Los Angeles, CA	93 (3)
Washington, DC	69 (2)
W. Palm Beach, FL	52 (2)
Philadelphia, PA	52 (2)
Chicago, IL	51 (2)
Boston, MA	51 (2)
Baltimore, MD	49 (2)
Ft. Lauderdale, FL	49 (2)
Houston, TX	46 (2)
Jersey City, NJ	43 (2)
Nassau-Suffolk, NY	39 (1)
Bergen-Passaic, NJ	27 (1)
New Haven, CT	27 (1)
Tampa-St. Petersburg, FL	26 (1)
Atlanta, GA	25 (1)
Jacksonville, FL	25 (1)
Middlesex, NJ	24 (1)
Monmouth-Ocean City, NJ	23 (1)
Detroit, MI	23 (1)
New Orleans, LA	20 (1)
Bridgeport, CN	20 (1)
Other standard metropolitan statistical areas	376 (13)
Rural/smaller metro. areas[a]	453 (16)
Total	2,786 (100)

[a] Includes data from rural and metropolitan areas that have populations of less than 500,000.

TABLE 1. *Risk factors associated with AIDS in children (less than 13 years of age) reported to the CDC (United States) as of December 31, 1990*

Risk factor	No. (%)
Perinatally acquired by mother's risk factor	2,327 (84)
IV drug user	1,163 (42)
Heterosexual contact	879 (32)
Transfusion recipient	47 (2)
Risk unknown	238 (8)
Transfusion-acquired	252 (9)
Hemophilia	139 (5)
Other/unknown	68 (2)
Total	2,786 (100)

TABLE 3. *Demographic characteristics of children (less than 13 years of age) with AIDS reported to CDC as of December 31, 1990 by transmission category, United States*

Demographic characteristic	Perinatal n = 2,327 [No. (%)]	Transfusion-acquired n = 252 [No. (%)]	Hemophilia n = 139 [No. (%)]	Unknown n = 68 [No. (%)]
Sex				
Female	1,158 (50)	90 (36)	3 (2)	34 (50)
Male	1,169 (50)	162 (64)	136 (98)	34 (50)
Race				
White	366 (16)	133 (53)	95 (68)	8 (12)
Black	1,326 (57)	56 (22)	18 (13)	39 (57)
Hispanic	617 (27)	58 (23)	23 (17)	21 (31)
Asian/Indian	10 (<1)	5 (2)	3 (2)	0
Unknown	8 (<1)	0	0	0
Age at diagnosis of AIDS				
Median	12 months	4.75 years	10 years	10 months
Range	1 month–11 years	4 months–12 years	13 months–12 years	1 month–12 years

The geographic distribution of transfusion-acquired and hemophilia-associated AIDS cases has been more diffuse compared with perinatally acquired cases. Whereas 57% of perinatally acquired cases come from New York, New Jersey, and Florida, 40 states have reported transfusion-acquired and/or hemophilia-associated cases and the top three states account for about 40% of the cases.

The age at diagnosis of AIDS in these three groups of children (perinatal, transfusion-acquired, and hemophilia) reflects the age at the time of infection and the incubation or latency period of the disease. Transmission of HIV from mothers to their infants takes place during gestation, labor and delivery, or (rarely) in the post partum period through breastfeeding (9). The median age at diagnosis of perinatally acquired AIDS cases reported to CDC was 12 months, and 80% of these cases were in children under age 3 years at the time of diagnosis. Because most children with transfusion-acquired AIDS were infected from blood transfusions in infancy, this disease has also largely affected infants and toddlers; however, nearly all cases being reported today received their contaminated transfusion at least 6 years ago, and thus are largely school-aged children. The median age for all reported children with transfusion-acquired AIDS is 4.75 years; the median age for those children diagnosed in 1989 and 1990 is 7.4 years. AIDS cases in children with hemophilia have largely been in those who were school-aged: their median age is 10 years (Table 3).

MODES OF TRANSMISSION IN CHILDREN

Perinatal Transmission

Evidence indicates that mothers can transmit HIV to their infants by three mechanisms: (1) through transplacental passage of the virus in utero; (2) through exposure to infectious maternal blood and vaginal secretions during labor and delivery; and (3) through breastfeeding. Prenatal transmission has been demonstrated by identification of the virus in fetal tissue and amniotic fluid (10–12). A dysmorphic syndrome has been reported, but not confirmed by carefully controlled studies, and remains controversial (13). Because the transmission patterns of HIV are quite similar to those of the hepatitis B virus, it is reasonable to assume that HIV can also be transmitted during the intrapartum period. However, the lack of highly sensitive and specific laboratory methods to diagnose infection has hindered our ability to document transmission via this route. Transmission through breastfeeding has been demonstrated in infants born to mothers who were infected post partum either through transfusions, or by heterosexual or IV drug use-associated transmission (14,15). Additionally, HIV has been isolated from breast milk (16).

Although transmission can occur through all these routes, the proportion of transmission attributable to each route is unknown. It is also unclear whether in utero transmission usually occurs early in gestation or in the third trimester. In the United States, in utero and/or intra partum transmission probably account for most perinatal transmissions, since very few HIV-infected drug-addicted mothers breastfeed their infants. In developing countries, nearly all women breastfeed their infants, but whether this contributes an additional risk of transmission in infants already exposed during pregnancy is unclear. The Italian Multicentre Study found a higher rate of transmission in breastfed infants compared with non-breast-fed infants, but this did not reach statistical significance (17). The French Collaborative Study Group found that transmission rates among breastfed infants were significantly higher compared with those who were not breastfed (18). However, in similar studies, both the European Collaborative Study and a perinatal study from Zaire did not find significant differences between the transmission rates in breastfed and non-breastfed infants (19,20). Although many developed countries, including the United States, have recommended that HIV-infected women refrain from breastfeeding (21,22), recommendations regarding breastfeeding for HIV-seropositive women in developing countries must be made in the context of the highly significant risks involved in formula feeding by women who may not have clean water for reconstituting powder or concentrate formula. In addition, many of these women cannot afford the formula. For these reasons, WHO has recommended that HIV-infected women in developing countries continue to breastfeed (23).

Several studies of HIV perinatal transmission have estimated the rate of transmission from mothers to infants. Although most larger studies have observed rates from 20% to 40% (17,18,24), one large study recently reported a rate of 13% (25). Studies of African women have found somewhat higher rates compared with studies of women from Europe and the United States (24). Maternal or infant (host) factors that influence the likelihood of transmission are under study. One such study found that women with lower CD4+ cell counts and more advanced disease were more likely to transmit to their infants (24). Because both the frequency of infected cells and the amount of virus in plasma are markedly increased in symptomatic patients compared with asymptomatic individuals (26,27), the greater amount of virus in the blood may be associated with increased transmission. To examine this possibility, virus quantitation studies comparing transmitting versus nontransmitting mothers need to be done.

Investigators have also focused on possible protective factors such as neutralizing antibody titers in the mothers and antibodies to epitopes of the V3 loop that contains the principal neutralizing domain of HIV. Three recent studies found that mothers with antibodies to certain epitopes of the V3 loop were less likely to transmit HIV to their infants (28–30). However, the studies used different methodologies (and therefore were not directly comparable), the sample sizes were small, and associations were found with different epitopes. In addition, other studies have not been able to confirm these findings with larger sample sizes (31,32). Nonetheless, these findings do raise the possibility of protective humoral immune factors that could be critical in preventing perinatal transmission and providing important clues for vaccine development. Further study is warranted.

The mechanism of in utero maternal–infant transmission is not known, but several hypotheses have been raised (33). Passage of HIV-infected maternal lymphocytes into the fetal circulation is one possibility. However, transplacental passage of maternal cells has been relatively rare in the murine model (34); thus, this mechanism seems somewhat unlikely. Direct infection of placental tissue and subsequent infection of fetal blood cells may be more likely. One study found that cells in the perimeter of the chorionic villi (possibly of trophoblastic origin), cells within the stroma [probably Hofbauer cells (placental macrophages)], and cells within the endothelial lining of blood vessels contained CD4+ receptors, the target site for virus attachment to cells (33). Another study examining placentas from three HIV-infected women found HIV-positive maternal decidual leukocytes, trophoblastic cells, villous mesenchymal cells (macrophages and endothelial cells), and embryonic blood cell precursors (35). HIV might also gain access to CD4− trophoblastic cells through phagocytosis (35). Study of the placenta and the role it plays in transmission of HIV from mothers to their infants/fetuses is an important area that requires further research.

Transfusion-associated Transmission

Transfusion of blood or blood components from an HIV-infected donor is a highly efficient mode of transmission. Over 90% of persons receiving an HIV-seropositive unit acquire the infection (36,37). Both cellular and plasma components of whole blood have transmitted HIV infection (38). Immunoglobulin preparations including Rh factor have not transmitted HIV because the fractionation process used to prepare these products effectively removes HIV by partitioning and inactivation (39).

CDC has estimated that approximately 12,000 transfusion recipients in the United States who survived their underlying disease acquired transfusion-associated HIV infection between 1978 and 1984 (40). Persons receiving multiple transfusions between 1978 and 1985 were at greater risk. HIV seroprevalence rates of 4–8% have been detected in leukemic (40), hemodialysis (41), and other patients receiving multiple transfusions during this period (42).

Since donor screening was implemented in March 1985, 13 adult/adolescent and 2 pediatric cases of AIDS following infection acquired from blood that was screened HIV negative have been reported to CDC as of January 1991. Ward et al. (5) estimated the rate of HIV infection in screened blood to be 0.003% (26/1,000,000 transfusions) (5). In a study of 4,163 cardiac surgery patients who were tested for HIV antibody before and after receiving blood transfusions, Cohen et al. (43) also found that the risk of transmission of HIV by transfusion of screened blood was 0.003% (30/1,000,000 units). Based on estimates of the chance that blood will be donated during the "window period" (time period shortly after HIV infection when antibody is not yet detectable), Cumming et al. (44) estimated that the transfused patient receiving the average transfusion (5.4 units) had odds of 1:28,000 of contracting HIV infection from the transfusions (44).

HIV has also been transmitted through transplantation of bone, kidney, liver, heart, pancreas, and possibly skin (45). HIV infection acquired through artificial insemination has also been reported, although the risk of acquiring infection following nonsexual exposure to infected semen is unclear. In one report from Australia, four of eight women artificially inseminated with cryopreserved semen became infected (46). However, in another report from New York City, 176 women were artificially inseminated with fresh semen from six donors later identified as HIV seropositive (47). Only 1 of 134 women tested was found to be HIV seropositive. The U.S. Public Health Service (45) recommends that all tissue and organ allograft donors as well as blood and semen donors be evaluated for risks associated with HIV infection and tested for HIV antibody.

Hemophilia-associated HIV Infection

Both factor VIII and factor IX concentrates have transmitted HIV (42). In the United States, up to 80% of persons with hemophilia receiving large-pool, non-heat-treated factor products from plasma donated before HIV screening have developed antibody to HIV (42). More severe hemophilia and greater factor usage have been associated with a greater risk of HIV infection. Persons with hemophilia treated exclusively with cryoprecipitate appear to have had a lower risk of exposure to HIV and subsequent infection (48).

Some investigators have speculated that, in some cases, persons with hemophilia may have become "immunized" by receiving HIV inactivated during the preparation or storage of unscreened, non-heat-treated factor products (49). However, in one study, 55 of 56 HIV-seropositive persons with hemophilia were also culture positive, indicating active infection (50).

Sexual transmission from HIV-infected men with hemophilia to their female sex partners, with subsequent perinatal transmission to their infants, is also a problem for these men and their families. Approximately 10–20% of the long-term female sex partners of HIV-infected men with hemophilia have acquired HIV infection through heterosexual contact (51). As of December 31, 1990, CDC had received reports of nine children with AIDS whose mothers acquired HIV infection from men with hemophilia.

Other Routes of Transmission

Early in the AIDS epidemic, concern was raised about transmission of HIV through casual contact in settings such as schools, daycare facilities, and families. However, evidence indicates that transmission in these settings is extremely rare or nonexistent. No cases of transmission within the school or daycare setting have been reported. Only 4% of the 161,073 AIDS cases reported to the CDC as of December 31, 1990, have not had an identifiable risk factor for infection, and special investigations of many of these cases have been completed and do not reveal transmission through casual contact (52). In at least 12 studies of over 800 family members of HIV-infected persons, transmission within families has not been found despite very close personal contact and sharing of items likely to be soiled with blood and body secretions of the infected family member (53–64).

Only one well-documented case of infant-to-mother transmission has been reported. This case involved a chronically ill child with a congenital intestinal abnormality whose mother was exposed extensively to the child's body fluids and blood while providing in-hospital nursing care for her child (65). She did not take precautions to avoid contact with her child's blood and body fluids.

The only reported case of possible household transmission occurred in a West German family and involved apparent sibling-to-sibling transmission (66). However, this case was reported in a brief letter with little indication of the extent of the investigation of the family or the nature of the contact between the two siblings. The authors concluded that the transmission occurred when the infected child bit the uninfected sibling; however, this seems unlikely since the bite was minor and did not break the skin.

Biting has received much attention as a possible mode of HIV transmission, but there is little evidence that biting transmits this virus. In a study of the family members of children with transfusion-associated HIV infection, nine HIV-infected children bit their contacts and seven contacts bit an HIV-infected child. There was no evidence of infection in the contacts (67). Similarly, no evidence of infection was found in 30 health care workers bitten or scratched by a brain-damaged adult with HIV infection (68), or in a woman who was bitten severely while attending an HIV-infected patient who was having a seizure (69). Further, four children bitten multiple times by an HIV-infected child over a 2-week period were seronegative 6 months after the incident (70). Transmission involving biting was suspected in one case of HIV infection in a woman who had been bitten by her infected IV-drug using sister during a fight. The infected sister's mouth was filled with blood at the time of the bite (71).

CDC and the American Academy of Pediatrics, as well as a number of state health and education departments, have recommended that most children with HIV infection be allowed to attend school and daycare (72–74). Concern has been raised regarding school and daycare attendance of infected infants and toddlers and neurologically handicapped children because of behaviors such as drooling, mouthing toys, incontinence, and biting. As the above discussion indicates, this concern is based more on theoretical grounds than actual evidence of transmission in these settings.

PREVENTION OF HIV INFECTION IN CHILDREN

Despite recent advances in therapy for HIV infection, there is no "cure." Prevention of infection is therefore paramount. Prevention of HIV infection in children requires prevention of infection in women of child-bearing age. Women can dramatically reduce their risk of HIV infection by using condoms during sexual intercourse and avoiding the use of IV drugs. However, changing behaviors in women already engaging in high-risk behavior and preventing high-risk behavior in adolescent women can be difficult. Public health programs and health care providers should educate and counsel women about the modes of transmission of HIV and provide them with the necessary skills and services needed for behavioral change, such as family planning and drug treatment services.

Strategies to prevent transmission from infected women to their children also need to be developed and implemented. Currently, the only effective means of preventing perinatal transmission is to prevent pregnancy, a strategy that may be unacceptable to many HIV-infected women whose desires to bear children outweigh the risk of transmission. HIV-infected women who are or want to become pregnant need to be carefully informed in a culturally and socially sensitive manner about the risks of transmission to their offspring, the risk of development of AIDS in HIV-infected children, the effects of HIV infection on pregnancy, the effects of pregnancy on the course of HIV infection, and the need to consider the future care of their children in the inevitable event of their death. Health care providers should recognize the right of the woman to choose between her reproductive options and should be supportive of her choice.

While some HIV-infected women will choose not to bear children, many will become pregnant by choice or because they are not taking precautions to prevent pregnancy. Therefore, to prevent perinatal transmission from these women to their infants, other strategies need to be developed. Clinical trials of zidovudine administered during pregnancy in hope of reducing the risk of perinatal transmission are under way. Other antiviral agents such as CD4-IgG (which blocks virus attachment to cells) and hyperimmune gammaglobulin have been proposed. HIV vaccines are also under development (75).

CONCLUSIONS

In only a few years, HIV infection has become a world-wide pandemic. Because the virus is primarily spread through sexual contact, devastating potential exists for the spread of infection to sexually active women and for transmission of the virus from these women to their children. The growing drug abuse problem and the associated sexual activity and prostitution in the United States will undoubtedly worsen the epidemic among women and children in this country.

The health, social, and financial consequences of this epidemic are staggering. WHO estimates that at least 11 million persons are infected with HIV world-wide (ref. 3 in chapter by Mastro et al.). Natural history studies indicate that most if not all of these persons will eventually develop AIDS. Because infected persons can remain asymptomatic and unaware of their risk of transmission for long periods of time, the potential for spread throughout populations is enormous.

To prevent this spread, health agencies world-wide should continue to develop effective prevention programs and commit the resources needed to implement and evaluate these efforts. Those concerned with the health of women and children need to insist on and ensure these policies.

REFERENCES

1. Kilbourne B, Buehler J, Rogers M. AIDS as a cause of death in children, adolescents, and young adults. *Am J Public Health* 1990;80:499–500.
2. CDC. Update: acquired immunodeficiency syndrome—United States, 1981–1990. *MMWR* 1991;40:358–63,369.
3. Gwinn M, Pappaioanou M, George JR, et al. Prevalence of HIV infection in childbearing women in the United States. *JAMA* 1991;265:1704–8.
4. Lui KJ, Lawrence DN, Morgan WM, Peterman TA, Haverkos HW, Bregman DJ. A model-based approach for estimating the mean incubation period of transfusion-associated acquired immunodeficiency syndrome. *Proc Natl Acad Sci USA* 1986;83:3051–5.
5. Ward JW, Holmberg SD, Allen JR, et al. Transmission of human immunodeficiency virus (HIV) by blood transfusions screened as negative for HIV antibody. *N Engl J Med* 1988;318:473–8.
6. CDC. Safety of therapeutic products used for hemophilia patients. *MMWR* 1988;37:441–50.
7. Freidman BA, Burns TL, Schork MA. *A study of national trends in transfusion practice.* National Heart, Lung, and Blood Institute contract NO1 HB-9-2920. Ann Arbor: The University of Michigan, 1980.
8. National Center for Health Statistics. *Advance report of final mortality statistics, 1987. Monthly vital statistics report,* vol 38, no 5, Suppl. Hyattsville, MD: Public Health Service, 1989.
9. Rogers MF. Perinatal HIV-1 infection. In: Kaslow RA, Francis DP, eds. *The epidemiology of AIDS.* New York: Oxford University Press, 1989;231–41.
10. Sprecher S, Soumenkoff G, Puissant F, Degueldre M. Vertical transmission of HIV in 15-week fetus. *Lancet* 1986;2:288–9.
11. Mundy DC, Schinazi RF, Gerber AR, Nahmias AJ, Randall HW. Human immunodeficiency virus isolated from amniotic fluid. *Lancet* 1987;2:459–60.
12. Jovaisas E, Koch MA, Schafer A, Stauber M, Lowenthal D. LAV/HTLV-III in 20-week fetus. *Lancet* 1985;2:1129.
13. Nicholas SW. Controversy: is there an HIV-associated facial dysmorphism? *Pediatr Ann* 1988;17:353–62.
14. Oxtoby MJ. Human immunodeficiency virus and other viruses in human milk: placing the issues in broader perspective. *Pediatr Infect Dis* 1988;7:825–35.
15. Hira SK, Mangrola UG, Mwale C, et al. Apparent vertical transmission of human immunodeficiency virus type 1 by breast-feeding in Zambia. *J Pediatr* 1990;117:421–4.
16. Thiry L, Sprecher-Goldberger S, Jonckheer T, et al. Isolation of

AIDS virus from cell-free breast milk of three healthy virus carriers. *Lancet* 1985;2:891–2.

17. Italian Multicentre Study. Epidemiology, clinical features, and prognostic factors of pediatric HIV infection. *Lancet* 1988;2: 1043–5.

18. Blanche S, Rouzioux C, Moscato MG, et al. A prospective study of infants born to women seropositive for human immunodeficiency virus type 1. *N Engl J Med* 1989;320:1643–8.

19. Ryder RW, Manzila T, Baende E, et al. Evidence from Zaire that breast-feeding by HIV-1-seropositive mothers is not a major route for perinatal HIV-1 transmission but does decrease morbidity. *AIDS* 1991;5:709–14.

20. The European Collaborative Study. Mother-to-child transmission of HIV infection. *Lancet* 1988;2:1039–42.

21. CDC. Recommendations for assisting in the prevention of perinatal transmission of human T-lymphotropic virus type III/lymphadenopathy-associated virus and acquired immunodeficiency syndrome. *MMWR* 1985;34:721–32.

22. Logan S, Newell M, Ades T, Peckham CS. Breast-feeding and HIV infection. *Lancet* 1988;1:1346.

23. World Health Organization. Breast-feeding/breast milk and human immunodeficiency virus (HIV). *Weekly Epidem Rec* 1987;62:245–6.

24. Ryder RW, Nsa W, Hassig SE, et al. Perinatal transmission of the human immunodeficiency virus type 1 to infants of seropositive women in Zaire. *N Engl J Med* 1989;320:1637–42.

25. The European Collaborative Study. Mother to child transmission of HIV infection. *Lancet* 1991;337:253–60.

26. Ho DD, Moudgil T, Alam M. Quantitation of human immunodeficiency virus type 1 in the blood of infected persons. *N Engl J Med* 1989;321:1621–5.

27. Schnittman SM, Greenhouse JJ, Psallidopoulos MC, et al. Increasing viral burden in CD4+ T cells from patients with human immunodeficiency virus (HIV) infection reflects rapidly progressive immunosuppression and clinical disease. *Ann Intern Med* 1990;113:438–43.

28. Goedert JJ, Mendez H, Drummond JE, et al. Mother-to-infant transmission of human immunodeficiency virus type 1: association with prematurity or low anti-gp 120. *Lancet* 1989;2:1352–4.

29. Rossi P, Moschese V, Broliden PA, et al. Presence of maternal antibodies to human immunodeficiency virus 1 envelope glycoprotein gp 120 epitopes correlates with the uninfected status of children born to seropositive mothers. *Proc Natl Acad Sci USA* 1989;86:8055–8.

30. Devash Y, Calvelli TA, Wood DG, Reagan KJ, Rubinstein A. Vertical transmission of human immunodeficiency virus is correlated with the absence of high affinity/avidity maternal antibodies to the gp120 principal neutralizing domain. *Proc Natl Acad Sci USA* 1990;87:3445–9.

31. Parekh BS, Shaffer N, Pau C-P, et al. Lack of correlation between maternal antibodies to V3 loop peptides of gp 120 and perinatal HIV-1 transmission. *AIDS* 1991;5:1179–84.

32. Durda P. Conference on Early Diagnosis of HIV Infection in Infants, Washington, DC, November 1990.

33. Maury W, Potts BJ, Rabson AB. HIV-1 infection of first-trimester and term human placental tissue: a possible mode of maternal-fetal transmission. *J Infect Dis* 1989;160:583–8.

34. Hunziker RD, Gambel P, Wegmann TG. Placenta as a selective barrier to cellular traffic. *J Immunol* 1984;133:667–71.

35. Lewis SH, Reynolds-Kohler C, Fox HE, Nelson JA. HIV-1 in trophoblastic and villous Hofbauer cells, and haematological precursors in eight-week fetuses. *Lancet* 1990;335:565–8.

36. Ward JW, Deppe DA, Samson S, et al. Risk of human immunodeficiency virus infection from blood donors who later developed the acquired immunodeficiency syndrome. *Ann Intern Med* 1987;106:61–2.

37. Donegan E, Stuart M, Niland JC, et al. Infection with human immunodeficiency virus type I (HIV-I) among recipients of antibody-positive blood donations. *Ann Intern Med* 1990;113:733–39.

38. Curran JW, Lawrence DN, Jaffe H, et al. Acquired immunodeficiency syndrome (AIDS) associated with transfusions. *N Engl J Med* 1984;310:69–75.

39. Centers for Disease Control. Lack of transmission of human immu-

nodeficiency virus through Rh$_0$ (D) immune globulin (human). *MMWR* 1987;36:728–9.

40. Centers for Disease Control. Human immunodeficiency virus infection in transfusion recipients and their family members. *MMWR* 1987;36:137–40.

41. Peterman TA, Lang GR, Mikos NJ, et al. HTLV-III/LAV infection in hemodialysis patients. *JAMA* 1986;255:2324–6.

42. Jason J, McDougal S, Holman RC, et al. Human T-lymphotropic retrovirus type III/lymphadenopathy-associated virus antibody. *JAMA* 1985;253:3409–15.

43. Cohen ND, Munoz A, Reitz BA, et al. Transmission of retroviruses by transfusion of screened blood in patients undergoing cardiac surgery. *N Engl J Med* 1989;320:1172–6.

44. Cumming PD, Wallace EL, Schorr JB, Dodd RY. Exposure of patients to human immunodeficiency virus through the transfusion of blood components that test antibody-negative. *N Engl J Med* 1989;321:941–6.

45. Centers for Disease Control. Semen banking, organ and tissue transplantation, and HIV antibody testing. *MMWR* 1988;37: 57–63.

46. Stewart GJ, Tyler JPP, Cunningham AL, et al. Transmission of HTLV-III virus by artificial insemination by donor. *Lancet* 1985;2:581–4.

47. Chiasson MA, Stoneburner RL, Joseph SC. Human immunodeficiency virus transmission through artificial insemination. *J Acquired Immune Deficiency Syndrome* 1990;3:69–72.

48. Kletzel M, Charlton R, Becton D, Berry DH. Cryoprecipitate: a safe factor VIII replacement. *Lancet* 1987;1:1093–4.

49. Eyster ME, Goedert JJ, Sarngadharan MG, Weiss SH, Gallo RC, Blattner WA. Development and early natural history of HTLV-III antibodies in persons with hemophilia. *JAMA* 1985;253:2219–23.

50. Jackson JB, Sannerud KJ, Hopsicker JS, Kwok SY, Edson JR, Balfour HH. Hemophiliacs with HIV antibody are actively infected. *JAMA* 1988;260:2236–9.

51. Kreiss JK, Kitchen LW, Prince HE, Kasper CK, Essex M. Antibody to human T-lymphotropic virus type III in wives of hemophiliacs: evidence for heterosexual transmission. *Ann Intern Med* 1985;102:623–6.

52. Castro KG, Lifson AR, White CR, et al. Investigations of AIDS patients with no previously identified risk factors. *JAMA* 1988;259:1338–42.

53. Thomas PA, Lubin K, Milberg J, Reiss R, Getchell J, Enlow R. Cohort comparison study of children whose mothers have acquired immunodeficiency syndrome and children of well inner city mothers. *Pediatr Infect Dis* 1987;6:247–51.

54. Friedland GH, Saltzman BR, Rogers MF, et al. Lack of household transmission of HTLV-III infection. *N Engl J Med* 1986;314: 344–9.

55. Jason JM, McDougal JS, Lawrence DN, Kennedy MS, Hilgartner M, Evatt BL. Lymphadenopathy-associated virus (LAV) antibody and immune status of household contacts and sexual partners of persons with hemophilia. *JAMA* 1986;255:212–5.

56. Kaplan JE, Oleske JM, Getchell JP, et al. Evidence against transmission of HTLV-III/LAV in families of children with AIDS. *Pediatr Infect Dis* 1985;4:468–71.

57. Lawrence DN, Jason JM, Bouhasin JD, et al. HTLV-III/LAV antibody status of spouses and household contacts assisting in home infusion of hemophilia patients. *Blood* 1985;66:703–5.

58. Redfield RR, Markham PD, Salahuddin SZ, et al. Frequent transmission of HTLV-III among spouse of patients with AIDS-related complex and AIDS. *JAMA* 1985;253:1571–3.

59. Berthier A, Chamaret S, Fauchet R, et al. Transmissibility of human immunodeficiency virus in haemophilic and non-haemophilic children living in a private school in France. *Lancet* 1986;2:598–601.

60. Brettler DB, Forsberg AD, Levine PH, Andrews CA, Baker S, Sullivan JL. Human immunodeficiency virus isolation studies and antibody testing. *Arch Intern Med* 1988;148:1299–1301.

61. Fischl MA, Dickinson GM, Scott GB, Klimas N, Fletcher MA, Parks W. Evaluation of heterosexual partners, children, and household contacts of adults with AIDS. *JAMA* 1987;257:640–4.

62. Peterman TA, Stoneburner RL, Allen JR, Jaffe HW, Curran JW. Risk of human immunodeficiency virus transmission from hetero-

sexual adults with transfusion-associated infections. *JAMA* 1988;259:55–8.

63. Romano N, De Crescenzo L, Lupo G, et al. Main routes of transmission of human immunodeficiency virus (HIV) infection in a family setting in Palermo, Italy. *Am J Epidemiol* 1988;128: 254–60.

64. Mann JM, Quinn TC, Francis H, et al. Prevalence of HTLV-III/LAV in household contacts of patients with confirmed AIDS and controls in Kinshasa, Zaire. *JAMA* 1986;256:721–4.

65. CDC. Apparent transmission of HTLV-III/LAV from a child to a mother providing health care. *MMWR* 1986;35:76–9.

66. Wahn V, Kramer HH, Voit T, Bruster HT, Scrampical B, Scheid A. Horizontal transmission of HIV infection between two siblings. *Lancet* 1986;2:694.

67. Rogers MF, White CR, Sanders R, et al. Lack of transmission of human immunodeficiency virus from infected children to their household contacts. *Pediatrics* 1990;85:210–4.

68. Tsoukas C, Hadjis T, Shuster J, Theberge L, Feorino P, O'Shaughnessy M. Lack of transmission of HIV through human bites and scratches. *J Acquired Immune Deficiency Syndromes* 1988;1: 505–7.

69. Drummond JA. Seronegative 18 months after being bitten by a patient with AIDS. *JAMA* 1986;256:2342–3.

70. Shirley LR, Ross SA. Risk of transmission of human immunodeficiency virus by bite of an infected toddler. *J Pediat* 1989;114:425–7.

71. [Anonymous]. Transmission of HIV by human bite. *Lancet* 1987;2:522.

72. Centers for Disease Control: education and foster care of children infected with human T-lymphotropic virus type III/lymphadenopathy-associated virus. *MMWR* 1985;34:517–21.

73. Task Force on Pediatric AIDS, American Academy of Pediatrics: pediatric guidelines for infection control of human immunodeficiency virus (acquired immunodeficiency virus) in hospitals, medical offices, schools, and other settings. *Pediatrics* 1988;82:801–7.

74. Rutherford GW, Oliva GE, Grossman M, et al. Guidelines for the control of perinatally transmitted human immunodeficiency virus infection and care of infected mothers, infants, and children. *West J Med* 1987;147:104–8.

75. Dolin R, Graham BS, Greenberg SB, et al. The safety and immunogenicity of a human immunodeficiency virus type 1 (HIV-1) recombinant gp160 candidate vaccine in humans. *Ann Intern Med* 1991;114:119–27.

76. Chin J, Sankaran G, Mann JM. Mother-to-infant transmission of HIV: an increasing global problem. In: Kessel E, Awan AK, eds. *Maternal and child care in developing countries.* Thun, Switzerland: Ott Publishers, 1989:299–306.

AIDS and Other Manifestations of HIV Infection,
Second Edition, Edited by Gary P. Wormser.
Published by Raven Press, Ltd., New York 1992.

CHAPTER 3

Epidemiology of HIV Infection and AIDS Outside of the United States

Timothy D. Mastro, Helene D. Gayle, and William L. Heyward

Through early 1991, 10 years after the recognition of acquired immunodeficiency syndrome (AIDS) in the United States, 366,455 cases of AIDS had been reported to the World Health Organization (WHO) from 162 countries in all regions of the world (1). However, due to substantial underreporting in many countries, these officially reported cases are thought to be only a fraction of the true number of AIDS cases, estimated to be closer to 1.5 million (2,3). Moreover, the epidemiology of human immunodeficiency virus (HIV) infection provides a more meaningful perspective on the pandemic. As of 1991, WHO estimated that, worldwide, 10 million adults had been infected with HIV-1; approximately 6 million of these adults were in sub-Saharan Africa, 2 million were in industrialized, Western countries (primarily North America and Western Europe), 1 million in Latin America, and perhaps 1 million in Asia. In addition, about 1 million children are estimated to have acquired HIV-1 infection perinatally (3). WHO projects that 15 million adults will have been infected with HIV-1 by 1995 (4).

The pandemic of HIV-1 infection and AIDS has been and will likely continue to be a volatile, dynamic process (5). The character of the epidemic in each country and population is in large part determined by the potential for groups of people to be exposed to HIV infection by the three documented modes of transmission: (1) by sexual intercourse (vaginal, anal, and oral); (2) parenterally, i.e., by injection, transfusion, or transplantation of HIV-infected blood, blood products, semen, tissues, or organs (including the sharing of drug-injecting equipment); and

(3) perinatally, from a woman to her fetus or infant (4). Whereas the epidemic in the United States and other industrialized, Western countries has predominantly affected homosexual/bisexual men and injecting drug users (IDUs), the principal mode of transmission in sub-Saharan Africa, where approximately 60% of the worldwide burden of HIV-1 infection has occurred, has been via heterosexual intercourse. In Latin America, the epidemic has manifested characteristics found in both Western and African countries. More recently, in Asia, the continent with 60% of the world's population, HIV-1 infection has begun to move rapidly, manifesting new combinations of these transmission characteristics.

In 1986, the retrovirus now known as HIV-2 was isolated in West Africa from persons with AIDS who were not infected with HIV-1 (6). Whereas the focus of HIV-2 infection remains in West Africa, persons infected with this virus have been reported from other parts of Africa, Europe, the Americas, and Asia (7–9). There is a growing understanding of the epidemiology and pathology of HIV-2 infection and the relationship of HIV-2 infection to the pandemic of HIV-1 infection and AIDS.

PATTERNS OF HIV INFECTION AND DISEASE

By 1988, three relatively distinct epidemiologic patterns of HIV-1 infection and disease could be distinguished (10–13). The patterns refer to both the predominant modes of HIV transmission and the time when extensive HIV transmission began. Since these patterns were defined, the progression of the epidemic in most regions of the world has diminished the distinctions among them. However, describing these patterns of HIV infection and disease is useful in understanding the early historical progression of the pandemic and comparing its impact on various regions and populations.

T. D. Mastro, H. D. Gayle, and W. L. Heyward: International Activity, Division of HIV/AIDS, National Center for Infectious Diseases, Centers for Disease Control, Atlanta, Georgia 30333.

Pattern I

Most transmission results from men having sex with men and the sharing of injecting equipment among IDUs. Extensive HIV-1 transmission probably began in the mid-1970s or early 1980s. Selected urban areas are most affected. Although sexual transmission is predominantly homosexual, limited heterosexual transmission occurs, particularly among the sexual partners of IDUs. The proportion of HIV-1 infections due to heterosexual transmission tends to increase over time. Perinatal transmission occurs primarily from female IDUs, female sex partners of male IDUs, and women from areas where heterosexual contact is the predominant transmission mode. Transmission from contaminated blood or blood products is not a continuing problem, but many persons were infected by this route before 1985. Pattern I is most typical of North America, Western Europe, Australia, New Zealand, and some areas of South America.

Pattern II

Transmission is primarily via heterosexual intercourse. Extensive HIV-1 transmission probably began in the early to late 1970s. The highest rates of HIV-1 infection occur among female prostitutes, their sexual contacts, and young adults in urban areas. Transfusion of HIV-infected blood is a continuing problem in many areas, and nonsterile needles and syringes pose an undetermined risk of transmission. Perinatal transmission is a growing problem in areas with high rates of HIV-1 infection among young women. Pattern II is found in sub-Saharan Africa and some Caribbean and Latin American countries.

Pattern III

This pattern was originally characterized by few reported AIDS cases and apparently low rates of HIV-1 transmission by all routes. However, the characteristics of pattern III are changing as the epidemic affects exposed populations in individual countries. HIV-1 infection was probably introduced in the early to mid-1980s; rates of HIV-1 infection vary widely, often with marked focalization. The dominant mode of transmission varies by country depending on behavioral practices and resulting exposure to HIV-1 infection. It is likely that areas of the world with this third pattern of HIV-1 infection will develop diverse subpatterns of infection. Pattern III was originally described in Asia, Oceania (minus Australia and New Zealand), the Middle East, North Africa, and Eastern Europe.

CASE DEFINITIONS OF AIDS

Epidemiologic surveillance of AIDS is needed to monitor the epidemic, to assess its impact, and to plan for the future. Before the discovery in 1983 that the virus now known as HIV-1 was the etiologic agent of AIDS (14,15) and before the development of serologic tests for HIV-1 antibody in 1985, surveillance was limited to cases of disease satisfying defined clinical criteria. The initial Centers for Disease Control (CDC) case definition for AIDS was developed in 1982 (16), later modified to include HIV serologic test results, and subsequently adopted by WHO (17–20). However, many of the clinical and pathologic conditions required to satisfy the CDC/WHO definition could not be diagnosed with the limited diagnostic and laboratory facilities available in many developing countries. There was a need for a workable case definition for use in surveillance and case reporting in developing countries.

In 1985, a simplified "WHO clinical case definition" of AIDS was developed in Bangui, Central African Republic (19,21). This clinical case definition was based on simple clinical signs and did not include HIV serologic test results (Table 1). The WHO clinical case definition was useful in improving surveillance in many sub-Saharan African countries. However, its positive predictive value for HIV-1 seropositivity in Africa was only 50–74% (22,23). The sensitivity in detecting HIV-related disease was 52–59% and the specificity in distinguishing disease not due to HIV infection was 78–90%. A clinical case definition was also developed for use with children in developing countries (Table 2) (19). This pediatric version of the WHO clinical case definition was reported

TABLE 1. *The World Health Organization ("Bangui") clinical case definition for AIDS in adults— for use in developing countries*

Absence of known causes of immunosuppression *and:*

  A. Generalized Kaposi's sarcoma *or* cryptococcal meningitis
      or
  B. At least two of the major signs associated with at least one minor sign

Major signs
  Weight loss ≥ 10% of body weight
  Chronic diarrhea > 1 month
  Prolonged fever > 1 month (intermittent or constant)

Minor signs
  Persistent cough for >1 month
  Generalized pruritic dermatitis
  Recurrent herpes zoster
  Oropharyngeal candidiasis
  Chronic progressive and disseminated herpes
    simplex infection
  Generalized lymphadenopathy

TABLE 2. *The World Health Organization ("Bangui") clinical case definition for AIDS in children— for use in developing countries*

Absence of known causes of immunosuppression *and* at least two of the major signs associated with at least two of the minor signs

Major signs
  Weight loss or abnormally slow growth
  Chronic diarrhea > 1 month
  Prolonged fever > 1 month

Minor signs
  Generalized lymphadenopathy
  Oropharyngeal candidiasis
  Repeated common infections (otitis, pharyngitis, etc.)
  Persistent cough
  Generalized dermatitis
  Confirmed maternal HIV-1 infection

to be difficult to apply in Africa because of a common inability to document weight loss or abnormal growth and to determine maternal HIV infection (24). The pediatric definition was found to have a positive predictive value of only 25–48% in Africa (25,26). Since 1985, HIV serologic testing has become more widely available, and HIV antibody testing has commonly been combined with the WHO clinical case definition for use in AIDS case surveillance. As a greater understanding of HIV infection and related diseases in developing countries (especially in Africa) is gained, further refinements of this definition will be possible. A newly proposed AIDS surveillance definition for use in Africa requires a positive test for HIV infection in association with a diagnosis of the wasting syndrome, tuberculosis, Kaposi's sarcoma, or debilitating neurologic disease (27).

In 1989, another simplified AIDS surveillance definition of AIDS was developed in Caracas, Venezuela, by a working group of the Pan American Health Organization for use in Latin America and the Caribbean where HIV serologic testing was generally available (28). A subsequent revision of this definition uses a point system for clinical findings and requires a positive HIV serologic test (Table 3) (29). This definition recognizes the prominent role of tuberculosis in the clinical picture of HIV-related disease in the countries for which it is intended.

CLINICAL MANIFESTATIONS

The reported clinical manifestations of HIV-related disease vary in different areas of the world. This probably results from true regional differences in the prevalence of specific opportunistic infections and malignant disorders related to HIV-1 infection as well as differences in the ability to diagnose these conditions reliably (22,30). In Africa, severe weight loss ("slim disease"), chronic diarrhea, and chronic fever, usually without specific etiologic diagnoses, are prominent in the presentation of AIDS (30). Whereas *Pneumocystis carinii* pneumonia is the most commonly diagnosed serious opportunistic infection in persons with AIDS in North America and Europe, this diagnosis is rarely made in Africa (30). Similarly, infections with nontuberculous mycobacteria, especially *Mycobacterium avium* complex, which are common in persons with AIDS in developed countries, have not been recognized as a substantial problem in Africa (31). Although both of these clinical conditions may be underdiagnosed in Africa, available evidence indicates that their true prevalence there is probably much lower than in North America (30,31).

The prevalence of neurologic complications of HIV-1 infection in most developing countries has also been incompletely explored, due in part to a lack of diagnostic facilities. A recent study in Kinshasa, Zaire, found neuropsychiatric abnormalities (including HIV-1-associated dementia complex and cryptococcal meningitis) in 43 (41%) of 104 HIV-infected hospital patients (32). This proportion is comparable to that reported for AIDS patients in North America (33).

Tuberculosis is probably the most commonly occurring opportunistic infection in persons infected with HIV-1 in Africa and Latin America (34,35). In many developing countries, about half of the adult population aged 20–40 years has been infected with *Mycobacterium tuberculosis;* they are at greatly increased risk for reactivation of tuberculosis when cell-mediated immunity declines following HIV-1 infection (35). The HIV/AIDS

TABLE 3. *The revised Pan American Health Organization ("Caracas") AIDS case definition*

Positive HIV serologic test and the absence of cancer or other cause of immunosuppression *plus* ≥ 10 cumulative points

Clinical feature	Points
Kaposi's sarcoma	10
Tuberculosis, noncavitary pulmonary or extrapulmonary	10
Tuberculosis, cavitary pulmonary or unspecified	5
Oral candidiasis or hairy leukoplakia	5
Herpes zoster, age < 60 years	5
Central nervous system dysfunction	5
Diarrhea for ≥1 month	2
Fever for ≥1 month	2
Cachexia or >10% weight loss	2
Asthenia for ≥1 month	2
Persistent dermatitis	2
Anemia, lymphopenia, or thrombocytopenia	2
Persistent cough or any pneumonia (except tuberculosis)	2
Lymphadenopathy ≥ 1 cm at ≥2 noninguinal sites for ≥1 month	2

epidemic has had a devastating effect on tuberculosis control efforts in many countries in Africa (34); for example, 35% of adult tuberculosis in Abidjan, Côte d'Ivoire, is attributable to HIV-1 and/or HIV-2 infection (36). Tuberculosis is also likely to be a prominent feature of the epidemic in Asia, given the magnitude of the burden of tuberculosis infection in this region even before the introduction of HIV infection (37).

Kaposi's sarcoma was endemic in tropical Africa before the emergence of the HIV/AIDS epidemic; however, the typical, endemic form of this neoplasm is relatively benign compared to the aggressive form related to HIV-1 infection (38,39). Whereas up to 40% of homosexual/bisexual men with AIDS in North America in the early 1980s were diagnosed with Kaposi's sarcoma (40), about 5–10% of African AIDS patients have this disease, closer to the proportion found in other North American HIV transmission groups (30,40).

EPIDEMIOLOGY BY REGION

Africa

Through early 1991, 92,922 cases of AIDS from 52 of 53 African countries had been reported to WHO (Table 4) (1). However, disease surveillance and reporting have been very incomplete, particularly before 1987 when few African countries routinely reported AIDS cases to WHO. It is generally accepted that the number of reported cases grossly underestimates the true number of AIDS cases. In early 1991, WHO estimated that approximately 800,000 adult AIDS cases had occurred in sub-Saharan Africa, more than half of the estimated global total. In addition, 90% of the estimated 500,000 pediatric cases resulting from perinatal transmission worldwide were thought to have occurred in Africa (3). Relatively few cases of AIDS have been reported from the countries of North Africa, but limited available data indicate that extensive HIV-1 transmission had occurred in some of these countries by 1990 (3).

Given the limitations of AIDS case reporting, the epidemiologic picture of the HIV/AIDS epidemic in Africa has been greatly enhanced by HIV seroprevalence surveys. WHO estimated the number of HIV-1 infections in sub-Saharan Africa to be 2.5 million in 1987 and 6 million in early 1991. In 1987, the areas most affected were several countries in East and Central Africa. By 1991, HIV-1 transmission had spread extensively to West and southern Africa, but countries in East and Central Africa remained the most severely affected (3).

The predominant mode of HIV-1 transmission in sub-Saharan Africa is heterosexual intercourse, accounting for more than 90% of infections in adults (3). However, transfusion of HIV-infected blood, notably to children with malaria-associated anemia, has been and remains a problem, accounting for up to 10% of new HIV infections (41–44). The transmission risk posed by medical injections is more difficult to quantify but accounts for an undetermined number of infections (45,46). The proportion of cases among young children resulting from perinatal transmission is increasing (47).

The prevalence of HIV-1 infection in countries of sub-Saharan Africa varies greatly. In urban Kampala, Uganda, in East Africa, the HIV-1 seroprevalence rate among pregnant women was 24% in 1987 (48,49) and by 1989 exceeded 20% in unselected blood donors (groups representing the general population) (50). Rates for the general population in rural areas ranged from 7% to 12% (49,50). The HIV-1 seroprevalence rate for urban adults without specific risk factors also exceeds 10% in Burundi, Rwanda, Zambia, Malawi, and Côte d'Ivoire, and exceeds 5% in Tanzania, Zaire, and the Central African Republic (51). Groups at especially high risk for HIV-1 infection in Africa include female prostitutes, sexually transmitted disease (STD) clinic patients, and, in some countries, male truck drivers. HIV-1 seroprevalence rates among these groups in Uganda in the late 1980s were 76–86%, 43–58%, and 32%, respectively (49–51). The HIV-1 seroprevalence rate among high-risk urban populations also exceeds 40% in Kenya, Rwanda, and Malawi, and exceeds 25% in Zaire, Tanzania, Zambia, Congo, and Ghana (51).

Data from Côte d'Ivoire have demonstrated the devastating effect that AIDS can have on a country within just a few years. In the late 1980s, epidemiologic studies in this West African country documented the rapid progression of the HIV/AIDS epidemic and assessed its impact on mortality. Although AIDS was first recognized in this country only in 1985, by 1988 in one urban hospital, 43% of adult patients were seropositive for HIV-1 and/or HIV-2 and AIDS accounted for 19% of medical admissions and 33% of medical deaths (52). By 1989, AIDS was reported to be the leading cause of deaths in adults in the capital city, Abidjan (53).

TABLE 4. *AIDS cases reported to WHO from African countries through May 1991; the ten countries reporting the most cases*

Country	Cases (cumulative)	Rate[a]
Uganda	21,719	123.4
Zaire	11,732	33.2
Kenya	9,139	36.0
Tanzania	8,163	31.4
Malawi	7,160	78.7
Côte d'Ivoire	6,836	56.5
Zimbabwe	6,716	64.0
Zambia	4,036	49.8
Rwanda	3,407	44.8
Burundi	3,305	59.0

[a] Cumulative per 100,000 1990 population (projected, U.S. Bureau of the Census).

Heterosexual Transmission of HIV-1

The predominance of heterosexual HIV transmission in Africa has generally resulted in a male-to-female ratio of HIV-1 infection and AIDS cases of approximately 1:1 (39,42,54). However, age-specific rates of disease vary by gender. For example, in Uganda, female AIDS cases outnumber male cases in the 15–24-year age group, whereas men outnumber women in the 30-year and older age group (55). In many countries the highest HIV-1 seroprevalence rates are in women aged 20–25 years and in men aged 25–35 years, reflecting sexual contact between older men and younger women (56).

A number of explanations for the relative efficiency of heterosexual transmission and the rapid spread of HIV-1 in sub-Saharan Africa have been proposed; however, a complete understanding is lacking. HIV-1 infection in Africa has been associated with increased numbers of heterosexual partners, a history of prostitution in women, and, for men, sexual contact with prostitutes (57–59). The role of STDs in augmenting the transmission of HIV-1 has received a great deal of attention. Genital ulcer disease and antibodies to *Haemophilus ducreyi* (the agent of chancroid) and herpes simplex virus type 2 have been associated with HIV-1 infection in both men and women in several studies (57,59–62). In addition, studies of female prostitutes in Zaire found HIV-1 infection to be associated with condylomata acuminata, cytologic evidence of human papilloma virus, purulent cervicitis, gonorrhea, chlamydial infections, and trichomoniasis (62,63). Thus, in African women, both ulcerative and nonulcerative STDs appear to be risk factors for HIV-1 infection. For men in Africa, lack of circumcision has been suggested as a risk factor for HIV infection, either independently or perhaps due to an association between genital ulcer disease and an intact foreskin (64,65).

Studies of HIV-1 transmission among married couples in Africa have found differing results. In Zaire, a large retrospective study of workers identified 239 married couples in which one or both members were HIV-1 seropositive; only 35 (15%) were both seropositive (59). The other 85% of couples remained discordant for HIV seropositivity despite repeated unprotected sex with spouses (59). Following an HIV-1 counselling program, condom use increased dramatically and a low HIV-1 seroconversion rate of 3.1/100 person-years of observation was documented (66). In contrast, in Kenya, an HIV seroconversion rate of 18% per year was found among the HIV-seronegative spouses of 65 seropositive persons (67). This high rate was documented despite counselling and condom usage rates of up to 54%. Seroconversion was not associated with STDs, cervical ectopy in women, or lack of circumcision in men (67). It remains to be thoroughly explained why the seroconversion rate in Kenya differs from that in Zaire and why it is so much greater than the rate of 0.2–4.8% per year found among female sex partners of HIV-infected hemophiliac men in North America and Europe (68,69).

Pediatric HIV Infection and AIDS

HIV infection in infants and children, primarily resulting from perinatal transmission, has accounted for about 15% of all HIV infections in Africa. WHO estimates that 10 million HIV-infected infants will have been born in Africa by the end of this century (3). The resulting increase in infant and child death from AIDS in the 1990s threatens to reverse the gains in child survival made over the past 20 years through improvements in programs for nutrition, immunization, and the control of malaria, diarrhea, and acute respiratory infections. Furthermore, by the year 2000, an estimated 3–5 million uninfected children will be orphaned when their HIV-infected parents die of AIDS (47,70). Rates of perinatal HIV-1 transmission in Africa, ranging from 39% to 52% (71–73), are comparable to but somewhat higher than rates in developed countries (74). Apparent transmission of HIV-1 from mothers to their infants during breast-feeding (75–78) poses a particular problem in Africa where, due to a lack of safe water, bottle feeding is associated with increased infant mortality (79). In 1987, WHO recommended that, where safe and effective alternatives were not available, biologic mothers should breastfeed their infants regardless of HIV-1 status (80). Subsequent analyses of limited available data weighing the risk of HIV-1 transmission via breastfeeding with the risks of bottle feeding in developing countries with poor sanitation supported these recommendations (81,82). A recent study from Rwanda documented HIV-1 seroconversion in four of ten breastfed children of mothers who seroconverted at least 6 months after delivery (78). Additional such data are needed to assess better the risk of HIV-1 transmission via breastfeeding in Africa.

HIV-2

HIV-2 infection remains closely associated with West Africa. In 1986, HIV-2 was first isolated from persons with AIDS in the West African countries of Guinea Bissau and the Cape Verde Islands (6). In 1985, persons in Senegal had been found to have what is now considered to be serologic evidence of HIV-2 antibody (7,83), and retrospective serologic studies indicate that persons from a number of West African countries became infected with HIV-2 as early as the 1960s (84). The seroprevalence of HIV-2 infection in low-risk urban populations has been found to be greater than 1.0% in the West African countries of Guinea Bissau, Cape Verde, Côte d'Ivoire, Sierra Leone, Mali, and Nigeria, and in the former Portuguese colonies of Angola and Mozambique

(7,51). The seroprevalence in high-risk urban populations has been reported to be greater than 10% in Guinea Bissau, Gambia, Côte d'Ivoire, Mali, Burkina Faso, and Angola (7,51). Reports of HIV-2 infection have come from several European countries, mostly among persons who have had some contact with persons from West Africa or former Portuguese colonies (7). Smaller numbers of persons with HIV-2 infection have been reported from the Americas, notably Brazil, and more recently from India (7–9).

Dual infection with HIV-1 and HIV-2 has been clearly demonstrated (85,86); however, serologic discrimination between the two infections may be problematic (87–89). Because of substantial homology for amino-acid sequence and genome of the two viruses, cross-reactivity between HIV-2 antibody and HIV-1 antigen (and the reverse) commonly occurs in serologic tests (7,86). Competitive enzyme-linked immunosorbent assays (ELISA) for antibodies to HIV-1 and HIV-2 and synthetic peptide immunoassays appear to be more specific in discriminating between the two infections (87,88,90). Newer serodiagnostic tests and criteria are evolving.

Available data indicate that HIV-2 shares the same modes of transmission as HIV-1 (91,92); however, data on the natural history and pathogenicity of HIV-2 relative to HIV-1 are less clear. In Guinea Bissau, epidemiologic investigations revealed excess mortality associated with HIV-2 seropositivity (compared to no HIV infection); the relative risk of dying for HIV-2-seropositive children was 61 and for adults 5 (91). Whereas studies in Côte d'Ivoire and Guinea Bissau indicate that advanced HIV-2 infection is associated with the same AIDS-defining symptoms and signs as HIV-1 (93–95), an ongoing prospective study of prostitutes in Senegal has found slower immunologic deterioration (as measured by CD4+ T cells) and progression to AIDS among persons with HIV-2 infection compared with persons with HIV-1 infection (96,97). Additional investigation is necessary to clarify further the epidemiology and pathogenicity of HIV-2.

The Americas (Outside the United States)

Through early 1991, 42,836 cases of AIDS from all 44 countries or territories in the Americas, excluding the United States, had been reported to WHO (1). By comparison, 174,893 U.S. AIDS cases had been reported to WHO, resulting in a cumulative rate of 70.5 cases/100,000 population. HIV-1 infection spread rapidly in this region in the 1980s, but the resulting geographic distribution of AIDS cases is not homogenous either among or within countries. The great diversity of the countries in this region has led to substantial variation in the patterns and rates of HIV-1 infection and AIDS (Table 5). Brazil has reported the largest number of cases, but the cumulative rate of AIDS is far higher in several other

TABLE 5. *AIDS cases reported to WHO from countries/islands in the Americas (outside the United States) through May 1991*

Country	Cases (cumulative)	Rate[a]
The ten countries reporting the most cases		
Brazil	17,337	11.3
Mexico	6,510	7.4
Canada	4,885	18.4
Haiti	3,086	48.2
Dominican Republic	1,506	20.6
Colombia	1,285	3.9
Honduras	1,133	21.4
Venezuela	1,061	5.4
Argentina	920	2.8
Trinidad and Tobago	736	56.6
The ten countries/islands with the highest rates of AIDS		
Bermuda	172	296.6
Bahamas	599	238.6
French Guiana	232	236.7
Barbados	192	73.8
Guadeloupe	195	56.7
Trinidad and Tobago	736	56.6
Martinique	177	53.2
Haiti	3,086	48.2
Honduras	1,133	21.4
Dominican Republic	1,506	20.6

[a] Cumulative per 100,000 1990 population (projected, U.S. Bureau of the Census).

small countries, mainly in the Caribbean islands. In the larger countries, HIV-1 infection is concentrated in urban areas (98).

Although several countries in the Americas have had comparable patterns of growth in the number of AIDS cases, the relative frequencies of sexual, parenteral, and perinatal transmission have varied markedly (99,100). Most South American countries experienced rapid spread of HIV-1 among homosexual men early in the epidemic. In some Caribbean and Latin American countries, including Brazil, Mexico, Haiti, Jamaica, and the Dominican Republic, many bisexual men were infected in this early phase; by the late 1980s, such men accounted for 15–25% of all AIDS cases (100–103). High rates of infection among bisexual men and, in some countries (notably Brazil), heterosexual IDUs have led to an increase in heterosexual transmission of HIV-1 to women (99,104). From the early 1980s to 1991, the proportion of reported AIDS cases resulting from heterosexual transmission increased in most Latin American countries, resulting in a decrease in the male-to-female ratios that ranged from 12:1 to 3:1 in most countries in the mid-1980s (98). In the Bahamas, the country with the second highest rate of AIDS, heterosexual transmission accounts for 73% of adult AIDS cases. Cocaine use (not by injection) was reported for 63% of adult cases and was commonly associated with prostitution and multiple sex partners (105). Thus, the epidemic in much of the Caribbean and Latin America has manifested epidemiologic characteristics of both pattern I and pattern II.

Transmission of HIV-1 among IDUs is a substantial problem in many countries in the Americas. In Bermuda, the country with the highest rate of AIDS cases, 58% of cases reported through 1988 were among IDUs (105). Although injecting drug use as a risk factor may be underreported in many countries, it appears to be prevalent in Argentina, Brazil, and Panama (98).

Parenteral transmission of HIV-1 from unscreened blood and the improper use of needles and syringes continues to be a problem in some countries (102). Inadequate blood screening procedures and the use of paid blood donors have resulted in an estimated 5–10% of all AIDS cases in some countries (98). In Mexico, HIV-1 transmission was documented as a result of poor aseptic technique in plasmapheresis centers using paid donors (106).

Increases in perinatal transmission of HIV-1 and pediatric AIDS cases have paralleled the increase in HIV-1 infection in women in several countries. In Haiti, the estimated HIV-1 transmission rate from mothers to their breastfed infants was 25% (107). Pediatric AIDS cases now account for 10% of all cases in the Caribbean, and 19% of cases in the Bahamas (99,105,108).

Between 1986 and 1989, Cuba implemented a program of mandatory, widespread HIV antibody testing, resulting in the evaluation of more than 5 million persons, approximately 75% of the adult population (109,110). The overall seroprevalence was 9/100,000; all but 1 of 434 infections were due to HIV-1 (110).

Europe

Through early 1991, 51,914 cases of AIDS from 28 of 29 European countries had been reported to WHO (Table 6) (1). The population groups predominantly affected are homosexual/bisexual men and IDUs. However, transmission patterns vary within the continent. In northern Europe, the majority of cases have been among homosexual/bisexual men. In contrast, in Italy and Spain, heterosexual IDUs account for >60% of cases of AIDS. As in the United States, the incidence of HIV-1 infection among homosexual men has decreased since the mid-1980s (3). Seroprevalence rates among IDUs vary greatly among European cities; large numbers of uninfected IDUs in many cities pose the potential for explosive transmission of HIV-1 through the sharing of injecting equipment.

In eastern Europe, outbreaks of nosocomial HIV-1 transmission have demonstrated the potential for epidemics resulting from the improper use of medical equipment. In Romania in 1990, a dramatic epidemic of AIDS, primarily among children less than 4 years of age living in public institutions, led to the infection of 1,000–

TABLE 6. *AIDS cases reported to WHO from European countries through May 1991; the ten countries reporting the most cases*

Country	Cases (cumulative)	Rate[a]
France	14,449	25.7
Italy	9,053	15.7
Spain	8,199	20.7
Germany	6,176	8.0
United Kingdom	4,454	7.8
Switzerland	1,778	26.9
Netherlands	1,683	11.3
Romania	1,331	5.7
Belgium	852	8.6
Denmark	784	15.4

[a] Cumulative per 100,000 1990 population (projected, U.S. Bureau of the Census).

2,000 children. Epidemiologic investigations indicated that HIV-1 transmission was due to the transfusion of unscreened blood and the improper use of needles and syringes to administer multiple therapeutic injections (111). In the USSR, a country with a very low HIV-1 seroprevalence of 1/100,000 (112), a nosocomial outbreak of HIV-1 infection affecting 152 children was attributed to the multiple use of syringes on hospital wards (113). An epidemiologic investigation of this outbreak indicated that HIV-1 infection was transmitted from infected infants to at least ten mothers, presumably via breastfeeding with cracked nipples; many HIV-infected infants had stomatitis with bleeding (113).

Asia

Through early 1991, only 1,088 cases of AIDS from 28 of 38 Asian countries had been reported to WHO (1). However, extensive spread of HIV-1 did not begin until the late 1980s in the most populous continent, and the small number of reported AIDS cases does not adequately reflect the dramatic increase in HIV-1 infection recently documented in some Asian countries.

Thailand serves as an example of the potential for rapid HIV-1 transmission in Asia. Although only 106 cases of AIDS have been reported to WHO from this Southeast Asian nation, HIV-1 infection has been documented in more than 26,000 persons, and it is estimated that more than 100,000 persons are actually infected (3). The epidemic in Thailand is described as having three waves. Before 1988, surveys had identified fewer than 200 HIV-infected persons. The first wave of infection occurred among IDUs. In early 1988, the HIV-1 seroprevalence among persons attending drug treatment centers in Bangkok, the capital, was 1%; by the end of 1988, this figure had risen to approximately 40% (114,115). The second wave of the epidemic was among female prostitutes (116). Between June 1989 and June 1990, the median province-specific HIV-1 seroprevalence among brothel prostitutes increased from 3.5% to 9.5% (117,118). More than 60% of some groups of low-price brothel prostitutes in northern Thailand have been found to be infected with HIV-1 (118). The third wave of the epidemic was detected among young, heterosexual men in 1990–1991. In the northern city of Chiang Mai, a study of male STD patients found 18% to be HIV-1 seropositive (119).

The dramatic epidemic in Thailand poses a danger for other Asian countries. Cross-border opiate traffic with Myanmar (Burma), Laos, and nearby China and related drug use and sharing of injecting equipment pose a risk for HIV-1 transmission in these countries. By late 1990, Chinese public health authorities had identified approximately 400 persons with HIV-1 infection. The great majority were from one region in western Yunnan province that shares a border with Myanmar; virtually all were injecting heroin users (personal communication: Dr. Timothy Dondero). Also, the migration of young women from Myanmar to northern Thailand to work as prostitutes will likely result in HIV-infected women returning to Myanmar.

In India, a country with a population of 850 million (larger than all of Africa), a sharp increase in HIV seroprevalence was noted in 1990 among female prostitutes, with estimated rates as high as 20–30% among the 100,000–200,000 female prostitutes in Bombay (3,120–122). As of 1991, it was estimated that 250,000 Indians were infected with HIV-1 (3). The potential for HIV transmission via transfused blood remains great. Professional blood donors meet over half the demand for blood from Indian hospitals, resulting in the sale of more than 5 million liters of blood annually (123). HIV-infected blood sellers in Delhi are predominantly single men with a history of multiple heterosexual partners (124). A survey in Bombay found the HIV seroprevalence to be 80% among some blood sellers (123). India recently suspended the manufacture of blood products because of the risk of HIV contamination and blood screening programs have been started in several cities. However, it is estimated that up to 95% of donated blood is not screened (123). As in Thailand, there has also been HIV-1 transmission among IDUs, with infection rates of over 50% in northeastern India (3).

Japan has reported only 374 AIDS cases, resulting in a very low cumulative rate of 0.3 cases/100,000 population. Many of these infections resulted from the transfusion of blood products before 1985 (3).

Oceania

Through early 1991, 97% of the 2,802 AIDS cases reported to WHO from this region were from Australia (2,494 cases) and New Zealand (229 cases). The pattern is similar to northern Europe, with homosexual men predominantly affected. A large proportion of the AIDS cases from other islands in this region resulted from the transfusion of HIV-infected blood products in the early to mid-1980s (3).

CONCLUSIONS AND THE FUTURE

After the first decade of the HIV/AIDS pandemic, the pace of transmission is increasing in much of the world. Even without further transmission, given the existing numbers of persons with HIV-1 and HIV-2 infection, the worst is yet to come in terms of the numbers of AIDS cases. Africa has already been devastated by the epidemic, and the coming years will bring an increased burden of AIDS-related death. As the Americas, Europe, and Africa began to come to terms with AIDS in the 1980s, Asia, with 3 billion people, will be the new arena for AIDS in the 1990s. India alone has more people than all of Africa, and extensive HIV transmission has only recently begun in this Asian country.

Epidemiologic data indicate that in developed, Western countries the majority of HIV-1 infections occurred during the early 1980s. The resulting peak incidence for AIDS cases and deaths is therefore expected to occur in the mid-1990s (4). By contrast, for the developing countries of Africa, Latin America, and Asia, available epidemiologic data predict continued high rates of transmission and increases in HIV seroprevalence. As a result, large increases in AIDS cases and deaths are expected during the next two decades (4). In most developing countries, AIDS is expected to become the leading cause of death in adults and one of the leading causes of infant and child mortality (4,47).

Although the epidemiology of HIV infection and AIDS portrays a grim picture of the pandemic, these data are important in guiding current interventions and actions for the future. Programs that can effectively reduce HIV transmission now will prevent large numbers of AIDS cases and deaths in the future.

REFERENCES

1. World Health Organization. *Global programme on AIDS update, AIDS cases reported to the Surveillance, Forecasting and Impact Assessment Unit (SFI)*. GPA/ER/CAS/91.06. Geneva: WHO, June 1991.
2. Palca J. The sobering geography of AIDS. *Science* 1991;252:372–3.
3. World Health Organization. *Global programme on AIDS: current and future dimensions of the HIV/AIDS pandemic—a capsule summary*. Geneva: WHO, April 1991.
4. Chin J. Present and future dimensions of the HIV/AIDS pandemic. VII International Conference on AIDS, Florence, Italy, June 17, 1991.
5. Mann JM. Global AIDS into the 1990s. *J AIDS* 1990;3:438–42.
6. Clavel F, Guetard D, Brun-Vezinet F, et al. Isolation of a new human retrovirus from West African patients with AIDS. *Science* 1986;233:343–6.

7. De Cock KM, Brun-Vézinet F. Epidemiology of HIV-2 infection. *AIDS* 1989;3[Suppl 1]:S89–S95.

8. Pieniazek D, Peralta JM, Ferriera JA, et al. Identification of mixed HIV-1/HIV-2 infections in Brazil by PCR. *AIDS* 1991;5:1293–99.

9. Rübsamen-Waigman H, Briesen HV, Maniar JK, Rao PK, Scholz C, Pfützner A. Spread of HIV-2 in Asia. *Lancet* 1991;337:550–1.

10. Mann JM, Chin J, Piot P, Quinn T. The international epidemiology of AIDS. *Sci Am* 1988;256:82–9.

11. Mann JM, Chin J. AIDS: a global perspective. *N Engl J Med* 1988;319:302–3.

12. Chin J, Mann JM. Global patterns and prevalence of AIDS and HIV infection. *AIDS* 1988;2[Suppl 1]:S247–S252.

13. Piot P, Plummer FA, Mhalu FS, Lamboray J-L, Chin J, Mann JM. AIDS: an international perspective. *Science* 1988;239:573–9.

14. Barré-Sinoussi F, Chermann JC, Rey F, et al. Isolation of a T-lymphotrophic retrovirus from a patient at risk for acquired immune deficiency syndrome (AIDS). *Science* 1983;220:868–71.

15. Gallo RC, Salahuddin SZ, Popovic M, et al. Frequent detection and isolation of cytopathic retroviruses (HTLV-III) from patients with AIDS and at risk for AIDS. *Science* 1984;224:500–3.

16. CDC. Update on acquired immune deficiency syndrome (AIDS)—United States. *MMWR* 1982;31:507–14.

17. CDC. Revision of the case definition of acquired immunodeficiency syndrome for national reporting—United States. *MMWR* 1985;34:373–5.

18. CDC. Revision of the CDC surveillance case definition for acquired immunodeficiency syndrome. *MMWR* 1987;36[Suppl]:1s–15s.

19. WHO. Acquired immunodeficiency syndrome (AIDS), CDC/WHO case definition for AIDS. *Weekly Epidemiol Rec* 1986;61:69–73.

20. WHO. Acquired immunodeficiency syndrome (AIDS), 1987 revision of CDC/WHO case definition for AIDS. *Weekly Epidemiol Rec* 1988;63:1–7.

21. WHO. Acquired immunodeficiency syndrome (AIDS). Workshop on AIDS in Central Africa, Bangui, October 22–25, 1985. *Weekly Epidemiol Rec* 1985;60:342.

22. Colebunders R, Mann JM, Francis H, et al. Evaluation of a clinical case-definition of acquired immunodeficiency syndrome in Africa. *Lancet* 1987;1:492–4.

23. De Cock KM, Colebunders R, Francis H, et al. Evaluation of the WHO clinical case definition for AIDS in rural Zaire. *AIDS* 1988;2:219–21.

24. Jackman J, Hedderwick S. Clinical case definition for AIDS in Africa. *Lancet* 1990;335:1456–7.

25. Colebunders RI, Greenberg A, Nguyen-Dinh P, et al. Evaluation of a clinical case definition of AIDS in African children. *AIDS* 1987;1:151–3.

26. Lepage P, van de Perre P, Dabis F, et al. Evaluation and simplification of the World Health Organization clinical case definition for paediatric AIDS. *AIDS* 1989;3:221–5.

27. De Cock KM, Selik RM, Soro B, Gayle H, Colebunders RL. AIDS surveillance in Africa: a re-appraisal of case definitions. *Br Med J* 1991;303:1186–88.

28. Pan American Health Organization. Working group on AIDS case definition. *PAHO Epidemiol Bull* 1990;10:9–11.

29. Weniger BG, Zacarías F, The Clinical AIDS Study Group, The Working Group on AIDS Case Definition. The new "Caracas" AIDS definition: a practical case surveillance tool developed for use in advanced developing countries. 7th International Conference on AIDS, Florence, Italy, 1991;WC96 (abst).

30. De Cock KM, Colebunders RL. Human immunodeficiency virus infection and AIDS. In: Strickland GT, ed. *Hunter's tropical medicine*. Philadelphia: WB Saunders, 1991:145–58.

31. Horsburgh CR. *Mycobacterium avium* complex infections in the acquired immunodeficiency syndrome. *N Engl J Med* 1991;324:1332–8.

32. Perriëns JH, Mussa M, Luabeya MK, et al. Neurological complications of HIV-1 seropositive internal medicine in patients in Kinshasa, Zaire. *J AIDS* [in press].

33. Levy MR, Bredesen DE. Central nervous system dysfunction in acquired immunodeficiency syndrome. *J AIDS* 1988;1:41–64.

34. Pitchenik AE. Tuberculosis control and the AIDS epidemic in developing countries. *Ann Intern Med* 1990;113:89–91.

35. Harries AD. Tuberculosis and human immunodeficiency virus in developing countries. *Lancet* 1990;335:387–90.

36. De Cock KM, Gnaore E, Adjorlolo G, et al. Risk of tuberculosis in patients with HIV-1 and HIV-II infections in Abidjan, Ivory Coast. *Br Med J* 1991;302:496–9.

37. Murray CJL, Styblo K, Rouillon A. Tuberculosis in developing countries: burden, intervention and cost. *Bull Int Union Against Tuberculosis Lung Dis* 1990;65:6–24.

38. Bayley AC, Downing RG, Cheingsong-Popov R, Tedder RS, Dalgleish AG, Weiss RA. HTLV-III serology distinguishes atypical and endemic Kaposi's sarcoma in Africa. *Lancet* 1985;1:359–61.

39. Quinn TC, Mann JM, Curran JW, Piot P. AIDS in Africa: an epidemiologic paradigm. *Science* 1986;234:955–63.

40. Beral V, Peterman TA, Berkelman RL, Jaffe HW. Kaposi's sarcoma among persons with AIDS: a sexually transmitted infection? *Lancet* 1990;335:123–8.

41. Greenberg AE, Nguyen-Dinh P, Mann JM, et al. The association between malaria, blood transfusions, and HIV seropositivity in a pediatric population in Kinshasa, Zaire. *JAMA* 1988;259:545–9.

42. N'Galy B, Ryder RW. Epidemiology of HIV infection in Africa. *J AIDS* 1988;1:551–8.

43. N'tita I, Mulanga K, Dulat C, et al. Risk of transfusion-associated HIV transmission in Kinshasa, Zaire. *AIDS* 1991;5:437–9.

44. Colebunders R, Ryder R, Francis H, et al. Seroconversion rate, mortality, and clinical manifestations associated with the receipt of human immunodeficiency virus-infected blood transfusion in Kinshasa, Zaire. *J Infect Dis* 1991;164:450–6.

45. Mann JM, Francis H, Davachi F, et al. Risk factors for human immunodeficiency virus seropositivity among children 1–24 months old in Kinshasa, Zaire. *Lancet* 1986;2:654–7.

46. Lepage P, van de Perre P. Nosocomial transmission of HIV in Africa: what tribute is paid to contaminated blood transfusions and medical injections. *Infect Control Hosp Epidemiol* 1988;9:200–3.

47. Chin J. Current and future dimensions of the HIV/AIDS pandemic in women and children. *Lancet* 1990;336:221–4.

48. Carswell JW, Lloyd G. Rise in prevalence of HIV antibodies recorded at an antenatal booking clinic in Kampala, Uganda. *AIDS* 1987;1:192–3.

49. Carswell JW. HIV infection in healthy persons in Uganda. *AIDS* 1987;1:223–7.

50. Goodgame RW. AIDS in Uganda—clinical and social features. *N Engl J Med* 1990;323:383–9.

51. Torrey BB, Way PO. *Seroprevalence of HIV in Africa: winter 1990.* CIR staff paper no. 55, May 1990. Washington, DC: Center for International Research, U.S. Bureau of the Census.

52. De Cock KM, Porter A, Odehouri K, et al. Rapid emergence of AIDS in Abidjan, Ivory Coast. *Lancet* 1989;2:408–11.

53. De Cock KM, Barrere B, Diaby L, et al. AIDS—the leading cause of adult death in the west African city of Abidjan, Ivory Coast. *Science* 1990;249:793–6.

54. Mann JM, Quinn TC, Francis H, et al. Prevalence of HTLV-III/LAV in household contacts of patients with confirmed AIDS and controls in Kinshasa, Zaire. *JAMA* 1986;256:721–4.

55. Berkley S, Naamara W, Okware S, et al. AIDS and HIV infection in Uganda—are more women infected than men? *AIDS* 1990;4:1237–42.

56. Potts M, Anderson R, Boily MC. Slowing the spread of human immunodeficiency virus in developing countries. *Lancet* 1991;338:608–13.

57. Kreiss JK, Koech D, Plummer FA, et al. AIDS virus infection in Nairobi prostitutes: spread of the epidemic to East Africa. *N Engl J Med* 1986;314:414–18.

58. Piot P, Plummer FA, Rey MA, et al. Retrospective seroepidemiology of AIDS virus infection in Nairobi prostitutes. *J Infect Dis* 1987;155:1108–12.

59. Ryder RW, Ndilu M, Hassig SE, et al. Heterosexual transmission of HIV-1 among employees and their spouses at two large businesses in Zaire. *AIDS* 1990;4:725–32.

60. Greenblatt RM, Lukehart SA, Plummer FA, et al. Genital ulceration as a risk factor for human immunodeficiency virus infection. *AIDS* 1988;2:47–50.

61. Cameron DW, Simonsen JN, D'Costa LJ. Female to male transmission of human immunodeficiency virus type 1: risk factors for seroconversion in men. *Lancet* 1989;2:403–7.

62. Nzila N, Laga M, Thiam MA, et al. HIV and other sexually transmitted diseases among female prostitutes in Kinshasa. *AIDS* 1991;5:715–21.

63. Laga M, Nzila N, Manoka AT, et al. Non-ulcerative sexually transmitted diseases (STDs) as risk factors for HIV infection. 6th International Conference on AIDS, San Francisco, 1990;ThC97 (abst).

64. Bongarts J, Reining P, Way P, Conant F. The relationship between male circumcision and HIV infection in African populations. *AIDS* 1989;3:373–7.

65. Tyndall M, Odhiambo P, Ronald AR, et al. The increasing seroprevalence of HIV-1 in males with other STDs in Nairobi, Kenya. 7th International Conference on AIDS, Florence, Italy, 1991;WC3117(abst).

66. Kamenga M, Ryder RW, Jingu M, et al. Evidence of marked sexual behaviour change associated with low HIV-1 seroconversion in 149 married couples with discordant HIV-1 serostatus: experience at an HIV counselling center in Zaire. *AIDS* 1991;5:61–7.

67. Moss G, Clemetson D, D'Costa LJ, et al. Despite safer sex practices after counselling, seroconversion is high among HIV serodiscordant couples in Nairobi, Kenya. 7th International Conference on AIDS, Florence, Italy, 1991;WC3119(abst).

68. Lusher JM, Operskalski EA, Aledort LM, et al. Risk of human immunodeficiency virus type 1 infection among sexual and nonsexual household contacts of persons with congenital clotting disorders. *Pediatrics* 1991;88:242–9.

69. Laurian Y, Peynet J, Verroust F. HIV infection in sexual partners of HIV-seropositive patients with hemophilia. *N Engl J Med* 1989;320:183.

70. Preble EA. Impact of HIV/AIDS on African children. *Soc Sci Med* 1990;31:671–80.

71. Ryder RW, Nsa W, Hassig SE, et al. Perinatal transmission of the human immunodeficiency virus type 1 to infants of seropositive women in Zaire. *N Engl J Med* 1989;320:1637–42.

72. Hira S, Kamanga J, Bhat GJ, et al. Perinatal transmission of HIV-1 in Lusaka, Zambia. *Br Med J* 1989;299:1250–2.

73. Lallemant M, Lallemant-Le Coeur S, Cheynier D, et al. Mother-child transmission of HIV-1 and infant survival in Brazzaville, Congo. *AIDS* 1989;3:643–6.

74. Oxtoby M. Perinatally acquired human immunodeficiency virus infection. *Pediatr Infect Dis J* 1990;9:609–19.

75. Ziegler JB, Cooper DA, Johnson RO, Gold J. Postnatal transmission of AIDS-associated retrovirus from mother to infant. *Lancet* 1985;1:896–8.

76. Colebunders RI, Kapita B, Nekwei W, et al. Breastfeeding and transmission of HIV. *Lancet* 1988;2:1487.

77. Hira SK, Manrola UG, Mwale C, et al. Apparent vertical transmission of human immunodeficiency virus type 1 by breast feeding in Zambia. *J Pediatr* 1990;117:421–4.

78. van de Perre P, Simonson A, Msellati P, et al. Postnatal transmission of human immunodeficiency virus type 1 from mother to infant. *N Engl J Med* 1991;325:593–8.

79. Pizzo PA, Butler KM. In the vertical transmission of HIV, timing may be everything. *N Engl J Med* 1991;325:652–4.

80. World Health Organization. Breast feeding/breastmilk and human immunodeficiency virus (HIV). *Weekly Epidemiol Rec* 1987;62:245–6.

81. Nicoll A, Killewo JZJ, Mgone C. HIV and infant feeding practices: epidemiological implications for sub-Saharan African countries. *AIDS* 1990;4:661–5.

82. Heymann SJ. Modeling the impact of breast-feeding by HIV-infected women on child survival. *Am J Public Health* 1990;80:1305–9.

83. Barin F, M'Boup S, Denis F, et al. Serologic evidence for virus related to simian T-lymphotrophic retrovirus III in residents of West Africa. *Lancet* 1985;2:1387–9.

84. Kawamura M, Yamazaki S, Ishikawa K, Kwofie TB, Tsujimoto H, Hayami M. HIV-2 in West Africa in 1966. *Lancet* 1989;1:385.

85. Rayfield M, De Cock KM, Heyward WL, et al. Mixed human immunodeficiency virus (HIV) infection in an individual: demon-stration of both HIV type 1 and type 2 proviral sequences by using polymerase chain reaction. *J Infect Dis* 1988;158:1170–6.

86. Evans LA, Moreau J, Odehouri K, et al. Simultaneous isolation of HIV-1 and HIV-2 from an AIDS patient. *Lancet* 1988;2:1389–91.

87. Caruso BMT, Dorizzi RM, Tagliaro F, et al. Rapid discrimination between HIV-1 and HIV-2 infection. *Lancet* 1989;2:1156–7.

88. De Cock KM, Porter A, Kouadio J, et al. Rapid and specific diagnosis of HIV-1 and HIV-2 infections: an evaluation of testing strategies. *AIDS* 1990;4:875–8.

89. De Cock KM, Porter A, Kouadio J, et al. Cross-reactivity on Western blots in HIV-1 and HIV-2 infections. *AIDS* 1991;5:859–63.

90. Tedder RS, O'Connor T, Hughes A, N'jie H, Corrah T, Whittle H. Envelope cross-reactivity in Western blot for HIV-1 and HIV-2 may not indicate dual infection. *Lancet* 1988;2:927–30.

91. Poulsen AG, Kvinesdal B, Aaby P, et al. Prevalence of and mortality from human immunodeficiency virus type 2 in Bissau, West Africa. *Lancet* 1989;1:827–31.

92. Gnaore E, De Cock KM, Gayle H, et al. Prevalence of and mortality from HIV type 2 in Guinea Bissau, West Africa. *Lancet* 1989;2:513.

93. Odehouri K, De Cock KM, Krebs JW, et al. HIV-1 and HIV-2 infection associated with AIDS in Abidjan, Côte d'Ivoire. *AIDS* 1989;3:509–12.

94. De Cock KM, Odehouri K, Colebunders RL, et al. A comparison of HIV-1 and HIV-2 infections in hospitalized patients in Abidjan, Côte d'Ivoire. *AIDS* 1990;4:443–8.

95. Nauclér A, Albino P, Da Silva AP, Andreasson PA, Andersson S, Biberfeld G. HIV-2 infection in hospitalized patients in Bissau, Guinea-Bissau. *AIDS* 1991;5:301–4.

96. Marlink R, Thior I, Dia MC, et al. Prospective study of the natural history of HIV-2. 7th International Conference on AIDS, Florence, Italy, 1991;TuC104(abst).

97. Siby T, Thior I, Marlink R, et al. Clinico-immunologic evaluation of HIV-2 infection in Senegal. 7th International Conference on AIDS, Florence, Italy, 1991;MB2438(abst).

98. Quinn TC, Narain JP, Zacarias FRK. AIDS in the Americas: public health priority for the region. *AIDS* 1990;4:709–24.

99. Narain JP, Hull B, Hospedales CJ, Mahabir S, Bassett DC. Epidemiology of AIDS and HIV infection in the Caribbean. *PAHO Bull* 1989;23:42–9.

100. Quinn TC, Zacarias FRK, St. John RK. AIDS in the Americas. *N Engl J Med* 1989;320:1006–7.

101. Koenig RE, Pittaluga J, Bogart M, et al. Prevalence of antibodies to the human immunodeficiency virus in Dominicans and Haitians in the Dominican Republic. *JAMA* 1987;257:631–4.

102. Pape JW, Liautaud B, Thomas F, et al. The acquired immunodeficiency syndrome in Haiti. *Ann Intern Med* 1985;103:674–8.

103. Murphy EL, Gibbs WN, Figueroa JP, et al. Human immunodeficiency virus and human T-lymphotrophic virus type I infection among homosexual men in Kingston, Jamaica. *J AIDS* 1988;1:143–9.

104. Cortes E, Detels R, Aboulafia D, et al. HIV-1, HIV-2, and HTLV-I infection in high-risk groups in Brazil. *N Engl J Med* 1989;320:953–8.

105. Bartholomew C, Cleghorn F. Retroviruses in the Caribbean. *PAHO Bull* 1989;23:76–80.

106. Avila C, Stetler HC, Sepulveda J, et al. The epidemiology of HIV transmission among paid plasma donors, Mexico City, Mexico. *AIDS* 1990;3:631–3.

107. Halsey NA, Boulos R, Holt E, et al. Transmission of HIV-1 infections from mothers to infants in Haiti. *JAMA* 1990;264:2088–92.

108. Figueroa JP. AIDS projections, a Jamaican perspective. *PAHO Bull* 1989;23:130–4.

109. Bayer R, Healton C. Controlling AIDS in Cuba. *N Engl J Med* 1989;320:1022–4.

110. Pérez-Stable EJ. Cuba's response to the HIV epidemic. *Am J Public Health* 1991;81:563–7.

111. Hersh BS, Popovici F, Apetrei R, et al. Acquired immunodeficiency syndrome in Romania. *Lancet* 1991;338:645–9.

112. Pokrovsky VV, Eramova I, Arzamastsev V, Nikonova V, Mozharova G. Epidemiologic surveillance for HIV-infection in the USSR in 1987–1989. 6th International Conference on AIDS, San Francisco, 1990;FC648(abst).

113. Pokrovsky VV, Kunetsova I, Eramova I. Transmission of HIV-infection from an infected infant to his mother by breast feeding. 6th International Conference on AIDS, San Francisco, 1990;ThC48(abst).

114. Uneklabh C, Phutiprawan T, Uneklabh T. Prevalence of HIV infection among Thai drug dependents. IV International Conference on AIDS, Stockholm, Sweden, 1988;5524 (abstr.).

115. Vanichseni S, Sonchai W, Plangsringarm K, Akarasewi P, Wright N, Choopanya K. Second seroprevalence survey among Bangkok's intravenous drug addicts (IVDA). V International Conference on AIDS, Montreal, Canada, 1989;TG023 (abstr.).

116. Siraprapasiri T, Thanprasertsuk S, Rodklay A, Srivanichakorn S, Sawanpanyalert P, Temtanarak J. Risk factors for HIV among prostitutes in Chiangmai, Thailand. *AIDS* 1991;5:579–82.

117. Ungchusak K, Thanprasertsuk S, Sriprapandh S, Pinichpongse S, Kunasol P. First national sentinel seroprevalence survey for HIV-1 infection in Thailand, June 1989. 6th International Conference on AIDS, San Francisco, June 1990;FC99(abst).

118. Ungchusak K, Thanprasertsuk S, Chokevivat V, Sriprapandh S, Pinichpongse S, Kunasol P. Trends of HIV spreading in Thailand detected by national sentinel seroprevalence. 7th International Conference on AIDS, Florence, Italy, 1991;MC3246(abst).

119. Kunanusont C, Weniger BG, Foy HM, Pruithithada N, Natpratan C. Modes of transmission for the high rate of HIV infection among male STD patients and male blood donors in Chiangmai, Thailand. 7th International Conference on AIDS, Florence, Italy, 1991;WC3086(abst).

120. [Anonymous]. India: prostitutes and the spread of AIDS. *Lancet* 1990;335:1332.

121. Singh YN, Malaviya AN. HIV prevention interventions among prostitutes of India: Delhi experience. 6th International Conference on AIDS, San Francisco, June, 1990;SC33 (abstr.).

122. Goldsmith MF. Rapid spread of pandemic in Asia dismays experts, spurs efforts to fight transmission. *JAMA* 1991;266:1048–9,1053.

123. Kandela P. India: HIV banks. *Lancet* 1991;338:436–7.

124. Chattopadhya D, Riley LW, Kumari S. Behavioural risk factors for acquisition of HIV infection and knowledge about AIDS among male professional blood donors in Delhi. *Bull WHO* 1991;69:319–23.

AIDS and Other Manifestations of HIV Infection,
Second Edition, Edited by Gary P. Wormser.
Raven Press, Ltd., New York © 1992.

CHAPTER 4

Introduction to Retroviruses

John M. Coffin

Over the last two decades, retroviruses have proved to be remarkably rewarding organisms for study. Quite apart from their role in important human diseases, these agents have provided researchers with incisive tools for probing the molecular basis of carcinogenesis, and have revealed novel and important mechanisms of information transfer. The intellectual impetus of the discovery of reverse transcriptase in 1970, and the financial impetus of the war on cancer in the early 1970's, combined to convert retrovirology from an arcane corner of virology to a major growth industry.

Not surprisingly, much of the early research emphasis was on unique features of retroviruses relevant to cancer, e.g., mechanisms of viral DNA and RNA synthesis as well as structure and function of viral and cellular oncogenes. Issues such as epidemiology, virion structure, immunology, and cytopathicity, among others, were not completely ignored, but received relatively little attention. The discovery that infection with a retrovirus, HIV, is intimately associated with the causation of AIDS has changed this emphasis dramatically, and has provided renewed impetus to studies that consider retroviruses as infectious pathogens rather than as transducing agents. Indeed, in the last few years, HIV has become the model retrovirus and a prime paradigm for retroviral infectious disease.

This chapter will provide background information on retrovirus–host cell interactions with an emphasis on virion and genome structure and molecular mechanisms of replication and pathogenesis. It is hoped that this will permit the nonretrovirologist to obtain a grasp of the subject adequate for understanding the current literature. Most of the general references are cited in several comprehensive works on the subject (1–3) as well as in

other recent chapters (4–9), which the interested reader is strongly encouraged to obtain.

DEFINITION

Retroviruses are most uniquely defined as those viruses with RNA genomes whose replication is via a DNA intermediate. In addition to this defining characteristic [the prefix retro refers to the use of a mechanism of information transfer (RNA to DNA) that is the reverse of the usual], retroviruses share many additional features, including the following.

1. The virion is always enveloped and contains a single type of surface glycoprotein spike as well as an internal, roughly spherical to roughly cylindrical core. The core contains the genome as well as several enzymes—most prominently *reverse transcriptase* (RT)—whose presence is readily, and (with care) unequivocally, detectable and diagnostic.

Other virion enzymatic activities invariably include a ribonuclease H used for DNA synthesis, an integrase (IN) protein needed for integration of viral DNA into cell DNA, and a protease (PR) used to generate the capsid proteins by cleavage of a precursor.

2. The retrovirus genome is unique in several respects. First, it is a 7–10-kb molecule of RNA structurally resembling eukaryotic mRNA with a 5' capping group and 3' polyadenylate sequence. Second, it is present in the virion in two copies. Thus, retroviruses are the only known diploid viruses. Third, it is always found in association with lower molecular weight RNAs, most notably a single molecule of tRNA that serves as a primer for DNA synthesis.

3. Finally, all major events in replication are unique to retroviruses. They include the following steps: synthesis of a double-stranded linear viral DNA copy of the genome in the cytoplasm of the infected cell by a process

J. M. Coffin: Department of Molecular Biology and Microbiology, Tufts University School of Medicine, Boston, Massachusetts 02111

that leads to the formation of long terminal repeats (LTRs); integration of viral DNA into cellular DNA in a regular way to form the *provirus,* and transcription of the provirus, using cellular machinery, to form new RNA genomes and mRNAs. Signals provided within the LTR stimulate (and sometimes regulate) the activity of the cellular transcription system. This cycle permits a more intimate association of replication with cellular function than in any other group of viruses.

NATURAL HISTORY

Retroviruses are widespread among vertebrates, and infectious virus has been isolated from fish, reptiles, birds, and mammals.

Particles morphologically resembling virions have been detected in lower phylogenetic classes as well, including insects and even tapeworms. Among mammals and birds virtually all species that have been examined sufficiently closely have yielded retroviruses. In a number of species such viruses are an important source of naturally occurring disease (Table 1). Although retroviruses were initially identified with malignancies, it is now apparent that they are associated with a wide variety of diseases, including malignant, degenerative, and immunologic. The type of disease produced by a given virus can often be influenced by the genetic makeup or age of the host, as well as by small changes in the viral structure. For example, some strains of avian leukosis (leukemia) virus (ALV) strains induce B lymphomas in most lines of chickens, but erythroleukemia in some other lines (10,11). Furthermore, only slightly different strains of ALV induce osteopetrosis whereas others lead to viremia, but no disease at all (12,13). Similarly, a relatively minor change in feline leukemia virus converts it from a virus that induces lymphoid malignancy to one that causes a fatal immunodeficiency resembling AIDS (14). Thus, even more than other viruses, the pathogenic spectrum of a given retrovirus isolate provides particularly poor criteria for classification.

Compared to many other viruses, retroviruses are transmitted from one host to another only very poorly. This low transmission rate no doubt reflects the lability of the virion. The half-life of the Rous sarcoma virus (RSV) in cell culture medium is on the order of a few hours, and all retroviruses are readily inactivated by mild detergent, gentle heating, drying, or moderately high or low pH. Thus, in many instances, transmission is by close physical contact involving exchange of blood or semen. In populations in which a virus is endemic, the major mode of transmission is often vertical, by infection of the offspring with virus produced by the mother e.g., via milk in mammals, or via the oviduct into the albumen of birds' eggs. A number of viruses have clearly special adaptations for this sort of existence. Mammary tumor virus, for example, is expressed at high levels in lactating mammary glands but at much lower levels in other tissue.

Most retrovirus infections are characterized by latency measured in months to years. Such long latent periods are what one would expect for a virus whose major modes of transmission are either vertical or via intimate contact, since a virus that killed its host before it could be transmitted would not persist in nature. Latency is also an inherent characteristic of retrovirus infection that inevitably involves integration of viral DNA into the host genome. Since a virus infection would be completely eliminated only by destruction of all infected cells, it is doubtful that this can be accomplished. All such infections, once established, are therefore likely to be permanent.

Retrovirus infection can even extend well beyond the life of a single infected host. Many species of vertebrates contain, as part of their genetic composition, inherited proviruses closely resembling those derived from infectious virus. These endogenous proviruses have been most intensively studied in chickens and mice (15,16),

TABLE 1. *Some retroviral diseases*

Species	Disease	Virus
Humans	T-cell leukemia/lymphoma	Human T-cell leukemia virus type I (HTLV-I)
	Acquired immunodeficiency syndrome (AIDS)	Human immunodeficiency virus (HIV)
Primates	Lymphoma	Gibbon ape leukemia virus (GALV)
Cattle	B-cell lymphoma	Bovine leukemia virus (BLV)
Sheep	Visna, Maedi	Visna
Goats	Arthritis, encephalitis	Caprine encephalitis virus (CaEV)
Horses	Anemia	Equine infectious anemia virus (EIAV)
Cats	T-cell lymphoma, immunodeficiency	Feline leukemia virus (FeLV)
	Immunodeficiency	Feline immunodeficiency virus (FIV)
Mice	T-cell lymphoma, paralysis, immunodeficiency; mammary carcinoma, T-cell lymphoma	Murine leukemia virus (MLV) Mouse mammary tumor virus (MMTV)
Chickens	B-cell lymphoma, erythroleukemia, osteopetrosis, wasting	Avian leukosis virus (ALV)

and have been found to be closely related to—and certainly derived from—exogenous viruses endemic to the same species. In general, they are very poorly expressed, due to secondary modification of the DNA (i.e., methylation). When expressed, many endogenous proviruses can give rise to complete infectious virus. In general, this virus is nonpathogenic. This nonpathogenicity presumably represents a specific adaptation to the endogenous lifestyle on the part of these viruses, since an endogenous virus that even slightly diminished the reproductive potential of its host would be rapidly lost. Although endogenous viruses are stably associated with a given host genome (the loss rate for such elements has been estimated

at 4×10^{-6} per generation) (17–19), their numbers and locations differ from individual host to host, indicating that they have been introduced relatively recently (postspeciation).

Both the retention of biological activity by endogenous proviruses and their structural characteristics indicate that they were derived by processes not greatly different from that of a normal virus life cycle, i.e., by infection of germ line cells with virus (usually derived from another endogenous provirus). There are, in eukaryotic genomes, numerous elements with provirus-like structures for which no virus has yet been found. These are collectively called "retrotransposons" (20–23), im-

TABLE 2. *Taxonomy of retroviruses*

Taxon	"Old taxonomy"	"New taxonomy"
Family	*Retroviridae*	*Retroviridae*
Subfamily	*Oncovirinae*	—[a]
Genus	Type C oncovirus	MLV-related viruses
Subgenus	Mammalian type C oncoviruses	Mammalian type C viruses
Species	MLV, FeLV, GALV, etc.	MLV, FeLV, GALV, etc.
Species	HTLV, BLV	—[b]
Subgenus	Reptilian type C oncoviruses	Reptilian type C viruses
Species	CSRV, VRV	CSRV, VRV
Subgenus	Avian type C oncoviruses	Retriculoendotheliosis viruses
Species	SNV, REV	SNV, REV
Species	ALV, RSV	—[b]
Genus	Type B oncovirus	Mammalian type B viruses
Species	MMTV	MMTV
Genus	Type D oncovirus	Type D viruses
Species	MPMV, SMRV	MPMV, SMRV
Genus	—[b]	ALV-related
Species	—[b]	ALV, RSV
Genus	—[b]	HTLV-BLV
Species	—[b]	HTLV-I, -II, BLV
Subfamily	*Lentivirinae*	—[a]
Genus	*Lentivirus*	*Lentivirus*
Subgenus	—	Ovine/caprine lentiviruses
Species	Visna, CAEV	Visna, CAEV
Subgenus	—	Equine lentiviruses
Species	EIAV	EIAV
Subgenus	—	Primate lentiviruses
Species	HIV, SIV	HIV, SIV
Subgenus	—	Feline lentiviruses
Species	FIV	FIV
Subgenus	—	Bovine lentiviruses
Species	BIV	BIV
Subfamily	*Spumavirinae*	—[a]
Genus	*Spumavirus*	*Spumavirus*
Species	HSRV, SRV	HSRV, SFV

[a] The subfamily level of classification is no longer used.

[b] These groups are no longer considered to be sufficiently similar to the mammalian type C viruses to be classified with them.

ALV, avian leukosis virus; BIV, bovine immunodeficiency virus; BLV, bovine leukemia virus; CAEV, caprine arthritis encephalitis virus; CSRV, corn snake retrovirus; EIAV, equine infectious anemia virus; FeLV, feline leukemia virus; FIV, feline immunodeficiency virus; GALV, gibbon ape leukemia virus; HIV, human immunodeficiency virus; HSRV, human spuma retrovirus; HTLV, human T-cell lymphotropic (leukemia) virus; MLV, murine leukemia virus; MMTV, mouse mammary tumor virus; MPMV, Mason-Pfizer monkey virus; REV, retriculoendotheliosis virus; RSV, Rous sarcoma virus; SFV, simian foamy virus; SIV, simian immunodeficiency virus; SNV, spleen necrosis virus; VRV, viper retrovirus.

plying that they move by reverse transcriptase but within the same cell, rather than passing in a virion from cell to cell.

TAXONOMY

For some time, the family Retroviridae was classified as shown in Table 2 under "Old taxonomy" (24). This classification was based principally on pathogenic and morphological characteristics and has been supplanted by the "New taxonomy" shown in the same table. By now, the nucleotide sequences of numerous retrovirus genomes have been determined including at least one representative of all listed taxa (25–28). Analysis of this wealth of information reveals that, within genera, the individual members are quite closely related in overall organization (refer to Fig. 2, for example) and sequence.

VIRION STRUCTURE AND ASSEMBLY

Virions of retroviruses are similar but not identical in appearance. All contain a capsid within a roughly spherical envelope with more or less visible spikes (or peplomers) of glycoproteins. The capsids vary somewhat in structure and the original classification system into B-, C-, and D-type particles is based on details of capsid morphology. (A particles are strictly intracellular forms.)

Lentiviruses [including human immunodeficiency virus (HIV)] have a different morphology. Where the typical A, B, C, and D particles contain roughly spherical capsids differing in the extent of condensation and location within the envelope, HIV and other lentiviruses have a distinctive oblong-shaped capsid.

Virions of retroviruses have a fairly simple protein composition, usually containing only eight or nine proteins. Because of the fragility of the internal structures, the details of the capsid organization are not well known. Figure 1 shows a set of electron micrographs displaying budding and mature virus and presents in schematic fashion what is currently known about virion structure. The virion structural genes and their products are listed in Table 3, and the distribution of sequences coding for the various retrovirus genes is shown in Fig. 2.

The surface glycoprotein spike consists of two proteins (29). The larger one (SU) contains the receptor binding activity and is necessary for specifying the initial interaction of the virus with the host cell.

The smaller transmembrane (TM) protein is joined to the larger by either a disulfide or a noncovalent bond and anchors the complex to the lipid envelope. The C-terminal end of the smaller protein spans the membrane and may interact with an internal virion protein. Such an interaction is not necessary for virion formation and may not always be necessary to ensure incorporation of the envelope protein into virions (30).

The SU glycoprotein contains the receptor binding activity. This interaction is of first importance in specifying the target animal and—in some cases (such as HIV)—the target cell to be infected (31–34). In the one case that has been genetically defined (ALV), receptor interaction specificity lies in roughly the middle third of the protein (35–37), but several analyses suggest a location nearer the C terminus of SU for HIV (38,39). The large glycoprotein also forms the major target for the immune response against virions and infected cells. Among different retroviruses it varies in apparent molecular weight from 60,000 to about 120,000, with the largest size found in HIV and other lentiviruses. Much of this variation is due to variable amounts of glycosylation: SU proteins of HIV isolates are predicted to contain about two dozen carbohydrate side chains (27). Much of the remaining difference in molecular weight of the large envelope protein of HIV compared to other retroviruses may be accounted for by about 125 amino acids in "hypervariable" regions (27). Both these features may be relevant to the survival of HIV in the face of an immune response (40–43), since the hypervariable regions might allow rapid antigenic variation and the glycosylation sites might mask potentially antigenic regions (for review see 44,45). Indeed, recent studies indicate that one of the hypervariable regions, known as the "V3 loop" (Fig. 3) contains a major determinant for recognition by neutralizing antibodies (46–49).

The envelope glycoproteins are the products of the *env* gene and their synthesis and processing are virtually identical among all retroviruses. The *env* gene products are translated from a spliced, subgenomic RNA and, like cellular glycoproteins, are synthesized on membrane-bound polyribosomes followed by removal of an N-terminal signal peptide. Glycosylation and transport occur via the usual cellular pathways through the endoplasmic reticulum and Golgi apparatus where cleavage (by a cellular enzyme) into the two subunits occurs. This cleavage is accomplished by a cellular enzyme at a recognition site of three or four basic amino acids. A structure of about 24 uncharged amino acid residues near the C terminus of the TM protein serves as a membrane anchor.

The internal proteins of the virion are all products of three genes, *gag, pro,* and *pol.* They are listed in Table 3. The *gag* (for group-specific antigen) gene contributes the bulk of structural proteins, which number three or four depending on the virus. The three invariant proteins are (from N to C terminus): (1) MA, a probable "matrix" protein that lies adjacent to the membrane and probably interacts with it (sometimes via an added fatty acid group) to mediate budding; (2) CA (major core shell protein), the largest gag product (p24 in HIV), which most likely forms the core shell visible in electron micrographs; and (3) NC, (for nucleoprotein), a small, basic, protein that is found in close association with the genome RNA and that is necessary for specific encapsida-

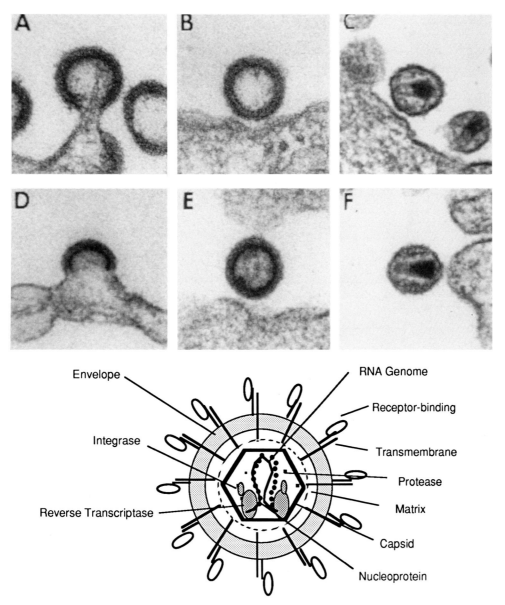

FIG. 1. The retrovirus virion. **Top:** Budding and mature virions. **A–C** and **D–F** show electron micrographs of cells producing HIV-1 and HIV-2, respectively. A and D show budding virions; B and E immature forms; and C and F mature forms. Note that the two viruses are morphologically indistinguishable. Micrographs courtesy of Dr. M Gonda.

    Bottom: This highly schematic figure shows the approximate locations of the various virion components common to all retroviruses. *MA,* matrix protein; *CA,* major core shell protein; *NC,* nucleoprotein; *PR,* protease; *RT,* reverse transcriptase; *IN,* endonuclease; *SU,* receptor binding protein; *TM,* transmembrane protein. MA, CA, NC, and PR are *gag* derived; RT and IN are *pol* derived; and SU and TM are *env* derived.

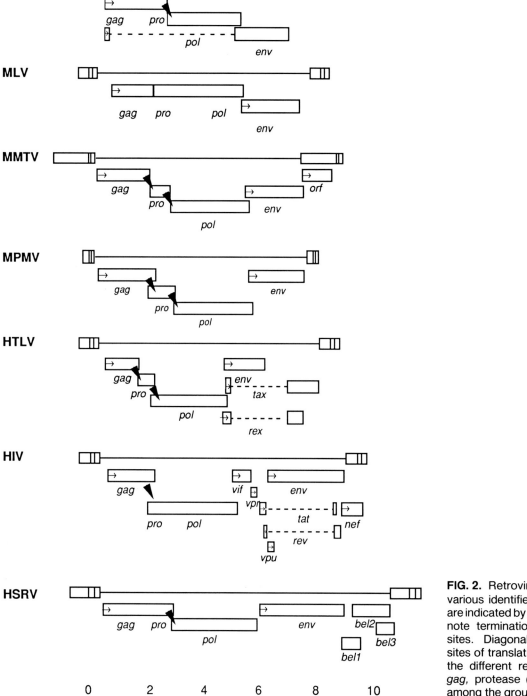

FIG. 2. Retrovirus reading frames. The various identified open reading frames are indicated by boxes. Dividing lines denote termination codons or cleavage sites. Diagonal arrowheads indicate sites of translational readthrough. Note the different relative positions of the *gag,* protease (*pro*), and *pol* domains among the groups of viruses. Note also the multiple use of the *env* region of HIV. See Table 2 for abbreviations.

TABLE 3. *Proteins of retrovirus virions*[a]

Current name	ALSV	Mammalian C-type	(B-type) MMTV	(B-type) D type	HTLV/BLV	Lenti
MA	p19	p15	p10	p10	p19/15	p15–17
?	p10	p12	p21	p18	NP[b]	NP[b]
CA	p27	p30	p27	p27	p24	p24–26
NC	p12	p10	p14	p14	p12	p7–11
PR	p15	p14	p13	—	p14	p17
RT	p68	p80	—	—	—	p66
IN	p32	p46	—	—	—	p32
SU	gp85	gp70	gp52	gp70	gp60	gp95–120
TM	gp37	p15E	gp36	gp22	gp30	gp41

[a] The order is 5′ to 3′ from top to bottom.
[b] Not present.
ALSV, avian leukosis/sarcoma virus; CA, major core shell protein; BLV, bovine leukemia virus; HTLV, human T-cell lymphotropic (leukemia) virus; IN, endonuclease; MA, matrix protein; MMTV, mouse mammary tumor virus; NC, nucleoprotein; PR, protease; RT, reverse transciptase; SV, receptor binding protein; TM, transmembrane protein.

tion of virion RNA (50–52) but that behaves in vitro as a nonspecific nucleic acid binding protein. NC proteins have a characteristic Cys-His sequence motif resembling that of Zn-binding proteins, but the interaction with Zn is unclear (51). Some, but not all, retroviruses have a fourth *gag* protein of unknown function located on the precursor between the matrix and capsid proteins.

The remaining virion proteins serve enzymatic, rather than structural, roles. The first of these is a protease (PR) encoded in the *pro* region C-terminal to the nucleic acid binding protein, and in various reading frames relative to *gag* and *pol* (Fig. 2). Finally, there are the two or three polypeptides (RT and IN) derived from the *pol* gene that carry out synthetic and nucleolytic events early in replication (synthesis of viral DNA and some steps necessary for integration). The functions of these are listed in Table 4.

The processing of *gag* and *pol* proteins is fairly well understood and is intimately connected with virion assembly and budding.

In all retroviruses, the *pro* and *pol* genes are expressed as a C-terminal extension of the *gag* precursor molecules. The synthesis and relative amounts of the precursors are determined by signals at the end of *gag* and/or

pro that specify translational bypassing, or "readthrough" of the usual translational stop signals (53,54). Both gene products are cleaved via the activity of the virion protease, which itself is part of the precursor, giving rise to the problem of how the protease itself is generated. The three-dimensional structures of both HIV and RSV PR proteins have recently been determined (55–58). This and other data (59–62) imply that the enzyme is an aspartic protease whose active site is formed by dimerization (63). Dimerization would require assembly of the *gag* precursor and thus prevent processing until the appropriate point in assembly. Once the initial cleavages take place, releasing active protease, the remaining cleavage would be relatively rapid. By this model, assembly and budding would be accomplished by *gag* and *gag–pol* precursors, ensuring both an appropriate balance of the virus proteins in virions as well as the absence of active reverse transcription complexes within the infected cell (see later). This scheme agrees with electron micrographic evidence showing that there is a significant structural rearrangement (from an open to a condensed core) shortly after budding.

The assembly and release of virions by budding is an unusual process in at least two respects. First, with most

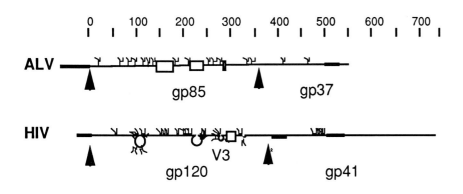

FIG. 3. The organization of *avian leukosis virus* (ALV) and HIV *env* proteins. In both cases the larger fragment is the receptor binding protein (SU); the smaller C-terminal protein (TM) contains the transmembrane region. The arrows represent cleavage sites; the open boxes, regions implicated in receptor binding; the branched symbols, sites of N-linked glycosylation; and the small loops regions of extensive variation in sequence.

TABLE 4. *Activities of* pol *gene products*

Product	Enzyme activity	Function
RT (reverse transcriptase)	DNA polymerase	Synthesis of viral DNA
	RNase H	Removal of genome and primers
IN (integrase)	Endonuclease	Removal of two bases from the end of the viral DNA
	Joining activity	Joining of viral and cellular DNA

retroviruses, assembly and budding occur simultaneously. Second, analysis of mutants shows that only a relatively small number of the virion proteins are required. Mutants lacking *pol, env,* and genome RNA still yield normal-appearing virions (except for the absence of surface projections). In fact, not even all of *gag* is required since mutants lacking the active PR and NC domains yield virus, albeit lacking in RNA and aberrant in appearance (64–66,52,67–70). Thus, the ability to form capsids and bud from a cell seems to reside in just the core and matrix proteins.

Nucleotide sequencing reveals that the *gag, pro,* and *pol* genes are directly adjoining and in various reading frames relative to one another. Expression of the appropriate relative amounts of the three nested precursors is accomplished by mechanisms that permit ribosomes to bypass termination signals at one or both of the junctions between the coding regions (53,54,71,72). In most cases, this suppression results from a shift in reading frame shortly before the terminator; in some cases readthrough occurs by insertion of a glutamine residue at a site corresponding to a termination signal (73). The frequency with which this aberration occurs determines the ratio of *gag, gag–pro,* and *gag–pol* precursor synthesized.

THE GENOME

As noted above, retrovirus genomes are synthesized and processed by the same mechanisms used for the synthesis of normal cell mRNA. Thus, the genomes physically resemble cell mRNAs: they have a sequence of about 200 A residues at their 3′ ends, a capping group of the usual sort at their 5′ end, and are further modified by the presence of methylated A residues at the sequence GACU (74,75). The overall organization of retrovirus genomes are similar one to another: the virion genes are always in the order *gag-pro-pol-env* and differ only in mechanism of readthrough expression of *pol* and disposition of the *pro* reading frame (Fig. 2). The function of additional reading frames is discussed below. In addition to the reading frames, all genomes contain a set of terminal regions essential for its function as a template for reverse transcription and for proper function (integration and transcription) of viral DNA (Fig. 4). From 5′ to 3′ these include:

R: A directly repeated sequence (12–250 bases; 98 in HIV) found adjacent to the poly (A) at the 3′ end. R serves a critical role during viral DNA synthesis to form a "bridge" for transfer of the growing chain from one end of the genome to the other.

U5: A unique sequence (80–200 bases) adjacent to R.

PB: The binding site for the tRNA primer that serves to initiate viral DNA synthesis soon after infection. The primer can be one of several different tRNAs (tRNA^{lys} in the case of HIV) and the primer binding site invariably consists of 18 bases perfectly complementary to the 3′ end of the tRNA.

Leader region: The sequence between PB and the beginning of *gag*. It usually contains two well-defined functions: a splice donor site for the generation of subgenomic mRNAs and a signal (sometimes called Ψ) that specifies assembly into virions presumably by specifically interacting with the NC domain of the *gag* precursor. The arrangement of these is usually a (5′) donor-packaging signal (3′) so that spliced mRNA's lack the signal and thus are not packaged.

Defined genome regions near the 3′ end include:

PP (for polypurine tract): A run of ten or more G and A residues that invariably mark the initiation site of plus-strand DNA synthesis, by providing a specific cleavage and primer site when present in an RNA–DNA hybrid.

U3: A unique region near the 3′ end varying in length from about 200 to 1,200 bases. Because it forms the upstream end of the LTR, U3 consists mostly of sequences relevant to initiation and regulation of transcription (see below).

R: Finally, the 3′ end of the genome contains a second copy of the repeated sequence identical to that of the 5′ end. Depending on the virus, either R or U3 contains a canonical signal (AAUAAA) for cellular systems that carry out cleavage and poly(A) addition to define the 3′ end of the genome.

In virions, the genome is invariably present in two copies joined to one another by base-pairing at multiple points, most strongly in a poorly defined region known as the "dimer linkage structure" near the 5′ end. The function of this unusual arrangement is not known with certainty; it has the effect of causing a very high frequency of recombination (76–78); an attractive

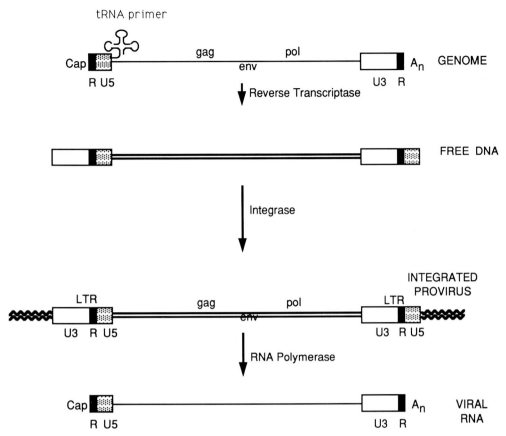

FIG. 4. Schematic outline of the retrovirus replication cycle. Single lines indicate RNA; double lines viral DNA (with LTR sequences boxed); and wavy lines show cell DNA around the integration site. (Courtesy of S. A. Herman).

idea is that the presence of two copies permits a high level of repair of damage to the relatively fragile single-stranded RNA.

REPLICATION

The replication of retroviruses can be divided into two phases. The first, including synthesis and integration of the provirus, is carried out principally by enzymes found in the virion; the second—including synthesis of progeny mRNAs and genomes is carried out entirely by cellular systems (Fig. 4). Given a virus that replicates in this fashion, the seemingly complex events of viral DNA synthesis can in fact be viewed as the simplest solution to two general problems.

First, all DNA polymerases (including reverse transcriptase) require a preexisting polymer to serve as primer for DNA synthesis. Second, cellular RNA polymerase II requires the presence of specific sequences upstream of the initiation site to provide important binding sites for transcription factors. Both of these problems dictate that the virus arrange a way to provide DNA sequences longer at the ends than the genome itself. The elegant solution achieved by the virus is to use the ability

of the reverse transcription system to change templates (or "jump") to synthesize a DNA molecule containing, as terminal repeats, sequences present only once near each end of the viral genome.

Initial Events

The entry of virus into cells requires interaction of the *env* protein with a specific receptor, since the lack of the receptor (or its blockage) reduces infectivity by 7 orders of magnitude or more. Penetration occurs by fusion of viral and cell membranes, mediated by the virion *env* protein. This fusion can take place either at the cell surface, or, depending on the virus and cell, following endocytosis or incorporation of the virion into a cellular vesicle (79). In the cases (such as HIV) in which entry is by direct fusion of virions with the cell membrane, a similar fusion can be mediated by interaction of *env* proteins on the surface of infected cells with receptors on an adjacent uninfected cell, leading to fusion of one cell with the other (80,81).

It is important to bear in mind that the subsequent early events do not require the synthesis of any virus-coded proteins and that they take place within some sort of (poorly defined) structure derived from the viral capsid (82,83). Most of these events are catalyzed by the virion enzymes encoded by the *pol* gene.

Viral DNA Synthesis

Synthesis of viral DNA occurs in the cytoplasm of infected cells. (By convention, the term provirus is reserved to the integrated form.) Space limitations preclude a complete description of this process here, so only highlights will be presented (6–9,84) (Fig. 5).

The overall process starts from a molecule of single-stranded RNA with the structure R-U5-genes-U3-R to a molecule of double-stranded DNA of the structure U3-R-U5-genes-U3-R-U5. The sequence U3-R-U5 thus constitutes the LTR. The ends of the LTR are defined by the sites of initiation of DNA synthesis. The first strand

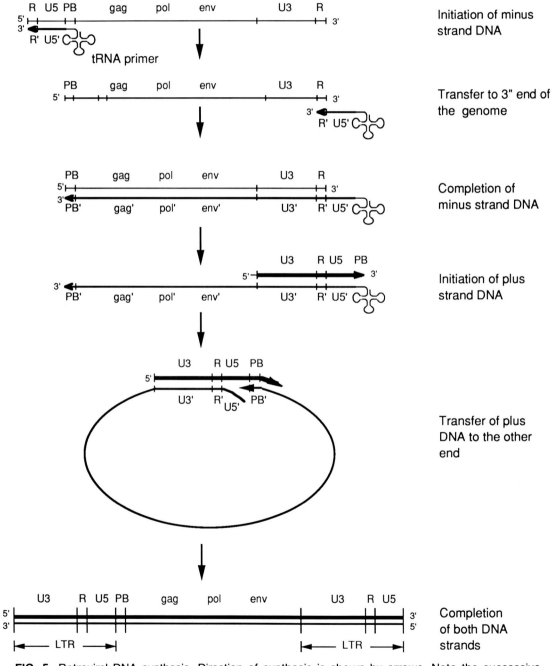

FIG. 5. Retroviral DNA synthesis. Direction of synthesis is shown by arrows. Note the successive "jumps" of reverse transcriptase, the first using the R sequence as a bridge, and the second using a copy of the primer binding (*PB*) site. (Courtesy of S. A. Herman).

synthesized (the minus strand) is initiated at the 3′ end of the tRNA primer and proceeds toward the 5′ end of the genome, and is thus a copy of U5 and R. When the 5′ end of the genome is reached, the RNase H removes the RNA just copied, and a new template primer pair is formed with the R at the 3′ end. This event constitutes the first jump, and permits completion of the minus strand. While this is happening, the RNase H activity is degrading the RNA template, except for the U_3 PP sequence, which is resistant, and creates a primer for plus strand synthesis using the U3-R portion of the minus strand DNA as template.

A second jump to the end of the minus strand then permits completion of both strands and formation of the LTRs.

Integration

The linear DNA molecules (probably still in association with capsid proteins) are transported to the nucleus.

The next event is integration of the viral DNA into that of the host (Fig. 6). The integration event is a regular and indispensable part of the replication cycle and is another characteristic that distinguishes retroviruses from all other families. Integration is a highly specific process, since the provirus is always joined in the same way to cellular DNA to provide a structure flanked by the LTRs. Invariably, there is a duplication of a short (four to six base) sequence of cell DNA and a loss of two bases at the exposed end of each LTR. The recent development of systems to study integration in vitro has led to a rapid increase in our understanding of the biochemical basis of this process (85–90) (Fig. 6). The principal reactions—all carried out by the IN protein—include: (1) removal of one or two bases from each 3′ end of the linear viral DNA molecule; (2) cleavage of the target DNA to leave four to six bases overhanging 5′ ends; and (3) joining of the 3′ end of the viral DNA to the 5′ ends of the target. Steps 2 and 3 are mechanistically coupled so that the energy derived from cleavage of the target is preserved to drive the joining reaction. The fill-in and

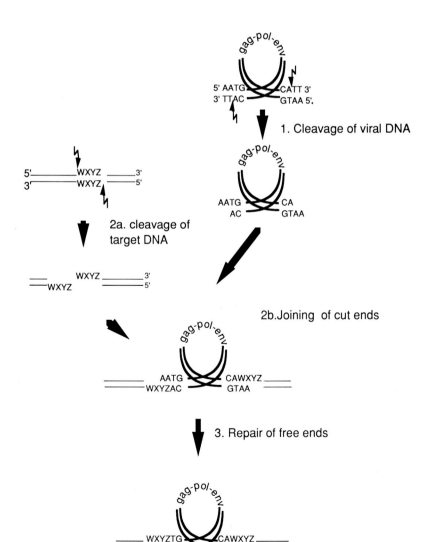

FIG. 6. A possible scheme for integration of viral DNA. Step 1, the removal of two bases from each end, is independent of the others; steps 2a and 2b are mechanistically linked. Steps 1 and 2 are catalyzed by integrase; step 3 is believed to be carried out by cellular repair systems. The heavy double lines show the two strands of DNA with the conserved sequence AATG . . . CATT at the ends. The lighter lines represent the cellular DNA target with WXYZ standing for any random sequence of bases.

repair of the resulting gaps (Fig. 6) is presumably accomplished by host cell repair systems.

Once integrated, the provirus is almost completely stable and is replicated regularly along with the cell DNA. There is no excision or direct transposition process, and loss of provirus (when it occurs) seems to be a consequence of random deletion events such as homologous recombination between the LTRs (17,91).

Expression

Once integrated, the provirus behaves as though it were a cellular gene; it serves as an efficient template for mRNA synthesis by RNA polymerase II. For this purpose, much of the U3 region of the LTR consists of sequences that resemble cellular signals for interaction with transcription and processing factors (Fig. 7).

5' of the initiation site for RNA synthesis (or "cap" site) are standard consensus signals for eukaryotic transcription: a TATA box about 24 bases upstream, and a CCAAT box about 80 bases upstream.

In addition there are more or less well-defined enhancer elements that can stimulate synthesis from a promoter in a relatively distance- and orientation-independent fashion. These are often present in multiple copies, as, for example, in the murine leukemia virus (MLV) LTR, which can contain a perfectly repeated sequence of about 70 base pairs in length containing identified binding sites for no less than six distinct factors (92), and HIV, which contains repeated binding sites for the sp1 transcription factor (93). The enhancer sequences can provide considerable biological specificity by affecting both the rate of virus replication (presum-

ably by regulating the rate of initiation of transcription) as well as the cell specificity of replication and pathogenesis. For example, the differential ability of various MLV strains to transform different cell types resides in relatively small sequence differences in the enhancer region of the LTR (94–96). Also, the availability of the NF-κB transcription factor is an important determinant of active transcription of the HIV LTR (97,98) and appears to be a major factor limiting expression (and hence, replication) of this virus to activated T cells and macrophages (99,100). In addition to specifying replication rate and tissue specificity, the LTR can also provide regulatory sequences. For example, the mammary tumor virus (MTV) U3 region contains sequences that respond to the action of glucocorticoid hormones, by binding hormone–receptor complex and stimulating transcription. Similarly, the human T-cell lymphtrophic virus types I and II (HTLV-I and -II) LTRs contain sequences that respond to the "transactivating" influence of the tax protein (see below).

In addition to specifying the initiation of transcription and hence the 5' end of the viral transcript, the LTR also specifies the 3' end of the RNA. As with most eukaryotic RNAs, synthesis of viral RNA almost certainly proceeds through the LTR into adjacent cell DNA and the primary transcript is then rapidly cleaved and polyadenylated to generate the final 3' end. A consensus addition signal (AAUAAA) is invariably found within either U3 or R, 16–20 bases upstream of the poly (A). Interestingly, this signal is not essential for replication (101) and a significant fraction of genomes can be derived from RNA polyadenylated at sites derived from adjoining host DNA (102).

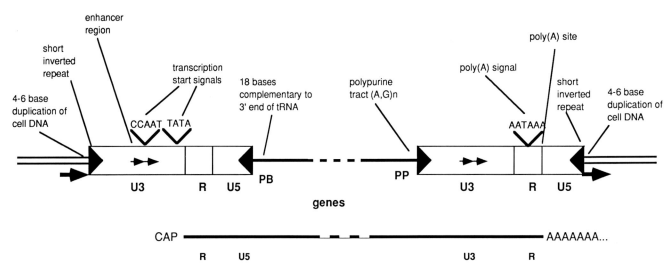

FIG. 7. Structural features of LTRs. The line at the bottom shows the beginning (5' end) and end (3' end) of the viral RNA. Note that although the LTRs are identical in sequence, the signals are only shown for the LTR in which they are important. Thus initiation signals are shown only in the 5' LTR; 3' processing signals only in the 5' LTR.

As shown in Fig. 7, the LTR thus contains a complex collection of signals used at various stages of virus replication. Despite the wide diversity of viruses and the virtually complete lack of sequence homology among different groups, all LTRs contain these signals and they can often be recognized by these features.

Transactivation

In many cases, expression of proviruses is accomplished entirely by factors and systems already in the cell prior to infection, for which the provirus and its transcript simply provide appropriate signals. Indeed, this property of the retrovirus infection cycle is crucial to the ability of some viruses to acquire oncogenes by exchanging host cell information for some or all of the coding sequence of the virus. This process would not be so readily feasible if these viruses required viral gene products for their expression. Some retroviruses, including HTLV and HIV, do not follow this rule. Rather, full expression of these viruses apparently requires the presence of one or more protein products of the virus genome itself. This phenomenon was first described with HTLV-I when it was found that reconstructed DNAs containing an HTLV-I LTR joined to a gene with a readily assayable product [chloramphenicol acetyl transferase, (CAT)] were expressed much more efficiently in HTLV-I in infected than in uninfected cells. This effect was found to be due to the protein encoded by the *tax* sequence encoded in the region between *env* and the LTR (103,104). This nuclear protein causes the level of viral transcripts to be greatly increased by affecting the rate of initiation of transcription via an indirect interaction with specific sequences in the U3 region of the LTR (104–106).

When the same sort of experiment is done with HIV (or other lentiviruses), a similar result is obtained: the expression of virus-like DNA constructs is greatly stimulated by prior infection of the cell (107). The effect of the relevant gene—now called *tat*—on HIV expression is superficially similar to that of *tax* on HTLV expression, but mechanistically very different. The essential region for *tat* interaction and binding is not in the DNA upstream of the transcription initiation site; rather it is in a RNA region called TAR, which lies in R, very near the 5′ end of the transcript (108). TAR is a highly structured region 50–60 bases in length that binds both *tat* and a cellular factor necessary for the effect (109,110). In addition to *tat*, specific enhancer sequences in the U3 are also required for transactivation (111). The mechanism of *tat* action is still strongly debated. Active hypotheses include: an "RNA enhancer" in which *tat* binding to *tar* interacts with transcription factors to increase initiation (112); and a variety of models in which the *tat–tar* inter-

action seems to stabilize the RNA synthesizing complex to prevent premature termination of transcription (113,114).

Genetic experiments show that transactivators are required for replication of HIV and HTLV; however, the role of transactivation in the life of these retroviruses remains to be clarified. Both types of viruses seem to have quiescent phases in infected individuals in which viral expression is difficult to detect. Transactivation may also allow higher levels of expression or a more rapid infection cycle than would be available with unmodified cell systems.

Processing

The viral RNA transcripts that are made have two distinct fates: they can become new genomes or they can serve as mRNA for the viral gene products. Most eukaryotic mRNAs are processed forms of the primary transcript that have been spliced—or cleaved and rejoined at specific signals (donors and acceptors)—to remove intervening sequences (introns). Retrovirus mRNAs follow this general rule, but with a twist. Only a fraction of the mRNA precursors are spliced to form subgenomic *env* (and sometimes other) mRNA. mRNA for the *gag, pro,* and *pol* genes is somehow protected from splicing and remains identical to the genome RNA. Clearly there must be a balance among these uses; too much or too little splicing would obviously be deleterious to virus replication. What determines this balance is, at present, not well understood. In the simpler virus groups, the inefficient use of splicing signals is almost certainly not due to the nature of the signals themselves or to any kind of direct regulation. Rather, it seems more likely that some structural feature of the RNA around the signals or within the *gag–pol* "intron" determines the efficiency of utilization of the *env* splice acceptor, since altering these sequences can drastically affect the relative amounts of spliced and unspliced mRNA (115–117).

With viruses of the lentivirus and HTLV-bovine leukemia virus (BLV) groups, there is also a more active control over the splicing process (118,106). Viruses of both groups encode a protein (*rev* and *rex*, respectively) that regulates the levels of unspliced (genomes and *gag-pro-pol* mRNA) and singly spliced (*env* mRNA) to multiply spliced (*rex, rev,* and transactivators) RNA (119–124). Although the *rex* and *rev* proteins are unrelated to one another and recognize unrelated viral sequences, they both seem to act by permitting viral RNA to bypass a cellular system that acts to prevent export from the nucleus of incompletely spliced RNAs (125,126). This similarity of function is emphasized by the fact that *rev* protein can substitute—at least inefficiently—for *rev* in appropriate assays (127). This regulatory mechanism acts to maintain the appropriate balance of virion to nonvirion proteins even with the more complex patterns of splicing exhibited in these virus groups.

Compared with the other well-studied retroviruses, which have only one spliced mRNA, HIV has a remarkably complex splicing pattern (128–130), in keeping with the additional open reading frames present on these viruses.

Other Genes

In addition to the genes whose products encode proteins involved in virion structure or activation of transcription and processing, some groups of viruses contain additional genes whose role in the virus life cycle remains to be fully clarified. In lentiviruses, there are at least four such genes, which vary somewhat from one species to another. These include:

nef. The *nef* gene product is a small, myristoylated protein localized on the inner face of the cell membrane that bears some resemblance to GTP-binding G proteins, like the *ras* protooncogene product (131,132). It is not essential for replication of lentiviruses in cell culture, and may inhibit their expression (133–135), although this point is controversial (136,137). An intact *nef* gene does seem to be required for efficient replication and disease induction by simian immunodeficiency virus (SIV) in monkeys (138).

vif. Virions produced in the absence of *vif* have reduced infectivity, possibly reflecting a role of this protein, which resembles a protease, in processing envelope proteins (139).

vpu. The *vpu* protein is found in the cytoplasm, and its presence seems to aid in the assembly of virions (140–144).

vpr. The *vpr* gene product is dispensable for replication, at least in some cell types (145,146). It is found in virions and may play a regulatory role early in infection (147,148). Like *vif, vpr* expression is dependent on *rev*, consistent with its role as a "late" gene (149,150).

One additional gene worthy of mention is a coding region located in the LTR of mouse mammary tumor virus (MMTV), formerly called *orf* (open reading frame) to indicate a lack of understanding of its function. The product of this region is not essential for replication of the virus, and although some workers had suggested that it had a regulatory role (151,152), its function has remained obscure. Recent evidence from a number of laboratories has shown that the *orf* region has a "superantigen" function, since its product can activate T cells expressing certain classes of receptor genes (153–158). While not required for replication in cell culture, this function may aid in the process of infection of the whole animal. Despite the present lack of mechanistic insight,

it has been proposed that this region be renamed *sag* (154,159).

PATHOGENESIS

Retroviruses can induce a wide variety of different diseases in natural and experimental hosts. As noted in a prior section, the pathological consequences of infection are various, including no disease; a variety of malignancies; various degenerative conditions; and probably also conditions with an autoimmune basis. Due to intense effort in the past few years, there has been considerable progress in understanding the cellular, molecular, and sometimes even the biochemical basis of these diseases. The molecular basis of retrovirus oncogenesis is probably best understood, although rapid progress is being made toward an understanding of the degenerative conditions associated with HIV and other cytopathic virus infections.

Malignancy

With the possible exceptions of the HTLV-BLV group (see below) and AIDS-associated malignancies, all retroviral carcinogenesis is mediated at least in part by the action of oncogenes (or *onc* genes). Oncogenes can be defined as nucleotide sequences that are derived from normal cellular genes (*c-onc* genes or protooncogenes) and that have been altered in some way to confer on their products the ability to transform certain normal cells into tumor cells.

The activation event that converts a protooncogene into an oncogene can be one of three fundamentally different types. First, all or part of the nucleotide sequence can be inserted into the viral genome, usually in place of viral genes. This rare set of events gives rise to rapidly transforming viruses such as RSV, Abelson murine leukemia virus, and simian sarcoma virus.

The second type of activation can occur following integration of a provirus into or near a protooncogene. This type of event, although it probably occurs less than once per million infected cells, can occur at high frequency per animal in certain circumstances, as in chickens infected with ALV or mice infected with MLV or MMTV. For example, integration within the *c-myc* gene is found in virtually all B-cell lymphomas induced by ALV, and in many T-cell lymphomas induced by MLV.

Third, similar or identical oncogenes can also apparently be activated by nonviral events. For example, chromosome breakage and rejoining may accomplish activation of *c-myc* in certain mouse and human lymphoid tumors, and point mutations can activate *ras* in spontaneous (or chemically induced) tumors.

Experience with retrovirally induced malignancies has

demonstrated that normal cells contain at least 20–30 different genes that can be activated into oncogenes. It seems that many (perhaps all) protooncogenes may be involved in the normal regulation of the cell cycle—in particular in the response of the cell to growth factors (160,161). There are two important—not mutually exclusive—differences between activated oncogenes and their cellular ancestors. First, their control is altered so that they are under the influence of viral rather than normal cellular transcriptional signals, leading to unregulated expression at higher levels and in inappropriate cell types. Second, they have frequently suffered mutations —such as deletions or point mutations in regulatory domains.

In contrast to the avian and murine viruses, carcinogenesis by HTLV and BLV does not seem to involve the action of typical oncogenes. These viruses do not contain cell-derived sequences, and there seems to be no similarity of integration regions between one tumor and the next, as would be expected for insertional activation. Rather, it has been suggested that carcinogenesis might be due to transactivation of cellular protooncogenes mediated by the *tax* gene product. A possible pair of targets for such transactivation is the T-cell growth factor interleukin-2 (IL-2), as well as the cell receptor for IL-2 (162–168). It could be imagined that overexpression of this protein could cause cells to be stimulated to divide in the complete absence of the usual IL-2 signal, but direct evidence for this mechanism remains scanty.

Cell killing

Although retrovirus infections need not lead to cell damage, the AIDS epidemic has forcefully brought home the importance of cytopathic infections in the biology of these viruses. At an organismal level, there are two distinct mechanisms for cell killing by retroviruses; direct cytopathic effects and immune surveillance against otherwise healthy cells expressing viral antigens. The latter interaction certainly occurs in some cases and may be of importance in "wasting" types of diseases associated with certain ALV infections. This issue has not yet been explored in great depth and is probably not important in AIDS.

Infection with a number of retroviruses—including HIV and even some oncoviruses—can lead to cell death in certain cell culture systems. Two fundamentally different mechanisms have been proposed, both of which may be important in HIV infection. The first mechanism involves apparent "overreplication" of the virus. It has been repeatedly noted that cells infected with cytopathic retroviruses have excessive amounts of unintegrated DNA—hundreds of copies as compared with one or a few copies in noncytopathic infections (169–172). Since retroviral DNA apparently does not contain sig-

nals for its own replication, the excess copies probably arise by repeated cycles of transcription–reverse transcription, either via complete infection cycles involving reinfection of a cell with virus produced by it, or by a "short-circuit" cycle involving reverse transcription of newly synthesized RNA. Two features of the "usual" replication cycle serve to prevent such effects. First, cleavage of the *gag* and *gag–pol* precursor proteins into an apparently active "mature" form does not take place until the virion is released (or about to be released) by the infected cell. Thus, an active reverse transcriptase-template complex seems never to be present within the cell. Second, expression of the *env* gene product at the cell surface confers a very high level of resistance to superinfection, preventing nascent viruses from reentering the same cell. Indeed, cytopathic variants of normally noncytopathic ALV strains differ specifically in the particular receptor utilized for infection (36,173), indicating that it may be more difficult to establish superinfection resistance with some retroviral receptors than others. In the case of HIV and most other cytopathic retroviruses, the mechanism of accumulation of viral DNA is not known.

Also not known is why excess viral DNA should be associated with cell killing. It may simply be that the excess of viral signals (such as binding sites for cellular transcriptional or translational factors) renders these factors unavailable to the cells for their own purposes. Alternatively, the DNA itself may be toxic or there may be a consequent high level of expression of some more toxic viral gene products.

An alternative cytopathic mechanism is based on the observation that HIV-infected cell cultures contain numerous multicellular syncytia comprised of large numbers of cells fused together. Such cells can apparently form by interaction of the *env* protein on the surface of an infected cell with the T4 protein of a neighboring uninfected cell, followed by membrane fusion analogous to that used for virus infection. This event has been observed directly on mixtures of T4-positive cells with cells expressing *env* protein (80,174). It has been proposed that this mechanism would permit a relatively small number of infected cells to do considerable damage by incapacitating a much larger number of CD4-positive uninfected cells. However, in cell culture cytopathic effects do not require cell fusion.

EVOLUTION

Although HIV has appeared as a human pathogen only very recently, there is every reason to believe that retroviruses have been around for at least a substantial fraction of vertebrate evolution.

Unlike most infectious agents, retroviruses have left "fossil" traces of prior association with their host in the form of endogenous proviruses in the germ line. Although the endogenous proviruses that can be readily expressed as infectious virus seem to be relatively recently acquired (at least postspeciation), recent experimentation has revealed additional, new classes of endogenous viruses in the DNA of several species, including humans (16,175–177). These are distantly related to the modern oncoviruses (such as murine leukemia virus) but are clearly of great antiquity, since they have suffered many point mutations, which would render their coding regions unusable, and even the LTRs (which should have been identical at the time of insertion) have diverged in sequence (177). Furthermore, the similarity of integration sites of some elements in humans and chimpanzees implies their presence prior to divergence of the species (178). Thus, the association, at least of oncoviruses, with human ancestors would seem to be quite long-standing, and to involve repeated waves of "endogenization" of proviruses.

Unfortunately, other groups of retroviruses such as lentiviruses do not seem to have left such distant traces in the germ line.

Although clearly very ancient, retroviruses are also capable of very rapid variation and adaptation to new niches, as evidenced by two recent examples. The first is the relatively frequent appearance of viruses containing oncogenes. These are presumably the consequence of a very rare series of events involving integration at specific sites and illegitimate recombination. Although the proportion of viruses containing an oncogene in a virus population could be substantially less than 10^{-10}, the consequence of infection of a single cell with such a virus is a readily visible tumor and a very large number of animals can be easily screened (by visiting a slaughterhouse or a veterinarian, for example). Because the horizontal transmission of retroviruses is very poor, viruses as virulent as the transforming viruses almost certainly die with the animal in which they arise. Thus, the laboratory can be considered the "new" niche to which these viruses have adapted.

The spread of HIV-1 and -2 into the human population represents a second example of recent retrovirus evolution. In both cases the virus is most likely a variant of much older viruses, which probably existed in Africa in association with a monkey population (179–183). It would seem likely that occasional infections of humans with these viruses had occurred throughout history, but conditions were not appropriate for their spread out of isolated pockets of infection. Their recent appearance throughout the world probably reflects changes in living conditions, including increased international travel.

It should be clear from the above discussion that retroviruses have adapted to a wide variety of niches, and have done so despite their very low rate of transmission and the lability of the virion. The adaptability of these viruses is intimately related to special features of the replication cycle. Retrovirus replication involves a fairly high frequency of both point mutations and rearrangements, and an extraordinarily high frequency of recombination. The former presumably reflects infidelity of the replication systems (probably both RNA polymerase and reverse transcriptase) and gives rise to about 0.1–1 error/replication cycle (184–187). The recombination frequency seems to be a consequence of the diploid genome of retroviruses and the ability of the reverse transcriptase system to change templates during replication (76,77,188).

The result of this "genetic flexibility" is a significant amount of genetic variation within even a closely related population of viruses. Different HIV isolates, for example, can differ by more than 10% from one another particularly in the *env* gene. The ability to generate this sort of variation may be important not only in allowing the viruses to adapt to new environments, but also to aid in survival in a particular host, as illustrated by the apparently rapid sequence and antigenic variation in HIV and some other retroviruses (27). It should be apparent that the rapid variability of these viruses is a major concern in developing strategies to deal with them. These issues will be more thoroughly covered in other chapters.

CONCLUSIONS

The outbreak of AIDS has provided renewed impetus to obtaining more extensive knowledge of retrovirus biology. It should be apparent that, although some areas are understood in considerable depth, such as the structure of the genome and the mechanism of viral DNA synthesis and integration, others remain quite obscure. As our understanding of the virology of AIDS has increased, many new and fascinating retrovirological problems have appeared, and many old problems (such as antigenic variation or mechanism of cell killing), which previously were relatively little studied, have moved into the forefront. Just as AIDS is quite different from all other infectious diseases, HIV is also quite different from all other retroviruses. Infection with this virus involves phenomena not seen before. Many questions remain unanswered, and the answers will be of both enormous practical and theoretical importance to understanding this devastating but fascinating disease.

REFERENCES

1. Swanstrom R, Vogt PK. *Retroviruses: strategies of replication.* Berlin: Springer-Verlag, 1990.
2. Weiss R, Teich N, Varmus H, Coffin J. *RNA tumor viruses.* Cold Spring Harbor, NY: Cold Spring Harbor Laboratory, 1984.
3. Weiss R, Teich N, Varmus H, Coffin J. *RNA tumor viruses.* Cold Spring Harbor, NY: Cold Spring Harbor Laboratory, 1985.
4. Coffin JM. Replication of retrovirus genomes. In: Domingo E, Holland JJ, Ahlquist P, eds. *RNA genetics,* vol II: *Retroviruses,*

viroids, and RNA recombination. Boca Raton, FL: CRC Press, 1988;3–22.

5. Coffin JM. Genetic variation in retroviruses. In: Kurstak E, Marusyk RG, Murphy FA, Van Regenmortel MHV, eds. *Applied virology research,* vol 2; *Virus variability, epidemiology, and control.* New York: Plenum, 1990;11–33.

6. Coffin JM. Retroviridae and their replication. In: Fields B, Knipe D, Chanock R, eds. *Virology,* 2nd ed. New York: Raven Press, 1990;1437–500.

7. Varmus H. Retroviruses. *Science* 1988;240:1427–35.

8. Varmus H, Brown P. Retroviruses. In: Howe M, Berg D, eds. *Mobile DNA.* Washington: ASM, 1989;53–108.

9. Varmus HE. Reverse transcription. *Sci Am* 1987;257:56–66.

10. Nilsen TW, Maroney PA, Goodwin RG, et al. c-erbB activation in ALV-induced erythroblastosis: novel RNA processing and promoter insertion result in expression of an amino-truncated EGF receptor. *Cell* 1985;41:719–26.

11. Robinson HL, Miles BD, Catalano DE, Briles WE, Crittenden LB. Susceptibility to erbB-induced erythroblastosis is a dominant trait of 151 chickens. *J Virol* 1985;55:617–22.

12. Aurigemma RE, Torgersen JL, Smith RE. Sequences of myeloblastosis-associated virus MAV-2(0) and UR2AV involved in the formation of plaques and the induction of osteopetrosis, anemia and ataxia. *J Virol* 1991;65:23–30.

13. Robinson HL, Reinsch SS, Shank PR. Sequences near the 5′ long terminal repeat of avian leukosis viruses determine the ability to induce osteopetrosis. *J Virol* 1986;59:45–9.

14. Overbaugh J, Donahue PR, Quackenbush SL, Hoover EA, Mullins JI. Molecular cloning of a feline leukemia virus that induces fatal immunodeficiency disease in cats. *Science* 1988;239:906–10.

15. Coffin JM. Endogenous viruses. In: Weiss R, Teich N, Varmus H, Coffin J, eds. *RNA tumor viruses.* Cold Spring Harbor, NY: Cold Spring Harbor Laboratory, 1982;1109–1204.

16. Stoye JP, Coffin JM. Endogenous viruses. In: Weiss R, Teich N, Varmus H, Coffin J, eds. *RNA tumor viruses.* Cold Spring Harbor, NY: Cold Spring Harbor Laboratory, 1985;357–404.

17. Copeland NG, Hutchinson KW, Jenkins. NA. Excision of the DBA ecotropic provirus in dilute coat-color revertants of mice occurs by homologous recombination involving the viral LTRs. *Cell* 1983;33:379–87.

18. Frankel WN, Stoye JP, Taylor BA, Coffin JM. A linkage map of endogenous murine leukemia proviruses. *Genetics* 1990;124:221–36.

19. Seperack PK, Strobel MC, Corrow DJ, Jenkins NA, Copeland NG. Somatic and germ-line reverse mutation rates of the retrovirus-induced dilute coat-color mutation of DBA mice. *Proc Natl Acad Sci USA* 1988;85:189–92.

20. Baltimore D. Retroviruses and retrotransposons: the role of reverse transcription in shaping the eukaryotic genome. *Cell* 1985;40:481–2.

21. Boeke JD. Retrotransposons. In: Domingo E, Holland JJ, Ahlquist P, eds. *RNA Genetics,* vol II: *Retroviruses, viroids, and RNA recombination.* Boca Raton, FL: CRC Press, 1988;59–103.

22. McClure MA. Retrotransposon evolution. *Mol Biol Evol* [submitted].

23. Temin HM. Reverse transcription in the eukaryotic genome: retroviruses, pararetroviruses, retro transposons, and retrotranscripts. *Mol Biol Evol* 1985;6:455–68.

24. Brown F, Atherton J, Knudson D. Classification and nomenclature of viruses (fifth report of the ICTV). *Intervirology* [in press].

25. Flugel RM, Rethwilm A, Maurer B, Darai G. Nucleotide sequence of the env gene and its flanking regions of the human spumaretrovirus reveals two novel genes. *EMBO J* 1987;6:2077–84.

26. Maurer B, Bannert H, Darai G, Flugel RM. Analysis of the primary structure of the long terminal repeat and the gag and pol genes of the human spumaretrovirus. *J Virol* 1988;62:1590–7.

27. Myers G, Rabson AB, Josephs SF, Smith TF, Berzofsky JA, Wong-Staal F. *Human retroviruses and AIDS 1990.* Los Alamos, NM: Los Alamos National Laboratory, 1990.

28. Van Beveren C, Coffin JM, Hughes S. Appendixes. In: Weiss R, Teich N, Varmus H, Coffin J, eds. *RNA tumor viruses.* Cold Spring Harbor, NY: Cold Spring Harbor Laboratory, 1985;559–1222.

29. Hunter R, Swanstrom R. Retrovirus envelope glycoproteins. In: Swanstrom R, Vogt PK, eds. *Retroviruses. Strategies of replication.* New York: Springer-Verlag, 1990;187–253.

30. Perez LG, Davis GL, Hunter E. Mutants of the Rous sarcoma virus envelope glycoprotein that lack the transmembrane anchor and cytoplasmic domains: analysis of intracellular transport and assembly into virions. *J Virol* 1987;61:2981–8.

31. Dalgleish AG, Beverly PCL, Clapham PR, Crawford DH, Greaves MF, Weiss RA. The CD4 (T4) antigen is an essential component of the receptor for the AIDS retrovirus. *Nature* 1984;312:763–7.

32. Klatzman D, Champagne E, Chamaret S, et al. T-lymphocyte T4 molecule behaves as the receptor for human retrovirus LAV. *Nature* 1984;312:767–8.

33. Maddon PJ, Dalgleish AG, McDougal JS, Claphap PR, Weiss RA, Axel R. The T4 gene encodes the AIDS virus receptor and is expressed in the immune system and the brain. *Cell* 1986;47:333–48.

34. Richardson JH, Edwards AJ, Cruickshank JK, Rudge P, Dalgleish AG. In vivo cellular tropism of human T-cell leukemia virus type 1. *J Virol* 1990;64:5682–7.

35. Bova CA, Olsen JC, Swanstrom R. The avian retrovirus env gene family: molecular analysis of host range and antigenic variants. *J Virol* 1988;62:75–83.

36. Dorner AJ, Coffin JM. Determinants for receptor interaction and cell killing on the avian retrovirus glycoprotein gp85. *Cell* 1986;45:365–74.

37. Dorner AJ, Stoye JP, Coffin JM. Molecular basis of host range variation in avian retroviruses. *J Virol* 1985;53:32–9.

38. Kowalski M, Potz J, Basiripour L, et al. Functional regions of the envelope glycoprotein of human immunodeficiency virus type 1. *Science* 1987;237:1351–5.

39. Willey RL, Smith DH, Lasky LA, et al. In vitro mutagenesis identifies a region within the envelope gene of the human immunodeficiency virus that is critical for infectivity. *J Virol* 1988;62:139–47.

40. Cheng-Mayer C, Quiroga M, Tung JW, Dina D, Levy JA. Viral determinants of human immunodeficiency virus type 1 T-cell or macrophage tropism, cytopathogenicity, and CD4 antigen modulation. *J Virol* 1990;64:4390–8.

41. Harada S, Kobayashi N, Koyanagi Y, Yamamoto N. Clonal selection of human immunodeficiency virus (HIV): serological differences in the envelope antigens of the cloned viruses and HIV prototypes (HTLV-III B, LAV, and ARV). *Virology* 1987;158:447–51.

42. Michel M-L, Mancini M, Sobczak E, et al. Induction of anti-human immunodeficiency virus (HIV) neutralizing antibodies in rabbits immunized with recombinant HIV-hepatitis B surface antigen particles. *Proc Natl Acad Sci USA* 1988;85:7957–61.

43. Weiss RA, Clapham PR, Weber JN, Dalgleish AG, Lasky LA, Berman PW. Variable and conserved neutralization antigens of human immunodeficiency virus. *Nature* 1986;324:572–5.

44. Coffin JM. Genetic variation in AIDS viruses. *Cell* 1986;46:1–4.

45. Sattentau QJ, Dalgleish AG, Weiss RA, Bevereley. PCL. Epitopes of the CD4 antigen and HIV infection. *Science* 1986;234:1120–3.

46. Epstein LG, Luiken C, Blumberg BM, et al. HIV-1 V3 domain variation in brain and spleen of children with AIDS: tissue-specific evolution within host-determined quasispecies. *Virology* 1991;180:583–90.

47. Griffiths JC, Berrie EL, Holdsworth LN, et al. Induction of high-titer neutralizing antibodies, using hybrid human immunodeficiency virus V3-Ty viruslike particles in a clinically relevant adjuvant. *J Virol* 1991;65:450–6.

48. Nara PL, Smit L, Dunlop N, et al. Emergence of viruses resistant to neutralization by V3-specific antibodies in experimental human immunodeficiency virus type 1 IIIB infection of chimpanzees. *J Virol* 1990;64:3779–91.

49. Scott CFJ, Silver S, Profy AT, et al. Human monoclonal antibody that recognizes the V3 region of human immunodeficiency virus gp120 and neutralizes the human T-lymphotropic virus type III$_{MN}$ strain. *Proc Natl Acad Sci USA* 1990;87:8597–601.

50. Fu X, Katz RA, Skalka AM, Leis J. Site-directed mutagenesis of

the avian retrovirus nucleocapsid protein pp12: mutation which affects RNA binding in vitro blocks viral replication. *J Biol Chem* 1988;263:2134–9.

51. Katz RA, Jentoff JE. What is the role of the Cys-His motif in retroviral nucleocapsid (NC) proteins? *Bioessays* [in press].

52. Meric C, Gouilloud E, Spahr P-F. Mutations in Rous sarcoma virus nucleocapsid protein p12 (NC): Deletions of Cys-His boxes. *J Virol* 1988;62:3228–3333.

53. Jacks T. Translational suppression in gene expression in retroviruses and retrotransposons. In: Swanstrom R and Vogt PK, eds. Retroviruses. Strategies of Replication. New York: Springer-Verlag, 1990;93–124.

54. Jacks T, Varmus HE. Expression of the Rous sarcoma virus pol gene by ribosomal frameshifting. *Science* 1985;230:1237–42.

55. Miller M, Jaskolski M, Mohana Rao JK, Leis J, Wlodawer A. Crystal structure of a retroviral protease proves relationship to aspartic protease family. *Nature* 1989;337:576–9.

56. Navia MA, Fitzgerald PMD, McKeever BM, et al. Three-dimensional structure of aspartyl protease from human immunodeficiency virus HIV-1. *Nature* 1989;337:615–20.

57. Skalka AM. Retroviral proteases: first glimpses at the anatomy of a processing machine. *Cell* 1989;56:911–13.

58. Weber IT, Miller M, Jaskolski M, Leis J, Skalka AM, Wlodawer A. Molecular modeling of the HIV-1 protease and its substrate binding site. *Science* 1989;243:928–31.

59. Hafenrichter R, Weiland F, Schneider J, Thiel H-J. Properties of retroviral protease responsible for *gag* precursor cleavage. *Virology* 1989;172:355–8.

60. Katoh I, Ikawa Y, Yoshinaka Y. Retrovirus protease characterized by a dimeric aspartic proteinase. *J Virol* 1989;63:2226–32.

61. Loeb DD, Hutchinson III CA, Edgell MH, Farmerie WG, Swanstrom R. Mutational analysis of human immunodeficiency virus type 1 protease suggests functional homology with aspartic proteinases. *J Virol* 1989;63:111–21.

62. Mous J, Heimer EP, LeGrice SFJ. Processing protease and reverse transcriptase from human immunodeficiency virus type 1 polyprotein in *Escherichia coli. J Virol* 1988;62:1433–6.

63. Oroszlan S, Luftig RB. Retroviral proteinases. In: Swanstrom R, Vogt PK, eds. *Retroviruses. Strategies of replication.* New York: Springer-Verlag, 1990;153–86.

64. Ashorn P, McQuade TJ, Thaisrivongs S, Tomasselli AG, Tarpley WG, Moss B. An inhibitor of the protease blocks maturation of human and simian immunodeficiency viruses and spread of infection. *Proc Natl Acad Sci USA* 1990;87:7472–6.

65. Katoh I, Yoshinaka Y, Rein A, Shibuya M, Odaka T, Oroszlan S. Murine leukemia virus maturation: protease region required for conversion from "immature" to "mature" core form and for virus infectivity. *Virology* 1985;145:280–92.

66. McQuade TJ, Tomasselli AG, Liu L, et al. A synthetic HIV-1 protease inhibitor with antiviral activity arrests HIV-like particle maturation. *Science* 1990;247:454–6.

67. Meric C, Spahr P-F. Rous sarcoma virus nucleic acid binding protein p12 is necessary for viral 70S RNA dimer formation and packaging. *J Virol* 1986;60:450–9.

68. Overton HA, McMillan DJ, Gridley SJ, Brenner J, Redshaw S, Mills JS. Effect of two novel inhibitors of the human immunodeficiency virus protease on the maturation of the HIV gag and gag-pol polyproteins. *Virology* 1990;179:508–11.

69. Peng C, Ho BK, Chang TW, Chang NT. Role of human immunodeficiency virus type 1-specific protease in core protein maturation and viral infectivity. *J Virol* 1989;63:2550–6.

70. Voynow SL, Coffin JM. Truncated gag-related proteins are produced by large deletion mutants of Rous sarcoma virus and form virus particles. *J Virol* 1985;55:79–85.

71. Jacks T, Madhani HD, Masiarz FR, Varmus HE. Signals for ribosomal frameshifting in the Rous sarcoma virus gag-pol region. *Cell* 1988;55:447–58.

72. Jacks T, Townsley K, Varmus HE, Majors J. Two efficient ribosomal frameshifting events are required for synthesis of mouse mammary tumor virus gag-related polyproteins. *Proc Natl Acad Sci USA* 1987;84:4298–302.

73. Yoshinaka Y, Katoh I, Copeland TD, Oroszlan SJ. Murine leukemia virus protease is encoded by the gag-pol gene and is synthesized through suppression of an amber termination codon. *Proc Natl Acad Sci USA* 1985;82:1618–22.

74. Csepany T, Lin A, Baldick CJ, Beemon K. Sequence specificity of N^6-adenosine methyltransferase. *J Biol Chem.* 1990;265:20117–22.

75. Kane SE, Beemon K. Precise localization of m6A in Rous sarcoma virus RNA reveals clustering of methylation sites: implications for RNA processing. *Mol Cell Biol* 1985;5:2298–2306.

76. Coffin JM. Structure, replication, and recombination of retrovirus genomes: some unifying hypotheses. *J Gen Virol* 1979;42:1–26.

77. Hu W-S, Temin HM. Retroviral recombination and reverse transcription. *Science* 1990;250:1227–33.

78. Hu WS, Temin HM. Genetic consequences of packaging two RNA genomes in one retroviral particle: pseudodiploidy and high rate of genetic recombination. *Proc Natl Acad Sci USA* 1990;87:1556–60.

79. Weiss RA. Experimental biology and assay of RNA tumor viruses. In: Weiss R, Teich N, Varmus H, Coffin J, eds. *RNA tumor viruses.* Cold Spring Harbor, NY: Cold Spring Harbor Laboratory, 1982;209–60.

80. Sodroski J, Goh WC, Rosen C, Campbell K, Haseltine WA. Role of the HTLV-III/LAV envelope in syncytium formation and cytopathicity. *Nature* 1986;322:470–74.

81. Stein BS, Gowda SD, Lifson JD, Pennhallow RC, Bensch KG, Engelman EG. pH-independent HIV entry into CD4-positive T cells via virus envelope fusion to the plasma membrane. *Cell* 1987;49:659–69.

82. Bowerman B, Brown PO, Bishop JM, Varmus HE. A nucleoprotein complex mediates the integration of retroviral DNA. *Genes Dev* 1989;3:469–78.

83. Farnet CM, Haseltine WA. Determination of viral proteins present in the human immunodeficiency virus type 1 preintegration complex. *J Virol* 1991;65:1910–15.

84. Varmus HE, Swanstrom R. Replication of retroviruses. In: Weiss R, Teich N, Varmus H, Coffin J, eds. *RNA tumor viruses.* Cold Spring Harbor, NY: Cold Spring Harbor Laboratory, 1985;74–134.

85. Brown PO. Integration of retroviral DNA. In: Swanstrom R, Vogt PK, eds. *Retroviruses. Strategies of replication.* New York: Springer-Verlag, 1990;19–48.

86. Brown PO, Bowerman B, Varmus HE, Bishop JM. Correct integration of retroviral DNA in vitro. *Cell* 1987;49:347–56.

87. Craigie R, Fujiwara T, Bushman F. The IN protein of Moloney murine leukemia virus processes the viral DNA ends and accomplishes their integration in vitro. *Cell* 1990;62:829–37.

88. Fujiwara T, Mizuuchi K. Retroviral DNA integration: structure of an integration intermediate. *Cell* 1988;54:497–504.

89. Lee YMH, Coffin JM. Efficient autointegration of avian retrovirus DNA in vitro. *J Virol* 1990;64:5958–65.

90. Lee YMH, Coffin JM. Relationship of avian retrovirus DNA synthesis to integration in vitro. *Mol Cell Biol* 1991;11:1419–30.

91. Stoye JP, Fenner S, Greenoak GE, Moran C, Coffin JM. Role of endogenous retroviruses as mutagens: the hairless mutation of mice. *Cell* 1988;54:383–91.

92. Speck NA, Baltimore D. Six distinct nuclear factors interact with the 75-base-pair repeat of the Moloney murine leukemia virus enhancer. *Mol Cell Biol* 1987;7:1101–10.

93. Jones KA, Kadonaga JT, Luciw PA, Tjian R. Activation of the AIDS retrovirus promoter by the cellular transcription factor. *Science* 1986;232:755–9.

94. Li Y, Golemis E, Hartley JW, Hopkins N. Disease specificity of nondefective Friend and Moloney murine leukemia viruses is controlled by a small number of nucleotides. *J Virol* 1987;61:693–700.

95. Rosen CA, Haseltine WA, Lenz J, Ruprecht R, Cloyd MW. Tissue selectivity of murine leukemia virus infection is determined by long terminal repeat sequences. *J Virol* 1985;55:862–66.

96. Stocking CR, Kollek, U. Bergholz, Ostertag W. Point mutations in the U3 region of the long terminal repeat of Moloney murine leukemia virus determine disease specificity of the myeloproliferative sarcoma virus. *Virology* 1986;153:145–9.

97. Bachelerie F, Alcami J, Arenzana-Seisdedos F, Virelizier J-L. HIV enhancer activity perpetuated by NF-κB induction on infection of monocytes. *Nature* 1991;350:709–12.

98. Bielinska A, Krasnow S, Nabel GJ. NF-κB-mediated activation of the human immunodeficiency virus enhancer: site of transcrip-

tional initiation is independent of the TATA box. *J Virol* 1989;63:4097–100.

99. Folks TM, Justement J, Kinter A, Dinarello CA, Fauci AS. Cytokine-induced expression of HIV-1 in a chronically infected promonocyte cell line. *Science* 1987;238:800–2.

100. Nabel G, Baltimore D. An inducible transcription factor activates human immunodeficiency virus expression in T cells. *Nature* 1987;326:711–13.

101. Swain A, Coffin JM. Polyadenylation at correct sites in genome RNA is not required for retrovirus replication or genome encapsidation. *J Virol* 1989;63:3301–6.

102. Herman SA, Coffin JM. Differential transcription from the long terminal repeats of integrated avian leukosis virus DNA. *J Virol* 1986;60:497–505.

103. Seiki M, Inoue JI, Takeda T, Yoshida M. Direct evidence that p-40x of human T-cell leukemia virus type I is a trans-acting transcriptional activator. *EMBO J* 1985;5:561–65.

104. Sodroski J, Rosen C, Goh WC, Haseltine W. A transcriptional activator protein encoded by the x-lor region of the human T-cell leukemia virus. *Science* 1985;228:1430–34.

105. Rosen CA, Sodroski JG, Haseltine WA. Location of cis-acting regulatory sequences in the human T-cell leukemia virus type I long terminal repeat. *Proc Natl Acad Sci USA* 1985;82:6502–6.

106. Varmus HE. Regulation of HIV and HTLV gene expression. *Genes Dev* 1988;2:1055–62.

107. Sodroski JG, Rosen C, Wong-Staal F, et al. Trans-acting transcriptional regulation of human T-cell leukemia virus type III long terminal repeat. *Science* 1985;227:171–3.

108. Sodroski J, Patarca R, Rosen C, Wong-Staal F, Haseltine W. Location of the trans-activating region on the genome of human T-cell lymphotropic virus type III. *Science* 1985;229:74–7.

109. Feng S, Holland EC. HIV-1 tat trans-activation requires the loop sequence within tar. *Nature* 1988;334:165–7.

110. Gatignol A, Buckler-White A, Berkhout B, Jeang K-T. Characterization of a human TAR RNA-binding protein that activates the HIV-1 LTR. *Science* 1991;251:1597–600.

111. Berkhout B, Gatignol A, Rabson AB, Jeang K-T. TAR-independent activation of the HIV-1 LTR: evidence that tat requires specific regions of the promoter. *Cell* 1990;62:757–67.

112. Sharp PA, Marciniak RA. HIV TAR: an RNA enhancer? *Cell* 1989;59:229–30.

113. Feinberg MB, Baltimore D, Frankel AD. The role of Tat in the human immunodeficiency virus life cycle indicates a primary effect on transcriptional elongation. *Proc Natl Acad Sci USA* 1991;88:4045–9.

114. Kao SY, Calman AF, Luciw PA, Peterlin BM. Anti-termination of transcription within the long terminal repeat of HIV-1 by tat gene product. *Nature* 1987;330:489–93.

115. Arrigo S, Beemon K. Regulation of Rous sarcoma virus RNA splicing and stability. *Mol Cell Biol* 1988;18:4858–67.

116. Katz RA, Kotler M, Skalka AM. cis-Acting intron mutations that affect the efficiency of avian retroviral RNA splicing: implications for mechanisms of control. *J Virol* 1988;62:2686–95.

117. Miller CK, Temin HM. Insertion of several different DNAs in reticuloendotheliosis virus strain T suppresses transformation by reducing the amount of subgenomic DNA. *J Virol* 1986;58:75–80.

118. Cullen BR, Greene WC. Regulatory pathways governing HIV-1 replication. *Cell* 1989;58:423–6.

119. Cullen BR. Trans-activation of human immunodeficiency virus occurs via a bimodal mechanism. *Cell* 1986;46:973–82.

120. Felber BK, Hadzopoulou-Cladaras M, Cladaras C, Copeland T, Pavlakis G. Rev protein of human immunodeficiency virus 1 affects the stability and transport of the viral mRNA. *Proc Natl Acad Sci USA* 1989;86:1495–9.

121. Inoue J-I, Yoshida M, Seiki M. Transcriptional (p40x) and posttranscriptional (p27x-III) regulators are required for the expression and replication of the leukemia virus type I genes. *Proc Natl Acad Sci USA* 1987;84:3363–57.

122. Itoh M, Inoue J, Toyoshima H, Akizawa T, Higashi M, Yoshida M. HTLV-1 *rex* and HIV-1 *rev* act through similar mechanisms to relieve suppression of unspliced RNA expression. *Oncogene* 1989;4:1275–9.

123. Seiki M, Inoue J-I, Kidaka M, Yoshida M. Two cis-acting elements responsible for posttranscriptional trans-regulation of gene expression of human T-cell leukemia virus type I. *Proc Natl Acad Sci USA* 1988;85:7124–8.

124. Sodroski J, Goh WC, Rosen C, Dayton A, Terwilliger E, Haseltine W. A second post-transcriptional trans-activator gene required for HTLV-III replication. *Nature* 1986;321:412–6.

125. Chang DD, Sharp PA. Regulation by HIV *rev* depends upon recognition of splice sites. *Cell* 1989;59:789–95.

126. Chang DD, Sharp PA. Messenger RNA transport and HIV rev regulation. *Science* 1990;249:614–15.

127. Rimsky L, Hauber J, Dukovich M, et al. Functional replacement of the HIV-1 rev protein by the HTLV-1 rex protein. *Nature* 1988;335:738–40.

128. Muesing MA, Smith DH, Cabradilla CD, Benton CV, Lasky LA, Capon DJ. Nucleic acid structure and expression of the human AIDS/lymphadenopathy retrovirus. *Nature* 1985;313:450–8.

129. Rabson AB, Daugherty DF, Venkatesan S, et al. Transcription of novel open reading frames of AIDS retrovirus during infection of lymphocytes. *Science* 1985;229:1388–90.

130. Schwartz S, Felber BK, Benko DM, Fenyo E-M, Pavlakis GN. Cloning and functional analysis of multiply spiced mRNA species of human immunodeficiency virus type 1. *J Virol* 1990;64:2519–29.

131. Kaminchik J, Bashan N, Pinchasi D, et al. Expression and biochemical characterization of human immunodeficiency virus type 1 nef gene product. *J Virol* 1990;64:3447–54.

132. Nebreda AR, Bryan T, Segade F, Wingfield P, Venkatesan S, Santos E. Biochemical and biological comparison of HIV-1 NEF and *ras* gene products. *Virology* 1991;183:151–9.

133. Ahmad N, Venkatesan S. Nef protein of HIV-1 is a transcriptional repressor of HIV-1 LTR. *Science* 1988;241:1481–5.

134. Cheng-Mayer C, Iannello P, Shaw K, Luciw PA, Levy JA. Differential effects of *nef* on HIV replication: implications for viral pathogenesis in the host. *Science* 1989;246:1629–32.

135. Maitra RK, Ahmad N, Holland SM, Venkatesan S. Human immunodeficiency virus type 1 (HIV-1) provirus expression and LTR transcription are repressed in NEF-expressing cell lines. *Virology* 1991;182:522–33.

136. Bachelerie F, Alcami J, Hazan U, et al. Constitutive expression of human immunodeficiency virus (HIV) nef protein in human astrocytes does not influence basal or induced HIV long terminal repeat activity. *J Virol* 1990;64:3059–62.

137. Kim S, Ikeuchi K, Byrn R, Groopman J, Baltimore D. Lack of a negative influence on viral growth by the nef gene of human immunodeficiency virus type I. *Proc Natl Acad Sci USA* 1989;86:9544–8.

138. Kestler HWI, Ringler DJ, Mori K, et al. Importance of the nef gene for maintenance of high virus loads and for development of AIDS. *Cell* 1991;65:651–62.

139. Guy B, Geist M, Dott K, Spehner D, Kieny M-P, Lecocq J-P. A specific inhibitor of cysteine proteases impairs a vif-dependent modification of human immunodeficiency virus type 1 env protein. *J Virol* 1991;65:1325–31.

140. Cohen EA, Terwilliger EF, Sodroski JG, Haseltine WA. Identification of a protein encoded by the vpu gene of HIV-1. *Nature* 1988;334:532–4.

141. Klimkait T, Strebel K, Hoggan MD, Martin MA, Orenstein JM. The human immunodeficiency virus type 1-specific protein *vpu* is required for efficient virus maturation and release. *J Virol* 1990;64:621–9.

142. Strebel K, Klimkait T, Maldarelli F, Martin MA. Molecular and biochemical analyses of human immunodeficiency virus type 1 vpu protein. *J Virol* 1989;63:3784–91.

143. Strebel K, Klimkait T, Martin MA. A novel gene of HIV-1, vpu, and its 16-kilodalton product. *J Virol* 1988;241:1221–3.

144. Terwilliger EF, Cohen EA, Lu Y, Sodroski JG, Haseltine WA. Functional role of human immunodeficiency virus type 1 vpu. *Proc Natl Acad Sci USA* 1989;86:5163–7.

145. Dedera D, Hu W, Vander Heyden N, Ratner L. Viral protein R of human immunodeficiency virus types 1 and 2 is dispensable for replication and cytopathogenicity in lymphoid cells. *J Virol* 1989;63:3205–8.

146. Hattori N, Michaels F, Fargnoli K, Marcon L, Gallo RC, Franchini G. The human immunodeficiency virus type 2 vpr gene is essential for productive infection of human macrophages. *Proc Natl Acad Sci USA* 1990;87:8080–4.

147. Cohen EA, Dehni G, Sodroski GJ, Haseltine WA. Human immunodeficiency virus vpr product is a virion-associated regulatory protein. *J Virol* 1990;64:3097–9.

148. Yu X-F, Matsuda M, Essex M, Lee T-H. Open reading frame vpr of simian immunodeficiency virus encodes a virion-associated protein. *J Virol* 1990;64:5688–93.

149. Garrett ED, Tiley LS, Cullen BR. Rev activates expression of the human immunodeficiency virus type 1 vif and vpr gene products. *J Virol* 1991;65:1653–7.

150. Schwartz S, Felber BK, Pavlakis GN. Expression of human immunodeficiency virus type 1 vif and vpr mRNAs is rev-dependent and regulated by splicing. *Virology* 1991;183:677–86.

151. Salmons B, Erfle V, Brem G, Gunzburg WH. *Naf,* a *trans*-regulating negative-acting factor encoded within the mouse mammary tumor virus open reading frame region. *J Virol* 1990;64:6355–9.

152. van Klaveren P, Bentvelzen P. Transactivating potential of the 3′ open reading frame of murine mammary tumor virus. *J Virol* 1988;62:4410–3.

153. Acha-Orbea H, Shakhov AN, Scarpellino L, et al. Clonal deletion of Vβ14-bearing T cells in mice transgenic for mammary tumour virus. *Nature* 1991;250:207–11.

154. Choi Y, Kappler JW, Marrack P. A superantigen encoded in the open reading frame of the 3′ long terminal repeat of mouse mammary tumour virus. *Nature* 1991;350:203–07.

155. Dyson PJ, Knight AM, Fairchild S, Simpson E, Tomonari K. Genes encoding ligands for deletion of Vβ11 T cells cosegregate with mammary tumour virus genomes. *Nature* 1991;349:531–2.

156. Frankel WN, Rudy C, Coffin JM, Huber BT. Linkage of Mls genes to endogenous mammary tumour viruses of inbred mice. *Nature* 1991;349:526–8.

157. Marrack P, Kushnir E, Kappler J. A maternally inherited superantigen encoded by a mammary tumor virus. *Nature* 1991;349:524–6.

158. Palmer E. Infectious origin of superantigens. *Curr Biol* 1991;1:74–6.

159. Coffin JM. Superantigens and endogenous retroviruses: a confluence of puzzles. [submitted].

160. Bishop JM. Molecular themes in oncogenesis. *Cell* 1991;64:235–48.

161. Hunter T. A thousand and one protein kinases. *Cell* 1987;50:823–9.

162. Ballard DW, Bohnlein E, Lowenthal JW, Wano Y, Franza BR, Greene WC. HTLV-I tax induces cellular proteins that activate κB element in the IL-2 receptor a gene. *Science* 1988;241:1652–5.

163. Greene WC, Leonard WJ, Wano Y, et al. Trans-activator gene of HTLV-II induces IL-2 receptor and IL-2 cellular gene expression. *Science* 1986;232:877–81.

164. Inoue J, Seiki M, Taniguchi T, et al. Induction of interleukin 2 receptor gene expression by p40ˣ encoded by human T-cell leukemia virus type 1. *EMBO J* 1986;5:2883–8.

165. Kanamori H, Suzuki N, Siomi H, et al. HTLV-1 p27 *rex* stabilizes human interleukin-2 receptor a chain mRNA. *EMBO J* 1990;9:4161–6.

166. Kronke M, Leonard WJ, Depper JM, Greene WC. Deregulation of interleukin-2 receptor gene expression in HTLV-I-induced adult T-cell leukemia. *Science* 1985;228:1215–7.

167. Leung K, Nabel GJ. HTLV-1 transactivator induces interleukin-2 receptor expression through an NF-κB-like factor. *Nature* 1988;333:776–8.

168. Maruyama M, Shibuya H, Harada H, et al. Evidence for aberrant activation of the interleukin-2 autocrine loop by HTLV-1-encoded p40x and T3/Ti complex triggering. *Cell* 1987; 48:343–50.

169. Donahue PR, Quackenbush SL, Gallo MV, et al. Viral genetic determinants of T-cell killing and immunodeficiency disease induction by the feline leukemia virus FeLV-FAIDS. *J Virol* 1991;65:4461–9.

170. Keshet E, Temin HM. Cell killing by spleen necrosis virus is correlated with a transient accumulation of spleen necrosis virus DNA. *J Virol* 1979;31:376–88.

171. Mullins JI, Chen CS, Hoover EA. Disease-specific and tissue-specific production of unintegrated feline leukaemia virus variant DNA in feline AIDS. *Nature* 1986;319:333–6.

172. Weller SK, Joy AE, Temin HM. Correlation between cell killing and massive second round superinfection by members of some subgroups of avian leukosis virus. *J Virol* 1980;33:494–506.

173. Weller SK, Temin HM. Cell killing by avian leukosis viruses. *J Virol* 1981;39:713–21.

174. Lifson JD, Reyes GR, McGrath MS, Stein BS, Engelman EG. AIDS retrovirus induced cytopathology: giant cell formation and involvement of CD4 antigen. *Science* 1986;232:1123–7.

175. Hehlmann R, Brack-Werner R, Leib-Mosch C. Human endogenous retroviruses. *Leukemia* 1988;2:167S–77S.

176. Mariani-Costantini R, Horn TM, Callahan R. Ancestry of a human endogenous retrovirus family. *J Virol* 1989;63:4982–5.

177. Repaske R, Steele PE, O'Neill RR, Rabson AB, Martin MA. Nucleotide sequence of a full-length human endogenous retroviral segment. *J Virol* 1985;54:764–72.

178. Steele PE, Martin MA, Rabson AB, Bryan T, O'Brien SJ. Amplification and chromosomal dispersion of human endogenous retroviral sequences. *J Virol* 1986;59:545–550.

179. Curran JW, Morgan WM, Hardy AM, Jaffe HW, Darrow WW, Dowdle WR. The epidemiology of AIDS: current status and future prospects. *Science* 1985;229:1352–7.

180. Essex M, Kanki PJ. The origins of the AIDS virus. *Sci Am* 1988;259:64–71.

181. Hoxie JA, Haggarty BS, Bonser SE, Rackowski JL, Shan H, Kanki PJ. Biological characterization of a simian immunodeficiency virus-like retrovirus (HTLV-IV): evidence for CD4-associated molecules required for infection. *J Virol* 1988;62:2557–68.

182. Huet T, Cheynier R, Meyerhans A, Roelants G, Wain-Hobson S. Genetic organization of a chimpanzee lentivirus related to HIV-1. *Nature* 1990;345:356–9.

183. Kanki PJ, Alroy J, Essex M. Isolation of T-lymphotropic retrovirus related to HTLV-III/LAV from wild-caught African green monkeys. *Science* 1985;230:951–4.

184. Coffin JM. Genetic variation in retroviruses. In: Kurstak E, Marusyk RG, Murphy FA, Regenmortel MHVV, eds. *Applied virology research,* vol 2: *Virus variability, epidemiology, and control.* New York: Plenum Press, 1990;11–33.

185. Coffin JM, Tsichlis PN, Barker CS, Voynow S. Variation in avian retrovirus genomes. *Ann NY Acad Sci* 1980;354:410–25.

186. Pathak VK, Temin HM. Broad spectrum of in vivo forward mutations, hypermutations and mutational hotspots in a retroviral shuttle vector after a single replication cycle: deletions and deletions with insertions. *Proc Natl Acad Sci USA* 1990;87:6024–8.

187. Pathak VK, Temin HM. Broad spectrum of in vivo forward mutations, hypermutations, and mutational hotspots in a retroviral shuttle vector after a single replication cycle: substitutions, frameshifts and hypermutations. *Proc Natl Acad Sci USA* 1990;87:6019–23.

188. Temin HM. Sex and recombination in retroviruses. *Trends Genet* 1991;7:71–4.

AIDS and Other Manifestations of HIV Infection,
Second Edition, Edited by Gary P. Wormser.
Published by Raven Press, Ltd., New York 1992.

CHAPTER 5

Pathogenesis of HIV-1 Infection

Howard E. Gendelman, Jan M. Orenstein, D. Chester Kalter,
and Chester Roberts

The human immunodeficiency virus (HIV), the etiologic agent of the acquired immunodeficiency syndrome (AIDS) (1–3), elicits a progressive and profound immunosuppression through a selective depletion of helper/inducer T lymphocytes (4–7). The consequences of viral replication in CD4+ T lymphocytes probably account for the immunosuppression. However, the virus-infected macrophage is also intimately involved in clinical manifestations of HIV infection. Aspects of disease revolve around replication of virus in tissue macrophages and are typified by central nervous system (CNS), lung, and lymphatic tissue pathology (8–17). The mechanism(s) by which HIV infection results in immunosuppression and other primary HIV disease manifestations will be a focus of this chapter.

LENTIVIRUS–HOST INTERACTIONS: AN OVERVIEW

Lentiviruses comprise a class of related retroviruses linked by their abilities to replicate continuously at a restricted rate in their host cells. Common features shared among lentiviruses include an incubation period of months to years, an insidious onset of clinical disease, and the inevitable induction of debilitating immunologic and CNS disease (18–21). The extent and nature of disease caused by lentiviruses varies from florid

tissue necrosis to mild immunopathology. Many virus-induced disease manifestations are mediated by the infected macrophage, the major if not exclusive virus target cell in tissue. Some lentiviruses also efficiently infect CD4+ T lymphocytes. Indeed, cats and primates manifest a significant immunosuppression caused by feline, simian and human immunodeficiency viral tropism for helper/inducer T cells. The list of lentiviruses is expansive indeed (22–24). These include HIV types 1 and 2 (1–3,25), the ruminant viruses, visna and caprine arthritis encephalitis viruses (18–21), equine infectious anemia virus (26), the simian immunodeficiency virus (SIV) (27–29), and the feline immunodeficiency virus (FIV) (30). All share similar biologic, morphologic, biochemical, and molecular features (22–24,31,32).

Lentiviruses are retroviruses. They have the potential to integrate their proviral DNA into host cell genomic DNA. This provides both an important means for escape from host immune surveillance and an avenue for viral mutation. Viral spread is species-specific, and restricted host-to-host transmission occurs only during exchange of body fluids. Productive viral gene expression is at low levels during any observed time period (33–35). The mechanisms surrounding persistent *in vivo* infection during long periods of subclinical infection are poorly understood but are thought to involve subversion of both nonspecific and specific immunologic responses. In several distinct ways, HIV is a typical lentivirus. Failure of production of high-titer neutralizing antibodies, antigenic drift of the viral envelope, and enhancement of viral infection with specific antibodies are examples of HIV's ability to subvert the many immune forces rallied against it (36–41). Ultimately, the end result of continual replication is a degenerative and inflammatory destruction of virus target tissues.

By ultrastructural observations, all lentiviruses are similar (42–45). The virion particle, 110 nm in diameter, has

H. E. Gendelman and D. C. Kalter: Department of Cellular Immunology, Walter Reed Army Institute of Research, Rockville, Maryland 20850; and Henry M. Jackson Foundation for the Advancement of Military Medicine, Washington, DC 20037.

J. M. Orenstein: Department of Pathology, George Washington University Medical Center, Washington, DC 20037.

C. Roberts: Department of Diagnostic Retrovirology, Walter Reed Army Institute of Research, Rockville, Maryland 20850.

a dense elongated central cylindrical core containing *gag* (group-specific antigen), structural elements, and two strands of an RNA genome of approximately 10 kb. Viral regulatory proteins and virus-encoded enzymes required for efficient replication (i.e., the reverse transcriptase and integrase) are also packaged into the virus particle. The size of the lentivirus genome is considerably larger than those of oncogenic retroviruses. The latter encode only structural proteins for *gag, env,* and *pol.* In contrast, HIV encodes for all the retroviral structural proteins as well as an additional six regulatory proteins. The virion is encased by a lipid envelope acquired as the virion buds from the surface of CD4+ T cells with envelope spike projections, or from vacuoles within an infected macrophage.

Biochemical similarities among lentiviruses include the large size and variability of the external viral envelope glycoprotein, the use of tRNA lysine as primers for reverse transcription, the presence of genes that upregulate viral gene expression (transactivating proteins), and other novel open reading frames in the genome (46–50). Homology of the *gag* and *pol* genes at the nucleotide level are present between HIV and other lentiviruses and attest to their molecular similarities.

HIV: LIFE CYCLE

The virion particle first binds to the host cell receptor, the human CD4 molecule, on the surface of helper/inducer T lymphocytes and monocytes. Evidence for the CD4 molecule as the HIV receptor abounds and includes the demonstration that CD4 and gp120, the major envelope glycoprotein of HIV, coprecipitate (51) (Fig. 1), that HIV infection of CD4+ cells is blocked by both soluble CD4 and monoclonal anti-CD4 antibodies (52,53), that non-virus-susceptible cells, e.g., HeLa cells (human cervical epithelial carcinoma) can be made HIV susceptible following transfection of CD4-expressing cDNAs (54), and that the HIV-1 gp120 envelope protein binds to CD4 with an extremely high affinity. After binding to the CD4 receptor the virus particle is internalized, it strips off its outer coat, and the RNA genome is released into the cytoplasm (55). The mechanism of postbinding viral entry into cells may occur by receptor-mediated endocytosis and/or pH-independent fusion of the viral transmembrane protein (gp41) with the cell membrane (56,57). Recent evidence strongly suggests that membrane fusion is the mechanism for virus entry. A hydrophobic amino-terminal domain of gp41 is thought to play a role as a fusion site for viral entry (58). This region of gp41 has amino-acid homology to fusion peptides of ortho- and paramyxoviruses. Once inside the cell, single-stranded viral genomic RNA is converted into double-stranded linear and/or circular DNAs (proviral DNA) by the virally encoded enzyme reverse tran-

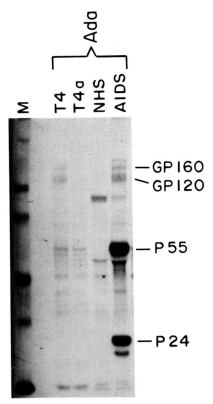

FIG. 1. gp120–CD4 interactions. Specific binding of the HIV envelope glycoprotein to CD4 is illustrated. Blood-derived monocytes were infected with HIV and cells metabolically labelled with ^{35}S methionine. Cell lysates were immunoprecipitated with pooled AIDS sera, uninfected normal human sera (NHS), and antibodies directed against the cell surface epitopes, T4 and T4a. Specific immunoprecipitation of the gp160 and gp120 envelope glycoproteins is shown.

scriptase (RT). Proviral DNA integration into host cell DNA provides one of a number of mechanisms for subversion of the host immunologic defenses. The process of integration is a reaction dependent upon the virally encoded endonuclease. HIV can also accumulate large levels of unintegrated DNA within infected cells. The role for unintegrated DNA is poorly understood but it may contribute to viral-induced cytopathicity (59–61). Proviral DNAs transcribe into viral genomic and messenger RNAs. Following transcription, viral mRNAs are appropriately spliced. Protein synthesis, processing, and virus assembly occur, with subsequent budding of mature virions from the surface of the infected cells (Fig. 2). Lentivirus infection in tissue culture systems results in a high proportion of productively infected cells with syncytium formation often leading to cell lysis (Figs. 3 and 4). The ultimate outcome of viral infection (latent versus productive) depends upon complex interactions between, viral, host regulatory proteins, and *cis*-acting sequences in the HIV genome. Indeed, productive HIV infection of both CD4+ T lymphocytes and monocytes requires cell activation and/or differentiation (62–64).

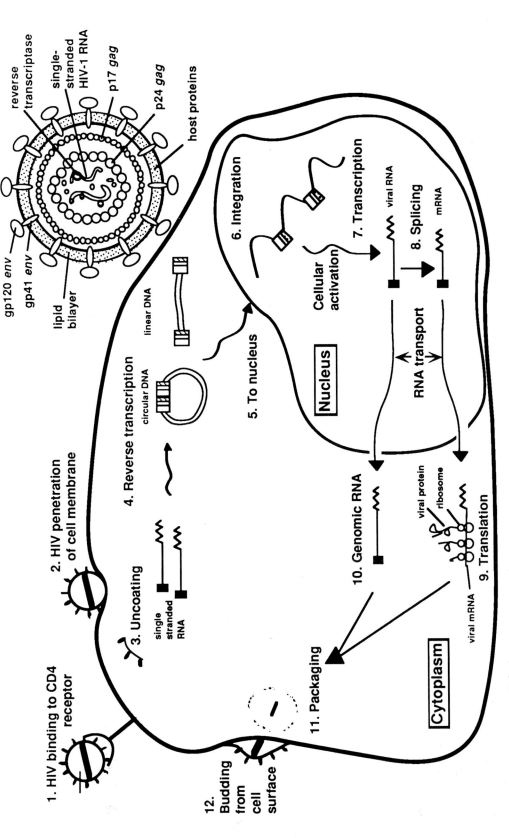

FIG. 2. The HIV life cycle. The viral particle attaches to the CD4 cell surface receptor and then enters and uncoats. Viral genomic RNA is reverse transcribed into cDNA and may integrate into the host genome. Host RNA polymerase II transcribes the provirus. The virus is assembled at or near the cell surface and then buds from the plasma membrane. The HIV virion is adapted from Greene (63).

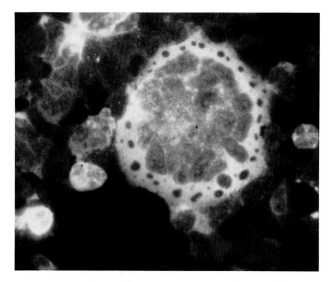

FIG. 3. Multinucleated giant cell formation following HIV infection of lymphoblasts. Peripheral blood mononuclear cells (PBMCs) were cultured with PHA/IL-2 and then infected with HIV at a multiplicity of infection (MOI) = 0.01. Following 7 days of infection, cells were harvested, cytocentrifuged, fixed in acetone, and then incubated with pooled AIDS patient sera. A viral antigen-positive syncytial cell is demonstrated.

If HIV DNA remains transcriptionally dormant, viral persistence ensues for the life of the cell or until cellular activation or stimulation leads to productive viral infection. Activation of viral gene expression may occur by several different signal mechanisms. Potential activators include other viral pathogens such as cytomegalovirus,

herpes simplex and hepatitis B viruses, phorbol esters, 5'-iodo-2'-deoxyuridine, ultraviolet irradiation, mitogens, anti-CD3 antibodies, and a variety of cytokines such as macrophage colony-stimulating factor (MCSF), granulocyte–macrophage colony-stimulating factor (GMCSF), interleukin (IL)-1β, IL-2, IL-4, IL-6, tumor necrosis factor (TNFα), transforming growth factor beta (TGFβ), and/or allogeneic stimulation from exposure to blood, semen, or microbial pathogens (65).

Viral persistence typified by latent integrated proviral DNA may continue indefinitely even through mitosis in bone marrow, lymph nodes, or other tissues. Daughter cells may be released into the circulation and disseminate virus (66). Components of the host immune response may be poorly equipped to control or eliminate such latently infected cells, especially if these cells have prolonged life spans as do progenitor cells in bone marrow or tissue macrophages. If productive infection does result, HIV-1 variants may arise as "escape mutants" from neutralizing antibodies (67). Indeed, HIV-1 isolates from chimpanzees immunized with gp120 and subsequently inoculated with virus demonstrate increased resistance over time to neutralization by the preexisting antibodies. Similarly, after acute infection with HIV-1 in humans, antibodies are demonstrated that neutralize only the initial HIV-1 isolate but not subsequent isolates (68). Similar events were described previously during lentivirus infection by visna, equine infectious anemia, and caprine arthritis encephalitis viruses (18,19). Thus the virus may adapt itself to changing immune pressure and thereby continue to replicate unimpeded through the course of infection.

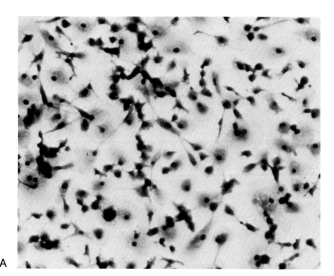
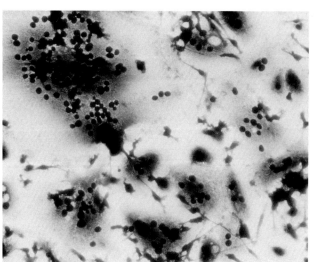

A   B

FIG. 4. HIV-induced syncytia formation in monocytes. Blood monocytes cultured in the presence of macrophage colony-stimulating factor (MCSF) were infected with HIV at a multiplicity of infection (MOI) = 0.01. Uninfected cells (**A**) and 7-day HIV-infected cells (**B**) are illustrated. Note the large number of nuclei in single cells and demonstrated in **b**.

HIV: GENOMIC ORGANIZATION

The HIV proviral genome has been well characterized. It is approximately 10 kb in length, and its organization has been deduced following analysis of the nucleotide sequence of recombinant proviral DNAs (Fig. 5) (46,47). HIV contains several genes common to all retroviruses including long terminal repeat sequences (*LTRs*), core proteins (*gag*), polymerase (*pol*), and envelope (*env*) genes. The HIV *LTRs* are 634 bp in length comprising regulatory segments for HIV replication. The U3, R, and U5 segments comprise the LTR. The U3 region contains the TATA box, upstream regulatory sequences including three binding sites for the transcriptional regulatory protein Sp1, and a core enhancer sequence (69). At the border of U3 and R is the mRNA initiation site. The target site for the positive regulatory effect of the viral *trans*-activating protein (*tat*), called TAR, is located within the R region. The polyadenylation signal, AAUAA, which is responsible for the addition of polyA residues at the 3′ end of viral RNAs, lies at the border of R and U5 sequences.

The *gag* gene encodes the group-specific antigens of all retroviruses, which are structural proteins forming the virion core. The *pol* gene encodes the viral protease, RT, endonuclease, and ribonuclease H. The viral protease p10 (70) cleaves the *gag* precursor p55 protein into its mature forms (p18, p24, and p16). Viral polypeptides, p51 and p64, have been shown to possess RT activity (71,72). This enzyme may be responsible not only for transcribing genomic RNA to proviral DNA but for the generation of large amounts of unintegrated HIV DNA unique to lentiviral infections. The p34 endonuclease (72) is encoded by the 3′ *pol* region and is responsible for the nucleolytic cleavages involved in the integration of HIV proviral DNA into host cell DNA. Ribonuclease destroys the genomic viral RNA following reverse transcription.

The *env* gene encodes the external envelope and transmembrane glycoproteins of the virus. A highly glycosylated precursor, gp160, undergoes proteolytic cleavage within infected cells to two mature proteins, an external *env* glycoprotein (gp120), which binds to the CD4 receptor on the cell membrane, and the transmembrane protein gp41, which anchors the gp120 to the virion particle (73–77). These are incorporated into progeny virions as oligomeric complexes. The linkage of gp120 and gp41 is noncovalent and does not involve disulfide bonds. Sub-

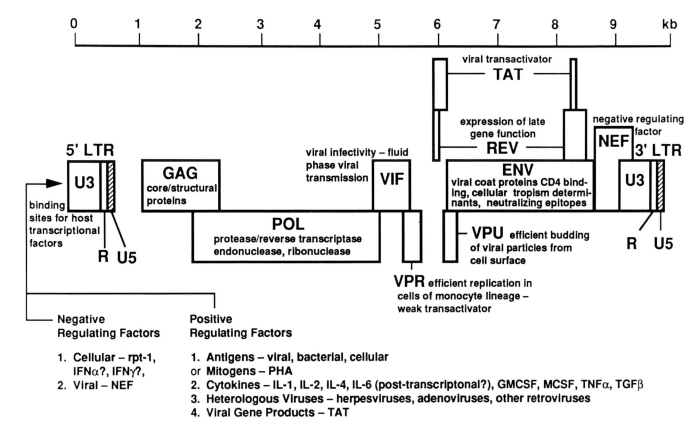

FIG. 5. The HIV-1 genome is flanked by long terminal repeats (*LTRs*). The proviral genes and the size and location of the open reading frames are shown. The genome contains the structural *env, pol,* and *gag* genes of all retroviruses and several regulatory genes whose identity and function are outlined.

sequent to viral binding to CD4+ lymphocytes, a fusion of viral and cellular membranes occurs via hydrophobic sequences present at the amino terminus of the gp41 (76). The *env* gene products also play important roles in producing syncytia formation and cytopathogenicity during HIV infections (77–82). The evasion of host immune surveillance mediated by the HIV *env* is related to its high degree of variability (83–86). This variability is associated with the very process of RT. The rate of nucleotide misincorporation by RT is > 10^{-4} per base per cycle and for a genome of about 10^4 bases (87), one base alteration occurs per genome per cycle. The variability of the *env* proteins help explain the emergence of escape mutants of the virus, the difficulties in design and implementation of vaccine strategies, and the abilities of the virus to evade host immune surveillance. Analyses of amino-acid sequences of the gp120s derived from different isolates of HIV reveal conserved and divergent domains (83–86). The conserved domains are important in viral binding to its receptor and provide nucleic acid sequences spanning the overlap of *env, tat,* and *rev* genes (83,84). Lasky et al. (76) demonstrated that monoclonal antibodies that blocked gp120–CD4 interactions mapped to a conserved region within *env.* In these studies, deletion of 12 amino acids (426–437) significantly altered *env*–CD4 interactions. Furthermore, antibodies directed against the CD4 binding domain neutralize infectivity of numerous HIV strains (group specificity). Divergent regions can share as little as 30–50% homology over 200 amino-acid domains.

Unlike the C-type retroviruses, HIV encodes three regulatory proteins, *tat* (*trans*-activator), *rev* (transition factor between early regulatory and late structural proteins), and *nef* (negative regulatory factor), as well as three other proteins involved in efficient viral replication, maturation, and release. The latter include *vif* (virion infectivity factor), *vpu* (viral protein U), and *vpr* (viral protein R) (87–96). The control of viral gene expression depends upon the interaction between cellular and virally encoded regulatory proteins.

The *tat* gene encodes a *trans*-activating protein of HIV, p14. This gene product augments HIV gene expression from the HIV *LTR* by increasing the rate of transcription, as well as increasing steady-state RNA levels by enhancing translation efficiency and/or functioning as an antiterminator or elongation factor of nascent HIV RNAs (88–92). Significant levels of HIV gene expression can only be achieved in the presence of *tat. Tat* activity is exerted through regulatory sequences located downstream of the transcriptional start site (untranslated 3' regions of the 5' *LTR* referred to as TAR). The *rev* protein encodes a second transactivating regulatory factor of HIV required for the proper processing of *gag* and *env* mRNAs and for the translation of their respective gene products (93,94). The *rev* protein controls the transition between the production of multiply spliced

early mRNAs and the longer late mRNAs by exerting effects on *cis*-acting negative regulatory factors. These negative acting regions have been mapped within the *gag* and *env* sequences. By binding to the *rev*-responsive element (RRE) within the *env* gene, *rev* allows efficient nuclear transport of the *gag–pol* and *env* mRNAs.

Unlike *tat* and *rev,* the *nef* protein is thought to downregulate HIV infection (95–97). The *nef* gene lies 3' to the end of *env* and extends into the U3 region of the 3'*LTR* and encodes a p27. Mutations in *nef* result in higher levels of virus replication, suggesting that this gene may have a negative regulatory role in HIV expression (96,97). The mechanism(s) of action, however, are poorly understood and more recent reports contest a downregulatory function of *nef* (98,99). The *vif* and *vpr* gene products are not absolutely required for assembly of virions or regulation of viral gene expression. However, proviruses that contain mutations in *vif* yield exceedingly low levels of infectious particles and infection can only be spread by cell-to-cell contact (100,101). This suggests a role for *vif* in cell-free spread of viral infections. The *vpu* protein is nonglycosylated and is thought to be associated with the inner surface of the cytoplasmic cell membrane (102). It is not essential for viral replication, but mutations in *vpu* result in decreased levels of virus and in an increase in cell-associated RT activity, possibly due to aberrant budding of viral particles into intracytoplasmic vesicles. *Vpr* is conserved in all HIV strains but is not absolutely required for infectivity in CD4+ T cells. A recent report suggests that *vpr* is required for efficient replication by HIV in cells of monocyte/macrophage lineage (103).

Although the genome of HIV-1 encodes several regulatory and structural genes of diverse function, proviral DNA contains a single transcriptional start site. Differential gene expression is regulated by gene-specific RNA splice events. Processed RNAs of *env, vif, vpr,* and *vpu* involve singly spliced transcripts whose major 5' *gag–pol* intron is deleted. RNAs of the regulatory genes *tat, rev,* and *nef* involve doubly spliced transcripts whose 3' *env* intron is deleted. Splicing events underlie mechanisms of viral latency and productive infection (104,105).

DIAGNOSIS OF HIV INFECTION

Infection by HIV occurs world-wide (106–108) and may be detected by a variety of serological, biochemical, virologic, and molecular assays outlined below (109–115).

Enzyme-Linked Immunosorbent Assay

A laboratory diagnosis of HIV-1 infection is established by enzyme-linked immunosorbent assay (ELISA) (109–111) and confirmed by Western blot (109) and/or other serologic tests. When screening ELISA is reactive but the confirmatory test nonreactive, the tested individual is designated HIV negative. The ELISA test employs a target viral lysate or protein placed onto an immobile matrix (e.g., a microtiter plate). Antibodies to HIV in patient sera are allowed to incubate with the test viral protein, and following washes to remove unbound antibodies, reactions are observed by capture of anti-human antibodies linked to an enzyme forming an insoluble color precipitate when mixed with a specific substrate. The color change is measured by a spectrophotometer. By comparing sample optical density (OD) to specific control panels, a sample may be scored as reactive or nonreactive. A major source for false-positive reactions in the ELISA test is the presence of nonviral cellular antigens in the cell lysate. This may be overcome by increasing the purity of the target viral preparations or through the use of recombinant HIV proteins.

Western Blot

Individual viral proteins are visualized in the Western blot assay. Here viral proteins are separated according to their molecular weights by polyacrylamide gel electrophoresis. Following electrophoresis the viral proteins are transferred onto nitrocellulose and then incubated with patient sera. After successive washes binding is demonstrated using capture anti-human antibodies linked to enzymes or by radioactive detection methods. The criteria for a reactive Western blot involves the demonstration of antibodies to at least two of three structural proteins of HIV (e.g., p24, p55, gp41, gp120/160) (109). The Western blot assay may be nondiagnostic in the face of a positive ELISA. If the patient is at risk for infection and the diagnosis is inconclusive, additional serological tests may be employed (e.g., radioimmunoprecipitation). Here viral and cellular proteins are radiolabeled with ^{35}S methionine. The radioactive proteins are reacted with patient sera bound to beads, nonreactive proteins are washed away, and the bound complexes are eluted and electrophoresed. Individual HIV proteins are visualized and compared with HIV standards.

Isolation of HIV from Peripheral Blood Mononuclear Cells

In select cases, serologically based test results are supplemented by virologic (112,113) and/or molecular assays (114,115). For example, a reactive antibody test in an infant's sera may in fact reflect passive transfer of maternal antibodies (114). A definitive diagnosis of HIV infection is made through rescue of infectious virus from the infant's peripheral blood mononuclear cells (PBMCs). PBMCs are isolated from heparinized blood by ficoll-hypaque gradient centrifugation. The isolated

cells are cocultivated with phytohemagglutinin (PHA) and IL-2 treated PBMCs from HIV-seronegative donors. RT activity and/or p24 viral antigens, an indicator of productive HIV infection, are measured in the supernatant fluids from the cocultures.

Polymerase Chain Reaction Amplification of HIV DNA

Polymerase chain reaction (PCR) is rapidly becoming a laboratory standard. Here, HIV-specific oligonucleotide primer pairs are used to amplify subgenomic DNAs from infected cells using a heat-stable DNA polymerase [*Thermus aquaticus* (Taq) polymerase]. The DNA amplification is performed in a thermal cycler programmed to denature, anneal, and extend the HIV DNAs. The PCR products are resolved on agarose gels and subsequently hybridized (for definitive identifications). This analysis is effective in amplifying viral DNAs from small numbers of infected cells (115). Because of the extraordinary sensitivity of this assay blind quality-control samples must be included into any testing algorithm.

HIV INFECTION IN THE HUMAN HOST: MODES OF IMMUNOSUPPRESSION

The hallmark of immunodeficiency in AIDS is a selective depletion of CD4+ helper/inducer T lymphocytes (7). The CD4+ T lymphocyte is a central cell in the immune response and closely regulates other immune cells, which include monocyte/macrophages, cytotoxic T cells, natural killer cells, and B cells. The interactions between CD4+ T cells and other immunoregulatory elements is mediated through cytokines and regulatory factors including IL-2, GMCSF, etc. that are trophic for lymphocytes as well as for other cells of the myeloid series. The selective loss of helper/inducer T cells during HIV infection results in opportunistic infections, neoplasms, and inevitably death of the virus-infected host. There are numerous postulated mechanisms for CD4+ T-lymphocyte depletion. These include direct cytotoxicity resulting from productive viral infection, and killing (116–118) from indirect mechanisms (119–133). In support of the former is the demonstration of high numbers of CD4+ T lymphocytes infected by HIV in blood (116–118). However, the number of productively infected cells in blood is low. HIV-specific RNA is detected in 1/10,000 to 1/1 million circulating leukocytes (33,116). Indeed, the paucity of viral RNA-expressing cells in blood makes other mechanisms for CD4+ T-lymphocyte depletion possible. The normal turnover of T lymphocytes in the body is rapid and one would expect that the T-cell pool would compensate for the numbers of productively infected and subsequently killed lymphocytes. Furthermore, the *in vivo* environment is not very conducive to supporting productive and efficient viral replication. In hematopoietic tissues, immature CD4+ progenitor cells continually divide but are poorly differentiated, while their circulating progeny are quiescent and respond to only a few specific activation signals. In lieu of these observations, indirect mechanisms for CD4+ T-cell destruction during disease are proposed by numerous investigators and supported by experimental analyses.

The high levels of accumulated unintegrated HIV DNA in infected cells may produce cytopathicity, based on the known association between unintegrated DNA and cell death in avian and spleen leukosis virus-infected cells (59,60). HIV does not usually allow superinfection, and the high numbers of latent PBMCs demonstrate on average one to two copies of proviral DNA (116). Alternatively, HIV may induce terminal differentiation of the infected T4 cell, leading to a shortened lymphocyte life span (119,120). This may occur, for example, by induction of host cell membrane permeability changes (121,122). Indeed, Lynn et al. (121) demonstrated that following productive HIV infection the cell membrane becomes more permeable to small cations and that phospholipid synthesis decreases. Furthermore, temporal studies have recently shown that acute HIV infection affects host-cell macromolecular synthesis and membrane function. However, there is no direct evidence for this mechanism *in vivo*. The observation that HIV infection of CD4+ HeLa cells results in cell lysis (54) opposes the notion that HIV cytopathicity is induced by terminal cell differentiation.

Mechanisms other than those mediated by viral replication may be operative.

1. The interactions between the CD4 molecule and the virus envelope protein (77–80,123) may play a prominent role in CD4+ T-lymphocyte cell death. Infected or uninfected CD4+ cells may be coated with free gp120, which could be recognized as foreign and then cleared by the immune system (120,124,125). This could explain the pancytopenia commonly seen in patients with AIDS. Interactions between the HIV envelope glycoprotein present on the surface of infected antigen-presenting cells (e.g., monocyte/macrophages or CD4+ T lymphocytes) and uninfected CD4+ cells could lead to the elimination of the latter (77–80). Indeed, productive *in vitro* HIV infection is typified by syncytia formation and often terminal cytopathicity (Fig. 3). The process of syncytia formation involves the HIV-infected cell and other uninfected CD4+ T lymphocytes (Fig. 3). During productive viral infection uninfected cells are recruited into syncytia through fusion of gp120 on the surface of infected cells and CD4 on uninfected cells (Fig. 4). The high level of HIV *env* glycoprotein on the surface of infected CD4+ lymphocytes results in cell fusion with neighboring uninfected CD4+ cells, leading to multinucleated giant cell formation and cell death. Thus, unin-

fected CD4+ cells are recruited into growing multinucleated giant cells through the interactions between the gp120 on the surface of infected cells and CD4 on the uninfected cells. In this regard, intracellular complexing of CD4 and *env* proteins may also play a role(s) in the cytopathogenicity induced by HIV infection (123). Leukocyte surface molecules also play roles in syncytia formation (126–128). Indeed, antibodies to adhesion molecules, especially integrin LFA-1, block syncytia (126). Furthermore, HIV infection can be delayed when antibodies to LFA-1 are kept in culture fluids blocking cell–cell contact (127,128). The fact that productive HIV infection can occur in LFA-1-deficient cells, leading to viable productively infected cells, supports the notion that the recruitment of CD4+ T lymphocytes into the syncytia precipitates their demise. Indeed, CD4 is rapidly downregulated following viral infection and non-CD4-expressing HIV-infected cells persist for long time periods despite demonstrably high levels of viral gene products (Fig. 6). Furthermore, viral species with defined biologic and molecular properties occur over time in infected individuals. HIV-1 isolates from asymptomatic carriers produce low levels of virus and syncytia (slow/low viruses) and those from patients with AIDS or AIDS-related complex (ARC) grow rapidly at high titers and induce syncytia (rapid/high) (129,130). These observations, in toto, would support a virus-induced mechanism for CD4+ T-lymphocyte depletion in AIDS. However, although multinucleated giant cells are commonly seen in HIV-infected cultures *in vitro,* it is important to point out that in only a minority of infected tissues, such as brain and spinal cord, can syncytia be demonstrated. Virus-induced syncytia in peripheral blood has never been demonstrated. Furthermore, syncytia formation occurs predominantly in specific cell lines, often at frequencies that do not involve the majority of the cell population. Most HIV-infected cells die without fusion. Moreover, monocytes and macrophages express CD4 on their surface and are not depleted but productively infected by virus. That HIV often does not induce significant cytopathic effects in monocytes strongly suggests that either the density of CD4 receptor expression is important in determining cytopathic effects or that gp120–CD4 interactions are not the sole determinant for viral cell killing. In support of the former hypothesis are studies demonstrating HIV-1 superinfection of human T-cell leukemia virus type I (HTLV-I)-transformed T-cell clones. Cell clones of either the CD4 or CD8 phenotype infected with HIV result in a productive infection; however, cytopathicity occurs only in the CD4+ clones (131). This cell death may be mediated through extracellular CD4–gp120 interactions or from the formation of intracellular toxic complexes of CD4 and the HIV envelope.

2. CD4+ lymphocyte depletion may involve the expression or alteration of cellular epitopes in virus-suscep-

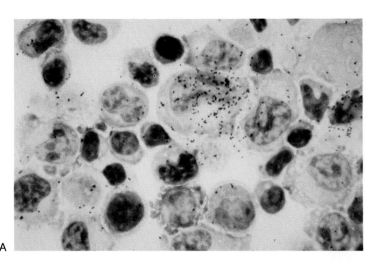

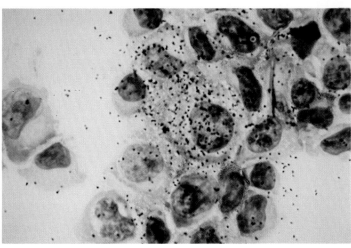

FIG. 6. Downmodulation of CD4 following productive HIV infection of lymphoblasts. PHA/IL-2-treated peripheral blood mononuclear cells (PBMCs) were infected with HIV HTLV-III$_b$ for 7 days. Cells were harvested, cytocentrifuged, fixed with 1% glutaraldehyde, and then stained with antibodies to CD4. Following the immunocytochemical assay the cell preparations were hybridized with HIV-specific single-stranded RNA probes (in situ hybridization). Silver grains indicative of HIV mRNA are seen in from cells staining negative for CD4 antigen (**A**). A replicate cell preparations is stained for HLA-DR and then hybridized with the HIV-specific RNA. Note dual HLA-DR- and HIV mRNA-labeled cell (**B**).

tible cells (132). Alteration in the HLA class II phenotype may occur in HIV-infected CD4+ T cells, thereby making them more susceptible to immune clearance. Here the HIV envelope binds to the CD4 molecule and may mimic a configuration of a portion of the class II major histocompatibility complex (MHC) antigen (132). Alternatively, viral epitopes expressed on the surface of immune-stimulated and virus-infected cells may precipitate their own demise. In this scenario, host antibody and cytotoxic lymphocyte responses against HIV-specific epitopes clear virus-infected CD4+ T lymphocytes (133).

3. HIV-infected lymphocytes may become more susceptible to superinfection by other pathogens. Cytomegalovirus (CMV) can abortively infect T cells and through dual CMV/HIV infection lead to an accelerated depletion of the CD4+ T lymphocyte (134).

4. HIV may preferentially infect a small population of precursor or memory cells that is responsible for growth of other CD4+ cells (7). This possibility has recently fallen into disfavor due to the inability to find infected precursor cells *in vivo*.

5. A selective depletion of a critical subset of CD4+ T lymphocytes (135) could result in the elimination of all cells carrying this phenotype. Subsets of CD4+ cells that recognize and respond to soluble antigen are selectively deficient in patients with AIDS. This deficiency occurs early in the course of disease and is quite common.

6. Substances released as a consequence of viral infection, such as soluble cell factors, viral proteins other than gp120, or other toxic elements, might ultimately destroy other CD4+ T lymphocytes (136–139).

ROLE OF MONOCYTES AND MACROPHAGES IN THE PERSISTENCE AND DISSEMINATION OF HIV INFECTIONS

Perhaps the most important shared property among lentiviruses involves target cell tropism. In each instance, infected monocytes and macrophages serve as a viral reservoir, evade host immune surveillance, initiate fulminant disease in specific target tissues, and serve as efficient host cells for the isolation and propagation of

HIV (140). In the infected human host, HIV has been demonstrated in, or recovered from, CD4+ T lymphocytes (116,117), monocytes in blood (15,16), and macrophages in brain (9,141–145), spinal cord (13) lung (11,146), skin (10), and lymphnodes (147). Infected alveolar macrophages may play an important role in the high incidence of *Pneumocystis carinii* pneumonia in

AIDS patients (146). Lymphocytic interstitial pneumonitis, spinal cord myelopathy, and AIDS-associated encephalopathy are all strongly associated with HIV-infected tissue macrophages.

During steady state, macrophages have critically important functions in providing antimicrobial defense for the host. Paradoxically, these scavenger cells perpetuate

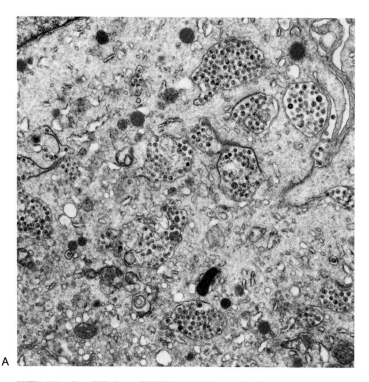

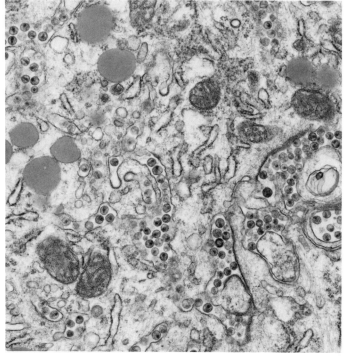

FIG. 7. Intracytoplasmic virion accumulation in HIV-infected monocytes. HIV-1 particles are seen within Golgi-derived vacuoles in a cultured monocyte (**A**) (×14,000). A portion of the cytoplasm of a multinucleated monocyte rich in HIV-1-containing vacuoles is illustrated (**B**). All stages of viral budding and release in addition to lipid vacuoles, swollen mitochondria, and disrupted membranes are seen.

viral persistence. Indeed, they represent the major tissue reservoir for HIV. The mechanisms of viral persistence in macrophages involve the presence of virus in intracytoplasmic vacuoles, which may provide an important means for escape from immune surveillance (148,149). HIV accumulates within Golgi-derived cytoplasmic vacuoles of macrophages (Fig. 7). Fusion with one another of small Golgi complex-derived vacuoles containing small numbers of virions, along with the continued budding of progeny virus into enlarging vacuoles, probably accounts for the increasing size of the vacuoles and the enlarging number of viral particles. This mechanism of viral assembly and virion accumulation contrasts with infection of CD4+ T lymphocytes (Fig. 8). Here the plasma membrane is the site of viral assembly; intravacuolar virus is only rarely identified in multinucleated cells.

The viral life cycle in monocytes and macrophages is regulated by physiological factors involved in maturation and differentiation of the cells from their precursors in bone marrow or blood (150,151). Bone marrow infection by HIV has not been conclusively identified. Furthermore, the number of monocytes expressing viral RNA in blood is very low. After these infected cells migrate from blood and mature into tissue macrophages, viral gene expression increases several thousand-fold and the virus life cycle goes to completion (e.g., mature virion particles are produced) (150). A similar phenomenon occurs *in vitro* as infected monocytes differentiate into macrophage-like cells. Not all mature macrophages in tissue are equally permissive for HIV infections. The specific susceptibility of tissues to the pathological process can be traced to permissiveness of local macrophage populations that support virus replication. In visna virus

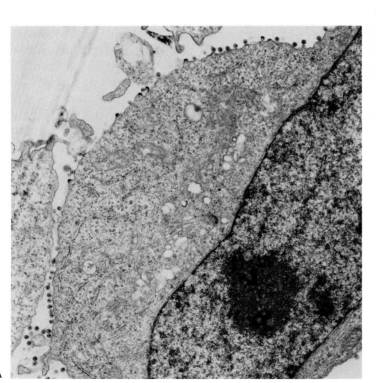

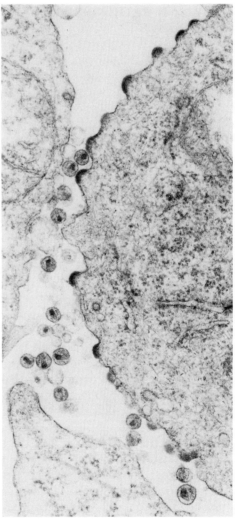

A

B

FIG. 8. Ultrastructural analysis of HIV-infected CD4+ T lymphocytes. Numerous HIV particles are demonstrated in association with the plasma membrane (**A**). In **B,** note the numerous virions in various stages of budding and release in association with the plasma membrane. This is in contrast to the intracytoplasmic accumulation of HIV previously demonstrated in monocytes.

infections, for example, brain and alveolar macrophages are highly permissive, but the mature Kupffer cells in liver, the histiocytes of connective tissue, or the Langerhans cells in skin all fail to support viral replication. Moreover, the lung and brain are primary sites for virus-induced lesions, while skin and liver tissues are not targets for pathological changes. These observations are consistent with the concept that genetically predetermined, cellular transcriptional factors (factors that vary with macrophage phenotype, maturation, and cell differentiation) may regulate viral gene expression and/or virus cell surface receptors. Indeed, cell activation is a necessary event for integration and provirally directed gene expression. Specific "cell activation" factors are probably only found in the subpopulations of macrophages that support viral replication and ultimately provide the molecular basis for the unique tissue tropism that underlies aspects of HIV pathogenesis (7,152–154).

BIOLOGY AND PATHOGENESIS OF CNS DISEASE

Whereas infection and ultimate loss of helper/inducer T lymphocytes accounts for immunosuppression and opportunistic infection, infection of macrophages serves as the basis for primary HIV disease. The CNS is a major tissue source for HIV and a primary site of disease during HIV infection. Although a number of AIDS-related opportunistic infections are described (toxoplasmosis, cryptococcosis, JC papovavirus infection, mycobacterial infection, etc.), HIV is a primary pathogen for induction of CNS disease (155–162). High levels of HIV gene products are detected in brain tissue by Southern blot, in situ hybridization, immunohistochemical, electron microscopic and viral isolation assays (163–167). Virus is expressed almost exclusively in cells of macrophage lineage (brain macrophages, microglia, and multinucleated giant cells), and in many cases up to 15% of brain macrophages express HIV-specific RNAs during disease (Figs. 9 and 10) (9). HIV enters the nervous system very early in infection and is probably carried there by monocytes from peripheral blood (160,167). Infection of cerebral endothelial cells may also occur and lead to blood–brain barrier permeability abnormalities, but clear evidence of *in vivo* HIV infection in these and other primary CNS cells (neurons, astrocytes, or oligodendrocytes) is lacking. Only tissue culture infections of these cell types have been demonstrated (168–170). This is underscored by experimental observations of explant cultures of adult human brains inoculated with HIV. In these culture systems, among the various cell types represented, viral replication occurs selectively in microglial macrophage cells (171). Furthermore, patients with the most severe clinical symptoms usually have the most intense pathology

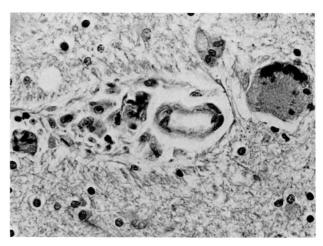

FIG. 9. CNS histopathologic changes in the AIDS dementia complex. A multinucleated macrophage, reactive astrocytes, and myelin pallor are illustrated.

and the highest levels of HIV infection in brain macrophages (160).

The CNS may be affected early in the course of HIV infection. Entry of HIV into the CNS may occur at the time of the primary seroconversion-related mononucleosis illness or during the subclinical phase of infection (172–178). Symptoms and signs of CNS disease soon after exposure to HIV include headache, encephalitis, aseptic meningitis, ataxia, or myelopathy. Laboratory evidence for early invasion of HIV into the brain includes: (1) inflammatory cells, cellular proteins and oligoclonal immunoglobulin bands in cerebrospinal fluid (CSF); (2) detectable levels of intrathecal antibodies to HIV; and (3) progeny HIV and viral antigens in CSF (163–165). Of all the laboratory tests, the recovery of virus from CSF of neurologically asymptomatic individuals at the time of, or subsequent to, seroconversion most strongly supports early virus invasion of the CNS (163,172).

An important question in the pathogenesis of CNS infection is whether productive HIV infection in brain macrophages induces disease or whether CNS disease is part of a broader metabolic dysfunction. Many investigators support the thesis that low-level infection of neurons and neuroglia produces the neurologic impairment associated with AIDS (179–181). Proposed theories of CNS dysfunction include a restricted noncytopathic infection of neurons and neuroglia, coexistence of opportunistic herpesvirus or fungal infections (182,183), growth factor blockade mediated by gp120, CNS toxicity related to cytokine secretion, and direct neuron killing by gp120. Low-level infection in neurons and glia may occur at levels capable of inducing cellular aberrations but below the sensitivity for detection by immunocytochemical and in situ hybridization assays. Numerous published reports indicate that cultured neuronal and astro-

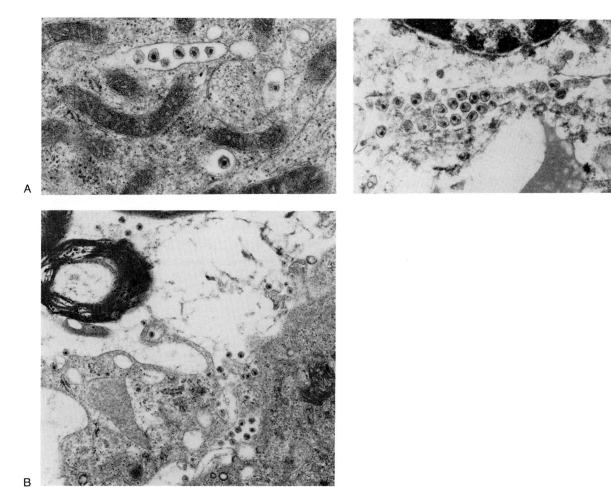

FIG. 10. The brain macrophage is the predominant cell in the central nervous system that supports HIV replication. The illustrated panels (**A and B**) are from a brain biopsy obtained from a patient with the AIDS dementia complex. **C** is from autopsy tissue from the spinal cord of a patient with AIDS-associated vacuolar myelopathy. **A** demonstrates several cytoplasmic vacuoles containing mature HIV particles within a brain macrophage. ×48,000. In **B,** numerous mature HIV virions are associated with the surface of a brain macrophage. ×25,000. In **C,** numerous HIV particles are associated with the surface of a macrophage within the spinal cord of a patient with vacuolar myelopathy. ×37,000.

glial cells support HIV replication (169,170). This infection may perturb their function and theoretically lead to the cognitive dysfunctions characteristic of AIDS dementia complex. Furthermore, previous work demonstrates that low levels of CD4 mRNA are present in astrocytic cell lines susceptible to HIV (170). This suggests that brain cells may be susceptible to HIV infection *in vivo.* Activation of viral infection in brain cells might occur during superinfection with herpesvirus or fungal pathogens. Indeed, several DNA-group viruses that may be present as opportunistic pathogens in brain are able to transactivate HIV LTR-directed gene expression (for example, CMV, herpes simplex type 1, and JC) (182,183). Other infectious processes seen in association with neurologic disease include fungal infection and toxoplasmosis, which could further upregulate viral replication by im-

mune stimulation. Coinfection with multiple interacting pathogens may act in a concerted fashion to augment HIV expression and precipitate disease. Once productive infection is established the precipitation of neurologic disease may be a consequence of toxicities elicited by viral proteins. For example, gp120 may antagonize normal vasoactive intestinal peptide (VIPergic) function in brain tissue (179). HIV has been found to mimic VIP binding activities. Other studies have demonstrated a more direct neurotoxicity of gp120. In these experiments gp120 induced neurotoxicity by increasing free Ca^{2+} in cultured neurons (180). The effect was prevented by Ca^{2+} channel antagonists. Recently, Sabatier et al. (181) demonstrated that intracerebroventricular injections of *tat* could induce toxic effects in rodents. Here, radiolabeled *tat* bound to rat brain synaptic nerve endings in a dose-dependent manner and induced a large depolarization modifying cell permeability. The neurotoxicity of *tat* was also demonstrated on glioma and neuroblastoma cells. Thus HIV gene products are directly toxic to primary neuronal cells and cell lines and may play a pivotal role in the pathogenesis of AIDS dementia complex.

Further studies suggest that secretory products from HIV-infected monocytes affect neuronal cell viabilities and function. As the macrophage is the predominant cell type productively infected by HIV in brain, investigators theorized that brain dysfunction was related in part or in whole to cell-coded toxins generated from HIV-infected macrophages (184–186). Indeed, macrophages play a preeminent role during both steady-state conditions and during inflammation in the regulation of tissue function. The regulatory role of macrophages is promulgated through release of many kinds of secretory molecules induced by different physiologic stimuli. Changes in the secretion or release of certain of these mediators could lead to disease and contribute to the symptomatology of HIV infection. For example, disordered secretion of the monokine TNF or cachectin has been postulated as the basis for "slim disease," a wasting syndrome unrelated to opportunistic infection and commonly seen in Africans with AIDS (184). Enhanced release of IL-1 or TNF could explain chronic fever in some AIDS patients. Both are endogenous pyrogens produced in monocytes. Chemotactic factors released from the infected monocytes could lead to infiltration of the brain with inflammatory cells and work in concert with other cytokines that directly precipitate disease by altering brain cell function. There is contradictory evidence, however, that blood monocytes and macrophages are depleted and/or functionally impaired in HIV infection (152–154,185,186). In one study, the number of Langerhans cells in the skin of patients with AIDS was reduced by 50% (185) but in other studies, no change in Langerhan cell numbers was observed (186). Published reports describe monocyte bactericidal activity and chemotaxis as either normal or defective (152–154). Monocyte secretion of IL-1 in the absence of exogenous stimuli was normal or elevated. One central problem in these analyses is that blood monocytes were the most frequently analyzed cell population. The short circulating half-life of monocytes of less than 30 hours, the unidirectional migration of these cells into tissues, and the low frequency of HIV infection *in vivo* suggest that they comprise a poor study population. In contrast, tissue macrophages play a preeminent role in HIV disease. The lack of evidence for cytolytic infection of neurons or neuroglia by HIV further suggests an indirect macrophage-mediated mechanism for CNS dysfunction. Indeed, recent studies suggest that disordered secretion of one or more monokines from HIV-infected monocyte/macrophages may initiate CNS cell damage. In one report, HIV-infected human monocytoid cells, but not infected human lymphoid cells, released toxic factors that destroyed chick and rat neurons in culture (187). The monocyte-produced neurotoxins were heat stable and protease resistant and acted by way of N-methyl-D-aspartate receptors. The authors hypothesized that the presence of chronically HIV-infected macrophages in brain continuously disrupt neurologic function through the release of neuron-killing factors until the death of the patient. Other reports refute these experimental observations (188).

The origin of HIV infection in the brain macrophage and the *in vivo* mechanisms underlying disease remain poorly understood. Infection may begin from activation or expansion of latent HIV infection of monocytes carried into the brain during cell maturation (the "Trojan horse" hypothesis) (9). Alternatively, but not mutually exclusive, is the concept that monocyte/macrophage infection occurs in brain by infection of microglia through contact with infected capillary endothelial cells or T lymphocytes. Whether cell-free virus crosses the blood–brain barrier or virus enters by way of infected monocytes or CD4+ T cells remains an open debate. Endothelial cells may provide a conduit of infection between blood and brain. Evidence that HIV enters the CNS through capillary endothelial cells is supported by an experimental model system for infection (144). Two weeks following SIV infection of macaques, inflammation and multinucleated giant cells could be demonstrated in the leptomeninges and brain parenchyma (around blood vessels). This finding suggests that entry is mediated through the choroid plexus, leptomeninges, and/or capillary endothelial cells.

Productive HIV replication in brain macrophages is influenced by cell maturational factors. The regulation of HIV gene expression by maturational and activation factors influences HIV gene synthesis acquired through cell activation/differentiation and may play a pivotal role in the permissive nature of the brain macrophage for HIV. For example, in the T-cell system, the mitogens phorbol myristate acetate and PHA positively stimulate HIV LTR-directed gene synthesis by increasing the synthesis of a cellular DNA binding protein, nuclear factor κB (NFκB) (189). In HIV-infected persons, leukocytes can be induced to produce infectious virus only after exposure to similar T-cell mitogens. The high percentage of HIV-infected brain macrophages suggests that these cells are already stimulated and have acquired the necessary transcriptional factors for sustained efficient viral replication.

CONCLUSIONS

Infection with HIV results in a persistent, productive infection in both CD4+ T cells and monocyte/macrophages despite a vigorous but ineffective host immune response. Distinct clinical syndromes result from viral infection in its principal target cells. T-cell infection and subsequent destruction result in immunosuppression and opportunistic infections while monocyte/macrophage infection leads to primary virus-induced disease, e.g., CNS disorders. Ultimately, most infected individuals develop both immunologic and neurologic abnormalities. The availability of future treatment and preventive measures for HIV infection will ultimately rely on a better understanding of the mechanisms of viral replication and modes of persistence in these principal target cells.

ACKNOWLEDGMENTS

The authors thank members of the HIV-Immunopathogenesis Program and the Military Medical Consortium for Applied Retroviral Research for helpful suggestions and continuing support, Ms. Victoria Hunter for excellent graphics, and Dr. Jim Hoxie for assistance with the immunoprecipitation experiment pictured in Fig. 1. Dr. H. E. Gendelman is a Carter-Wallace Fellow of the Johns Hopkins University School of Public Health and Hygiene. The views expressed in this article do not necessarily reflect those of the United States Army or the Department of Defense.

REFERENCES

1. Barre-Sinoussi F, Chermann JC, Rey F, et al. Isolation of a T-lymphotropic retrovirus from a patient at risk for acquired immune deficiency syndrome (AIDS). *Science* 1983;220:868–71.
2. Popovic M, Sarngadharan MG, Read E, Gallo RC. Detection, isolation, and continuous production of cytopathic retroviruses (HTLV-III) from patients with AIDS and pre-AIDS. *Science* 1984;224:497–500.
3. Levy JA, Hoffman AD, Kramer SM, et al. Isolation of lymphocytopathic retroviruses from San Francisco patients with AIDS. *Science* 1984;225:840–2.
4. Gottlieb MS, Schroff R, Schanker HM, et al. *Pneumocystis carinii* pneumonia and mucosal candidiasis in previously healthy homosexual men: evidence of a new acquired cellular immunodeficiency. *N Engl J Med* 1981;305:1425–31.
5. Bowen DL, Lane HC, Fauci AS. Immunopathogenesis of the acquired immunodeficiency syndrome. *Ann Intern Med* 1985;103:704–9.
6. Popovic M, Read-Connole E, Gartner S. Biological properties of HTLV-III/LAV: a possible pathway of natural infection in vivo. *Ann Inst Pasteur Immunol* 1986;137,D:413–7.
7. Fauci AS. The human immunodeficiency virus: infectivity and mechanisms of pathogenesis. *Science* 1988;239:617–22.
8. Gartner S, Markovits P, Markovitz DM, et al. The role of mononuclear phagocytes in HTLV-III/LAV infection. *Science* 1986;233:215–9.
9. Koenig S, Gendelman HE, Orenstein JM, et al. Detection of AIDS virus in macrophages in brain tissue from AIDS patients with encephalopathy. *Science* 1986;233:1089–93.
10. Tschacler E, Groh V, Popovic M, et al. Epidermal Langerhans cells—a target for HTLV-III/LAV infection. *J Invest Dermatol* 1987;88:233–7.
11. Salahuddin SZ, Rose RM, Groopman JE, et al. Human T lymphotropic virus type III infection of human alveolar macrophages. *Blood* 1986;68:281–4.
12. Gendelman HE, Orenstein JM, Martin MA, et al. Efficient isolation and propagation of human immunodeficiency virus on CSF-1 stimulated human monocytes. *J Exp Med* 1988;167:1428–41.
13. Eilbott DJ, Peress N, Burger H, et al. Human immunodeficiency virus expression and replication in macrophages in the spinal cords of AIDS patients with myelopathy. *Proc Natl Acad Sci USA* 1989;86:3337–41.
14. Gendelman HE, Orenstein JM, Baca LM, et al. Editorial review: the macrophage in the persistence and pathogenesis of HIV infection. *AIDS* 1989;3:475–95.
15. Schuitemaker H, Kootstra NA, Goede REY, et al. Monocytotropic human immunodeficiency virus type 1 (HIV-1) variants detectable in all stages of HIV-1 infection lack T-cell line tropism and syncytium-inducing ability in primary T-cell culture. *J Virol* 1991;65:356–63.
16. McElrath MJ, Steinman RM, Cohn AZ. Latent HIV-1 infection in enriched populations of blood monocytes and T cells from seropositive patients. *J Clin Invest* 1991;87:27–30.
17. Price RW, Brew B, Sidtis J, et al. The brain in AIDS: central nervous system HIV-1 infection and AIDS dementia complex. *Science* 1988;239:586–92.
18. Narayan O, Cork LC. Lentiviral diseases of sheep and goats: chronic pneumonia leukoencephalomyelitis and arthritis. *Rev Infect Dis* 1985;7:89–98.
19. Haase AT. Pathogenesis of lentivirus infections. *Nature* 1986;322:130–6.
20. Narayan O, Clements JE. Biology and pathogenesis of lentiviruses of ruminant animals. In: Wong-Staal F, Gallo RC, eds. *Retrovirus biology—an emerging role in human disease.* New York: Marcel Dekker. 1987;117–40.
21. Narayan O, Clements JE. Biology and pathogenesis of lentiviruses. *J Gen Virol* 1989;70:1617–39.
22. Gonda MA, Wong-Staal F, Gallo RC, et al. Sequence homology and morphologic similarity of HTLV III and visna virus, a pathogenic lentivirus. *Science* 1985;227:173–7.
23. Chiu IM, Yaniv A, Dahlberg JE. Nucleotide sequence evidence for relationship of AIDS retrovirus to lentiviruses. *Nature* 1985;317:366–8.
24. Rabson AB, Martin MA. Molecular organization of the AIDS retrovirus. *Cell* 1985;40:477–80.
25. Guyader M, Emerman M, Sonigo P, et al. Genome organization and transactivation of the human immunodeficiency virus, type 2. *Nature* 1987;326:662–9.
26. Cheevers WP, McGuire TC. Equine infectious anemia virus: immunopathogenesis and persistence. *Rev Infect Dis* 1985;7:83–8.
27. Daniel MD, Letvin NL, King NW, et al. Isolation of T-cell tropic HTLV-III-like retrovirus from macaques. *Science* 1985;228:1201–4.
28. Kanki PJ, McLane MF, King NW, Jr, et al. Serologic identification and characterization of a macaque T-lymphotropic retrovirus closely related to HTLV-III. *Science* 1985;228:1199–201.
29. Letvin NL, Daniel MD, Sehgal PK, et al. Induction of AIDS-like disease in macaque monkeys with T-cell tropic retrovirus STLV-III. *Science* 1985;230:71–3.
30. Pederson NC, Ho EW, Brown ML, Yamamoto JK. Isolation of a T-lymphotropic virus from domestic cats with an immunodeficiency-like syndrome. *Science* 1987;235:790–3.
31. Sonigo P, Alizon M, Staskus K, et al. Nucleotide sequence of the visna lentivirus: relationship to the AIDS virus. *Cell* 1985;42:369–82.
32. Stephens RM, Casey JW, Rice NR. Equine infectious anemia virus *gag* and *pol* genes: relatedness to visna and AIDS virus. *Science* 1986;231:589–94.
33. Harper ME, Marselle LM, Gallo RC, Wong-Staal F. Detection of lymphocytes expressing human T-lymphotropic virus type III in lymph nodes and peripheral blood from infected individuals by in situ hybridization. *Proc Natl Acad Sci USA* 1986;83:772–6.
34. Narayan O, Kennedy-Stoskopf S, Zink CM. Lentivirus-host interactions: lessons from visna and caprine arthritis-encephalitis viruses. *Ann Neurol* 1988;23[Suppl]:S95–S100.
35. Gendelman HE, Leonard JM, Dutko FJ, et al. Immunopathogenesis of human immunodeficiency virus infection in the central nervous system. *Ann Neurol* 1987;23[Suppl]:S78–S81.
36. Clements JE, Pedersen FS, Narayan O, Haseltine WA. Genomic

changes associated with antigenic variation of visna virus during persistent infection. *Proc Natl Acad Sci USA* 1980;77:4454–8.

37. Narayan O, Clements JE, Kennedy-Stoskopf S, Royal R. Mechanisms of escape of visna lentiviruses from immunological control. *Contrib Microbiol Immunol* 1987;8:60–76.
38. Kennedy-Stoskopf S, Narayan O. Neutralizing antibodies to visna lentivirus: mechanism of action and possible role in virus persistence. *J Virol* 1986;59:37–44.
39. Francis DP, Petricciani JC. The prospects for and pathways toward a vaccine for AIDS. *N Engl J Med* 1985;313:1586–90.
40. Hahn BH, Shaw GM, Taylor ME, et al. Genetic variation in HTLV-III/LAV over time in patients with AIDS or at risk for AIDS. *Science* 1986;232:1548–53.
41. Ho DD, Sarnagaharan MG, Hirsch MS, et al. Human immunodeficiency virus neutralizing antibodies recognize several conserved domains on the envelope glycoproteins. *J Virol* 1987;61:2024–8.
42. Bouillant AMP, Becker SAW. Ultrastructural comparison of oncovirinae (type C), spumavirinae, and lentivirinae: three subfamilies of retroviridae found in farm animals. *J Natl Cancer Inst* 1984;72:1075–84.
43. Dahlberg JE, Gaskin JM, Perk K. Morphological and immunological comparison of caprine arthritis encephalitis and ovine progressive pneumonia viruses. *J Virol* 1981;39:914–9.
44. Gonda MA, Charman HP, Walker JL, Coggins L. Scanning and transmission electron microscopic study of equine infectious anemia virus. *Am J Vet Res* 1978;39:731–40.
45. Munn RJ, Marx PA, Yamamoto JK, Gardner MB. Ultrastructural comparison of the retroviruses associated with human and simian acquired immunodeficiency syndromes. *Lab Invest* 1985;53:194–9.
46. Wain-Hobson S, Sonigo P, Danos P, Cole S, Alizon M. Nucleotide sequence of the AIDS virus LAV *Cell* 1985;40:9–17.
47. Ratner L, Haseltine W, Patarca R, et al. Complete nucleotide sequence of the AIDS virus, HTLV-III. *Nature* 1985;313:277–84.
48. Starcich B, Ratner L, Josephs SF, et al. Characterization of long terminal repeat sequences of HTLV-III. *Science* 1985;227:538–40.
49. Muesing MA, Smith DH, Cabradilla CD, et al. Nucleic acid structure and expression of the human AIDS/lymphadenopathy retrovirus. *Nature* 1985;313:450–8.
50. Sanchez-Pescador R, Power MD, Barr PJ, et al. Nucleotide sequence and expression of an AIDS-associated retrovirus (ARV-2). *Science* 1985;227:484–92.
51. McDougal JS, Kennedy MS, Sligh JM, et al. Binding of HTLV-III/LAV to T4+ T cells by a complex of the 110K viral protein and the T4 molecule. *Science* 1986;231:382–5.
52. Dalgleish AG, Beverley PCL, Clapham PR, et al. The CD4(T4) antigen is an essential component of the receptor for the AIDS retrovirus. *Nature* 1984;312:763–7.
53. Klatzmann D, Champagne E, Chamaret S, et al. T-lymphocyte T4 molecule behaves as the receptor for human retrovirus LAV. *Nature* 1984;312:767–8.
54. Maddon PJ, Dalgleish AG, McDougal JS. The T4 gene encodes the AIDS virus receptor and is expressed in the immune system and the brain. *Cell* 1986;47:333–48.
55. Varmus H. Retroviruses. *Science* 1988;240:1427–35.
56. Dales S, Hanafusa H. Penetration and intracellular release of the genomes of avian RNA tumor viruses. *Virology* 1972;50:440–58.
57. Stein BS, Gowda SD, Lifson JD, et al. pH-independent HIV entry into CD4-positive T cells via virus envelope fusion to the plasma membrane. *Cell* 1987;49:659–68.
58. Bedinger P, Moriarty A, von Borstel RC, et al. Internalization of the human immunodeficiency virus does not require the cytoplasmic domain of CD4. *Nature* 1988;229:1402–5.
59. Weller SK, Joy AE, Temin HM. Correlation between cell killing and massive second-round superinfection by members of some subgroups of avian leukosis virus. *J Virol* 1980;33:494–506.
60. Keshet E, Temin HM. Cell killing by spleen necrosis virus is correlated with a transient accumulation of spleen necrosis virus DNA. *J Virol* 1979;31:376–88.
61. Shaw, GM, Hahn BH, Arya SK, Groopman JE, Gallo RC, Wong-Staal F. Molecular characterization of human T-cell (lymphotropic) virus type III in the acquired immune deficiency syndrome. *Science* 1984;226:1165–71.

62. McCune JM. HIV-1: the infective process in vivo. *Cell* 1991;64:351–63.
63. Greene WC. Mechanisms of disease: the molecular biology of human immunodeficiency virus type 1 infection. *N Engl J Med* 1991;324:308–17.
64. Nabel G, Baltimore D. An inducible transcription factor activates expression of human immunodeficiency virus in T cells. *Nature* 1987;326:711–3.
65. Rosenberg ZF, Fauci AS. The immunopathogenesis of HIV infection. *Adv Immunol* 1989;47:377–431.
66. Gendelman HE, Narayan O, Molineaux S, et al. Slow persistent replication of lentiviruses: role of macrophages and macrophage precursors in bone marrow. *Proc Natl Acad Sci USA* 1985;82:7086–90.
67. Nara P, Smit T, Dunlop JM, et al. Emergence of viruses resistant to neutralization by V3-specific antibodies in experimental human immunodeficiency virus type 1 IIIb infection of chimpanzees. *J Virol* 1990;64:3779–91.
68. Albert J, Abrahamsson B, Nagy K, et al. Rapid development of isolate-specific neutralizing antibodies after primary HIV-1 infection and consequent emergence of virus variants which resist neutralization by autologous sera. *AIDS* 1990;4:107–12.
69. Garcia JA, Harrich E, Soultarakis E, et al. Human immunodeficiency virus type 1 LTR TATA and TAR region sequences required for transcriptional regulation. *EMBO J* 1989;8:765–79.
70. Lillehoj EP, Salazar FHR, Mervis RJ et al. Purification and structural characterization of the putative gag-pol protease of human immunodeficiency virus. *J Virol* 1988;62:3053–8.
71. Veronese FD, Copeland TD, DeVico AL, et al. Characterization of highly immunogenic p66/p51 as the reverse transcriptase of HTLV-III/LAV. *Science* 1986;231:1289–91.
72. Lightfoote MM, Coligan JE, Folks TM, et al. Structural characterization of reverse transcriptase and endonuclease polypeptides of the acquired immunodeficiency syndrome retrovirus. *J Virol* 1986;60:771–5.
73. McKeating JA, Willey RL. Structure and function of the HIV envelope. *AIDS (Lond)* 1989;3[Suppl]:S35–S41.
74. DiMarzo Veronese F, DeVico AL, Copeland TD, Oroszlan S, Gallo RC, Sarngadharan MG. Characterization of gp41 as the transmembrane protein coded by the HTLV-III/LAV envelope gene. *Science* 1985;229:1402–4.
75. Fisher AG, Ratner L, Mitsuya H, et al. Infectious mutants of HTLV-III with changes in the 3′ region and markedly reduced cytopathic effects. *Science* 1986;233:655–9.
76. Lasky LA, Nakamura G, Smith DH, et al. Delineation of a region of the human immunodefiency virus type 1 gp120 glycoprotein critical for interaction with the CD4 receptor. *Cell* 1987;50:975–85.
77. Lifson JD, Reyes GR, McGrath MS, et al. AIDS retrovirus induced cytopathology: giant cell formation and involvement of CD4 antigen. *Science* 1986;232:1123–7.
78. Sodroski J, Goh WC, Rosen C, et al. Role of the HTLV-III/LAV envelope in syncytium formation and cytopathicity. *Nature* 1986;322:470–4.
79. Lifson JD, Feinberg MB, Reyes GR, et al. Induction of CD4-dependent cell fusion by the HTLV-III/LAV envelope glycoprotein. *Nature* 1986;323:725–8.
80. Lifson J, Coutre S, Huang E, Engleman E. Role of envelope glycoprotein carbohydrate in human immunodeficiency virus (HIV) infectivity and virus-induced cell fusion. *J Exp Med* 1986;164:2101–6.
81. Robey WG, Safai B, Oroszlan S, et al. Characterization of envelope and core structural gene products of HTLV-III with sera from AIDS patients. *Science* 1985;228:593–5.
82. Allen JS, Coligan JE, Barin F, et al. Major glycoprotein antigens that induce antibodies in AIDS patients are encoded by HTLV-III. *Science* 1985;228:1091–4.
83. Willey RL, Rutledge RA, Dias S, et al. Identification of conserved and divergent domains within the envelope gene of the acquired immunodeficiency syndrome retrovirus. *Proc Natl Acad Sci USA* 1986;83:5038–42.
84. Starcich BR, Hahn BH, Shaw GM, et al. Identification and characterization of conserved and variable regions in the envelope

gene of HTLV-III/LAV, the retrovirus of AIDS. *Cell* 1986;45:637–48.

85. Alizon M, Wain-Hobson S, Montagnier L, Sonigo P. Genetic variability of the AIDS virus: nucleotide sequence analysis of two isolates from African patients. *Cell* 1986;46:63–74.

86. Wain-Hobson S. HIV genome variability in vivo. *AIDS* 1989;3[Suppl 1]:S13–S18.

87. Roberts JD, Bebenek K, Kunkel TA. The accuracy of reverse transcriptase from HIV-1. *Science* 1988;242:1171–3.

88. Arya SK, Guo C, Josephs SF, Wong-Staal F. Transactivator gene of human T-lymphotropic virus type III (HTLV-III). *Science* 1985;229:69–73.

89. Sodroski J, Patarca R, Rosen C, Wong-Staal F, Haseltine W. Location of the trans-activating region on the genome of human T-cell lymphotropic virus type III. *Science* 1985;229:74–7.

90. Fisher AG, Feinberg MB, Josephs SF, et al. The trans-activator gene of HTLV-III is essential for virus replication. *Nature* 1986;320:367–71.

91. Rosen CA, Sodroski JG, Goh WC, et al. Post-transcriptional regulation accounts for the trans-activation of the human T-lymphotropic virus type III. *Nature* 1986;319:555–9.

92. Cullen BR. Trans-activation of human immunodeficiency virus occurs via a bimodal mechanism. *Cell* 1986;46:973–82.

93. Sodroski J, Goh WC, Rosen C, et al. A second post-transcriptional trans-activator gene required for HTLV-III replication. *Nature* 1986;321:412–7.

94. Feinberg MB, Jarrett RF, Aldonvini A, et al. HTLV-III expression and production involve complex regulation at the levels of splicing and translation of viral RNA. *Cell* 1986;46:807–17.

95. Luciw PA, Cheng-Mayer C, Levy JA. Mutational analysis of the human immunodeficiency virus: the orf-B region down-regulates virus replication. *Proc Natl Acad Sci USA* 1987;84:1434–8.

96. Ahmad H, Venkatesan S. Nef protein of HIV-1 is a transcriptional repressor of HIV-1 LTR. *Science* 1988;241:1481–5.

97. Niederman TMJ, Thielan BJ, Ratner L. Human immunodeficiency virus type 1 negative factor is a transcriptional silencer. *Proc Natl Acad Sci USA* 1989;86:1128–32.

98. Hammes SR, Dixon EP, Malim MH, et al. Nef protein of human immunodeficiency virus type 1: evidence against its role as a transcriptional inhibitor. *Proc Natl Acad Sci USA* 1989;86:9549–53.

99. Kim S, Ilkeuchi K, Byrn R, et al. Lack of a negative influence on viral growth by the nef gene of human immunodeficiency virus type 1. *Proc Natl Acad Sci USA* 1989;86:9544–8.

100. Strebel K, Daugherty D, Clouse K, et al. The HIV "A" (sor) gene product is essential for virus infectivity. *Nature* 1987;328:728–30.

101. Fisher AG, Ensoli B, Ivanoff L, et al. The sor gene of HIV-1 is required for efficient virus transmission in vitro. *Science* 1987;237:888–92.

102. Strebel K, Klimkait T, Maldarelli F, Martin MA. Molecular and biochemical analysis of human immunodeficiency virus type 1 vpu protein. *J Virol* 1989;63:3784–91.

103. Hattori N, Michales F, Fargnoli K, et al. The human immunodeficiency virus type 2 *vpr* gene is essential for productive infection of human macrophages. *Proc Natl Acad Sci USA* 1990;87:8080–4.

104. Kim S, Bryn R, Groopman J, Baltimore D. Temporal aspects of DNA and RNA synthesis during human immunodeficiency virus infection: evidence for differential gene expression. *J Virol* 1989;63:3708–13.

105. Guatelli JC, Gingeras TR, Richman DD. Alternative splice acceptor utilization during human immunodeficiency virus type 1 infection of cultured cells. *J Virol* 1990;64:4093–8.

106. Piot P, Plummer FA, Mhalu FS, et al. AIDS: an international perspective. *Science* 1988;239:573–9.

107. Curran JW, Jaffe HW, Hardy A, et al. Epidemiology of HIV infection and AIDS in the United States. *Science* 1988;239:610–6.

108. Winkelstein W Jr, Piot P. Epidemiology overview. *AIDS* 1989;3[Suppl 1]:S51–S52.

109. Burke DS. Laboratory diagnosis of human immunodeficiency virus infection. In: Judson FN, ed. *Clinics in laboratory medicine,* vol 9. New York: WB Saunders, 1989;369–92.

110. Beneson AS, Peddecord KM, Hoghern LK, et al. Reporting the results of human immunodeficiency tests. *JAMA* 1990;262:3435–40.

111. Croxson T, Mathur-Wagh U, Handwerger S, et al. Prognostic significance of quantitative levels of HIV p24 binding capacity in HIV infection. *AIDS Res Hum Retroviruses* 1990;6:455–63.

112. Special Report, CDC: Interpretation and use of the Western blot assay for serodiagnosis of human immunodeficiency virus type 1 infections. *Lab Med* 1990;21:174–7.

113. Coombs R, Gjerset G, Nikora B, et al. Isolation of human immunodeficiency virus (HIV) from the peripheral blood lymphocytes (PBL) and plasma of asymptomatic and symptomatic HIV seropositive hemophiliacs. *CDC AIDS Weekly* 1988;4:17.

114. Jendis JB, Tomasik Z, Hunziker U, et al. Evaluation of diagnostic tests for HIV infection in infants born to HIV-infected mothers in Switzerland. *AIDS* 1988;2:273–81.

115. Abbott MA, Poiesz BJ, Byren BC et al. Enzymatic gene amplification: qualitative and quantitative methods for detecting proviral DNA amplified in vitro. *J Infect Dis* 1988;158:1158–69.

116. Schnittman SM, Psallidopoulos MC, Lane HC, et al. The reservoir for HIV-1 in peripheral blood is a T cell that maintains expression of CD4. *Science* 1989;245:305–8.

117. Ho DD, Moudgil T, Alam M. Quantitation of human immunodeficiency virus type 1 in the blood of infected persons. *N Engl J Med* 1989;321:1621–5.

118. Brinchmann JE, Albert J, Vartdal F. Few infected CD4+ T cells but a high proportion of replication-competent provirus copies in asymptomatic human immunodeficiency virus type 1 infection. *J Virol* 1991;65:2019–23.

119. Zagury D, Bernard J, Leonard R, et al. Long-term cultures of HTLV-III-infected T cells: a model of cytopathology of T-cell depletion in AIDS. *Science* 1986;231:850–3.

120. Klatzmann D, Gluckman JC. HIV infection: facts and hypotheses. *Immunol Today* 1986;7:291–6.

121. Lynn WS, Tweedale A, Cloyd MW. Human immunodeficiency virus (HIV-1) cytotoxicity: perturbation of the cell membrane and depression of phospholipid synthesis. *Virology* 1988;163:43–51.

122. Cloyd MW, Lynn WS. Perturbation of host-cell membrane is a primary mechanism of HIV cytopathology. *J Virol* 1991;181:500–11.

123. Hoxie JA, Alpers JD, Rackowski J, et al. Alterations in T4(CD4) protein and mRNA synthesis in cells infected with HIV. *Science* 1986;234:1123–7.

124. McDougal JS, Mawle A, Cort SP, et al. Role of T cell activation and expression of the T4 antigen. *J Immunol* 1985;135:3151–62.

125. Ho DD, Pomerantz RJ, Kaplan JC. Pathogenesis of infection with human immunodeficiency virus. *N Engl J Med* 1987;317:278–86.

126. Hildreth JEK, Orentas RJ. Involvement of a leukocyte adhesion receptor (LFA-1) in HIV-induced syncytium formation. *Science* 1989;244:1075–8.

127. Valetin A, Lundin K, Patarroyo M, Asjo B. The leukocyte adhesion glycoprotein CD18 participates in HIV-1-induced syncytia formation in monocytoid and T cells. *J Immunol* 1990;144:934–7.

128. Pantaleo G, Butini L, Graziosi C, et al. Human immunodeficiency virus (HIV) infection in CD4+ T lymphocytes genetically deficient in LFA-1: LFA-1 is required for HIV-mediated cell fusion but not for viral transmission. *J Exp Med* 1991;173:511–4.

129. Cheng-Mayer C, Seto D, Tateno M, Levy JA. Biologic features of HIV-1 that correlate with virulence in the host. *Science* 1988;240:80–2.

130. Fenyo EM, Morfeldt-Manson L, Chiodi F, et al. Distinct replicative and cytopathic characteristics of human immunodeficiency virus isolates. *J Virol* 1988;333:278–80.

131. DeRossi A, Franchini G, Aldonvini A, et al. Differential response to the cytopathic effects of human T-cell lymphotropic virus type III (HTLV-III)-superinfection in T4+ (helper) and T8+ (suppressor) T-cell clones transformed by HTLV-I. *Proc Natl Acad Sci USA* 1986;83:4297–4301.

132. Ziegler JL, Stites DP. Hypothesis: AIDS is an autoimmune disease directed at the immune system and triggered by a lymphotropic retrovirus. *Clin Immunol Immunopathol* 1986;41:305–14.

133. Stricker RB, McHugh TM, Moody DJ, et al. An AIDS-related

cytotoxic autoantibody reacts with a specific antigen on stimulated CD4+ T cells. *Nature* 1987;327:710–3.

134. Schrier RD, Nelson JA, Oldstone MBA. Detection of human cytomegalovirus in peripheral blood lymphocytes in a natural infection. *Science* 1985;230:1048.

135. Schnittman SM, Lane HC, Greenhouse J, et al. Preferential infection of CD4+ memory T cells by human immunodeficiency virus type 1: evidence for a role in the selective T cell functional defects observed in infected individuals. *Proc Natl Acad Sci USA* 1990;87:6058–62.

136. Giulian D, Vaca K, Noonan CA. Secretion of neurotoxins by mononuclear phagocytes infected with HIV. *Science* 1990;250:1593–6.

137. Merrill JE, Koyanagi Y, Chen ISY. Interleukin 1 and tumor necrosis factor a can be induced from mononuclear phagocytes by human immunodeficiency virus type 1 binding to the CD4 receptor. *J Virol* 1989;63:4404–8.

138. Ratner L, Polmar SH, Paul N, Ruddle N. Cytotoxic factors secreted by cells infected by human immunodeficiency virus type I. *AIDS Res Hum Retroviruses* 1987;3:147–55.

139. Margolick DJ, Volkman DJ, Folks TM, Fauci AS. Amplification of HTLV-III/LAV infection by antigen-induced activation of T cells and direct suppression by virus of lymphocyte blastogenic responses. *J Immunol* 1987;138:1719–23.

140. Narayan O, Zink C. Role of macrophages in lentivirus infections. In: Perk K, ed. *Immunodeficiency disorders and retroviruses.* New York: Academic Press, 1987;128–48.

141. Stoler MH, Eskin TA, Benn S, et al. Human T-cell lymphotropic virus type III infection of the central nervous system—a preliminary in situ analysis. *JAMA* 1986;256:2360–4.

142. Wiley CA, Schrier RD, Nelson JA, et al. Cellular localization of human immunodeficiency virus infection within the brains of acquired immune deficiency syndrome patients. *Proc Natl Acad Sci USA* 1986;83:7089–93.

143. Vazeux R, Brousse N, Jarry A, et al. AIDS subacute encephalitis; identification of HIV-infected cells. *Am J Pathol* 1987;126:403–10.

144. Michaels J, Sharer LR, Epstein LG. Human immunodeficiency virus type 1 (HIV-1) infection of the nervous system: a review. *Immunodeficiency Rev* 1988;1:71–104.

145. Gabuzda DH, Ho DD, de al Monte SM, et al. Immunohistochemical identification of HTLV-III antigen in brains of patients with AIDS. *Ann Neurol* 1986;20:289–95.

146. Chayt KJ, Harper ME, Marselle LM, et al. Detection of HTLV-III RNA in lungs of patients with AIDS and pulmonary involvement. *JAMA* 1986;256:2356–9.

147. Le Tourneau A, Audouin J, Diebold J, et al. LAV-like viral particles in lymph node germinal centers in patients with the persistent lymphadenopathy syndrome and the acquired immunodeficiency syndrome-related complex: an ultrastructural study of 30 cases. *Hum Pathol* 1986;17:1047–51.

148. Orenstein JM, Meltzer MS, Phipps T, Gendelman HE. Cytoplasmic assembly and accumulation of human immunodeficiency virus types 1 and 2 in recombinant human colony-stimulating factor-1-treated human monocytes: an ultrastructural study. *J Virol* 1988;62:2578–86.

149. Ringler DJ, Hunt RD, Desrosiers RC, et al. Simian immunodeficiency virus-induced meningoencephalitis: natural history and retrospective study. *Ann Neurol* 1988;23:S101–S107.

150. Gendelman HE, Narayan O, Kennedy-Stoskopf S, et al. Tropism of sheep lentiviruses for monocytes: susceptibility to infection and virus gene expression increases during maturation of monocytes to macrophages. *J Virol* 1986;58:67–74.

151. Gendelman HE, Narayan O, Kennedy-Stoskopf S, et al. Slow virus macrophage interactions: characterization of a transformed cell line of sheep alveolar macrophages that express a marker for susceptibility to ovine-caprine lentivirus infections. *Lab Invest* 1984;51:547–55.

152. Bender BS, Davidson BL, Kline R, Brown C, Quinn T. Role of the mononuclear phagocyte system in the immunopathogenesis of human immunodeficiency virus infection and the acquired immunodeficiency syndrome. *Rev Infect Dis* 1988;10:1142–54.

153. Roy S, Wainberg MA. Role of the mononuclear phagocyte system in the development of acquired immunodeficiency syndrome (AIDS). *J Leuk Biol* 1988;43:91–7.

154. Pauza CD. HIV Persistence in monocytes leads to pathogenesis and AIDS. *Cell Immunol* 1988;112:414–9.

155. Navia BA, Jordan BD, Price RW. The AIDS dementia complex: I. Clinical features. *Ann Neurol* 1986;19:517–24.

156. Navia BA, Cho E-S, Petito CK, Price RW. The AIDS dementia complex: II. Neuropathology. *Ann Neurol* 1986;19:525–35.

157. de la Monte SM, Ho DD, Schooley RT, et al. Subacute encephalomyelitis of AIDS and its relation to HTLV-III infection. *Neurology* 1987;37:562–9.

158. Levy RM, Bredesen DE, Rosenblum ML. Opportunistic central nervous system pathology in patients with AIDS. *Ann Neurol* 1988;23[Suppl]:S7–S12.

159. Snider WD, Simpson MD, Nielsen S, et al. Neurological complications of acquired immune deficiency syndrome: analysis of 50 patients. *Ann Neurol* 1983;14:403–18.

160. Price RW, Sidtis J, Rosenblum M. The AIDS dementia complex: some current questions. *Ann Neurol* 1988;23[Suppl]:S27–S33.

161. Navia BA, Price RW. The acquired immunodeficiency syndrome dementia complex as the presenting or sole manifestation of human immunodeficiency virus infection. *Arch Neurol* 1987;44:65–9.

162. Gabuzda DH, Hirsch MS. Neurologic manifestations of infection with human immunodeficiency virus. Clinical features and pathogenesis. *Ann Intern Med* 1987;107:383–91.

163. Ho DD, Rota TR, Schooley RT, et al. Isolation of HTLV-III from cerebrospinal fluid and neural tissue of patients with neurologic syndromes related to the acquired immunodeficiency syndrome. *N Engl J Med* 1985;313:1493–7.

164. Goudsmit J, Wolters EC, Bakker M, et al. Intrathecal synthesis of antibodies to HTLV-III in patients without AIDS or AIDS related complex. *Br Med J* 1986;292:1231–4.

165. Levy JA, Shimabukuro J, Hollander H, et al. Isolation of AIDS-associated retroviruses from cerebrospinal fluid and brain of patients with neurological symptoms. *Lancet* 1985;2:586–8.

166. Epstein LG, Sharer LR, Goudsmit J. Neurological and neuropathological features of human immunodeficiency virus infection in children. *Ann Neurol* 1988;23[Suppl]:S19–S23.

167. Shaw GM, Harper ME, Hahn BH, et al. HTLV-III infection in brains of children and adults with AIDS encephalopathy. *Science* 1985;227:177–82.

168. Pumarola-Sune T, Navia BA, Cordon-Cardo C, et al. HIV antigen in the brains of patients with the AIDS dementia complex. *Ann Neurol* 1987;21:490–6.

169. Cheng-Mayer C, Rutka JT, Rosenblum ML, et al. Human immunodeficiency virus can productively infect cultured human glial cells. *Proc Natl Acad Sci USA* 1987;84:3526–30.

170. Funke I, Hahn A, Rieber EP, Weiss E, Reithmuller G. The cellular receptor (CD4) of the human immunodeficiency virus is expressed on neurons and glial cells in human brain. *J Exp Med* 1987;165:1230–5.

171. Watkins BA, Dorn HH, Kelly WB, et al. Specific tropism of HIV-1 for microglial cells in primary human brain cultures. *Science* 1990;249:549–53.

172. Grant I, Atkinson JH, Hesselink JR, et al. Evidence for early CNS involvement in AIDS and other HIV infections. *Ann Intern Med* 1987;107:828.

173. Cooper DA, Gold J, Maclean P, et al. Acute AIDS retrovirus infection: Definition of a clinical illness associated with seroconversion. *Lancet* 1985;1:537–40.

174. Hollander H, Stringari S. Human immunodeficiency virus-associated meningitis: clinical course and correlations. *Am J Med* 1987;83:813–6.

175. Ho DD, Sarngadharan MG, Resnick L, et al. Primary human T-lymphotropic virus type III infection. *Ann Intern Med* 1985;103:880–3.

176. Griffin DE, McArthur JC, Cornblath DR. Neopterin and interferon-gamma in serum and cerebrospinal fluid of patients with HIV associated neurologic disease. *Neurology* 1991;4:69–74.

177. Bredesen DE, Messing R. Neurological syndromes heralding the acquired immune deficiency syndrome. *Ann Neurol* 1983;14:141.

178. McArthur JC, Cohen BA, Farzedegan H, et al. Cerebrospinal fluid abnormalities in homosexual men with and without neuropsychiatric findings. *Ann Neurol* 1988;23[Suppl]:S34–S37.

179. Brenneman DE, Westbrook GL, Fitzgerald SP, et al. Neuronal

cell killing by the envelope protein of HIV and its prevention by vasoactive intestinal peptide. *Nature* 1989;335:639–42.

180. Dreyer EB, Kaiser PK, Offermann JT, Lipton SA. HIV-1 coat protein neurotoxicity prevented by calcium channel antagonists. *Science* 1990;248:364–7.

181. Sabatier J-M, Vives E, Mabrouk K, et al. Evidence for neurotoxic activity of tat from human immunodeficiency virus type 1. *J Virol* 1991;65:961–7.

182. Gendelman HE, Phelps W, Fiegenbaum L, et al. Transactivation of the human immunodeficiency virus long terminal repeat sequence by DNA viruses. *Proc Natl Acad Sci USA* 1986;83: 9759–63.

183. Mosca JD, Bednarik DP, Raj NBK, et al. Herpes simplex virus type-1 can reactivate transcription of latent human immunodeficiency virus. *Nature* 1987;325:67–70.

184. Serwadda D, Mugerwa RD, Sewankambo N, et al. Slim disease: a new disease in Uganda and its association with HTLV-III infection. *Lancet* 1985;2:849–52.

185. Belsito DV, Sanchez MR, Baer RL, et al. Reduced Langerhans' cell Ia antigen and ATPase activity in patients with the acquired immunodeficiency syndrome. *N Engl J Med* 1984;310:1279–82.

186. Kanitakis J, Marchand C, Su H, et al. Immunohistochemical study of normal skin of HIV-1-infected patients shows no evidence of infection of epidermal Langerhans' cells by HIV. *AIDS Res Hum Retroviruses* 1989;5:293–302.

187. Giulian D, Vaca K, Noonan CA. Secretion of neurotoxins by mononuclear phagocytes infected with HIV-1. *Science* 1991;250:1593–6.

188. Bryant H, Burgess S, Gendelman HE, et al. Neuronotropic activity associated with monocyte growth factors and products of stimulated monocytes. In: Frederickson RCA, ed. *Peripheral signalling of the brain in neuroimmune and cognitive function.* Toronto: Hogrefe and Huber, [in press].

189. Nabel G, Baltimore D. An inducible transcription factor activates expression of human immunodeficiency virus in T cells. *Nature* 1987;326:711–3.

AIDS and Other Manifestations of HIV Infection,
Second Edition, Edited by Gary P. Wormser.
Raven Press, Ltd., New York © 1992.

CHAPTER 6

Viral Cofactors in the Pathogenesis of HIV Disease

Jeffrey Laurence

The average interval between human immunodeficiency virus (HIV) infection of an adult through sexual intercourse or blood transfusion and development of clinical acquired immunodeficiency syndrome (AIDS) is 10 and 5 years, respectively (1,2). The basis for such a prolonged period of clinical latency, and for the great variability in incubation periods among ostensibly similar hosts, is unclear. Several factors to accommodate such differences have been proposed, such as genetic susceptibility, viral strain diversity, age, development of HIV *env* variations after initial infection, and amount and route of the initial viral inoculum.

The thesis of this chapter is that intermittent activation of HIV expression in latently infected cells, by direct or indirect involvement of other viruses, plays a role in determining the rate of development of HIV-related disease. It is proposed that the slow but relentless progression of immunologic dysfunction and clinical symptomatology characteristic of HIV infection is not because HIV is an intrinsically slow-growing retrovirus, but is rather dependent upon the complex nature of viral gene regulation and interactions among the virus, the target cell, the infected cell, and the host, networks susceptible to modulation by infectious cofactors. This chapter updates material presented by the author in two more extensive reviews (3,4), and introduces a new concept of the virus as superantigen.

EXTENT OF HIV INFECTION IN VIVO

Early in the course of HIV infection absolute numbers of CD4+ T lymphocytes may be within normal limits while many measures of cellular immunity are markedly perturbed. This was initially puzzling as, by the limits of

in situ hybridization, <1 in 10,000 circulating or lymph node-associated mononuclear cells were reported to contain HIV transcripts (5). Recent data indicate, however, that much greater numbers of cells may be chronically infected in vivo, persisting as stationary cell intermediates from which HIV may be induced. Using DNA amplification techniques such as the polymerase chain reaction (PCR), the frequency of infected peripheral CD4+ T lymphocytes in AIDS patients is shown to be at least 1% (6), while in asymptomatic HIV-seropositive individuals it ranges from 0.04% to 1.3% (7). Circulating monocytes do not appear to act as such a reservoir for HIV. For example, using similar techniques one group reported HIV proviral DNA in only 2 of 14 peripheral monocyte samples from HIV-seropositive individuals (6), while another found HIV sequences in all of 27 CD4+ T-cell samples, but in only 2 of 20 monocyte samples (8). This lineage may be an important source of infectious virus in other body compartments. For example, in cerebrospinal fluid, a large percentage of macrophages may be HIV infected, although the ratio of unintegrated to integrated provirus is tenfold higher when compared with CD4+ peripheral T cells (9).

Quantitation of HIV-1 RNA in the peripheral blood of HIV-infected individuals at various stages of disease (10) and direct comparisons of HIV proviral DNA and RNA transcripts by PCR (11) reveal a progressive rise in HIV expression with advancing stages of HIV infection. As shown in Table 1, while proviral DNA was detectable in virtually all HIV-seropositive individuals, there was a trend toward finding higher levels of RNA transcripts in those at more advanced stages of HIV infection. Clearly, longitudinal studies with several samples from each individual are needed to investigate this question fully, but (as a first approximation) increases in HIV RNA may reflect, and perhaps predict, progression of clinical

---

J. Laurence: Department of Medicine, Cornell University Medical College, New York, New York 10021.

TABLE 1. *PCR of DNA and RNA in blood samples grouped according to clinical status at time of collection*

Clinical symptom	T-helper cell (1 μl)	Serum p24 antigen[a]	PCR DNA	PCR RNA
Seropositive				
None	ND	—	ND	—
None	240	—	+	+
None	1,097	—	+++	—
LAS	638	—	−	−
LAS	308	—	+	−
LAS	164	0.119	+	−
LAS	799	—	+	+
LAS	576	—	+	+
LAS	432	—	++	−
LAS	251	—	++	−
LAS	357	0.413	++	+
LAS	244	—	++	+
LAS	ND	0.130	ND	++
LAS	ND	0.802	ND	++
LAS	159	0.319	++	++
LAS	143	—	+++	+
LAS	236	0.314	+++	+++
AIDS	162	—	+	+
AIDS	170	—	+	++
AIDS	525	—	++	−
AIDS	87	—	+++	++
Seronegative				
None	ND	—	−	−

[a] Optical density (A_{492}) of serum antigen assay; only numbers for HIV-positive samples (>0.115) are shown.

[b] +++, ++, +, and − denote high level, intermediate level, low level, and background level, respectively, for relative intensities of oligomer restriction fragment observed in autoradiogram.

AIDS, acquired immunodeficiency syndrome; LAS, lymphadenopathy syndrome; ND, not done; PCR, polymerase chain reaction.

Data derived from Hart et al. (11).

symptoms. These results have recently been extended by findings that increases in plasma viremia (12,13), or HIV transcribing cells detectable by in situ hybridization and laser scanning microscopy (14), may be harbingers of clinical progression. But what leads to such a productive viral infection?

CLINICAL EVIDENCE FOR INVOLVEMENT OF VIRAL COFACTORS

Clinical surveys of virus infections in relationship to HIV induction are difficult to evaluate, as there is a high incidence of seropositivity for most of the candidate viruses among both HIV-infected and sexually active control populations. Serologic studies suggest that herpes simplex virus type 2 (HSV-2) infection is a risk factor for subsequent or concurrent HIV-1 infection (15), but these data give little indication of mechanism. Indeed, HSV-2 may simply facilitate transmission of HIV-1, as it causes visible blistering, erosion, and bleeding of penile, rectal, and vaginal mucosa, and HIV-1 has been isolated from such genital ulcers (16).

Anecdotal reports suggest that concurrent infection with HIV-1 and cytomegalovirus (CMV) produces an atypically severe syndrome. In one preliminary survey primary CMV infection of HIV-seropositive individuals led to a more rapid decline in CD4+ T cell counts than in HIV-seropositive controls unexposed to CMV (17). The overall average decline in CD4+ T cells in HIV-seropositive asymptomatic individuals is about 85 cells/mm^3/year, while in HIV-seropositive CMV converters it was 170 cells/mm^3/year. In another study of 108 HIV-infected hemophiliacs, the risk of advanced HIV disease in CMV-seropositive individuals was 2.5 times that of a similar CMV-seronegative cohort ($p = 0.02$) (18), albeit such a correlation was not recognized by others (19).

Human herpesvirus 6 (HHV-6) is a novel human herpesvirus that has recently received much attention. Although it can infect myriad types of hematopoietic and neuroglial cells, it is primarily tropic and cytopathic in vitro for CD4+ T lymphocytes (20). No apparent serologic distinction between HIV-seronegative and HIV-seropositive groups at various stages of disease has been found, and previous exposure to HHV-6 does not predispose to or affect the course of HIV infection (21). However, differences in expression of HHV-6 may be more pertinent to interactions between HHV-6 and HIV. In situ hybridization of lymph nodes from HIV-seropositive persons revealed HHV-6 in 88%, with an estimated frequency of positive cells of 0.01% (22). In contrast, while 60% of HIV-seronegative individuals with malignant lymphoma are HHV-6 seropositive, only 2% (3/246) had HHV-6 DNA in their lymph nodes (23). These data suggest that HIV may be associated with the activation of HHV-6.

Viruses with more restricted distributions have been more clearly defined clinically as cofactors in HIV expression. Human T-cell lymphotropic virus type I (HTLV-I) was implicated in enhancement of progression to AIDS in a small pilot study in Trinidad. Of 34 asymptomatic HIV-seropositive homosexual men, 9% progressed to AIDS in 3.5 years if infected with HIV-1 alone, whereas 50% ($p = 0.03$) did so if dually infected (24). Recently, two other independent reports have confirmed that HTLV-I or -II can hasten the clinical progression of HIV (25,26). Other viral infections are being pursued in large clinical surveys of HIV seropositive individuals. Hepatitis B virus (HBV) infection, although it can stimulate enhancer regions of HIV in vitro as discussed below, is unrelated to acquisition of HIV-1 infection or more rapid progression of immune deficiency or clinical symptoms (27). It may, however, be a cofactor for malignancy in these individuals, similar to links between cervical and anal carcinoma and papillomaviruses (28), and Epstein-Barr Virus (EBV) and malignant lymphomas (reviewed in ref. 3) in AIDS.

POTENTIAL MECHANISMS FOR VIRAL COFACTORS IN HIV INFECTION BASED ON IN VITRO MODELS

Latency is defined by establishment of a virus in its host, typically for prolonged periods in the absence of symptomatology, followed by occasional episodes of a lytic replicative cycle accompanied by obvious pathology. As such, viral persistence represents an evasion of the host's immune surveillance network. There are two essential elements in the establishment of latency: unique components of viral structure, including *trans*-acting transcriptional activator proteins and their *cis*-responsive targets; and immune responses that are ineffectual in recognizing and clearing viral particles and virus-infected cells.

Infection of resting cells may produce one form of HIV latency, maintained in the absence of necessary cellular factors, with the majority of proviral DNA unintegrated and stably maintained for prolonged periods. Encounters with appropriate stimuli could then result in cell proliferation and a permissive infection. Return of these cells into the resting G_0 state may then establish a second latent form, with integrated but quiescent HIV provirus (29). Subsequent exposure to antigen or cytokines, perhaps induced by viral infections, or to heterologous viral *trans*-acting proteins themselves, could then promote viral reactivation. By this scheme, a viral "cofactor" implies an in vivo activation signal. It would have two critical roles: conversion of a latent or chronic infection to a productive one, and generation of a susceptible population of target cells to facilitate viral spread. These two roles are examined below.

Control of HIV Replication and Cellular Activation

Two groups have recently completed an elegant series of in vitro experiments to define controls on HIV replication at the level of T-cell activation and proviral integration (30,31). Contrary to earlier reports (32), resting T cells can be infected by HIV, although a block to virus replication exists in these cells (30,31). In the absence of immune or viral activation, the number of activated peripheral CD4+ T cells is very low; such cells could not present a frequent target for initial HIV infection. In addition, there is a block to viral integration in resting T cells, with proviral DNA maintained exclusively extrachromosomally. The cytoplasm of these cells contain circular HIV molecules with ligated long terminal repeat (LTR)/LTR junctions. (The significance of LTR sequences will become apparent as they are discussed later on in the context of *trans*-acting factors.) Proviral circles were able to persist in cells in vitro for at least 2 weeks. It was not possible to induce ("rescue") virus from resting T cells harboring such extrachromosomal HIV (30). Un-

like their activated counterparts, infected T cells also maintain their CD4 surface receptors, and are not incorporated efficiently into syncytia (32). Thus, cytopathic effects of HIV-1 replication may be restricted to infected T cells in the activated state. [This does not mean that extrachromosomal viral nucleic acid in resting cells is transcriptionally silent, albeit the types of transcripts made are controversial (30,31).] Subsequent activation of infected resting cells appears to permit provirus integration and virus production within 48 hours.

This model is presented schematically in Fig. 1. Viral cofactors, here represented by HTLV-I and -II, could serve either as a mitogenic stimulus to T-cell activation and HIV integration or, at a later stage, to enhance HIV replication via mechanisms described below. Whether or not the unintegrated HIV genome in quiescent cells can be completely reverse transcribed is controversial. However, it does appear that HIV DNA in these cells is labile, leading to the possibility that it could be completely degraded (31). This process could lead to a self-restricting type of infection, essentially removing infectious virus from the host. Evidence that this may occur in clones of HIV-infected human B cells in vitro supports this intriguing possibility (33).

Viral Cofactors and Transcriptional Regulation

For HIV, as for other mammalian retroviruses, regulatory elements—promoters and enhancers located primarily in the LTR of the proviral DNA—are recognized by host factors, thereby influencing the virus' growth potential in cells of divergent type and state of differentiation. In HIV, both cellular and viral proteins exert their influence, directly or indirectly, on DNA sequences located near the point of RNA initiation, the "cap" site. Transcription via RNA polymerase II is dependent on an initiation complex that forms near this point.

A common motif among these pathways is the enhancer nucleic acid sequence nuclear factor κB (NFκB). NFκB is a potent *cis*-acting regulatory sequence first noted in the κ light chain immunoglobulin promoter, and now known to be present in regulatory sequences for the interleukin-2 receptor alpha subunit (Tac) and in CMV, as well as in HIV. At least four NFκB proteins bind to these enhancer elements and are referred to by their molecular weight in kilodaltons: p50, p55, p75, and p85; all are structurally related to the *v-rel* oncogene (34). In HIV-infected cells, the 50-kd cellular protein has been shown to bind to specific sequences in the HIV LTR. In so doing, it can markedly upregulate transcription initiated by the HIV *trans*-acting protein Tat, encoded by its *tat* gene. The p50 NFκB cellular protein is usually complexed to a 65-kd protein, as well as to one of two forms of an inhibitory protein, either the 37-kd IkB-α or the 45-kd IkB-β, which inhibits its activity (29). Phosphory-

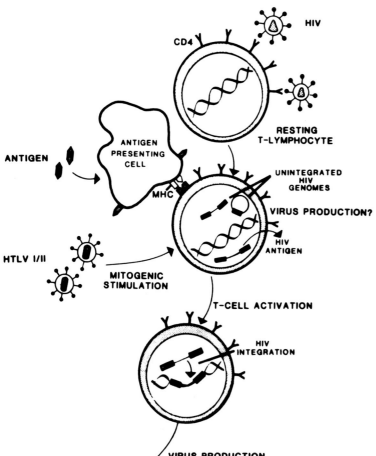

FIG. 1. Proposed scheme for infection of resting CD4+ T lymphocytes with HIV, and induction of HIV from such a reservoir. Following HIV infection of quiescent T cells, proviral DNA is maintained in an extrachromosomal state (linear and circular forms are depicted). These transcriptionally active forms may contribute to the HIV antigen pool, although this point is controversial. Viral integration may occur upon cellular activation mediated through viral cofactors such as human T-cell leukemia virus and (*HTLV*)-*I* -*II*. Unrestricted viral replication could then follow, with superinfection by HIV, and cytopathic effects. From Stevenson et al. (30).

lation of IkB by protein kinase C may release the active species from its inactive cytosolic form and permit translocation of NFκB to the nucleus (35). Such activation by protein kinases, inducing NFκB expression, may be one method by which mitogenic stimulation, either via antigen recognition or viral infection, serves as a cofactor for the regulation of HIV. This hypothesis is illustrated in the first part of Fig. 2.

Alternatively, viruses may encode their own *trans*-acting factors, which can activate HIV expression through specific sequences in the HIV LTR (36). This process is illustrated in Fig. 2 by the E1A transforming protein of adenovirus. The ability to *trans*-activate HIV in vitro has similarly been demonstrated for all of the herpesviruses—CMV, EBV, HSV-1 and -2, and HHV-6 (reviewed in refs. 3 and 4)—as well as HBV (37), HTLV-I and -II (38), and papovaviruses (39,40). Some of the sites in the HIV-LTR that appear to be important for the various viral factors are illustrated in Fig. 3.

Of course, such direct mechanisms would require coinfection of a single cell with HIV and the viral cofactor. Using double-labeling in situ techniques, it was shown that CMV and HIV can coinfect the same cell in vivo, at least in the central nervous system. This coinfection of HIV harboring cells by CMV is a common event, occurring with a frequency > 10% (41). Such dual infection of monocytes and T cells can upregulate the level of HIV

produced (42) as well as enhance cytopathicity (43). These phenomena are not always straightforward, however. For example, while there is general agreement that HHV-6 sequences can activate the HIV LTR, in some systems coinfection with HHV-6 leads to an inhibition, rather than stimulation, of HIV replication (44,45).

Under most circumstances, however, dual infection will still be a rare event. Instead, cofactor viruses may induce cytokines that then activate HIV in latently infected cells. Active HIV replication may, in turn, enhance secretion of these same cytokines in a positive feedback loop, further facilitating the spread of HIV. This has been demonstrated in vivo with factors induced by EBV or CMV infection of monocytes (46). Alternatively, mammalian retroviruses may stimulate selected cells by acting as "superantigens." Superantigens are molecules capable of bridging major histo-compatibility complex class II molecules with T cells bearing certain T cell receptor V_β (variable region of the β chain of this dimeric molecule) gene products. This interaction may lead to cell activation, lymphokine secretion, and upregulation of viral replication. Data from our laboratory (J. Laurence et al.) suggest that HIV-1 can act in this manner.

Finally, viruses may serve as cofactors by altering receptor biology. The high-affinity receptor for HIV is CD4. However, alternate low-affinity receptors also ap-

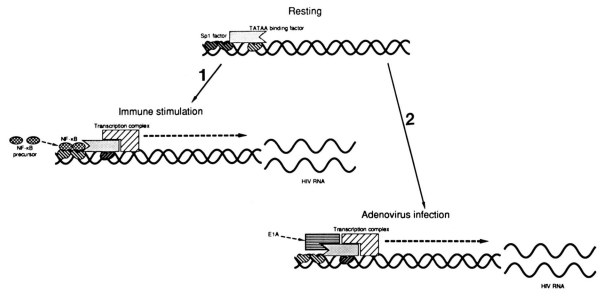

FIG. 2. Alternate pathways for activation of HIV at the level of transcription. **1:** Induction of HIV mRNA in activated CD4+ T cells may be mediated by NF𝑘B, as its precursor form is induced upon mitogenic or antigenic stimulation (e.g., viral). **2:** Viruses may serve directly as cofactors for transcriptional activation of HIV through its long terminal repeat (LTR), acting on regions apart from NF𝑘B, as illustrated here for the adenovirus EIA protein. Modified from Nabel (36).

pear to exist, enabling uptake of HIV into cells that lack detectable surface CD4 or CD4 transcripts. These include Fc-γ and complement (CR3) receptors. If Fc receptor-mediated HIV infection is significant in vivo, induction of these molecules by herpesviruses on target cells (47) should be considered another means by which HIV and herpesviruses interact. Indeed, human lung fibroblasts can be rendered susceptible to HIV by CMV-induced Fc receptor expression (48). Phenotypic mixtures of viral pseudotypes, by which the nucleic acid of one virus becomes encapsidated by proteins from an unrelated virus, have also been reported between HIV and HSV-1 (49) and between HIV and HTLV-I and -II (50). Such hybrid progeny could alter cell tropisms, providing a brief window by which HIV can extend its host range or escape neutralization. A summary of the potential means by which viruses could serve as co-factors for the enhancement of cytopathology by HIV is given in Table 2.

Potential for Therapeutic Intervention

Attempts to block acquisition or reactivation of herpetic infections might inhibit facilitation of HIV transmission through prevention of anogenital or oral ulcerations. However, as most HIV-seropositive individuals show evidence of prior herpesvirus infections, and up to 20% of HIV seropositive intravenous drug users are already coinfected with HTLV-II (51), primary prevention is often not possible. Methods to intervene, directly or indirectly, in HIV–viral cofactor interactions may be feasible. Inhibition of active HIV replication with antiviral nucleoside analogs such as zidovudine [3'-azido-3'-deoxythymidine (AZT)] might be coupled with control of active herpesvirus replication and induction of cellular lymphoproliferation with drugs such as ganciclovir, phosphonoformate, and acyclovir; blockade of induction of latent HIV infection by anti-protein kinase C

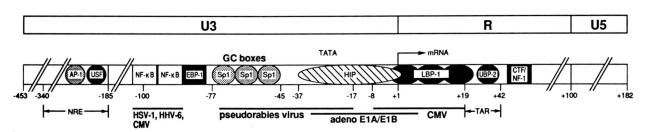

FIG. 3. Regulatory elements of the HIV-1 LTR, with regions important for transactivation by viral factors. *CMV,* cytomegalovirus; *HHV-6,* human herpersvirus 6; *HSV-1,* herpes simplex virus 1; *NRE,* negative regulatory element; *TAR, trans*-acting response element, the binding site for the *tat* gene product. Modified from Barry et al. (40).

TABLE 2. *Summary of mechanisms by which viruses may serve as cofactors in HIV pathogenesis*

Induction of proliferation in resting, latently infected cells via mitogenic, antigenic or superantigen stimulation
Coinfection, directly stimulating transcriptional regulators of HIV
Induction of cytokines or stress molecules (e.g., heat shock protein), which act on transcriptional regulators of HIV or facilitate syncytium formation
Upregulation of HIV receptors
Formatin of viral pseudotypes with altered host tropism

agents and anticytokine monoclonal antibodies; and inhibition of viral release by α-interferon.

In vitro, protein kinase C antagonists H-7 (52,53), staurosporine (53), tamoxifen (54), and scavengers for reactive oxidative intermediates such as N-acetyl-L-cysteine (55) inhibit stimulation of the HIV LTR and upregulation of HIV virions from chronically infected cell lines. These agents may act by inhibiting induction of regulatory molecules such as NFκB, or interacting with negative regulating elements in the HIV LTR (54,55). Prevention of the binding of NFκB and other activation factors to viral enhancer sequences, by way of peptides, chelating agents, or "antisense" oligonucleotides, is also being evaluated. In terms of cytokine activation, transforming growth factor beta (TGF-β) potently suppresses the upregulation of HIV expression in chronically infected cell lines stimulated with interleukin-6, granulocyte–monocyte colony-stimulating factor, or endotoxin-activated monocyte supernatants (56), and antitumor necrosis factor/cachexin (anti-TNF-α) antibodies have similar effects (57). Other inhibitors of TNF-α such as pentoxifylline (58) are already being evaluated in HIV-infected individuals. Should the HIV-associated superantigen phenomenon prove important *in vivo,* methods of blocking interactions with the pertinent V$_{\beta}$-expressing CD4+ T cells could be utilized, a concept proven feasible in animals affected by bacterial superantigens. There is a pressing need to devote increased resources to exploring such means for blocking activation of latent HIV, interfering with the acquisition and replication of those viruses or their induced cytokines. The ultimate goal is development of a chronic therapy for asymptomatic HIV-seropositive individuals.

REFERENCES

1. Lui K-J, Darrow WW, Rutherford GW III. A model-based estimate of the mean incubation periods for AIDS in homosexual men. *Science* 1988;240:1333–5.
2. Costagliola D, Mary J-Y, Brouard N, Laporte A, Valleron A-J. Incubation time for AIDS from French transfusion-associated cases. *Nature* 1989;338:768–9.
3. Laurence J. Molecular interactions among herpesviruses and human immunodeficiency viruses. *J Infect Dis* 1990;162:338–46.
4. Laurence J. Herpesviruses as co-factors in the immunopathogenesis of AIDS. *Dev Med Virol* 1990;6:249–88.
5. Harper ME, Masselle LM, Gallo RC, Wong-Staal F. Detection of lymphocytes expressing human T lymphotropic virus type III in lymph nodes and peripheral blood from infected individuals by in situ hybridization. *Proc Natl Acad Sci USA* 1986;83:772–6.
6. Schnittman SM, Psallidopoulos MC, Lane HC, et al. The reservoir for HIV-1 in human peripheral blood is a T cell that maintains expression of CD4. *Science* 1989;244:305–7.
7. Psallidopoulos MC, Schnittman SM, Thompson LM III, et al. Integrated proviral human immunodeficiency virus type 1 is present in CD4+ peripheral blood lymphocytes in healthy seropositive individuals. *J Virol* 1989;63:4626–44.
8. Spear GT, Chin-Yih O, Kessler HA, Moore JC, Schochetman G, Landay AL. Analysis of lymphocytes, monocytes, and neutrophils from human immunodeficiency virus (HIV)-infected persons for HIV DNA. *J Infect Dis* 1990;162:1239–44.
9. Pang S, Koyanagi Y, Miles S, Wiley C, Vinters HV, Chen ISY. High levels of unintegrated HIV-1 DNA in brain tissue of AIDS dementia patients. *Nature* 1990;343:85–9.
10. Solomon R, Thompson J, Gillespie D. Quantitation of HIV-1 RNA in blood cells of ARC and AIDS patients. *J Clin Lab Anal* 1989;3:282–6.
11. Hart C, Spira T, Moore J, et al. Direct detection of HIV RNA expression in seropositive subjects. *Lancet* 1988;2:596–9.
12. Ho DD, Moudgil T, Alam M. Quantification of human immunodeficiency virus type 1 in the blood of infected persons. *N Engl J Med* 1989;321:1621–5.
13. Coombs RW, Collier AC, Allain JP, et al. Plasma viremia in human immunodeficiency virus infection. *N Engl J Med* 1989;321:1626–31.
14. Lewis DE, Minshall M, Wray NP, Paddock SW, Smith LC, Crane MM. Confocal microscopic detection of human immunodeficiency virus RNA producing cells. *J Infect Dis* 1990;162:1373–8.
15. Holmberg SD, Stewert JA, Gerber AR, et al. Prior herpes simplex virus type 2. Infection as a risk factor for HIV infection. *JAMA* 1988;259:1048–50.
16. Kreiss JK, Coombs R, Plummer F, et al. Isolation of human immunodeficiency virus from genital ulcers in Nairobi prostitutes. *J Infect Dis* 1989;160:380–4.
17. Smith K. Am Soc Microbiol, Anaheim, CA, May, 1990.
18. Webster A, Lee CA, Cook DG, et al. Cytomegalovirus infection and progression towards AIDS in hemophiliacs with human immunodeficiency virus. *Lancet* 1989;2:63–5.
19. Goedert JJ. AIDS in subjects with hemophilia. *N Engl J Med* 1990;322:1234.
20. Takahashi K, Sonoda S, Higashi K, et al. Predominant CD4+-lymphocyte tropism of human herpesvirus 6-related virus. *J Virol* 1989;63:3161–3.
21. Spira TJ, Bozeman LH, Sanderlin KC, et al. Lack of correlation between human herpesvirus-6 infection and the course of human immunodeficiency virus infection. *J Infect Dis* 1990;161:567–70.
22. Krueger GRF, Koch B, Raman A, et al. Antibody prevalence to HBLV (human herpesvirus-6, HHV-6) and suggestive pathogenicity in the general population and in patients with immune deficiency syndromes. *J Virol Methods* 1988;21:125–31.
23. Josephs SF, Buchbinder A, Streicher HZ, et al. Detection of human B-lymphotropic virus (human herpesvirus 6) sequences in B cell lymphoma tissue of three patients. *Leukemia* 1988;2:132–5.
24. Bartholomew C, Blattner W, Cleghorn F. Progression to AIDS in homosexual men co-infected with HIV and HTLV-I in Trinidad. *Lancet* 1987;2:1469.
25. Hattori T, Koito A, Takatsuki K, et al. Frequent infection with human T-cell lymphotropic virus type I in patients with AIDS, but not in carriers of human immunodeficiency virus type 1. *J AIDS* 1989;2:272–6.
26. Weiss SH, French J, Holland B, et al. HTLV-I, -II coinfection is significantly associated with risk for progression to AIDS among

HIV seropositive drug abusers. 6th International Conference on AIDS, Montreal, Canada, June 1989; ThAO23 (abst).

27. Solomon RE, van Raden M, Kaslow RA, et al. Association of hepatitis B surface antigen and core antibody with acquisition and manifestations of human immunodeficiency virus type 1 (HIV-1) infection. *Am J Public Health* 1990;80:1475–8.

28. Caussy D, Goedert JJ, Palefsky J, et al. Interaction of human immunodeficiency and papilloma viruses: association with anal epithelial abnormality in homosexual men. *Int J Cancer* 1990;46:214–9.

29. Cullen BR, Green WC. Regulatory pathways governing HIV-1 replication. *Cell* 1989;58:423–6.

30. Stevenson M, Stanwick TL, Dempsey MP, Lamonica LA. HIV-1 replication is controlled at the level of T cell activation and proviral integration. *EMBO J* 1990;5:1551–60.

31. Zack JA, Arrigo SJ, Weitsman SR, Go AS, Haislip A, Chen ISY. HIV-1 entry into quiescent primary lymphocytes: molecular analysis reveals a labile, latent viral structure. *Cell* 1990;61:213–22.

32. Gowda SD, Stein BS, Mohagheghpour H, Benike CJ, Engleman EG. Evidence that T cell activation is required for HIV-1 entry in CD4+ T lymphocytes. *J Immunol* 1989;142:773–80.

33. Dahl KE, Burrage T, Jones J, Miller G. Persistent nonproductive infection of Epstein-Barr virus-transformed human B lymphocytes by human immunodeficiency virus type 1. *J Virol* 1990;64:1771–83.

34. Ballard DW, Walker WH, Doerre S, et al. The v-*rel* oncogene encodes a kB enhancer binding protein that inhibits NFκB function. *Cell* 1990;63:803–14.

35. Zabel U, Baeurele PA. Purified human IkB can rapidly dissociate the complex of the NFκB transcription factor with its cognate DNA. *Cell* 1990;61:255–65.

36. Nabel GJ. Activation of human immunodeficiency virus. *J Lab Clin Med* 1988;111:495–500.

37. Twu J-S, Rosen CA, Haseltine WA, Robinson WS. Identification of a region within the human immunodeficiency virus type 1 long terminal repeat that is essential for transactivation by the hepatitis B virus gene X. *J Virol* 1989;63:2857–60.

38. Greene WC, Bohnlein E, Ballard DW. HIV-1, HTLV-I and normal T-cell growth: transcriptional strategies and surprises. *Immunol Today* 1989;10:272–8.

39. Gendelman HE, Phelps W, Feigenbaum L, et al. Trans-activation of the human immunodeficiency virus long terminal repeat sequence by DNA viruses. *Proc Natl Acad Sci USA* 1986;83:9759–63.

40. Barry PA, Pratt-Lowe E, Peterlin BM, Luciw PA. Cytomegalovirus activates transcription directed by the long terminal repeat of human immunodeficiency virus type 1. *J Virol* 1990;64:2932–40.

41. Nelson JA, Reynolds-Kohler C, Oldstone MBA, Wiley CA. HIV and HCMV coinfect brain cells in patients with AIDS. *Virology* 1988;165:286–90.

42. Skolnik PR, Kosloff BR, Hirsch MS. Bidirectional interactions between human immunodeficiency virus type 1 and cytomegalovirus. *J Infect Dis* 1988;157:508–14.

43. Casareale D, Fiala M, Chang CM, Cone LA, Macarski ES. Cytomegalovirus enhances lysis of HIV-infected T lymphoblasts. *Int J Cancer* 1989;44:124–30.

44. Levy JA, Larday A, Lennette ET. Human herpesvirus 6 inhibits human immunodeficiency virus type 1 replication in cell culture. *J Clin Microsc* 1990;28:2362–4.

45. Carrigan DR, Knox KK, Tapper MA. Suppression of human immunodeficiency virus type 1 replication by human herpesvirus-6. *J Infect Dis* 1990;162:844–51.

46. Clouse KA, Robbins PB, Fernie B, Ostrove JM, Fauci AS. Viral antigen stimulation of the production of human monokines capable of regulating HIV-1 expression. *J Immunol* 1989;143:470–5.

47. Johansson PJH, Hardela FA, Sjoquist J, Schroder AK, Christensen P. Herpes simplex 1-induced Fc receptor binds to the C gamma-C gamma 3 interface region of IgG in the area that binds staphylococcal protein A. *Immunology* 1989;66:8–13.

48. Mckeating JA, Griffiths PD, Weiss RA. HIV susceptibility conferred to human fibroblasts by cytomegalovirus-induced Fc receptor. *Nature* 1990;343:659–61.

49. Zhu Z, Chen SSL, Huang AS. Phenotypic mixing between human immunodeficiency virus and vesicular stomatitis virus or herpes simplex virus. *J AIDS* 1990;3:215–9.

50. Lusso P, Lori F, Gallo RC. CD4-independent infection by human immunodeficiency virus type 1 after phenotypic mixing with human T-cell leukemia viruses. *J Virol* 1990;64:6341–4.

51. Lee H, Swanson P, Shorty W, Zack JA, Rosenblatt JD, Chen ISY. High rate of HTLV-II infection in seropositive i.v. drug abusers in New Orleans. *Science* 1988;244:471–5.

52. Tong-Starkson SE, Luciw PA, Peterlin BM. Signalling through T lymphocyte surface proteins, TCR/CD3 and CD38, activates the HIV-1 long terminal repeat. *J Immunol* 1989;142:702–7.

53. Laurence J, Sikder SK, Jhaveri S, Solomon JE. Phorbol ester-mediated induction of HIV-1 from a chronically infected promonocyte clone: blockade by protein kinase inhibitors and relationship to *tat*-directed *trans*-activation. *Biochem Biophys Res Commun* 1990;166:349–57.

54. Laurence J, Cooke H, Sikder SK. Effect of tamoxifen on regulation of viral replication and human immunodeficiency virus (HIV) long terminal repeat-directed transcription in cells chronically infected with HIV-1. *Blood* 1990;75:696–703.

55. Staal FJT, Roederer M, Herzenberg LA. Intracellular thiols regulate activation of nuclear factor kB and transcription of human immunodeficiency virus. *Proc Natl Acad Sci USA* 1990;87:9943–7.

56. Fauci AS. Cytokine regulation of HIV expression. *Lymphokine Res* 1990;9:527–31.

57. Poli G, Bressler P, Kinter A, et al. Interleukin 6 induces human immunodeficiency virus expression in infected monocytic cells alone and in synergy with tumor necrosis factor α by transcriptional and post-transcriptional mechanisms. *J Exp Med* 1990;172:151–8.

58. Fazely F, Dezube BJ, Allen-Ryan J, Pardee AB, Ruprecht RM. Pentoxifylline (trental) decreases the replication of the human immunodeficiency virus type 1 in human peripheral blood mononuclear cells and in cultured T cells. *Blood* 1991;77:1653–9.

AIDS and Other Manifestations of HIV Infection,
Second Edition, Edited by Gary P. Wormser.
Raven Press, Ltd., New York © 1992.

CHAPTER 7

Virologic and Biologic Features of HIV-2

Phyllis J. Kanki

The history of retrovirology began with the discovery and characterization of animal retroviruses in inbred strains of mice and chickens. Subsequent studies of these agents led to the first descriptions of oncogenes and their role in cancer development. Retroviruses were also discovered in a variety of outbred animal species including cats, cows, monkeys, and others. In many of these animal systems the retrovirus infection resulted in the development of a variety of cancers. Studies of retroviruses in outbred animal systems demonstrated the broad spectrum of disease that these agents were capable of producing.

In 1980, Gallo and colleagues (1) reported the isolation of the first human retrovirus, human T-cell leukemia virus [now termed human T-lymphotropic virus (HTLV-I)]. HTLV-I is widely believed to play an etiologic role in the development of adult T-cell leukemia/lymphoma and also tropical spastic paraparesis (2,3). HTLV-II is closely related to HTLV-I and was first isolated from a T-cell variant form of hairy cell leukemia; its definitive role in human cancer or disease is still under investigation (4). Polymerase chain reaction (PCR) technology and type-specific serology have allowed the distinction of these closely related HTLVs, and a more precise picture of the epidemiology and geographic distribution of these viruses is now becoming apparent (5,6). Soon after the discovery of HTLV-I and HTLV-II, a closely related simian virus, simian T-lymphotropic virus (STLV-I), was described by Miyoshi and colleagues (7). STLV-I is now known to infect most species of Old World monkeys and great apes (8). Similar to its human counterpart, this virus is capable of in vitro lymphocyte immortalization and in vivo has been linked with spontaneous lymphoid malignancy in the simian host (9). Molecular genetic studies indicate that STLV-I

and HTLV-I are closely related and sequence analysis of the STLV-I genome shows close to 95% homology with similar genomic organization (10).

In the early 1980s, the acquired immunodeficiency syndrome (AIDS) was first described as a clinical and epidemiological entity. It is now well recognized that AIDS is caused by an exogenous human retrovirus termed human immunodeficiency virus type 1 (HIV-1) (11,12). The complexities of HIV-1 extend from the intricate genetic machinery that finely controls virus replication to the panorama of clinical and epidemiological features of this viral infection in humans (13). The identification of new human retroviruses linked to significant disease promoted renewed interest in the search for other animal and human retroviruses. Early in 1985, a related virus, simian immunodeficiency virus (SIV), was found in immunodeficient macaque monkeys. SIV was found to have major viral antigens that were similar and cross-reactive with the viral antigens of HIV-1 (14). SIV is known to induce immunosuppression in most Asian macaque species and thus represents an excellent animal model for the study of immunodeficiency virus pathogenesis. However, SIV in its natural hosts, the African green monkey, mangabey, and perhaps other African primates, appears to infect significant numbers of these species and yet to be relatively nonpathogenic (14–18). The existence of a simian relative of HIV-1 found in large numbers of naturally infected African primates suggested the possibility that people might also be susceptible to infection with a SIV-related virus (14,15,19).

In 1985, a new human T-lymphotropic retrovirus was discovered in Senegal, West Africa (19,20). We observed antibodies in healthy Senegalese that demonstrated strong reactivity to the *env, gag,* and *pol* antigens of SIV. When reacted with HIV-1, these same serum samples showed only weak cross-reactive antibodies to the *gag* and *pol* antigens. It was therefore recognized that these individuals had been exposed to a virus more closely related to SIV and more distantly related to the proto-

P. J. Kanki: Department of Cancer Biology, Harvard School of Public Health and the Harvard AIDS Institute, Boston, Massachusetts 02115.

type AIDS virus, HIV-1 (19,20). Subsequently, Clavel and colleagues (21) demonstrated similar SIV antibody reactivity in two AIDS patients originating from West Africa. This new human retrovirus has now been termed human immunodeficiency virus type 2 (HIV-2) (22). Various strain names have been given to HIV-2, including lymphadenopathy virus (LAV)-2, SBL-6669, and HTLV-4 (ST). It is now believed that these are all the same virus type. All HIV-2 strains thus far identified are serologically cross-reactive and therefore, most serology-based studies are not thought to be strain specific (22–25).

VIROLOGY

Both HIV-1 and HIV-2 are human lentiviruses with a number of similar virologic properties. Both viruses have a target cell tropism for CD4+ T lymphocytes and a propensity for establishing latent infections. Like other retroviruses, the HIVs are single positive-strand RNA viruses with particles approximately 100 nm in diameter. Virions have a characteristic dense, cylindrical protein core that encases the genomic RNA molecules and viral enzymes (reverse transcriptase, integrase, and protease). This ultrastructural morphology is indistinguishable from other animal lentiviruses and distinct from type C retroviruses including HTLV (26). The binding of the envelope of HIV to the CD4 molecule is only a first step in viral entry, with subsequent fusion events that appear to require both viral envelope and other cellular factors (27,28). HIV-2 isolates have demonstrated tropism for cells bearing the CD4 marker, similar to both HIV-1 and SIV. Blocking studies with recombinant soluble CD4 have verified that SIV and HIV-2, like HIV-1, bind via their external envelope glycoprotein, gp120, to a common cellular receptor, the differentiation antigen CD4 (29–31). It is of interest that HIV-2 has a lower binding affinity for the CD4 receptor as compared with HIV-1 (31).

Once inside the cell, the processes of reverse transcription and integration occur. The HIV replication cycle is unique, with a complex array of various viral-encoded factors that regulate both positively and negatively on the level of virus expression. This culminates in the final steps of virus assembly, maturation, and release, similar to other retroviruses. HIV replication is closely linked to the death of the CD4+ cell. This cytopathicity is a hallmark of HIV infection and has been studied extensively both in vitro and in vivo. In vitro studies of HIV-2 isolates by a number of laboratories have described differences in cytopathicity of HIV-2 as compared with HIV-1 (32–34). In comparison with HIV-1, HIV-2 isolates demonstrate decreased cell killing, less syncytial cell formation, reduced virus replication, and differences in interaction with CD4, in some cases related to the clinical stage of the HIV-2-infected individual (32–34).

The antigenic relatedness of both SIV and HIV-2 to the prototype HIV-1 virus prompted both the discovery and further classification of these related viruses (14,19,20,23). Subsequent genetic analysis confirmed the relationships indicated by antigenic studies, demonstrating that HIV-2 was more closely related to SIV than to HIV-1 (approximately 40% nucleotide homology) (35–37). Similar to HIV-1, restriction site polymorphism and sequence data indicate variability among HIV-2 strains (38,39). As more sequence data have become available from various HIV-2 and SIV strains, it has also become apparent that no branching order of divergence can be specified and that these virus types may in fact share a common ancestor (40). Sequence variability of structural genes such as env and gag has been similar between HIV-2 and HIV-1, with greater variability in the env genes. Interestingly, regulatory gene sequences are more variable among HIV-2 isolates compared with HIV-1 (41).

The overall genomic organizations of HIV-1 and HIV-2/SIV are similar except for the presence of the unique gene termed vpx found in both HIV-2 and SIV (36,37) and the vpu gene unique to HIV-1. The major viral antigens of HIV-2 have been identified by immunoblot and radioimmunoprecipitation analysis; they bear striking similarity and cross-reactive epitopes with the viral antigens of HIV-1 (19,23,41,42). The gag-encoded products include a p55 myristylated precursor, a major core protein, p24–26, and an amino-terminal myristylated gag protein, p15 (14,20,23). The pol-encoded proteins, readily distinguished by immunoblot and radioimmunoprecipitation of virus preparations, include a p64, p53, and p34 (endonuclease) (14,23,42). The gag and pol genes are well conserved for both HIVs and SIV (36,37). The gag- and pol-encoded proteins exhibit broad serological cross-reactivity. It is the presence of cross-reactive antigens primarily from the gag and pol genes that enables the frequent detection of HIV-2 antibodies in HIV-1 serologic assays.

The most highly immunogenic antigens are the env-related glycoproteins, which include a gp160 precursor polyprotein, the mature envelope glycoprotein, gp120, and the transmembrane gp32–40. There appears to be polymorphism in the env-related glycoproteins, similar to what has been previously observed in different strains of HTLV-I (23,43,44). The env genes of HIV-1 and HIV-2 show less conservation at a genetic and antigenic level, whereas HIV-2 and SIV show a high degree of conservation. Sequence analysis of several HIV-2 and SIV strains has demonstrated a stop codon in the middle of the open reading frame encoding the transmembrane protein (36,37); this finding explains the smaller transmembrane protein size that is seen with certain HIV-2 isolates (33,43). It is not known whether the presence of two different sized transmembrane proteins in in vitro cell systems indicates a mixture of virus strains or one virus strain capable of modulating expression of the transmembrane stop codon. Furthermore, the in vivo significance of this unique property of HIV-2 and SIV isolates is unknown.

Nucleotide sequence comparison between HIV-1 and HIV-2 or SIV has revealed similar conserved domains scattered throughout the entire envelope gene, including the proposed CD4-binding site of gp120 (36,37,40). Variable domains show multiple point mutations and deletions. At the amino-acid level, there is approximately 50% homology between the env-encoded products of HIV-1 and HIV-2. It is still not known whether some of the conserved domains of the env gene are immunogenic and/or capable of eliciting a cross-protective response to both virus types. Virus neutralization studies have shown that a high proportion of HIV-2-positive sera are capable of cross-neutralizing HIV-1 isolates in addition to neutralizing HIV-2 isolates (45,46). The degree to which HIV-1-positive sera can cross-neutralize HIV-2 isolates remains controversial. (45,46). Ljundgren and coworkers have reported a lack of cross-reaction between HIV-1 and HIV-2 in antibody-dependent cellular cytotoxicity (ADCC) studies (47).

The human and primate immunodeficiency viruses share a number of unique properties when compared with other known human and animal retroviruses. One of these unique features includes the complex genetic structure that encodes for the typical structural proteins of the virus as well as for at least six regulatory genes. Present data suggest that the function of these genes is complex, with positive and negative feedback loops that affect virus replication, viral transcription, and viral translation (13). For instance, functional evidence of tat activity has been shown for HIV-2 and SIV, similar to and cross-reactive with HIV-1 tat (48,37). It appears that with appropriate serologic assays, specific antibodies can be detected to all of the known HIV-1 gene products in infected individuals, although at varying rates (49–54). It is not known if differential responses to these viral antigens are important in the pathogenesis of HIV infection, or if they can be utilized as prognostic markers for disease progression.

The regulatory gene products common to both HIV-1 and HIV-2 include vif (p23), tat (p14), rev (p19), nef (p27), and vpr (p18). In addition, HIV-1 has a unique regulatory gene product, vpu (p15), and HIV-2 has a unique regulatory gene product, vpx (p16) (54,55). The regulatory gene products of HIV-2 have been identified by sequence analysis and in many cases can be assayed in conventional immunoblot or radioimmunoprecipitation (RIP)–sodium dodecyl sulfate/polyacrylamide gel electrophoresis (SDS/PAGE) (e.g., nef, tat, and vpx) (56). Little is currently known regarding the immunogenicity of HIV-2 regulatory proteins in vivo. Our preliminary data suggest that they are less uniformly immunogenic, similar to the HIV-1 system. These less immunoreactive

serologic markers may not be useful for serodiagnosis but might assist in discriminating virus types or active from passive antibodies in mother–infant pairs.

vpx is a regulatory gene unique to HIV-2 and SIV, and is absent in HIV-1 (55). We have analyzed a number of HIV-2 strains that productively make virus to determine the expression of vpx antigen using radioimmunoprecipitation of cysteine-labeled whole-cell homogenates reacted with heterologous goat antisera raised to recombinant vpx. Our results indicate that despite roughly equivalent reverse transcriptase levels and expression of structural gene products, there is discernible variation in the expression of vpx among various HIV-2 isolates (57). Yu et al. (58) have described studies suggesting that vpx mutants may be more cytolytic than wild-type virus in certain T-cell lines. Continued analysis of the function of these regulatory genes and correlation with in vivo events may provide important clues on the mechanisms of pathogenicity employed by HIV viruses.

SERODIAGNOSIS

The close antigenic relationship of HIV-1 and HIV-2 has created new problems for serologic diagnosis. Currently employed HIV-1 immunoassays demonstrate variable sensitivity for detecting HIV-2 antibody, depending on the testing format and antigen preparation used (59,60). HIV-1 recombinant-based and/or competition-type assays are frequently more type-specific and therefore do not readily detect HIV-2 antibody-positive samples. In contrast, many of the commonly used commercial first-generation HIV-1 antibody enzyme-linked immunosorbent assays (ELISAs) detected over 80% of HIV-2-positive samples (60). The latter results can be attributed to the fact that HIV-2 antibody-positive sera frequently contain high-titer antibodies directed at the cross-reactive epitopes that exist between the virus types. A number of assays formatted like ELISAs are currently being developed to screen for both virus types. These tests if employed in a serodiagnostic algorithm will require further immunoblot analysis of both HIV-1 and HIV-2 antigens or type-specific synthetic peptide assays to confirm virus type. Current recommendations for immunoblot diagnostic criteria require the presence of antibodies directed at two env-encoded proteins ± gag- or pol-encoded proteins for specific virus type diagnosis (61).

In Burkina Faso and Côte d'Ivoire significant rates of infection with both HIV-1 and HIV-2 are seen in risk populations (62,63). In these countries a number of individuals were found who possess antibodies with strong reactivity to the env antigens, particularly the gp120, of both HIV-1 and HIV-2 (62,63). This type of serologic profile has been termed "dual reactive." "Dual-reactive" sera are defined as sera that are reactive with equal intensity to the envelope antigens of both HIV-1 and HIV-2. This pattern may be indicative of atypical cross-reactivity between HIV-1 and HIV-2, the presence of an intermediate-type virus, dual infection, or dual exposure to both virus types. Dual infection by both HIV-1 and HIV-2 has been confirmed by virus isolation (64) and PCR techniques (65) on a small number of individuals with this "dual-reactive" serologic profile. It is still not known what proportion of these "dual reactives" are actually dual infections or just cases of cross-reactivities between virus types. Positive anti-*vpx* and anti-*vpu* reactivity may be a convenient alternate serologic means of diagnosing dual infection/exposure (54,55). In addition, a number of recombinant-based or synthetic peptide-based assays are currently under evaluation to distinguish these virus types better with serologic techniques. However, the gold standard for these assays is virus isolation and/or PCR techniques that are difficult to perform for large numbers of specimens (61).

EPIDEMIOLOGY IN WEST AFRICA

HIV-2 was given its name to indicate its close relationship to HIV-1, the prototype AIDS virus, based on similarities in cell tropism, major antigenic cross-reactivity, and genetic properties including a similar genome structure and significant nucleotide homology. Seroepidemiologic studies have demonstrated significant rates of HIV-2 infection in West Africa, and case reports from developed countries indicate that the spread of HIV-2 through international travel is ongoing (66–77). Despite the similarities of HIV-2 to HIV-1 from a virological standpoint, many aspects of the comparative epidemiology of these two human retroviruses are still incompletely understood. As we learn more about the biology of HIV-1, we improve our ability to predict future consequences and devise realistic interventions aimed at slowing the AIDS epidemic. It is therefore of critical importance to understand better the biology and clinical significance of HIV-2 infection and evaluate its potential as a second AIDS-causing virus.

GEOGRAPHIC DISTRIBUTION

Seroepidemiologic studies have demonstrated significant rates of HIV-2 infection in West Africa with negligible rates in Central and East Africa where HIV-1 is most prevalent. We have conducted serosurveys on over 21,000 serum samples representing ten West African nations and seven Central or East African nations (66,69–72). All serum samples were tested by immunoblot for antibodies to both HIV-2 and HIV-1; the results for several West African countries are shown in Table 1. Selected sentinel groups from urban populations were sampled with recognition that such data would not be

TABLE 1. *Seroprevalence of HIV-1 and HIV-2 in West African sentinel populations*[a]

Country	HIV status	Control (%)	Risk (%)
Senegal (n = 10,200)	HIV-2	0.9	8.0
	HIV-1	0.07	1.7
	HIV-2/HIV-1	0.0	0.3
Guinea (n = 458)	HIV-2	0.9	0
	HIV-1	0.6	0
	HIV-2/HIV-1	0	0
Guinea Bissau (n = 1,209)	HIV-2	9.0	64
	HIV-1	0	0
	HIV-2/HIV-1	0	0
Mauritania (n = 356)	HIV-2	0	0
	HIV-1	0	0
	HIV-2/HIV-1	0	0
Burkina Faso (n = 1,022)	HIV-2	0.5	16.4
	HIV-1	0.2	4.8
	HIV-2/HIV-1	0	2.7
Côte d'Ivoire (n = 1,103)	HIV-2	0.4	12.8
	HIV-1	2.7	8.9
	HIV-2/HIV-1	0	3.7
Benin (n = 923)	HIV-2	0.3	3.5
	HIV-1	0.3	4.2
	HIV-2/HIV-1	0	0
Cameroon (n = 546)	HIV-2	0	0
	HIV-1	0	0
	HIV-2/HIV-1	0	0
Cape Verde (n = 1,342)	HIV-2	0.8	1.0
	HIV-1	0.08	1.0
	HIV-2/HIV-1	0	0
Gambia (n = 212)	HIV-2		5.7
	HIV-1		0
	HIV-2/HIV-1		0

[a] All 17,371 samples were collected between 1985 and 1988 from urban centers and tested by immunoblot for both HIV-1 and HIV-2. HIV-2/HIV-1+ were confirmed by RIP-SDS/PAGE. Control populations included blood donors, pregnant women, and hospital personnel. Risk populations were defined as female prostitutes and male STD patients.

representative of the general population but would, nonetheless, provide information on the general distribution patterns of HIV-2 infection and identify particular population groups that would be useful study populations for more in-depth epidemiologic studies.

In West Africa, cross-sectional seroepidemiologic surveys conducted in major urban centers of most countries have demonstrated variable but significant rates of HIV-2 infection in all countries (66–77). In general, the prevalence of HIV-2 was higher than that of HIV-1 in each West African country surveyed when either control healthy or sexually active groups were examined. However, HIV-1 was more frequent in AIDS patients or suspect cases, even in areas where HIV-2 was more prevalent than HIV-1 (66–68,77). Our studies demonstrate a widely varied prevalence of HIV-2 among West African countries ranging from 0% to 9% in blood donor populations. Sexually active risk groups such as female prostitutes and male clients attending a sexually transmitted disease (STD) clinic showed higher rates of HIV-2 and HIV-1 infection. HIV-1 and HIV-2 infections were seen at significant rates in urban centers of both Burkina Faso and Côte d'Ivoire (62,63,68). In contrast, we and others have reported on relatively low rates of HIV-2 in other parts of sub-Saharan Africa (69,76). A notable exception to this finding, however, are the significant rates of both HIV-1 and HIV-2 reported in Angola and Mozambique, both former Portugese colonies similar to Guinea Bissau in West Africa (74,75).

HIV-2 infection appears to be rare outside of Africa at the present time. The HIV-2-infected individuals who have been detected in Europe and the United States usually had connections to West Africa (70,71,76). Limited studies conducted in the United States failed to identify HIV-2 in individuals from typical high-risk groups for HIV-1, such as homosexual/bisexual men, hemophiliacs, and intravenous drug users (70). Identified cases of HIV-2 have included both asymptomatic individuals and patients with AIDS. It is likely that increased international travel will enhance the spread of HIV-2 outside of West Africa.

TRANSMISSION

In our previous studies, HIV-2 prevalence was higher in sexually active risk groups such as female prostitutes and sexually transmitted disease patients when compared with healthy control populations (62,66). In some urban centers of West Africa the prevalence of HIV-2 in female prostitutes ranged from 15% to 64%. All individuals in our studies were examined at the time of serum sampling and were found to be without signs or symptoms of AIDS. The prevalence ratio of sexually active risk groups compared with control populations was 7.4 ($\chi^2 = 297$, $p < 0.0001$). Therefore, like HIV-1, HIV-2 appears to be heterosexually transmitted in Africa.

HIV-2 is also believed to be transmitted by mother-to-infant contact, like HIV-1. However, a large prospective study of HIV-2 perinatal transmission has not been done. Individual case reports indicate that: (1) like HIV-1, passive transfer of maternal antibodies complicates HIV-2 diagnosis in infants (78) and (2) low numbers of reported perinatally acquired HIV-2 infection make even approximate estimates of rates of transmission difficult. A better understanding of this mode of transmission is critical in a geographic area where the virus is already known to have infected sexually active adults at high rates (2–40%). Data from such studies will be important in projections of the impact of HIV-2 infection on the population in general and will aid in targeting interventions to prevent the spread of this virus.

Preliminary data from two perinatal prospective studies of 16 children born to HIV-2-positive mothers and followed for over 9 months indicate that none of the infants had HIV-2 antibodies that persisted after 9 months (79,80). Other studies have sought to evaluate perinatal transmission indirectly by studying children born to mothers currently known to be HIV-2 seropositive. Poulson et al. (68) tested 18 children (<3 years of age) born to 15 such mothers; none of the 18 children was found to be HIV-2 seropositive. These results do not, however, preclude the possibility that HIV-2-infected infants had been born and died prior to the survey or that the mothers were infected subsequent to giving birth. Nonetheless, these studies may imply a low perinatal transmission rate of HIV-2.

A recent cross-sectional study of children and their mothers in Abidjan, Côte d'Ivoire, suggests that there are differences in rates of transmission of HIV-1 and HIV-2 (81). All infants (15 months of age) found to be positive also had currently seropositive mothers. Although passive antibodies would still be present in many of these infants, it was of interest to note that 66% (35/53) of infants born to HIV-1-positive mothers were HIV-1 positive, whereas only 30% (3/10) of infants born to HIV-2-positive mothers were positive. Among children (ages 15–71 months), 14 of 30 (47%) HIV-1-positive children were concordant with their mothers, whereas, 1 of 12 (8%) children of HIV-2-seropositive mothers was HIV-2 positive. Again, although this study does not directly measure perinatal transmission rate, it does provide support to other studies suggesting that the efficiency of perinatal transmission for HIV-2 may be less than that of HIV-1.

In terms of clinical disease, most identified HIV-2-positive children have been healthy (78,81). Two related cases have shown clinical abnormalities including generalized lymphadenopathy (7-year-old girl) or generalized lymphadenopathy and diarrhea (her 20-month-old brother) (82). The sparsity of case reports and the lack of any case-control or prospective studies make definitive conclusions difficult at this time. As can be seen, both the transmission and natural history of HIV-2 in pediatric populations are areas in need of further study. Inasmuch as HIV-1 infection in pediatric populations is a distinct entity and more rapidly progressive than in adults, the study of HIV-2 infection in infants may contribute to our overall understanding of the pathobiology of HIV-2 versus HIV-1.

DISEASE ASSOCIATION

The health status of individuals from whom virus has been isolated is but one means of assessing the pathogenic potential of a virus. HIV-2 has been isolated both from healthy individuals and from AIDS patients originating in West Africa, and a number of case reports or case series on HIV-2 AIDS have been published (83–86). However, these types of studies do not provide evidence for a temporal relationship between exposure to HIV-2 and the development of AIDS (72); they lack comparable data on controls, and are prone to publication bias. Nevertheless, such studies have been instrumental in demonstrating the association of AIDS with HIV-2 infection.

Despite many similarities in the clinical picture of HIV-1 and HIV-2 AIDS cases, a longer incubation period for the development of full-blown AIDS has been reported among HIV-2-infected individuals (87–89). Studies conducted in France of HIV-2-infected blood donors and recipients of their blood products have documented 14–16 years of HIV-2 infection without signs of immunodeficiency (88,90). In addition, two of three HIV-2-positive AIDS cases reported by Brun-Vezinet and colleagues (84) were still alive and stable 3 years after the diagnosis of AIDS. In a comparison of the outcome of HIV-1 versus HIV-2 AIDS cases, Le Guenno (91) reported a 6-month survival advantage among a small number of HIV-2 AIDS cases compared with HIV-1 cases at the military hospital in Senegal. This increase seemed important, since the average survival of an HIV-1 AIDS case in the same hospital was only approximately 6 months. Gody et al. (89) have also reported improved survival among a larger group of HIV-2 AIDS cases in Côte d'Ivoire.

Clinical examination of over 62 HIV-2-infected West African prostitutes failed to demonstrate an increase in AIDS-related signs or symptoms or generalized lymphadenopathy compared with prostitutes seronegative for HIV-2 infection (92). This finding contrasts with similar studies conducted on Nairobi prostitutes with HIV-1 infection, in which a large proportion (54%) were found to have generalized lymphadenopathy on physical examination (93). Likewise, in Rwandese HIV-1-infected prostitutes, clinical examination revealed generalized lymphadenopathy in 83% and signs or symptoms suggestive of HIV-like disease in 38% (94).

Taken together, these reports seem to indicate possible differences between HIV-1 and HIV-2, in the length of the incubation period from initial infection to AIDS and a somewhat better outcome among HIV-2 AIDS patients. It therefore appears that the natural history and clinical course of HIV-2-infected individuals may differ significantly from that of HIV-1.

NATURAL HISTORY

Since the discovery of HIV-2, we have been involved in a prospective study of registered female prostitutes in Senegal (92,95,96). Through serology for HIV-1 and HIV-2 and questionnaire data, we have been able to assess risk determinants for both virus types in these sexually active women (96). Among 1,275 female prostitutes from Dakar, HIV-2 seropositivity was associated with many years of sexual activity and a history of scari-

fication, whereas HIV-1 infection correlated with a shorter duration of prostitution and a history of hospitalization. Among 278 female prostitutes from Ziguinchor, HIV-2 seroprevalence was associated with Guinea Bissau nationality and multiple years of sexual activity. Among 157 female prostitutes from Kaolack, HIV-2 seroprevalence was associated with a long period of sexual activity and lack of condom usage. These findings demonstrate that risk determinants for HIV-2 and HIV-1 may differ even within the same self-identified high-risk population. Further studies are clearly needed to assess which sexual practices are more directly associated with acquisition of HIV.

Critical to our understanding of the biology of HIV-2 is the assessment of this virus's ability to induce AIDS. Prospective studies of this subject have been difficult to conduct even with HIV-1 infection. It is clear, however, that the simple comparison of selected AIDS patients with either HIV-1 or HIV-2 is not sufficient to draw conclusions regarding the natural history of these viral infections (72). The determination of differences in the natural history of HIV-2 as compared with HIV-1 infection requires the study of individuals over time. Our ongoing prospective study of asymptomatic HIV-2-infected persons in Senegal is now in its sixth year (92,97,98). With a rate of follow-up of over 90%, we have observed a difference in outcome between HIV-2- and HIV-1-infected individuals. Among 166 HIV-2-seropositive women followed for 399 person-years, one has developed AIDS and one ARC. In contrast, of 24 HIV-1-seropositive women followed for 61 person-years, we have observed 2 AIDS and 2 ARC cases. This translates to a 12-fold greater relative risk for development of AIDS among HIV-1-infected individuals. Also, there were fewer abnormal clinical or immunologic parameters among HIV-2 seropositives than might have been expected in a similar group of HIV-1-infected persons (98).

These data suggest that the pathogenic potential of these two immunodeficiency viruses differ. Some have argued that the apparent low level of disease progression in this cohort may be due to the more recent introduction of HIV-2 infection in this population. This seems unlikely since many of the women were known to have been infected since the beginning of the study in 1985, and incidence data indicate that the rate of new HIV-2 infection is quite minimal. Retrospective studies conducted in populations of Dakar, Senegal, in the mid-1970s also demonstrate that HIV-2 was present at least 18 years ago. Furthermore, we have found that the HIV-2 seroprevalence rate among seropositive female prostitutes in Dakar increases with age (66). In prostitutes over the age of 50 years the HIV-2 seroprevalence rate was close to 100%. This age-specific seroprevalence curve is indicative of an endemic virus present in the population for at least several generations. This finding is also consistent with the relatively high rates of HIV-2 infection found in healthy adult control populations.

Our prospective serologic study of female prostitutes in Senegal allowed direct measurement of the seroincidence of both HIV-2 and HIV-1. Although the incidence of HIV-2 infection had been assumed to be similar to that of HIV-1 (99), our findings indicate that the rates of new infection are dissimilar. The cumulative incidence of HIV-2 infection over the 6-year period was 8.6/1,000 person-years, with little fluctuation over the study period. In contrast, the HIV-1 incidence in the same population increased tenfold, suggesting a rapid influx of HIV-1 infection and a relatively stable incidence of HIV-2, the more prevalent virus type. These observations are supportive of the hypothesis that HIV-2 is not a new infectious agent in this population and that its spread via sexual transmission is relatively constant. Mathematical modeling of the data from our studies has indicated that the infectivity of HIV-1 is approximately four times that of HIV-2 per sexual act (100). HIV-2 transmission in this cohort of sexually active women is 1% per year, which is low compared with that of HIV-1 prostitute cohorts in East Africa in whom a seroconversion rate of up to 50–70% per year has been observed (101). Similarly, the estimated doubling time (assuming constant incidence) for HIV-1 prevalence within our cohort is shorter (2–3 years) than that of HIV-2 (10 years) (99).

Therefore, the results of epidemiologic and prospective clinical studies indicate that the pathogenicity of HIV-2 is not identical to that of HIV-1. Additional studies are necessary to define further the natural history and clinical significance of HIV-2 infection. This will be critical to health policy decisions in many West African countries where HIV-2 infection is common, as well as in other parts of the world where this virus is sure to become more widespread. As public health officials worldwide become involved in detection of HIV-2-infected individuals, up-to-date information on the biology of HIV-2 and its potential for disease will be important for counseling those found to be infected.

CONCLUSIONS

Since the discovery of a second human immunodeficiency virus in 1985, considerable progress has been made in understanding the virology and epidemiology of this new agent. Despite numerous similarities in virologic structure and function, certain unique genes and differences in virus–cell interactions have been noted. Although HIV-2 has been found predominantly in West Africa, its spread world-wide is currently being documented. It is widely believed that the modes of transmission of HIV-1 and HIV-2 are similar, but the comparative rates of viral transmission may be more important. Incidence data indicate that HIV-2 may spread through heterosexual transmission more slowly than HIV-1. Studies of perinatal transmission of HIV-2 also indicate that the transmissibility of HIV-2 may differ from that of

HIV-1. In summary, despite a number of similarities between HIV-2 and HIV-1, important differences also exist. These include differences in risk determinants for sexually active populations, distinct incidence patterns of infection, and a prolonged induction period for the development of AIDS. The virologic determinants and mechanisms for these apparent biological differences are still unknown. However, an understanding of how HIV-2 differs from HIV-1 at a host level is essential for interpretations of comparative virologic studies. We are hopeful that such comparative studies will yield important information on the pathogenic mechanisms employed by HIV viruses and lead the way to the development of effective interventions for the prevention of AIDS. Our understanding of the complexity of this ever-expanding family of human retroviruses has increased dramatically over the past few years. A more complete appreciation of the in vitro and in vivo correlates of pathogenicity will allow for further progress in understanding pathogenic mechanisms of retrovirally induced disease. It is hoped that such insights will provide important direction in our studies to prevent and control retrovirally induced diseases world-wide.

ACKNOWLEDGMENTS

This work results from the Inter-University Convention for the Research of AIDS and other Viral Induced Diseases (Dakar, Tours, Limoges, and Harvard). The research was supported in part by DAMD 17-87-C-7072 and 17-90-0138.

REFERENCES

1. Poiesz BJ, Ruscetti AF, Gazdar AF, Bunn PA, Minna JD, Gallo RC. Detection and isolation of type C retrovirus particles from fresh and cultured lymphocytes of patients with cutaneous T-cell lymphoma. *Proc Natl Acad Sci USA* 1980;77:7415–9.
2. Wong-Staal F, Gallo RC. The family of human T-lymphotropic leukemia viruses: HTLV-I as the cause of adult T-cell leukemia and HTLV-III as the cause of acquired immunodeficiency syndrome. *Blood* 1985;55:253–63.
3. Gessain A, Vernant JC, Maurs L, et al. Antibodies to human T-lymphotropic virus type-I in patients with tropical spastic paraparesis. *Lancet* 1985;2:407–9.
4. Kalyanaramen VS, Sarngadharan MG, Robert-Guroff M, et al. A new subtype of human T-cell leukemia virus (HTLV-II) associated with a T-cell variant of hairy cell leukemia. *Science* 1982;218:517–23.
5. Ehrlich GD, Glaser JB, LaVigne K, et al. Prevalence of human T-cell leukemia/lymphoma virus (HTLV) type II infection among high-risk individuals: type-specific identification of HTLVs by polymerase chain reaction. *Blood* 1989;74:1658–64.
6. Chen YA, Lee TH, Wiktor S, et al. Type-specific antigens for serological discrimination of HTLV-I and HTLV-II infection. *Lancet* 1990;336:1153–5.
7. Miyoshi I, Yoshimoto S, Fujishita M, et al. Natural adult-T-cell leukemia virus infection in Japanese monkeys. *Lancet* 1982;2:658.
8. Miyoshi I, Fujishita M, Taguchi H, et al. Natural infection in non-human primates with adult T-cell leukemia virus or a closely related agent. *Int J Cancer* 1983;32:333.

9. Homma T, Kanki PJ, Hunt RD, et al. Lymphoma in macaques: association with virus of human T-lymphotropic virus family. *Science* 1984;225:716–8.

10. Watanabe T, Seiki M, Tsujimoto H, Miyoshi I, Hayami M, Yoshida M. Sequence homology of the simian retrovirus genome with human T-cell leukemia virus type 1. *Virology* 1985;144:59–65.

11. Barre-Sinoussi F, Chermann JC, Rey F, et al. Isolation of a T-lymphotropic retrovirus from a patient at risk for acquired immune deficiency syndrome (AIDS) *Science* 1983;220:868–71.

12. Popovic M, Sarngadharan M, Read E, et al. Detection, isolation, and continuous production of cytopathic retroviruses (HTLV-III) from patients with AIDS and pre-AIDS. *Science* 1984;224:497–500.

13. Wong-Staal, F. Human immunodeficiency viruses and their replication. In: Fields BN, Knipe DM, et al., eds. *Virology,* 2nd ed. New York: Raven Press, 1990;1529–43.

14. Kanki PJ, McLane MF, King NW Jr, et al. Serological identification and characterization of a macaque T-lymphotropic retrovirus closely related to HTLV-III. *Science* 1985;228:1199–201.

15. Kanki PJ, Kurth R, Becker W, Dreesman G, McLane MF, Essex M. Antibodies to simian T-lymphotropic virus type III in African green monkeys and recognition of STLV-III viral proteins by AIDS and related sera. *Lancet* 1985;2:1330–2.

16. Murphy-Corb M, Martin LN, Rangan SRS, et al. Isolation of an HTLV-III related retrovirus from macaques with simian AIDS and its possible origin in asymptomatic mangabeys. *Nature* 1986;321:435–37.

17. Fultz PN, McClure HM, Anderson DC, Swenson RB, Anand R, Srinivasan A. Isolation of a T-lymphotropic retrovirus from naturally infected sooty mangabey monkeys (*Cercocebus atys*). *Proc Natl Acad Sci USA* 1986;83:5286–90.

18. Benveniste RE, Arthur LO, Tsai C, et al. Isolation of a lentivirus from a macaque with lymphoma. Comparison with HTLV-III/LAV and other lentiviruses. *J Virol* 1986;60:483–90.

19. Barin F, M'Boup S, Denis F, Kanki P, Allan JS, Lee TH, Essex M. Serological evidence for virus related to simian T-lymphotropic retrovirus III in residents of west Africa. *Lancet* 1985;2:1387–9.

20. Kanki PJ, Barin F, M'Boup S, et al. New human T-lymphotropic retrovirus related to simian T-lymphotropic virus type III (STLV-IIIAGM). *Science* 1986;232:238–43.

21. Clavel F, Guetard D, Brun-Vezinet F, et al. Isolation of a new human retrovirus from West African patients with AIDS. *Science* 1986;233:343–6.

22. Biberfeld G, Brown F, Esparza J, et al. Meeting report, WHO working group on characterization of HIV-related retroviruses: criteria for characterization and proposal for a nomenclature system. *AIDS* 1987;1:189–90.

23. Kanki PJ, Essex M, Barin F. Antigenic relationships between HTLV-3/LAV, STLV-3, and HTLV-4. In: Chanock R, Brown F, Lerner R, Ginsberg H, eds. *Vaccines 87.* Cold Spring Harbor, NY: Cold Spring Harbor Press, 1987;185–87.

24. Albert J, Bredberg U, Chiodi F, et al. A new human retrovirus isolate of West African origin (SBL-6669) and its relationship to HTLV-IV, LAV-II, and HTLV-IIIB. *AIDS Res Hum Retroviruses* 1987;3:3–10.

25. Kanki PJ. West African human retroviruses related to STLV-III. *AIDS* 1987;I:141–5.

26. Gonda MA, Braun MJ, Clements JE, et al. HTLV-III shares sequence homology with a family of pathogenic lentiviruses. *Proc Natl Acad Sci USA* 1986;83:4007–11.

27. Dalgleish A, Berverly P, Clapham P, et al. The CD4 (T4) antigen is an essential component of the receptor for the AIDS retrovirus. *Nature* 1984;312:763–6.

28. Maddon PJ, Dalgleish AG, McDougal JS, Clapham PR, Weiss RA, Axel R. The T4 gene encodes the AIDS virus receptor and is expressed in the immune system and the brain. *Cell* 1986;47:333–48.

29. Sattentau QJ, Clapham PR, Weiss RA, et al. The human and simian immunodeficiency viruses HIV-1, HIV-2 and SIV interact with similar epitopes on their cellular receptor, the CD4 molecule. *AIDS* 1988;2:101–5.

30. Clapham PR, Weber JN, Whitby JN, et al. Soluble CD4 blocks the infectivity of diverse strains of HIV and SIV for T cells and monocytes but not for brain and muscle cells. *Nature* 1989;337:368–70.

31. Moore JP. Simple methods for monitoring HIV-1 and HIV-2 gp120 binding to soluble CD4 by enzyme-linked immunosorbent assay: HIV-2 has a 25-fold lower affinity than HIV-1 for soluble CD4. *AIDS* 1990;4:297–305.

32. Evans LA, Moreau J, Odehouri K, et al. Characterization of a noncytopathic HIV-2 strain with unusual effects on CD4 expression. *Science* 1988;240:1522–5.

33. Kong LI, Lee SW, Kappes JC, et al. West African HIV-2-related human retrovirus with attenuated cytopathicity. *Science* 1988;240:1525–9.

34. Albert J, Naucler A, Bottiger B, et al. Replicative capacity of HIV-2, like HIV-1, correlates with severity of immunodeficiency. *AIDS* 1990;4:291–5.

35. Franchini G, Collalti E, Arya SK, et al. Genetic analysis of a new subgroup of human and simian T-lymphotropic retroviruses: HTLV-IV, LAV-2, SBL6669, and STLV-III AGM *AIDS Res Hum Retroviruses* 1987;3:11–7.

36. Franchini G, Gurgo C, Guo HG, et al. Sequence of simian immunodeficiency virus and its relationship to the human immunodeficiency viruses. *Nature* 1987;328:539–43.

37. Guyader M, Emerman M, Sonigo P, Clavel F, Montagnier L, Alizon M. Genome organization and transactivation of the human immunodeficiency virus type 2. *Nature* 1987;326:662–9.

38. Zagury JF, Franchini G, Reitz M, et al. Genetic variability between HIV-2 isolates is comparable to the variability among HIV type 1. *Proc Natl Acad Sci USA* 1988;85:5941–5.

39. Tristem M, Mansinho K, Champalimaud JL, Ayres L, Karpas A. Six new isolates of human immunodeficiency virus type 2 (HIV-2) and the molecular characterization of one (HIV-2$_{CAM2}$). *J Gen Virol* 1989;70:479–84.

40. Kirchoff F, Jentsch KD, Bachmann B, et al. A novel proviral clone of HIV-2: biological and phylogenetic relationships to other primate immunodeficiency viruses. *Virology* 1990;177:305–11.

41. Allan JS, Kanki PJ. Identification of the nef product in HIV-2 and SIV, in preparation.

42. Allan JS, Coligan JE, Lee TH, et al. Immunogenic nature of a *pol* gene product of HTLV-III/LAV. *Blood* 1987;69:331–3.

43. Kanki PJ, Barin F, Essex M. Antibody reactivity to multiple HIV-2 isolates. 4th International Conference on AIDS, Stockholm, Sweden, June, 1988.

44. Lee TH, Homma T, Schultz K, et al. Antigens expressed by human T-cell leukemia virus transformed cells. In: Gallo RC, Essex M, Gross L, eds. *Human T-cell leukemia viruses.* Cold Spring Harbor, NY: Cold Spring Harbor Press, 1984;111–20.

45. Weiss RA, Clapham PR, Weber JN, et al. HIV-2 antisera cross-neutralize HIV-1. *AIDS* 1987;2:95–100.

46. Bottiger B, Karlsson A, Andreasson PA, Naucler A, Costa CM, Biberfeld G. Cross-neutralizing antibodies against HIV-1 (HTLV-IIIB and HTLV-IIIRF) and HIV-2 (SBL-6669 and a new isolate SBL-K135). *AIDS Res Hum Retroviruses* 1989;5:525–32.

47. Ljundgren K, Chiodi F, Biberfeld G, Norrby E, Jondal M, Fenyo EM. Lack of cross-reaction in antibody dependent cellular cytotoxicity between human immunodeficiency virus (HIV) and HIV-related West African strains. *J Immunol* 1988;140:602–5.

48. Arya SK, Beaver B, Jagodzinski L, et al. New human and simian HIV-related retroviruses possess functional transactivator (*tat*) gene. *Nature* 1987;328:548–50.

49. Essex M, Allan J, Kanki P, et al. Antigens of human T-lymphotropic virus type III/lymphadenopathy-associated virus. *Ann Intern Med* 1985;103:700–3.

50. Lee TH, Coligan JE, Allan JS, McLane MF, Groopman JE, Essex M. A new HTLV-III/LAV protein encoded by a gene found in cytopathic retroviruses. *Science* 1986;231:1546–9.

51. Allan JS, Coligan JE, Lee TH, et al. A new HTLV-III/LAV encoded antigen detected by antibodies from AIDS patients. *Science* 1985;230:810–3.

52. Arya SK, Gallo RC. Three novel genes of human T-lymphotropic virus type III: immune reactivity of their products with sera from acquired immune deficiency syndrome patients. *Proc Natl Acad Sci USA* 1986;83:2209–13.

53. Franchini G, Robert-Guroff M, Aldovini A, et al. Spectrum of

natural antibodies against five HTLV-III antigens in infected individuals: correlation of antibody prevalence with clinical status. *Blood* 1987;69:437–41.

54. Matsuda Z, Chou MJ, Matsuda M, et al. Human immunodeficiency virus type 1 has an additional coding sequence in the central region of the genome. *Proc Natl Acad Sci USA* 1988;85:6968–72.

55. Yu XF, Ito S, Essex M, Lee TH. A naturally immunogenic virion-associated protein specific for HIV-2 and SIV. *Nature* 1988;335:262–5.

56. Essex M, Kanki PJ, Barin F, Chou MJ, Lee TH. Immunogenicity of HIV-1 and HIV-2 antigens and relationship to disease development. In: Girard M, Vallette L, eds. *2nd Colloque des Cent Gardes 1987.* 1988;219–20.

57. Kanki PJ, Samuels K, Hailman E, et al. Confirmation of HIV-2 infection by recombinant env peptides, vpx reactivity and HIV-2 specific PCR. V International Conference on AIDS in Africa, Kinshasa, Zaire, 1990.

58. Yu X-F, Yu QC, Essex M, et al. The vpx gene of simian immunodeficiency virus facilitates efficient viral replication of fresh lymphocytes and macrophages. *J Virol* 1991;65:5088–91.

59. Denis F, Leonard G, Sangare A, et al. Comparison of ten HIV enzyme immunoassays for detection of antibody to HIV-2 in West African sera. *J Clin Microbiol* 1988;26:1000–4.

60. Kanki PJ, M'Boup S, Hernandez-Avila M, Essex M. Ability of HIV-I ELISAs to detect HIV-2 positive sera. 3rd International Conference of AIDS and Associated Cancers in Africa, Arusha, Tanzania, September, 1988.

61. WHO. HIV-2 Working Group: criteria for HIV-2 serodiagnosis, Marseilles, France, October, 1989.

62. Kanki PJ, M'Boup S, Ricard D, et al. Human T-lymphotropic virus type 4 and the human immunodeficiency virus in West Africa. *Science* 1987;236:827–31.

63. Denis F, Barin F, Gershey-Damet GM, et al. Prevalence of human T-lymphotropic retroviruses type III (HIV) and type IV in Ivory Coast. *Lancet* 1987;1:408–11.

64. Evans LA, Moreau J, Odehouri K, et al. Simultaneous isolation of HIV-1 and HIV-2 from an AIDS patient. *Lancet* 1988;2:1389–91.

65. Rayfield M, DeCock K, Heyward W, et al. Mixed human immunodeficiency virus (HIV) infection in an individual: demonstration of both HIV type 1 and type 2 proviral sequence by using polymerase chain reaction. *J Infect Dis* 1988;158:1170–6.

66. Kanki PJ, Marlink R, Siby T, Essex M, M'Boup S. Biology of HIV-2 infection in West Africa. In: Papas T, ed. *Gene regulation and AIDS.* Portfolio Publishing Company of Texas, 1990; 255–72.

67. Gnaore E, De Cock KM, Gayle H, et al. Prevalence of and mortality from HIV type 2 in Guinea Bissau, West Africa. *Lancet* 1989;2:513.

68. Poulsen AG, Aaby P, Frederiksen K, et al. Prevalence of and mortality from human immunodeficiency virus type-2 in Bissau, West Africa. *Lancet* 1989;1:827–30.

69. Kanki PJ, Allan J, Barin F, et al. Absence of antibodies to HIV-2/HTLV-4 in six Central African nations. *AIDS Res Hum Retroviruses* 1987;3:317–22.

70. Couroce AM. HIV-2 in blood donors and in different risk groups in France. *Lancet* 1987;1:1151.

71. CDC. Update: HIV-2 infection—United States. Current trends. *MMWR* 1989;38:572–80.

72. Romieu I, Marlink R, Kanki P, M'Boup S, Essex M. HIV-2 link to AIDS in West Africa. *J AIDS* 1990;3:220–30.

73. Zohoun I, Bigot A, Sankale JL, Bjorkman A, M'Boup S, Kanki PJ. Prevalence of HIV-1 and HIV-2 in Benin. 4th International Conference on AIDS, Stockholm, Sweden, June, 1988.

74. Bottiger B, Berggren I, Leite J, et al. Prevalence of HIV and HTLV-IV infections in Angola. 2nd International Conference on AIDS and Associated Cancers in Africa, Naples, Italy, September, 1987.

75. Barreto J, Ingold L, Dela Cruz F, et al. HIV prevalence in Mozambican blood donors. 4th International Conference on AIDS, Stockholm, Sweden, June, 1988.

76. Horsburgh CR, Holmberg SD. The global distribution of human immunodeficiency virus type 2 (HIV-2) infection. *Transfusion* 1988;28:192–5.

77. De Cock KM, Brun-Vezinet F. Epidemiology of HIV-2 Infection. *AIDS* 1989;3[Suppl 1]:S89–95.

78. Matheron S, DeMaria H, Dormont D, et al. HIV-2 Infection in mother-infant couples. 4th International Conference on AIDS, Stockholm, Sweden, June, 1988.

79. Andreasson PA, Dias F, Goudiaby JMT, Naucler A, Biberfield G. HIV-2 infection in prenatal women and vertical transmission of HIV-2 in Guinea-Bissau. 4th International Conference on AIDS in Africa, Marseilles. France, October, 1989.

80. Hojlyng N, Kvinesdal BB, Molbak K, Aaby P. Vertical transmission of HIV-2; does it occur? 4th International Conference on AIDS in Africa. Marseilles, France, October, 1989.

81. Ouattara SA, Gody M, Rioche M, et al. Blood transfusions and HIV infections (HIV1, HIV2/LAV2) in Ivory Coast. *J Trop Med Hyg* 1988;91:212–5.

82. De Cock KM, Odehouri K, Moreau J, et al. Rapid emergence of AIDS in Abidjan, Ivory Coast. *Lancet* 1989;2:408–10.

83. Clavel F, Mansinho K, Chamaret S, et al. Human immunodeficiency virus type 2 infection associated with AIDS in West Africa. *N Engl J Med* 1987;316:1180–5.

84. Brun-Vezinet F, Rey MA, Katlama C, et al. Lymphadenopathy-associated virus type 2 in AIDS and AIDS-related complex. *Lancet* 1987;1:128–32.

85. Rey MA, Girard PM, Harzic M, Madjar JJ, Brun-Vezinet F, Saimot AG. HIV-1 and HIV-2 double infection in French homosexual male with AIDS-related complex (Paris, 1985). *Lancet* 1987;1:388–9.

86. Ayanian JZ, Maguire JH, Marlink RG, Essex M, Kanki PJ. HIV-2 infection in the United States. *N Engl J Med* 1989;320:1422–3.

87. Saimot AG, Matheron S, Brun-Vezinet F. Manifestations cliniques de l'infection HIV-2. *Méd Maladies Infect* 1988; Spécial Decembre:707–12.

88. Ancelle R, Bletry O, Baglin AC, Brun-Vezinet F, Rey MA, Godeau P. Long incubation period for HIV-II infection. *Lancet* 1987;1:688–9.

89. Gody M, Ouattara SA, de The G. Clinical experience in relation to HIV-1 and HIV-2 infection in rural hospital in Ivory Coast, West Africa. *AIDS* 1988;2:433–6.

90. Dufoort G, Couroux AM, Ancell-Park R, Bletry O. No clinical signs 14 years after HIV-2 transmission via blood transfusion. *Lancet* 1988;2:510.

91. LeGuenno B, Sarthou JL, Berlioz C, et al. Comparison of HIV1 and HIV2 infections in a hospital in Dakar, Senegal. 4th International Conference on AIDS, Stockholm, Sweden, June, 1988.

92. Marlink R, Ricard D, M'Boup S, et al. Clinical, hematological, and immunological evaluation of individuals exposed to human immunodeficiency virus type 2 (HIV-2). *Aids Res Hum Retroviruses* 1988;4:137–48.

93. Kreiss JK, Koech D, Plummer FA, et al. AIDS virus infection in Nairobi prostitutes: spread of the epidemic to East Africa. *N Engl J Med* 1986;314:414–8.

94. Van de Pierre P, Clumeck N, Carael M, et al. Female prostitutes, a risk group for infection by the human T-cell lymphotropic virus type III. *Lancet*. 1985;2:524–7.

95. Kanki PJ. Clinical significance of HIV-2 infection in West Africa. In: Volberding P, Jacobson M, eds. *1989 AIDS clinical reviews.* New York: Marcel Dekker, 1989;95–108.

96. Kanki PJ, M'Boup S, Marlink R, et al. Prevalence and risk determinants of HIV-2 and HIV-1 in West African female prostitutes [submitted].

97. Marlink R, M'Boup S, Kanki PJ, et al. Reduced virulence of HIV-2 as compared to HIV-1 [submitted].

98. Marlink R, Thior I, Siby T, et al. The natural history of HIV-2 infection. 5th International Conference on AIDS in Africa, Kinshasa, Zaire, October, 1990.

99. Kanki P, M'Boup S, Marlink R, et al. Direct measurement of incidence of HIV-1 and HIV-2 in female prostitutes in Senegal. 7th International Conference on AIDS, Florence, Italy, June, 1991.

100. Donnelly C, Leisenring W, Sandberg S, et al. Comparison of transmission rates of HIV-1 and HIV-2 in a cohort of prostitutes in Dakar, Senegal. *Bull Math Bio* [in press].

101. Simonsen JN, Plummer FA, Ngugi EN, et al. HIV infection among lower socioeconomic strata prostitutes in Nairobi. *AIDS* 1990;4:139–44.

AIDS and Other Manifestations of HIV Infection,
Second Edition, Edited by Gary P. Wormser.
Raven Press, Ltd., New York © 1992.

CHAPTER 8

Laboratory Detection of Human Retroviral Infection

Stanley H. Weiss

The characterization in 1984 of a new human retrovirus, the human immunodeficiency virus (HIV), is the foundation for understanding the acquired immunodeficiency syndrome (AIDS) epidemic (1–3). The evidence is overwhelming that HIV infection is necessary for a person to develop AIDS (4–6). The spectrum and natural history of retroviral infection remain the subject of vigorous research efforts (5,6).

In 1988 a nomenclature committee suggested that the term human immunodeficiency virus be used for this generic class of viruses (6a), rather than lymphadenopathy-associated virus (LAV) or human T-lymphotropic virus type III (HTLV-III) (1,7). Significant genetic variations occur among HIV strains (8–10). Nearly all HIV infection in the United States is due to HIV type 1 (HIV-1), but in other parts of the world such as West Africa, HIV type 2 (HIV-2) predominates (11,12). For these reasons biologicals derived from specific isolates should specify the viral strain of origin (e.g., HTLV-IIIB), and tests based upon HIV reagents should reference the precise sources.

The methods and limitations of assays to detect evidence of HIV exposure are reviewed. An approach to the rational use and interpretation of these tests is provided. Given the increasing attention to the HTLV family of viruses (13), a separate section below discusses tests for these agents. Recent developments are highlighted at the end of the chapter.

APPROACHES TO THE DETECTION OF INFECTIOUS AGENTS

A laboratory measure that directly detects the presence of an infectious agent is highly desirable. For some agents, such as hepatitis B virus (HBV), large quantities of viral antigen are produced during active infection and tests that effectively measure viral antigen are available. For many other viral agents, however, antigen may not be directly detectable even during active infection (14).

The presence or absence of antibodies (humoral response) is one way to detect whether or not a host response to the agent has occurred. The presence of antibodies should not be interpreted as indicating resolution of infection; many viruses are characterized by persistence. Retroviruses, such as HTLV and HIV, can integrate within the viral genome (DNA) of the host cell. Thus, in theory the presence of antibodies could be a marker of: (1) past but resolved, (2) latent, or (3) active infection. It is uncertain whether or not continual viral expression must occur to sustain antibody production over a prolonged time, e.g., by periodically or continuously rechallenging the immune system. Prospective epidemiologic serologic studies indicate that once an adult has produced HIV antibodies ("seropositive"), complete loss of antibodies ("seroreversion") is rare (15) and virus can usually be recovered from seropositive persons. HIV antibodies are therefore generally interpreted as evidence of persistent infection, not resolution of past infection. The exception is the infant less than 18 months of age whose mother was HIV seropositive at delivery (16). IgG antibodies can cross the placenta to high titer, and may then take many half-lives to decay to an undetectable level. Serological results based on cord blood thus give useful data on maternal, but not newborn infection.

S. H. Weiss: Division of Infectious Disease Epidemiology, Department of Preventive Medicine and Community Health, University of Medicine and Dentistry of New Jersey - New Jersey Medical School, Newark, New Jersey 07107.

Recent studies suggest that only about one-half of newborns who were initially seropositive are actually HIV infected. Prospective studies indicate that only about 30% of all children born to seropositive mothers are infected with HIV. Specialized HIV tests are therefore particularly informative for young children. Specialized tests are also important to detect persons who are infected but antibody negative ("seronegative").

ANTIBODY DETECTION

The enzyme-linked immunosorbent assay (ELISA) was previously successfully employed for detecting antibodies to HTLV (17). This background was important in developing serologic assays for HIV (18,19), leading to the development of a prototype HIV ELISA that was reproducible, sensitive, and specific (20). The research breakthrough enabling production of purified HIV type HTLV-IIIB in large quantities was integral to the development of these assays (2).

Several commercial companies were licensed by the Food and Drug Administration (FDA) for marketing HIV type 1 antibody ELISA kits to screen donated blood products in the United States in 1985. These kits were also utilized at "alternative tests sites," where persons who considered themselves at increased risk for HIV infection could be tested voluntarily (21). Testing for HIV is now widely available from commercial laboratories, although some states (such as New York) have strictly regulated test availability, and many states now require that positive HIV test results be confidentially reported with personal identifiers to the state department of health.

As of 1991, the FDA had licensed HIV antibody screening assays from nine vendors, one HIV antibody confirmation assay (Western blot), and one HIV antigen detection assay. However, some of these tests are no longer being manufactured. There are multiple other unlicensed assays that are sold for "research use" as well as others that are used only "in house" by commercial or research laboratories.

Although the intended purposes in the blood bank and clinical/diagnostic settings are similar, the practical applications are quite different. In the former situation, the goal is to screen out any blood that is potentially infected with HIV—it is critical to minimize false negatives in order to ensure a continuing safe supply of blood products. In the latter clinical instance, the primary purpose is to counsel persons correctly concerning whether or not they are infected.

Medical and nonmedical considerations concerning AIDS and the HIV epidemic have led to a perceived impact for HIV testing that is far greater than for most other laboratory tests. HIV testing is also perceived as an invasive procedure in our society. Fears concerning the medical implications of reactive test results and a potential social risk in the event of a break in confidentiality have foundation (3). False-positive results similarly raise special concern. A written informed consent procedure in advance of testing was initially recommended in 1985, prior to HIV ELISA licensure, to address these issues (3), and is now used by many to document pretest discussions.

Predictive Value

One should note that sensitivity and specificity as defined by the epidemiologist for laboratory tests (Table 1) reflect aspects of the test configuration as defined by the manufacturer, and remain constant for all approved uses. Alternative interpretive criteria or cut-off values will affect the sensitivity and specificity (20).

Much more important to the users, in practice, are the positive and negative predictive values. These will vary depending upon the (estimated) "true" positivity proportion in the population being tested; ideally, a gold standard would be employed to determine this proportion (Table 1). When dealing with an individual patient, the predictive values depend upon the *prior probability of infection* [*seropositivity*] or (analogously) the *prior probability of disease* (22), which represents an estimate of the relevant population proportion. A *pretest probability* assessment is required whenever test results are to be interpreted meaningfully.

TABLE 1. *Epidemiologic assessment of tests: definitions*

Sensitivity[a]—the probability that a test result will be positive if infection is present
Specificity[a]—the probability that a test result will be negative if infection is not present
Gold (reference) standard—A definitive means of categorization, widely accepted by experts in the field, for absolutely defining the presence or absence of a condition (such as HIV infection)
Silver (criterion) standard—The best currently available (or the accepted) standard, which is expected to be superseded as technology advances; used as an interim reference standard when a gold standard either does not exist or is otherwise unavailable

[a] Laboratory personnel frequently use these terms differently, with the terms applied to detection and strength of a "test signal" (e.g., titer) rather than the epidemiologic, statistical definitions above.

LABORATORY DETECTION / 97

Although health care professionals who order HIV tests have become increasing familiar with these tests, it is highly desirable for the laboratory report to provide the clinician with considerable guidance concerning the implications and limitations of the results. Further consultation with the laboratory (or blood bank) director, infectious disease specialist, or other expert may be particularly important in circumstances of an "unexpected" result. Such experts should be able to assist the clinician in employing standard principles of decision theory to apply the battery of licensed and unlicensed (research) tests appropriately and efficiently to a given situation.

Confidentiality concerns may severely limit the information that is routinely provided to the testing laboratory by the referring professional. Since clinical data impact on the pretest probability assessment and thus on the predictive value of a test, such direct discussions may help resolve the clinical interpretation of putatively "indeterminate" results. The types of tests and considerations regarding them are discussed in depth below.

Comparison of Screening Assays

The ELISA was the first HIV antibody detection procedure to be licensed in the United States. The first generation of commercial antibody kits had sensitivities and specificities (see Table 1 for definitions; cf. ref. 20 for formulae) of approximately 98% (23,24). However, comparative data on the antibody ELISA kits were limited and complicated by the absence of a generally accepted gold (or even silver) standard (Table 1). Licensure required correct identification of sera in an FDA test panel, but the panel was limited in extent and was designed as but one of several essential minimum requirements. Different manufacturers have used different panels of sera in their evaluations. Therefore, apparent observed differences may merely reflect differences in patient selection and not true differences among the tests.

Lacking an established reference laboratory standard, a prototype HIV assay was assessed on the basis of clinical-epidemiologic considerations, which included a panel of sera drawn from healthy blood donors prior to the AIDS epidemic who were considered "true negatives" (20). In contrast, the subsequent FDA assessment of vendor products relied upon current blood donors (22,25,26). Since some current donors are HIV infected, the operative assumption that "all blood donors are true negatives" on which this FDA methodology is based, is known to be false. Unfortunately, this leads to the paradoxical situation that perfect specificity (no false positives) would be attained only for a test that detected absolutely *no* positives among current blood donors. A test that was *never* positive would have perfect specificity

(but zero sensitivity). Comparison of tests by "the numbers" alone, for these reasons, could lead to highly misleading conclusions and undesirable results.

In the absence of gold standards, the true sensitivity and specificity for the detection of HIV antibodies remain somewhat imprecise. Furthermore, these assays primarily detect IgG, not IgM or IgA antibodies. HIV antigenemia and/or IgM antibodies can sometimes precede the expression of IgG antibodies, reflecting an eminently plausible biologic scenario. Thus, even if an IgG assay were perfectly sensitive for such antibodies, some persons truly infected with HIV would not be detected by the serologic tests for HIV IgG antibody. The frequency, duration, and importance of this (IgG) seronegative window remain the subject of investigation (27,28).

Test Performance

Receiver operator characteristic (ROC) curve analysis is a useful method for comparing the performance of assays when congruent definitions of sample groups have been provided, and for assessing claims of vendor improvement. Such analysis, for example, would show that a purportedly improved prototype ELISA (29) in fact apparently had poorer performance than a predecessor assay (20).

False ELISA Reactivity

The first-generation HIV ELISA kits used purified disrupted whole virus. Purification included an attempt to remove (human or bacterial) cellular contaminants in the manufacturing process. High-titer HLA-antibody sera demonstrated limitations on first-generation preparation purity, for those tests in which HIV was grown in human cell lines, such as H9/HTLV-IIIB. Evaluation of the prototype HIV ELISA raised the potential issue of false-positive reactions on the basis of HLA class II reactivity, although there was very little such reactivity with the prototype assay itself, reflecting high antigen purity (20,30). Problems associated with false HLA reactivity were noted subsequent to licensure for at least two first-generation commercial assays (31,32). Methods to reduce HLA reactivity were developed (33), and the second generation of HIV ELISAs had improved specificity. With the advent of viral components produced through recombinant methods in bacteria such as *Escherichia coli* (34), it became evident that analogous issues also arise for these tests. It is suspected that persons such as intravenous drug users who are repetitively exposed to bacterial pathogens, and hence to the ubiquitous *E. coli,* may have particularly high rates of false reactivity on such recombinant assays.

Manufacturers generally recommend that their kits be

used on fresh sera. Repetitive freezing and thawing of sera increases the probability of false-positive reactions (reflecting decreased specificity, usually primarily due to weak reactives), and may potentially also decrease sensitivity. If sera are heated in an attempt to inactivate virus as a laboratory biosafety measure, both assay sensitivity and specificity are impaired for several of the commercial screening assays.

Analysis of specific clinical conditions that have given difficulties for certain tests in practice, and knowledge concerning the design of these tests (and thus the theoretical problems) can help guide the discriminating laboratory manager in judiciously evaluating the results from a commercial assay (Table 2).

Control Assays

HIV antibody detection tests generally involve the use of preparations containing one or more HIV antigens.

An analogous assay may be run in parallel with comparable reagents but excluding HIV antigen, providing a comparison (control) assay for the evaluation of reactivity. Absence of reactivity on the control assay in the face of reactivity on the primary assay implies that the reactivity is related to HIV itself, i.e., is a true positive. This technique has been effectively utilized in research evaluation studies of ELISA (e.g., the proprietary H9 control plate), immunofluorescence, and Western blot methods, and serves routinely as a parallel control in radioimmunoprecipitation as well as in direct viral detection methods.

While reactivity in the control assay indicates the presence of some reactivity to nonviral constituents (e.g., related to HLA antibodies or antinuclear antibodies), it cannot rule out the possibility of concomitant true reactivity. Thus, false positivity cannot be presumed and alternative HIV assays may need to be employed to discriminate between true and false positivity. Similarly, it is erroneous to utilize tests that directly detect conditions associated with false reactivity (e.g., HLA antibodies) to

---

TABLE 2. *Evaluation of potential sources of error with HIV ELISA screening tests*

I. Dichotomous interpretation of results
  The test is actually a continuous measurement: the chance of misclassification varies with the relative test reactivity strength of the sample. Thus, if the test result is merely classified as negative/positive, information is lost. As an alternative, results may be classified as:
  A. Non-reactive.
  B. "Gray zone positive," weakly reactive, or borderline.
  C. Reactive.
  D. Strongly reactive.
II. Procedural error
  A. Physical mixing up of specimens during testing (retesting correctly labeled sera would reveal a discrepancy).
  B. Subsequent incorrect linkage of test results (testing of a newly acquired specimen from the same subject would reveal a discrepancy).
III. Technical error during testing
  A. Erroneous dilution (or omission) of sera or reagents.
  B. Splashing during test sera or reagent addition, or pipet contamination.
  C. Washing errors.
  D. Incorrect absorbance measurement (e.g., wrong wavelength; bubbles on wet plate or scratches on plate; equipment or electronic malfunction).
IV. Test kit error
  A. Variability in kit reactivity (related to vendor quality control).
  B. Instability or deterioration of reagents.
V. False-positive results
  Although some occur in association with certain clinical conditions, specific confirmatory tests are important. Recognized problems include:
      1. HLA-antibodies: (particularly related to the viral purification process of some early test kits; pose a diagnostic question for multiparous women and others with repeated HLA exposures).
      2. Repetitive freeze/thaws (e.g., some stored sera).
      3. Other retroviruses.
      4. Heating of sera.
      5. Autoantibodies (e.g., ? antinuclear antibodies as in systemic lupus erythematosus, or antimitochondrial antibodies).
      6. Hypergammaglobulinemia, "sticky sera" (e.g., specimens from Africa).
      7. Acute or inflammatory phase responses after vaccination (263, 264); see section "Recent Developments."
VI. False-negative results
  A. HIV-specific antibodies may decline as a function of severity of HIV-related immune dysfunction.
  B. Viremic patients without (IgG) antibodies—including those persons recently exposed/infected.
  C. Hypogammaglobulinemia (including congenital conditions) as a variant of B above.
  D. States of antigen excess.
  E. ? Heating of sera.

rule out true positivity (30,32). In summary, a control assay assists in data interpretation but should not be relied upon as an independent confirmation assay.

Reactivity Strength

The whole-virus ELISA detects reactivity to any of a variety of viral components. AIDS patients with opportunistic infections have been shown to be significantly less reactive by ELISA than AIDS patients with Kaposi's sarcoma (20). This finding probably reflects the observation that during the course of HIV infection, humoral immunity is also impaired, resulting in decreased levels of specific HIV antibody. Persons with HIV-associated lymphadenopathy tend to be very strongly reactive by ELISA, as well as by immunofluorescence (35), suggesting a strong humoral response.

The relative titers of viral component-specific antibodies vary over time in individuals. This can lead to systematic differences in ELISA reactivity and detection rates among varying populations or patient groups. Furthermore, in some persons HIV antigen may be produced in sufficient quantity to form immune complexes with corresponding HIV antibodies, and may sometimes reduce antibody reactivity strength to the extent of false-negative antibody test results. In several panels of sequential sera from seroconverters, antibody to p24 was the first to be routinely detected by Western blots or monoclonal reagents. In late stages of HIV infection, given the existence of a spectrum of viral antigens, immunologic reactivity usually persists to at least some components. In early infection, the phenomena of immune complex formation may contribute to the *seronegative window*.

Special Problems

Studies undertaken in Africa suggested the occurrence of nonspecific, weak HIV ELISA reactivity, particularly among persons with high antibody titers against species of malaria (36). The specificity issues noted above certainly apply to Africa as well. Additionally, the apparently nonspecific association with malaria in some early studies there (36) may have been partly related to an insufficient accounting for the interval temporal changes that can occur during the development of research assays (37). This also highlights the dilemma of interpretations of low-level ("weakly reactive result") reactivity on a screening test, in the absence of confirmatory assays.

Subsequent investigators have also found African sera to be unusually reactive on ELISAs (38). This finding would be consistent with the hypothesis that the higher immunoglobulin levels observed in this population may, in effect, systematically shift the standardization curve for African as compared with U.S. and European sera.

Since a competitive ELISA outperformed other screening methodologies in some research studies of African sera (39), there may be selected circumstances for specialized approaches.

Exposure to other related retroviruses, human and/or nonhuman, may also explain some of the low-level reactivities in regions such as Africa. The finding of very low titer antibodies to HIV in stored sera from Uganda is consistent with such a possibility (40). Infrequently, high-titer HTLV-I antibodies can lead to falsely reactive HIV screening results (20), perhaps relating to p24 *gag* protein cross-reactivity (41). With the continuing discovery of additional retroviruses, ongoing research is likely to clarify these cross-reactivity issues gradually.

Other Screening Tests

Alternative screening methods besides ELISA have been developed, for example, dot-blots and latex agglutination formats. The latter can yield results in seconds (42), analogous to some home pregnancy kits. Early developmental work indicated frequent pro-zone phenomena, in which sera with high levels of HIV antibody gave false-negative results. Dilution of sera both identified and resolved this problem, but the sensitivity and specificity have remained below that of the ELISAs. Thus, these kits are recommended only when sophisticated laboratories are impractical or very rapid preliminary results are very valuable. Tests based on panels of monoclonal antibodies, which might be constituted as "dipsticks", have usually been utilized for confirmation rather than screening purposes.

The reference body fluid for antibody testing is blood, either serum or plasma. Antibodies may also be reliably detected in urine, both with research assays and with minor modification in the performance of commercial assays (43–46). The relatively acellular nature of a clean-catch urine in the absence of genital or bacterial urinary tract infections may balance the apparently lower titer of antibody, to enable the attainment of a reasonable sensitivity/specificity tradeoff. Detection of HIV antibody in saliva has been somewhat more problematical (47–49). One speculation is that proteins or other substances in saliva may bind to HIV antibodies, impairing detection.

Although serological tests for IgM and for IgA antibodies have been developed, technical problems have apparently so far limited their usefulness. IgM and IgA do not cross the placenta, so particular attention has been placed on their use in neonatal diagnosis. However, some negative HIV IgM tests during the first month of life have occurred in children subsequently shown to be HIV infected. Such false-negative results could represent instances of HIV transmission during the birth process itself (49a), rather than prepartum. Thus the misclassification may ultimately represent biological rather than simply technical phenomena, although the latter explanation has been the most widely presumed.

ANTIBODY CONFIRMATION ASSAYS

Immunofluorescence

Antibodies against viruses are commonly detected in clinical laboratories by indirect immunofluorescence assays (IFA). For HIV, IFA has been primarily utilized as a research tool and, in some laboratories, for "confirmation" testing. Acetone-fixed HIV-infected and-uninfected (control) cells are typically applied to slides or isolated wells, incubated with test sera, and counterstained (e.g., with fluorescein-conjugated anti-human IgG). A dilution series of a given serum is usually run to assess strength (titer) of reactivity. The reactions are viewed microscopically as a fluorescent stain.

The fluorescent staining pattern, when read by a skilled observer, is quite informative. Antinuclear antibody and antimitochondrial antibody reactivity patterns may be causes of non-HIV reactivity. Furthermore, the titration endpoints of the reactions on infected and uninfected cells can be compared. This information is then synthesized as a positive or negative result. There is significant potential for observer bias in these subjective assessments. Reactions against both infected and uninfected cells may suggest nonspecific reactivity. However, such an IFA pattern might also occur concomitantly with a true HIV-specific antibody, such as in high-risk persons with high anti-HLA titers (30).

Spectrum of HIV Antibodies

Several confirmation assays enable the visualization of specific antibody reactivities. With the sequencing of the nucleic acid structure of several isolates of HIV, the functional structure of this RNA virus was rapidly unveiled. The HIV genome includes several open reading frames related to essential viral components, including: (1) *gag*—the viral core; (2) *pol*—the enzymes reverse transcriptase (which is essential in creating a DNA copy of the viral RNA) and endonuclease; (3) *env*—the envelope of the virus, including the glycoprotein (gp) membrane; and (4) *tat*—a *trans*-acting protein related to the control of viral replication. Serologic studies using cloned monoclonal reagents (50–52), along with predictions based on the viral genome, have provided an evolving picture of the nature of the various component viral proteins of HIV-1 (Table 3). (The gene product sizes for HIV-2 differ somewhat; see refs. 53 or 54, and Table 3). These components vary in inherent immunogenicity, and may be produced to varying degrees during the course of infection. Antibodies to some viral components, e.g., the HIV-1 regulatory gene *tat* (14 kd), are not detected by standard techniques.

Western Blot and Radioimmunoprecipitation

Western Blot

While the disrupted whole-virus ELISA detects HIV antibodies, the precise spectrum of component antibodies is not demonstrated. The Western blot (also known as the immunoblot) procedure has become a mainstay in confirmation, since it readily permits visualization of the component antibody reactivities (18,19) (Fig. 1).

Preparation of the Western blot begins with purification of HIV from culture materials, followed by dissociation of the concentrated HIV with detergent. In early assays these steps involved the selective loss of some viral components such as gp120/gp160. The material is then resolved by polyacrylamide gel electrophoresis, so that the components are separated by their molecular weights, and then electrophoretically transferred to a support medium such as nitrocellulose paper. Individual strips are reacted with test or control sera, and then developed to reveal bands where the serum antibodies have bound to the resolved viral proteins. The development process involves either photographic plates to reveal radioactivity (e.g., a strip radioimmunoassay) (55) or chemical incubation (e.g., the biotin–avidin technique). The

TABLE 3. *Major genes and gene products of HIV-1, HIV-2, and HTLV*

Gene	Gene products[a]		
	HIV-1	HIV-2	HTLV
Group-specific antigen/core (*gag*)	p17, p24, p40, p55	p16, p26, p56	p19, p24, p28, p53
Polymerase (*pol*)[b]	p31, p51, p66	p34, p53, p68	
Envelope (*env*)	gp41, gp120, gp160	gp36/41, gp80, gp105/125, gp140	gp46, gp62/68
Miscellaneous			p38*tax*, p21*env*,[c] p42*gag*[d]

[a] Represented by p (protein) or gp (glycoprotein), plus the approximate molecular weight of the antigen in kilodaltons.
[b] Endonuclease and reverse transcriptase.
[c] Produced in high titer by recombinant methods.
[d] p42 is tentatively classified as *gag*.

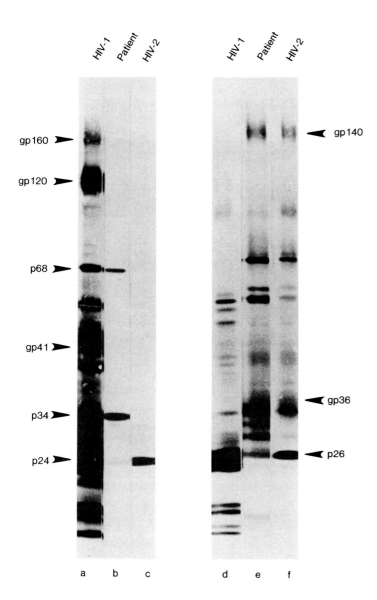

FIG. 1. Western blot analysis of serum samples from an HIV-1-infected patient (HIV-1 control), an AIDS patient with PCR-confirmed HIV-2 infection (53), and an HIV-2-infected patient (HIV-2 control) using HIV-1 antigens (**lanes a–c**) or HIV-2 antigens (**lanes d–f**). Reactivity and cross-reactivity of sera from HIV-1- and HIV-2-infected patients are demonstrated in the *gag* (p24/p26), *pol* (p31/p34 and p66/p68), and *env* (gp41/gp36 and gp160/gp140) gene products. From Lombardo et al. (53).

latter approach gained commercial favor due to the shorter processing time and the elimination of radioactive materials, and it received FDA licensure in 1987. Second-generation Western blots reveal the larger envelope components gp120 and gp160. Several alternative criteria have been proposed for HIV-1 Western blot interpretation (Table 4).

Radioimmunoprecipitation

The radioimmunoprecipitation assay (RIPA) requires HIV to be grown in cell culture in the presence of a radioactive label, purified, and disrupted (56–58). Standard techniques lead to poor labeling of gp41, but lentil-lectin enhancement or alternative radiolabels may be

TABLE 4. *Criteria for "confirmed positive" HIV-1 Western blot result*

Organization	Minimum band pattern required
DuPont-Biotech[a]	p24 *and* p31 *and* (gp41 *or* gp120/160)
Consortium for Retrovirus Serology Standardization (104)	(p24 *or* p31) *and* (gp41 *or* gp120/160)
American Red Cross (103)	At least one band from *each* gene product group: *gag and pol1 and env*
Association of State and Territorial Public Health Laboratory Directors (ASTPHLD) (105)[b]	Any *two* of: p24, gp41, *or* gp120/160

[a] Food and Drug Administration-licensed DuPont Western blot package insert from 1987. Test is currently manufactured by Cambridge Biotech.

[b] The Centers for Disease Control continues to support this prior recommendation (258).

utilized if gp41 detection by RIPA is desired. The material is reacted with the test serum, isolated by precipitation, fully washed, resolved electrophoretically, and developed to analyze the radioactivity pattern. The entire process takes several days to over 1 week and requires considerable technical skill. Since RIPA reliably detects gp120 and gp160 antibodies, it was the reference standard for these large-envelope antibodies until Western blots were improved. RIPA analysis routinely includes a comparison against control material from a radiolabeled cell culture that was grown without HIV, to differentiate cellular from viral reactivity.

Utilization and Interpretation

The great confirmatory powers of Western blot and RIPA lie in their ready demonstration of the specific HIV-related antibodies and in the pattern itself. When classic patterns are present, positivity is a virtual certainty (Table 4). When several related antibodies are detected, the pattern still has high predictive value. Thus the Western blots that detect gp120 and gp160 are helpful in classifying potentially ambiguous sera. In some lots of Western blot reagents, the gp120 and gp160 bands may not be sufficiently separated to appear as clearly independent bands.

A broad gp41 Western blot band was initially accepted as adequate confirmation of sera from a person at high risk of HIV. It was also clearly necessary to have further confirmatory evidence for sera from very low-risk group sera. Since a solitary sharp (thin) Western blot band at p40 was likely to indicate reactivity unrelated to HIV, an experienced virologist and laboratory were crucial in making this critical but subjective distinction during the first years of HIV testing. As in other areas of medicine, adequate training in subtle differences can be essential.

Greater experience and the extension of testing to many labs revealed that significant variations in Western blot reactivity were observed in practice, with results not infrequently discordant compared with those from reference Western blot laboratories (59). Thus aberrant findings clearly required follow-up (60). Such problems led to calls for more formalized and restrictive interpretation of Western blots (Table 4). In some states, only a single centralized lab is permitted to perform testing to help ensure quality control.

In the absence of gp41 on Western blot, there initially was widespread agreement that the combination of p24 and pr53*gag* (by RIPA) provided reliable confirmation. However, the interpretation of Western blots with isolated reactivities was highly controversial (61). When single bands were noted as the sole reactivity, in some instances subsequent testing of follow-up sera showed clear-cut broad reactivities—suggesting that the initial result was consistent with early HIV infection (62).

Some data suggested that p24 core antibody frequently preceded envelope antibodies.

However, persons with solitary p24 bands may be found among historic blood donor sera (20) and instances of prolonged persistent p24 reactivity in low-risk subjects have been noted. This persistent reactivity pattern can be associated with a relatively sharp (i.e., atypical) p24 region. Whereas the initial Centers for Disease Control (CDC) Western blot interpretative criteria accepted p24 alone as sufficient for Western blot confirmation of sera that were repeatedly reactive by ELISA, retrovirologists now routinely treat such Western blot patterns as equivocal. Thus, in some early epidemiologic studies, some persons may have been misclassified.

The observed sequence of development of HIV antibodies is dependent upon the inherent technical sensitivities of the assays employed as well as the biology of infection. Thus, although gp41 antibody may be absent on Western blot, other *env* antibodies such as gp120/160 may be detected. Some sera that have appeared to have antibodies solely to the p24 core antigen can also be shown to have *env* reactivity with RIPA and other newer assays. Commercial HIV antibody assays have tended to detect p24 antibody first in seroconverters.

The interpretation of other Western blot and RIPA patterns in terms of specificity and sensitivity for HIV infection remains uncertain (25,63,64). Persons without evidence of HIV antibodies or with unusual Western blot reactivity patterns have sometimes been found to be HIV infected by culture (25,65) or had positive polymerase chain reaction (PCR) results (66,67), as discussed below.

HIV-2 AND HIV-1

The initial serologic studies in West Africa that found reactivity to a second, related HIV were based on cross-reactivity to simian retroviruses; indeed, HTLV-IV represented a simian contaminant, not a human retrovirus (68,69). Isolation and characterization of LAV-2 led to the acceptance of HIV-2 as a virus distinct from HIV-1, but controversy existed regarding pathogenicity. Most persons infected with HIV-2 appeared to be healthy in several of the initial serosurveys in Africa.

In 1988 the first instance of HIV-2 infection in the United States was confirmed (70). This case helped to confirm the fact that HIV-2, at least in some persons, can cause clinical AIDS (71). This and other cases highlighted the limitation of some HIV-1 screening tests for the detection of HIV-2 infection (53). Serologic discrimination of HIV-1 and HIV-2 can be difficult (72), so that confirmation by PCR is helpful (53,53a,b) and has been utilized to demonstrate apparent coinfection with both HIV-1 and HIV-2. Competitive ELISAs have also been proposed (73). Specific synthetic peptides may also help discriminate between HIV-1 and HIV-2 (69,74). The size of the HIV-1 and HIV-2 antigens also differs somewhat (see Table 3), so that Western blot and RIPA prepared with the respective viruses can also provide some assistance (53,54,64,75). Because of the serological cross-reactivities between HIV-1 and HIV-2 (Fig. 1), in certain populations it is difficult to ascertain whether an individual is infected with HIV-1, HIV-2, or a new viral type, or whether the individual is infected simultaneously with multiple viruses (75). More specific tests such as viral isolation or molecular probes (e.g., PCR) are necessary to distinguish between infections with these viruses in some populations (75a).

Given the very low prevalence of HIV-2 in countries such as the United States, screening assays that detect both HIV-1 and HIV-2 have been developed to reduce screening costs (76–78). Contrary to some theoretical expectations, the sensitivity of the combined assays is comparable to many of the individual HIV assays. Additional cases of HIV-2 infection have been documented in the United States (79). The FDA has licensed Genetic Systems to sell an ELISA that detects HIV-2. Ongoing seroepidemiologic studies by the CDC, the FDA, and the blood bank industry are monitoring the utility of implementation of HIV-2 assays. The long-term follow-up of indeterminate HIV-2 confirmation tests has received some attention (80). The FDA appears likely to mandate the use of combined HIV-1 and HIV-2 screening tests by blood banks in the United States during 1992. Multiple vendors are refining such tests.

OTHER ANTIBODY TESTS

Neutralizing Antibodies

Some HIV antibodies have neutralizing properties in vitro, e.g., inhibition of syncytial formation (81–84). The protective role, if any, of the antibodies detected by these methods remains to be determined (85,85a). These research assays have found particular application in HIV vaccine developmental efforts (86). Antibodies to purified thymosin α-1 also show some evidence of neutralizing capability in vitro, which may be related to the hormone's similarity to HIV p17 (87). An unconfirmed report has linked the presence of specific antibody to lack of mother-to-child transmission (88,88a,88b).

The principal neutralizing domain of HIV appears to be in the V3 hypervariable region of the envelope (the "loop") (89–94), although other viral regions may also prove to be important. A small amount of variation, either in the loop (95) or outside it, can affect neutralization. The reactivity pattern to various neutralizing sera may be useful in classifying viral strains (96,97). These issues are under active investigation (98–102).

If tests for neutralizing antibody to HIV prove clinically important, new diagnostic assays can be anticipated in future years.

INTERPRETATION OF HIV ELISA RESULTS

It is essential to estimate the probability of infection *prior* to testing (the *pretest probability*), in order to interpret a test result appropriately, whatever the purpose—whether it be clinical, counseling, or research. This estimate dramatically impacts upon the attained predictive value after testing (or *posttest probability*).

In the absence of any information to gauge pretest probability, as in the blinded laboratory, the positive predictive value can be maximized (and false positives minimized) by using extremely conservative classification criteria. This is done at the expense of classifying many samples as *indeterminate*. In part, this explains the rationale for the conservative Western blot criteria chosen by the FDA and the vendor for the Western blot package insert, and the similar American Red Cross criteria (103) (Table 4). The use of such criteria is analogous to the assumption that the pretest probability is very low.

Gray Zone

Many laboratories utilize additional cut-off points compared to a vendor's recommendation (package insert), since simple dichotomization may be misleading (Table 2). Indeed, during clinical trials (pre-FDA approval) or postlicensure marketing, many vendors bring in-house both reactive specimens and those with somewhat lesser reactivity. A threshold of 10%, and occasionally even 20%, below the standard cut-off is chosen; gray zone (weakly reactive) results are defined as those between this threshold and the standard cut-off.

Epidemiologic assessment of HIV tests confirmed early that with increasing reactivity (higher absorbances) on the HIV ELISA, the likelihood of true positivity monotonically increased; similarly, with lower ELISA reactivity the likelihood of true negativity increased (20). Furthermore, reducing the ELISA cut-off value will provide higher sensitivity but lower specificity for a given assay configuration than would be obtained with a higher cut-off value (20). These properties enable an end-user to develop and tailor, when appropriate, interpretative criteria alternative to those criteria specified in a package insert, so that the test can be meaningfully extended to additional testing situations.

The nature and degree of further evaluation, and the ultimate clinical interpretation, vary as a function of the strength of ELISA reactivity and the pretest assessment.

Persons at High Risk

When the prior probability is high (as for persons at high risk from hyperendemic regions), the positive predictive value of a reactive or strongly reactive ELISA is extremely high (Table 2). Although a confirmation assay, such as a Western blot, may give an "indeterminate" result based on simple application of some generic criteria (Table 4), alternative interpretative schema or tests can often be used to confirm the diagnostic impression. In this circumstance, categorization by either the Consortium for Retrovirus Serology Standardization (104) or the Association of State and Territorial Public Health Laboratory Directors (ASTPHLD) (105) criteria is clearly preferable to the conservative generic package insert criteria.

A weakly reactive screening result requires further testing to obtain confirmation if the Western blot is not clearly positive. Thus the actual absorbance values, and not simply a reactive/nonreactive result, should be routinely obtained from the testing laboratory.

A nonreactive result from a high-risk patient has only a moderate negative predictive value in this situation: it is important to rule out technical or procedural error (Table 2), recheck the clinical history, and possibly employ alternative and/or more sensitive assays. A surprising negative result should not be accepted as final without further evaluation, since it has a significant chance of being wrong in this circumstance (i.e., a false-negative result). For example, consider a U.S. patient with clinical AIDS who has a negative HIV screening test. If the person were originally from West Africa, specific evaluation for HIV-2 would be warranted—grounded both on epidemiology and decision theory (53,70).

Persons at Low Risk

For a well person at very low HIV risk, such as a blood donor, the negative predictive value of a nonreactive ELISA result is extremely high. In the event of a reactive result, procedural or technical error should be ruled out (Table 2), since many will be false positives. Thus, standard blood bank policy for a reactive result is to repeat the test in duplicate. Many will be clearly negative with near zero absorbance values on both repeat tests. Given the very low pretest estimate, the overwhelming likelihood is an erroneous first result. However, if the donor's history raised any suspicion of risk, which would revise the pretest estimate upwards, additional testing by another methodology would be warranted. A repetitively reactive result is likely to be a true positive, but multiple confirmatory tests may be necessary to attain an acceptable positive predictive value. For example, an indeterminate Western blot may be clarified by other tests or by clinical follow-up. The related finding, that most persons with persistently indeterminate Western blots appear to be uninfected with HIV (106,107), is consistent with these expectations based upon decision analysis considerations.

Care must be taken, however, when interpreting the results from a sequence of tests. Assays are generally not strictly independent, since one source of bias may simultaneously affect multiple laboratory techniques. Pure Bayesian analysis, which assumes strictly independent tests, will therefore lead to overestimation of predictive values.

A weakly reactive result often suggests the need for clinical reassessment, and thus further discussion with the subject. If there is a possibility that the result reflects an early seroconversion, repeat antibody testing in several weeks might clarify an equivocal result. Alternatively, other diagnostic tests may be done immediately, e.g., Western blot, antigen assays, or other direct viral detection methods, or screening assays from other vendors. If the individual has a condition associated with false-positive reactions, a negative direct confirmatory test (e.g., Western blot) is strong evidence for true negativity.

Among low-risk persons, the repeat clinical history may continue to indicate no risk behaviors or exposures, which means that the pretest probability remains extremely low. In this circumstance, even an initial positive confirmatory test implies only a low positive predictive value; further evaluation may be appropriate, e.g., by reference research laboratories.

IMMUNOLOGIC DETECTION

Before the discovery of HIV, the diagnosis of AIDS relied upon clinical criteria (108–115). Early studies also characterized immunologic impairment, particularly low CD4 counts, comparatively elevated CD8 counts, and a low CD4/CD8 ratio. Persons without AIDS, but who had similar risk behaviors as those with AIDS, frequently also had similar abnormalities. These and other immunologic tests were useful in epidemiologic studies to examine risk factors associated with the epidemic (116–123). The advent of HIV serology indicated that these tests remained useful for staging patients, but confirmed the expectation that they were not sufficiently accurate to be used to predict for individual persons whether or not they were infected with HIV (124–131).

Helper T-cell defects occur early in HIV infection (132–134). Lymphokine production can be used to detect antigenic peptide recognition by T-helper lymphocytes, in symptomatic and asymptomatic persons known to be infected with HIV (135,136). These tests are also useful to monitor the response of persons receiving prototype vaccinations against HIV (G. M. Shearer, personal communication). HIV type 1-specific T-helper cell responses have been reported in HIV-seronegative individuals (137). Several investigators have found similar results in studies of persons at high risk of exposure (G.

M. Shearer, unpublished data; S. H. Weiss, unpublished data). One person with this immunologic profile, who was under prospective study, subsequently seroconverted (138). Further studies and follow-up will be necessary to interpret these findings, which: (1) may be nonspecific, (2) may represent an immunologic response following exposure without latent infection, and/or (3) may indicate early evidence of HIV infection in seronegative persons.

DIRECT HIV DETECTION METHODS

Several methods of direct detection are summarized in Table 5 (including some key limitations of the methods) and are reviewed below.

In Situ Hybridization

The technique of *in situ* hybridization offers a direct approach for localization of HIV nucleic acid sequences in cellular preparations (139–141). The limited proportion of infected cells *in vivo,* the low viral sequence copy number per cell, and the need to examine slide preparations by hand with light microscopy limit its application outside highly sophisticated research laboratories. Recent studies demonstrate higher proportions of infected cells than reported in the early studies. It is uncertain whether these differences reflect an improved technique versus an artefact related to stage of HIV illness in the early reports.

Antigen Assays

Parenteral needlestick injuries among health care and laboratory workers exposed to HIV have led to HIV transmission only infrequently (5), (142–144). This suggested that the usual infectious titer of HIV in peripheral blood was much lower than for hepatitis B virus. An HIV antigen assay therefore needs to be extraordinarily sensitive to be useful. *In vitro* hybridization experiments, which indicated that HIV-infected cells are rare in blood,

brain, and lung (139–141), also suggested that detection of HIV antigen in tissue homogenates would likely require sensitive assays. Massive viremia appears to be unusual. Sensitive *in vitro* HIV antigen detection systems have been developed (145–149). Rigorous assessment of such assays in terms of specificity and reproducibility remains limited. Demonstration that an assay specifically measures viral antigen is a challenging task, in so far as there are no independent laboratory criteria. The specificity of a given assay is likely to prove greater in an acellular sterile body fluid such as cerebrospinal fluid.

The clinical utility of antigen assays has so far been limited. Circulating HIV p24 antigen may precede detectable HIV antibodies and thereafter become nondetectable, only to reappear in some persons with severe clinical immunosuppression (149–150a). Antigen may have some value in evaluating response to therapy.

In regions where HIV transmission and seroconversion rates are high, and confidential self-exclusion programs are too nonspecific or otherwise of limited value, screening of blood for HIV antigen may be warranted (150b). In the United States, screening HIV-seronegative blood donors for antigen appears to detect many more false positives than true positives, so that blood banks have not routinely utilized this as a screening tool (150c,d).

Recent studies indicate that an acidification step in the p24 antigen assay can lead to detection of antigen in a higher percentage of HIV-seropositive persons (151). This acidification step disrupts immune complexes that exist between p24 antibody and antigen, but it also reduces total p24 antigen as evidenced by neutralization. Innovations by Abbott Laboratories (151), Ortho Diagnostic Systems (152), and Coulter appear especially promising, and may widen the scope of application for antigen assays.

Tissue Culture

HIV virus isolation by cell culture involves the use of carefully selected permissive cell lines (such as some malignant T-cell lines) or cocultivation with fresh, normal

TABLE 5. *Direct viral detection methods and limitations*

Method	Limitations
Viral p24 (core) antigen	Often not detectable; limited by latency and immune complex formation; latter may be partly overcome with acidification techniques (see text)
In vitro propagation (viral culture)	Variable success rates; generally qualitative; viral strains cultured may be highly selected
Southern blot or *in situ* hybridization for viral nucleic acid	Sensitivity limited by the number of infected cells
Polymerase chain reaction (PCR)	Prone to false positives due to contamination; false-negative results possible with viral variants (259), if a variable region is amplified, or limited number of cells (see text)
Ligase chain reaction (LCR)	Still under development (see text) (260–261)

lymphocytes that have been stimulated with mitogens and maintained with T-cell growth factor (and sometimes α-interferon) (1,2,153). Viral isolates with a propensity for growth in specific lines, e.g., monocyte/macrophage lines, have been described, and may reflect differences in the cellular biology among different strains of HIV (154–157). Culture enhances viral titer and permits detection by other assays (158). Retroviruses can be detected by testing the culture at periodic intervals for specific Mg^{2+}-dependent reverse transcriptase activity in the medium and/or viral antigen detection (as described above). These findings are then further confirmed by detection of viral antigens within the cultured cells, such as by electron microscopy and/or by in situ use of monoclonal reagents.

Positive cultures may indicate either active or latent HIV infective states. These culture methods require advanced technology within the context of adequate provisions for biosafety and are not feasible beyond the research setting. The cost is great, and the laboratory equipment and skilled research technicians are extremely limited. The limited sensitivity and the difficulty of performing HIV cultures do not allow widespread use for the determination of HIV carrier states.

Polymerase Chain Reaction

Gene amplification, utilizing the PCR technology developed by Cetus, has opened new vistas in the detection of infectious agents. The methodology can be used to amplify either DNA or RNA (159–163). The principles have been reviewed recently in depth, and are outside the scope of this chapter (161,164).

For DNA amplification by PCR, synthetic oligonucleotide primers complimentary to the region bordering each side of the area of interest are used. Efficiency considerations lead to the design of primers 15–35 bases in length. The region chosen for detection and amplification requires some care; for example, sequences in which hairpin turns or loops can form need to be avoided.

Theoretically, the nucleotide area of interest will double with each cycle; in practice, 80–90% efficiency is often achieved. This exponential doubling leads to sufficient amounts of DNA to be amenable for many forms of analysis. Probes for the amplified region aid in detec-

tion. Amplifying proviral integrated HIV within the human genome is analogous to finding successfully the proverbial needle in a haystack. Examples of HIV primer probes have been reviewed (161).

False-negative PCR results can occur for technical reasons. Heparin, for example, can inhibit PCR (165). ACD solution is the preferred anticoagulant for specimen collection, especially when cells will not be processed and extensively washed, to reduce false negatives. Biologic reasons for false negatives include (1) genomic variation in HIV (259): the nucleotides flanking a presumed constant region may vary (primer failure) or the amplified region may vary (probe failure); and (2) virus exists below the detectable level.

False-positive PCR results have raised even greater concern (166). The exponential amplification carries great risk of inadvertent contamination, which may vary from gross contamination to amounts consistent with aerosol passage, as may occur with simply flicking open a specimen tube cap near an adjacent specimen (Table 6).

When the number of expected copies produced by PCR approaches one (or less), then statistical considerations (which can be modeled as a Poisson distribution) predict the likelihood of PCR positivity. With very low original copy number in a sample, PCR can be anticipated to be positive only some of the time. When a positive result is not consistently confirmed, it can be difficult to determine whether this represents a true positive with low copy number (e.g., few infected cells in a terminal, severely CD4-depleted AIDS patient, or perhaps a seronegative person at high exposure risk) versus aerosol contamination.

In devising a commercial PCR diagnostic center, Roche has built a facility in North Carolina to minimize the risk of contamination (167). Since carryover has been identified as a major cause of contamination, separate rooms for reagent preparation, specimen preparation, PCR set-up, and analysis exist. Movement of materials only proceeds forward to the next self-contained room, never backwards. It seems likely that FDA licensure of PCR detection methods will become a reality in the near future.

False-positive results may be further minimized by requiring that the PCR be positive on two or more gene products. PCR reactivity on only one gene would be

TABLE 6. *Degrees of polymerase chain reaction contamination*

Classification	Volume of contaminant (μl)	Approximate no. of copies PCR product produced after 30 cycles
Spill or gross contamination	1–100	10^7–10^9
Smudge	10^{-4}–0.1	10^3–10^6
Aerosol	10^{-9}–10^{-5}	0.01–100

Adapted from McCreedy et al. (167).

classified as indeterminate, and would require further investigation to clarify its meaning. Viral variation or defective viruses, or insufficient sample material, may contribute to indeterminate results. In preliminary HIV PCR trials by the Roche facility, indeterminate HIV PCR results have been rare (167).

PCR may be performed on fresh or cultured lymphocytes. Obviously, in either case virus siblings (variants) that differ in the primer region will not be amplified. In addition, conformational or related issues may lead to varying efficiency in replication for different sibling variants, which may give rise to large differences in relative copy number over many PCR cycles. Subject to the above caveats, on fresh material the results will reflect the underlying HIV sibling distribution. Since defective retrovirus variants may be among those amplified, and at least in theory might be the only HIV detected, a positive PCR result (particularly in a seronegative individual) does not necessarily indicate active infection. If the cells are cultured first, then only viruses capable of *in vitro* replication will be detected, and the relative ability to replicate in culture will heavily influence the distribution of viral variants that are detected. This latter methodology is thus inferior when attempting to understand molecular epidemiologic events and sibling evolution.

Potential uses of PCR include

1. Confirmation of serologic results (168–172), examination of other bodily fluids (173,174) or stored material (175), and staging (176)
2. Resolution of indeterminate Western blots (107)
3. Resolution of infective status in infants (177–182a)
4. Reassurance of persons at low HIV risk (183,184)
5. Screening for retroviral infection risk (185)
6. Identification of latent infection in seronegative persons at HIV risk (66,186–196c)
7. Quantitation of viral load (151,170,197)
8. Detection of defective or aberrant retroviruses (198)
9. Evaluation of viral variation (199–203a,259).

Many of the these applications are still being refined, and remain the subject of considerable controversy (203b). In particular, experts are divided concerning the typical explanation for positive PCR results in seronegative persons, given the widely varying results referenced in the reports above, with viewpoints ranging from: (1) false positive to (2) transient infection with clearing to (3) latent infection. In part, this controversy reflects our still emerging understanding of the biology of retroviral infection.

DIAGNOSIS OF HTLV

HTLV-I was the first human retrovirus to be discovered (204), followed shortly by HTLV-II (205). The development of the HIV ELISA methodology was aided by the developmental work that had been done for the HTLV-I ELISA (17,20). The discovery of the second instance of HTLV-II infection, in an intravenous drug user who died of *Pneumocystis carinii* pneumonia prior to the discovery of HIV, was prompted by atypical reactivity on the existing HTLV-I diagnostic tests and required viral isolation to prove its near identity to the HTLV-II Mo prototype (206). It is not surprising that there are many similarities in the diagnostic modalities for HTLV and HIV. This section highlights the differences.

In 1988, a blood screening program for HTLV-I was instituted in the United States utilizing ELISAs licensed by the FDA (207,208). These assays are based on HTLV-I-infected cell lysates as the source of capture antigen, but can detect antibodies to both HTLV-I and HTLV-II due to antigenic cross-reactivity (206,209,210). These assays do not differentiate between HTLV-I and HTLV-II. Other promising assays in development have not yet been widely evaluated (211–214a).

HIV-1 can be cultured to much higher titers than HTLV-I, so that the antigen preparation for the whole-virus ELISA can be purified more easily for HIV than for HTLV. Cellular contamination of the viral preparation leads to cross-reactivity and nonspecific (false-positive) reactions more frequently for HTLV than HIV. Serologic assays for HTLV antigen have been used to monitor HTLV cell cultures, but have not found clinical application since measurable cell-free HTLV concentrations have not been detected in peripheral blood. This absence of significant cell-free virus is in contrast to HIV, and may help explain some of the differences in epidemiologic transmission patterns.

That many persons infected with HTLV have only low titers of antibody further complicates the picture. In contrast, the titers for HIV antibody tend to be relatively high. Thus the HTLV ELISA is both less sensitive and less specific than a comparable HIV ELISA. The impaired specificity makes confirmatory testing absolutely essential for HTLV (210).

In Japan, a particle agglutination test has been used for HTLV-I screening with good success (215,216). Recent improvements aid in the detection of low-titer antibodies by particle agglutination (217), an issue particularly relevant to the detection of asymptomatic HTLV-I carriers.

If a confirmatory test can not detect antibody titers as weak as the screening test can detect, some true positives will be unconfirmed and categorized erroneously as negative. This situation frequently occurs with HTLV (but not HIV) diagnostics. Much care must be taken in interpreting HTLV results, both when counseling patients and when reading the literature critically.

Western blots are particularly poor HTLV confirmatory tests. Sera rarely react with HTLV *env* products. If both *gag* and *env* reactivity are required for confirmation, a Western blot alone will confirm few sera (218).

Commercially available Western blots used for confirmation of ELISA-reactive specimens among intravenous drug users within the United States may be indeterminate or negative in a majority of individuals (219–222). In addition, the relative titers of HTLV-specific proteins vary greatly depending upon both the cell line and HTLV variant used to produce HTLV for the test kit (S. H. Weiss, unpublished observations).

For these reasons, some investigators have used RIPA to confirm indeterminate HTLV Western blot patterns. This approach is flawed, since even Western blot negative sera should be tested by RIPA. However, RIPA frequently cannot detect low-titer antibody, so Western blot plus RIPA confirmation schema will miss some true positives. RIPA is also limited to select research laboratories. In summary, standard Western blots have limited utility, and can not play the same role as they do in HIV diagnostics.

Competitive ELISAs can be used to confirm HTLV screening results, and to categorize whether the infection is due to HTLV-I or HTLV-II (209). Although extraordinarily time-consuming, this approach was the first to demonstrate high rates of HTLV infection in a cohort of U.S. intravenous drug users, and also the first to show HTLV-II seroprevalence rates that exceeded HTLV-I (209,223).

Immunofluorescence was used in many early HTLV studies either for screening or for confirmation of ELISA results (224,225). When HTLV-II-infected cells, in addition to an assay with HTLV-I infected cells, are used for immunofluorescence, in light of the existence of high HTLV-II seroprevalence in the United States, only a few additional sera were actually confirmed (210,226). Many HTLV-II sera, including the Mo HTLV-II prototype, react well on HTLV-I assays, including immunofluorescence. Immunofluorescence patterns consistent with antinuclear antibodies (ANA) were also seen frequently among intravenous drug users. Since true infection simultaneous with ANA is possible, interpretation in this high-risk group is difficult.

HTLV-II p24 antibodies can strongly cross-react with HTLV-I p24 antigen (41), so that a radioimmunoassay (RIA) utilizing purified HTLV-I p24 has been suggested as an alternative HTLV confirmatory test (227). However, HTLV-II may tend to give systematically lower reactivity than HTLV-I on this HTLV-I-based assay (S. H. Weiss, unpublished data). Given all these problems with the standard assays, an alternative approach was suggested in 1987 utilizing concomitant reactivity on an HTLV-I ELISA, an HTLV-I p24 RIA, and on either an HTLV-I or HTLV-II immunofluorescence assay (210). The rates of HTLV infection reported in that study were quite high. Subsequent studies, nevertheless, indicated that these criteria were too strict, and underestimated true seroprevalence (228,229).

Serologic tests for HTLV-II have generally used HTLV-I based reagents, which may have impaired sensitivity for detection of HTLV-II. The HTLV screening tests licensed by the FDA were evaluated using reference panels composed only of HTLV-I sera. Given the high prevalence of HTLV-II in some geographic regions, the HTLV-I-based tests may not be adequate (229,212).

The advent of a Western blot spiked with recombinant p21*env* protein holds promise as a new confirmatory test, which may be able to differentiate HTLV-I from HTLV-II reliably (221,229,230) (Fig. 2). Other serologic approaches, such as peptide assays, also hold promise (231–238c).

PCR has proved extremely useful in confirming HTLV infection, and delineating the type of HTLV (229,239–243). It is reasonable to expect that different primer pairs will have different sensitivities for identification of HTLV-I or HTLV-II infection within given populations (229). Differences in PCR amplification efficiency have been noted for HTLV primer pairs SK 43/44 and SK 110/111 (B. McCreedy, unpublished observations). Primer set SK 43/44 and probe SK 45 appear to yield better results following amplification of low copy number HTLV DNA than does the primer pair SK 110/111 and probes SK 112 and SK 188. Further research is this area is necessary (229).

In addition, nucleotide sequence diversity and the issue of defective or incomplete retroviral elements may need to be considered. Little is known about sequence diversity among HTLV-II isolates. However, deleted HTLV-I proviruses have been shown to exist in fresh leukemic cells of patients with adult T-cell leukemia–lymphoma syndrome (244,245). Recently Hall and colleagues found deleted HTLV-I provirus in HTLV ELISA-seronegative patients with mycosis fungoides (198). Some analyses of HTLV ELISA-reactive cohorts by means of PCR have found 12–24% of the HTLV infection nontypeable (242,246), although others found almost all specimens to be typeable with the newer primers and probes (229). The ability to detect all HTLV-II-infected individuals by ELISA screening assays, or to confirm infection by Western blot or PCR, may therefore be limited by sequence diversity and possibly proviral deletions. Further characterization of optimal PCR primer pairs, ELISA and Western blot capture antigens (230), and possible newer serological assays [such as the use of synthetic peptides (237,238b)] should be a focus of future research. In addition, HTLV-I capture antigens in ELISA screening assays and standard Western blot may be inappropriate for use in the United States, Italy (247), Argentina (248), Panama (249,250), and other regions where HTLV-II has been demonstrated.

One study has linked sexual transmission of HTLV-I with the presence of anti-HTLV-I tax antibody (251). Thus, selective assays may be important in further defining epidemiologic transmission characteristics. For HIV, studies of specific antibody patterns have been contro-

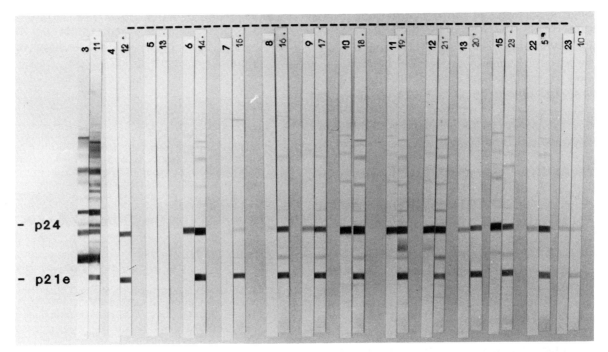

FIG. 2. HTLV Western blots. Paired western blot results comparing standard Biotech/DuPont strips with the Cambridge Biotech strips containing added recombinant p21*env* protein. The major bands represented are p24 and p21*env*. Strips 3 and 11 were incubated with HTLV-I-positive control serum, strips 4 and 12 with HTLV-II-positive control serum, and strips 5 and 13 with control serum negative for HTLV-I and HTLV-II. All remaining pairs represent individuals from a study of intravenous drug users in New Jersey (229) who were HTLV-ELISA-(Abbott Laboratories) reactive and confirmed by PCR to represent HTLV-II infection. Figure courtesy of Paul E. Palumbo, MD, Steven S. Alexander, PhD, and Stanley H. Weiss, MD.

versial with respect to prediction of transmission (88). More work in this area for HTLV is also necessary.

Currently, multiple assays are necessary to define accurately the prevalence of HTLV-I and -II in a given population. Further work is required for the development of assays that are highly sensitive and specific. Recent studies suggest that HTLV-II may have immunologic and health consequences (228,252–256a), as does HTLV-I (13,257). Specific laboratory assays will be important tools in further clarifying the epidemiology of HTLV-II. These newer approaches, in combination with an ELISA that includes HTLV-II antigens, hold great promise for improving HTLV diagnostics.

The commercial HTLV Western blot commonly used by blood banks to confirm repeat HTLV ELISA reactivity is inadequate for confirmation of HTLV-II infection. Since counseling of donors by blood banks is done when ELISA results are confirmed, the sensitivity and specificity of the confirmatory tests are critical. The conventional Western blot should be replaced or supplemented by other easily performed assays, particularly in geographic regions where the prevalence of HTLV-II represents a significant proportion of the HTLV serologic reactivity (212,213).

RECENT DEVELOPMENTS

The ligase chain reaction (LCR) has promise as a new technique for amplifying DNA (260, 261). LCR, like PCR, uses oligonucleotides that anneal to specific, complementary sequences on the target DNA to be amplified. LCR appears to have significant potential to produce quantitative results and to be automated. In contrast to PCR, in theory LCR will only amplify stretches of DNA that have the entire exact sequence utilized. Thus LCR essentially combines both an amplification and a detection step. Specific DNA alleles can be selectively amplified by LCR or special application of PCR methodology (262). Initial commercial emphasis for LCR may be for the detection of infectious agents that exhibit little inherent variation, which would capitalize on the specificity of LCR as a screening or confirmation test. PCR currently has greater speed and sensitivity compared to LCR (260). LCR technology will be an active area of research that has significant potential for widespread use in laboratory DNA diagnostics.

In December 1991, a test kit manufacturer informed the FDA of a phenomenon of multiple false-positive reactions (263), possibly linked to influenza vaccination.

These blood donors were repetitively reactive on screening tests for HIV-1, HTLV-I, and the newly licensed and implemented hepatitis C virus screening kits, but negative by a variety of confirmatory assays. The problem was found to extend to kits made by other manufacturers. The detection of this phenomenon was aided by the simultaneous use by blood banks of test kits for three different infectious agents, pinpointing that the lack of specificity might be an indicator of a more general problem.

Preliminary data suggest that, in part, the phenomenon is related to an acute or inflammatory phase response that may be due to acute phase reactants (263, 264). It is associated with a variety of immunizations, including tetanus and hepatitis B, not just influenza. Although several of the affected assays use goat antihuman IgG, sera from some of the individuals exhibiting this phenomenon bind to bare beads or plates, indicative of a "stickiness" attribute not related to a specific antigen, and thus it is not virus specific.

Preliminary data from a CDC pilot study suggest that about 35% of the multiple reactors among blood donors had some vaccination in the prior 2 weeks, significantly more compared to this history in only 12% of the control donors. The majority of the multiple reactors had no apparent risk factor. The peak influenza vaccination season began in October 1991, when approximately 12% reported recent vaccination. Of those, multiple false-positive reactions occurred in 0.4%. This contributed a total of 0.05% to a preexisting background false positive rate of 0.17%, leading to a total false positive rate for HIV-1 of 0.22% among blood donors. In at least some individuals, the false reactivity is transient (263). Extensive further evaluation of the phenomenon of false positive reactivity is ongoing (264).

CONCLUSIONS

The armamentarium of HIV and HTLV detection systems has continued to grow rapidly. Testing alternatives will steadily move from the research bench to the clinical laboratory. The judicious choice of these tools will depend upon an increased understanding of the dynamics of retroviral infection, critical head-to-head comparison testing, and cost–benefit decision analyses. Further development and evaluation are warranted for direct HIV detection methods as well as for other immunologic tests of HIV exposure, and for serologic detection and confirmation of HTLV infection.

ACKNOWLEDGMENTS

I thank Debbie Fields and Karen McGirt for their expert assistance in manuscript preparation. This work was supported in part by the New Jersey State Department of Health (grants 90-195-AIDS and 91-105-AIDS), the Foundation of UMDNJ (grant 15-89), and NIH Biomedical Research Support grant (2-507-RR05393).

REFERENCES

1. Gallo RC, Salahuddin SZ, Popovic M, et al. Frequent detection and isolation of cytopathic retroviruses (HTLV-III) from patients with AIDS and at risk for AIDS. *Science* 1984;224:500–3.
2. Popovic M, Sarngadharan MG, Read E, Gallo RC. Detection, isolation, and continuous production of cytopathic retroviruses (HTLV-III) from patients with AIDS and pre-AIDS. *Science* 1984;224:497–500.
3. Landesman SH, Ginzburg HM, Weiss SH. The AIDS epidemic. *N Engl J Med* 1985;312:521–5.
4. Blattner WA. Blattner and colleagues respond to Duesberg. *Science* 1988;241:514–7.
5. Weiss SH, Biggar RJ. The epidemiology of human retrovirus-associated illnesses. *Mt Sinai J Med* 1986;53:579–91.
6. Melbye M. The natural history of human T lymphotropic virus-III infection: the cause of AIDS. *Brt Med J* 1986;292:5–12.
6a.Coffin J, Haase A, Levy JA, et al. Human immunodeficiency viruses. *Science* 1986;223:697.
7. Barre-Sinoussi F, Chermann JC, Rey F, et al. Isolation of a T-lymphotropic retrovirus from a patient at risk for acquired immune deficiency syndrome (AIDS). *Science* 1983;220:868–71.
8. Hahn BH, Shaw GM, Taylor ME, et al. Genetic variation in HTLV-III/LAV over time in patients with AIDS or at risk for AIDS. *Science* 1986;232:1548–53.
9. Saag MS, Hahn BH, Gibbons J, et al. Extensive variation of human immunodeficiency virus type 1 in vivo. *Nature* 1988;334:440–4.
10. Wain-Hobson S. HIV genome variability in vivo. *AIDS* 1989;3[Suppl 1]:s13–s18.
11. Brun-Vezinet F, Katlama C, Ceuninck D, et al. Lymphadenopathy associated virus type 2 (LAV-2)—seroepidemiological study in Cape Verde islands. 3rd International Conference on AIDS, Washington, DC, 1987.
12. Kanki P, M'Boup S, Barin F, et al. HTLV-IV and HTLV-III/HIV in West Africa. 3rd International Conference on AIDS, Washington, DC, June 1987.
13. Blattner WA. Epidemiology of HTLV-I and associated diseases. In: Blattner WA, ed. Human retrovirology: HTLV. New York: Raven Press, 1990;251–65.
14. Dodd RY. Donor screening and epidemiology. *Prog Clin Biol Res* 1985;182:389–405.
15. Farzadegan H, Polis MA, Wolinsky SM, et al. Loss of human immunodeficiency virus type 1 (HIV-1) antibodies with evidence of viral infection in asymptomatic homosexual men. *Ann Intern Med* 1988;108:785–90.
16. CDC. Classification system for human immunodeficiency virus (HIV) infection in children under 13 years of age. *MMWR* 1987;36:225–35.
17. Saxinger WC, Gallo RC. Application of the indirect enzyme-linked immunosorbent assay microtest to the detection and surveillance of human T-cell leukemia-lymphoma virus. *Lab Invest* 1983;49:371–7.
18. Sarngadharan MG, Popovic M, Bruch L, Schupbach J, Gallo RC. Antibodies reactive with human T-lymphotropic retroviruses (HTLV-III) in the serum of patients with AIDS. *Science* 1984;224:506–8.
19. Schupbach J, Popovic M, Gilden RV, Gonda MA, Sarngadharan MG, Gallo RC. Serological analysis of a subgroup of human T-lymphotropic retroviruses (HTLV-III) associated with AIDS. *Science* 1984;224:503–5.
20. Weiss SH, Goedert JJ, Sarngadharan MG, et al. Screening test for HTLV-III (AIDS agent) antibodies: specificity, sensitivity, and applications. *JAMA* 1985;253:221–5.
21. CDC. Additional recommendations to reduce sexual and drug abuse-related transmission of human T-lymphotropic virus type III/lymphadenopathy-associated virus. *MMWR* 1986;35:152–5.

22. Weiss SH, Goedert JJ. Screening for HTLV-III antibodies: the relation between prevalence and positive predictive value and its social consequences. *JAMA* 1985;253:3397.
23. Marwick C. Use of AIDS antibody test may provide more answers. *JAMA* 1985;253:1694–9.
24. Sivak SL, Wormser GP. Predictive value of a screening test for antibodies to HTLV-III. *Am J Clin Pathol* 1986;85:700–3.
25. Petricciani JC, Seto B, Wells M, Quinnan G, McDougal JS, Bodner AJ. An analysis of serum samples positive for HTLV-III antibodies. *N Engl J Med* 1985;313:47–8.
26. CDC. Results of human T-lymphotropic virus type III test kits reported from blood collection centers—United States, April 22 —May 19, 1985. *MMWR* 1985;34:375–6.
27. Marlink RG, Allan JS, McLane MF, Essex M. Low sensitivity of ELISA testing in early HIV infection. *N Engl J Med* 1987;315:1549.
28. Salahuddin SZ, Groopman JE, Markham PD, et al. HTLV-III in symptom-free seronegative persons. *Lancet* 1984;2:1418–20.
29. Carlson JR, Bryant ML, Hinrichs SH, et al. AIDS serology testing in low- and high-risk groups. *JAMA* 1985;253:3405–8.
30. Weiss SH, Mann DL, Murray C, Popovic M. HLA-DR antibodies and HTLV-III antibody ELISA testing. *Lancet* 1985;2:157.
31. Kuhnl P, Seidl S, Holzberger G. HLA DR4 antibodies cause positive HTLV-III antibody ELISA results. *Lancet* 1985;1:1222–3.
32. Hunter JB, Menitove JE. HLA antibodies detected by ELISA HTLV-III antibody kits. *Lancet* 1985;2:397.
33. Arthur LO, Bess JW Jr, Heffner Barrett C, et al. Removal of HLA DR antigens from HTLV-III preparations using immunoaffinity chromatography. *J Cell Biochem* 1986;10A[Suppl]:226 (abst).
34. Chang TW, Kato I, McKinney S, et al. Detection of antibodies to human T-cell lymphotropic virus-III (HTLV-III) with an immunoassay employing a recombinant *Escherichia coli*-derived viral antigenic peptide. *Biotechnology* 1985;3:905–9.
35. Kaminsky LS, McHugh T, Stites D, et al. High prevalence of antibodies to AIDS-associated retrovirus in AIDS and related conditions but not in other disease states. *Proc Natl Acad Sci USA* 1985;82:5535–9.
36. Biggar RJ, Gigase PL, Melbye M, et al. ELISA HTLV retrovirus antibody reactivity associated with malaria and immune complexes in healthy Africans. *Lancet* 1985;2:520–3.
37. Blaser MJ, Cohn DL, Cody H, et al. Counterimmunoelectrophoresis for detection of human serum antibody to HTLV-III. *J Immunol Methods* 1986;91:181–6.
38. Gazzolo L, Robert-Guroff M, Jennings A, et al. Type-I and type-III HTLV antibodies in hospitalized and out-patient Zairians. *Int J Cancer* 1985;36:373–8.
39. Melbye M, Njelesani EK, Bayley A, et al. Evidence for heterosexual and clinical manifestations of human immunodeficiency virus infection and related conditions in Lusaka, Zambia. *Lancet* 1986;2:1113–5.
40. Saxinger WC, Levine P, Dean AG, et al. Evidence for exposure to HTLV-III in Uganda prior to 1973. *Science* 1985;227:1036–8.
41. Mann DL, DeSantis P, Mark G, et al. HTLV-I-associated B-cell CLL: indirect role for retrovirus in leukemogenesis. *Science* 1987;236:1103–6.
42. Carlson JR, Mertens SC, Yee JL, et al. Preliminary communication: rapid, easy and economical screening test for antibodies to the human immunodeficiency virus. *Lancet* 1987;1:361–2.
43. Cao Y, Friedman-Kien AE, Chuba JV, Mirabile M, Hosein B. IgG antibodies to HIV-1 in urine of HIV-1 seropositive individuals. *Lancet* 1988;1:831–2.
44. Connell JA, Parry JV, Mortimer PP, et al. Preliminary report: accurate assays for anti-HIV in urine. *Lancet* 1990;335:1366–9.
45. Desai S, Bates H, Michalski FJ. Detection of antibody to HIV-1 in urine. *Lancet* 1991;337:183–4.
46. Reagan KJ, Lile CC, Book GW, Devash Y, Winslow DL, Bincsik A. Use of urine for HIV-1 antibody screening. *Lancet* 1991;335:358–9.
47. Shoeman RL, Pottathil R, Metroka C. Antibodies to HIV in saliva. *N Engl J Med* 1989;320:1145–6.
48. Archibald DW, Cole GA. In vitro inhibition of HIV-1 infectivity by human salivas. *AIDS Res Hum Retroviruses* 1990;6:1425–32.
49. Major CJ, Read SE, Coates RA, et al. Comparison of saliva and blood for human immunodeficiency virus prevalence testing. *J Infect Dis* 1991;163:699–702.
49a. Goedert JJ, Duliege A-M, Amos CI, Felton S, Biggar RJ, The International Registry of HIV-exposed Twins. High risk of HIV-1 infection for first-born twins. *Lancet* 1991;338:1471–5.
50. DiMarzo Veronese F, Copeland TD, DeVico AL, et al. Characterization of highly immunogenic p66/p51 as the reverse transcriptase of HTLV-III/LAV. *Science* 1986;231:1289–91.
51. Wright CM, Felber BK, Paskalis H, Paslakis GN. Expression and characterization of the trans-activator of HTLV-III/LAV virus. *Science* 1986;234:988–92.
52. DiMarzoVeronese F, Sarngadharan MG, Rahman R, et al. Monoclonal antibodies specific for p24, the major core protein of human T-cell leukemia virus type III. *Proc Natl Acad Sci USA* 1985;82:5199–202.
53. Lombardo JM, Horsburgh CR, Denny TN, et al. Evaluation of an atypical HIV type 1 antibody: serologic pattern leading to detection of HIV type 2 infection in North America. *Arch Pathol Lab Med* 1989;113:1245–9.
53a. Pieniazek D, Peralta JM, Ferreira JA, et al. Identification of mixed HIV-1/HIV-2 infections in Brazil by polymerase chain reaction. *AIDS* 1991;5:1293–9.
53b. Busch MP. The need for rigorous molecular epidemiology. *AIDS* 1991;5:1379–80.
54. Parekh BS, Pau C-P, Granade TC, et al. Oligomeric nature of transmembrane glycoproteins of HIV-2: procedures for their efficient dissociation and preparation of western blots for diagnosis. *AIDS* 1991;5:1009–13.
55. Towbin H, Staehelin T, Gordon J. Electrophoretic transfer of proteins from polyacrilamide gels to nitrocellulose sheets: procedures and some applications. *Proc Natl Acad Sci USA* 1979;82:4350–4.
56. Robey WG, Safai B, Oroszlan S, et al. Characterization of envelope and core structural gene products of HTLV-III with sera from AIDS patients. *Science* 1985;228:593–5.
57. Barin F, McLane MF, Allan JS, Lee TH, Groopman JE, Essex M. Virus envelope protein of HTLV-III represents the major target antigen for antibodies in AIDS patients. *Science* 1985;228:1094–6.
58. Allan JS, Coligan JE, Barin F, et al. Major glycoprotein antigens that induce antibodies in AIDS patients are encoded by HTLV-III. *Science* 1985;228:1091–3.
59. CDC. Update: serologic testing for HIV-1 antibody—United States, 1988 and 1989. *MMWR* 1990;39:380–3.
60. Saag MS, Britz J. Asymptomatic blood donor with a false positive HTLV-III western blot. *N Engl J Med* 1986;314:118.
61. Carlson JR, Hinrichs SH, Levy NB, et al. Evaluation of commercial AIDS screening test kits. *Lancet* 1986;1:1388.
62. Biggar RJ, Johnson BK, Musoke SS, et al. Severe illness associated with appearance of antibody to human immunodeficiency virus in an African. *Br Med J* 1986;293:1210–1.
63. Esteban JI, Shih JW-K, Tai C-C, Bodner AJ, Kay JWD, Alter HJ. Importance of western blot analysis in predicting infectivity of anti-HTLV-III/LAV positive blood. *Lancet* 1985;2:1083–6.
64. Schulz TF, Oberhuber W, Schmidt B, et al. Serological discrimination between HIV-1 and HIV-2. *Lancet* 1988;2:162–3.
65. Ward JW, Grindon AJ, Feorino PM, Schable C, Parvin M, Allen JR. Laboratory and epidemiologic evaluation of an enzyme immunoassay for antibodies to HTLV-III. *JAMA* 1986;256:357–61.
66. Imagawa DT, Lee MH, Wolinsky SM, et al. Human immunodeficiency virus type 1 infection in homosexual men who remain seronegative for prolonged periods. *N Engl J Med* 1989;320:1458–62.
67. Wolinsky SM, Rinaldo CR, Kwok S, et al. Human immunodeficiency virus type 1 (HIV-1) infection a median of 18 months before a diagnostic western blot: evidence from a cohort of homosexual men. *Ann Intern Med* 1989;111:961–72.
68. Hirsch VM, Olmsted RA, Murphey-Corb M, Purcell RH, Johnson PR. An African primate lentivirus (SIVsm) closely related to HIV-2. *Nature* 1989;339:389–92.
69. Baillou A, Janvier B, Mayer R, et al. Site-directed serology using synthetic oligopeptides representing the C-terminus of the external glycoproteins of HIV-1, HIV-2, or SIV$_{mac}$ may distinguish subtypes among primate lentiviruses. *AIDS Res Hum Retroviruses* 1991;7:767–71.
70. Weiss SH, Lombardo J, Michaels J, et al. AIDS due to HIV-2 infection—New Jersey. *MMWR* 1988;37:33–35.

71. Kloser PC, Mangia AJ, Leonard J, et al. HIV-2 associated AIDS in the USA: the first case. *Arch Intern Med* 1989;149:1875–7.

72. Marquart K-H, Muller HAG. Different serological HIV-2 results in three HIV-1-infected men from the Gambia. *Infection* 1989;17:63–4.

73. Simon F, Meana A, Rinaldi R, et al. HIV-1 competitive ELISA for serological diagnosis of HIV-2 positivity. *AIDS* 1990;4:1169–70.

74. Broliden PA, Ruden U, Ouattara AS, et al. Specific synthetic peptides for detection of and discrimination between HIV-1 and HIV-2 infection. *J Acquired Immune Deficiency Syndrome* 1991;4:952–8.

75. Holzer T, Allen RG, Heynen CA, et al. Discrimination of HIV-2 infection from HIV-1 infection by Western blot and radioimmunoprecipitation assay. *AIDS Res Hum Retroviruses* 1990;6:515–24.

75a.Grankvist O, Bredberg-Raden U, Gustafsson A, et al. Improved detection of HIV-2 DNA in clinical samples using a nested primer-based polymerase chain reaction. *J AIDS* 1992;5:286–93.

76. Abiola PO, Parry JV, Mortimer PP. Sensitivity for anti-HIV-2 of combined HIV antibody kits. *Lancet* 1990;336:1386–7.

77. Myrmel H, Holm-Hansen C, Haukenes G. Evaluation of two rapid tests for the detection of HIV-1/HIV-2 antibodies. *AIDS* 1990;4:1164–6.

78. Das PC, Smit Sibinga CT. Combined HIV-1/2 assay kits. *Lancet* 1991;337:125–6.

79. CDC. Update: HIV-2 infection—United States. *MMWR* 1989;108:785–90.

80. Pepin J, Dalby M, Gaye I, Berry N, Whittle H. Long-term follow-up of subjects with an indeterminate HIV-2 western blot. *AIDS* 1991;5:1274–5.

81. Robert-Guroff M, Brown M, Gallo RC. HTLV-III-neutralizing antibodies in patients with AIDS and AIDS-related-complex. *Nature* 1985;316:72–4.

82. Weiss RA, Clapham PR, Cheingsong-Popov R, et al. Neutralization of human T-lymphotropic virus type III by sera of AIDS and AIDS-risk patients. *Nature* 1985;316:69–71.

83. Faulkner-Valle GP, De Rossi A, Gassa OD, Chieco-Bianchi L. LAV/HTLV-III neutralizing antibodies in the sera of patients with AIDS, lymphadenopathy syndrome and asymptomatic seropositive individuals. *Tumori* 1986;72:219–24.

84. Evans DJ, McKeating J, Meredith JM, et al. An engineered poliovirus chimaera elicits broadly reactive HIV-1 neutralizing antibodies. *Nature* 1989;339:385–8.

85. Wang CY, Looney DJ, Walfield AM, et al. Long-term high-titer neutralizing activity induced by octameric synthetic HIV-1 antigen. *Science* 1991;254:285–8.

85a.Wiseman G, Rubinstein A, Martinez P, Lambert S, Devash Y, Goldstein H. Cellular and antibody responses directed against the HIV-1 principal neutralizing domain in HIV-1-infected children. *AIDS Res Hum Retroviruses* 1991;7:839–45.

86. Wiseman G, Rubinstein A, Martinez P, Lambert S, Devash Y, Goldstein H. Cellular and antibody responses directed against the HIV-1 principal neutralizing domain in HIV-1-infected children. *AIDS Res Hum Retroviruses* 1991;7:839–45.

87. Sarin PS, Sun DK, Thornton AH, Naylor PH, Goldstein AL. Neutralization of HTLV-III/LAV replication by antiserum to thymosin-alpha-1. *Science* 1986;232:1135–7.

88. Goedert JJ, Drummond JE, Minkoff HL, et al. Mother-to-infant transmission of human immunodeficiency virus type 1: association with prematurity or low anti-gp120. *Lancet* 1989;2:1531–4.

88a.Devash Y, Calvelli TA, Wood DG, Reagan KJ, Rubinstein A. Vertical transmission of human immunodeficiency virus is correlated with the absence of high-affinity/avidity maternal antibodies to the gp120 principal neutralizing domain. *Proc Natl Acad Sci USA* 1990;87:3445–9.

88b.Parekh BS, Shaffer N, Pau C-P, et al. Lack of correlation between maternal antibodies to V3 loop peptides of gp120 and perinatal HIV-1 transmission. *AIDS* 1991;5:1179–84.

89. Nara PL, Goudsmit J. Sequence invariance and conformational dependence of the V3 region during the early emergence of HIV-1 neutralization escape mutants: a model of humoral V3-specific selection and deletion. In: Girard M, Valette L, eds. *Retroviruses of human A.I.D.S. and related animal diseases: Quatrième Colloque des Cent Gardes.* Paris: Pasteur Vaccins, 1989;203–215.

90. Goudsmit J. Genomic divergence within the coding sequence for the principal neutralization epitope of HIV-1. In: Girard M, Valette L, eds. *Retroviruses of human A.I.D.S. and related animal diseases: Quatrième Colloque des Cent Gardes.* Paris: Pasteur Vaccins, 1989;55–60.

91. Goudsmit J, Kuiken CL, Nara PL. Linear versus conformational variation of V3 neutralization domains of HIV-1 during experimental and natural infection. *AIDS* 1989;3:s119–s123.

92. Javaherian K, Langlois AJ, McDanal C, et al. Principal neutralizing domain of the human immunodeficiency virus type 1 envelope protein. *Proc Natl Acad Sci USA* 1989;86:6768–72.

93. LaRosa GJ, Davide JP, Weinhold K, et al. Conserved sequence and structural elements in the HIV-1 principal neutralizing determinant. *Science* 1990;249:932–5.

94. LaRosa GJ, Weinhold K, Profy AT, et al. Conserved sequence and structural elements in the HIV-1 principal neutralizing determinant: further clarifications. *Science* 1991;253:1146.

95. Ivanoff LA, Looney DJ, McDanal C, et al. Alteration of HIV-1 infectivity and neutralization by a single amino acid replacement in the V3 loop domain. *AIDS Res Hum Retroviruses* 1991;7:595–603.

96. Carrow EW, Vujcic LK, Glass WL, et al. High prevalence of antibodies to the gp120 V3 region principal neutralizing determinant of HIV-1$_{MN}$ in sera from Africa and the Americas. *AIDS Res Hum Retroviruses* 1991;7:831–8.

97. Kodama T, Burns DPW, Silva DP, DiMarzoVeronese F, Desrosiers RC. Strain-specific neutralizing determinant in the transmembrane protein of simian immunodeficiency virus. *J Virol* 1991;65:2010–8.

98. Devash Y, Rusche JR, Nara PL. Methods for analysis of biologically functional antibodies to the HIV-1 gp120 principal neutralizing domain (PND). *HIV Vaccines* 1991; [in press].

99. Golding B, Golding H, Preston S, et al. Production of a novel antigen by conjugation of HIV-1 to *Brucella abortus*: studies of immunogenicity, isotype analysis, T-cell dependency, and syncytia inhibition. *AIDS Res Hum Retroviruses* 1991;7:435–6.

100. Ho DD, McKeating JA, Li XL, et al. Conformational epitope on gp120 important in CD4 binding and human immunodeficiency virus type 1 neutralization identified by a human monoclonal antibody. *J Virol* 1991;65:489–93.

101. Moore JP, Weiss RA. Passive primate protection. *Nature* 1991;352:376–7.

102. Zwart G, Landedijk H, van der Hoek L, et al. Immunodominance and antigenic variation of the principal neutralization domain of HIV-1. *Virology* 1991;181:481–9.

103. Sandler SG, Dodd RY, Gang CT. Diagnostic tests for HIV infection. In: DeVita VT, Hellman S, Rosenberg SA, eds. *AIDS: etiology, diagnosis, treatment, and prevention.* Philadelphia: JP Lippincott, 1988;121–36.

104. Consortium for Retrovirus Serology Standardization. Serological diagnosis of human immunodeficiency virus infection by western blot testing. *JAMA* 1988;260:674–9.

105. CDC. Interpretation and use of the western blot assay for serodiagnosis of human immunodeficiency virus type 1 infections. *MMWR* 1989;38[Suppl 7]7:1–7.

106. Jackson JB, MacDonald KL, Cadwell J, et al. Absence of HIV infection in blood donors with indeterminate western blot tests for antibody to HIV-1. *N Engl J Med* 1990;322:217–22.

107. Celum CL, Coombs RW, Lafferty W, et al. Indeterminate human immunodeficiency virus type 1 western blots: seroconversion risk, specificity of supplemental tests, and an algorithm for evaluation. *J Infect Dis* 1991;164:656–64.

108. Siegal FP, Lopez C, Hammer GS, et al. Severe acquired immunodeficiency in male homosexuals, manifested by chronic perianal ulcerative herpes simplex lesions. *N Engl J Med* 1981;305:1439–44.

109. Gottlieb MS, Schroff R, Schanker HM, et al. *Pneumocystis carinii* pneumonia and mucosal candidiasis in previously healthy homosexual men: evidence of a new acquired cellular immunodeficiency. *N Engl J Med* 1981;305:1425–31.

110. Masur H, Michelis MA, Greene JB, et al. An outbreak of community-acquired *Pneumocystis carinii* pneumonia: initial manifestation of cellular immune dysfunction. *N Engl J Med* 1981;305:1431–8.

111. CDC. *Pneumocystis* pneumonia—Los Angeles. *MMWR* 1981;30:250–2.
112. CDC. Kaposi's sarcoma and *Pneumocystis* pneumonia among homosexual men—New York City and California. *MMWR* 1981;30:305–8.
113. CDC. A cluster of Kaposi's sarcoma and *Pneumocystis carinii* pneumonia among homosexual male residents of Los Angeles and Orange counties, California. *MMWR* 1982;31:305–7.
114. CDC. Possible transfusion-associated acquired immune deficiency syndrome (AIDS)—California. *MMWR* 1982;31:652–4.
115. Masur H, Michelis MA, Wormser GP, et al. Opportunistic infection in previously healthy women: initial manifestation of a community-acquired cellular immunodeficiency. *Ann Intern Med* 1982;97:533–9.
116. Goedert JJ, Neuland CY, Wallen WC, et al. Amyl nitrite may alter lymphocytes in homosexual men. *Lancet* 1982;1:412–6.
117. Eyster ME, Goedert JJ, Poon M-C, Preble OT. Acid-labile alpha interferon: a possible preclinical marker for the acquired immunodeficiency syndrome in hemophilia. *N Engl J Med* 1983;309:583–6.
118. Biggar RJ, Melbye M, Ebbesen P, et al. Low T-lymphocyte ratios in homosexual men: epidemiologic evidence for a transmissible agent. *JAMA* 1984;251:1441–6.
119. Preble OT, Eyster ME, Goedert JJ. Acid-labile alpha interferon. *N Engl J Med* 1984;310:923–4.
120. Lane HC, Masur H, Edgar LC, Whalen G, Rook AH, Fauci AS. Abnormalities of B-cell activation and immunoregulation in patients with the acquired immunodeficiency syndrome. *N Engl J Med* 1983;309:453–8.
121. Fauci AS, Macher AM, Longo DL, et al. Acquired immunodeficiency syndrome: epidemiologic, clinical, immunologic, and therapeutic considerations. *Ann Intern Med* 1984;100:92–106.
122. Shearer GM. Allogeneic leukocytes as a possible factor in induction of AIDS in homosexual men. *N Engl J Med* 1983;308:223–4.
123. Moll B, Emeson EE, Butkus Small C, Friedland GH, Klein RS, Spigland I. Inverted ratio of inducer to suppressor T-lymphocyte subsets in drug abusers with opportunistic infections. *Clin Immunol Immunopathol* 1982;25:417–23.
124. Goedert JJ, Sarngadharan MG, Biggar RJ, et al. Determinants of retrovirus (HTLV-III) antibody and immunodeficiency conditions in homosexual men. *Lancet* 1984;2:711–6.
125. Melbye M, Biggar RJ, Ebbesen P, et al. Seroepidemiology of HTLV-III antibody in Danish homosexual men: prevalence, transmission, and disease outcome. *Brt Med J* 1984;289:573–5.
126. Eyster ME, Goedert JJ, Sarngadharan MG, Weiss SH, Gallo RC, Blattner WA. Development and early natural history of HTLV-III antibodies in persons with hemophilia. *JAMA* 1985;253:2219–23.
127. Dobozin BS, Judson FN, Cohn DL, et al. The relationship of cellular immunity to antibodies to HTLV-III in homosexual men. *Cell Immunol* 1986;98:156–71.
128. Shine D, Moll B, Emeson E, et al. Serologic, immunologic, and clinical features of parenteral drug users from contrasting populations. *Am J Drug Alcohol Abuse* 1987;13:401–12.
129. Horsburgh CR, Davis KC, Hasiba V, et al. Altered immunity in hemophilia correlates with presence of antibody to HTLV-III. *J Clin Immunol* 1986;6:37–42.
130. Fuchs D, Unterweger B, Hausen A, et al. Anti-HIV-1 antibodies, anti-HTLV-I antibodies and neopterin levels in parenteral drug addicts in the Austrian Tyrol. *J Acquired Immune Deficiency Syndrome* 1988;1:65–6.
131. Feibnegger G, Spira TJ, Fuchs D, Werner-Felmayer G, Dierich MP, Wachter H. Individual probability for onset of full-blown disease in patients infected with human immunodeficiency virus type 1. *Clin Chem* 1991;37:351–5.
132. Shearer GM, Clerici M. Early T-helper cell defects in HIV infection. *AIDS* 1991;5:245–53.
133. Lane HC, Depper JM, Greene WC, Whalen G, Waldmann TA, Fauci AS. Qualitative analysis of immune function in patients with the acquired immunodeficiency syndrome: evidence for a selective defect in soluble antigen recognition. *N Engl J Med* 1985;313:79–84.
134. Pahwa S, Pahwa R, Saxinger C, Gallo RC, Good RA. Influence of the human T-lymphotropic virus/lymphadenopathy-associated virus on functions of human lymphocytes: evidence for immuno-

suppressive effects and polyclonal B-cell activation by banded viral preparations. *Proc Natl Acad Sci USA* 1985;82:8198–202.
135. Clerici M, Stocks NI, Zajac RA, et al. Interleukin-2 production used to detect antigenic peptide recognition by T-helper lymphocytes from asymptomatic HIV-seropositive individuals. *Nature* 1989;339:383–5.
136. Lucey DR, Melcher GP, Hendrix CW, et al. Human immunodeficiency virus infection in the U.S. Air Force: seroconversions, clinical staging, and assessment of a T helper cell functional assay to predict change in CD4+ T cell counts. *J Infect Dis* 1991;164:631–7.
137. Clerici M, Berzofsky JA, Shearer GM, Tacket CO. Exposure to human immunodeficiency virus type 1-specific T helper cell responses before detection of infection by polymerase chain reaction and serum antibodies. *J Infect Dis* 1991;164:178–82.
138. Clerici M, Berzofsky JA, Shearer GM, Tacket CO. T-helper cell assays detect exposure to HIV-1 antigen earlier than demonstration of infection by serum antibodies or polymerase chain reaction. 7th International Conference on AIDS, Florence, Italy, 1991;42 (abst).
139. Harper ME, Marselle LM, Gallo RC, Wong-Staal F. Detection of HTLV-III-infected lymphocytes in lymph nodes and peripheral blood from AIDS patients by in situ hybridization. *Proc Natl Acad Sci USA* 1986;83:772–6.
140. Chayt KJ, Harper ME, Marselle LM, et al. Detection of HTLV-III RNA in lungs of patients with AIDS and pulmonary involvement. *JAMA* 1986;256:2356–9.
141. Stoler MH, Eskin TA, Benn S, Angerer RC, Angerer LM. Human T-cell lymphotropic virus type III infection of the central nervous system: a preliminary in situ analysis. *JAMA* 1986;256:1260–4.
142. Weiss SH, Saxinger WC, Rechtman D, et al. HTLV-III infection among health care workers: association with needle-stick injuries. *JAMA* 1985;254:2089–93.
143. Moss A, Osmond D, Bacchetti P, et al. Risk of seroconversion for acquired immunodeficiency syndrome (AIDS) in San Francisco health workers. *J Occup Med* 1986;28:821–4.
144. Weiss SH. HIV infection and the healthcare worker. *Med Clin North Am* 1992;76:269–80.
145. Saxinger WC, Rose A. FDA/NIH/CDC workshop: experience with HTLV-III antibody testing—update on: screening, laboratory and epidemiologic correlations. 1985 (unpublished).
146. Paul DA, Falk LA. Detection of HTLV-III antigens in serum. *J Cell Biochem* 1986;10A[Suppl]:224.
147. Falk L, Paul D, Knigge M. Detection of HTLV-III antigens in lysates of peripheral blood/lymph node mononuclear cells. *J Cell Biochem* 1986;10A[Suppl]:200.
148. Hedenskog M, Ward B, Dewhurst S, et al. Testing for AIDS retrovirus (HTLV-III/LAV) antibodies and antigens by indirect immunofluorescence. *J Cell Biochem* 1986;10A[Suppl]:201 (abst).
149. Goudsmit J, DeWolf F, Paul DA, et al. Expression of human immunodeficiency virus antigen (HIV-Ag) in serum and cerebrospinal fluid during acute and chronic infection. *Lancet* 1986;2:177–80.
150. Allain JP, Laurian Y, Paul DA, Senn D. Members of the AIDS-haemophilia French Study Group: serologic markers in early stages of human immunodeficiency virus infection in hemophiliacs. *Lancet* 1986;2:1233–6.
150a. Phillips AN, Lee CA, Elford J, et al. p24 antigenaemia, CD4 lymphocyte counts and the development of AIDS. *AIDS* 1991;5:1217–22.
150b. Chiewsilp P, Isarangkura P, Poonkasem A, Iamsilp W, Khamenketkran M, Stabunswadigan S. Risk of transmission of HIV by seronegative blood. *Lancet* 1991;338:1341.
150c. Busch MP, Taylor PE, Lenes BA, et al. Screening of selected male blood donors for p24 antigen of human immunodeficiency virus type 1. *N Engl J Med* 1990;323:1308–12.
150d. Busch MP, Mosley JW, Alter HJ, Epstein JS. Case of HIV-1 transmission by antigen-positive, antibody-negative blood. *N Engl J Med* 1991;325:1175.
151. Henrard DR, Mehaffey WF, Allain J-P. A sensitive viral capture assay for detection of plasma viremia in HIV-infected individuals. *AIDS Res Hum Retroviruses* 1992; [in press].
152. Rolon N, Hill T, Kissinger R, Sito A, Geltosky J, Britz J. HIV recombinant antigen neutralization assay: a supplemental test to ELISA and western blot. 1991 (unpublished).

153. Salahuddin SZ, Markham PD, Popovic M, et al. Isolation of infectious human T-cell leukemia/lymphotropic virus type III (HTLV-III) from patients with acquired immunodeficiency syndrome (AIDS) or AIDS-related complex (ARC) and from healthy carriers: a study of risk groups and tissue sources. *Proc Natl Acad Sci USA* 1985;82:5530–4.

154. Weiss SH, Goedert JJ, Gartner S, et al. Risk of human immunodeficiency virus (HIV-1) infection among laboratory workers. *Science* 1988;239:68–71.

155. Gartner S, Markovits P, Markovitz DM, Kaplan MH, Gallo RC, Popovic M. The role of mononuclear phagocytes in HTLV-III/LAV infection. *Science* 1986;233:215–9.

156. Gartner S, Markovits P, Markovitz DM, Betts RF, Popovic M. Virus isolation from and identification of HTLV-III/LAV-producing cells in brain tissue from a patient with AIDS. *JAMA* 1986;256:2365–71.

157. Streicher HZ, Joynt RJ. HTLV-III/LAV and the monocyte/macrophage. *JAMA* 1986;256:2390–1.

158. Jackson JB, Coombs RW, Sannerud K, Rhame FS, Balfour HH Jr. Rapid and sensitive viral culture method for human immunodeficiency virus type 1. *J Clin Microbiol* 1988;26:1416–8.

159. Byrne BC, Li JJ, Sninsky J, Poiesz B. Detection of HIV-1 RNA sequences by in vitro DNA amplification. *Nucleic Acids Res* 1988;16:4165.

160. Ou C-Y, Kwok S, Mitchell SW, et al. DNA amplification for direct detection of HIV-1 in DNA of peripheral blood mononuclear cells. *Science* 1988;239:295–7.

161. Muul LM. Current status of polymerase chain reaction assays in clinical research of human immunodeficiency virus infection. In: DeVita VT, Hellman S, Rosenberg SA, eds. *AIDS update 3.* Philadelphia; JB Lippincott, 1990;1–19.

162. Hart C, Spira T, Moore J, et al. Direct detection of HIV RNA expression in seropositive subjects. *Lancet* 1988;2:596–9.

163. Erlich HA, Gelfand D, Sninsky JJ. Recent advances in the polymerase chain reaction. *Science* 1991;252:1643–51.

164. Schochetman G, Sninsky JJ. Direct detection of human immunodeficiency virus infection using the polymerase chain reaction. In: Schochetman G, George JR, eds. *AIDS testing: methodology and management issues.* New York: Springer-Verlag, 1991; 90–110.

165. Holodniy M, Kim S, Katzenstein D, Konrad M, Groves E, Merigan TC. Inhibition of human immunodeficiency virus gene amplification by heparin. *J Clin Microbiol* 1991;29:676–9.

166. Kwok S, Higuchi R. Avoiding false positives with PCR. *Nature* 1989;339:237–8.

167. McCreedy BJ, Chimera JA, Callaway TH. Detection of HIV in clinical samples using polymerase chain reaction amplification. In: *Abstracts of the 119th annual meeting of the American Public Health Association.* 1991;119:302 (abst).

168. Horsburgh CR Jr, Ou C-Y, Jason J, et al. Concordance of polymerase chain reaction with human immunodeficiency virus antibody detection. *J Infect Dis* 1990;162:542–5.

169. Lifson AR, Stanley M, Pane J, et al. Detection of human immunodeficiency virus DNA using polymerase chain reaction in a well-characterized group of homosexual and bisexual men. *J Infect Dis* 1990;161:436–9.

170. Hsia K, Spector SA. Human immunodeficiency virus DNA is present in a high percentage of CD4+ lymphocytes of seropositive individuals. *J Infect Dis* 1991;164:470–5.

171. Shoebridge GI, Barone L, Wing-Simpson A, et al. Assessment of HIV status using the polymerase chain reaction in antibody-positive patients and high-risk antibody-negative haemophiliacs. *AIDS* 1991;5:221–4.

172. McElrath MJ, Steinman RM, Cohn ZA. Latent HIV-1 infection in enriched populations of blood monocytes and T cells from seropositive patients. *J Clin Invest* 1991;87:27–30.

173. Mermin JH, Holodniy M, Katzenstein DA, Merigan TC. Detection of human immunodeficiency virus DNA and RNA in semen by the polymerase chain reaction. *J Infect Dis* 1991;164:769–72.

174. Shaunak S, Albright RE, Bartlett JA. Amplification of human immunodeficiency virus provirus from cerebrospinal fluid: results of long-term clinical follow-up. *J Infect Dis* 1991;164:818.

175. Santa G, Schneider C. RNA extracted from paraffin-embedded human tissues is amenable to analysis by PCR amplification. *BioTechniques* 1991;11:304–8.

176. Schechter MT, Neumann PW, Weaver MS, et al. Low HIV-1 proviral DNA burden detected by negative polymerase chain reaction in seropositive individuals correlates with slower disease progression. *AIDS* 1991;5:373–9.

177. Rogers MF, Ou C-Y, Rayfield M, et al. Use of the polymerase chain reaction for early detection of the proviral sequences of human immunodeficiency virus in infants born to seropositive mothers. *N Engl J Med* 1989;320:1649–54.

178. Tudor-Williams G. Early diagnosis of vertically acquired HIV-1 infection. *AIDS* 1991;5:103–5.

179. Gupta P, Brady M, Raab M, Urbach A. Detection of human immunodeficiency virus by virus culture and polymerase chain reaction in children born to seropositive mothers. *J Acquired Immune Deficiency Syndrome* 1991;4:1004–6.

180. Young KKY, Nelson RP, Good RA. Discordant human immunodeficiency virus infection in dizygotic twins detected by polymerase chain reaction. *Pediatr Infect Dis J* 1990;9:454–6.

181. De Rossi A, Ades AE, Mammano F, et al. Antigen detection, virus culture, polymerase chain reaction, and in vitro antibody production in the diagnosis of vertically transmitted HIV-1 infection. *AIDS* 1991;5:15–20.

182. Scarlatti G, Lombardi V, Plebani A, et al. Polymerase chain reaction, virus isolation and antigen assay in HIV-1-antibody-positive mothers and their children. *AIDS* 1991;5:1173–8.

182a.Scarlatti G, Lombardi V, Plebani A, et al. Polymerase chain reaction, virus isolation and antigen assay in HIV-1 antibody positive mothers and their children. *AIDS* 1991;5:1173–8.

183. Wormser GP, Joline C, Bittker S, Forseter G, Kwok S, Sninsky JJ. Polymerase chain reaction for seronegative health care workers with parenteral exposure to HIV-infected patients. *N Engl J Med* 1989;321:1681–2.

184. Raffanti S, Svenningsson A, Resnick L. Determination of HIV-1 status of discarded sharps: polymerase chain reaction using minute quantities of blood. *JAMA* 1990;264:2501.

185. Busch MP, Eble BE, Khayam-Bashi H, et al. Evaluation of screened blood donations for human immunodeficiency virus type 1 infection by culture and DNA amplification of pooled cells. *N Engl J Med* 1991;325:1–5.

186. Imagawa DT, Lee MH, Visscher B, Dudley J, Detels R. Human immunodeficiency virus type 1 infection in homosexual men who remain seronegative for prolonged periods. *N Engl J Med* 1989;321:1681.

187. Imagawa D, Detels R. HIV-1 in seronegative homosexual men. *N Engl J Med* 1991;325:1250–1.

188. Hewlett IK, Laurian Y, Epstein J, Hawthorne CA, Ruta M, Allain J-P. Assessment by gene amplification and serological markers of transmission of HIV-1 from hemophiliacs to their sexual partners and secondarily to their children. *J Acquired Immune Deficiency Syndrome* 1990;3:714–20.

189. Lefrere J-J, Moriotti M, Ferrer-Le-Coeur F, Rouger P, Noel B, Bosser C. PCR testing in HIV-1 seronegative haemophilia. *Lancet* 1990;336:1386.

190. Mariotti M, Lefrere J-J, Noel B, et al. DNA amplification of HIV-1 in seropositive individuals and in seronegative at-risk individuals. *AIDS* 1990;4:633–7.

191. Shoebridge GI, Gatenby PA, Nightingale BN, et al. Polymerase chain reaction testing of HIV-1 seronegative at-risk individuals. *Lancet* 1990;336:180–1.

192. Wormser GP, Rabkin CS, Joline C. Frequency of nosocomial transmission of HIV infection among health care workers. *N Engl J Med* 1988;319:307–8.

193. Hooper C. Eavesdropping on rare 'silent' HIV-1 infection. *J NIH Res* 1991;3:71–6.

194. Lee T-H, El-Amad Z, Reis M, et al. Absence of HIV-1 DNA in high-risk seronegative individuals using high-input polymerase chain reaction. *AIDS* 1991;5:1201–7.

195. Nielsen C, Teglbjaerg LS, Pedersen C, Lundgren JD, Nielsen CM, Vestergaard BF. Prevalence of HIV infection in seronegative high-risk individuals examined by virus isolation and PCR. *J Acquired Immune Deficiency Syndrome* 1991;4:1107–11.

196. Sheppard HW, Dondero D, Arnon J, Winkelstein W Jr. An evaluation of the polymerase chain reaction in HIV-1 seronegative men. *J Acquired Immune Deficiency Syndrome* 1991;4:819–23.

196a.Ensoli F, Fiorelli V, Mezzaroma I, et al. Plasma viraemia in seronegative HIV-1-infected individuals. *AIDS* 1991;5:1195–9.

196b.Jason J, Ou C-Y, Moore JL, et al. Prevalence of human immunodeficiency virus type 1 DNA in hemophilic men and their sex partners. *J Infect Dis* 1989;160:789–94.

196c.Lee T-H, El-Amad Z, Reis M, et al. Absence of HIV-1 DNA in high-risk seronegative individuals using high-input polymerase chain reaction. *AIDS* 1991;5:1201–7.

197. Holodniy M, Katzenstein DA, Sengupta S, et al. Detection and quantification of human immunodeficiency virus RNA in patient serum by use of the polymerase chain reaction. *J Infect Dis* 1991;163:862–6.

198. Hall WW, Liu CR, Schneewind O, et al. Deleted HTLV-I provirus in blood and cutaneous lesions of patients with mycosis fungoides. *Science* 1991;253:317–20.

199. Agius G, Kolesnitchenko V, Snart R, Zagury JF, Laaroubi K, Zagury D. Variable stringency hybridization of polymerase chain reaction amplified HIV-1 DNA fragments. *J Virol Methods* 1990;30:141–50.

200. Villinger F, Powell JD, Jehuda-Cohen T, et al. Detection of occult simian immunodeficiency virus SIVsmm infection in asymptomatic seronegative nonhuman primates and evidence for variation in SIV gag sequence between in vivo- and in vitro-propagated virus. *J Virol* 1991;65:1855–62.

201. McNeary T, Westervelt P, Thielan BJ, et al. Limited sequence heterogenicity among biologically distinct human immunodeficiency virus type I isolates from individuals involved in a clustered infectious outbreak. *Proc Natl Acad Sci USA* 1990;87:1917–21.

202. CDC. Possible transmission of human immunodeficiency virus to a patient during an invasive dental procedure. *MMWR* 1990;39:489–92.

203. Kleim JP, Ackermann A, Brackmann HH, Gahr M, Schneweis KE. Epidemiologically closely related viruses from hemophilia B patients display high homology in two hypervariable regions of the HIV-1 env gene. *AIDS Res Hum Retroviruses* 1991;7:417–21.

203a.Cichutek K, Norley S, Linde R, et al. Lack of HIV-1 V3 region sequence diversity in two haemophiliac patients infected with a putative biologic clone of HIV-1. *AIDS* 1991;5:1185–7.

203b.Koup RA, Ho DD. Immunosilent HIV-1 infection: intrigue continues. *AIDS* 1991;5:1263.

204. Poiesz BJ, Ruscetti FW, Gazdar AF, Bunn PA, Minna JD, Gallo RC. Detection and isolation of type-C retrovirus particles from fresh and cultured lymphocytes of patients with cutaneous T-cell lymphoma. *Proc Natl Acad Sci USA* 1980;77:7415–9.

205. Kalyanaraman VS, Sarngadharan MG, Robert-Guroff M, et al. A new subtype of human T-cell leukemia virus (HTLV-II) associated with a T-cell variant of hairy cell leukemia. *Science* 1982;218:571–3.

206. Hahn BH, Popovic M, Kalyanaraman VS, et al. Detection and characterization of an HTLV-II provirus in a patient with AIDS. In: *Acquired immune deficiency syndrome.* New York: Alan R. Liss, Inc., 1984;73–81.

207. CDC. Licensure of screening tests for antibody to human T-lymphotropic virus type I. *MMWR* 1988;37:736–40-5–7.

208. Barnes DM. HTLV-I: to test or not to test. *Science* 1988;242:372–3.

209. Robert-Guroff M, Weiss SH, Giron JA, et al. Prevalence of antibodies to HTLV-I, -II, and -III in intravenous drug abusers from an AIDS endemic region. *JAMA* 1986;255:3133–7.

210. Weiss SH, Ginzburg HM, Saxinger WC, et al. Emerging high rates of human T-cell lymphotropic virus type I (HTLV-I) and HIV infection among U.S. drug abusers (DA). 3rd International Conference on AIDS Washington, DC, June, 1987.

211. Kline RL, Brothers T, Halsey N, Boulos R, Lairmore MD, Quinn TC. Evaluation of enzyme immunoassays for antibody to human T-lymphotropic viruses type I/II. *Lancet* 1991;337:30–3.

212. Wiktor SZ, Pate EJ, Weiss SH, et al. Sensitivity of HTLV-I antibody assays for HTLV-II. *Lancet* 1991;338:512–3.

213. Hartley TM, Malone GE, Khabbaz RF, Lal RB, Kaplan JE. Evaluation of a recombinant human T-cell lymphotropic virus type I (HTLV-I) p21E antibody detection enzyme immunoassay as a supplementary test in HTLV-I/II antibody testing algorithms. *J Clin Microbiol* 1991;29:1125–7.

214. Lal RB, Rudolph DL, Lairmore MD, et al. Serologic discrimination of human T cell lymphotropic virus infection by using a synthetic peptide-based enzyme immunoassay. *J Infect Dis* 1991;163:41–6.

214a.Viscidi RP, Hill PM, Li S, et al. Diagnosis and differentiation of HTLV-I and HTLV-II infection by enzyme immunoassays using synthetic peptides. *J Acquired Immune Deficiency Syndrome* 1991;4:1190–8.

215. Hinuma Y, Nagata K, Hanaoka M. Adult T-cell leukemia antigen in an ATL cell line and detection of antibodies to the antigen in human sera. *Proc Natl Acad Sci USA* 1981;78:6476–80.

216. Ikeda M, Fujino R, Matsui T. A new agglutination test for serum antibodies to adult T-cell leukemia virus. *Gann* 1984;75:845–8.

217. Okayama A, Ishizaki J, Tachibana N, Tsuda K, Essex M, Mueller N. The particle agglutination (PA) assay and its use in detecting lower titer HTLV-I antibodies. In: Blattner WA, ed. *Human retrovirology: HTLV.* New York: Raven Press, 1990;401–7.

218. Hartley TM, Khabbaz RF, Cannon RO, Kaplan JE, Lairmore MD. Characterization of antibody reactivity to human T-cell lymphotropic virus types I and II using immunoblot and radioimmunoprecipitation assays. *J Clin Microbiol* 1990;28:646–50.

219. Lee HH, Weiss SH, Brown LS, et al. Patterns of HIV-I and HTLV-I/II in intravenous drug abusers from the Middle Atlantic and Central Regions of the USA. *J Infect Dis* 1990;162:347–52.

220. Biggar RJ, Buskell-Bales Z, Yakshe PN, Caussy D, Gridley G, Seeff L. Antibody to human retroviruses among drug users in three east coast American cities, 1972–1976. *J Infect Dis* 1991;163:57–63.

221. Wiktor SZ, Alexander SS, Shaw GM, et al. Distinguishing between HTLV-1 and HTLV-II by western blot. *Lancet* 1990;335:1533.

222. Cantor KP, Weiss SH, Goedert JJ, Battjes RJ. HTLV-I/II seroprevalence and HIV/HTLV coinfection among U.S. intravenous drug users. *J Acquired Immune Deficiency Syndrome* 1991;4:460–7.

223. Weiss SH, Blattner WA, Ginzburg HM, et al. Retroviral antibodies in parenteral drug users (PDU) from an AIDS endemic region. Program of Abstracts of the 25th Interscience Conference on Antimicrobiol Agents Chemotherapy 1985;25:228(abst).

224. Essex M, McLane MF, Lee TH, et al. Antibodies to cell membrane antigens associated with human T-cell leukemia virus in patients with AIDS. *Science* 1983;220:859–62.

225. Essex M, McLane MF, Lee TH, et al. Antibodies to human T-cell leukemia virus: membrane antigens (HTLV-MA) in hemophiliacs. *Science* 1983;221:1061–4.

226. Weiss SH, Saxinger WC, Ginzburg HM, Mundon FK, Blattner WA. Human T-cell lymphotropic virus type I (HTLV-I) and HIV prevalences among U.S. drug abusers. Proceedings of ASCO, 1987;6:4(abst).

227. Alvord WG, Drummond JE, Arthur LO, et al. A method for predicting individual HIV infection status in the absence of clinical information. *AIDS Res Hum Retroviruses* 1988;4:295–304.

228. Weiss SH, Klein C, French J, Palumbo P, Blattner W, Altman R. Mortality associated with human T-cell lymphotropic virus type 2 (HTLV-2) infection in intravenous drug abusers. 7th International Conference on AIDS, Florence, Italy, 1991.

229. Palumbo P, Weiss SH, McCreedy BJ, et al. Evaluation of HTLV in a cohort of intravenous drug users. *J Infect Dis* 1992; [in press].

230. Lipka JJ, Santiago P, Chan L, et al. Modified western blot assay for confirmation and differentiation of human T cell lymphotropic virus type I and II. *J Infect Dis* 1991;164:400–3.

231. Chen Y-M, Lee T-H, Wiktor SZ, et al. Type-specific antigens for serological discrimination of HTLV-I and HTLV-II infection. *Lancet* 1990;336:1153–5.

232. Lillehoj EP, Alexander SS, Dubrule CJ, et al. Development and evaluation of an HTLV-I serologic confirmatory assay incorporating a recombinant envelope polypeptide. *J Clin Microbiol* 1990;28:2653–8.

233. Hall WW, Kaplan MH, Salahuddin SZ, et al. Concomitant infections with human T-cell leukemia viruses (HTLVs) and human immunodeficiency virus (HIV): identification of HTLV-II infection in intravenous drug abusers (IVDAs). In: Blattner WA, ed. *Human retrovirology: HTLV.* New York: Raven Press, 1990;115–27.

234. Hjelle B, Scalf R, Swenson S. High frequency of human T-cell leukemia-lymphoma virus type II infection in New Mexico blood

donors: determination by sequence-specific oligonucleotide hybridization. *Blood* 1990;76:450–4.

235. Rosenblatt JD, Zack JA, Chen ISY, Lee H. Recent advances in detection of human T-cell leukemia viruses type I and type II infection. *Nat Immun Cell Growth Regul* 1990;9:143–9.

236. Chen Y-MA, Essex M. Identification of a recombinant HTLV-II envelope protein for serological detection of HTLV-II carriers. *AIDS Res Hum Retroviruses* 1991;7:453–7.

237. Horal P, Hall WW, Svennerholm B, et al. Identification of type-specific linear epitopes in the glycoproteins gp46 and gp21 of human T-cell leukemia viruses type I and type II using synthetic peptides. *Proc Natl Acad Sci USA* 1991;88:5754–8.

238. Lal RB, Heneine W, Rudolph DL, et al. Synthetic peptide-based immunoassays for distinguishing between human T-cell lymphotropic virus type I and type II infections in seropositive individuals. *J Clin Microbiol* 1991;29:2253–8.

238a. Lal R, Brodine S, Kazura J, Mbidde-Katonga E, Yanagihara R, Roberts C. Sensitivity and specificity of a recombinant transmembrane glycoprotein spiked western immunoblot for serological confirmation of HTLV type 1 and type 2 infection. *J Clin Microbiol* 1992;30:296–9.

238b. Blomberg J, Robert-Guroff M, Blattner WA, Pipkorn R. Type- and group-specific continuous antigenic determinants of HTLV. Use of synthetic peptides for serotyping of HTLV-I and -II infection. *J AIDS* 1992;5:294–302.

238c. Hall WW, Takahashi H, Liu C, et al. Multiple isolates and characteristics of human T-cell leukemia virus type II. *J Virol* 1992;66:2456–63.

239. Lee H, Swanson P, Shorty VS, Zack JA, Rosenblatt JD, Chen ISY. High rate of HTLV-II infection in seropositive IV drug abusers in New Orleans. *Science* 1989;244:471–5.

240. Ehrlich GD, Greenberg S, Abbott MA. Detection of human T-cell lymphoma/leukemia viruses. In: Innis MA, Gelfand DH, Sninsky JJ, White TJ, eds. *PCR protocols: a guide to methods and applications*. San Diego: Academic Press, Inc., 1990;325–6.

241. Kwok S, Gallo D, Hanson C, McKinney N, Poiesz B, Sninsky JJ. High prevalence of HTLV-II among intravenous drug abusers: PCR confirmation and typing. *AIDS Res Hum Retroviruses* 1990;6:561–5.

242. Smith D, Mann E, Anderson E, Canavaggio M, Lee H. Comparison of HTLV-I/II infection by serology and PCR. 7th International Conference on AIDS, Florence, Italy, 1991.

243. De BK, Srinivasan A. Multiple primer pairs for the detection of HTLV-I by PCR. *Nucleic Acids Res* 1989;17:2142.

244. Kobayashi N, Hatanaka M. Molecular aspects of human T-cell leukemia virus type I (HTLV-I). *Cancer Res* 1986;1:64–95.

245. Korber B, Okayama A, Donnelly R, Tachibana N, Essex M. Polymerase chain reaction analysis of defective human T-cell leukemia virus type I proviral genomes in leukemic cells of patients with adult T-cell leukemia. *J Virol* 1991;65:5471–6.

246. Khabbaz RF, Harter D, Lairmore M, et al. Human T lymphotropic virus type II (HTLV-II) infection in a cohort of New York intravenous drug users: an old infection? *J Infect Dis* 1991;163:252–6.

247. Varnier OE, Lillo F, Alexander SS, Forbis RM, Present W, Lazzarin A. HTLV seroreactivity in Italian intravenous drug addicts is primarily due to HTLV-II infection. *JAMA* 1991;265:597.

248. Bouzas MB, Muchinik G, Zapiola I, et al. Human T cell lymphotropic virus type II infection in Argentina. *J Infect Dis* 1991;164:1026–7.

249. Reeves WC, Saxinger C, Brenes MM, et al. Human T-cell lymphotropic virus type I (HTLV-I) seroepidemiology and risk factors in metropolitan Panama. *Am J Epidemiol* 1988;127:532–9.

250. Lairmore MD, Jacobson S, Gracia F, et al. Isolation of human T-cell lymphotropic virus type 2 from Guaymi Indians in Panama. *Proc Natl Acad Sci USA* 1990;87:8840–4.

251. Chen Y-M, Okayama A, Lee T-H, Tachibana N, Mueller N, Essex M. Sexual transmission of human T-cell leukemia virus type I associated with the presence of anti-Tax antibody. *Proc Natl Acad Sci USA* 1991;88:1181–6.

252. Weiss SH, French J, Holland B, Parker M, Lin-Greenberg A, Altman R. HTLV-I/II co-infection is significantly associated with risk for progression to AIDS among HIV+ intravenous drug abusers. 5th International Conference on AIDS, Montreal, Canada, 1989.

253. Wiktor SZ, Jacobson S, Weiss SH, et al. Spontaneous lymphocyte proliferation in HTLV-II infection. *Lancet* 1991;337:327–8.

254. DeShazo RD, Chadha N, Morgan JE, et al. Immunologic assessment of a cluster of asymptomatic HTLV-I-infected individuals in New Orleans. *Am J Med* 1989;86:65–70.

255. Kira J-I, Koyanagi Y, Hamakado T, Itoyama Y, Yamamoto N, Goto I. HTLV-II in patients with HTLV-I-associated myelopathy. *Lancet* 1991;338:64–5.

256. Kiyokawa T, Yamaguchi K, Nishimura Y, Yoshiki K, Takatsuki K. Lack of anti-HTLV-II seropositivity in HTLV-I-associated myelopathy and adult T-cell leukaemia. *Lancet* 1991;338:451.

256a. Hjelle B, Appenzeller O, Mills R, et al. Chronic neurodegenerative disease associated with HTLV-II infection. *Lancet* 1992;339:645–6.

257. Welles SL, Mueller N, Tachibana N, et al. Decreased eosinophil numbers in HTLV-I carriers. *Lancet* 1991;337:987.

258. CDC. Interpretive criteria used to report western blot results for HIV-1-antibody testing—United States. *MMWR* 1991;40:692–5.

259. Candotti D, Jung M, Kerouedan D, et al. Genetic variability affects the detection of HIV by polymerase chain reaction. *AIDS* 1991;5:1003–7.

260. Weiss R. Hot prospect for new gene amplifier: Ligase chain reaction, a combination DNA amplifier and genetic screen, could do for DNA diagnostics what PCR has done for basic molecular biology. *Science* 1991;254:1272–3.

261. Barany F. Genetic disease detection and DNA amplification using cloned thermostable ligase. *Proc Natl Acad Sci, USA* 1991;88:189–93.

262. Ii S, Minnerath S, Ii K, Dyck PJ, Sommer S. Two-tiered DNA-based diagnosis of transthyretin amyloidosis reveals two novel point mutations. *Neurology* 1991; 41:893–8.

263. Food and Drug Administration. Open meeting transcript of the Vaccine and Related Biologic Products Advisory Committee of the Food and Drug Administration, January 30, 1992. Bethesda, MD: Miller Reporting Company, Inc., 1992;1–176.

264. Food and Drug Administration. Open meeting transcript of the Blood Products Advisory Committee of the Food and Drug Administration, March 12–13, 1992. Bethesda, MD: C.A.S.E.T. Associates, Ltd., 1992; 1–450.

*AIDS and Other Manifestations of HIV Infection,
Second Edition,* Edited by Gary P. Wormser.
Raven Press, Ltd., New York © 1992.

CHAPTER 9

Animal Models for HIV Infection and Disease

Patricia N. Fultz

Following the initial recognition that the acquired immunodeficiency syndrome (AIDS) was caused by an infectious agent, the first proposed use of animals was for attempting to identify the pathogenic microorganism responsible for the disease. Various species of small laboratory animals and nonhuman primates were inoculated with material from AIDS patients in hope of reproducing the disease syndrome and amplifying the infectious organism. All of these attempts failed (1) with the exception of experimental inoculation of chimpanzees (*Pan troglodytes*) with tissue samples (2,3) and, soon thereafter, with the (at that time) putative causative agent, human immunodeficiency virus (HIV) (3,4). In the 7 years since the initial failed attempts to infect other species with HIV, investigators have been successful in developing alternative animal models. Results obtained with the various model systems have proved valuable in gaining insights into all aspects of HIV-induced disease, including natural history and mechanisms of pathogenesis at both the biologic and molecular level. Although model systems have been used in only a limited number of drug studies to date, it is expected that more in vivo analyses will be undertaken in animals as the number of candidate therapeutic drugs increases. In the area of vaccine development, however, animal models have already provided significant contributions, the most important of which was the demonstration that protective immunity against retrovirus infections could be elicited by vaccination, an achievement that many had previously considered to be almost impossible. The chimpanzee, due to its unique susceptibility to infection by low doses of prototype HIV strains, has played and will continue to play a major role in development of vaccines against HIV. This chapter will provide an overview of animal models for HIV infection that are currently available, focusing on the relative importance of each as they relate to pathogenesis, therapeutic intervention, and vaccines.

PATHOGENESIS AND NATURAL HISTORY OF INFECTION

In general, the pathophysiology of HIV infection in humans (see references 5 and 6 for reviews) can be briefly summarized as follows. An acute disease syndrome occurs during the first month after primary infection and is accompanied by high levels of viral replication manifested as viremia and antigenemia. Antibodies to HIV *gag*- and *env*-encoded proteins can be detected as early as 1–2 weeks after onset of symptoms of acute infection, but generally seroconversion occurs within 2–3 months. Concomitant with increasing antibody titers, the viremia and antigenemia fall to low or undetectable levels, suggesting immune-mediated clearance of virus. Following a prolonged interval of months to years, in which the virus establishes a chronic infection or appears latent, replication of the virus increases, again detected by viremic and antigenemic episodes, perhaps due to periodic stimulation of the immune system by intercurrent infections or inflammatory responses. During this period (or preceding it), the immune system deteriorates as absolute numbers and percentages of CD4+ lymphocytes decline, and the infected person develops an increasing number of clinical problems, including opportunistic infections and malignancies, which ultimately result in death. It is not clear whether the immune system malfunctions as a result of HIV infection per se or in concert with specific cofactors. This latter point is just one of many questions that can be addressed experimentally with appropriate animal model systems.

HIV Infection of Chimpanzees

Following the initial demonstrations in 1984 (2,4), it was soon established that chimpanzees could be repro-

P. N. Fultz: Department of Microbiology, University of Alabama at Birmingham School of Medicine, Birmingham, Alabama 35294.

ducibly infected with the lymphadenopathy-associated virus (LAV)-1$_{BRU}$ and human T-lymphotropic virus (HTLV)-IIIB isolates of HIV-1 (7,8), and that virus could be recovered from peripheral blood mononuclear cells (PBMC) upon almost all attempts by cocultivation with mitogen-stimulated normal human PBMC (9). Despite the fact that more than 100 chimpanzees have been experimentally infected with various isolates of HIV-1, some for more than 8 years, none of the animals has developed symptoms of AIDS or AIDS-related complex (ARC). This observation, however, may be an artifact because all HIV-infected chimpanzees are housed in strict isolation facilities with little opportunity for exposure to multiple pathogens. If repeated stimulation of the immune system or a specific pathogen as cofactor is required for progression to disease, then it is reasonable to assume that housing animals in isolation will lengthen the asymptomatic period. Prolonged lymphadenopathy in a chimpanzee has been reported twice; both cases occurred during the first year of infection and resolved spontaneously after several months (2,10). A recent report describes extended CD4+ lymphocytopenia and thrombocytopenia in a chimpanzee that had been infected for about 5 years and had been exposed to three different HIV-1 isolates (11). This finding provides suggestive evidence that, given sufficient time, chimpanzees may develop disease. Even though HIV infection of chimpanzees will never be a model for pathogenesis, it does provide an excellent model of asymptomatic infections in humans and has already proved to be important in vaccine development (see below).

Although no acute disease syndrome has been observed, other early events following HIV infection of chimpanzees closely parallel those that occur in humans (7–9,12). Initial high levels of virus replication with viremia and antigenemia decrease as HIV-specific humoral immunity develops. The humoral immune response includes antibodies to all of the major proteins encoded by the HIV genome, type-specific neutralizing antibodies that broaden over time to react with more diverse strains (8,13,14), and antibodies that function in antibody-dependent cellular cytotoxicity (A. Mawle, personal communication) and antibody-dependent complement mediated cytotoxicity reactions (15). HIV-infected chimpanzees also develop cell-mediated proliferative responses to HIV and purified HIV antigens (16,17), and cytotoxic T-lymphocyte activity that, at least for *gag* antigens, appears to be restricted by the major histocompatibility complex (11). HIV-1-infected chimpanzees, like humans, have been shown to have CD8+ lymphocytes that suppress replication of HIV-1 (11,18). Despite the presence of multiple immune response mechanisms that appear to restrict HIV replication, the virus is not eliminated, analogous to what occurs in humans. During long-term infection of chimpanzees, HIV has been isolated frequently from PBMC, from cells obtained by lymph node biopsies, and from bone marrow (unpublished data), but rarely from plasma as cell-free virus (7,9,19,20), which is consistent with the presence of high levels of neutralizing antibodies.

Several theories have been proffered to explain the failure of HIV-infected chimpanzees to develop disease. These include the following: (1) HIV is not cytopathic for chimpanzee CD4+ lymphocytes, and chimpanzee macrophages are not infected by HIV (20); (2) chimpanzee PBMC do not support cell-to-cell transmission of HIV, i.e., lack of syncytia formation between HIV gp120 on infected cells and the chimpanzee CD4 molecule on uninfected cells (21); (3) HIV-infected chimpanzees do not, but humans do, have cytotoxic lymphocytes that lyse uninfected CD4+ lymphocytes (22); and (4) normal chimpanzees, but not humans, have CD8+ lymphocytes that suppress replication of HIV-1 (18). Many of the observations on which the above conclusions were based may be isolate specific, i.e., they may be true for some HIV-1 strains, but not others. The benign course of HIV infection in chimpanzees cannot be explained by differences in cell tropism or virus–cell interactions. At least some HIV-1 isolates with which chimpanzees are infected replicate efficiently in vitro in both chimpanzee CD4+ lymphocytes and bone marrow macrophages and are cytopathic for CD4+ lymphocytes (23,24). The suggestion that CD8+ cells in chimpanzees are responsible for the differential pathogenesis in chimpanzees and humans does not appear valid since it has been reported (25) that normal HIV-seronegative persons also have CD8+ lymphocytes with the ability to suppress HIV-1 replication. Furthermore, since fusion of HIV-infected cells does not appear to be the major mechanism for cell killing by HIV, it still appears reasonable that failure of chimpanzees to develop disease may be a function of time and multiple perturbations of the immune system, as discussed above.

HIV-1-infected chimpanzees, therefore, appear to be excellent models for assessing the roles of specific and nonspecific immunity in maintenance of the asymptomatic state and for studying cofactors in disease. The validity of the chimpanzee as a model for human HIV infection is supported by the fact that HIV can be transmitted in these animals by the same routes as in humans: intravenously (2,7,8), via mucous membranes (19), and in utero (26), but not by casual contact (27). PBMC from chimpanzees were recently shown to be permissive for replication of human herpes virus 6 (HHV-6) (28), a virus for which coexistence and replication in the same cell as HIV-1 has been demonstrated (29). Thus, it might be worthwhile to develop HHV-6 infection of chimpanzees as a model to study the interactions of these two viruses in vivo.

HIV-2 Infection of Monkeys

Although a limited number of studies have been done to assess the pathogenicity of HIV-2 in nonhuman primate species, it is apparent that HIV-2 infection of monkeys results, at best, in a persistent asymptomatic infection similar to that of HIV-1 infection of chimpanzees. Attempts to infect rhesus macaques (*Macaca mulatta*) (30–35), cynomolgus monkeys (*M. fascicularis*) (35,36), African green monkeys (*Cercopithecus aethiops*) (34), mangabey monkeys (*Cercocebus atys*) (32), baboons (30,32), and a chimpanzee (unpublished data) with various isolates of HIV-2 have resulted in long-term persistent infections in all of the simian species except the African green monkeys. In the baboons and chimpanzee, infection appeared to be transient. Putkonen et al. (36) successfully infected three of four cynomolgus monkeys with the HIV-2$_{SBL-K135}$ isolate and Stahl-Hennig et al. (35) infected six of six cynomolgus monkeys with the HIV-2$_{ben}$ isolate. Infection of two rhesus macaques by an infectious molecular clone, HIV-2$_{sbl/isy}$, also resulted in persistently low antibody titers and recovery of virus during the first few months after inoculation (34). In general, inoculation of high doses of virus has resulted in less than 100% successful infections, which were characterized by relatively low, but persistent, antibody levels. The ability to isolate infectious virus from PBMC was variable, with more failures than successes. These data suggest a very low level of virus replication, which may be a reflection of the apparent differences in pathogenicity and natural history between HIV-1 and HIV-2 (37). No HIV-2-infected animal has developed signs of disease reminiscent of AIDS or ARC, despite the fact that some of the animals have been infected for up to 5 years (unpublished data). Because of the lack of disease in HIV-2-infected monkeys, this model will only prove valuable for pathogenesis studies if pathogenic strains are generated upon serial passage in vivo or if infectious molecular clones can be manipulated such that they are rendered pathogenic. Furthermore, unless an HIV-2 isolate can be adapted such that it infects a simian species reproducibly following inoculation of a low dose of virus, this model will have only limited usefulness in studies to assess efficacy of antiviral treatments and vaccines.

SIV Infection of Macaques and Other Simian Species

In contrast to the limitations of the HIV-chimpanzee and HIV-2-simian systems, simian immunodeficiency virus (SIV) infection of macaques has proved an excellent model for defining the natural history and mechanisms of pathogenicity of T-lymphotropic lentiviruses. This appears to be true only for those isolates of SIV that belong to the HIV-2/SIV$_{smm}$/SIV$_{mac}$ subgroup and does not include those isolates designated SIV$_{agm}$ (38), SIV$_{mnd}$ (39), or SIV$_{syk}$ (40), none of which has been shown to induce disease either in their natural hosts or in experimentally infected animals (41,42). Thus, infection of various monkey species with these last three viruses provides additional model systems for asymptomatic infection and, perhaps more importantly, for gaining insight

into protective mechanisms. Identification of specific immune responses or virus–host cell interactions that might be responsible for the observed lack of pathogenicity of these viruses might suggest prophylactic or therapeutic approaches to HIV infections. A possible explanation for failure of SIV$_{smm}$ and SIV$_{agm}$ to induce disease in their natural hosts, sooty mangabeys and African green monkeys, respectively, is the finding that neither of these viruses are cytopathic for CD4+ cells from mangabeys (43) or African green monkeys (42). Whether other factors are important in maintenance of asymptomatic infections requires additional study.

Experimental infection of several macaque species, including rhesus, pig-tailed, and cynomolgus monkeys, can be readily achieved by intravenous inoculation (44–50) or application of virus to mucosal surfaces (51). In general, SIV-infected macaques respond to infection much the same as HIV-infected humans and chimpanzees. Soon after infection, high levels of virus and viral antigen can be detected in serum. These decline, sometimes to undetectable levels, as SIV-specific antibodies are produced. The ability to isolate virus from PBMC and from plasma of infected animals appears to be correlated directly with disease. That is, high titers of plasma viremia and antigenemia are more frequently detected in those animals that develop disease more rapidly and present with more frequent clinical signs of disease (48,50). Some animals that die less than 6 months after SIV inoculation never produce detectable antibodies to the virus (46,48).

More recent studies have shown that SIV-infected macaques develop virus-specific cell-mediated responses. Cytotoxic T lymphocytes (CTL) specific for inactivated SIV (52) and for purified SIV *gag* and *env* antigens (53–55) have been reported. In addition, the presence of *gag*-specific CTL appeared to be correlated with increased survival (53). The CTL activity was mediated by CD8+ lymphocytes and was restricted by major histocompatibility antigens. As has been demonstrated for HIV-infected humans and chimpanzees, SIV-infected macaques also harbor CD8+ lymphocytes that can suppress both replication and recovery of virus from PBMC in culture (56,57).

Although the latent periods between exposure and development of disease vary both with species of macaque and specific virus isolates, most animals ultimately develop an AIDS-like disease very similar to that observed in humans. Disease in macaques is characterized, in part, by rash, enterocolitis, encephalitis, B-cell lymphomas, weight loss, lymphadenopathy, and opportunistic infections, including cytomegalovirus, *Pneumocystis carinii,* and *Mycobacterium avium-intracellulare* (44, 58–61; for review, see reference 60). Hematologic abnormalities, such as hypergammaglobulinemia, thrombocytopenia, loss of CD4+ lymphocytes, and elevated levels of soluble interleukin (IL)-2 receptors, also have been documented, just as in human AIDS patients (59,60).

Because of the many similarities in virologic and immunologic parameters and in disease manifestations between HIV infection of humans and SIV infection of macaques, this model system is proving useful for detailed analyses of pathogenesis and natural history. It is hoped that these studies will lead to the identification of the following: protective immune responses for T-lymphotropic lentiviruses; specific factors that influence disease progression; and viral determinants of pathogenicity. In addition, several groups are attempting to develop macaque models for studying maternal/fetal transmission of SIV, which, if successful, would be important in devising strategies for preventing transmission of HIV from pregnant women to their infants.

Infections with Immunodeficiency-Like Lentiviruses

Subsequent to the isolation of the HIVs and SIVs, immunodeficiency-like viruses from two other mammalian species were identified: bovine immunodeficiency-like virus (BIV) from cattle (62) and feline immunodeficiency virus (FIV) from cats (63). The major *gag* antigen of BIV, but not that of FIV, has epitopes cross-reactive with the p24 *gag* of HIV, but both of these viruses infect a broader range of cell types than do HIV or SIV. While BIV apparently does cause persistent lymphocytosis, lymphadenopathy, lesions in the central nervous system (CNS), progressive weakness, and emaciation in infected cattle (62), it is unlikely that this model system will be utilized widely due to the obvious impediments of size of the animals and lack of required facilities.

Infection of cats with FIV, however, offers the advantage of a small animal that is readily available. While disease or immunologic abnormalities induced by FIV in pathogen-free cats appears limited, at least within the first 2 years after inoculation, naturally infected cats often develop immunologic abnormalities and chronic symptoms, including those indicative of CNS disease (64), that ultimately lead to an AIDS-like illness (65–67). Pedersen et al. (68) found that coinfection of cats with FIV and another retrovirus, feline leukemia virus (FeLV), greatly potentiated the course of FIV-induced disease and resulted in death 6–8 weeks after inoculation of the viruses. Thus, this model may be valuable in identifying potential cofactors for development of AIDS-like disease.

Infection of Small Animals with HIV

Although early attempts to infect small animals with HIV-1 were not successful, two groups subsequently showed that rabbits could be infected with some isolates of HIV-1 (69,70). However, attempts to refine the model so that it would be suitable for experimental manipulation have not been successful. At this time it appears that HIV infection of rabbits is not a viable model system.

There is substantial evidence that HIV cannot replicate in murine cells. However, transplantation of human adult PBMC or fetal lymphoid tissue into mice with the SCID (severe combined immunodeficient) mutation results in hu-PBL-SCID and SCID-hu mice, respectively, that can be infected by HIV-1 (71,72). These animals do not develop ARC or AIDS, but do exhibit early manifestations of HIV infection. Their usefulness for pathogenesis studies is therefore limited. The use of transgenic mice expressing various HIV-1 genes or other genes under control of the HIV-1 long terminal repeat (LTR) also may provide useful, but limited, information concerning the possible role(s) of specific HIV-1-encoded genetic information in pathogenesis (73–76). To illustrate the potential usefulness of transgenic mice, animals with the *tat* gene in their germ line developed dermal lesions that resembled Kaposi's sarcoma (73) and the F1 progeny of a transgenic mouse carrying the entire HIV-1 provirus uniformly developed disease and died by 25 days after birth (74). However, due to an environmental malfunction, all of these transgenic founder mice were lost.

Infections with Other Lentiviruses

Prior to the identification of the HIVs and SIVs, the classic lentiviruses—visna/maedi of sheep, caprine arthritis–encephalitis virus of goats, and equine infectious anemia virus of horses—were used to define the pathogenesis of, and immunologic responses to, viruses associated with long-term progressive disease (for reviews, see references 77 and 78). Although these viruses cause diseases distinct from those induced by the immunodeficiency viruses, there are similarities in virus–host interactions, including cell tropisms and immune responses, that can be used as models for understanding the pathogenesis of lentiviruses.

THERAPEUTIC INTERVENTION IN INFECTION

HIV infections basically manifest in three ways: asymptomatic infection, ARC, or AIDS. Ideally, the goal is to prevent progression from the asymptomatic state to ARC or AIDS, but for those persons who are already in the latter categories, effort must be directed at halting or, if possible, reversing disease progression. Thus, testing innovative approaches to new therapies requires animal model systems that exhibit the same spectrum of clinical presentations seen in human patients. Even though some model systems may not provide an accurate reflection of human disease, they still can provide useful background data, especially if they are cost efficient and utilize animals that require less specialized husbandry skills than more relevant models. A consensus of opinion has been reached that supports the use of small animal models, when appropriate, in initial tests of new drugs and treatment regimens. If circumstances warrant further testing prior to phase 1 human trials, then nonhuman primate models should be employed.

Model Systems for Asymptomatic Infection

Infection of several nonhuman primate species with various HIVs or SIVs results in long-term persistent infections comparable to the asymptomatic stage of human HIV infection. As discussed above, these include HIV-1 infection of chimpanzees, HIV-2 infection of macaques, SIV_{agm} infection of African green monkeys, and SIV_{smm} infection of mangabeys. Since these infections rarely, if ever, progress to AIDS, analysis of virus-specific immunity may lead to the identification of protective immune responses or, alternatively, of factors important in virus–host interactions that allow the virus and host to establish a symbiotic relationship. Initial studies of SIV_{agm} infection in African green monkeys (79) and SIV_{smm} in sooty mangabeys (80) revealed that SIV-specific neutralizing antibodies were usually not detectable, which suggests that neutralization of cell-free virus is not an important mechanism in preventing disease progression. This hypothesis is supported by the observation that sooty mangabeys have high levels of SIV, yet do not develop disease (50).

Another aspect of asymptomatic infection that must be addressed with animal models relates to the question: what factors influence the transition from asymptomatic infection to disease? Associated questions include, for example: is the transition preceded by increased viral expression? HIV-1 infection of chimpanzees and HIV-2 infection of macaques are excellent models to address these questions because there is suggestive evidence that: (1) chimpanzees may develop disease symptoms as length of time of infection and exposure to other pathogens increase (11); and (2) antigen-specific and nonspecific immune stimulation increases virus load, at least transiently (81). Identification of specific cofactors for progression to disease in either of these models might have a major impact on management of persons with asymptomatic HIV infections. Using the FIV cat model, Pedersen et al. (68) provided support for this idea by showing that FIV-induced disease progression is hastened by intercurrent infection with another virus, FeLV.

Model Systems for Therapeutic Intervention in ARC or AIDS

The obvious choice for testing antiviral drugs and to develop therapies to intervene in the course of HIV-induced disease is the SIV-macaque model. This is primarily because SIV infection of macaques elicits the entire spectrum of disease stages seen in HIV-infected persons, and many of the opportunistic infections that are observed during SIV infection are the same as those that are prevalent in HIV-infected persons. In addition, SIV and HIV replication is controlled by similar complex regulatory genes. Rapid assessment of therapeutic efficacy of drugs targeted to interfere in virus replication is possible using an SIV_{smm} variant ($SIV_{smmPBj14}$), which induces acute disease and death in pig-tailed macaques within 1 or 2 weeks after inoculation (82). Although the disease course is greatly accelerated relative to other SIV strains, many features of the acute disease, such as loss of CD4+ cells, resemble those observed during long-term persistent infections with other isolates. Finally, the SIV-macaque model is valuable for testing new therapeutic intervention strategies against unrelated microbial pathogens during concurrent infection with an immunodeficiency virus. Although the possibilities for application of the SIV-macaque model are limitless, its use is constrained by the expense, housing facilities, and trained personnel required for performing experimental studies with monkeys.

Several reasonable alternatives to the SIV-macaque model are available for testing new drugs for antiretroviral properties in vivo. These include infection of cats with either FIV or FeLV and various murine models. The FIV reverse transcriptase enzyme has been shown in vitro to be inhibited by 3'-azido-3'-deoxythymidine (AZT) and phosphonoformate to the same extent as HIV-1 (83). Therefore, the ability of a particular drug to prevent FIV replication and infection may be a reliable indicator of efficacy against HIV. Using the FeLV-cat system, Tavares et al. (84) showed that AZT could prevent infection with FeLV when therapy was initiated within 7 days of inoculation. However, because FeLV is a type-C retrovirus with less complicated regulatory mechanisms than the lentiviruses, FIV would appear to be the virus of choice in feline systems. Furthermore, crucial immunologic reagents, such as monoclonal antibodies to feline T-cell antigens, have been and are being generated, which will enhance the utility of this model.

Although no murine lentiviruses have been identified, primary in vivo screening of antiretroviral drugs can be performed with various type-C oncornaviruses that induce an AIDS-like disease in mice. These include the LP-BM5 murine leukemia virus (MuLV) (85), which also induces B-cell immunoblastic lymphomas (86), the Duplan strain of MuLV (87), Rauscher MuLV (RLV) (88), and the neurotropic Cas-Br-E strain (89). The utility of these model systems has been demonstrated with chronic AZT treatment of mice infected with various MuLVs (88–90). When AZT was tested in these models, it effectively suppressed viremia and disease development, not only in adult mice but also in offspring of pregnant animals (91). While the use of murine models is cost effective and rapid and allows for quantitative analyses, limitations exist. Constraints are based on the facts that: (1) type C viruses do not contain the novel regulatory genes found in lentiviruses; and (2) the pharmacokinetics of some drugs may differ in mice and humans. One murine system, however, overcomes these limitations: the hu-PBL-SCID or SCID-hu mice. McCune et al. (92) demonstrated suppression, but not complete inhibition of HIV replication in AZT-treated SCID-hu mice. The SCID-hu model has the advantage of using HIV as the infecting virus, but is limited in that protection against disease cannot be analyzed. Depending on the novelty or mechanism of action of antivirals that are effective in murine models, additional information on the efficacy of promising drugs could be obtained from subsequent testing in nonhuman primate models or in phase 1 human clinical trials.

DEVELOPMENT OF EFFICACIOUS VACCINES

As with trials of new therapeutic approaches to disease prevention, there is no substitute for animal models in the development of vaccines and for trials of vaccine efficacy. Even though some prototype vaccines have apparently protected macaques and chimpanzees from infection with cell-free virus (see below), the requirement that an HIV vaccine protect absolutely from infection is probably unrealistic. However, vaccination against HIV may limit initial replication and dissemination of the virus, which could influence the rate at which the infection progresses to disease. It is also possible that prior immunization might result in establishment of lifetime infections yet prevent progression to disease. Because of the inherent nature of retroviruses and the fact that they can remain latent as proviruses for extended periods, it is imperative that vaccine candidates be tested in animal models prior to phase III clinical trials in humans. Even though it is preferable to utilize HIV itself, the fact that only chimpanzees can be reliably infected with HIV-1 is restrictive, due to the expense and limited availability of these animals. An accepted strategy for the generation of an efficacious HIV vaccine is to develop, test, and refine prototype SIV vaccines as models for HIV vaccines, which would be tested in chimpanzees before going into phase III trials.

SIV/HIV-2-Macaque Models

Several groups have successfully protected macaques from infection with cell-free SIV by immunization with inactivated whole virus prepared from the same strain as that used for the challenge virus inoculum (93–95). Protection was observed with low (1–10 animal infectious doses), but not high (10^3–10^6 animal infectious doses), challenge doses of SIV. More recently, Stott et al. (96) showed that vaccination of macaques with inactivated SIV-infected cells also protected against challenge with a low dose of homologous SIV. Although the immune mechanisms responsible for preventing infection are not

known, protection did not correlate with the presence of high levels of neutralizing antibodies. These studies demonstrated conclusively, however, that it was possible to prevent low doses of cell-free SIV from establishing infection by vaccination with whole virus or virus-infected cells.

Because HIV is transmitted by parenteral exposure or via mucosal surfaces, vaccines must be able to prevent infection by both routes. As discussed above, SIV infection of macaques can be established by intravenous injection or by application of virus to the genital mucosa (51). An initial attempt to demonstrate vaccine efficacy against infection via mucosal surfaces failed to protect four of four animals from infection with 100–1,000 animal infectious doses (97). Vaccinated animals challenged in parallel by the intravenous route also were not protected, but vaccination appeared to delay disease progression in the latter group. In related studies, prior infection with a live, attenuated strain of SIV (98) or with HIV-2 (99) did not prevent superinfection with pathogenic SIV, but did prevent early disease. The fact that HIV-2 protected against disease consequences associated with SIV suggests that some protection against heterologous virus strains can be achieved by vaccination. (For reviews of SIV vaccine studies, see chapter by Gardner and Luciw and ref. 100.)

HIV-Chimpanzee Model

The ultimate test for efficacy of any HIV-1 vaccine candidate is to determine whether it can protect against infection in chimpanzees. After the initial attempts to protect chimpanzees by immunization with recombinant vaccinia virus expressing gp160 env (10) or with the purified gp120 envelope glycoprotein (101,102) failed, the prospects of an effective HIV vaccine seemed remote. The successful protection of macaques from SIV infection with inactivated whole virus, however, led to renewed efforts to demonstrate protection in chimpanzees. Two groups now have reported protection of chimpanzees from intravenous challenge with 10 to 40 chimpanzee infectious doses of HIV-1$_{HTLV-IIIB}$. Immunogens consisted of whole inactivated virus, purified gp120, gp160, p18 gag, p27 nef, or p23 vif, peptides representing the V3 loop, i.e., the principal neutralizing determinant, or various combinations of these; all of these antigens were derived from the LAV-1$_{BRU}$ or HTLV-IIIB isolates. Berman et al. (103) reported protection of two chimpanzees immunized with gp120 formulated in alum; however, immunization with gp160 failed to protect two other animals. Girard et al. (104) demonstrated apparent protection in three chimpanzees that were immunized with various combinations of HIV antigens.

Two observations that may be of significance were made in the latter study. First, boosting of the immune response with purified V3 peptides elicited high titers of neutralizing antibodies that persisted for at least 1 year. Whether antibodies to the V3 loop are required for protection has not been established, but the study by Berman and colleagues (103) and a study by Emini et al. (105) provide supporting evidence that these antibodies may be important. In the Emini study, in vitro incubation of HIV-1 with serum containing antibodies to the V3 loop prevented infection of a chimpanzee, whereas incubation with serum lacking these particular antibodies failed to inhibit infection. Second, a chimpanzee that appeared to be protected by multiple criteria, including failure to isolate virus from PBMC and lymph node cells, failure to detect HIV-1 DNA by polymerase chain reaction using nested primers, and failure to detect an anamnestic antibody response, proved to be harboring latent virus. At $7\frac{1}{2}$ months after challenge and on subsequent attempts, virus was isolated from PBMC and bone marrow cells. Similar occurrences were documented in two SIV macaque trials (93,94). These latter observations underscore not only the insidious nature of HIV and SIV, but also the need for long-term follow-up of all vaccinated and challenged animals before conclusions can be made about the ability of a vaccine to protect absolutely against infection.

As in the SIV-macaque model, the identity of the protective response(s) in chimpanzees has not been established. Analysis of humoral and cell-mediated immune responses elicited by the various immunogens has not revealed specific correlates to protection. It is clear, however, that the major envelope glycoprotein, gp120, is sufficient. That gp120 is also necessary was suggested by a study in which immunization with the purified p55 *gag* precursor protein failed to protect the one chimpanzee that was challenged (106). Furthermore, passive transfer of high titers of purified HIV-1 neutralizing antibodies to chimpanzees failed to prevent infection when the animals were challenged with 100 chimpanzee 50% infectious doses (107). Thus, it is possible that both humoral and cell-mediated responses are required for maximum protection against cell-free virus. Since HIV-1 is highly cell associated and can remain latent for extended periods with little or no detectable viral replication, future critical experiments must assess the ability of candidate vaccines to protect against challenge with cell-associated virus. Thus, the HIV-chimpanzee model, as well as the SIV-macaque model, will continue to provide valuable information regarding the possibility of generating an effective HIV-1 vaccine for humans.

Other Models

While the SIV-macaque and HIV-chimpanzee model systems must be used as the final tests for efficacy of prototype HIV vaccines, it is possible that useful information can be gained from small animal models. Relevant information regarding efficacy, the identification of protective immune responses, and theoretical approaches to novel vaccine designs could be obtained with the FIV-cat system. In addition, reconstituting SCID mice with cells from persons receiving candidate HIV vaccines in phase 1 clinical trials may be useful in assessing whether the vaccines elicit appropriate immune responses that have the ability to prevent or inhibit infection of the human cells in an in vivo situation.

CONCLUSIONS

The importance of animal model systems in dissecting the pathogenesis of, and in developing effective therapies and vaccines for, infectious diseases cannot be overestimated. Because the immune system is highly complex and incompletely understood, no alternative method exists for defining all interactions between a pathogen and its host. Factors that facilitate or prevent progression to disease as a consequence of HIV infection are even more complicated because HIV infects CD4+ lymphocytes and monocyte/macrophages, both of which play important and often critical roles in immune defense. Although a few differences between SIV infection of monkeys and HIV infection of humans have been observed, overall this model has proved extremely valuable in defining mechanisms of pathogenesis, in assessing efficacy of new chemo- and immunotherapeutic approaches to limit HIV-induced disease, and in developing effective vaccines to prevent transmission of HIV. HIV infection of chimpanzees will never be a model for disease, even if chimpanzees ultimately develop symptoms similar to ARC or AIDS, but the ability of potential vaccines to protect chimpanzees from infection will continue to be the gold standard in HIV vaccine development. Small animal models, such as FIV infection of cats and HIV infection of SCID-hu or hu-PBL-SCID mice, also will be valuable because they provide the opportunity for large-scale screening of new drugs. Animal model systems are an expensive component of medical research, but the information gained from their use is invaluable.

REFERENCES

1. Morrow WJW, Wharton M, Lau D, Levy JA. Small animals are not susceptible to human immunodeficiency virus infection. *J Gen Virol* 1987;68:2253–7.
2. Alter HJ, Eichberg JW, Masur H, et al. Transmission of HTLV-III infection from human plasma to chimpanzees: an animal model for AIDS. *Science* 1984;226:549–52.
3. Gajdusek DC, Gibbs CJ Jr, Rodgers-Johnson P, et al. Infection of chimpanzees by human T-lymphotropic retroviruses in brain and other tissues from AIDS patients. *Lancet* 1985;1:55–6.
4. Francis DP, Feorino PM, Broderson JR, et al. Infection of chimpanzees with lymphadenopathy-associated virus. *Lancet* 1984;2:1276–7.

5. Fauci AS. The human immunodeficiency virus: infectivity and mechanisms of pathogenesis. *Science* 1988;239:617–22.

6. Lifson AR, Rutherford GW, Jaffe HW. The natural history of human immunodeficiency virus infection. *J Infect Dis* 1988; 158:1360–7.

7. Fultz PN, McClure HM, Swenson RB, et al. Persistent infection of chimpanzees with human T-lymphotropic virus type-III/lymphadenopathy-associated virus: a potential model for acquired immunodeficiency syndrome. *J Virol* 1986;58:116–24.

8. Nara PL, Robey WG, Arthur LO, et al. Persistent infection of chimpanzees with human immunodeficiency virus: serological responses and properties of reisolated viruses. *J Virol* 1987; 61:3173–80.

9. Fultz PN, McClure HM, Swenson RB, Anderson DC. HIV infection of chimpanzees as a model for testing chemotherapeutics. *Intervirology* 1989;30(S1):51–8.

10. HU S-L, Fultz PN, McClure HM, et al. Effect of immunization with a vaccinia-HIV *env* recombinant on HIV infection of chimpanzees. *Nature* 1987;328:721–3.

11. Fultz PN, Siegel RL, Brodie A, et al. Prolonged CD4+ lymphocytopenia and thrombocytopenia in a chimpanzee persistently infected with HIV-1. *J Infect Dis* 1991;163:441–7.

12. Goudsmit J, Smit L, Krone WJA, et al. IgG response to human immunodeficiency virus in experimentally infected chimpanzees mimics the IgG response in humans. *J Infect Dis* 1987;155: 327–31.

13. Goudsmit J, Debouck C, Meloen RH, et al. Human immunodeficiency virus type 1 neutralization epitope with conserved architecture elicits early type-specific antibodies in experimentally infected chimpanzees. *Proc Natl Acad Sci USA* 1988;85:4478–82.

14. Goudsmit J, Thiriart C, Smit L, Bruck C, Gibbs CJ. Temporal development of cross-neutralization between HTLV-IIIB and HTLV-III RF in experimentally infected chimpanzees. *Vaccine* 1988;6:229–32.

15. Nara PL, Robey WG, Gonda MA, Carter SG, Fischinger PJ. Absence of cytotoxic antibody to human immunodeficiency virus-infected cells in humans and its induction in animals after infection or immunization with purified envelope glycoprotein gp120. *Proc Natl Acad Sci USA* 1987;84:3797–801.

16. Eichberg JW, Zarling JM, Alter HJ, et al. T-cell responses to human immunodeficiency virus (HIV) and its recombinant antigens in HIV-infected chimpanzees. *J Virol* 1987;61:3804–8.

17. Morrow WJW, Homsy J, Eichberg JW, et al. Long-term observation of baboons, rhesus monkeys, and chimpanzees inoculated with HIV and given periodic immunosuppressive treatment. *AIDS Res Hum Retroviruses* 1989;5:233–45.

18. Castro BA, Walker CM, Eichberg JW, Levy JA. Suppression of human immunodeficiency virus replication by CD8+ cells from infected and uninfected chimpanzees. *Cell Immunol* 1991;132: 246–55.

19. Fultz PN, McClure HM, Daugharty H, et al. Vaginal transmission of human immunodeficiency virus (HIV) to a chimpanzee. *J Infect Dis* 1986;154:896–900.

20. Nara P, Hatch W, Kessler J, Kelliher J, Carter S. The biology of human immunodeficiency virus-1 IIIB infection in the chimpanzee: in vivo and in vitro correlations. *J Med Primatol* 1989;18:343–55.

21. Camerini D, Seed B. A CD4 domain important for HIV-mediated syncytium formation lies outside the virus binding site. *Cell* 1990;60:747–54.

22. Zarling JM, Ledbetter JA, Sias J, et al. HIV-infected humans, but not chimpanzees, have circulating cytotoxic T lymphocytes that lyse uninfected CD4+ cells. *J Immunol* 1990;144:2992–8.

23. Kannagi M, Yetz JM, Letvin NL. In vitro growth characteristics of simian T-lymphotropic virus type III. *Proc Natl Acad Sci USA* 1985;82:7053–7.

24. Watanabe M, Ringler DJ, Fultz PN, MacKey JJ, Boyson JE, Letvin NL. A chimpanzee-passaged human immunodeficiency virus isolate is cytopathic for chimpanzee cells but does not induce disease. *J Virol* 1991;65:3344–8.

25. Brinchmann JE, Gaudernack G, Vartdal F. CD8+ T cells inhibit HIV replication in naturally infected CD4+ T cells. Evidence for a soluble inhibitor. *J Immunol* 1990;144:2961–6.

26. Eichberg JW, Lee DR, Allan JS, et al. In utero infection of an infant chimpanzee with HIV. *N Engl J Med* 1988;319:722–3.

27. Fultz PN, Greene C, Switzer W, Swenson B, Anderson D, McClure HM. Lack of transmission of human immunodeficiency virus from infected to uninfected chimpanzees. *J Med Primatol* 1987;16:341–7.

28. Lusso P, Markham PD, DeRocco SE, Gallo RC. In vitro susceptibility of T lymphocytes from chimpanzees (*Pan troglodytes*) to human herpesvirus 6 (HHV-6): a potential animal model to study the interactions between HHV-6 and human immunodeficiency virus type 1 in vivo. *J Virol* 1990;64:2751–8.

29. Lusso P, Ensoli B, Markham PD, et al. Productive dual infection of CD4+ T lymphocytes by HIV-1 and HHV-6. *Nature* 1989;337:370–3.

30. Letvin NL, Daniel MD, Sehgal PK, et al. Infection of baboons with HIV-2. *J Infect Dis* 1987;156:406–7.

31. Fultz PN, Switzer W, McClure HM, Anderson D, Montagnier L. Simian models for AIDS: SIV/SMM and HIV-2 infection of macaques. In: Ginsberg H, Brown F, Lerner RA, Chanock RM, eds. *Vaccines 88*. New York: Cold Spring Harbor Laboratory, 1988;167–170.

32. Nicol I, Flamminio-Zola G, Dubouch P, et al. Persistent HIV-2 infection of rhesus macaque, baboon, and mangabeys. *Intervirology* 1989;30:258–67.

33. Dormont D, Livartowski J, Chamaret S, et al. HIV-2 in rhesus monkeys: serological, virological, and clinical results. *Intervirology* 1989;30(S1):59–65.

34. Franchini G, Markham P, Gard E, et al. Persistent infection of rhesus macaques with a molecular clone of human immunodeficiency virus type 2: evidence of minimal genetic drift and low pathogenic effects. *J Virol* 1990;64:4462–7.

35. Stahl-Hennig C, Herchenroder O, Nick S, et al. Experimental infection of macaques with HIV-2$_{ben}$, a novel HIV-2 isolate. *AIDS* 1990;4:611–7.

36. Putkonen P, Bottiger B, Warstedt K, Thorstensson R, Albert J, Biberfeld G. Experimental infection of cynomolgus monkeys (*Macaca fascicularis*) with HIV-2. *J Acquired Immune Deficiency Syndrome* 1989;2:366–73.

37. Romieu I, Marlink R, Kanki P, M'Boup S, Essex M. HIV-2 link to AIDS in West Africa. *J Acquired Immune Deficiency Syndrome* 1990;3:220–30.

38. Ohta Y, Masuda T, Tsujimoto H, et al. Isolation of simian immunodeficiency virus from African green monkeys and seroepidemiologic survey of the virus in various non-human primates. *Int J Cancer* 1988;41:115–22.

39. Tsujimoto H, Cooper RW, Kodama T, et al. Isolation and characterization of simian immunodeficiency virus from mandrills in Africa and its relationship to other human and simian immunodeficiency viruses. *J Virol* 1988;62:4044–50.

40. Emau P, McClure HM, Isahakia M, Else JG, Fultz PN. Isolation from African Sykes' monkeys (*Cercopithecus mitis*) of a lentivirus related to human and simian immunodeficiency viruses. *J Virol* 1991;65:2135–40.

41. Gravell M, London WT, Hamilton RS, Stone G, Monzon M. Infection of macaque monkeys with simian immunodeficiency virus from African green monkeys: virulence and activation of latent infection. *J Med Primatol* 1989;18:247–54.

42. Honjo S, Narita T, Kobayashi R, et al. Experimental infection of African green monkeys and cynomolgus monkeys with a SIV$_{AGM}$ strain isolated from a healthy African green monkey. *J Med Primatol* 1990;19:9–20.

43. Fultz PN, Anderson DC, McClure HM, Dewhurst S, Mullins JI. SIVsmm infection of macaque and mangabey monkeys: correlation between in vivo and in vitro properties of different isolates. *Dev Biol Standard* 1990;72:253–8.

44. Letvin NL, Daniel MD, Sehgal PK, et al. Induction of AIDS-like disease in macaque monkeys with T-cell tropic retrovirus STLV-III. *Science* 1985;230:71–3.

45. Kannagi M, Kiyotaki M, Desrosiers RC, et al. Humoral immune responses to T cell tropic retrovirus simian T lymphotropic virus type III in monkeys with experimentally induced acquired immune deficiency-like syndrome. *J Clin Invest* 1986;78:1229–36.

46. Daniel MD, Letvin NL, Sehgal PK, et al. Long-term persistent infection of macaque monkeys with the simian immunodeficiency virus. *J Gen Virol* 1987;68:3183–9.

47. Benveniste RE, Morton WR, Clark EA, et al. Inoculation of baboons and macaques with simian immunodeficiency virus/Mne,

a primate lentivirus closely related to human immunodeficiency virus type 2. *J Virol* 1988;62:2091–101.

48. Zhang J, Martin LN, Watson EA, et al. Relationship of antibody responses and viral antigenemia to SIV/delta-induced immunodeficiency disease in the rhesus monkey. *J Infect Dis* 1988;158:1277–86.

49. Putkonen P, Warstedt K, Thorstensson R, et al. Experimental infection of cynomolgus monkeys (*Macaca fascicularis*) with simian immunodeficiency virus (SIVsm). *J Acquired Immune Deficiency Syndrome* 1989;2:359–65.

50. Fultz PN, Stricker RB, McClure HM, Anderson DC, Switzer WM, Horaist C. Humoral response to SIV/SMM infection in macaque and mangabey monkeys. *J Acquired Immune Deficiency Syndrome* 1990;3:319–29.

51. Miller CJ, Alexander NJ, Sutjipto S, et al. Genital mucosal transmission of simian immunodeficiency virus: animal model for heterosexual transmission of human immunodeficiency virus. *J Virol* 1989;63:4277–84.

52. Vowels BR, Gershwin ME, Gardner MB, Ahmed-Ansari A, McGraw TP. Characterization of simian immunodeficiency virus-specific T-cell-mediated cytotoxic response of infected rhesus macaques. *AIDS* 1989;3:785–92.

53. Miller MD, Lord CI, Stallard V, Mazzara GP, Letvin NL. The *gag*-specific cytotoxic T lymphocytes in rhesus monkeys infected with the simian immunodeficiency virus of macaques. *J Immunol* 1990;144:122–8.

54. Yamamoto H, Miller MD, Tsubota H, et al. Studies of cloned simian immunodeficiency virus-specific T lymphocytes. *gag*-specific cytotoxic T lymphocytes exhibit a restricted epitope specificity. *J Immunol* 1990;144:3385–91.

55. Yamamoto H, Miller MD, Watkins DI, et al. Two distinct lymphocyte populations mediate simian immunodeficiency virus envelope-specific target cell lysis. *J Immunol* 1990;145:3740–6.

56. Kannagi M, Chalifoux LV, Lord CI, Letvin NL. Suppression of simian immunodeficiency virus replication *in vitro* by CD8+ lymphocytes. *J Immunol* 1988;140:2237–42.

57. Tsubota H, Lord CI, Watkins DI, Morimoto C, Letvin NL. A cytotoxic T lymphocyte inhibits acquired immunodeficiency syndrome virus replication in peripheral blood lymphocytes. *J Exp Med* 1989;169:1421–34.

58. Baskin GB, Murphey-Corb M, Watson EA, Martin LN. Necropsy findings in rhesus monkeys experimentally infected with cultured simian immunodeficiency virus (SIV)/delta. *Vet Pathol* 1988;25:456–67.

59. McClure HM, Anderson DC, Fultz PN, Ansari AA, Lockwood E, Brodie A. Spectrum of disease in macaque monkeys chronically infected with SIV/SMM. *Vet Immunol Immunopathol* 1989;21:13–24.

60. Letvin NL, King NW. Immunologic and pathologic manifestations of the infection of rhesus monkeys with simian immunodeficiency virus of macaques. *J Acquired Immune Deficiency Syndrome* 1990;3:1023–40.

61. Feichtinger H, Putkonen P, Parravicini C, et al. Malignant lymphomas in cynomolgus monkeys infected with simian immunodeficiency virus. *Am J Pathol* 1990;137:1311–5.

62. Gonda MA, Braun MJ, Carter SG, et al. Characterization and molecular cloning of a bovine lentivirus related to human immunodeficiency virus. *Nature* 1987;330:388–91.

63. Pedersen NC, Ho EW, Brown ML, Yamamoto JK. Isolation of a T-lymphotropic virus from domestic cats with an immunodeficiency-like syndrome. *Science* 1987;235:790–3.

64. Dow SW, Poss ML, Hoover EA. Feline immunodeficiency virus: a neurotropic lentivirus. *J Acquired Immune Deficiency Syndrome* 1990;3:658–68.

65. Yamamoto JK, Sparger E, Ho EW, et al. Pathogenesis of experimentally induced feline immunodeficiency virus infection in cats. *Am J Vet Res* 1988;49:1246–58.

66. Ackley CD, Yamamoto JK, Levy N, Pedersen NC, Cooper MD. Immunologic abnormalities in pathogen-free cats experimentally infected with feline immunodeficiency virus. *J Virol* 1990;64:5652–5.

67. Siebelink KHJ, Chu I-H, Rimmelzwaan GF, et al. Feline immunodeficiency virus (FIV) infection in the cat as a model for HIV infection in man: FIV-induced impairment of immune function. *AIDS Res Hum Retroviruses* 1990;6:1373–8.

68. Pedersen NC, Torten M, Rideout B, et al. Feline leukemia virus infection as a potentiating cofactor for the primary and secondary stages of experimentally induced feline immunodeficiency virus infection. *J Virol* 1990;64:598–606.

69. Filice G, Cereda PM, Varnier OE. Infection of rabbits with human immunodeficiency virus. *Nature* 1988;335:366–9.

70. Kulaga H, Folks T, Rutledge R, Truckenmiller ME, Gugel E, Kindt TJ. Infection of rabbits with human immunodeficiency virus 1. A small animal model for acquired immunodeficiency syndrome. *J Exp Med* 1989;169:321–6.

71. Namikawa R, Kaneshima H, Lieberman M, Weissman IL, McCune JM. Infection of the SCID-hu mouse by HIV-1. *Science* 1988;242:1684–6.

72. Mosier DE, Gulizia RJ, Baird SM, Wilson DB, Spector DH, Spector SA. Human immunodeficiency virus infection of human-PBL-SCID mice. *Science* 1991;251:791–4.

73. Vogel J, Hinrichs SH, Reynolds RK, Luciw PA, Jay G. The HIV *tat* gene induces dermal lesions resembling Kaposi's sarcoma in transgenic mice. *Nature* 1988;335:606–11.

74. Leonard JM, Abramczuk JW, Pezen DS, et al. Development of disease and virus recovery in transgenic mice containing HIV proviral DNA. *Science* 1988;242:1665–70.

75. Khillan JS, Deen KC, Yu S-H, Sweet RW, Rosenberg M, Westphal H. Gene transactivation mediated by the TAT gene of human immunodeficiency virus in transgenic mice. *Nucleic Acids Res* 1988;16:1423–30.

76. Leonard J, Khillan JS, Gendelman HE, et al. The human immunodeficiency virus long terminal repeat is preferentially expressed in Langerhans cells in transgenic mice. *AIDS Res Hum Retroviruses* 1989;5:421–30.

77. Haase AT. Pathogenesis of lentivirus infections. *Nature* 1986;322:130–6.

78. Narayan O, Clements JE. Biology and pathogenesis of lentiviruses. *J Gen Virol* 1989;70:1617–39.

79. Norley SG, Kraus G, Ennen J, Bonilla J, Konig H, Kurth R. Immunological studies of the basis for the apathogenicity of simian immunodeficiency virus from African green monkeys. *Proc Natl Acad Sci USA* 1990;87:9067–71.

80. Fultz PN, Gordon TP, Anderson DC, McClure HM. Prevalence of natural infection with SIVsmm and STLV-1 in a breeding colony of sooty mangabey monkeys. *AIDS* 1990;4:619–25.

81. Fultz PN, Gluckman J-C, Muchmore E, Girard M. Immune stimulation results in transient increases in infected cells in HIV-infected chimpanzees. *AIDS Res Hum Retroviruses* 1992;8:in press.

82. Fultz PN, McClure HM, Anderson DC, Switzer WM. Identification and biologic characterization of an acutely lethal variant of simian immunodeficiency virus from sooty mangabeys (SIV/SMM). *AIDS Res Hum Retroviruses* 1989;5:397–409.

83. North TA, North GLT, Pedersen NC. Feline immunodeficiency virus, a model for reverse transcriptase-targeted chemotherapy for acquired immune deficiency syndrome. *Antimicrob Agents Chemother* 1989;33:915–9.

84. Tavares L, Roneker C, Johnston K, Lehrman SN, deNoronha F. 3′-Azido-3′-deoxythymidine in feline leukemia virus-infected cats: a model for therapy and prophylaxis of AIDS. *Cancer Res* 1987;47:3190–4.

85. Yetter RA, Buller RML, Lee JS, et al. CD4+ T cells are required for development of a murine retrovirus-induced immunodeficiency syndrome (MAIDS). *J Exp Med* 1988;168:623–35.

86. Klinken SP, Fredrickson TN, Hartley JW, Yetter RA, Morse HC III. Evolution of B cell lineage lymphomas in mice with a retrovirus-induced immunodeficiency syndrome, MAIDS. *J Immunol* 1988;140:1123–31.

87. Aziz DC, Hanna Z, Jolicoeur P. Severe immunodeficiency disease induced by a defective murine leukaemia virus. *Nature* 1989;338:505–8.

88. Ruprecht RM, O'Brien LG, Rossoni LD, Nusinoff-Lehrman S. Suppression of mouse viraemia and retroviral disease by 3′-azido-3′-deoxythymidine. *Nature* 1986;323:467–9.

89. Sharpe AH, Jaenisch R, Ruprecht RM. Retroviruses and mouse embryos: a rapid model for neurovirulence and transplacental antiviral therapy. *Science* 1987;236:1671–4.

90. Portnoi D, Stall AM, Schwartz D, Merigan TC, Herzenberg LA, Basham T. Zidovudine (azido dideoxythymidine) inhibits

characteristic early alterations of lymphoid cell populations in retrovirus-induced murine AIDS. *J Immunol* 1990;144:1705–10.

91. Sharpe AH, Hunter JJ, Ruprecht RM, Jaenisch R. Maternal transmission of retroviral disease and strategies for preventing infection of the neonate. *J Virol* 1989;63:1049–53.

92. McCune JM, Namikawa R, Shih C-C, Rabin L, Kaneshima H. Suppression of HIV infection in AZT-treated SCID-hu mice. *Science* 1990;247:564–6.

93. Desrosiers RC, Wyand MS, Kodama T, et al. Vaccine protection against simian immunodeficiency virus infection. *Proc Natl Acad Sci USA* 1989;86:6353–7.

94. Murphey-Corb M, Martin LN, Davison-Fairburn B, et al. A formalin-inactivated whole SIV vaccine confers protection in macaques. *Science* 1989;246:1293–7.

95. Carlson JR, McGraw TP, Keddie E, et al. Vaccine protection of rhesus macaques against simian immunodeficiency virus infection. *AIDS Res Hum Retroviruses* 1990;6:1239–46.

96. Stott EJ, Chan WL, Mills KHG, et al. Preliminary report: protection of cynomolgus macaques against simian immunodeficiency virus by fixed infected-cell vaccine. *Lancet* 1990;2:1538–41.

97. Sutjipto S, Pedersen NC, Miller CJ, et al. Inactivated simian immunodeficiency virus vaccine failed to protect rhesus macaques from intravenous or genital mucosal infection but delayed disease in intravenously exposed animals. *J Virol* 1990;64:2290–7.

98. Marthas ML, Sutjipto S, Higgins J, et al. Immunization with a live, attenuated simian immunodeficiency virus (SIV) prevents early disease but not infection in rhesus macaques challenged with pathogenic SIV. *J Virol* 1990;64:3694–700.

99. Putkonen P, Thorstensson R, Albert J, et al. Infection of cyno-

molgus monkeys with HIV-2 protects against pathogenic consequences of a subsequent simian immunodeficiency virus infection. *AIDS* 1990;4:783–89.

100. Gardner MB. Vaccination against SIV infection and disease. *AIDS Res Hum Retroviruses* 1990;6:835–46.

101. Berman PW, Groopman JE, Gregory T, et al. Human immunodeficiency virus type 1 challenge of chimpanzees immunized with recombinant envelope glycoprotein gp120. *Proc Natl Acad Sci USA* 1988;85:5200–4.

102. Arthur LO, Bess JW, Waters DJ, et al. Challenge of chimpanzees (*Pan troglodytes*) immunized with human immunodeficiency virus envelope glycoprotein gp120. *J Virol* 1989;63:5046–53.

103. Berman PW, Gregory TJ, Riddle L, et al. Protection of chimpanzees from infection by HIV-1 after vaccination with recombinant glycoprotein gp120 but not gp160. *Nature* 1990;345:622–5.

104. Girard M, Kieny M-P, Pinter A, et al. Immunization of chimpanzees confers protection against challenge with human immunodeficiency virus. *Proc Natl Acad Sci USA* 1991;88:542–6.

105. Emini EA, Nara PL, Schleif WA, et al. Antibody-mediated in vitro neutralization of human immunodeficiency virus type 1 abolishes infectivity for chimpanzees. *J Virol* 1990;64:3674–8.

106. Emini EA, Schlief WA, Quintero JC, et al. Yeast-expressed p55 precursor core protein of human immunodeficiency virus type 1 does not elicit protective immunity in chimpanzees. *AIDS Res Hum Retroviruses* 1990;6:1247–50.

107. Prince AM, Horowitz B, Baker L, et al. Failure of a human immunodeficiency virus (HIV) immune globulin to protect chimpanzees against experimental challenge with HIV. *Proc Natl Acad Sci USA* 1988;85:6944–8.

AIDS and Other Manifestations of HIV Infection,
Second Edition, Edited by Gary P. Wormser.
Raven Press, Ltd., New York © 1992.

CHAPTER 10

Simian Retroviruses

Murray B. Gardner and Paul A. Luciw

Simian retroviruses are classified within four different subfamilies, the oncoviruses (type C), the type D retroviruses, the lentiviruses (type E), and the spumaviruses (type F) (Table 1). This chapter will review the salient biology of each of these viral subfamilies in the order given. Emphasis will be on the type D retrovirus and lentivirus subfamilies because of their etiologic association with simian acquired immunodeficiency syndrome (AIDS). Simian immunodeficiency virus (SIV) is genetically related to the human immunodeficiency virus (HIV), and experimental infection of captive macaques with SIV produces a progressive and fatal immunodeficiency similar to AIDS in humans; thus this primate lentivirus is proving to be useful and essential for AIDS vaccine development and for antiviral drug research.

ONCOVIRUSES

Oncoviruses were the target of extensive research done in the 1970s seeking to identify cancer-causing retroviruses in animals and humans. Several comprehensive reviews of this subfamily of type C retroviruses have been previously published (1–3). Type C viruses are divided into two major groups depending on whether their route of transmission is endogenous or exogenous under natural conditions.

Endogenous Type C Primate Viruses

Evidence became available in the early 1970s that retroviral genes were present in the genomic DNA of many mammalian species, including primates (4). Many of these isolates were obtained by cocultivation of primate

cell cultures with cells of candidate permissive host species. Most of these endogenous viruses were not infectious for cells of their species of origin, i.e., they had a xenotropic host range. The endogenous viruses appeared to be well conserved in evolution and to represent part of the natural inheritance of these species. It was assumed that the endogenous viral genes were evolutionarily conserved relics of ancient infections by exogenous retroviruses, primarily of the same animal species. This phenomenon was apparently accounted for by the discovery of the viral enzyme reverse transcriptase, which provided the mechanism for converting the complete RNA genome of exogenous retroviruses into double-stranded DNA (5,6). Another viral enzyme, the integrase, functioned to insert this proviral information, more or less at random, into the chromosomal DNA of somatic and, on rarer occasions, germ cells. It was discovered that: (1) not only did all chickens and mice contain such retroviral (then called RNA tumor virus) information in their cellular genomes, but all mammals did as well; (2) endogenous viral genes coding for core proteins, envelope glycoproteins, and the enzyme reverse transcriptase were under independent regulation; and (3) the endogenous viral genes were expressed in many instances in the absence of virus production. In certain inbred strains of chickens and mice, the inherited endogenous genes became activated to form complete viruses, which were infectious for their own species' cells (i.e., ecotropic host range) and eventually caused thymic lymphomas in the AKR and related mouse strains. The viral oncogene hypothesis (7) that guided much of cancer virus research in the 1970s was based on this idea: that activation of endogenous virogenes included oncogenes that led to cancer. However, this generalization, although of tremendous heuristic value, did not prove entirely accurate. All of the endogenous virogenes in outbred mammals were subsequently shown to be nonpathogenic and oncogenes were determined to be normal cellular growth-promoting

M. B. Gardner and P. A. Luciw: Department of Medical Pathology and California Primate Research Center, University of California, Davis, California 95616.

TABLE 1. *Simian retroviruses*

Virus subfamily	Host	Exogenous	Endogenous	Pathogenic
Oncovirus (Type C)				
	Tree shrew		TRV-1	No
	Baboons		BaEV	No
	Macaques		Mac-1; MMC-1	No
	Colobus		CPC-1	No
	Owl monkey		OMC-1	No
	Gibbon apes	GaLV		Lymphoma
	Wooly monkey	SSAV/SSV		Sarcoma
	African monkeys and apes	STLV-I		Lymphoma
	Macaques	STLV-I		No
Type D				
	Macaques	SRV 1–5 (MPMV)		SAIDS
	Langur		Po 1-Lu	No
	Squirrel monkey		SMRV	No
Lentivirus (type E)				
	African monkeys (natural hosts)	SIV		No
	Macaques (experimental host)	SIV		SAIDS
Spumavirus (type F)				
	African and Asian monkeys, apes, and chimpanzees	SFV		No
	Squirrel, spider, and capuchin monkeys	SFV		No

BaEV, baboon endogenous virus; CPC-1, colobus monkey endogenous virus, strain 1; GaLV, gibbon ape leukemia virus; Mac-1, stumptail macaque endogenous virus, strain 1; MMC-1, rhesus macaque endogenous virus, strain 1; MPMV, Mason-Pfizer monkey virus (SRV-3); OMC-1, owl monkey endogenous virus, strain 1; Po-1-Lu, Langur (*Presbytis*) endogenous virus; SAIDS, simian AIDS; SFV, simian foamy virus; SIV, simian immunodeficiency virus; SMRV, squirrel monkey endogenous retrovirus; SRV, simian type D retroviruses, strains 1–5; SSAV/SSV, simian sarcoma associated virus/simian sarcoma virus; STLV-I, simian T-lymphotropic virus, strain 1; TRV, tree shrew endogenous virus, strain 1.

genes that indeed could be activated or transduced by exogenous type C retroviruses (8). Although a number of useful roles for endogenous virogenes were postulated, it has not been possible as yet to demonstrate a biologic function for these genes in primates.

Baboon Endogenous Virus

The first endogenous type C virus isolate of primate origin, baboon endogenous virus (BaEV), was recovered from a baboon placenta (9). Subsequently, many independent but closely related isolates were obtained from diverse normal adult and embryonic tissues of several different species of baboons. Like most other endogenous viruses, these could only be grown in permissive cells of certain species different from the species of origin. This prototype endogenous primate type C virus became a useful tool for probing the evolutionary relationship of various primates. Sequences related to those of the baboon virus were found in all other Old World monkeys, with the degree of relatedness determined by the evolutionary distance between species (10). BaEV was not shown to have oncogenic or other biologic activity. Its function, if any, remains unknown. Quite surprisingly, BaEV was partially related to the endogenous feline type C virus RD114. Since RD114 DNA was not present in the genomic DNA of most members of the cat family, it was concluded that BaEV spread from ancestral baboons to ancestors of the domestic cat about 5 million years ago. Several other similar examples were noted of suspected cross-species transmission of endogenous type C viruses among animals in evolutionary times (11). However, currently it has been very difficult to document transpecies spread of any animal retrovirus, endogenous or exogenous, under natural conditions. An important exception is the inadvertent infection of Asian macaques in primate centers by the exogenous lentivirus (SIV) from certain African monkeys, an event that causes simian AIDS (12) (see below).

Subsequently, six other primate retroviruses were isolated and characterized, making a total of seven distinct genetically transmitted endogenous retrovirus groups in primates (13). These newer isolates included type C virions from a stumptail macaque and an owl monkey and type D viruses from the squirrel monkey and a langur monkey. The endogenous type D virus of Asian langurs may have been the source, via transpecies infection in distant times, of the exogenous type D retroviruses that cause AIDS in Asian macaques. Like BaEV, these other endogenous primate retroviruses have no known biologic role. Apart from the baboon and owl monkey these endogenous retroviral genes are powerfully repressed at the cellular level in their primate hosts and are only rarely expressed as complete virus particles. In recent years a number of sequences related to murine and primate retrovirus reverse transcriptase genes have been found by polymerase chain reaction (PCR) analysis in human genomic DNA (14). Some of these sequences are related to human T-lymphotropic virus I (HTLV-I) and to other previously described human endogenous proviral DNAs. As in nonhuman primates the significance of these human endogenous proviral sequences remains unknown.

Gibbon Ape Leukemia Virus and Simian Sarcoma Virus

The first exogenous primate type C virus [gibbon ape leukemia virus (GaLV)] was isolated from several captive gibbon apes that developed spontaneous leukemia (15). About the same time a closely related virus called simian sarcoma virus (SSV) was recovered from a pet wooly monkey with a spontaneous fibrosarcoma (16). GaLV was then shown to be fairly common in captive gibbon apes and to be spread horizontally and congenitally as a purely exogenous virus (17). Molecular hybridization analysis suggested that it might have been acquired in the evolutionary past by transpecies infection with an endogenous type C virus of feral Asian mice (11). By contrast, SSV was found only in the one wooly monkey, i.e., it was neither endogenous nor exogenous in this species. Because the GaLV-infected gibbon ape and SSV-infected wooly monkey had frequent physical contact in the same household and because the GaLV and simian sarcoma-associated or helper virus (SSAV) were so closely related, it was logical to assume that SSV was derived from GaLV by transpecies infection. The sarcoma-inducing property of SSV was later shown to be caused by the transduction of the *sis* oncogene (β chain of platelet-derived growth factor) from the wooly monkey genomic DNA by prior infection with the SSAV (18). This was a rare one-time event, and still represents the only example of a sarcoma virus isolated from a solid tumor of a nonhuman primate. Experimental studies of SSV cell transformation and induction of sarcomas or gliomas in marmosets were very helpful in elucidating the molecular mechanisms underlying its rapid oncogenicity, e.g., defectivity of sarcoma viruses, rescue by helper type C viruses (such as SSAV), and transduction of the *sis* oncogene (1).

Because GaLV occurs naturally in gibbon apes in captivity, it is assumed to occur in gibbon apes in the wild, but this has not been studied. GaLV was isolated on several occasions and at different locations from cases of spontaneous malignant lymphoma or granulocytic leukemia occurring in captive gibbon apes (19). Subsequently, the virus was also isolated from healthy seropositive carriers. The virus causes a systemic blood-born (cell-associated and cell-free) infection of multiple tissues; virus can be readily isolated from many organs. It has a wide in vitro host range for a number of nonhematopoietic cell types of diverse species and is nontransforming and noncytopathic. All of the GaLV isolates are closely related to each other, but individual isolates can be distinguished by highly sensitive immunologic or nucleic acid hybridization assays. Experimental transmission studies showed that the GaLV isolates were very stable and could induce the same tumor (e.g., granulocytic leukemia with a latent period of 6–14 months) as that seen in the animal from which the virus was initially isolated. Infectious molecular clones of GaLV are not available for in vivo pathogenicity study. Natural transmission of GaLV was documented several times in captive gibbon apes but the route of spread is not known (17). Congenital transmission was also observed. Neutralizing antibodies were protective against fulminating viremia and subsequent development of tumors. Despite extensive surveys, and numerous false alarms, GaLV infection of humans has never been found (20). In the late 1970s the gibbon ape colonies were disbanded and studies of GaLV and SSV have largely ceased.

Simian T-Lymphotropic Virus, Type I

Naturally occurring infection with simian T-lymphotropic virus, type 1 (STLV-I), which is closely related to HTLV-I (21), is highly prevalent in African and Asian nonhuman primates (22–25). Serosurveys indicate that STLV-I is a common infection (10–60%) in Cercopithecoidea, particularly in African green monkeys (*Cercopithecus aethiops*), baboons (*Papio* spp.), and macaques. Infection is frequent in feral monkeys as well as in captive monkeys in primate centers (26) and zoos (27). An increasing seropositivity rate with increasing age suggests that the virus is horizontally spread, and epidemiological observations suggest that sexual transmission may account for much of this spread. Seroepidemiologic studies have found no evidence for transmission of STLV-I from monkeys to humans (26). These simian retroviruses have the same genetic constitution—*gag, pol, env, tax,* and long terminal repeat (LTR)—as HTLV-I, and all of these sequences are highly homologous (90–95%) with those of HTLV-I (21). Furthermore, like HTLV-I, STLV-I can immortalize cultured T cells (22). Although most of the STLV-infected monkeys are healthy, the occurrence of an adult T-cell leukemia (ATL), identical to ATL in humans, has been documented in one infected African green monkey (28). Despite a report to the contrary (29), STLV-I has not been linked to lymphomas in macaques. Therefore, the leukemogenic potential of STLV is analogous to that of HTLV-I.

In contrast to HTLV-I infection of humans, STLV infection of monkeys has not been linked to immunosuppression or neurologic disease. Nevertheless, STLV has a natural history and biology in nonhuman primates that is very similar to HTLV-I in humans. Therefore, it could serve as an excellent surrogate for HTLV-I infection of humans except that, like HTLV-I infection, the ATL incidence is so low (≤1%) and the latent period so long (many years) that it can not be used as a practical experimental model for studies focused on neoplasia. However, it is important to screen African and Asian monkeys in primate centers for infection with this virus because it could be an important cofactor in studies with SIV or other viruses. A national reference laboratory has been established to perform this service for primate facilities in the United States and to monitor animal handlers for possible cross-species infection (26). Results from this laboratory confirm that infection with STLV-I is rather common in macaques at different centers without evidence for spread of this virus to humans in contact with the infected animals.

Cynomolgus monkeys (*M. fascicularis*) have been used in attempts to develop an HTLV-I vaccine. In one experiment (30), four monkeys were immunized with a recombinant HTLV-I *env* gene product produced in *E. coli,* and challenged with live MT-2 cells, a high HTLV-I producer cell line. After challenge, all four control non-immunized monkeys were infected, whereas all four of the immunized monkeys were protected. Protection correlated best with vaccine induction of specific antibody against envelope glycoproteins (gp68 and gp46) of HTLV-I including high titered syncytial inhibiting neutralizing antibody. In a second study (31), three monkeys were immunized with an HTLV-I *gag* and *env* subunit vaccine and challenged with an STLV-I-infected cell line. After challenge the two controls were infected, while the three vaccinates were apparently uninfected. However, an increase in antibody titers in the vaccinates after challenge suggests that they had been transiently infected. Protection correlated with induction of HTLV-I and to a lesser extent STLV-I syncytial inhibition antibody and cytotoxic T lymphocytes (CTL) against STLV-I-infected cells. Thus, as previously shown in murine and feline type C virus systems (32), vaccine protection against this subfamily of retroviruses under specific laboratory conditions also extends to the primate type C viruses.

TYPE D RETROVIRUSES

The type D retrovirus subfamily is indigenous to Asian macaques in which they are nononcogenic but po-

tentially immunosuppressive (33,34). Several serotypes called simian retroviruses (SRV) 1–5 have been described at different primate centers. These exogenous viruses may cause a profound T- and B-cell depletion and a fatal immunodeficiency syndrome resembling human AIDS in its terminal stages. For this reason the immunosuppressive disease induced by type D retrovirus was initially called simian AIDS (SAIDS), but now this term is generally restricted to the fatal immunosuppressive disease caused by SIV. SIV is more closely related to HIV than is SRV, and type D-related viruses have not as yet been found in humans. Therefore research on SIV is considered more relevant to AIDS and has largely replaced research on SRV.

Epidemiology

Since 1985 type D retroviruses have been identified as the causative agents of a naturally occurring infectious immunodeficiency disease in eight species of macaques at five of the seven primate centers in the United States (34). The centers affected with this disease are the New England, California, Oregon, Washington, and Wisconsin centers. The Yerkes and Delta primate centers in the southeastern United States are currently spared this problem. Infection appears to be highly prevalent in Asian macaques in captivity and these species are the natural hosts of the type D retrovirus subfamily. Type D retrovirus infection has been found in healthy feral macaques in India but the prevalence of infection with the different serotypes in these feral animals remains to be determined. The type D retroviruses are related to the endogenous retrovirus (PO-1-Lu) of the spectacled langur (*Presbytis obscuris*), another Asian monkey from which it may have had its evolutionary origin (35). Although similar to each other in ultrastructural features, the type D particles are morphologically distinct from HIV and SIV particles (36). The original type D retrovirus isolated from macaques in 1970 was called Mason-Pfizer monkey virus (MPMV) (37). A serologic survey of U.S. primate centers in the mid-1970s indicated that about 25% of all macaques had antibody reacting to MPMV; this observation revealed the wide-spread distribution of this infection in captive macaques before the 1980s (38). Extensive serologic surveys of humans, including primate center animal handlers, over the last two decades has shown no proof of type D retrovirus infection despite some unconfirmed observations to the contrary (20). Many putative human type D retrovirus isolates were found to be contaminants of MPMV growing in HeLa cells. All of the contemporary type D isolates associated with simian AIDS are related to MPMV but are distinct envelope variants falling into five major serotypes. SRV-1 is the serotype in macaques at the California and New England Primate Centers, and the SRV-2 serotype is present in macaques at the Oregon and Washington Primate Centers. The original MPMV is the third distinct serotype, now known to be present in macaques at the Wisconsin Primate Center. Experimental transmission of MPMV in the early 1970s led to death in many infant rhesus monkeys from a wasting syndrome with thymic atrophy, profound neutropenia, anemia, lymphoid depletion, and opportunistic infections (39). The features of this immunosuppressive syndrome were the same as those observed in the early 1980s. Reisolation and experimental transmission of MPMV from its initial source, a frozen sample of the spontaneous rhesus mammary carcinoma, confirmed the earlier observation that this virus, like SRV-1 and SRV-2, was immunosuppressive and apparently nononcogenic (40). Each of these three type D retrovirus serotypes (SRV-1, SRV-2, and SRV-3) has been molecularly cloned and totally sequenced (41–43), and fatal simian AIDS has been induced with an infectious molecular clone of SRV-1 (44). Two further type D serotypes, SRV-4 and SRV-5, have been found in macaques at the University of California, Berkeley, and at the primate center in Beijing, China. Serial epidemiologic and virologic surveys have shown that type D retroviruses are the primary cause of almost all cases of spontaneous SAIDS in each of the five centers where endemic infection with these viruses exist (34). However, variations in disease severity and clinical manifestations with the different SRV serotypes and the different species of macaques at each center, have been observed under conditions of both natural and experimental exposure. The SRV-2 serotype is particularly associated not only with immunosuppression, but with a proliferative disorder termed retroperitoneal fibromatosis (RF), which has features in common with Kaposi's sarcoma (45–47).

Before the causative retrovirus (i.e., SRV-1) was identified, a cage exposure experiment was begun to prove the infectious nature of the disease at the California Primate Research Center in an outdoor corral (NC-1) in which many deaths from simian AIDS had occurred (48). Nineteen of 23 (83%) healthy tracer juvenile rhesus died of a fatal immunosuppressive disease within 9 months of introduction into the resident affected population. In contrast, 21 healthy sentinel juvenile rhesus placed in the same outdoor enclosure but denied physical contact with the SAIDS affected group by a 10-foot-wide buffer zone remained healthy and seronegative for $2\frac{1}{2}$ years. Thus direct physical contact was required for spread of the disease. The most likely route of natural transmission is by percutaneous inoculation of virus-containing saliva via biting and scratching (49). Following the isolation of SRV-1 from affected rhesus in NC-1 and the development of appropriate serologic and virologic assays for its detection, it was found that all monkeys with SAIDS in NC-1 were persistently infected with this type D retrovirus. All of the healthy "sentinel" monkeys located within the same enclosure but denied physical contact with the affected animals were free of infectious SRV-1 and antiviral antibody. In NC-1 the specific mortality rate from simian AIDS was higher in juveniles than in adults, and the overall prevalence of SRV-1 antibody in all ages ranged from 68% to 85%. Passive maternal immunity to SRV-1 may have protected some of the infants. Antibody prevalence increased with age; essentially all animals over 3 years of age were seropositive. Seroconversion was found to be a poor indicator of active infection; about 50% of virus-positive juveniles had no antibody detectable by enzyme-linked immunosorbent assay (ELISA). In disease-free breeding colonies of rhesus monkeys the prevalence of SRV-1 antibody was only 4% by ELISA.

Repeated viral isolations from all animals in NC-1 revealed the following patterns of infection: (1) SRV-1 viremia with clinical SAIDS; (2) transient viremia with clinical recovery; (3) intermittent viremia suggesting reactivation of latent infection; (4) viremia in a 1-day-old infant, suggesting transplacental transmission; and (5) persistent viremia and virus shedding in several healthy animals. In a retrospective epidemiologic analysis, one healthy carrier in NC-1 was linked by direct physical contact to 34 cases of SAIDS over a 3-year period (49). SAIDS was experimentally transmitted to two juvenile rhesus by inoculation of SRV-1-containing saliva from this adult female monkey. Although SRV-1 could be isolated from peripheral blood mononuclear cells (PBMC) and most body secretions of infected animals, the most plentiful source of virus was the saliva, which was the major natural route of virus transmission. The transmission of SRV in semen has not been evaluated. Although SRV-1 is present in vaginal secretions, the female-to-male sexual transmission of this virus also remains undetermined. Perinatal transmission of SRV-1 transplacentally or via milk appears to occur infrequently.

Clinical Features

The clinical features of SAIDS induced by type D retrovirus include generalized lymphadenopathy, splenomegaly, fever, weight loss, diarrhea, anemia, lymphopenia, granulocytopenia, and thrombocytopenia. Necrotizing gingivitis (NOMA) is occasionally observed. Despite the striking depletion of peripheral blood cellular elements, the bone marrow is frequently hypercellular. Electrophoresis of sera of ill animals reveals hypoproteinemia, hypoalbuminemia, and hypogammaglobulinemia. Numerous bacterial, protozoan, and viral superinfections have been identified including cytomegalovirus (CMV) and leukocyte-associated herpesvirus infections. Disseminated CMV has been the most frequent opportunistic infection (50). Concentrations of IgG, IgA, and IgM are decreased but complement component C3 is not changed and C4 is increased (51). The absolute lymphocyte count decreases but the OKT4/OKT8 ratio remains unchanged when compared with controls reflecting an absolute decrease in both helper and suppressor T cells. Thus, in comparison with human AIDS and SIV-induced SAIDS, an inverted T-cell helper/suppressor ratio is not found in disease induced by the type D retrovirus. A decreased response to mitogens [concanavalin A (con A), phytohemagglutinin (PHA)] and to allogeneic lymphoid cells occurs early and becomes more severe near death. Response to the mitogen PWM is variable. Interleukin-2 causes a complete or partial restoration of the response to the mitogens con A and PHA. The virally induced mechanism underlying these profound hematological disturbances is unknown.

A major difference between SRV and SIV or HIV is the broader immunosuppressive effect of the type D retrovirus on both T and B cells, with a consequent depression of both T- and B-cell function (52). This difference is correlated with the broader tropism of the type D retrovirus for both T and B cells in vitro compared with the more restricted T4 tropism of HIV and SIV. Unlike SIV and HIV infection of macaques and humans, respectively, SRV does not cause hypergammaglobulinemia, which is consistent with the histologic absence of plasma cells and the early impairment of B-cell function. Other differences between type D retrovirus disease and SIV- or HIV-induced AIDS include an absence of *Pneumocystis carinii* as a common opportunistic infection and the infrequent occurrence of Kaposi's sarcoma (unless

retroperitoneal fibrosis is the simian counterpart). The major similarities and differences between SRV and SIV are listed in Table 2.

Experimental Transmission

Experimental transmission of SRV-1, using virus grown in tissue culture media, confirmed the virulence of this virus, as previously indicated by the natural cage exposure observations and by experimental inoculations of infected blood and tissue homogenates (53). Intravenous inoculation of SRV-1 into 14 juvenile (9–11 months) rhesus led to the same spectrum of clinical disease as seen naturally in NC-1. All animals became infected, six died acutely 7–20 weeks after inoculation, six remained persistently infected up to 1 year after inoculation, and two developed neutralizing antibody, became nonviremic, and remained healthy after 1 year. Monkeys dying acutely had a high level of persistent viremia and no serum antibody response by ELISA, whereas monkeys with a more indolent clinical course had a low-grade viremia and only a transient initial antibody response to the major core antigen (p27) (54). Monkeys that never became ill and were either nonviremic or transiently viremic developed high levels of serum antibody including neutralizing antibody to the virus envelope. Thus, in the SRV SAIDS model system, disease resistance can be correlated with humoral antibody levels and neutralizing activity. These observations further establish the etiologic role of SRV-1 in this fatal immuno-

TABLE 2. *Comparison of simian retrovirus (SRV) and simian immunodeficiency virus (SIV)*

Similarities
    Exogenous lymphotropic retroviruses that induce fatal immunodeficiency in macaques after a long incubation period
    Pathogenic molecular clones have been derived
    Persistent infection despite host immune response
    Length of survival correlates with vigor of antiviral antibody response
    Low levels of virus expression *in vivo;* predominantly cell associated
    Neurotropic
    Syncytia induction *in vitro*
    Inefficient transmission by close physical contact with body secretions
    Not transmitted to humans
    Infection can be prevented by immunization with inactivated whole virus vaccines

Differences
    SIV does not cause disease in its natural host, i.e., African monkeys; SRV does cause disease in its natural host, i.e., Asian macaques
    SIV is genetically more closely related to HIV than is SRV
    SIV is more virulent for macaques than is SRV
    SRV neutralizing antibody can allow for recovery from infection; SIV neutralizing antibody does not allow for recovery from infection
    SIV uses the CD4 receptor; SRV has a different unidentified receptor and wider cell tropism
    SIV envelope mutates more rapidly than SRV
    SIV causes neuropathology; SRV does not
    SIV is more T-cell cytopathic than SRV
    SRV is transmitted by saliva; SIV is probably transmitted sexually
    SRV readily spreads among macaques; SIV does not

suppressive disease. Conclusive proof of this etiology came later with the induction of an identical, fatal disease using molecularly cloned infectious SRV-1 (44), and the prevention of this disease with an SRV-1 vaccine (55).

Pathology

At necropsy, affected animals show severe depletion of lymphocytes in both germinal centers and paracortical regions of lymph nodes, as well as an absence of plasma cells. The histopathology of lymph nodes is virtually indistinguishable from that of lymph nodes in the terminal stage of human AIDS (50). The distribution of SRV-1 in tissues of infected macaques was studied by virus isolation, electron microscopy (EM), immunohistochemistry, and molecular hybridization (56). Virus could be isolated from PBMC, plasma, serum, urine, saliva, lymph nodes, tears, breast milk, cerebrospinal fluid, and vaginal secretions of sick monkeys as well as some healthy carriers. Separation of peripheral blood T and B cells by panning and fluorescent cell sorting indicated that animals with SAIDS harbored infectious type D retrovirus in both T and B cells but more in T4 cells than in T8 cells (52). Virus was also detected in macrophages but not in mature neutrophils or platelets. Macrophage and neutrophil function was not impaired early in the course of disease (57). Serial titrations suggested that only 0.1– 1% of lymphocytes was infected in peripheral blood. Testing of the susceptibility of normal macaque lymphocytes to infection with SRV in vitro was possible but was difficult because of the inability to establish long-term cultures of macaque lymphocytes. SRV-1 will grow in established human T-cell lines such as HUT 78, as well as in certain Epstein Barr virus (EBV)-transformed human B cells, such as Raji cells. The ability of simian type D retroviruses to induce syncytia in Raji cells is the basis for an infectious virus assay (58), and serum inhibition of such syncytia is the basis for a neutralizing antibody assay (59). Apart from syncytia, the virus has no direct cytolytic effect and it is nontransforming. OKT4 antibodies do not block infection of Raji cells. The receptor for the type D retrovirus is unknown, but it must be present widely on different cell types. The receptor gene for the simian type D retroviruses in human cells has recently been localized to chromosome 19; it is unrelated to other known surface markers (60).

By immunohistochemistry with a monoclonal antibody to the SRV-1 transmembrane glycoprotein (gp20), viral protein was identified in cells of salivary gland, lymph node, spleen, thymus, and choroid plexus, but not in the brain parenchyma of SAIDS monkeys (56). Viral antigen was commonly detected in germinal centers of lymph node and spleen, and viral particles were seen by EM at the same locations, apparently in association with antigen-processing dendritic reticulum cells. The amount of viral antigen increased as the disease progressed, and it appeared predominantly in the perifollicular capillary endothelial cells of the spleen. The only other in vivo site where abundant virus particles were detected by EM was the salivary glands. Southern blot analysis has revealed SRV-1 DNA in lymph nodes, salivary gland, and brain, and SRV-2 DNA in lymph nodes, spleen, PBMC, and retroperitoneal fibromatosis tissues, but not in skeletal muscle or liver of affected macaques (47). By in situ hybridization, SRV-1 RNA was detected in salivary gland and brain parenchyma of rhesus monkeys without overt neurological symptoms. A finding of SRV-1 nucleic acid in the absence of detectable core antigen or neuropathology in the brain of monkeys suggested viral latency in the central nervous system (CNS). A partial transcriptional block to SRV expression in the brain parenchyma was suggested by the observation that very few cells were positive by in situ hybridization for viral RNA, seemingly too few to account for the signal seen by Southern blot for viral DNA. The cell types infected have not been identified, and macrophages or giant cells characteristic of HIV-infected human brains (61,62) or SIV-infected macaque brain (63) have not been seen. No evidence of reactivation of type D virus from this latent state in the CNS has been observed over several years of observation. Despite the evidence for latency, cell-free SRV-1 could be isolated from the cerebrospinal fluid of over 50% of neurologically normal monkeys with SRV SAIDS. A few scattered epithelial cells in the choroid plexus appear to be the source of cell-free virus in the cerebrospinal fluid (56).

SRV Genetic Structure

SRV-1, SRV-2, and SRV-3 (MPMV) have been molecularly cloned and sequenced (41–43). All three viruses have a similar genetic organization, with four separate translation frames encoding the group-specific antigen (gag), protease (prt), RNA-dependent DNA polymerase (pol), and envelope glycoprotein (env). The prt genes of all SRV-1–3 and of HTLV-II, bovine leukosis virus (BLV), murine mammary tumor virus (MMTV), and hamster intracisternal A particles are in separate translational frames from the gag and pol genes. Computer sequence analysis indicates that a segment of the prt gene has been transposed between SRV-1 and visna virus (64). Each type D retrovirus utilizes tRNA lysine as a primer for minus strand DNA synthesis. Visna virus, MMTV, HIV-1, and SIV also utilize tRNA lysine as primer. However, the simian type D viruses have a markedly different genetic organization from HIV and SIV and lack extensive homology with these viruses. Transactivation of long terminal repeat (LTR) sequence-mediated gene expression is not a property of type D retrovirus replication (65). Each type D retrovirus has a *gag* precursor polypeptide cleaved by the *prt* enzyme into six proteins identified as p10, pp18, p12, p14, p27, and p4 (66,67). A comparison of amino-acid mismatches based on nucleotide sequences shows that SRV-1 is more closely related to MPMV than is SRV-2. Whereas the *gag, prt, pol* and C-terminal *env* domains of the three viruses differ only by 5–15%, the externally located N-terminal domains differ by 17% in comparison between SRV-1 and MPMV, and by 42% between SRV-1 and SRV-2. The LTRs of SRV-1 and MPMV are 88% homologous; SRV-2 shows 70% LTR homology with either virus. In keeping with their distinct neutralization serotypes, SRV-1 and SRV-2 show more envelope amino-acid variation ($\geq$40%) than seen so far among different HIV-1 isolates ($\leq$25%).

Control of SRV

At the California Primate Research Center, it was possible to eliminate type D retrovirus infection in group-housed monkeys by a serial test (antiviral antibodies and virus isolation) and removal program (68). Experimental type D infection was also prevented by an SRV-1 vaccine (55). This vaccine was prepared with sucrose gradient-purified formalin-inactivated whole virus combined with the adjuvant threonyl muramyl dipeptide (MDP-Syntex). The vaccine was shown to be free of residual infectious virus and was given (1 mg virus protein/dose) intramuscularly to six naive juvenile rhesus at 18, 15, and 9 weeks prior to challenge with a lethal dose of SRV-1. Six matched control animals received adjuvant only. Four weeks after the third immunization, the six vaccinates had SRV-1 antibody titers ranging from 1:40 to 1:370. None of the adjuvant controls seroconverted to SRV-1. By the seventh day postchallenge all six unvaccinated animals were viremic with SRV-1. Four of these animals remained viremic and died after $2\frac{1}{2}$–11 months. One vaccinated monkey had transient viremia 7 days postchallenge but was virus negative by day 14. The other five vaccinates were completely protected from viremia, and all six vaccinates were protected from persistent viremia. All six vaccinated monkeys have remained clinically healthy for 2 years following challenge. Protection was thus complete, indicating that a killed whole virus (SRV-1) vaccine can prevent this fatal immunosuppressive retroviral disease in macaques. These findings were confirmed at the Washington Primate Center where macaques were protected against SRV-2 challenge infection by immunization with a vaccinia virus vector expressing the SRV-2 envelope (69). Recently, it has been shown at the California Primate Research Center that rhesus monkeys immunized with either an SRV-1 vaccinia envelope or an SRV-3 (MPMV) vaccinia enve-

lope construct develop cross-neutralizing antibody and are protected against challenge infection with SRV-1 (M. Gardner et al., unpublished data). This cross-protection between SRV-1 and SRV-3 is not surprising in view of their fairly close genetic relationship and partial cross-neutralization. However, a polyvalent vaccine may be needed to protect against both SRV-1 and SRV-2 infection because these are more distantly related neutralization serotypes.

In summary, simian type D retroviruses and the associated fatal immunosuppressive disease are highly prevalent and account for over 99% of the morbidity and mortality from spontaneous SAIDS in macaque colonies at various primate centers (34). SRV disease differs from SIV- and HIV-induced AIDS in that both resistance to and recovery from infection appears to be correlated with the presence of neutralizing antibodies, and SRV is not as restricted to or cytopathic for T4 cells. Despite the difference between type D retrovirus and SIV or HIV infection, the highly reproducible and rapid experimental transmission of SRV disease along with the short time required for viral detection in vitro (7–10 days) makes this an attractive primate model for studying the mechanism of fatal immune suppression from an acquired retrovirus. The availability of molecularly cloned and sequenced viruses representing each of the first three type D retrovirus serotypes, and the ability to produce fatal simian AIDS with molecularly cloned SRV-1, are further attractive attributes of this model, allowing possible identification of the critical virus genes involved in pathogenesis. Because of their broad cellular tropism and lack of cytopathic effect, these type D viruses might serve as useful vectors for gene therapy experiments in the future.

SIMIAN IMMUNODEFICIENCY VIRUSES

Epidemiology

The SIV constitute a family of naturally occurring lentiviruses indigenous to certain simian species in Africa (70,71). In their natural African simian hosts, these viruses apparently cause no disease. By contrast, accidental or inadvertent infection of macaques with certain strains of SIV causes a persistent infection, with eventual death from an AIDS-like disease showing many parallels to human AIDS (72). African nonhuman primates found to harbor the viruses asymptomatically include various species of African green monkeys (*Cercopithecus aethiops*), sooty mangabeys (*Cercocebus atys*), and mandrills (*Papio sphinx*). Sequence analysis of these isolates reveals this to be a very large and heterogeneous family of lentiviruses with considerable heterogeneity within a monkey species and extensive divergence between monkey species (73,74). The envelope variation between SIV isolates from a single species appears to be at least as much as occurs between HIV-1 isolates (≤25%), and the variation between species may possibly be as great as that between HIV-1 and HIV-2 (≤50%). The African monkey lentiviruses can thus be divided into at least three major groups: the African green monkey group, the mandrill group, and the sooty mangabey group. The sooty mangabey SIV isolates are more closely related to the SIV isolates from macaques in primate centers and to HIV-2 human isolates (75,76). The close similarity between SIV from sooty mangabeys and SIV from macaques, together with the knowledge that SIV is not indigenous in Asian macaques, suggests that SIV in macaques was acquired accidentally by cross-species spread (? doctors' needles) from sooty mangabeys, or closely related species, in U.S. primate centers.

It is not understood why these viruses fail to cause disease in their natural African simian host. Compared with HIV-1-infected humans and SIV-infected macaques, the primate lentiviruses are present in the natural host as a productive infection in the same cell types, namely CD4+ lymphocytes and macrophages, and elicit a similar immunologic response (77). However, SIV is not cytopathic in its natural host. Thus, resistance to virus-induced cytopathology at the cellular level appears to be one major factor in explaining the lack of pathogenicity in the natural host. Cellular immunity, particularly that mediated by CD8+ lymphocytes, may also play a critical role (78).

SIV isolates from African green monkeys and mandrills are less closely related to SIV_{mac}, SIV_{sm}, or HIV-2 and are about equidistant from HIV-1 and HIV-2 (71,73,74). This suggests that SIV may have existed in these African monkey species for a long time. On the other hand, the closer similarity of SIV_{mac}, SIV_{sm}, and HIV-2 (75,76) suggests that HIV-2 may represent a rare example of cross-species infection with SIV_{sm}, probably in recent times (i.e., 30–200 years). The evolutionary source of HIV-1, however, remains an enigma because of the marked sequence dissimilarity between HIV-1 and any of the existing SIVs. However, a recent chimpanzee isolate of SIV (SIV_{cpz}) is more closely related to HIV-1 than HIV-2 and may represent this missing link (79).

Since 1984 SIV has been isolated from four species of macaques (*Macaca mulatta, M. arctoides, M. fascicularis,* and *M. nemestrina*) from five U.S. primate centers (New England, Delta, Yerkes, California, Washington) and from sooty mangabeys (*C. atys*) at three of these centers (Delta, Yerkes, California) (34). Based on serological and molecular comparison, these SIV isolates appear quite similar one to the other, although differences are apparent at the peptide mapping, restriction map, and sequence levels. The prototype SIV isolates from rhesus, pigtailed, and stumptailed macaques are called SIV_{mac} (72), SIV_{mne} (80), and SIV_{stm} (34), respectively,

and SIV from sooty mangabeys is called SIV_{sm} with strain designation, e.g., $SIV_{smDelta670}$ (81,82). These SIV strains have been used to infect macaques experimentally and cause simian AIDS (also called SAIDS). SIV isolates from African monkeys have generally not been as pathogenic for macaques, although simian AIDS was induced in pigtailed macaques after a long latent period by one SIV_{agm} isolate (83). It is very likely that the pathogenic strains of SIV from macaques or sooty mangabeys in primate centers represent variant strains that have become adapted to macaques. In the natural host these potentially virulent variants are presumably suppressed by as yet undefined factors, e.g., CD8+ suppressor cells.

Experimental Transmission

All species of macaques appear to be vulnerable to infection with SIV_{mac}, SIV_{mne}, or macaque-adapted SIV_{sm}, and the age of the animal is not a critical factor (34,70). Virtually 100% of inoculated animals become persistently infected from about 2 weeks after inoculation until death. Virus can be readily isolated from PBMCs, plasma, lymph nodes, spleen, salivary gland, and other tissues. The number of CD4 lymphocytes decreases soon after infection and then plateaus at ≤1,000/ mm³, until progressively decreasing to less than 400/ mm³ shortly before death. Proliferative responses to T-cell-dependent B-cell mitogens, such as PWM, are markedly diminished before the CD4 cell count is markedly reduced. The virus uses the same CD4 receptor as does HIV on human T cells, and it can be blocked with the same monoclonal antibodies. One to 3 weeks after inoculation and prior to the onset of immunosuppression, SIV-infected macaques, like some HIV-infected humans, develop a transient skin rash (84). Immunohistochemical evidence suggests that this rash may be the consequence of injury of SIV-infected Langerhans cells by cytotoxic T cells. The main clinical features of SIV infection of macaques are wasting, with a loss of 15–60% of body weight and persistent diarrhea. Lymph nodes may be initially enlarged, but they soon atrophy and show hyalinized germinal centers and a paucity of follicles. Immunohistochemical staining of lymph nodes in early stages reveals a decrease in T4 cells and an increase in both T8 and B cells. Opportunistic infections include adenovirus infection, cytomegalovirus infection, papovavirus [simian virus 40 (SV40)] infection, candidiasis, cryptosporidiosis, and trichomoniasis. Encephalopathy with brain histology showing macrophages and giant cells containing lentivirus particles is a prominent finding, particularly in animals that mount a weak antibody response and have a greater amount of virus in tissues (85). The histologic appearance of brain is indistinguishable from that described in human AIDS (62,63). The probability of inoculated animals surviving infection correlates directly with the strength of the antibody response (86). Animals who die rapidly have low antibody responses that recognize only the viral envelope protein, and show a progressive decline both in total plasma immunoglobulin level and in number of T4 cells. Longer survivors remain persistently infected but have higher antibody titers to both core and envelope proteins, an increased total plasma immunoglobulin levels, and a slower reduction in T4 cells. However, neutralizing antibody levels, as measured by the classical infectivity assays, do not in general correlate well with survival.

The reliable and highly reproducible infection of macaques with SIV_{mac} or closely related strains, for example, SIV_{mne} and SIV_{sm}, is an ideal model for studies of disease pathogenesis, antiviral drug testing, immunotherapy, and vaccination. In addition, standardized stocks of these viruses with dose titrations in vitro and in vivo, using standardized assay systems and reagents, are now available at several primate centers. Studies indicating successful genital mucosal transmission of SIV_{mac} suggest that this may be a useful model for heterosexual transmission of HIV (87). An acutely lethal variant of SIV_{sm} (PBj14) has been derived, which may be useful for rapid antiviral drug screening and vaccine studies (88). Induction of simian AIDS with a molecular clone of SIV indicates that this virus is both necessary and sufficient for inducing a fatal AIDS-like disease (89). In addition, this molecular clone of SIV, along with the construction and in vivo testing of recombinant and mutant viruses, will facilitate identification of viral determinants of pathogenesis.

Genetic Organization and Regulation

SIV has a complex genetic organization that includes genes for virion precursor proteins (i.e., *gag, pol,* and *env*) as well as accessory genes, some of which regulate viral gene expression in infected cells (90,91). Most investigations have focused on the *gag, pol,* and *env* genes; genetic and sequence similarities of SIV with HIV-1 indicate that the virion proteins of both virus groups have similar properties (92). Various SIV isolates as well as HIV-2 encode a gene designated *vpx,* which encodes a protein that is packaged into virus particles (93,94). HIV-1 does not encode an open reading frame for the *vpx* gene. A precise role for *vpx* has not yet been established, although analysis of genetically engineered HIV-2 mutants reveals that *vpx* is dispensable for viral replication in tissue culture cells (93,94).

The LTR is 453 bp long and is found at each end of the proviral configuration; signals for integration and regulation of viral gene expression are encoded in the SIV LTR (95). Transcriptional promoter elements in the LTR are a TATA box for initiation of viral RNA synthesis and several upstream elements, which include an enhancer sequence recognized by the cellular nuclear factor κ B

(NFkB) (96–99). Cell activation signals that function through the NFkB site to augment viral gene expression may be important for converting a latent infection to a state of active viral replication (100).

A regulatory gene found in all simian and human lentiviruses is the transactivator (*tat*) (100,101,102). The target (TAR) for *tat* is a sequence downstream from the cap site in the U5 portion of the LTR that folds into a stem–loop structure (98,100–103). The mechanism of *tat* function may involve both initiation of transcription as well as elongation of newly initiated transcripts; these effects may be mediated by cellular proteins that interact with *tat* (104). A posttranscriptional transactivator, designated the regulator of viral expression (*rev*), functions to shift viral replication from an early phase characterized by synthesis of spliced messages for viral regulatory proteins to a late phase in which unspliced and singly spliced (*env*) messages for virion proteins accumulate (105). *rev* may function by promoting transport of unspliced and singly spliced viral messages and by affecting the host cell's splicing mechanism. A target element responsive to *rev* (RRE) is a sequence about 200 bases long that adopts a secondary structure that is important for recognition by *rev* (106,107). The negative effector gene (*nef*) is encoded by an open reading frame that extends from the end of *env* into the 3' LTR (108,109). *nef* is dispensable for viral replication in a variety of tissue culture cells (110,111). Some studies support the notion that *nef* downregulates viral gene expression; however, other studies show that deletion of *nef* has no effect on viral replication in tissue culture cells (112). Recent analysis of SIV_{mac} molecular clones in experimentally infected rhesus macaques has shown that the *nef* gene is important for high virus load and pathogenesis (113).

A model for regulation of lentivirus gene expression with an early and a late phase takes into account the properties of viral regulatory genes (101). Early after infection, a low level of transcription produces double-spliced *tat* and *rev* messages. After accumulation of both *tat* and *rev* proteins, the splicing pattern changes so that synthesis of messages (unspliced and singly spliced mRNA) for virion structural proteins predominates. *nef* may play a role by acting through sequences in the upstream portion of the LTR to suppress viral transcription and thus maintain virus in a latent stage (109).

Primate lentiviruses also encode other accessory genes whose functions in viral replication are under current investigation. The viral infectivity factor (*vif*) has been studied in the HIV-1 system (114). *vif* appears to play a role in production of infectious virus particles, perhaps by functioning at a step in virion assembly (115). *vif*-like genes as well as *rev*-like genes are conserved in lentiviral evolution since these genes are encoded by the known primate lentiviruses and the animal lentiviruses such as visna-maedi virus of sheep and equine infectious anemia virus (92). Genetic studies in the HIV-1 system have shown that both *vif* and *rev* are required for efficient virus replication. A small gene, designated *vpr,* has been shown to augment expression directed by the LTR (116). Interestingly, *vpr* is dispensable for SIV replication since virus with a deletion mutation in this gene productively infects tissue culture cells (117).

SIV in nonhuman primates offers critically important opportunities to determine the role of various viral genes in viral transmission, distribution, latency, and persistence, and in patterns of pathogenesis. Several strains of SIV recovered from molecularly cloned viral genomes have been shown to cause fatal disease in experimentally infected macaques (89,118). Some molecular clones of SIV yield virus that is infectious for macaques but appears not to cause disease for 2 years (119,120). Thus it is feasible to identify viral determinants of pathogenesis by analysis of (1) site-specific mutations introduced into cloned viral genomes; and (2) recombinant genomes constructed between SIV strains that show distinct biological properties either in tissue culture systems (e.g., macrophage tropism) or in vivo (e.g., pathogenic potential). In addition, it may be informative to construct recombinant genomes between SIV and HIV-1 and/or HIV-2 to investigate the roles of specific HIV genes in viral replication and pathogenesis in nonhuman primates.

HIV-2 INFECTION OF MACAQUES

Macaques can usually be transiently infected with one or another strain of HIV-2 (121–123). Cynomolgus macaques seem especially susceptible to this infection. Most animals seroconvert and virus may be isolated from the PBMC from several weeks to several months after inoculation. More than 50% of cynomolgus macaques inoculated with the HIV-2$_{6669}$ strain develop a persistent infection but, with one possible exception, no disease has occurred in any animal up to 24 months after infection. Molecular clones of HIV-2 have also been inoculated into rhesus monkeys but, despite persistent infection, disease has not yet been induced (124). Therefore, HIV-2 infection of macaques appears to be a potentially useful vaccine model with many of the same attributes as HIV-1 infection of chimpanzees but with considerably more economic and practical benefits. Recently an inactivated whole HIV-2 vaccine has protected cynomolgus macaques against challenge infection with this virus (125).

VACCINES

Vaccines against Experimental SIV Infection of Macaques

During the past 2 years successful vaccine protection against SIV has been reported by five groups (126–130) using relatively crude inactivated whole virus preparations under special laboratory conditions, by one group using native envelope glycoproteins (131), and by one group using a mixture of four recombinant envelope peptides (132). The vaccines have protected against challenge with low-dose, 10–200 animal infectious doses (ID), with the homologous virus given as cell-free inoculations either intramuscularly (IM) or intravenously (IV). In all trials, 100% of the nonvaccinated control monkeys became persistently infected with the challenge virus beginning 2 weeks after inoculation. Higher challenge doses ($>10^3$ ID) have not been protected against by any SIV vaccine, nor was genital mucosal challenge infection prevented in one vaccine experiment (133). Virus for the vaccine was grown in human T-cell lines, whereas, to maintain maximum virulence, the live virus for challenge was grown in fresh human or rhesus T cells. Successful vaccines were achieved by inactivating the whole virus with formalin, β-propiolactone, or detergent. Sucrose gradient purification was used in two of the successful whole virus vaccines and column chromatography in two other vaccine formulations. The amount of virus antigen used to confer protective immunity ranged from 500 μg to 2.8 mg, and the schedule of immunizations consisted of a maximum of five inoculations over a 13-month period to a minimum of 4 inoculations over a 4-month interval. With each vaccine the antibody levels declined rapidly after each boost and challenge was done at the height of the immune response, 2–4 weeks after the final boost. In vaccine-protected monkeys, antiviral antibodies declined after challenge, reaching minimal levels by 4–6 months postchallenge. Preliminary results suggest that vaccinated monkeys remain protected for only a relatively short time after the last boost. In one study (103), two of four SIV-vaccinated monkeys were susceptible to challenge infection with 10 ID of the same virus 8 months after the last boost, and, in another study (129), one of four monkeys was susceptible to infection with the same dose at 4 months after the last boost. The adjuvant used in most of the studies was MDP (Syntex), although other successful vaccines were formulated with incomplete Freund's adjuvant or Quil A. There was no systemic or local adverse reactions to any of the inactivated whole virus vaccines and none of these vaccine preparations contained residual live virus based on thorough in vitro and in vivo assays done prior to challenge.

Each of the whole virus vaccines contained virus proteins from the core (p55, p25, p17) as well as the outer (gp120) and transmembrane envelope (gp32). The transmembrane envelope was truncated (gp32) from its native form (gp46) by propagation of the virus in human T-cell lines (104). During virus purification SIV, like other lentiviruses, loses much of its envelope. However, because of ill-defined tissue culture variables, some stocks of SIV retain more envelope than others. Perhaps for this reason a significant amount (2.3% and 8.5%) of gp120 was preserved in two vaccine preparations in which it was measured (127,128). The vaccines induced antibody to all the major structural proteins of the virus, and titers (particularly to the p27 antigen) were similar to those seen after experimental infection. However, vaccine-induced neutralizing antibody levels were several-fold less than titers observed during infection as measured by classical all-or-none infectivity tests in tissue culture systems. In one study (128), vaccine-protected monkeys before challenge showed a generally higher titer of envelope antibodies as measured by ELISA and Western blot and of neutralizing antibodies based on a sensitive syncytial inhibition assay. Interestingly, sera from protected monkeys in this experiment also showed a selective binding to a synthetic peptide (Sp1) representing a portion of the SIV_{mac} putative V3 loop (134). The V3 loop of HIV-1 has been shown to be an immunodominant domain responsible for strong type-specific neutralization (135). However, in the other two successful SIV vaccine studies (126, 127) in the United States, some of the nonprotected animals also had antibody reactivity to SIV Sp1, and neutralizing antibody titers did not correlate as well with antibody reactivity to this peptide. Immunization of goats with the SIV_{mac} V3 loop peptide linked to tetanus toxoid induced a high titer (1:640) of syncytial neutralizing antibody (T. Palker, personal communication); whether this will also occur in rhesus monkeys and protect against SIV challenge infection is unknown. However, this approach was successful in stimulating high-titered anti-HIV neutralizing antibodies in rhesus monkeys (136). In summary, although the SIV V3 region apparently contains an important neutralizing determinant, other neutralizing sites must also participate in protective immunity. In view of the correlation also seen between vaccine protection against HIV-1 in chimpanzees and binding of antibody to the HIV-1 V3 loop, it seems all the more important that this envelope domain be included as part of a successful AIDS vaccine strategy.

Initial results indicate that vaccine protection has been obtained against two strains of SIV (SIV_{mac} and $SIV_{smDelta}$) that differ by about 17% in outer envelope nucleotide sequences and by about 10% in amino acid sequences (137). The putative V3 loop is nearly homologous in these two strains of SIV, which may account for this cross-protection. Cross-protection of SIV_{mac}-vaccinated monkeys against challenge infection with HIV-2 (125) or of HIV-2-infected monkeys against challenge infection with SIV_{sm} (138), has not been possible, probably because these strains are too divergent.

The mechanism of vaccine protection in these studies remains unsettled. It is most likely that neutralizing antibody directed at the V3 loop and other sites has reached the minimal level necessary to inactivate relatively low doses of cell-free challenge virus, before transient or latent infection can be established. It is not known whether these challenge doses of SIV are representative of the amount of HIV involved in transmission of this virus to humans through sexual or intravenous exposures. However, humans are certainly exposed to cell-associated as

well as cell-free virus. Although the level of vaccine-induced neutralizing antibody was several-fold less than that generally reached during the course of infection, this antibody level apparently functions more effectively in preventing the establishment of infection than in eliminating virus once infection is established. The absence of covert infection in the vaccine-protected monkeys is supported by the lack of an anamnestic antibody response after challenge, by the failure to detect viral nucleic acid in blood or tissues (bone marrow, lymph nodes) using PCR, and by the failure to transmit infectious virus to naive monkeys by blood transfusion or lymph node extracts. However, in the first two SIV vaccine studies (126,127), breakthroughs of infectious virus occurred in two apparently protected monkeys, one at 5 months and the other at 7 months after challenge, both accompanied at that time by an anamnestic antibody response. These two monkeys went on to develop simian AIDS. Clearly, only prolonged follow-up will determine whether the other vaccine-protected monkeys are completely free of latent virus. These findings contrast with prior experience with the successful type C and type D retrovirus vaccines, in which protection could be achieved against much higher challenge doses ($> 10^6$ ID) and in which transient infection and anamnestic antibody response after challenge could usually be demonstrated in the protected animals. Nevertheless, these results show that it is possible to protect macaques against low challenge doses with homologous virus given IV or IM by immunization with inactivated whole SIV vaccines. Important questions remaining to be answered with the inactivated whole, or future subunit, SIV or HIV-2 vaccines in macaques are the duration of protection and the extent of protection against heterologous virus strains, mucosal infection, and cell-associated virus challenge. The role of cellular immune mechanisms [such as antibody-mediated cell cytotoxicity (ADCC) and CTL] in vaccine protection remains to be determined. It seems likely that vaccine induction of memory T and B cells, as well as cell-mediated immunity, will be required for long-lasting immunity and protection against cell-associated virus infection (139). No evidence as yet suggests that the current SIV or HIV-2 vaccines meet all of these requirements. A recent review covers the current status of SIV vaccine research (140).

Other Vaccine Approaches

A modified live virus vaccine was developed from an attenuated molecular clone of SIV_{mac} (141). After a transient infection with this virus, monkeys remained latently infected, seropositive, and healthy for over $2\frac{1}{2}$ years. Nevertheless, they became productively superinfected after challenge with high-dose 10^3 ID of virulent parental SIV. However, these monkeys survived much longer (up to 3 years) than most of the infected control monkeys. This attenuated viral vaccine is now being tested against low challenge doses of SIV given systemically and by genital mucosal routes. A lectin lentil column-purified glycoprotein-enriched gp120 vaccine of SIV$_{sm}$ protected two of four macaques against 10 ID of live virus, whereas a core-enriched (lentin lectil flow-through) vaccine of this same virus failed to protect against the same challenge dose (131). These observations further support the importance of the SIV envelope as a protective immunogen. SIV$_{mac}$ vaccinia recombinant expressing *env* plus *gag* proteins failed to protect against IV challenge with 200 ID of the homologous virus (142) despite inducing higher titers of neutralizing antibody than seen in animals protected with the inactivated whole virus vaccine. This disquieting result may possibly be explained by the monotypic nature of the vaccine DNA as compared with the multitypic DNA in the challenge virus, or perhaps the immunogenicity of the immunodominant domains in the vaccinia SIV construct was not sufficiently preserved. Inhibition, but not complete protection against SIV$_{mne}$ infection, was observed in three of three macaques after immunization with a mixture of four recombinant SIV$_{mne}$ envelope peptides expressed as β-galactosidase fusion proteins in *E. coli* (132). These peptides were selected based on analogy with immunodominant regions of the HIV-1 envelope (143) and included two peptides from the extracellular gp120 and two peptides from the transmembrane gp32. Animals showing the strongest protection had the highest neutralizing antibody titer before challenge. The peptides used were from different regions of the SIV envelope than the putative V3 loop, indicating the presence of several other B-cell neutralization epitopes in the SIV envelope. This is the only example so far of the use of recombinant envelope peptides in the SIV model of vaccine protection. Vaccine protection was also recently achieved in the HIV-1 chimpanzee system using a recombinant gp120 immunogen and protection correlated best with neutralizing antibodies directed at the HIV-1 V3 loop (144). Macaques at the University of California, Davis are now being immunized with SIV$_{mac}$ with recombinant gp130 expressed in mammalian cells (145) and in vaccinia virus vectors (T. Yilma, personal communication), and plans are being made to immunize macaques with a mixture of synthetic peptides representing the SIV$_{mac}$ envelope V3 loop combined with other B- and T-cell epitopes (T. Palker, personal communication), and with genetically defective SIV pseudovirions (L. Arthur, personal communication). How successful these novel vaccine approaches will be compared with the results obtained with inactivated whole virus remains to be seen.

ANTIVIRAL AGENTS AGAINST SIV

Animal models represent an essential link in the development of antiviral drugs for human illness. The principal target of HIV antiviral therapy in humans is the viral reverse transcriptase (RT) enzyme. However, virtually every step in the replication of HIV (or SIV) can serve as a target for a new therapeutic intervention (146). Such targets include the CD4 receptor and the viral *tat* and protease genes. Six of the anti-reverse transcriptase drugs were found to inhibit SIV replication completely in vitro in highly permissive B- and T-cell lines (147), and the RT of SIV was shown to have the same in vitro kinetics of 3'-azido-3'-deoxythymidine (AZT) inhibition as HIV-1 (148). Uninfected macaques have been used for pharmacokinetic and toxicity studies with several of the dideoxynucleosides, with responses similar to what has been observed in humans (149–151). AZT has been shown to cross the placenta readily but not to accumulate in the fetus when administered to near-term pregnant macaques (152). A few studies in SIV-infected macaques have examined the in vivo effect of anti-HIV agents on immunologic function or SIV expression. First to be tested was recombinant soluble human CD4, which caused a beneficial effect on virus expression accompanied by an improvement in bone marrow function but only while being administered (50 days) (153). In another study (154), soluble CD4 caused no toxicity at doses of <40 mg/kg/day, but antibodies to it were formed in cynomolgus monkeys. Very recently, it was reported that rhesus CD4 autoantibodies stimulated by the antigenically closely related human CD4 accounted for the anti-SIV effect (N. Letvin, personal communication). The hazards of bypassing animal models and using only the conventional laboratory-adapted virus strains and cell lines for antiviral drug testing were recently emphasized by the finding that much higher concentrations of recombinant soluble CD4 are required to neutralize primary HIV-1 isolates as compared with laboratory strains of HIV-1 (155). CD4 immunotoxins such as the CD4-*Pseudomonas* exotoxin hybrid protein (156) inhibit SIV and HIV-2 as well as HIV-1 in cell culture and are now being tested in the macaque model. AZT, dideoxycytidine (ddC), [9-(2-phosphyonylmethoxyethyl adenine] (PMEA), and foscarnet have all been shown to have a beneficial prophylactic effect on SIV by reducing SIV infectivity levels and delaying disease, or decline of CD4 cells, if given to SIV-infected monkeys before or soon after infection (157,158). However, little or no effect was observed when these agents were given therapeutically after infection was established. More specifically, AZT given in a dose of 100 mg/kg/day to rhesus monkeys starting 1–8 hours prior to IV challenge with 10–50 ID$_{50}$ of SIV$_{sm}$ did not prevent infection but did slightly suppress viremia and delay the fall in CD4 cells (158). Recent anecdotal reports indicate that prophylaxis with AZT soon after human exposure to HIV-1 also fails to prevent infection (159,160). The SIV macaque model should be particularly useful for basic investigations on the side effects of antiviral drug action and on the pathogenicity of drug-resistant mutants of SIV (161). These kinds of studies are now timely because of the ability to induce simian AIDS with molecular clones of SIV (89,118). This model will also aid in the selection of candidate antiretroviral drugs or combinations of drugs, and in the evaluation of efforts to block vertical transmission of the virus. The genital mucosal route for experimental transmission of SIV is a suitable model for antiviral drug testing, as illustrated by studies demonstrating partial inhibition of SIV vaginal infection by the spermicide nonoxynol-9 (162). As yet, the SIV model has not been used to study the effects of therapy with immunomodulators (e.g. interferon) or to evaluate treatment directed at either opportunistic infections (e.g. cytomegalovirus) or lymphomas that may develop in infected macaques, analogously to HIV infection of humans.

Based on Salk's hypothesis (163), several studies have been done in this model to test the efficacy of postinfection immunotherapy with inactivated SIV vaccines. The first used a γ-irradiated whole SIV vaccine with incomplete Freund's adjuvant given once, 4 months after infection (164). Another study used a glutaraldehyde-fixed, whole-virus-infected cell vaccine with Quil-A as adjuvant, given 4, 8, 12, and 36 weeks after infection (98). The third used a formalin-inactivated whole SIV vaccine given with MDP administered every month for 11 months starting 1 month after infection (165). None of these experiments, the last still in progress, has yet shown any detectable change in virus titer, immune status, or clinical course, even though the inactivated whole virus vaccines were successful in protecting naive monkeys against challenge infection. Initial efforts at prophylaxis using passive immunization in this model with immunoglobulin from infected monkeys also failed to show an antiviral effect and may even have enhanced infection (M. MacKenzie, personal communication). An attempt is now under way to assess passive immunization with immunoglobulin from monkeys protected with an SIV vaccine. Passive immunization with sera from HIV-2 vaccine-protected monkeys appears to have protected one of four HIV-2-challenged cynomolgus macaques (166). The SIV and HIV-2 macaque models are thus providing excellent opportunities to explore further the feasibility of passive as well as active immunization.

SIMIAN FOAMY VIRUSES

Simian foamy viruses (SFV), members of the spumavirus subfamily of retroviruses, are found in a variety of animal species, including cats, hamsters, cows, and humans (167). Nonhuman primates known to harbor multiple strains (serotypes) of these viruses include promisians, macaques, African green monkeys, baboons, apes, and chimpanzees. The foamy viruses are highly cytopathic in cell culture and are broadly infectious for different cell types, including cultured epithelial, fibroblast, and lymphoid cells. In their natural host these viruses cause a persistent latent infection in the presence of neutralizing antibody and have been isolated from several organs and tissues including lymph nodes, brain, and peripheral blood leukocytes. Interestingly, these viruses have not been causatively linked to any disease in any species (168), although a serologic association with subacute thyroiditis in humans and chronic arthritis in cats has been suggested (169,170). Rabbits experimentally infected with SFV appeared to become immunosuppressed (171). The major significance of these viruses until now has been the annoying cytopathic effect that they cause in vitro. Because they are retroviruses with reverse transcriptase activity, foamy viruses are apt to cause confusion in the search for other potentially pathogenic retroviruses such as SRV, SIV, or STLV.

The genome of simian foamy virus type 1 (SFV-1), an isolate obtained from a rhesus macaque, has been molecularly cloned, completely sequenced, and compared with the sequences of the cloned human foamy virus (HFV) (172). The genomes of SFV-1 and HFV are closely related, with about 80% homology in the *pol* genes and about 70% homology in the *env* gene. The SFV-1 LTR is usually long (1,621 bp) and shows about 85% homology with HFV in the R and U5 regions but considerable divergence in the U3 region (25% homology). The SFV-1 genome encodes two large open reading frames (ORFs) beyond the *env* gene that show homology to corresponding ORFs of HFV. One of these ORFs (*TAF*) in SFV has recently been shown by transient expression assays in vitro to encode the transcriptional transactivator that acts on a target element in the U3 portion of the LTR. The function of the second ORF in SFV remains to be determined. Based on analogies with the simian lentiviruses and oncoviruses, SIV and STLV, respectively, the second ORF is likely to be a posttranscriptional transactivator with a function like *rev* and *rex*. An understanding of the regulation of spumavirus gene expression will help answer the question of the molecular mechanisms that control retrovirus latency and replication in the host animal. These studies may also uncover a cofactor role for these viruses in diseases such as simian or human AIDS.

REFERENCES

1. Deinhard F. Biology of primate lentiviruses. In: Klein G, ed. *Viral oncology.* New York: Raven Press, 1980;1–431.
2. Gardner MB. Historical background. In: Stephenson R, ed. *Molecular biology of RNA tumor viruses.* New York: Academic Press, 1980;1–46.
3. Weiss R, Teich N, Varmus H, Coffin J, eds. *RNA tumor viruses.* New York: Cold Spring Harbor Laboratory Press, 1980;1–1281.
4. Coffin J. Endogenous viruses. In: Weiss R, Teich N, Varmus H, Coffin J (eds). *RNA tumor viruses.* New York: Cold Spring Harbor Laboratory Press, 1980;1109–203.

5. Temin HM, Mizutani S. RNA-dependent DNA polymerase in virions of Rous sarcoma virus. *Nature* 1970;226:1211–3.
6. Baltimore D. RNA-dependent DNA polymerase in virions of RNA tumor viruses. *Nature* 1970;226:1209–11.
7. Huebner RJ, Todaro GJ. Oncogenes of RNA tumor viruses as determinants of cancer. *Proc Natl Acad Sci USA* 1969;64: 1087–94.
8. Bishop JM. Viral oncogenes. *Cell* 1987;42:23–38.
9. Benveniste RE, Lieber MM, Livingston DM, Sherr CJ, Todaro GJ, Kalter SS. Infectious C-type virus isolated from a baboon placenta. *Nature* 1974;248:17–20.
10. Benveniste RE, Todaro GJ. Evolution of type C virus genes: I. Nucleic acid from baboon type C virus as a measure of divergence among primate species. *Proc Natl Acad Sci USA* 1974;71:4513–8.
11. Todaro GJ. Interspecies transmission of mammalian retroviruses. In: Stephenson JR, ed. *Molecular biology of RNA tumor viruses.* New York: Academic Press, 1980;47–76.
12. Gardner MB, Luciw PA. Animal models of AIDS. *FASEB J* 1989;3:2593–2606.
13. Bryant ML, Sherr CJ, Sen A, Todaro GT. Molecular diversity among five different endogenous primate retroviruses. *J Virol* 1978;28:300–13.
14. Shih A, Misra R, Rush MG. Detection of multiple, novel reverse transcriptase coding sequences in human nucleic acids: relation to primate retroviruses. *J Virol* 1989;63:64–75.
15. Kawakami TG, Huff GD, Buckley PM, Dungworth DL, Snyder SP. C-type virus associated with gibbon lymphosarcoma. *Nature* 1972;235:170–1.
16. Theilen GH, Gould D, Fowler M, Dungworth DC. C-type virus in tumor tissue of a wooly monkey (*Lagorthrix* spp.) with fibrosarcoma. *J Natl Cancer Inst* 1971;47:881–9.
17. Kawakami TG, Sun L, McDowell TS. Natural transmission of gibbon ape leukemia virus. *J Natl Cancer Inst* 1978;61:1113–5.
18. Robbins KC, Devare SG, Aaronson SA. Molecular cloning of integrated simian sarcoma virus: genomic organization of infectious DNA clones. *Proc Natl Acad Sci USA* 1981;78:2918–22.
19. Kawakami TG, Kallias GV Jr, Holmberg C. Oncogenicity of gibbon ape type C myelogenous leukemia virus. *Int J Cancer* 1980;25:641–6.
20. Gardner MB, Rasheed S, Shimizu S, et al. Search for RNA tumor virus in humans. In: Hiatt HH, Watson JD, Winsten JA, eds. *Cold Spring Harbor Conferences on Cell Proliferation,* vol 4. New York: Cold Spring Harbor Laboratory Press, 1977;1235–1251.
21. Watanabe S, Seiki M, Tsujimoto H, Miyoshi I, Hayami M, Yoshida M. Sequence homology of the simian retrovirus genome with human T-cell leukemia virus type I. *Virology* 1985;144:59–65.
22. Miyoshi I, Fujishita M, Taguchi H, Matsubayashi K, Miwa N, Tanioka Y. Natural infection in non-human primates with adult T-cell leukemia virus or a closely related agent. *Int J Cancer* 1983;32:333–6.
23. Hunsmann G, Schneider J, Schmitt J, Yamamoto N. Detection of serum antibodies to adult T-cell leukemia virus in non-human primates and in people from Africa. *Int J Cancer* 1983;32:329–32.
24. Voevodin AF, Lapin BA, Yakovleva LA, Ponomaryeva TI, Oganyan TE, Razmadze EN. Antibodies reacting with human T-lymphotropic retrovirus (HTLV-I) or related antigens in lymphomatous and healthy hamadryas baboons. *Int J Cancer* 1985;36:579–84.
25. Ishida T, Yamamoto K, Shotake T, Nozawa K, Hayami M, Hinuma Y. A field study of infection with human T-cell leukemia virus among African primates. *Microbiol Immunol* 1986;30: 315–21.
26. Lairmore MD, Lerche NW, Schultz KT, et al. Prevalence of SIV, STLV-I, and type D retrovirus antibodies in captive rhesus macaques and investigation of immunoblot reactivity to SIV p27 in human and rhesus monkey sera. *AIDS Res Hum Retroviruses* 1990;6:1233–8.
27. Lowenstine LJ, Pedersen NC, Higgins J, et al. Seroepidemiologic survey of captive Old World nonhuman primates from North American zoos and vivaria for antibodies to human and simian retroviruses and isolation of a lentivirus from sooty mangabeys (*Cercocebus atys*). *Int J Cancer* 1986;38:563–74.
28. Tsujimoto H, Seiki M, Nakamura H, et al. Adult T-cell leukemia-like disease in monkey naturally infected with simian retrovirus related to human T-cell leukemia virus type I. *Jpn J Cancer Res* 1985;76:911–4.
29. Homma T, Kanki PJ, King NW, et al. Lymphoma in macaques: association with virus of human T lymphotrophic family. *Science* 1984;225:716–8.
30. Nakamura H, Hayami M, Ohta Y, et al. Protection of cynomolgus monkeys against infection by human T-cell leukemia virus type-I by immunization with viral *env* gene products produced in *Escherichia coli. Int J Cancer* 1987;40:403–7.
31. Dezzutti CS, Frazier DE, Olsen RG. Efficacy of an HTLV-1 subunit vaccine in prevention of a STLV-1 infection in pig-tailed macaques. *Dev Biol Standard* 1990;72:287–96.
32. Gardner MB, Petersen N, Marx P, Henrickson R, Luciw P, Gilden R. Vaccination against viral induced animal tumors. In: Reif AE, Mitchell MS, eds. *Immunity to cancer.* New York: Academic Press, 1990;605–17.
33. Gardner MB, Marx PA. Simian acquired immunodeficiency syndrome. In: Kline G, ed. *Advances in viral oncology,* vol 5. New York: Raven Press, 1985;57–81.
34. Gardner MB, Luciw P, Lerche N, Marx P. Non-human primate retrovirus isolates and AIDS. In: Perk K, ed. *Immunodeficiency disorders and retroviruses.* New York: Academic Press, 1988;32:171–226.
35. Benveniste RE, Todaro GJ. Evolution of primate oncornaviruses: an endogenous virus from langurs (*Presbytis* spp.) with related virogene sequences in other Old World monkeys. *Proc Natl Acad Sci USA* 1977;74:4557–761.
36. Munn RJ, Marx PA, Yamamoto JK, Gardner MB. Ultrastructural comparison of the retroviruses associated with human and simian acquired immunodeficiency syndrome. *Lab Invest* 1985;53:194–5.
37. Chopra HS, Mason MN. A new virus in a spontaneous mammary tumor of a rhesus monkey. *Cancer Res* 1970;30:2081–6.
38. Fine DL, Arthur LO. Expression of natural antibodies against endogenous and horizontally transmitted macaque retroviruses in captive primates. *Virology* 1981;112:49–61.
39. Fine DL, Landon JC, Pienta RJ, et al. Responses of infant rhesus monkeys to inoculation with Mason-Pfizer monkey virus materials. *J Natl Cancer Inst* 1975;54:651–8.
40. Bryant ML, Gardner MB, Marx PA, et al. Immunodeficiency in rhesus monkeys associated with the original Mason-Pfizer monkey virus. *J Natl Cancer Inst* 1986;77:957–65.
41. Power MD, Marx PA, Bryant ML, Gardner MB, Barr PJ, Luciw PA. The nucleotide sequence of a type D retrovirus, SRV-1, etiologically-linked with the simian acquired immunodeficiency syndrome. *Science* 1986;231:1567–72.
42. Thayer RM, Power MD, Bryant ML, Gardner MB, Barr PJ, Luciw PA. Sequence relationships of type D retroviruses which cause simian acquired immunodeficiency syndrome. *J Virol* 1987;157:317–29.
43. Sonigo P, Barker C, Hunter E, Wain-Hobson S. Nucleotide sequence of Mason-Pfizer monkey virus: an immunesuppressive D-type retrovirus. *Cell* 1986;45:375–85.
44. Heidecker-Fanning G, Lerche NW, Lowenstine LJ, et al. Induction of simian acquired immune deficiency syndrome (SAIDS) with a molecular clone of a type D SAIDS retrovirus. *J Virol* 1987;61:3066–71.
45. Giddens WE, Tsai CA, Morton WR, Ochs HD, Knitter GH, Blakey GA. Retroperitoneal fibromatosis and acquired immunodeficiency syndrome in macaques. *Am J Pathol* 1985;119: 253–63.
46. Tsai CC, Giddens WE Jr, Ochs HD, et al. Retroperitoneal fibromatosis and acquired immunodeficiency in macaques: clinical and immunologic studies. *Lab Animal Sci* 1986;2:119–25.
47. Bryant ML, Marx PA, Shiigi SN, Wilson BJ, McNulty WP, Gardner MB. Distribution of type D retrovirus sequences in tissues of macaques with simian acquired immune deficiency and retroperitoneal fibromatosis. *Virology* 1986;150:149–60.
48. Lerche NW, Marx PA, Osborn KG, et al. Natural history of endemic type D retrovirus infection and acquired immune deficiency syndrome in group-housed rhesus monkeys. *J Natl Cancer Inst* 1987;79:847–54.

49. Lerche NW, Osborn KG, Marx PA, et al. Inapparent carriers of simian AIDS type D retrovirus and disease transmission with saliva. *J Natl Cancer Inst* 1986;77:489–96.

50. Osborn KG, Prahalada S, Lowenstine LJ, Gardner MB, Maul DH, Henrickson RV. The pathology of an epizootic of acquired immunodeficiency in rhesus macaques. *Am J Pathol* 1984;114:94–103.

51. Maul DH, Miller CH, Marx P, et al. Immune defects in simian acquired immunodeficiency syndrome. *Vet Immunol Immunopathol* 1984;8:201–14.

52. Maul DH, Zaiss CP, MacKenzie MR, Shiigi SM, Marx PA, Gardner MB. Simian retrovirus D serogroup 1 has a broad cellular tropism for lymphoid and nonlymphoid cells. *J Virol* 1988;62:1768–73.

53. Maul DH, Lerche NW, Osborn KG, et al. Pathogenesis of simian AIDS in rhesus macaques inoculated with type D retroviruses. *Am J Vet Res* 1986;47:863–8.

54. Kwang H-S, Pedersen NC, Lerche NW, Osborn KG, Marx PA, Gardner MB. Viremia, antigenemia and serum antibodies in rhesus macaques infected with simian retrovirus, type I and their relationship to disease course. *Lab Invest* 1987;56:591–7.

55. Marx PA, Pedersen N, Lerche N, et al. Prevention of simian acquired immune deficiency syndrome with a formalin-inactivated type D retrovirus vaccine. *J Virol* 1986;60:431–5.

56. Lackner AA, Rodriguez MH, Bush CE, et al. Distribution of a macaque immunosuppressive type D retrovirus in neural, lymphoid, and salivary tissues. *J Virol* 1988;62:2134–42.

57. LeGrand EK, Donovan RM, Marx PA, et al. Monocyte function in rhesus monkeys with simian acquired immune deficiency syndrome. *Vet Immunol Immunopathol* 1985;10:131–46.

58. Daniel MD, King NW, Letvin NL, Hunt RD, Sehgal PK, Desrosiers RC. A new type D retrovirus isolated from macaques with an immunodeficiency syndrome. *Science* 1984;223:602–5.

59. Marx PA, Osborn KG, Maul DH, et al. Isolation of a new serotype of simian acquired immune deficiency syndrome type D retrovirus from celebes black macaques (*Macaca nigra*) with immune deficiency and retroperitoneal fibromatosis. *J Virol* 1985;56:571–8.

60. Sommerfelt MA, Williams BP, McKnight A, Goodfellow PN, Weiss RA. Localization of the receptor gene for type D simian retroviruses on human chromosome 19. *J Virol* 1990;64:6214–20.

61. Sharer LR, Epstein LG, Cho E-S, et al. Pathologic features of AIDS encephalopathy in children: evidence for LAV/HTLV-III infection of brain. *Hum Pathol* 1986;17:271–84.

62. Wiley CA, Schrier RD, Nelson JR, Lampert PW, Oldstone MBA. Cellular localization of human immunodeficiency virus infection within the brains of acquired immune deficiency syndrome patients. *Proc Natl Acad Sci USA* 1986;83:7089–93.

63. Letvin NL, King NW. Immunologic and pathologic manifestations of the infection of rhesus monkeys with simian immunodeficiency virus of macaques. Review. *J Acquired Immune Deficiency Syndrome* 1990;3:1023–40.

64. McClure MA, Johnson MS, Doolittle RF. Relocation of a protease-like gene segment between two retroviruses. *Proc Natl Acad Sci USA* 1987;84:2693–7.

65. Thielan BJ, Hunter E, Desrosiers RC, Ranter L. *Trans*-activator of long terminal repeat sequences-mediated gene expression is not a property of type D retrovirus replication. *J Gen Virol* 1987;68:2265–70.

67. Hendersen LE, Sowder R, Smythers G, Benveniste RE, Oroszlan S. Purification of N-terminal amino acid sequence comparisons of structural proteins from retrovirus-D/Washington and Mason-Pfizer monkey virus. *J Virol* 1985;55:778–87.

68. Lerche NW, Marx PA, Gardner MB. Elimination of type D retrovirus infection from group housed rhesus monkeys using serial testing and removal. *Lab Anim Sci* 1990;141:123–7.

69. Hu S-L, Zarling JM, Chinn J. Protection of macaques against simian AIDS by immunization with a recombinant vaccina virus expressing the envelope glycoproteins of simian type D retrovirus. *Proc Natl Acad Sci USA* 1989;86:7213–7.

70. Desrosiers RC, Letvin NL. Animal models for acquired immunodeficiency syndrome. *Rev Infect Dis* 1987;9:438–46.

71. Gardner MB, Luciw PA. Simian immunodeficiency viruses and their relationship to the human immunodeficiency viruses. *AIDS* 1988;2[Suppl 1]:S3–S10.

72. Letvin NL, Daniel MD, Sehgal PK, et al. Introduction of AIDS-like disease in macaque monkeys with T-cell tropic retrovirus STLV-III. *Science* 1985;230:71–3.

73. Miura T, Tsujimoto H, Fukasawa M, Ohta Y, Honjo S, Hayami M. Genetic analysis and infection of SIVagm and SIVmnd. *J Med Primatol* 1989;18:255–9.

74. Johnson PR, Gravell M, Allan J, et al. Genetic diversity among simian immunodeficiency virus isolates from African green monkeys. *J Med Primatol* 1989;18:271–7.

75. Hirsch VM, Olmstead RA, Murphey-Corb M, Purcell RH, Johnson PR. SIV from sooty mangabeys: an African non-human primate lentivirus closely related to HIV-2. *Nature* 1989;339:389–92.

76. Benveniste RE, Raben D, Hill RW, et al. Molecular characterization and comparison of simian immunodeficiency virus isolates from macaques, mangabeys, and African green monkeys. *J Med Primatol* 1989;18:287–303.

77. Fultz PN, Anderson DC, McClure HM, Dewhurst S, Mullins JI. SIVsmm infection of macaque and mangabey monkeys: correlation between *in vivo* and *in vitro* properties of different isolates. *Dev Biol Standard* 1990;72:253–8.

78. Kannagi M, Chalifoux LV, Lord CT, Letvin NL. Suppression of simian immunodeficiency virus replication *in vitro* by CD8+ lymphocytes. *J Immunol* 1988;140:2237–42.

79. Huet T, Cheynier R, Meyerhans A, Roelants G, Wain-Hobson S. Genetic organization of a chimpanzee lentivirus related to HIV-1. *Nature* 1990;345:356–9.

80. Benveniste RE, Arthur LO, Tsai C-C, et al. Isolation of a lentivirus from a macaque with lymphoma. Comparison with HTLV III/LAV and other lentiviruses. *J Virol* 1986;60:483–90.

81. Murphey-Corb M, Martin LN, Rangan SRS, et al. Isolation of an HTLV-III-related retrovirus from macaques with simian AIDS and possible origin in asymptomatic mangabeys. *Nature* 1986;321:435–7.

82. Fultz PV, McClure HM, Anderson DC, Swenson RB, Anand R, Srinivasan A. Isolation of T-lymphotropic retroviruses from naturally infected sooty mangabey monkeys (*Cerocebus atys*). *Proc Natl Acad Sci USA* 1986;83:5286–90.

83. Gravell M, London W, Hamilton RS, Stone G, Monzon M. Infection of macaque monkeys with simian immunodeficiency virus from African green monkeys: virulence and activation by latent infection. *J Med Primatol* 1989;18:247–54.

84. Ringler DJ, Hancock WW, King NW, et al. Immunophenotypic characterization of the cutaneous exanthem of SIV-infected rhesus monkeys. *Am J Pathol* 1987;126:199–207.

85. Ringler DJ, Hunt RD, Desrosiers RC, Daniel MD, Chalifoux LV, King NW. Simian immunodeficiency virus induced meningoencephalitis: natural history and retrospective study. *Ann Neurol* 1987;23[Suppl]:S101–7.

86. Kannagi M, Kiyotaki M, Desrosiers RC, et al. Humoral immune responses to T cell tropic retrovirus STLV-III in monkeys with experimentally induced AIDS-like syndrome. *J Clin Invest* 1986;78:1229–36.

87. Miller CJ, Alexander NJ, Sutjipto S, et al. Genital mucosal transmission of simian immunodeficiency virus: an animal model for the heterosexual transmission of HIV. *J Virol* 1989;63:4277–84.

88. Fultz PN, McClure HM, Anderson DC, Switzer WM. Identification and biologic characterization of an acutely lethal variant of simian immunodeficiency virus from sooty mangabeys (SIV/SMM). *AIDS Res Hum Retroviruses* 1989;5:397–409.

89. Kestler H, Kodama T, Ringler D, et al. Induction of AIDS in rhesus monkeys by molecularly cloned simian immunodeficiency virus. *Science* 1990;248:1109–12.

90. Chakrabarti L, Guyader M, Alizon M, et al. Sequence of simian immunodeficiency virus from macaque and its relationship to other human and simian retroviruses. *Nature* 1987;328:543–7.

91. Franchini G, Gurgo C, Guo H-G, et al. Sequence of simian immunodeficiency virus and its relationship to the human immunodeficiency viruses. *Nature* 1987;328:539–42.

92. Myers G, Rabson AB, Josephs SF, Smith TF, Wong-Staal F. Human retroviruses and AIDS 1990: a compilation and analysis of

nucleic acid and amino acid sequences. Appendix 1. Los Alamos, NM: Los Alamos National Laboratory, 1990.

93. Henderson LE, Sowder RC, Copeland TD, Benveniste RE, Oroszlan S. Isolation and characterization of a novel protein (x-orf product) from SIV and HIV-2. *Science* 1988;241:199–201.

94. Kappes JC, Morrow CD, Lee SW, et al. Identification of a novel retroviral gene unique to human immunodeficiency virus type 2 and simian immunodeficiency virus SIVmac. *J Virol* 1988;62:3501–5.

95. Varmus H, Brown P. Retroviruses. In: Berg H, Howe M, eds. *Mobile DNA* Washington, DC: ASM Press, 1990;53–108.

96. Nabel G, Baltimore D. An inducible transcription factor activates expression of human immunodeficiency virus in T cells. *Nature* 1987;326:711–3.

97. Anderson MG, Clements JE. Comparison of the transcriptional activity of the long terminal repeats of simian immunodeficiency viruses $SIV_{mac}251$ and $SIV_{mac}239$ in T-cell lines and macrophage cell lines. *J Virol* 1991;65:51–60.

98. Arya SK. Human and simian immunodeficiency retroviruses: activation and differential transactivation of gene expression. *AIDS Res Hum Retroviruses* 1988;4:175–86.

99. Renjifo B, Speck NA, Wyand S, Hopkins N, Li Y. *cis*-Acting elements in the U3 region of a simian immunodeficiency virus. *J Virol* 1990;64:3130–4.

100. Peterlin BM, Luciw PA. Molecular biology of HIV (review). *AIDS* 1990;2[Suppl 1]:29–40.

101. Cullen BR, Greene WC. Regulatory pathways governing HIV-1 replication. *Cell* 1989;58:423–6.

102. Sharp PA, Marciniak RA. HIV TAR: an RNA enhancer? *Cell* 1989;59:229–30.

103. Vigilanti GA, Mullins JI. Functional comparison of transactivation by simian immunodeficiency virus from rhesus macaques and human immunodeficiency virus type 1. *J Virol* 1988;62:4523–32.

104. Dingwall C, Ernberg I, Gait MJ, et al. HIV-1 *tat* protein stimulates transcription by binding to a U-rich bulge in the stem of the TAR RNA structure. *EMBO J* 1990;9:4145–53.

105. Chang DD, Sharp PA. Regulation of HIV rev depends upon recognition of splice sites. *Cell* 1989;59:789–95.

106. Malim M, Bohnlein S, Fenrick R, Le SY, Maizel JV, Cullen BR. Functional comparison of the rev transactivators encoded by different primate immunodeficiency virus species. *Proc Natl Acad Sci USA* 1989;886:8222–6.

107. Le S-Y, Malim MH, Cullen BR, Maizel JV. A highly conserved RNA folding region coincident with the rev response element of primate immunodeficiency viruses. *Nucleic Acids Res* 1990;18:1613–23.

108. Colombini S, Arya SK, Reitz MS, Jagodzinski L, Beaver B, Wong-Staal F. Structure of simian immunodeficiency virus regulatory genes. *Proc Natl Acad Sci USA* 1989;86:4813–7.

109. Ahmad N, Venkatesan S. *Nef* protein of HIV-1 is a transcriptional repressor of HIV-1 LTR. *Science* 1988;241:1481–5.

110. Luciw PA, Cheng-Mayer C, Levy JA. Mutational analysis of the human immunodeficiency virus. The orf-B region downregulates virus replication. *Proc Natl Acad Sci USA* 1987;84:1434–8.

111. Terwilliger E, Sodroski JG, Rosen CA, Haseltine WA. Effects of mutations within the 3' *orf* open reading frame region of human T-cell lymphotropic virus type III (HTLV-III/LAV) on replication and cytopathogenicity. *J Virol* 1986;60:754–60.

112. Cullen BR. The positive effect of the negative factor. *Nature* 1991;351:698–9.

113. Kestter HW, Ringter DJ, Mori K, et al. Importance of the *nef* gene for maintenance of high virus loads and for development of AIDS. *Cell* 1991;651–62.

114. Zack JA, Arrigo SJ, Chen ISY. Control of expression and cell tropism of human immunodeficiency virus type 1. *Adv Virus Res* 1990;38:125–46.

115. Strebel K, Daugherty D, Clouse K, et al. The HIV 'A' (*sor*) gene product is essential for virus infectivity. *Nature* 1987;328:728–30.

116. Cohen EA, Terwilliger EF, Jalinoos Y, Proulx J, Sodroski JG, Haseltine WA. Identification of HIV-1 vpr production and function. *J AIDS* 1990;3:11–8.

117. Yu X-F, Matsuda M, Essex M, Lee T-H. Open reading frame *vpr* of simian immunodeficiency virus encodes a virion-associated protein. *J Virol* 1990;64:5688–93.

118. Dewhurst S, Embretson JE, Anderson DC, Mullins JI, Fultz PN. Sequence analysis and acute pathogenicity of molecularly cloned $SIV_{SMM-PBj14}$. *Nature* 1990;345:636–40.

119. Naidu YM, Kestler HW, Li Y, et al. Characterization of infectious molecular clones of simian immunodeficiency virus (SIV_{mac}) and human immunodeficiency virus type 2: persistent infection of rhesus monkeys with molecular cloned SIV_{mac}. *J Virol* 1988;62:4691–6.

120. Marthas ML, Banapour B, Sutjipto S, et al. Rhesus macaques inoculated with molecularly cloned simian immunodeficiency virus. *J Med Primatol* 1989;18:311–9.

121. Nicol I, Flamminio-Zola G, Dubouch P, et al. Persistent HIV-2 infection of rhesus macaque, baboon, and mangabeys. *Intervirology* 1989;30:258–67.

122. Dormont D, Livartowski J, Chamaret S, et al. HIV-2 in rhesus monkeys: serological, virological and clinical results. *Intervirology* 1989;30:59–65.

123. Stahl-Hennig C, Herchenroder O, Nick S, et al. Experimental infection of macaques with HIV-2$_{ben}$, a novel HIV-2 isolate. *AIDS* 1990;4:611–7.

124. Franchini G, Markham P, Gard E, et al. Persistent infection of rhesus macaques with a molecular clone of human immunodeficiency virus type 2: evidence of minimal genetic drift and low pathogenetic effects. *J Virol* 1990;64:4462–7.

125. Putkonen P, Thorstensson R, Walther L, et al. Vaccine protection against HIV-2 infection in cynomolgus monkeys. *AIDS Res Hum Retroviruses* 1990;7:271–7.

126. Desrosiers R, Wyand M, Kodama T, et al. Vaccine protection against simian immunodeficiency virus infection. *Proc Natl Acad Sci USA* 1989;86:6353–7.

127. Murphey-Corb M, Martin L, Davison-Fairburn B, et al. A formalin-inactivated whole SIV vaccine confers protection in macaques. *Science* 1989;246:1293–7.

128. Carlson JR, McGraw TP, Keddie E, et al. Vaccine protection of rhesus macaques against simian immunodeficiency virus infection. *AIDS Res Hum Retroviruses* 1990;6:1239–46.

129. Stott EJ, Chan WL, Mills K, et al. Preliminary report: protection of cynomolgus macaques against simian immunodeficiency virus by fixed infected cell vaccine. *Lancet* 1990;336:1538–41.

130. Cranage MP, Cook N, Thompson A, et al. Protection of rhesus macaques from infection with SIV_{mac} using a formalin inactivated whole virus preparation. AIDS Directed Programme, 4th Annual Workshop, University of Exeter, September 24–26, 1990; (abst 83).

131. Murphey-Corb M, Martin L, Davison-Fairburn B, et al. A formalin-killed whole SIV vaccine, but not DOC-disrupted glycoprotein and gag subunit preparation protects rhesus monkeys following challenge with a 10 ID 50 dose of live virus. Abstract. 21st Congress of AIDS, Annecy, France, 1989; (abst).

132. Shafferman A, Jahrling P, Benveniste RE, et al. Immunization of macaques with a vaccine of HIV-based, conserved SIV envelope peptides. *Proc Natl Acad Sci USA* 1991;88:7126–30.

133. Sutjipto S, Pedersen N, Gardner MB, et al. Inactivated whole simian immunodeficiency virus fails to protect rhesus macaques from intravenous or genital mucosal infection but delays the subsequent disease course of intravenously challenged-exposed animals. *J Virol* 1990;64:2290–7.

134. Gardner MB, Carlson JR, Rosenthal A, et al. SIV protection of rhesus monkeys. *Biotechnol Ther* (Repligen) 1991;2:9–19.

135. LaRosa GJ, Davide JD, Weinhold K, et al. Conserved sequence and structural elements in the HIV-1 principal neutralization determinant. *Science* 1990;249:932–5.

136. Hart MK, Palker TJ, Matthews TJ, et al. Synthetic peptides containing T and B cell epitopes from human immunodeficiency virus envelope gp120 induce anti-HIV proliferative responses and high titers of neutralizing antibodies in rhesus monkeys. *J Immunol* 1990;145:2677–85.

137. Murphey-Corb M, Gardner M, Davison-Fairburn B, Martin L. Immunization with an inactivated whole SIV vaccine blocks viral infection and/or replication after challenge with a genetically distinct strain of virus. 3rd Annual Meeting of the National Coopera-

tive Vaccine Development Groups for AIDS, October 1–5, Clearwater, FL, 1990; (abst).

138. Putkonen P, Thorstensson R, Albert J, et al. Infection of cynomolgus monkeys with HIV-2 protects against pathogenic consequences of a subsequent simian immunodeficiency virus infection. *AIDS* 1990;4:783–9.

139. Ada GL. The immunological principles of vaccination. *Lancet* 1990;335:523–6.

140. Gardner MB, Stott J. Progress in the development of SIV vaccines. Review In: *AIDS 1990*;4(suppl 1):S137–41.

141. Marthas ML, Sutjipto S, Higgins J, et al. Immunization with a live, attenuated simian immunodeficiency virus (SIV) prevents early disease but not infection in rhesus macaques challenged with pathogenic SIV. *J Virol* 1990;64:3694–700.

142. Desrosiers RC, Sehgal P, Kodama T, et al. Use of simian immunodeficiency virus for AIDS vaccine research. 21st Congress of AIDS, Annecy, France, 1989; (abst).

143. Shafferman A, Lennox J, Grosfeld H, Sadoff J, Redfield R, Burke DS. Patterns of antibody recognition of selected conserved amino acid sequences from the HIV envelope in sera from different stages of HIV infection. *AIDS Res Hum Retroviruses* 1989;5:33–9.

144. Berman PW, Gregory TH, Riddle L, et al. Protection of chimpanzees from infection by HIV-1 after vaccination with recombinant glycoprotein gp120 but not gp160. *Nature* 1990;345:622–5.

145. Haigwood NC, Nara P, Scandella C, et al. Development of HIV and SIV envelope-based subunit vaccines: use of native glycoproteins in primates. International Conference on Advances in AIDS Vaccine Development, 3rd Annual Meeting of the NCVDG for AIDS, October 1–5, Clearwater, FL, 1990; (abst).

146. Mitsuya H, Yarchoan R, Broder S. Molecular targets for AIDS therapy. *Science* 1990;249:1533–44.

147. Tsai CC, Follis K, Yarnell M, Deaver LE, Benveniste R, Sager PR. In vitro screening for antiretroviral agents against simian immunodeficiency virus (SIV). *Antiviral Res* 1990;14:87–98.

148. Wu JC, Chernow M, Boehme RE, et al. Kinetics and inhibition of reverse transcriptase from human and simian immunodeficiency viruses. *Antimicrob Agents Chemother* 1988;32:1887–90.

149. Good SS, Hoble CS, Crouch R, Johnson RC, Rideout JL, DeMiranda P. Isolation and characterization of an ether glucuronide of zidovudine, a major metabolite in monkeys and humans. *Drug Metab Dispos* 1990;18:321–6.

150. Kaul S, Dandekar KA, Pittman KA. Analytical method for the quantification of 2'3' didehydro 3' deoxythymidine, a new anti human immunodeficiency virus (HIV) agent by high performance liquid chromatography (HPLC) and ultraviolet (UV) detection in rat and monkey plasma. *Pharmacol Res* 1989;6:895–9.

151. Russell JW, Whiterock VJ, Marrero D, Klink LJ. Disposition in animals of a new anti HIV agent: 2'3' didehydro 3'dideoxythymidine. *Drug Metab Dispos* 1990;18:153–7.

152. Lopez-Anaya A, Unadkat JD, Schumann LA, Smith AL. Pharmacokinetics of zidovudine (azidothymidine). I. Transplacental transfer. *J Acquired Immune Deficiency Syndrome* 1990;3:959–64.

153. Watanabe M, Reimann KA, DeLong PA, Liu T, Fisher RA, Letvin NC. Effect of recombinant soluble CD4 in rhesus monkeys infected with simian immunodeficiency virus of macaques. *Nature* 1989;337:267–70.

154. Bugelski PJ, Fong KLL, Salleveld HA, et al. Preclinical development of recombinant soluble T4. S96. 3rd International Conference on Antiviral Research, Brussels, Belgium April 22–27, 1990. *Antiviral Res* 1990;S109.

155. Daar ES, Li XL, Mougdil T, Ho DD. High concentrations of recombinant soluble CD4 are required to neutralize primary human immunodeficiency virus type 1 isolates. *Proc Natl Acad Sci USA* 1990;87:6574–8.

156. Berger EA, Clouse KA, Chaudhary VK, et al. CD4-pseudomonas exotoxin hybrid protein blocks the spread of human immunodeficiency virus infection *in vitro* and is active against cells expressing the envelope glycoproteins from diverse primate immunodeficiency retroviruses. *Proc Natl Acad Sci USA* 1989;86:9539–43.

157. Lundgren B, Ljundahl Stahle E, Wahren B, Norrby E, Oberg B. Antiviral effects of AZT, foscarnet and DDC in SIV-infected macaques (*Macaca fascicularis*). International TNO Meeting on Animal Models in AIDS, Maastricht, The Netherlands, 1989; (abst).

159. Lange JMA, Boucher CAB, Hollack CEM, et al. Failure of zidovudine prophylaxis after accidental exposure to HIV-1. *N Engl J Med* 1990;322:1375–7.

160. Looke DFM, Grove DI. Failed prophylactic zidovudine after needlestick injury [Letter]. *Lancet* 1989;335:1280.

161. Richman DD. Zidovudine resistance of human immunodeficiency virus. *Rev Infect Dis* 1990;12:S507–S512.

162. Miller CJ, Alexander NJ, Sutjipto S, Joye SM, Marx PA. Effect of virus dose and nonoxynol-9 on the genital transmission of SIV in rhesus macaques. *J Med Primatol* 1990;19:401–9.

163. Salk J. Prospects for the control of AIDS by immunizing seropositive individuals. *Nature* 1987;327:473–6.

164. Gardner MB, Jennings M, Carlson JR, et al. Postexposure immunotherapy of simian immunodeficiency virus (SIV) infected rhesus with an SIV immunogen. *J Med Primatol* 1989;18:321–8.

165. Murphy-Corb M, Davison-Fairburn B, Ohkawa S, Martin L, Baskin G. Immunization of healthy SIV-infected macaques with a formalin inactivated whole virus vaccine has no apparent effect on disease progression and survival. 8th Annual Symposium on Nonhuman Primate Models for AIDS, New Orleans, LA, 1990; (abst 39).

166. Putkonen P, Thorstensson R, Ghavamzadeh L, et al. Prevention of HIV-2 and SIV$_{sm}$ infection by passive immunization in cynomolgus monkeys. *Nature* 1991;352:436–38.

167. Hooks JJ, Detrick-Hooks B. Spumavirinae: foamy virus group infections. Comparative aspects and diagnosis. In: Kurstak E, Kurstak C, eds. *Comparative diagnosis of viral disease*. New York: Academic Press, 1981;599–618.

168. Weiss RA. Foamy retroviruses. A virus in search of a disease. *Nature* 1988;333:497–8.

169. Pedersen NC, Pool RR, O'Brien T. Feline chronic progressive polyarthritis. *Am J Vet Res* 1980;41:522–35.

170. Stancek D, Stancekova M, Janotka M, Hnilica P, Oravec D. Isolation and some serological and epidemiological data on the viruses recovered from patients with subacute thyroiditis de Quervain. *Med Microbiol Immunol* 1975;161:133–44.

171. Hooks JJ, Detrick-Hooks B. Simian foamy virus-induced immunosuppression in rabbits. *J Gen Virol* 1979;44:383–90.

172. Mergia A, Luciw PA. Replication and regulation of primate foamy viruses. *Virology* 1991;184:475–82.

AIDS and Other Manifestations of HIV Infection,
Second Edition, Edited by Gary P. Wormser.
Raven Press, Ltd., New York © 1992.

CHAPTER 11

Immunodeficiency in HIV-1 Infection

Robert C. Bollinger and Robert F. Siliciano

Infection with the human immunodeficiency virus type 1 (HIV-1) (1,2) initiates a complex and fascinating series of host–virus interactions, the ultimate consequence of which is profound impairment of the host immune system. The extraordinary complexity of the host–virus interactions in HIV-1 infection results in part from the fact that HIV-1 infects two cell types that are involved in virtually all immune responses, CD4+ T lymphocytes and cells of the monocyte–macrophage lineage. The trophism of HIV-1 for these cells is due to the high affinity of the HIV-1 envelope protein (gp120) for the cell surface glycoprotein CD4 (3–6), which is expressed at high levels on cells of the CD4+/CD8− T-cell subset and at lower levels on monocytes and macrophages (7). How virus infection of these cell types leads to immunodeficiency is the central question in AIDS immunology.

The acquired immunodeficiency syndrome (AIDS) (8–12) resulting from HIV-1 infection is characterized by numerous immunologic abnormalities, the most prominent of which are severe quantitative and qualitative defects in the CD4+ T-lymphocyte compartment. In their initial clinical studies describing an acquired immunodeficiency condition in homosexual men, Gottlieb et al. (10) noted that affected individuals had a decreased concentration of CD4+ T cells in the peripheral blood. Subsequently, prospective studies have shown that much of the decline in CD4+ T-cell counts occurs during the incubation period between initial infection and the development of symptoms. In adults, the average length of this incubation period is 8–10 years. Opportunistic infections usually do not occur until the level of CD4+ T cells has dropped below 200 cells/mm^3. Several studies have shown that the degree of loss of CD4+ T cells is an excellent predictor of progression to AIDS (13–16). These findings suggest that the loss of CD4+ T

R. C. Bollinger and R. F. Siliciano: Department of Medicine, Johns Hopkins University School of Medicine, Baltimore, Maryland 21205.

cells is central to the development of clinical immunodeficiency. In addition to the quantitative defects in the CD4+ T-cell compartment, HIV-1-infected individuals also show defects in the functional capacity of the surviving CD4+ T-cell population (17).

The major immunologic defects found in AIDS patients are summarized in Table 1. Although the numerical and functional defects in the CD4+ T-cell compartment are particularly dramatic, functional defects in other cell types also occur in the disease. This chapter will consider recent advances in understanding the molecular mechanisms by which HIV-1 infection produces immunodeficiency, focusing in particular on quantitative and qualitative defects in the CD4+ T-cell compartment. Two questions will be considered in detail. First, what causes the loss of CD4+ T cells in HIV-1 infection? Second, what factors are responsible for the functional defects observed in those CD4+ T cells that are not depleted? Defects in B-cell function will also be considered. Defects in macrophage function are discussed elsewhere in this volume. For a comprehensive discussion of the earlier work on the immunology of HIV-1 infection, the reader is referred to several excellent reviews (18–21).

HOST–VIRUS INTERACTION IN HIV-1 INFECTION: THE IMMUNE RESPONSE TO HIV-1

The immunologic abnormalities in HIV-1-infected individuals must be viewed in the context of the ongoing immune response to HIV-1. In infected individuals, immunodeficiency develops despite the presence of readily detectable B- and T-lymphocyte responses to HIV-1. In fact, in many ways, HIV-1 is a highly immunogenic virus. Virtually all infected individuals develop antibody responses to several of the protein products of the HIV-1 genome, notably the envelope glycoproteins (22,23). Even more striking is the finding that most infected indi-

TABLE 1. *Immunologic defects in AIDS*

Cell type	Defect	Diagnostic tests	Mechanism
CD4+ T cell	Depletion of CD4+ T cells	Decreased CD4+ T cell count, decreased CD4+/CD8+ ratio, lymphopenia, decreased DTH responses	See text
	Intrinsic functional defects	Decreased proliferative responses to mitogen or antigen, decreased helper responses, decreased lymphokine production, decreased DTH responses	See text
CD8+ T cell	Decreased HIV-specific CTL	Decreased HIV-specific CTL	Decreased help?; viral escape?
B cell	Polyclonal B-cell activation	Hypergammaglobulinemia, increased spontaneous PFC, increased spontaneous proliferation	Viral proteins?; EBV, CMV?
	Poor antigen-specific B-cell responses	Poor response to immunization	Helper defect, intrinsic B-cell defect?
	B-cell malignancies		Chronic B-cell activation?; EBV?; decreased immunologic surveillance?
NK cell	Cellular defect	Decreased ADCC activity of cells	Unknown
	Humoral defect	Decreased ADCC activity of serum	B cell defects, viral escape
Macrophages	Decreased chemotaxis Decreased phagocytosis		Unknown

ADCC, antibody-dependent cellular cytotoxicity; CMV, cytomegalovirus; CTL, cytolytic T lymphocytes; DTH, delayed-type hypersensitivity; EBV, Epstein-Barr virus; NK, natural killer; PFC, plaque-forming cells.

viduals also have very high levels of virus-specific cytolytic T-lymphocyte (CTL) activity (24–26). The frequency of HIV-1-specific CTL in the peripheral blood of seropositive individuals is sufficiently high that cytolytic activity can be detected in freshly isolated peripheral blood mononuclear cell preparations without any in vitro restimulation (24). Given that HIV-1 infection generally induces vigorous B- and T-lymphocyte responses, it is important to consider whether these responses exert beneficial antiviral effects.

With respect to the humoral response, this issue has been addressed in in vitro studies of the neutralization of HIV-1 by sera from infected individuals (27,28). In general, levels of neutralizing antibodies are low even when high levels of antibodies to HIV-1 envelope glycoproteins are present. Most neutralizing antibodies recognize an epitope located in the third hypervariable region of HIV-1 gp120 (29–31), which is part of a loop between Cys residues at positions 301 and 336 (32). (Numbering for gp120 residues refers to the HIVBRU sequence, beginning with the first Met residue in the *env* open reading frame.) This principal neutralizing determinant (PND) has a conserved β-turn flanked on either side by variable residues. Current evidence suggests that this region of gp120 is involved in fusion events following the binding of virions to CD4+ cells rather than in the binding reaction itself. Mutations in the PND decrease the capacity of the envelope protein to mediate membrane fusion

events, but such mutations do not affect binding to CD4 (33). Regions of gp120 that appear to be involved in binding to CD4 have been identified in site-directed mutagenesis (34,35) and monoclonal antibody blocking studies (35,36). These residues are located closer to the C-terminal region of gp120 and do not overlap the PND.

There are several possible explanations for the failure of neutralizing antibodies to halt disease progression. One is that the virus can spread by direct cell-to-cell transmission. Recent work by Gupta and coworkers (37) suggests that HIV-1 infection can spread in an in vitro culture system even in the presence of zidovudine and neutralizing antibody. This process is inhibitable by anti-CD4 and may represent spread of genomic viral RNA from infected to uninfected cells during reversible CD4-dependent membrane fusion events. Another potential reason is that the neutralization of viral infectivity in vivo is more difficult than in in vitro assays because of the much higher concentrations of infectable target cells in in vivo sites such as lymph nodes (38). If this is the case, high-titer neutralizing antibodies may be required to prevent infection and/or disease progression. A third explanation for the failure of neutralizing antibodies to prevent disease progression is that antienvelope antibodies may in some cases facilitate the uptake of HIV-1 by cells that express Fc receptors, such as monocytes and macrophages (39,40). This effect has been demonstrated in vitro but its in vivo significance remains to be established. Finally, as is discussed in the next section, the failure of neutralizing antibodies to prevent disease progression may be due to the continuous emergence of neutralization-resistant variants, which is a reflection of the striking propensity of HIV-1 to undergo genetic change. Late in the course of disease, there is also most likely a declining capacity to mount de novo antibody responses to new antigenic determinants. Polyclonal B-cell activation with concomitant hypergammaglobulinemia is a consistent part of the clinical picture of HIV-1 infection. At the same time, AIDS patients have greatly diminished antibody responses to novel and recall antigens both because of decreased T-cell help and because of intrinsic B-cell abnormalities (41). One might, therefore, expect that late in the disease course infected individuals would have a decreased capacity to generate antibodies to newly emergent, neutralization-resistant variants.

With regard to the CTL response, HIV-1-specific CD8+ CTL are readily detected in healthy seropositive individuals and are sometimes detected in patients with AIDS (24–26). Interestingly, a report by Plata and colleagues (25) suggests that the frequency of cells capable of giving rise to HIV-1 env-specific CTL is unusually high even in seronegative individuals. There is considerable current interest in whether these cells exert a beneficial antiviral effect by lysing infected T cells and macrophages. CTL isolated from infected individuals have been shown to lyse HIV-1-infected macrophages (25) and CD4+ T cells (26) in vitro. The lysis of infected macrophages is of particular importance given the evidence that such cells represent a reservoir for HIV-1 in infected individuals (42–44). CD8+ T cells from HIV-1-infected donors have also been shown to suppress virus replication in infected cultures through a major histocompatibility complex (MHC)-restricted mechanism (45–47). The frequency of HIV-1-specific CTL has been shown in some studies to decline as the clinical and immunological status of the patient deteriorates (26,48), perhaps as a result of the fact that HIV-1-specific CTL in infected individuals are contained within an expanded population of CD8+/DR+ T cells that are poorly clonogenic (48). Although further longitudinal studies will be needed to determine whether the drop in levels of virus-specific CTL is causally related to disease progression, it is quite likely that the CD8+ HIV-1-specific CTL response exerts a significant antiviral effect in vivo and is therefore beneficial to the host. Such a mechanism, while limiting the spread of infection, probably also contributes to CD4+ T-cell depletion through the destruction of infected cells. Again, the emergence of viral variants with changes in epitopes recognized by CTL may permit viral escape from this component of the immune response.

In summary, vigorous B- and CD8+ T-cell responses to HIV-1 have been demonstrated in infected individuals. Although such responses ultimately fail to control the infection, they may delay the onset of symptomatic disease for a period of years. The ability of the virus to evade these responses through genetic change, coupled with the progressive virus-induced destruction of CD4+ T-cell compartment, eventually leads to immunodeficiency.

SEQUENCE VARIABILITY IN HIV-1

HIV-1 exhibits a striking degree of genomic heterogeneity that is evident when the nucleotide sequences of viral isolates from different infected individuals are compared (49–54). This heterogeneity arises in part from the fact the HIV-1 reverse transcriptase has a high error rate (1/1,700–1/4,000 nucleotides) (55,56). Even distinct molecular clones of HIV-1 obtained from a single infected individual show sequence heterogeneity (57–59). Although viral clones from a given individual are more closely related to each other than to HIV-1 clones from other infected individuals, the level of genetic heterogeneity that occurs within a given individual is sufficient to produce variants with significantly different biological properties (60,61). Of the protein products of the HIV-1 genome, the envelope glycoprotein gp120 shows by far the most sequence variability. There is considerable current interest in the issue of whether or not this natural variation may contribute to the pathogenesis of AIDS by permitting the in vivo selection of variant viral clones that are not recognized by existing neutralizing antibodies or virus-specific CTL. In other lentivirus systems, including visna virus infection in sheep and equine infectious anemia virus infection in horses, the emergence of viral variants resistant to neutralizing antibodies has been well documented (62). For HIV-1, neutralization-resistant variants have been obtained in vitro in infected cultures maintained in the presence of neutralizing antibody (63). In addition, neutralization-resistant variants have been isolated from gp120-immunized chimpanzees infected with HIV-1 (64). Although sera from infected individuals are not highly type-specific in neutralization, subtle changes in env sequence can dramatically affect neutralization by such sera (65).

With respect to viral escape from the host CTL response, the rapid emergence of viral variants with changes in CTL epitopes has been demonstrated recently in lymphocytic choriomeningitis virus infections of T-cell receptor transgenic mice, in which CTL expressing a particular virus-specific T-cell receptor are present at high frequency (66). The viral variants that were isolated had sequence changes in the epitope recognized by this receptor. The changes were shown to interfere with recognition of processed viral antigen by the receptor. HIV-1 sequence variability may in principle affect T-cell recognition of viral proteins at two levels: the binding of the processed viral antigen to the relevant MHC molecule and the recognition of the resulting peptide–MHC complex by the T-cell antigen receptor (67,68). This problem has been analyzed for class II-restricted human CTL specific for the HIV-1 envelope protein. In the case of some epitopes, a considerable degree of naturally occurring sequence variability can be tolerated without loss of binding to the presenting MHC molecule (67), although for other epitopes even a single conservative substitution at a critical residue can prevent recognition in the context of the relevant MHC molecule (69).

The propensity of HIV-1 to undergo rapid genetic change may not only lead to the emergence of variants resistant to predominant antibody or CTL responses, but may also lead to the emergence of variants with different replication rates, host cell ranges, and cytopathic potential. This important aspect of HIV-1 pathogenesis is discussed in a subsequent section.

QUANTITATIVE ASPECTS OF HIV-1 INFECTION OF CD4+ T CELLS

In considering the mechanisms responsible for the quantitative and qualitative defects in the CD4+ T-cell compartment in HIV-1 infection, it is important to note at the outset that this compartment is heterogeneous with respect to several critical parameters. *Although HIV-1 exhibits trophism for CD4+ cells, only a very small proportion of the CD4+ T cells in an HIV-1-seropositive individual are infected at any given time.* Therefore, the CD4+ T-cell compartment consists of a small number of infected cells and a much larger number of noninfected cells. In addition, CD4+ T cells differ in their states of activation and prior history of antigen exposure. Each of these factors is important in understanding the effects of HIV-1 on the CD4+ T-cell compartment.

Table 2 lists potential mechanisms for CD4+ T-cell depletion in HIV-1 infection. CD4+ T-cell depletion can be viewed in terms of a virus-induced alteration in cell kinetics within this compartment. In infected individ-

TABLE 2. *Mechanisms for CD4+ depletion in HIV-1 infection*

A. Decreased production
B. Loss of HIV-1-infected CD4+ T cells
   1. Direct viral cytopathic effects
      a. Syncytium formation
      b. Syncytium-independent cytopathic effects
   2. Destruction by immunologic mechanisms
      a. CD8+ cytolytic T lymphocytes (CTL)
      b. CD4+ CTL
      c. Antibody-dependent cellular cytotoxicity (ADCC)
C. Loss of noninfected CD4+ T cells
   1. Syncytium formation
   2. gp120-dependent cytolysis by CD4+ CTL
   3. gp120-dependent ADCC

uals, the rate of CD4+ T-cell loss exceeds the rate at which CD4+ T cells are produced through thymic differentiation and/or clonal expansion of peripheral CD4+ T cells. CD4+ T cells may be lost through a number of potential mechanisms, some of which operate on infected cells. Interestingly, there are other mechanisms for CD4+ T-cell depletion that operate on noninfected cells.

Before considering mechanisms for CD4+ T-cell destruction, the possibility that the production of CD4+ T cells is decreased in HIV-1 infection will be discussed. Rates of CD4+ T-cell production are not readily measured in humans, but pathologic examination of thymuses from AIDS patients suggests that HIV-1 infection accelerates the thymic involution that normally occurs with age (70). The mechanism is unclear. Tremblay et al. (71) have shown that thymocytes can be infected with HIV-1 in vitro. Thymocytes obtained from children undergoing cardiac surgery can be infected following activation with the mitogen phytohemagglutinin (PHA). However, it is possible that under these conditions the principal target cells for infection are the mature CD4+/CD8− thymocytes. Recently in vitro infections of thymocyte subpopulations separated by flow cytometry have been carried out. Using a sensitive polymerase chain reaction (PCR) assay, the double-positive (CD4+/CD8+) subpopulation, which gives rise to both the CD4+ and CD8+ T cell lineages, was shown to contain HIV-1 DNA 2 days after exposure to virus (72). Even the CD3−/CD4−/CD8− thymocyte subpopulation, which gives rise to the double-positive cells, was found to contain HIV-1 DNA. Infection of these cells may reflect low-level expression of CD4 (73). In vitro infection of progenitor cells from human bone marrow has also been reported (74). It remains to be determined whether infection of T-cell precursors occurs in vivo, and, if so, whether such infections have an important role in CD4+ T-cell depletion. HIV-1 provirus is not detected in B lymphocytes (75), suggesting that stable infection of bone marrow progenitor cells either does not occur in vivo or does not lead to vertical transmission of the virus to progeny cell populations. Similarly, HIV-1 provirus is not detected in circulating CD8+ T-cells, suggesting that stable infection of double-negative or double-positive thymocytes either does not occur in vivo or does not lead to vertical transmission of the virus to mature T cells.

Most of the current evidence suggests that accelerated CD4+ T-cell loss, rather than decreased CD4+ T-cell production, is the critical factor in CD4+ T-cell depletion. Analysis of mechanisms for the destruction of mature CD4+ T cells requires an understanding of the extent to which viral infection of this population of cells occurs in vivo. Studies of the frequency of HIV-1 infected T cells are summarized below and in Table 3. In an important early study, Harper et al. (76) established that in AIDS-related complex (ARC) and AIDS patients,

TABLE 3. *Frequency of HIV-1-infected cells in natural infection*

Stage of disease	Method of detection[a]	Type of infected cells detected[b]	Frequency of infected cells[c]	Ref.
AIDS, ARC	ISH	Active	<1/10,000 PBMC	76
AIDS	ISH	Active	1/1,000 CD4+ T	75
AIDS	FIA	Productive	1/170,000 PBMC	80
AIDS	LDC	Active + latent	1/1,600 CD4+ T	75
Asymptomatic	LDC	Active + latent	1/50,000 PBMC	79
ARC	LDC	Active + latent	1/370 PBMC	79
AIDS	LDC	Active + latent	1/450 PBMC	79
CDC II	PCR	Active + latent	1/22,00 PBMC	78
CDC IV	PCR	Active + latent	1/2,000 PBMC	78
Asymptomatic	PCR	Active + latent	1/2,800 PBMC	77
AIDS	PCR	Active + latent	1/100 CD4+ T	75

[a] Methods of detection include in situ hybridization (ISH), focal immunoassay (FIA), limiting dilution culture (LDC), and polymerase chain reaction (PCR).

[b] In situ hybridization detects actively infected cells producing viral mRNA. FIA detects infected cells producing infectious virions. Limiting dilution culture, if carried out under conditions favoring activation of HIV-1 gene expression in latently infected cells, detects both actively and latently infected cells capable of giving rise to infectious virus. PCR detects cells carrying HIV-1 DNA sequences, including both actively and latently infected cells.

[c] Frequencies vary widely between different individuals in the same stage of disease. For purposes of comparison, the geometric mean frequencies are tabulated. PBMC, peripheral blood mononuclear cells.

AIDS, acquired immuno-deficiency syndrome; ARC, AIDS-related complex; CDC, Centers for Disease Control; HIV-1, human immunodeficiency virus type 1.

the frequency of cells expressing HIV-1 RNA as detected by in situ hybridization was extremely low, generally <1/10,000 and often <1/100,000 mononuclear cells in the lymph nodes and peripheral blood. It is perhaps more useful to consider these figures in the form of the fraction of CD4+ that is actively infected. Almost all of the infected cells in peripheral blood are CD4+ T cells (75). Assuming that CD4+ T cells comprise 10% of the peripheral blood mononuclear cells (PBMC) in AIDS patients (values from 1% to 25% are observed in different patients), a frequency of 1 actively infected cell per 10,000 PBMC represents 1 actively infected cell in 1,000 CD4+ T cells. This figure agrees well with results of another more recent in situ hybridization study of CD4+ T cells purified from the peripheral blood of AIDS patients by fluorescence-activated cell sorting (75). The in situ hybridization approach does not detect cells that are in a latent stage of infection. Such cells contain integrated HIV-1 proviral DNA but do not actively transcribe viral genes. Several recent studies have employed PCR to quantitate HIV-1 proviral DNA (75,77,78). This method detects latently infected cells as well as those that are actively infected. In different PCR studies, estimates of the frequency of infected cells among PBMC range from 1/2,800 to 1/21,500 in asymptomatic individuals.

Two other approaches to the quantitation of infected cells have been described. End-point dilution culture has been used to detect the precursor frequency of HIV-1 infected cells (79). This technique gave a lower estimate (1/50,000) of the frequency of infected PBMC in asymptomatic seropositive individuals. A sensitive focal immu-

noassay has also been used to detect PBMC releasing infectious virions. Without in vitro PHA stimulation, productively infected cells were detected in 6/97 (6%) seropositive individuals (80). The frequency of infected cells was <1/170,000 PBMC.

With progression to AIDS, the frequency of infected cells increases by a factor of 10–100. PCR studies suggest that the frequency of infected cells is about 1/2,000 PBMC (78). Limiting dilution culture gives a higher frequency, about 1/400 PBMC (79). PCR analysis of CD4+ T cells purified from the PBMC of AIDS patients by sorting gives a frequency of 1/100 CD4+ T cells (75). The results of these studies, taken together with results from in situ hybridization analysis of actively infected cells, suggest that most of the infected cells are in a latent stage of infection at any given time.

T-CELL ACTIVATION AND HIV-1 INFECTION

Analysis of the mechanism of CD4+ T-cell depletion also requires an understanding of the relationship between T-cell activation and HIV-1 infection. It has been generally stated that HIV-1 can infect both resting and activated CD4+ T cells, although HIV-1 replication occurs much more readily in activated T cells (81–83). Recently, molecular aspects of HIV-1 infection of resting T cells have been analyzed in detail. Zack and colleagues (84) used PCR to follow the molecular course of HIV-1 infection of resting peripheral blood CD4+ T cells. The initial stages of reverse transcription of viral RNA were shown to occur in both resting and activated T cells.

However, in resting cells, the process did not proceed to completion. Replication intermediates in the form of unintegrated viral DNA were detected and were shown to be labile, with a $t_{\frac{1}{2}}$ of about 1 day. Stevenson and colleagues (85) have also analyzed the interaction of HIV-1 with resting T cells. Interestingly, they found that unintegrated viral DNA persisted in cells for several weeks. This unintegrated viral DNA was also shown to be transcriptionally active, giving rise to *gag* and *env* gene products but not infectious virus (86). Thus, it appears that when HIV-1 binds to resting CD4+ T cells, which constitute the vast majority of circulating CD4+ T cells, the genomic RNA is delivered to the cytoplasm and initial stages of reverse transcription occur. However, unless the infected cell is activated by antigen, stable integration and productive infection do not occur.

These results help to explain the low frequency of infected cells in spite of the presence of continuous viremia throughout the course of infection. Recent studies by Ho et al. (79) and Coombs et al. (87) have shown that cell-free infectious virus is present in the plasma of infected individuals throughout the course of the infection. Estimates of the mean plasma titers were 25–30 tissue culture infectious dose (TCID)/ml for individuals in the asymptomatic phase of infection and rose to 320–3,500 in AIDS patients. Free virus present in the plasma and extracellular fluid is likely to interact with resting CD4+ T cells, which represent the most numerous population of susceptible cells in the blood and tissues. The work of Zack et al. (84) and Stevenson et al. (85,86) indicates that interactions between free virus and resting T cells does not lead to stable or productive infections unless the infected cells encounter antigen before the replication intermediates decay. Activated T cells, which are present at lower frequency, can become stably and/or productively infected upon initial encounter with the virus. These findings emphasize the importance of antigen-induced T-cell activation in the pathophysiology of HIV-1 infection.

Although HIV-1 infection of resting T cells does not lead to stable infection, viral sequences can be detected by PCR in CD4+ T cells that have the surface phenotype of naive T cells (88). Presumably these cells have not been previously activated by antigen. It is unclear whether HIV-1 DNA detected in these cells represents unintegrated viral DNA or integrated provirus present as the result of low-efficiency stable infection of immature or naive resting CD4+ T cells. Additional studies are needed to determine whether the interaction of HIV-1 with resting T cells in vivo can result in stable integration of HIV-1 provirus.

The state of T-cell activation also influences viral gene expression in infected cells (81–83). This is partly because host cell nuclear factors involved in antigen-induced T-cell activation, including nuclear factor κB (NFκB), interact with the HIV-1 long terminal repeat (LTR) and upregulate viral gene expression (89,90). Certain cytokines may also induce viral gene expression in latently infected T cells. Studies by Poli and colleagues have established that tumor necrosis factor-α (TNF-α), a monocyte/macrophage and T-cell-derived cytokine, and the related lymphocyte-derived cytokine TNF-β can dramatically increase HIV-1 gene expression in chronically infected human T-lymphocytic and promonocytic cell lines (91). Whether or not the same is true of resting, latently infected T cells in vivo remains to be determined.

CYTOPATHIC EFFECTS OF HIV-1 ON INFECTED CD4+ T CELLS

Under some experimental conditions, HIV-1 infection of susceptible cell types in vitro results in death of the infected cell population. The initial finding that HIV-1 was cytopathic for CD4+ T cells (2) led to the notion that direct cytopathic effects of the virus on infected cells produced the CD4+ T-cell depletion that is characteristic of HIV-1 infection in humans. Two general types of HIV-1-induced cytopathic effects have been observed in vitro. In some experimental systems, syncytia or multinucleated giant cells form by the fusion of infected cells expressing envelope protein and noninfected cells expressing CD4 (92,93). Syncytium formation as a mechanism for CD4+ depletion is discussed below. There are also cytopathic effects that operate at the level of individual infected cells, that is, under some conditions, HIV-1-infected T cells appear to die from the infection independent of any cell–cell fusion events (94,95). Although the actual molecular mechanism for single cell killing by HIV-1 is unclear, several potential mechanisms have been analyzed experimentally and are discussed in this section.

One mechanism for syncytium-independent cytopathic effects involves the accumulation of unintegrated viral DNA. The presence of high levels of unintegrated viral DNA derived by reverse transcription of RNA molecules from newly infecting virions has been associated with cytopathic effects in in vitro infections by avian retroviruses (96,97) and in in vivo infections by feline retroviruses (98). In addition, high levels of unintegrated viral DNA have also been observed in infections by other lentiviruses such as visna virus (99). Shaw and colleagues (100) detected unintegrated viral DNA in HIV-1-infected cell lines and in peripheral blood and lymph node lymphocytes from AIDS patients. More recently, Chen and colleagues (101) have used PCR to assay for unintegrated viral DNA in PBMC and in brain tissue from AIDS patients. Interestingly, higher ratios of unintegrated to integrated DNA were observed in samples of brain tissue from patients with HIV-1 encephalitis than in PBMC from these patients. Although unintegrated DNA was detected in PBMC samples, it was not clear whether this DNA actually produced cytopathic effects.

Factors controlling the accumulation of unintegrated

viral DNA have been analyzed in several recent studies. Temporal aspects of the production of unintegrated viral DNA have been monitored in in vitro infections of the H-9 T-cell line (102). Unintegrated viral DNA is first detected in infected cells at about 4 hours postinfection and increases dramatically at about 30 hours as a result of reinfection by virus produced in the first cycle of infection. After peaking at 50–80 hours postinfection, the amount of unintegrated viral DNA begins to decline. By this time, sufficient envelope protein is present in infected cells to block all of the CD4 molecules so that further reinfection is prevented. In H-9 cells, the level of unintegrated viral DNA at this peak was estimated to be a minimum of 20 copies/cell. This level of unintegrated viral DNA was not toxic to the cells. In another study, Richman and colleagues (103) found that in in vitro infections of the CEM T-cell line by HIV-1, accumulation of unintegrated HIV-1 DNA occurred as a result of the reinfection of previously infected cells and was associated with cell killing, predominantly through syncytium formation (103). Thus, following initial infection, viral replication and reinfection occur before interference is established by downregulation of CD4. Stevenson and colleagues (95) have shown that CEM cells expressing the HIV-1 env gene following transduction with a retroviral vector, acquired a cytolysis-resistant phenotype characterized by low surface expression of CD4 and subsequent resistance to second round infection and failure to accumulate high levels of unintegrated viral DNA. Interestingly, induction of viral replication by the phorbolester TPA resulted in syncytium-independent cytolysis. Taken together, these studies demonstrate that accumulation of unintegrated viral DNA involves a reinfection or superinfection process that is regulated by CD4 expression. Higher levels of unintegrated viral DNA are associated with cytopathic effects, but the mechanism is unclear. Unintegrated viral DNA itself may be toxic. Alternatively, it may be transcribed (86), giving rise to viral gene products (including envelope protein) that cause cell killing via syncytium-dependent or -independent mechanisms. It is also possible that a high level of unintegrated viral DNA is a functionally insignificant indicator of high-level virus infection. Another critical question is whether unintegrated viral DNA can accumulate in infected cells in vivo to a sufficient extent to produce cytopathic effects.

A second potential mechanism for HIV-1-induced single cell killing involves the envelope glycoprotein and, in particular, the interaction of this protein with CD4. Susceptibility to cytopathic effects appears to be related to levels of CD4 expression. For example, cells of the monocyte/macrophage lineage, which express low levels of CD4, can be infected by HIV-1 but generally do not show cytopathic effects (42–44). In addition, the level of expression of CD4 by subclones of the monocytic line U937 is correlated with susceptibility of the clones to HIV-1-induced cytopathic effects (104). In an interesting

recent study, Koga and colleagues (105,106) have analyzed the cytopathic effects resulting from env gene expression using a transfection system with an inducible promoter. CD4+ and CD4− sublines of U937 and the T-cell tumor line Jurkat were transfected with a vector carrying the HIV-1 env gene under the control of the metallothionein promoter. Cytopathic effects were observed upon induction of env gene expression only in the CD4+ sublines, suggesting that env gene expression is not in itself toxic to the cell. Rather, it is the coexpression of gp160 and CD4 that produced cytopathic effects at the single cell level. In these studies intracellular complexes of CD4 and gp160 were observed. In addition, in CD4+ U937 cells, accumulations of envelope protein at the nuclear pores were noted, leading to the proposal that the CD4–gp160 complexes that accumulated at the nuclear pores produced cytopathic effects by interfering with the transport of molecules between the nucleus and the cytoplasm. Whether such complexes localize to nuclear pores in infected T cells was not determined. In any event, these studies demonstrate that in CD4+ cells, cytopathic effects can result from the expression of the HIV-1 env gene in the absence of other viral genes (except rev, which is necessary for env expression).

In another interesting recent study, the envelope protein has been implicated in HIV-1-induced cytopathic effects at the single cell level. Stevenson and colleagues (107) carried out successive infections of the cytolysis-sensitive MT-4 T-cell line and isolated surviving cells from each round of infection. This approach led to the amplification of an HIV-1 variant with a normal capacity for replication and syncytium formation but a reduced ability to mediate single cell killing. The critical differences responsible for the loss of cytopathic potential were mapped to the envelope gene. Two amino-acid substitutions were present in the gp120 subunit, each of which produced the loss of a conserved glycosylation site. In another study, Kowalski and colleagues (108) have shown that mutations in the amino terminus of gp41 lead to a loss of syncytium formation and single cell killing without affecting viral replication. Thus, subtle differences in the envelope protein can affect cytopathic potential. It is important to note that the naturally occurring variability in HIV-1 genomic sequence has also been shown to affect cytopathic potential. As is discussed below, not all HIV-1 isolates induce cytopathic effects in infected cells.

IMMUNE DESTRUCTION OF INFECTED CD4+ T CELLS

Another potential mechanism for the loss of CD4+ T cells in HIV-1 infection involves the destruction of such cells by components of the immune system, particularly CD8+ CTL. Cytolytic activity specific for the HIV-1 envelope proteins has been detected in freshly isolated, unfractionated PBMC from healthy seropositive individuals and AIDS patients (24–26,109). While a portion of this lytic activity may represent non-MHC-restricted antibody-dependent cellular cytotoxicity (ADCC), there is clearly an MHC-restricted component mediated by *env*-specific CTL. This is a remarkable finding given that virus-specific CTL responses are generally demonstrable only after an in vitro restimulation step, which is needed to expand specific clones. CTL specific for HIV-1 *pol* (110), *gag* (111), and *nef* (112) gene products have also been reported.

Two additional mechanisms for the immune destruction of HIV-1-infected CD4+ T cells should be mentioned. First, CD4+ CTL specific for the HIV-1 envelope protein can lyse HIV-1-infected T cells (113,114). We have shown that such CD4+ CTL constitute a part of the normal immune response to the envelope protein, and they have also been cloned from the cerebrospinal fluid of AIDS patients with neurological disorders (115). The ability of these cells to lyse HIV-1-infected T cells reflects an unexpected antigen-processing reaction in which the envelope protein synthesized within infected cells is processed for association with class II MHC gene products (113,114). The potential role of CD4+ CTL in the pathophysiology of HIV-1 infection is discussed below. Second, infected cells may be destroyed in vivo by CD16+ effector cells through ADCC. This process is dependent upon circulating anti-gp120 antibodies. Sera from infected humans will promote lysis of HIV-1-infected target cells by CD16+ effector cells from normal donors (116,117). In some (116–118) but not all (119) studies, the ADCC-promoting activity in sera from AIDS patients was lower than that in sera from healthy seropositive individuals. The target antigen for this ADCC reaction appears to be gp120 since ADCC against CD4+ target cells that have been preincubated with purified gp120 is also observed (120). In addition, Koup and colleagues (119) have recently used vaccinia vectors to express separately HIV-1 *env* and *gag* proteins in target cells. ADCC activity in sera from infected hemophiliacs was directed only at *env* determinants (119). Freshly isolated PBMC (121) and purified CD16+ cells (122) from infected individuals mediated gp120-specific, non-MHC-restricted lysis of target cells expressing gp120, suggesting that in vivo arming of CD16+ effector cells with anti-gp120 occurs. This gp120-specific ADCC provides a mechanism not only for the destruction of HIV-1-infected cells in vivo, but also for the depletion of noninfected CD4+ T cells that have taken up free gp120 by virtue of its high-affinity binding to CD4 (120).

RELATIONSHIP BETWEEN HIV-1 INFECTION AND CD4+ T-CELL DEPLETION

A central question in AIDS immunology is whether the destruction of HIV-1-infected cells by direct viral cytopathic effects and by immunologic mechanisms can, in concert, account for the CD4+ T-cell depletion that is the characteristic feature of this infection. The bulk de-

pletion of the CD4+ T-cell compartment that occurs as the disease progresses must be reconciled with two other observations. First, at any given time only a very small fraction of the CD4+ T cells are infected. This is particularly true during the asymptomatic period when bulk CD4+ T-cell depletion is occurring. Second, at any given time, most of the infected cells are not expressing viral genes.

The loss of HIV-1-infected cells as a result of direct viral cytopathic effects or from immune destruction is most likely to occur in the setting of active infection when viral genes are being transcribed. HIV-1 gene expression depends upon the interaction of inducible host nuclear factors with the HIV-1 LTR. This transcriptional activation is intimately associated with antigen-induced activation of the T cell. Therefore, depletion of CD4+ T cells by cytopathic effects of the virus or by immune destruction of infected cells requires that each depleted T cell be exposed to both virus and antigen. Figure 1 presents a hypothetical scheme summarizing the interactions between HIV-1, CD4+ T cells, and antigen during the course of HIV-1 infection. Resting noninfected T cells represent by far the largest subpopulation in the CD4+ T cell compartment. These resting cells may be naive (1°) or memory (2°) cells. As is discussed below, viral DNA sequences are found mainly in the memory T cells. Interaction of resting T cells with HIV-1 leads to abortive infection unless antigen is encountered before the replication intermediate (unintegrated viral DNA) decays. Infection may also occur following antigen-induced activation. In this case, the cells are highly susceptible to infection and to HIV-1-induced cytopathic effects as well as immune destruction. In the absence of additional antigen stimulation, activated 1° T cells can return to a resting state as memory (2°) cells. Destruction by viral cytopathic effects or immunologic mechanisms requires another round of antigen stimulation. At any given time, most of the CD4+ T cells are present in the resting noninfected compartments. As the disease progresses, the number of cells in the resting infected compartments increases. The level of actively infected cells is never very high, because such cells are either rapidly killed or return to a quiescent, latently infected state. In summary, because of the association between HIV-1 gene expression and T-cell activation, antigen is postulated to play a critical role in CD4+ T-cell depletion. Whether it is possible to account for the bulk depletion of the CD4+ T-cell compartments by the antigen-dependent mechanisms shown in Fig. 1 is still unclear. Subsequent sections of this chapter present other mechanisms to account for CD4+ T-cell depletion.

MECHANISMS FOR THE DEPLETION OF NONINFECTED CD4+ T CELLS

In HIV-1 infection, there are several interesting reactions that can potentially cause the loss of noninfected

Thymus

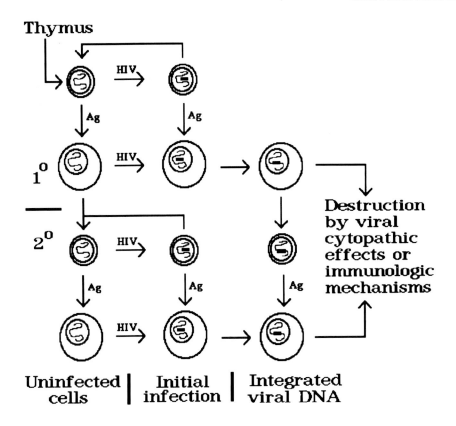

Destruction by viral cytopathic effects or immunologic mechanisms

| Uninfected cells | Initial infection | Integrated viral DNA |

FIG. 1. Hypothetical scheme for the interaction of CD4+ T cells with antigen (Ag) and human immunodeficiency virus type 1 (HIV-1) in natural infection. Antigen stimulation of resting CD4+ T cells (small cells) induces blast transformation giving rise to activated cells (large cells), which can eventually revert to a resting state in the absence of further antigen stimulation. Infection of resting T cells results in reverse transcription of viral genomic RNA giving rise to viral DNA, which either decays or becomes physically integrated into the host chromosome depending on the state of activation of the T cell. Primary T cells (1°) are T cells before or during initial response to antigen. Secondary (2°) T cells are T cells that have been previously exposed to antigen.

CD4+ T cells. In early studies of HIV-1 infection of susceptible cell lines in vitro, the formation of multinucleated giant cells was noted. Subsequent studies showed that infected cells expressing gp120 could fuse with non-infected cells expressing CD4 (92,93). Inclusion of non-infected CD4+ T cells in short-lived syncytia provides a potential mechanism for CD4+ T-cell depletion. The process of syncytium formation involves membrane fusion events initiated by the interaction of gp120 and CD4 on opposing cell surfaces. Recent studies suggest that the cell adhesion molecule LFA-1 also plays an obligatory role in the cell–cell fusion reactions that generate syncytia (123–125).

The extent to which syncytium formation contributes to CD4+ T-cell depletion in vivo is unclear. In pathologic studies of lymph nodes and spleen from infected individuals, giant cells are observed only rarely (70). In addition, not all HIV-1 isolates induce syncytia in vitro. Isolates from different infected individuals show variation in biological properties including rates of replication in vitro, ability to infect various T-cell and monocyte-macrophage cell lines, ability to induce syncytia, and ability to induce cytopathic effects (60,61,126). In a given individual, the capacity of HIV-1 isolates to induce cytopathic effects in vitro increases with disease progression. Levy and colleagues (60) have shown that in a small series of seropositive individuals followed over time isolates obtained before the onset of symptoms were not cytopathic whereas isolates taken subsequent to the onset of symptoms showed the capacity to induce either syncytia or balloon degeneration in infected cultures.

Other studies have shown that isolates with the capacity to induce syncytia emerge with disease progression in certain individuals, although in many cases progression to AIDS is not accompanied by a transition from non-syncytia-inducing (NSI) to syncytia-inducing (SI) phenotype (127). High in vitro replication rates appear to correlate with the SI phenotype and with rapid CD4+ T-cell loss in vivo. The precise role of syncytium formation in the pathogenesis of immunodeficiency in HIV-1 infection remains to be clarified.

Other mechanisms for the destruction of noninfected CD4+ T cells have been proposed. A report from Zarling et al. (128) suggests that PBMC from HIV-1-infected individuals have a high degree of cytolytic activity for PHA-activated CD4+ T cells from most normal and HIV-1-infected allogeneic donors. Such activity seems to be mediated by cells with the surface phenotype of normal cytolytic T cells (CD3+/CD4−/CD8+/CD16−/TCRα − β+). This highly unusual type of lytic activity is not detected in PBMC from seronegative individuals. Unfortunately, since the cells responsible for this activity have not yet been isolated and cloned, the significance of the observed lytic activity is unclear at the present time.

Two other mechanisms for the destruction of noninfected CD4+ T cells depend upon the release of gp120 from the surface of infected cells or HIV-1 virions and the subsequent binding of shed gp120 to CD4+ T cells. The noncovalent association between gp120 and gp41 is readily disrupted, and gp120 can thus be shed from infected cells (129,130) at rates that vary among different HIV-1 isolates (131). Shed gp120 would then be expected to bind to CD4+ T cells by virtue of the high-affinity gp120–CD4 interaction. Weinhold and colleagues (120) have shown that CD4+ T cells that have taken up free gp120 can be destroyed by an ADCC mechanism that depends on the presence of anti-gp120 antibodies. This reaction is observed at gp120 concentrations as low as 6×10^{-10} M (132). In principle, it can operate on both resting and activated CD4+ T cells.

Our laboratory has shown that free gp120 can bind to CD4 on activated human CD4+ T cells and then be internalized and processed for association with class II MHC molecules (133). We have also demonstrated that gp120-specific CD4+ CTL comprise a significant portion of the normal human T-cell response to gp120 and that these cells can readily lyse activated autologous CD4+ T cells that have taken up and processed free gp120, regardless of whether or not the target cells are infected with HIV-1. This cytolytic reaction proceeds even when target cells are exposed to very low concentrations of gp120 ($<10^{-10}$ M). Thus one of the most significant consequences of the existence of CD4+, gp120-specific CTL may be the involvement of such cells in the fundamental pathophysiologic feature of AIDS, the severe depletion of the CD4+ subset of T lymphocytes. The elucidation of this novel pathway for the depletion of noninfected CD4+ T cells was dependent upon the discovery that T cells can process protein antigens that have bound with high affinity to a T-cell surface structure. Similar observations have been recently made by Lanzavecchia and colleagues (134). Blocking studies with anti-CD4 and soluble CD4 have demonstrated that T-cell uptake of gp120 is totally dependent upon an initial interaction between gp120 and CD4. Activated CD8+ T cells can readily present peptide fragments of gp120 to gp120-specific CTL (133). However, CD8+ T cells lack a specific focusing mechanism for taking up intact gp120 and therefore are not generally susceptible to destruction by CD4+, gp120-specific CTL.

The in vivo significance of this CD4+ CTL-mediated pathway relative to other proposed pathways for CD4+ T-cell destruction (such as lytic infection and syncytium formation) remains to be established. One important factor is clearly the amount of gp120 shed in infected individuals. In this regard, it should be noted that the autocytolytic mechanism described above can operate even when the concentration of gp120 is below the kd of the gp120–CD4 interaction, indicating that uptake and processing of only a small number of gp120 molecules may be sufficient to render a T cell susceptible to lysis. Recent results from our laboratory suggest that this processing pathway is highly dependent upon the state of activation of the target T cell and occurs efficiently only in highly activated cells (135). In addition, this pathway can be inhibited by anti-gp120 antibodies that are present in the plasma of infected individuals (135).

The pathway for CD4+ cell depletion described above is of particular interest because it accounts for the deple-

tion of precisely those clonal T-cell specificities that are directed at frequently encountered ubiquitous opportunistic pathogens such as *Candida albicans* and at pathogens that coinfect HIV-1-infected individuals such as cytomegalovirus, Epstein-Barr virus, and herpes simplex virus. Given the findings presented above, one can imagine that activated CD4+ T lymphocytes responding appropriately to such organisms may be selectively destroyed by CD4+ gp120-specific CTL as a consequence of gp120 uptake by their own surface CD4 molecules. This unique type of "innocent bystander" effect may deplete critical helper T-cell clonal specificities, thus exposing the host to a myriad of opportunistic infections.

CD4+ CTL specific for the envelope protein can also participate in several other interesting reactions, which are summarized in Fig. 2. Although viral proteins synthesized in infected cells are generally processed for association with class I MHC gene products and subsequent recognition by CD8+ CTL (136), we have found that HIV-1-infected cells can be lysed by class II MHC-restricted, CD4+ CTL (114). The mechanism by which the envelope protein is processed in infected cells for association with class II MHC gene products and subsequent recognition by CD4+ CTL is unclear. We have recently shown that delivery of the envelope protein to the cellular compartment where processing takes place requires that the protein be translocated into the rough endoplasmic reticulum and remain anchored to the lumenal/extracellular membrane face (113). One possible explanation is that this novel processing reaction involves expression of the envelope protein on the cell surface followed by reinternalization and processing in an endocytic compartment.

We have also shown that human CD4+ CTL specific for the HIV-1 envelope protein can release TNF-α. The production of this lymphokine by *env*-specific T cells is potentially important for several reasons. First, TNF-α is an important general mediator of inflammation. Second, TNF-α and TNF-β have recently been shown to induce HIV-1 gene expression in latently infected T-cell

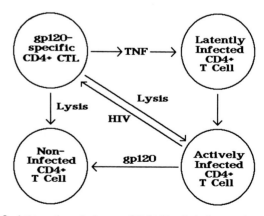

FIG. 2. Interactions between CD4+ T cells in human immunodeficiency virus type 1 (HIV-1) infection. CTL, cytotoxic T lymphocytes; TNF, tumor necrosis factor.

and monocytic cell lines (91). It is possible that the amount of TNF-α released is sufficient to induce latently infected cells in the same microenvironment to upregulate HIV-1 gene expression. Finally, TNF-α may be involved in the mechanism of cytotoxicity by CD4+ CTL. Analysis of the biological role of CD4+, gp120-specific CTL is further complicated by the fact that these CTL can be infected by HIV-1 (137). Because of the extraordinary complexity of the series of the interactions outlined in Fig. 2, additional studies will be needed to determine whether the CD4+ CTL specific for the envelope protein have net beneficial effects for the host. Interestingly, such cells can be induced in seronegative individuals by immunization with soluble gp120 or gp160.

FUNCTIONAL DEFECTS IN CD4+ T CELLS

In addition to the quantitative depletion of CD4+ T cells that occurs during the course of HIV-1 infection, there are also qualitative defects in the function of the surviving CD4+ T cells (Table 4). In a pivotal early study, Lane and colleagues showed that unfractionated PBMC from AIDS patients showed decreased responsiveness to the mitogens PHA and pokeweed mitogen (PWM) (17). However, when purified CD4+ T cells were tested, responses were not significantly different from responses of cells from uninfected donors, suggesting that the lower response seen with unfractionated PBMC from patients was simply due to a lower percentage of CD4+ T cells. Most importantly, purified CD4+ T cells from AIDS patients did show a marked defect in responsiveness to soluble antigen presented by monocytes (17). This defect was shown to be intrinsic to the T cell and did not occur at the level of the antigen-presenting cell (20).

There are conflicting studies dealing with the question of when during the course of HIV-1 infection this functional defect becomes manifest. In some studies, T-cell proliferative responses to soluble recall antigens are spared until immediately before the onset of AIDS

(138,139). However, the CD4+ T-cell help needed for the in vitro generation of antiinfluenza CTL responses is defective in some healthy HIV-1-seropositive individuals (140). Healthy seropositive individuals also show significantly decreased proliferative responses to immobilized anti-CD3 antibodies (141). This has been attributed to selective depletion of memory CD4+ T cells that normally account for much of this response (142, see below).

The mechanism for the decreased responsiveness of CD4+ T cells to soluble antigens is of great interest. One possibility is that the functional defects in surviving CD4+ T cells actually reflect the fact that responsive cells are preferentially deleted. This possibility is discussed in the next section.

SUBSETS OF CD4+ CELLS IN HIV-1 INFECTION

Recent evidence suggests that human CD4+ T cells can be divided into subsets based on the expression of certain plasma membrane proteins (reviewed in 143). For example, adult peripheral blood CD4+ T lymphocytes can be subdivided into two subsets based on expression of CD29, CD45RA, and CD45RO (144,145). CD29, recognized by monoclonal antibody 4B4 (144), is the 130-kd β subunit of VLA1-6 and the fibronectin receptor. CD45RA, recognized by monoclonal antibody 2H4 (146), is a 220-kd isoform of a plasma membrane protein, the T200 leukocyte common antigen (LCA), which has a cytoplasmic domain with phosphatase activity. CD45RO is a 180-kd isoform of the LCA generated by alternative mRNA splicing. Careful analysis of the levels of expression of a number of cell surface proteins has shown that naive T cells have the phenotype CD29^{low}, CD45RO−, CD45RA+. In contrast, memory cells have the phenotype CD29^{high}, CD45RO+, CD45RA− (147). In addition, naive cells are LFA-1^{low}, LFA-3−, whereas memory cells are LFA-1^{high}, LFA-3+. Memory cells also express higher levels of CD2 and CD44. Thus, activation appears to result in the upregulation of a number of cell surface proteins involved in cell adhesion reactions including LFA-1, LFA-3, CD2, CD44, and CD29, as well as a shift in the form of CD45 expressed from CD45RA to CD45RO. It should be noted that none of these proteins is unique to CD4+ T cells.

Studies by Schnittman et al. (148) indicate that naive and memory CD4+ subsets differ in susceptibility to HIV-1 infection both in vivo and in vitro. Following short-term in vitro infection with HIV-1, memory cells contained four- to tenfold more HIV-1 DNA than naive cells. When naive and memory subsets of peripheral blood CD4+ T cells were isolated from HIV-1-seropositive individuals, memory CD4+ cells again showed four- to tenfold higher levels of HIV-1 DNA by PCR analysis. The memory subset shows a loss of anti-

TABLE 4. *Mechanisms for functional defects in CD4+ T cells*

A. Defects in HIV-1-infected T cells
   1. Preferential infection, depletion, or inactivation of CD4+ memory T cells
   2. Decreased expression of CD4
   3. Defects in signaling through the T-cell antigen receptor
B. Functional defects in noninfected CD4+ T cells
   1. Infection and inactivation during an antigen-driven response through interaction with infected APC
   2. Suppressive effects of HIV-1 proteins, especially gp120
   3. Effects of binding of gp120 and anti-gp120
   4. Anti-class II antibodies
   5. Downregulation of class II expression on APC
   6. Cytokine effects (i.e., TGFβ)

APC, antigen-presenting cells; HIV-1, human immunodeficiency virus type 1; TGFβ, tranforming growth factor beta.

CD3 responsiveness in HIV-1 infection. Proliferative responses to the recall antigen tetanus toxoid, which are mediated by memory cells, are also decreased in seropositive individuals. Schnittman et al. (148) proposed that the preferential infection of memory cells involves interactions between the CD4-associated kinase p56^{lck} and the phosphatase CD45 following binding of HIV-1 virions to CD4, although current evidence suggests that binding of intact virions or free gp120 to CD4 does not result in signal transduction (see below). Because memory CD4+ cells show a quantitatively greater susceptibility to HIV-1 infection, they might be expected to show more rapid elimination during the course of HIV-1 infection. Some (142,149–151) but not other (13) studies suggest that there is a preferential loss of memory cells from the peripheral blood of seropositive individuals, although both subsets show profound depletion in AIDS patients.

Preferential infection of CD4+ subsets has also been demonstrated in simian immunodeficiency virus (SIV) infection of macaques. In primates, CD44 shows a bimodal distribution among peripheral blood T cells. Activated T cells are CD44^{high} (152). Following SIV infection of macaques, CD44^{high} CD4+ T cells are preferentially infected and deleted (153). In the human, CD44 has a unimodal distribution on CD4+ T cells and the amount of CD44 does not appear to be related to susceptibility to HIV-1 infection (148).

As was discussed above, there is considerable reason to believe that antigen plays a critical role in driving CD4+ T cells into states in which they are susceptible to infection by HIV-1 and subsequent destruction by viral cytopathic effects or immune mechanisms. It is, therefore, reasonable that frequently activated cells would be depleted first. The selective loss of memory cells can account for the decreased responsiveness of CD4+ T cells from AIDS patients to recall antigens. In addition, there are several other mechanisms that may contribute to the hyporesponsiveness of CD4+ T cells in HIV-1 infection. These mechanisms are summarized in Table 4 and are discussed in the next section.

OTHER MECHANISMS FOR DEFECTS IN CD4+ T-CELL FUNCTION

The CD4+ T-cell compartment in infected individuals contains only a small percentage of infected cells. There are several reasons why these HIV-1-infected cells might respond poorly to antigen stimulation. Most of these cells are in the latent stage of infection. In the case of latently infected cells, activation with antigen may also activate viral gene expression, exposing the cell to viral cytopathic effects and to destruction by immune mechanisms. In the case of noninfected cells, activation with antigen renders the T cell highly susceptible to infection, particularly if the antigen-presenting cell is an HIV-1-infected macrophage. Mann and colleagues (154)

have shown that macrophages infected in vitro with HIV-1 can present antigen to T cells and that the encounter results in transfer of infection to the responding T-cell population in a process that is dependent upon T-cell activation.

Infected cells that are actively expressing viral genes at the time of encounter with antigen are even less likely to be able to respond successfully. Active HIV-1 infection of CD4+ T cells results in a dramatic decrease in cell surface expression of CD4 (4,5,155). Normally, CD4 plays a critical role in T-cell activation by virtue of its association with class II MHC gene products on the surface of the antigen-presenting cells (156), and its participation in signal transduction through association with the tyrosine kinase p56^{lck} (157,158). Thus, decreased CD4+ expression may render the T cell functionally inert. The decrease in CD4 expression also has the effect of facilitating the release of infectious virions by preventing reuptake. Several mechanisms for the decrease in cell surface CD4 appear to be involved including the formation of intracellular complexes between CD4 and gp160 (95). Willey and colleagues (159) have shown that gp160 itself is transported to the cell surface very inefficiently. As a result, complexes of CD4 and gp160 are retained in the endoplasmic reticulum (160). In addition, decreases in the level of CD4 mRNA (161) and posttranscriptional mechanisms affecting CD4 biosynthesis (162,163) have also been described. Salmon et al. (161) have shown that in acute in vitro infections of normal human CD4+ lymphoblasts, surface CD4 molecules may be initially blocked by gp120. As is discussed below, gp120 binds to a site on CD4 that appears to overlap the site at which CD4 interacts with class II MHC molecules, rendering the CD4 molecules functionally inactive. Subsequently, after a few days, decreases in the surface expression of CD4 are noted, due to formation of intracellular complexes of gp160 and CD4 and to decreases in the level of CD4 mRNA. Other cell surface proteins, including class I (164) and class II (165) MHC gene products, may also be downregulated in HIV-1-infected cells. Infected T cells also show impaired signal transduction through the T-cell receptor, as evidenced by decreased Ca^{2+} fluxes following triggering with anti-CD3 antibodies (166).

Although HIV-1-infected CD4+ T cells do not respond normally to stimulation through the antigen receptor, infected cells represent only a small fraction of the total CD4+ T-cell population. It is, therefore, unclear why T-cell populations from AIDS patients respond so poorly to antigen stimulation. A number of hypotheses have been put forward. Several of them involve the potential immunosuppressive effects of HIV-1 proteins released from infected cells. In evaluating the inhibitory effects of these proteins, several questions should be considered.

1. Can the suppressive entity be identified directly in seropositive individuals?

2. If so, is it present at sufficiently high concentrations to mediate suppressive effects?

3. Is there a reasonable mechanistic explanation for the suppressive effects?

4. Do anti-HIV antibodies abrogate the effect?

In most cases, the answers to these important questions are not yet available.

The best studied case of immunosuppression by an HIV-1 gene product is that of the effect of HIV-1 gp120 on CD4+ T-cell responses. Chirmule and colleagues (167) have shown that purified gp120 can inhibit the proliferative responses of a CD4+, tetanus toxoid-specific T-cell clone at doses below 1×10^{-10} M. In this study, early events in signal transduction were shown to be inhibited by gp120. Weinhold and colleagues (132) have also observed that gp120 can inhibit the proliferative and cytotoxic responses of antigen-specific CD4+ T-cell clones. One explanation for the inhibitory effects of gp120 is that it prevents the interaction of CD4 with its ligand on the target cell, MHC class II. The interaction of CD4+ T cells with cell-size lipid vesicles bearing class II MHC molecules can be inhibited by gp120, although higher concentrations are required (4×10^{-8} M) (168). Similarly, the interaction of CD4-transfected COS cells with class II-bearing B cells can be completely inhibited by 2×10^{-7} M gp120 (169). These results are consistent with mutagenesis studies indicating that the regions of CD4 that interact with gp120 also appear to be involved in interactions with MHC class II, although the class II binding site on CD4 appears to be larger and more complex than the gp120 binding site (169). Another possibility is that the binding of gp120 to CD4 transmits signals that interfere with activation through the T-cell antigen receptor, as is seen with anti-CD4 antibodies (170). Center and colleagues (171) have reported that treatment of resting human T cells with partially purified gp120 increases intracellular levels of inositol triphosphate and Ca^{2+}, induces expression of the IL2 receptor, and initiates a chemotactic response. In other studies, increases in intracellular Ca^{2+} have not been noted following binding of gp120 (172,173) or HIV-1 virions (173). Interestingly, binding of gp120 and then anti-gp120 to CD4+ peripheral blood T cells can inhibit the increases in intracellular Ca^{2+} seen after T-cell receptor cross-linking (172). The effect was observed at gp120 concentrations as low as 1×10^{-10} M and with sera from 14 of 14 AIDS patients. Critical to evaluating the potential in vivo role of any of these mechanisms is the question of whether the amount of gp120 released in the local microenvironment is sufficient to induce the relevant effect, a question that is difficult to answer at the present time.

Peptides derived from the gp41 subunit of the envelope protein have also been associated with immunosuppression (174–176). A sequence in the extracellular domain of gp41 has homology to immunosuppressive sequences previously identified in murine and feline retrovirus transmembrane proteins. Immunosuppression by synthetic peptides representing this region of gp41 is only observed at relatively high peptide concentrations and usually requires coupling of the peptides to protein carriers. For these reasons, the in vivo significance of these observations remains unclear. In particular, it is unclear how gp41, an integral membrane protein, could be released into the extracellular fluid, and whether sufficient concentrations are present to mediate the effect in vivo. It is also unclear whether antienvelope antibodies, which are present in the circulation in relatively high titer in most if not all infected individuals, would abrogate these immunosuppressive effects given that the immunosuppressive epitope overlaps a major B-cell epitope in gp41.

Nanomolar concentrations of the HIV-1 regulatory protein Tat have recently been shown to inhibit T-cell proliferative responses to recall antigens but not to mitogens (177). Interestingly, Tat can enter cells from the extracellular environment in a functionally active form (177).

Autoantibodies have also been invoked as potential mediators of immunosuppression in HIV-1 infection. Antibodies directed at the extracellular portion of CD4 can be detected in 10% of HIV-1-infected individuals (178). Golding and colleagues (179) have shown that 36% of AIDS patients have antibodies that react with a pentapeptide sequence from the cytoplasmic portion of gp41 (residues 837–844) that is homologous to a portion of the $\beta1$ domain of HLA-DR and -DQ gene products. These antibodies were shown to inhibit the proliferative responses of normal CD4+ T cells to tetanus toxoid and alloantigen and to mediate the destruction of class II-bearing cells by an ADCC mechanism (180). Finally, Levy and colleagues (181) have described an autoantibody present in the sera of most AIDS patients, but not healthy seropositive individuals, that recognized an 18-kd T-cell surface protein. It is currently unclear whether the various types of autoantibodies described above have any functional significance in vivo.

DEFECTS IN B-CELL FUNCTION

In addition to the effects on CD4+ T cells described above, infection with HIV-1 results in dramatic effects on B-lymphocyte function (reviewed in ref. 182). Normal absolute numbers of circulating B cells are found in HIV-1-infected individuals. However, there are three major lines of evidence suggesting that HIV-1 infection results in abnormalities in B-cell function. First, there is strong evidence for an increased degree of B-cell activation in infected individuals. Second, despite ongoing B-cell activation, antibody responses to specific immunogens are very poor, particularly in patients with AIDS. Finally, there is evidence of altered regulation of Epstein-

Barr virus (EBV) infection of B lymphocytes in HIV-1-infected individuals. Each of these topics is discussed in more detail below.

Increased B-cell activation occurs early in the disease process as evidence by high levels of antibody-producing B cells and by hypergammaglobulinemia (41,183,184). There is a higher than normal percentage of immature B cells and an increased number of activated B cells (185). The increased number of activated B cells seen in AIDS patients has been suggested as a marker of disease progression (185). Spontaneous in vitro B-cell proliferation is also characteristic of HIV-1 infection (41,186). Circulating immune complexes (187–190) can be detected in the sera of AIDS patients. Also part of the clinical picture of HIV-1 infection is immune complex-associated pathology including autoimmune thrombocytopenia (191) and anemia (192). The polyclonal B-cell activation seen in HIV-1 infection is often termed "spontaneous," although there is some evidence that much of the hypergammaglobulinemia actually results from a strong humoral response to HIV itself (193). Other proposed mechanisms for nonspecific B-cell activation in HIV-1 infection include direct effects of HIV-1 virions or HIV-1 proteins (194–196) as well as activation mediated by EBV (see below).

The polyclonal B-cell activation seen in HIV-1 infection is found in conjunction with decreased in vivo humoral responses to specific antigens. In an important early study (41), Fauci and colleagues demonstrated that AIDS patients had reduced responses to a T-independent B-cell mitogen *Staphylococcus aureus* Cowan strain, indicating an intrinsic B-cell defect. Healthy seropositive individuals also show B-cell functional defects, including failure to produce immunoglobulin in response to pokeweed mitogen in the presence of adequate allogeneic T-cell help (141). There is also impaired antibody production after antigenic challenge. Responses to pneumococcal vaccine antigens (197) are impaired, as are responses to natural infections with *Giardia lamblia* (198), *Toxoplasma gondii* (199), *Coccidioides immitis* (200), and cytomegalovirus (201). The molecular mechanisms underlying the functional defects and the spontaneous activation are unknown. Recent work suggests that overproduction of transforming growth factor beta (TGF-β) may be associated with suppression of humoral responses in HIV-1 infection (202).

The role of EBV in the B-cell abnormalities seen in HIV-1 infection is of interest given the decreased regulation of EBV infection in HIV-1-infected individuals (203–205) and the increased risk of B-cell malignancies (206,207). EBV is a well known in vitro polyclonal B-cell activator (208). Although coinfected B cells can be isolated from HIV-1-positive individuals and although EBV-transformed B cells have been shown to support HIV-1 growth in vitro, the role of EBV as a cofactor in AIDS-associated B-cell malignancies has recently been challenged by the observation that some non-Hodgkin's lymphomas in these patients lack the EBV genome (194,209,210).

Recent studies suggest that the polyclonal B-cell activation seen in HIV-1 infection may contribute to the pathophysiology of the disease through a novel cytokine-dependent mechanism. Activated human B cells release TNF-α and IL-6. Both cytokines can induce HIV-1 replication in the latently infected promonocytic cell line U1. In addition, TNF-α induces HIV-1 replication in the chronically infected human T-cell line ACH-2 (91). Without additional in vitro activation, B lymphocytes purified from HIV-1-infected individuals with hypergammaglobulinemia release sufficient amounts of TNF-α and IL-6 to induce HIV-1 replication in these chronically infected cell lines (211). Thus, the polyclonal B-cell activation seen in infected individuals may contribute to the spread of virus because cytokines released by activated B cells can activate HIV-1 replication in latently infected cells.

CONCLUSIONS

HIV-1 infection initiates an extraordinarily complex set of host–virus interactions that ultimately destroy the CD4+ T-cell compartment of the immune system. Considerable progress has been made in in vitro analysis of the numerous potential immunologic and virologic mechanisms by which HIV-1 can induce immunodeficiency. Critical areas for future research include an analysis of which of the many potential mechanisms outlined above are actually responsible in vivo for the quantitative and qualitative defects in CD4+ T cells observed in HIV-1 infection. This will depend on the development of methods for monitoring these processes in vivo in natural infection in humans or in the closely related SIV model in macaques. Research in this direction is likely to be critical for the design of new therapeutic approaches and for the development of AIDS vaccines.

REFERENCES

1. Barre-Sinoussi F, Chermann JC, Rey F, et al. Isolation of a T-lymphocyte retrovirus from a patient at risk for acquired immune deficiency syndrome. *Science* 1983;220:868–70.
2. Popovic M, Sarngadharan MG, Read E, Gallo RC. Detection, isolation, and continuous production of cytopathic retroviruses (HTLV-III) from patients with AIDS and pre-AIDS. *Science* 1984;224:497–500.
3. Dalgleish AG, Beverley PCL, Clapham PR, Crawford DH, Greaves MF, Weiss RA. The CD4 (T4) antigen is an essential component of the receptor for the AIDS retrovirus. *Nature* 1984;312:763–7.
4. Klatzmann D, Champagne E, Chamaret S, et al. T-lymphocyte T4 molecule behaves as the receptor for human retrovirus LAV. *Nature* 1984;312:767–8.
5. McDougal JS, Kennedy MS, Sligh JM, Cort SP, Mawle A, Nich-

olson JKA. Binding of HTLV-III/LAV to T4$^+$ T cells by a complex of a 110K viral protein and the T4 molecule. *Science* 1986;231:382–5.

6. Maddon PJ, Dalgleish AG, McDougal JS, Clapham PR, Weiss RA, Axel R. The T4 gene encodes the AIDS virus receptor and is expressed in the immune system and the brain. *Cell* 1986;47:333–48.

7. Moscicki RA, Amento EP, Krane SM, Kurnick JT, Colvin RB. Modulation of surface antigens of a human monocyte cell line, U937, during incubation with T-lymphocyte conditioned medium: detection of T4 antigen and its presence on normal blood monocytes. *J Immunol* 1983;131:743–8.

8. Gottlieb, MS, Schanker HM, Fan PT, et al. *Pneumocystis* pneumonia–Los Angeles. *MMWR* 1981;30:250–2.

9. Friedman-Klein A, Laubenstein L, Marmor M, et al. Kaposi's sarcoma and *Pneumocystis* pneumonia among homosexual men —New York City and California. *MMWR* 1981;30:305–8.

10. Gottlieb MS, Schroff R, Schanker HM, et al. *Pneumocystis carinii* pneumonia and mucosal candidiasis in previously healthy homosexual men: evidence of a new acquired cellular immunodeficiency. *N Engl J Med* 1981;305:1425–31.

11. Masur H, Michelis MA, Greene JB, et al. An outbreak of community acquired *Pneumocystis carinii* pneumonia: initial manifestation of cellular immune dysfunction. *N Engl J Med* 1981;305:1431–8.

12. Siegal FP, Lopez C, Hammer GS, et al. Severe acquired immunodeficiency in male homosexuals, manifest by chronic perianal ulcerative herpes simplex lesions. *N Engl J Med* 1981;305:1439–44.

13. Giorgi JV, Detels R. T-cell subset alterations in HIV-infected homosexual man: NIAID multicenter AIDS cohort study. *Clin Immunol Immunopathol* 1989;52:10–8.

14. Polk BF, Robin F, Brookmeyer R, et al. Predictors of the acquired immunodeficiency syndrome developing in a cohort of seropositive homosexual men. *N Engl J Med* 1987;316:61–6.

15. Goedert JJ, Biggar RJ, Melbye M, et al. Effect of T4 count and cofactors on the incidence of AIDS in homosexual men infected with human immunodeficiency virus. *JAMA* 1987;257:331–4.

16. Moss AR, Bacchetti P, Osmond D. et al. Seropositivity for HIV and the development of AIDS or AIDS related condition: three year follow up of the San Francisco General Hospital cohort. *Br Med J* 1988;296:745–50.

17. Lane HC, Depper JM, Greene WC, Whalen G, Waldmann TA, Fauci AS. Qualitative analysis of immune function in patients with the acquired immunodeficiency syndrome: evidence for a selective defect in soluble antigen recognition. *N Engl J Med* 1985;313:79–84.

18. Ho DD, Pomerantz RJ, Kaplan JC. Pathogenesis of infection with human immunodeficiency virus. *N Engl J Med* 1987;317:278–86.

19. Rosenberg ZF, Fauci AS. The immunopathogenesis of HIV infection. *Adv Immunol* 1989;46:377–405.

20. Koenig S, Fauci AS. AIDS: immunopathogenesis and immune response to the human immunodeficiency virus. In: DeVita V, Hellman S, Rosenberg SA, eds. *AIDS*, 2nd ed. Philadelphia: JB Lippincot Co, 1988.

21. McCune MJ. HIV-1: the infective process in vivo. *Cell* 1991;64:351–63.

22. Allan JS, Coligan JE, Barin F, et al. Major glycoprotein antigens that induce antibodies in AIDS patients are encoded by HTLV-III. *Science* 1985;228:1091–3.

23. Barin F, McLane MF, Allan JS, Lee TH, Groopman JE, Essex M. Virus envelope protein of HTLV-III represents major target antigen for antibodies in AIDS patients. *Science* 1985;228:1094–6.

24. Walker BD, Chakrabarti S, Moss B. et al. HIV-specific cytotoxic T lymphocytes in seropositive individuals. *Nature* 1987;328:345–8.

25. Plata F, Autran B, Martins LP, et al. AIDS virus-specific cytotoxic T lymphocytes in lung disorders. *Nature* 1987;328:348–51.

26. Hoffenbach A, Langlade-Demoyen P, Dadaglio G, et al. Unusually high frequencies of HIV-specific cytotoxic lymphocytes in humans. *J Immunol* 1989;142:452–61.

27. Robert-Guroff M, Brown M, Gallo RC. HTLV-III-neutralizing antibodies in patients with AIDS and AIDS-related complex. *Nature* 1985;316:72–5.

28. Weiss RA, Clapham PR, Cheingsong-Popov R, et al. Neutralization of HTLV-III by sera of AIDS and AIDS-risk patients. *Nature* 1985;316:69–72.

29. Rusche JR, Javaherian K, McDanal C, et al. Antibodies that inhibit fusion of human immunodeficiency virus-infected cells bind a 24-amino acid sequence of the viral envelope gp120. *Proc Natl Acad Sci USA* 1988;85:3198–202.

30. Palker TJ, Clark ME, Langlois AJ, et al. Type-specific neutralization of human immunodeficiency virus with antibodies to *env*-encoded synthetic peptides. *Proc Natl Acad Sci USA* 1988;85:1932–6.

31. Goudsmit J, Debouck C, Meloen RH, et al. Human immunodeficiency virus type 1 neutralization epitope with conserved architecture elicits early type-specific antibodies in experimentally infected chimpanzees. *Proc Natl Acad Sci USA* 1988;85:4478–82.

32. Leonard CK, Spellman MW, Riddle L, Harris RJ, Thomas JN, Gregory TJ. Assignment of intrachain disulfide bonds and characterization of potential glycosylation sites of the type 1 recombinant human immunodeficiency virus envelope glycoprotein (gp120) expressed in Chinese hamster ovary cells. *J Biol Chem* 1990;265:10373–82.

33. Freed EO, Myers DJ, Risser R. Identification of the principal neutralizing determinant of human immunodeficiency virus type 1 as a fusion domain. *J Virol* 1991;65:190–4.

34. Kowalski M, Potz J, Basiripour L, et al. Functional regions of the envelope glycoprotein of human immunodeficiency virus type 1. *Science* 1987;37:1351–5.

35. Lasky LA, Nakamura G, Smith DH, et al. Delineation of a region of the human immunodeficiency virus type 1 gp120 glycoprotein critical for interaction with the CD4 receptor. *Cell* 1987; 50:975–85.

36. Dowbenko D, Nakamura G, Feenie, et al. Epitope mapping of the human immunodeficiency virus type 1 gp120 with monoclonal antibodies. *J Virol* 1988;62:4703–11.

37. Gupta P, Balachandran R, Ho M, Enrico A, Rinaldo C. Cell-to cell transmission of human immunodeficiency virus type 1 in the presence of azidothymidine and neutralizing antibody. *J Virol* 1989;63:2361–5.

38. Layne SP, Spouge JL, Dembo M. Quantifying the infectivity of human immunodeficiency virus. *Proc Natl Acad Sci USA* 1989;86:4644–8.

39. Takeda A, Tuazon C, Ennis FA. Antibody-enhancement of infection by HIV-1 via Fc receptor-mediated entry. *Science* 1988;242:580–3.

40. Homsy J, Meyer M, Tateno M, Clarkson S, Levy JA. The Fc and not CD4 receptor mediates antibody enhancement of HIV infection in human cells. *Science* 1989;244:1357–60.

41. Lane HC, Masur H, Edgar LC, Whalen G, Rook AH, Fauci AS. Abnormalities of B-cell activation and immunoregulation in patients with the acquired immunodeficiency syndrome. *N Engl J Med* 1983;309:453–8.

42. Ho DD, Rota TR, Hirsch MS. Infection of monocyte/macrophages by human T lymphotropic virus type III. *J Clin Invest* 1986;77:1712–20.

43. Gartner S, Markovits P, Markovitz DM, Kaplan MH, Gallo RC, Popovic M. The role of mononuclear phagocytes in HTLV-III/ LAV infection. *Science* 1986;233:215–9.

44. Nicholson JKA, Gross GD, Callaway CS, McDougal JS. In vitro infection of human monocytes with T lymphotropic virus type III/lymphadenopathy-associated virus (HTLV-III/LAV). *J Immunol* 1986;137:323–9.

45. Walker CM, Moody DJ, Stites DP, Levy JA. CD8+ lymphocytes can control HIV infection in vitro by suppressing virus replication. *Science* 1986;234:1563–6.

46. Trubota H, Lord CI, Watkins DI, Moumoto C, Letvin NL. A cytotoxic T lymphocyte inhibits acquired immunodeficiency syndrome virus replication in peripheral blood lymphocytes. *J Exp Med* 1989;169:1421–34.

47. Kannagi M, Masuda T, Hattori T, et al. Interference with human immunodeficiency virus (HIV) replication by CD8+ T cells in peripheral blood leukocytes of asymptomatic HIV carriers in vitro. *J Virol* 1990;64:3399–406.

48. Pantaleo G, De Maria A, Koenig S, et al. CD8+ T lymphocytes of patients with AIDS maintain normal broad cytolytic function despite the loss of human immunodeficiency virus-specific cytotoxicity. *Proc Natl Acad Sci USA* 1990;87:4818–22.

49. Wong-Staal F, Shaw GM, Hahn BH, et al. Genomic diversity of human T-lymphotropic virus type III (HTLV-III). *Science* 1985;229:759–62.

50. Benn S, Rutledge R, Folks T, et al. Genomic heterogeneity of AIDS retroviral isolates from North America and Zaire. *Science* 1985;230:949–51.

51. Hahn BH, Gonda MA, Shaw GM, et al. Genomic diversity of the acquired immune deficiency syndrome virus HTLV-III: different viruses exhibit greatest divergence in their envelope genes. *Proc Natl Acad Sci USA* 1985;82:4813–7.

52. Willey RL, Rutledge RA, Dias S, et al. Identification of conserved and divergent domains within the envelope gene of the acquired immunodeficiency syndrome retrovirus. *Proc Natl Acad Sci USA* 1986;83:5038–42.

53. Starcich BR, Hahn BH, Shaw GM, et al. Identification and characterization of conserved and variable regions in the envelope gene of HTLV III/LAV, the retrovirus of AIDS. *Cell* 1986;45:637–48.

54. Alizon M, Wain-Hobson S, Montagnier L, Sonigo P. Genetic variability of the AIDS virus: nucleotide sequence analysis of two isolates from African patients. *Cell* 1986;46:63–74.

55. Roberts JD, Bebenek K, Kunkel TA. The accuracy of reverse transcriptase from HIV-1. *Science* 1988;242:1171–3.

56. Preston BD, Poiesz BJ, Loeb LA. Fidelity of HIV-1 reverse transcriptase. *Science* 1988;242:1168–71.

57. Hahn BH, Shaw GM, Tayler ME, et al. Genetic variation in HTLV-III/LAV over time in patients with AIDS or at risk for AIDS. *Science* 1986;232:1548–53.

58. Saag MS, Hahn BH, Gibbons J, et al. Extensive variation of human immunodeficiency virus type-1 *in vivo*. *Nature* 1988;334:440–4.

59. Meyerhans A, Cheynier R, Alabert J, et al. Temporal fluctuations in HIV quasispecies in vivo are not reflected by sequential HIV isolations. *Cell* 1989;58:901–10.

60. Cheng-Mayer C, Seto D, Tateno M, Levy JA. Biologic features of HIV-1 that correlate with virulence in the host. *Science* 1988;240:80–2.

61. Fisher AG, Ensoli B, Looney D, et al. Biologically diverse molecular variants within a single HIV-1 isolate. *Nature* 1988;334:440–7.

62. Clements JE, Gdovin SL, Montelaro RC, Narayan O. Antigenic variation on lentiviral diseases. *Annu Rev Immunol* 1988;6:139–59.

63. Reitz MS Jr, Wilson C, Naugle C, Gallo RC, Robert-Guroff M. Generation of a neutralization resistant variant of HIV-1 is due to selection for a point mutation in the envelope gene. *Cell* 1988;54:57–63.

64. Nara PL, Smit L, Dunlop N, et al. Emergence of viruses resistant to neutralization by V3-specific antibodies in experimental human immunodeficiency virus type 1 IIIB infection of chimpanzees. *J Virol* 1990;64:3779–91.

65. Looney DJ, Fisher AG, Putney SD, et al. Type-restricted neutralization of molecular clones of human immunodeficiency virus. *Nature* 1988;241:357–9.

66. Pircher H, Moskophidis D, Rohrer U, Burki K, Hengartner H, Zinkernagel RM. Viral escape by selection of cytotoxic T cell-resistant virus variants *in vivo*. *Nature* 1990;346:629–33.

67. Callahan KM, Fort M, Obah EA, Reinherz ER, Siliciano RF. Genetic variability in HIV-1 gp120 affects interactions with HLA molecules and T cell receptors. *J Immunol* 1990;144:3341–6.

68. Takahashi H, Houghten R, Putney SC, et al. Structural requirements for class I MHC molecule-mediated antigen presentation and cytotoxic T cell recognition of an immunodominant determinant of the human immunodeficiency virus envelope protein. *J Exp Med* 1989;170:2023–35.

69. Hammond SA, Obah E, Stanhope P, et al. Characterization of a conserved T cell epitope in HIV-1 gp41 recognized by vaccine-induced human cytolytic T cells. *J Immunol* 1991;146:1470–7.

70. Macher AM, De Vinatea ML, Angritt P, Tuur SM, Reichert CM. Pathologic features of patients infected with the human immunodeficiency virus. In: DeVita V, Hellman S, Rosenberg SA, eds. *AIDS,* 2nd ed. Philadelphia: JB Lippincott Co, 1988;155–184.

71. Tremblay M, Numazaki K, Goldman H, Wainberg MA. Infection of human thymic lymphocytes by HIV-1. *J Acquired Immune Deficiency Syndromes* 1990;3:356–60.

72. Schnittman SM, Denning SM, Greenhouse JJ, et al. Evidence for susceptibility of intrathymic T-cell precursors and their progeny carrying T-cell antigen receptor phenotypes $TCR\alpha\beta^+$ and $TCR\gamma\delta^+$ to human immunodeficiency virus infection: a mechanism for CD4+ (T4) lymphocyte depletion. *Proc Natl Acad Sci USA* 1990;87:7727–31.

73. Wu L, Scollay R, Egerton M, Pearse M, Spangrude GJ, Shortman K. CD4 expressed on the earliest T-lineage precursor cells in the adult murine thymus. *Nature* 1991;349:71–4.

74. Folks TM, Kessler SW, Orenstein JM, Justement JS, Jaffe ES, Fauci AS. Infection and replication of HIV-1 in purified progenitor cells of normal human bone marrow. *Science* 1988;242:919–22.

75. Schnittman SM, Psallidopoulos C, Lane HC, et al. The reservoir for HIV-1 in human peripheral blood is a T cell that maintains expression of CD4. *Science* 1989;245:305–8.

76. Harper ME, Marselle LM, Gallo RC, Wong-Staal F. Detection of lymphocytes expressing human T-lymphotropic virus type III in lymph nodes and peripheral blood from infected individuals by in situ hybridization. *Proc Natl Acad Sci USA* 1987;83:772–6.

77. Psallidopoulos MC, Schnittman SM, Thompson LM, et al. Integrated proviral human immunodeficiency virus type 1 is present in CD4+ peripheral blood lymphocytes in healthy seropositive individuals. *J Virol* 1989;63:4626–31.

78. Simmonds P, Balfe P, Peutherer JF, Ludlam CA, Bishop JO, Brown AJL. Human immunodeficiency virus-infected individuals contain provirus in small numbers of peripheral blood mononuclear cells and at low copy number. *J Virol* 1990;64:864–72.

79. Ho DD, Moudgil T, Alam M. Quantitation of human immunodeficiency virus type 1 in the blood of infected persons. *N Engl J Med* 1989;321:1621–5.

80. Chesebro B, Wehrly K, Metcalf J, Griffin DE. Use of a new CD4-positive HeLa cell clone for direct quantitation of infectious human immunodeficiency virus from the blood of AIDS patients. *J Infect Dis* 1991;163:64–70.

81. McDougal JS, Mawle A, Cort SP, et al. Cellular tropism of the human retrovirus HTLV-III/LAV. I. Role of T cell activation and expression of the T4 antigen. *J Immunol* 1985;135:3151–62.

82. Zagury D, Bernard J, Chenier R, Feldman M, Sarin P, Gallo RC. Immune induction of T cell death in long term HTLV-III-infected cultures. A cytopathogenic model for AIDS T cell depletion. *Science* 1985;231:850–3.

83. Margolick JB, Volkman DJ, Folks TM, Fauci AS. Amplification of HTLVIII/LAV infection by antigen-induced activation of T cells and direct suppression by virus of lymphocyte blastogenic responses. *J Immunol* 1987;138:1719–23.

84. Zack JA, Arrigo SJ, Weitsman SR, Go AS, Haislip A, Chen ISY. HIV-1 entry into quiescent primary lymphocytes: molecular analysis reveals a labile, latent viral structure. *Cell* 1990;61:213–22.

85. Stevenson M, Stanwick TL, Dempsey MP, Lamonica CA. HIV-1 replication is controlled at the level of T cell activation and proviral integration. *EMBO J* 1990;9:1551–60.

86. Stevenson M, Haggerty S, Lamonica CA, et al. Integration is not necessary for expression of human immunodeficiency virus type 1 protein products. *J Virol* 1990;64:2421–5.

87. Coombs RW, Collier AC, Allain J-P, et al. Plasma viremia in human immunodeficiency virus infection. *N Engl J Med* 1989;321:1626–31.

88. Schnittman SM, Lane HC, Greenhouse J, Justement JS, Baseler M, Fauci AS. Preferential infection of CD4+ memory T cells by human immunodeficiency virus type 1: evidence for a role in the selective T-cell functional defects observed in infected individuals. *Proc Natl Acad Sci USA* 1990;87:6058–62.

89. Nabel G, Baltimore D. An inducible transcription factor activates expression of human immunodeficiency virus in T cells. *Nature* 1987;326:711–3.

90. Greene WC. Regulation of HIV-1 gene expression. *Annu Rev Immunol* 1990;8:453–75.

91. Folks TM, Clouse KA, Justement J, et al. Tumor necrosis factor

α induced expression of human immunodeficiency virus in a chronically infected T-cell clone. *Proc Natl Acad Sci USA* 1989;86:2365–8.

92. Lifson JD, Feinberg MB, Reyes GR, et al. Induction of CD4-dependent cell fusion by the HTLV-III/LAV envelope glycoprotein. *Nature* 1986;323:725–8.
93. Sodroski J, Goh WC, Rosen C, Campbell K, Haseltine WA. Role of the HTLV-III/LAV envelope in syncytium formation and cytopathicity. *Nature* 1986;322:470–4.
94. Somasudaran M, Robinson HL. A major mechanism of human immunodeficiency virus-induced cell killing does not involve cell fusion. *J Virol* 1988;61:3114–9.
95. Stevenson M, Meier C, Mann AM, Chapman N, Wasiak A. Envelope glycoprotein of HIV induces interference and cytolysis resistance in CD4+ T cells: mechanism for persistence in AIDS. *Cell* 1988;53:483–96.
96. Keshnet E, Temin H. Cell killing by spleen necrosis virus is correlated with a transient accumulation of spleen necrosis virus DNA. *J Virol* 1979;31:376–88.
97. Weller S, Joy A, Temin H. Correlation between cell killing and massive second-round superinfection by members of some subgroups of avian leukosis virus. *J Virol* 1980;33:494–506.
98. Mullins J, Chen C, Hoover E. Disease-specific and tissue-specific production of unintegrated feline leukemia virus variant DNA in feline AIDS. *Nature* 1986;319:333–6.
99. Haase AT, Brahic M, Carroll D, et al. Visna: an animal model for studies of virus persistence. In: Stevens JG, et al., eds. *Persistent viruses.* New York: Academic Press, 1978;643–54.
100. Shaw GM, Hahn BH, Arya SK, Groopman JE, Gallo RC, Wong-Staal F. Molecular characterization of human T-cell leukemia (lymphotropic) virus type III in the acquired immune deficiency syndrome. *Science* 1984;226:1165–71.
101. Pang S, Koyanagi Y, Miles S, Wiley C, Vinters HV, Chen ISY. High levels of unintegrated HIV-1 DNA in brain tissue of AIDS dementia patients. *Nature* 1990;343:85–9.
102. Kim S, Byrn R, Groopman J, Baltimore D. Temporal aspects of DNA and RNA synthesis during human immunodeficiency virus infection: evidence for differential gene expression. *J Virol* 1989;63:3708–13.
103. Pauza CD, Galindo JE, Richman DD. Reinfection results in accumulation of unintegrated viral DNA in cytopathic and persistent human immunodeficiency virus type 1 infection of CEM cells. *J Exp Med* 1990;172:1035–42.
104. Asjo B, Ivhed I, Gidlund M, et al. Susceptibility to infection by the human immunodeficiency virus correlates with T4 expression in a parental monocytoid cell line and its subclones. *Virology* 1987;157:359–64.
105. Koga Y, Sasaki M, Yoshida H, Wigzell H, Kimura G, Nomoto K. Cytopathic effect determined by the amount of CD4 molecules in human cell lines expressing envelope glycoprotein of HIV. *J Immunol* 1990;144:94–102.
106. Koga Y, Sasaki M, Nakamura K, Kimura G, Nomoto K. Intracellular distribution of the envelope glycoprotein of human immunodeficiency virus and its role in the production of cytopathic effect in CD4+ and CD4− human cell lines. *J Virol* 1990;64:4661–71.
107. Stevenson M, Haggerty S, Lamonica C, Mann AM, Meier C, Wasiak A. Cloning and characterization of human immunodeficiency virus type 1 variants diminished in the ability to induce syncytium-independent cytolysis. *J Virol* 1990;64:3792–803.
108. Kowalski M, Bergeron L, Dorfman T, Haseltine W, Sodroski W. Attenuation of human immunodeficiency virus type 1 cytopathic effect by a mutation affecting the transmembrane envelope glycoprotein. *J Virol* 1991;65:281–91.
109. Koenig S, Earl P, Pail D, et al. Group-specific, major histocompatibility complex class I-restricted cytotoxic responses to human immunodeficiency virus 1 (HIV-1) envelope proteins by cloned peripheral blood T cells from an HIV-1-infected individual. *Proc Natl Acad Sci USA* 1988;85:8638–42.
110. Walker BD, Flexner C, Paradis TJ, et al. HIV-1 reverse transcriptase is a target for cytotoxic T lymphocytes in infected individuals. *Science* 1988;240:64–6.
111. Nixon DF, Townsend ARM, Elvin JG, Rizza CR, Gallwey J, McMicheal AJ. HIV-1 gag-specific cytotoxic T lymphocytes de-

fined with recombinant vaccinia virus and synthetic peptides. *Nature* 1988;336:484–7.
112. Koenig S, Fuerst TR, Wood LV, et al. Mapping the fine specificity of a cytolytic T cell response to the HIV-1 *nef* protein. *J Immunol* 1990;145:127–35.
113. Polydefkis M, Koenig S, Flexner C, et al. Anchor-sequence dependent endogenous processing of the HIV-1 envelope glycoprotein gp160 for CD4+ T cell recognition. *J Exp Med* 1990;171:875–88.
114. Orentas RJ, Hildreth JKE, Obah E, et al. An HIV envelope protein vaccine induces CD4+ human cytolytic T cells active against HIV-infected cells. *Science* 1990;248:1234–7.
115. Sethi KK, Naher H, Stroehmann I. Phenotypic heterogeneity of cerebrospinal fluid-derived HIV-specific and HLA-restricted cytotoxic T-cell clones. *Nature* 1988;335:178–80.
116. Rook AH, Lane HC, Folks T, McCoy S, Alter H, Fauci AS. Sera from HTLV-III/LAV antibody-positive individuals mediate antibody-dependent cellular cytotoxicity against HTLV-III/LAV-infected T cell. *J Immunol* 1987;138:1064–7.
117. Ljunggren K, Bottiger B, Biberfeld G, Karlson A, Fenyo EM, Jondal M. Antibody-dependent cellular cytotoxicity-inducing antibodies against human immunodeficiency virus. Presence at different clinical stages *J Immunol* 1987;139:2263–7.
118. Tyler DS, Stanley SD, Nastala CA, et al. Alterations in antibody-dependent cellular cytotoxicity during the course of HIV-1 infection. Humoral and cellular defects. *J Immunol* 1990;144:3375–84.
119. Koup RA, Sullivan JL, Levine PH, et al. Antigenic specificity of antibody-dependent cell-mediated cytotoxicity directed against human immunodeficiency virus in antibody-positive sera. *J Virol* 1989;63:584–90.
120. Lyerly HK, Matthews TJ, Langlois AJ, Bolognesi DP, Weinhold KJ. Human T-cell lymphotropic virus IIIb glycoprotein (gp120) bound to CD4 determinants on normal lymphocytes and expressed by infected cells serves as target for immune attack. *Proc Natl Acad Sci USA* 1987;84:4601–5.
121. Riviere Y, Tanneau-Salvador F, Regnault A, et al. Human immunodeficiency virus-specific cytotoxic responses of seropositive individuals: distinct types of effector cells mediate killing of targets expressing *gag* and *nef* proteins. *J Virol* 1989;63:2270–7.
122. Tyler DS, Nastala CL, Stanley SD, et al. Gp120 specific cellular cytotoxicity in HIV-1 seropositive individuals. Evidence for circulating CD16+ effector cells armed in vivo with cytophilic antibody. *J Immunol* 1989;142:1177–82.
123. Hildreth JEK, Orentas RJ. Involvement of a leukocyte adhesion receptor (LFA-1) in HIV-induced syncytium formation. *Science* 1989;244:1075–8.
124. Valentin A, Lundin K, Patarroyo M, Asjo B. The leukocyte adhesion glycoprotein CD18 participates in HIV-1-induced syncytia formation in monocytoid and T cells. *J Immunol* 1990;144:934–8.
125. Pantaleo G, Butini L, Graziosi C, et al. Human immunodeficiency virus (HIV) infection in CD4+ T lymphocytes genetically deficient in LFA-1: LFA-1 is required for HIV-mediated cell fusion but not for viral transmission. *J Exp Med* 1991;173:511–4.
126. Fenyo EM, Morfeldt-Manson L, Chiodi F, et al. Distinct replicative and cytopathic characteristics of human immunodeficiency virus isolates. *J Virol* 1988;62:4414–9.
127. Tersmette M, Gruters RA, de Wolf F, et al. Evidence for a role of virulent human immunodeficiency virus (HIV) variants in the pathogenesis of acquired immunodeficiency syndrome: studies on sequential HIV isolates. *J Virol* 1989;63:2118–25.
128. Zarling JM, Ledbetter JA, Sias J, et al. HIV-infected humans, but not chimpanzees, have circulating cytotoxic T lymphocytes that lyse uninfected CD4+ T cells. *J Immunol* 1990;144:2992–8.
129. Kieny M, Rautmann G, Schmitt D, et al. AIDS virus env protein expressed from a recombinant vaccinia virus. *Bio/Technology* 1986;4:790–5.
130. Gelderbloom HR, Hausmann EHS, Ozel M, Pauli G, Koch MA. Fine structure of human immunodeficiency virus and immunolocalization of structural proteins. *Virology* 1987;156:171–6.
131. McKeating JA, McKnight A, Moore JP. Differential loss of envelope glycoprotein gp120 from virions of human immunodefi-

ciency virus type 1 isolates: effects on infectivity and neutralization. *J Virol* 1991;65:852–60.

132. Weinhold KJ, Lyerly HK, Stanley SD, Austin AA, Matthews TJ, Bolognesi DP. HIV-1 gp120-mediated immune suppression and lymphocyte destruction in the absence of viral infection. *J Immunol* 1989;142:3091–7.

133. Siliciano RF, Lawton T, Knall C, et al. Analysis of host-virus interactions in AIDS with anti-gp120 human T cell clones: effect of HIV sequence variation and a mechanism for CD4+ cell depletion. *Cell* 1988;54:561–75.

134. Lanzavecchia A, Roosnek E, Gregory T, Berman P, Abrignani S. T cells can present antigens such as HIV gp120 targeted to their own surface molecules. *Nature* 1988;334:530–32.

135. Polydefkis M, Stanhope P, Siliciano RF. Unpublished results.

136. Morrison LA, Lukacher AE, Braciale VL, Fan D, Braciale TJ. Differences in antigen presentation to MHC class I- and class II-restricted influenza virus-specific cytolytic T lymphocyte clones. *J Exp Med* 1986;163:903–12.

137. Orentas RJ, Hildreth JKE, Siliciano RF. Unpublished observations.

138. Giorgi JV, Fahey JL, Smith DC, et al. Early effects of HIV on CD4+ lymphocytes in vivo. *J Immunol* 1987;138:3725–30.

139. Gurley RJ, Ikeuchi K, Byrn RA, Anderson K, Groopman JE. CD4+ lymphocyte function with early human immunodeficiency virus infection. *Proc Natl Acad Sci USA* 1989;86:1993–7.

140. Shearer GM, Bernstein DC, Tung KSK, et al. A model for the selective loss of major histocompatibility complex self-restricted T cell immune responses during the development of acquired immune deficiency syndrome (AIDS). *J Immunol* 1986;137:2514–21.

141. Miedema F, Chantal Petit AJ, Terpstra FG, et al. Immunological abnormalities in human immunodeficiency virus (HIV)-infected asymptomatic homosexual men. HIV affects the immune system before CD4+ helper T cell depletion occurs. *J Clin Invest* 1988;82:1908–14.

142. van Noesel CJM, Gruters RA, Terpstra FG, Schellekens PTA, van Lier RAW, Miedema F. Functional and phenotypic evidence for a selective loss of memory T cells in asymptomatic human immunodeficiency virus-infected men. *J Clin Invest* 1990;86:293–9.

143. Cerottini J-C, MacDonald HR. The cellular basis of T-cell memory. *Annu Rev Immunol* 1989;7:77–89.

144. Morimoto C, Letvin NL, Boyd AW, et al. The isolation and characterization of the human helper inducer T cell subset. *J Immunol* 1985;134:3762–9.

145. Akbar AN, Terry L, Timms A, Beverley PCL, Janossy G. Loss of CD45R and gain of UCHL1 reactivity is a feature of primed T cells. *J Immunol* 1988;140:2171–8.

146. Morimoto C, Letvin NL, Distaso JA, Aldrich WR, Schlossman SF. The isolation and characterization of the human suppressor inducer T cell subset. *J Immunol* 1985;134:1508–15.

147. Sanders ME, Makgoba MW, Sharrow SO, et al. Human memory T lymphocytes express increased levels of three cell adhesion molecules (LFA-3, CD2, and LFA-1) and three other molecules (UCHL1, CDw29, and Pgp-1) and have enhanced IFN-γ production. *J Immunol* 1988;140:1401–7.

148. Schnittman SM, Lane HC, Greenhouse J, Justement JS, Baseler M, Fauci AS. Preferential infection of CD4+ memory T cells by human immunodeficiency virus type 1: evidence for a role in the selective T-cell functional defects observed in infected individuals. *Proc Natl Acad Sci USA* 1990;87:6058–62.

149. de Martini RM, Turner RR, Formanti SC, et al. Peripheral blood mononuclear cell abnormalities and their relationship to clinical course in homosexual men with HIV infection. *Clin Immunol Immunopathol* 1988;46:258–71.

150. Fletcher MA, Azen SP, Adelsberg B, et al. Immunophenotyping in a multicenter study: the transfusion safety study experience. *Clin Immunol Immunopathol* 1989;52:38–47.

151. De Paoli P, Battistin S, Crovatto M, et al. Immunologic abnormalities related to antigenaemia during HIV-1 infection. *Clin Exp Immunol* 1988;74:317–20.

152. Willerford DM, Hoffman PA, Gallatin WM. Expression of lymphocyte adhesion receptors for high endothelium in primates.

153. Gallatin WM, Gale MJ Jr, Hoffman PA, et al. Selective replication of simian immunodeficiency virus in a subset of CD4+ lymphocytes. *Proc Natl Acad Sci USA* 1989;86:3301–5.

154. Mann DL, Gartner S, Le Sane F, Buchow H, Popovic M. HIV-1 transmission and function of virus-infected monocytes/macrophages. *J Immunol* 1990;144:2152–8.

155. Hoxie JA, Alpers JD, Raackowski JL, et al. Alterations in T4 (CD4) protein and mRNA synthesis in cells infected with HIV. *Science* 1986;234:1123–5.

156. Doyle C, Strominger JL. Interaction between CD4 and class II MHC molecules mediates cell adhesion. *Nature* 1987;330:256–9.

157. Barber EK, Dasgupta JD, Schlossman SF, Trevillyan JM, Rudd CE. The CD4 and CD8 antigens are coupled to a protein-tyrosine kinase (p56lck) that phosphorylates the CD3 complex. *Proc Natl Acad Sci USA* 1989;86:3277–81.

158. Veillette A, Bookman MA, Horak EM, Samelson LE, Bolen JB. Signal transduction through the CD4 receptor involves the activation of the internal membrane tyrosine-kinase p56lck. *Nature* 1989;338:257–9.

159. Willey RL, Bonifacino JS, Potts BJ, Martin MA, Klausner RD. Biosythesis, cleavage, and degradation of the human immunodeficiency virus 1 envelope glycoprotein gp160. *Proc Natl Acad Sci USA* 1988;85:9580–4.

160. Crise B, Buonocore L, Rose JK. CD4 is retained in the endoplasmic reticulum by the human immunodeficiency virus type 1 glycoprotein precursor. *J Virol* 1990;64:5585–93.

161. Salmon P, Olivier R, Riviere Y, et al. Loss of CD4 membrane expression and CD4 mRNA during acute human immunodeficiency virus replication. *J Exp Med* 1988;168:1953–69.

162. Stevenson M, Zhang X, Volsky DJ. Down regulation of cell surface molecules during noncytopathic infection of T cells with human immunodeficiency virus. *J Virol* 1987;61:3741–8.

163. Yuille MAR, Hugunin M, John P, et al. HIV-1 infection abolishes CD4 biosynthesis but not CD4 mRNA. *J Acquired Immune Deficiency Syndromes* 1988;1:131–7.

164. Kerkau T, Schmitt-Landgraf R, Schimpl A, Wecker E. Downregulation of HLA class I antigens in HIV-1-infected cells. *AIDS Res Hum Retroviruses* 1989;6:613–20.

165. Petit AJC, Terpstra FG, Miedema F. Human immunodeficiency virus infection down-regulates HLA class II expression and induces differentiation in promonocytic U937 cells. *J Clin Invest* 1987;79:1883–9.

166. Linette GP, Hartzman RJ, Ledbetter JA, June CH. HIV-1-infected T cells show a selective signaling defect after perturbation of CD3/antigen receptor. *Science* 1988;241:573–6.

167. Chirmule N, Kalyanaraman VS, Oyaizu N, Slade HB, Pahwa S. Inhibition of functional properties of tetanus antigen-specific T-cell clones by envelope glycoprotein gp120 of human immunodeficiency virus. *Blood* 1990;75:152–9.

168. Rosenstein Y, Burakoff SJ, Herrmann SH. HIV-gp120 can block CD4-class II MHC-mediated adhesion. *J Immunol* 1990;144:526–31.

169. Clayton LK, Sieh M, Pious DA, Reinherz ER. Identification of human CD4 residues affecting class II MHC vs HIV-1 gp120 binding. *Nature* 1989;339:548–51.

170. Bank I, Chess L. Perturbation of the T4 molecule transmits a negative signal to T cells. *J Exp Med* 1985;162:1294–303.

171. Kornfield H, Cruikshank WW, Pyle SW, Berman JS, Center DM. Lymphocyte activation by HIV-1 envelope glycoprotein. *Nature* 1988;335:445–8.

172. Mittler RS, Hoffmann MK. Synergism between HIV gp120 and gp120-specific antibody in blocking human T cell activation. *Science* 1989;245:1380–2.

173. Horak ID, Popovic M, Horak EM, et al. No T-cell tyrosine protein kinase signalling or calcium mobilization after CD4 association with HIV-1 or HIV-1 gp120. *Nature* 1990;348:557–60.

174. Ruegg CL, Monell CR, Strand M. Inhibition of lymphoproliferation by a synthetic peptide with sequence identity to gp41 of human immunodeficiency virus type 1. *J Virol* 1989;63:3257–60.

175. Cianciolo GJ, Bogerd H, Snyderman R. Human retrovirus-re-

lated synthetic peptides inhibit T lymphocyte proliferation. *Immunol Lett* 1988;19:7–13.

176. Chanh TC, Kennedy RC, Kanda P. Synthetic peptides homologous to HIV transmembrane glycoprotein suppress normal human lymphocyte blastogenic response. *Cell Immunol* 1988;111:77–86.
177. Viscidi RP, Mayur K, Lederman HM, Frankel AD. Inhibition of antigen-induced lymphocyte proliferation by Tat protein from HIV-1. *Science* 1989;246:1606–8.
178. Kowalski M, Ardman B, Basiripour L, et al. Antibodies to CD4 in individuals infected with human immunodeficiency virus type 1. *Proc Natl Acad Sci USA* 1989;86:3346–50.
179. Golding H, Robey FA, Gates FT, et al. Identification of homologous regions in human immunodeficiency virus 1 gp41 and human MHC class II β1 domain. *J Exp Med* 1988;167:914–23.
180. Golding H, Shearer GM, Hillman K, et al. Common epitope in human immunodeficiency virus (HIV) I-GP41 and HLA class II elicits immunosuppressive autoantibodies capable of contributing to immune dysfunction in HIV I-infected individuals. *J Clin Invest* 1989;83:1430–5.
181. Stricker RB, McHugh TM, Moody DJ, et al. An AIDS-related cytotoxic autoantibody reacts with a specific antigen on stimulated CD4+ T cells. *Nature* 1987;327:710–3.
182. Amadori A, Chieco-Bianchi L. B cell activation and HIV-1 infection: deeds and misdeeds. *Immunol Today* 1990;11:374–9.
183. Crawford DH, Weller I, Iliescu V. Polyclonal activation of B cells in homosexual men. *Lancet* 1984;2:536–8.
184. Sieber G, Tecihmann H, Ludwig WD. B-cell function in AIDS. *Blut* 1985;51:143–4.
185. Martine-Maa O, Crabb E, Mitsuyasu RT, Fahey JL, Giorgi JV. Infection with the human immunodeficiency virus (HIV) is associated with an in vivo increase in B lymphocyte activation and immaturity. *J Immunol* 1987;138:3720–4.
186. Mizuma H, Litwin S, Zolla-Pazner S. B cell activation in HIV infection: relationship of spontaneous immunoglobulin secretion to various immunologic parameters. *Clin Exp Immunol* 1988;71:410–416.
187. McDougal JS, Hubbard M, Nicholson JKA, et al. Immune complexes in the acquired immunodeficiency syndrome (AIDS): relationship to disease manifestation, risk group, and immunologic deficit. *J Clin Immunol* 1985;4:130–5.
188. Euler HH, Kern P, Loffler H, et al. Precipitable immune complexes in healthy homosexual men, acquired immune deficiency syndrome and related lymphadenopathy syndrome. *Clin Exp Immunol* 1985;59:267–75.
189. Lightfoot M, Folks T, Redfield R, et al. Circulating IgA immune complexes in AIDS. *Immunol Invest* 1985;14:341–5.
190. Bost KL, Hahn BH, Saag MS, Shaw GM, Weigent DA, Blalock JE. Individuals infected with HIV possess antibodies against IL-2. *Immunology* 1988;65:611–5.
191. Stricker RB, Abrams DI, Corash L, Shuman MA. Target platelet antigen in homosexual men with immune thrombocytopenia. *N Engl J Med* 1985;313:1375–80.
192. McGinniss MH, Macher AM, Rook AH, Alter HJ. Red cell autoantibodies in patients with acquired immune deficiency syndrome. *Transfusion* 1986;26:405–9.
193. Amadori A, Zamarchi R, Ciminale V, et al. HIV-1-specific B cell activation. A major constituent of spontaneous B cell activation during HIV-1 infection. *J Immunol* 1989;143:2146–52.
194. Montagnier L, Gruest J, Chamaret S, et al. Adaption of lymph-

195. Pahwa S, Pahwa R, Saxinger C, et al. Influence of the human T-lymphotropic virus/lymphadenopathy-associated virus on functions of human lymphocytes: evidence for immunosuppressive effects and polyclonal B-cell activation by banded viral preparations. *Proc Natl Acad Sci USA* 1986;83:9124–8.
196. Schnittman SM, Lane HC, Higgins SE, et al. Direct polyclonal activation of human B lymphocytes by the acquired immune deficiency syndrome virus. *Science* 1986;233:1084–6.
197. Janoff EN, Douglas JM, Gabriel AT, et al. Class-specific antibody response to pneumococcal capsular polysaccharides in men infected with human immunodeficiency virus type 1. *J Infect Dis* 1988;158:983–9.
198. Janoff EN, Smith PD, Blaser MJ. Acute antibody responses to *Giardia lamblia* are depressed in patients with AIDS. *J Infect Dis* 1988;157:798–804.
199. Luft DJ, Conley R, Remington J. Outbreak of central nervous system toxoplasmosis in Western Europe and North America. *Lancet* 1983;1:781–3.
200. Roberts CJ. Coccidioidomycosis in acquired immune deficiency syndrome. Depressed humoral as well as cellular immunity. *Am J Med* 1984;76:734–6.
201. Dylewski J, Chan S, Merigan TC. Absence of detectable IgM antibody during cytomegalovirus disease in patients with AIDS. *N Engl J Med* 1983;309:493–7.
202. Kekow J, Wachsman W, McCutchan JA, Gross WL, Zachariah M, Carson DA, Lotz M. Transforming growth factor-β and suppression of humoral responses in HIV infection. *J Clin Invest* 1991;87:1010–16.
203. Birx DL, Redfield RR, Tosato G. Defective regulation of Epstein-Barr virus infection in patients with acquired immunodeficiency syndrome (AIDS) or AIDS-related disorders. *N Engl J Med* 1986;314:874–9.
204. Sumaya CV, Boswell RN, Ench Y. Enhanced serological and virological findings of Epstein-Barr virus in patients with AIDS and AIDS-related complex. *J Infect Dis* 1986;154:864–70.
205. Rinaldo CR, Kingsley LA, Lyter DW, et al. Association of HTLV-III with Epstein-Barr virus infection and abnormalities of T lymphocytes in homosexual men. *J Infect Dis* 1986;154:556–61.
206. Ziegler JL, Miner RC, Rosenbaum E. Outbreak of Burkitt's like lymphoma in homosexual men. Clinical and immunologic findings. *Lancet* 1982;2:631–3.
207. Levine AM, Meyer PR, Begandy MK. Development of B cell lymphoma in homosexual men. Clinical and immunologic findings. *Ann Intern Med* 1984;100:7–13.
208. Pearson G. Epstein-Barr virus: immunology. In: Klein G, ed. *Viral oncology.* Raven Press; New York, 1980;739–68.
209. Casareale D, Sinangil F, Hedenskog M, et al. Establishment of retrovirus-, Epstein-Barr virus-positive B-lymphocytoblastoid cell lines derived from individuals at risk for acquired immune deficiency syndrome (AIDS). *AIDS Res* 1984;1:253–70.
210. Shiramizu B, McGrath MS. Molecular pathogenesis of AIDS-associated non-Hodgkin's lymphoma. *Hematol Oncol Clin North Am* 1991;5:323–30.
211. Rieckmann P, Poli G, Kerle JH, Fauci AS. Activated B lymphocytes from human immunodeficiency virus-infected individuals induce virus expression in infected T cells and a premonocytic cell line, U1. *J Exp Med* 1991;173:1–5.

AIDS and Other Manifestations of HIV Infection,
Second Edition, Edited by Gary P. Wormser.
Raven Press, Ltd., New York © 1992.

CHAPTER 12

Serological Factors Associated with HIV Infection

Russell H. Tomar

Human immunodeficiency virus (HIV) infection is clinically latent for years before the diagnosis of acquired immunodeficiency syndrome (AIDS) is evident. The CD4 lymphocyte level is the best studied and most accepted single assay for monitoring the course of infection and the response to therapy. However, it is quite variable and alone leaves much to be desired in determining the course of infection in any one person. Thus, additions to or substitutions for CD4 counts would be welcome. Several host-derived markers have been studied. These have provided insight into the pathogenesis of AIDS and have helped to guide and measure therapeutic interventions.

This chapter will concentrate on six markers: β-2 microglobulin, neopterin, soluble interleukin-2 (IL-2) receptors, antilymphocyte antibodies, paraproteins, and inhibitors of lymphocyte proliferation. Measurement of the first two provide similar predictive values; the last four have been investigated in some detail in our laboratory. Other less well studied factors will be mentioned only briefly. For more details on antilymphocyte antibodies, paraproteins, and serum inhibitors, the reader is referred to reference 1.

β-2 MICROGLOBULIN

β-2 Microglobulin is a 11,800-dalton polypeptide that appears to be the primordial precursor of the immunoglobulin domain. It is coded for on chromosome 15(q21-22). It serves as the light or nonspecific structural chain of class I antigens of the human major histocompatibility complex (MHC). β-2 Microglobulin is present throughout the body on most nucleated cells but in greatest density on lymphoid cells and especially T lympho-

cytes (2). Its function is unknown but there is some recent information suggesting a role in presenting antigens to T cells through its interactions with the antigen-specific MHC chain (3,3a).

Since both polyclonal and monoclonal antibodies to β-2 microglobulin are readily available, many immunoassays have been devised to measure the soluble form of this protein. Radioimmunoassays, enzyme-linked immunoassays, and fluorescence polarization immunoassays are all commercially available. Reference values among assays differ somewhat. Measurement of serum β-2 microglobulin has proved useful in some transplantation centers in monitoring the development of organ rejection and its reversal (4). Serum β-2 microglobulin is often elevated in inflammatory disorders such as rheumatoid arthritis (5), systemic lupus erythematosus (SLE) (6), Sjögren's syndrome (7), and Crohn's disease (8) and in lymphoproliferative disorders including multiple myeloma (9,10), B-cell lymphoma (11), and chronic lymphocytic leukemia (12).

Zolla-Pazner and her associates (13) were among the first to suggest that serum β-2 microglobulin determinations might be useful as a surrogate marker for AIDS before HIV had been isolated and an anti-HIV test developed. Many studies have confirmed that serum β-2 microglobulin increases in HIV infection. Most investigations indicate that levels increase as the disease progresses (14–21). In one study, serum β-2 microglobulin decreased in conjunction with clinical improvement on zidovudine therapy (22). Levels in the cerebrospinal fluid (CSF) may be determined and are often increased in HIV infection of the CNS, especially in those individuals with dementia (23–25). There are relatively few comparisons of the predictive value of β-2 microglobulin with neopterin, and either or both with CD4 lymphocyte counts. The information that is available suggests that

R. H. Tomar: University of Wisconsin Hospitals and Clinics, Madison, Wisconsin 53792.

β-2 microglobulin may be slightly less reliable than neopterin and that neither is quite as reliable as CD4 values (15,25). The assay is available in kit form and is relatively easy to perform and certainly less costly than determination of the CD4 cell count.

NEOPTERIN

Neopterin is emerging as an excellent marker of both macrophage activation and infection by HIV. Neopterin is produced in activated macrophages from guanosine triphosphate (GTP) during the biosynthesis of tetrahydrobiopterin. γ-Interferon has been shown to be an excellent neopterin producer as it activates macrophages (26). Urinary and serum neopterin levels increase concurrently with the appearance of a number of malignancies (27).

Neopterin may be measured in serum or other body fluids such as urine or CSF by either high-performance liquid chromatography (HPLC) or immunoassay, but is generally done by radioimmunoassay. Urinary levels of neopterin mirror serum values, and in most cases either may be measured (27–30).

Serum neopterin is increased in HIV-infected individuals when compared with healthy heterosexuals, uninfected homosexual men, or uninfected intravenous drug users. In addition, the level of neopterin appears to increase as HIV infection progresses (27,31–36).

Although there is evidence for local production of neopterin, cerebrospinal values of neopterin are closely related to those in serum. At the time of this writing, it is not clear if CSF levels increase in AIDS dementia (36).

Use of neopterin measurements adds to the predictive value of CD4 cell counts. Neopterin alone may be a slightly more powerful predictor of clinical course than β-2 microglobulin alone, although the difference may not be clinically significant (15). Some evidence suggests that neopterin alone is a better discriminator than CD4 lymphocyte counts alone (34). Determination of neopterin levels is only now coming into greater use in the United States, and we can expect further clarification of its role in defining the course of HIV infection.

SOLUBLE INTERLEUKIN-2 RECEPTORS

IL-2, a cytokine produced by T lymphocytes, plays a pivotal role in the proliferation of T lymphocytes and the differentiation of natural killer cells and B cells. After appropriate contact with antigen or mitogen, T lymphocytes secrete IL-2. At the same time, these cells also express the natural receptor for IL-2. The IL-2 receptor is composed of two polypeptides, a 55,000 MW chain (also known as Tac) and a 75,000 MW chain. Together these two chains form the high-affinity IL-2 receptor. Tac is

sometimes referred to as the low-affinity receptor (37,38).

The key determinants for cell proliferation are the amount of IL-2 in the surrounding millieu and the amount of IL-2 receptor on the cell surface. After IL-2 binds to its receptor, the complex is thought to be internalized, releasing a soluble form of Tac (sIL-2R) into the serum or medium. It is not clear if sIL-2R is actually derived from the 55-kd polypeptide or is produced independently, partially digested, and released as a 40–45-kd substance. IL-2 binds with great affinity to sIL-2R and the latter can be shown to inhibit the effects of the cytokine (39,40).

sIL-2R is found in supernates of activated T lymphocytes and, in lesser quantities, B lymphocytes and monocytes (40–42). Several centers have found measurement of serum sIL-2R to be of use in monitoring organ rejection or the effectiveness of therapy of selected tumors (38). In addition, serum sIL-2R may be increased in patients with non-Hodgkin's lymphoma, rheumatoid arthritis, SLE, and Sjögren's syndrome (43–45).

Soluble IL-2 receptors may be measured by immunological techniques, most commonly by enzyme immunosorbent assays. At least two commercial assays are available. We exploited the assay developed by Dr. David Nelson and his colleagues that uses two monoclonal antibodies against somewhat different epitopes of sIL-2R and builds a complex sandwich on plastic (41,46).

Several groups have confirmed our finding that sIL-2R is increased in the serum of individuals infected with HIV (46–50). We found this elevation early in the course of HIV infection and in a few patients even prior to the detection of a positive antibody test for HIV. Unfortunately, the assay is not specific for HIV and was also found to be increased—although at a lower serum level —in those at increased risk to become infected with HIV. We interpret this to mean that if significant immune activation takes place, sIL-2R is likely to be elevated in serum. In a series of in vitro experiments, we could find no increase of sIL-2R in supernates of activated lymphocytes from HIV-positive subjects. Furthermore, an increase in T lymphocytes expressing surface Tac is not common in HIV infection (51,52). Thus, the cellular origin of sIL-2R in AIDS is not likely to be T lymphocytes. Several investigators have now demonstrated that the most likely source of serum sIL-2R in HIV infection is the monocyte/macrophage (53,54).

Investigators do not agree on whether or not sIL-2R increases as HIV-related immunodeficiency progresses (15). Our data suggest that this is not the case (49). Moreover, the predictive value of serum sIL-2R versus other markers is not settled. We found it of lesser use than absolute CD4 counts or serum inhibitors (see below). However, we did not compare it with neopterin or β-2 microglobulin in predictive value and some workers believe it to be similar to β-2 microglobulin (15). CSF measurement for sIL-2R has not been consistently predictive of either systemic or CNS HIV infection (55,56).

While sIL-2R may bind and thus inactivate IL-2, there is no evidence supporting a pathogenetic role in the development of AIDS.

ANTILYMPHOCYTE ANTIBODIES

Antilymphocyte antibodies (ALA) is a rather generic term for antibodies against a number of different determinants expressed on lymphocytes. Thus, ALA may be classified as against a particular cell type or subset, a specific determinant that may also be present on other cells, or even a specific cell. ALA are most commonly seen in individuals receiving heterologous tissues such as transplant and blood products and pregnant women. The most important determinant in these cases seems to be against antigens of the major histocompatibility locus (57).

ALA have been described in several pathological states including primary immunodeficiency states and (most prominently) SLE (57,58). The significance of this finding is controversial, possibly because of differences in methodology and in classification of SLE. ALA have also been used therapeutically, i.e., generally murine monoclonal ALA against a specific tumor target. Interestingly, anti-murine ALA sometimes develop that interfere with the efficacy of ALA (59). It is more difficult to demonstrate human anti-human ALA, but at least in theory these might exist and influence the immune response. This background is supplied to emphasize the dearth of knowledge about ALA and about their role in the physiology and pathology of the immune system.

To date, virtually all ALA assays use as targets lymphocytes that are exposed to serum containing putative ALA. The method of readout varies from microcytotoxicity to double-labeled immunofluorescence. The results that one obtains from the various methods are usually, but not always, confirmatory. The sensitivities and specificities vary not only with the general method but with the specific laboratory protocols. We have used microcytotoxicity as well as single- and double-labeled immunofluorescence on freshly prepared lymphocytes, lymphocytes separated into several T- and B-cell components, and T- and B-cell lines. Results are comparable but by no means identical (1,60).

In 1981, we discovered that the sera of patients with AIDS had ALA when we sought a simplistic reason for the characteristic low lymphocyte counts. We used a microcytotoxicity assay adopted from the histocompatibility laboratory. Our first three patients demonstrated ALA against CD8, CD4, and B cells. In a collaborative study with Dr. Tom Spira at the Centers for Disease Control

(CDC), we successfully identified nine of ten subjects with *Pneumocystis carinii* pneumonia or Kaposi's sarcoma (KS). We found that none of the ten sera from healthy heterosexuals was positive but that two of the five other "controls" had ALA. Later we were told that both of these men developed AIDS and that our lone false negative turned out to have classical KS and was HIV negative (61).

While we developed more sophisticated procedures utilizing flow cytometry and immunofluorescence, the basic information remained the same, i.e., many HIV-infected persons had ALA, and there appeared to be no single lymphocyte or set of lymphocytes preferentially involved. ALA appear in the serum some time after infection with HIV but before the development of AIDS (49). Several groups have confirmed the presence of ALA in HIV-infected patients (62–66). However, there remains some controversy about the specificity of the target cell (64,65,67). We looked for such specificity in several different ways: by separating cells positively and negatively and using both immunofluorescence and microcytotoxicity; by using double-labeled immunofluorescence; and by determining ALA against a number of T- and B-cell lines (60). We have not ruled out the possibility that antibodies are developed against a single, or more likely, a series of epitopes that have broad distribution, such as class II antigens of the MHC. Others have suggested this and it remains an attractive hypothesis (67).

ALA appear later than sIL-2R in the serum of HIV-infected individuals. There is a theoretical reason for ascribing a role in pathogenesis to ALA but this remains speculative.

PARAPROTEINS

In this instance, we define *paraprotein* as monoclonal or oligoclonal immunoglobulins of restricted heterogeneity. Most commonly the term paraprotein brings to mind multiple myeloma or Waldenström's macroglobulinemia or monoclonal gammopathy of unknown significance. These proteins are generally present in rather large quantities and by themselves may cause pathological consequences. In the first two conditions, they are the products of malignant cells that themselves cause harmful effects.

The paraproteins seen in HIV-infected individuals resemble more those seen in some primary immunodeficiencies and occasionally in other conditions. They are present in small quantities—and are thus often difficult to identify—and are likely the result of immune dysfunction rather than a truly malignant cell. However, as in the case of CSF oligoclonal immunoglobulins in multiple sclerosis, these serum paraproteins may also serve as a marker of disease and provide further evidence of the immunological apoplexy seen in AIDS.

The most common methods of seeking paraproteins are serum electrophoresis, immunoelectrophoresis, and immunofixation. The sensitivity of these methods varies with the medium, the titer of antisera used, the sensitivity of the detection system, and the experience of the operator. In general, immunofixation is the most sensitive for detecting small quantities of paraproteins. There are other methods that may be even more sensitive such as capillary electrophoresis or isoelectric focusing, but these are not commonly used in clinical laboratories.

We and others have found that a significant number of individuals infected with HIV demonstrate serum paraproteins (68–72). This occurs after the initial phases of infection, and the amount and number of subjects with positive findings does not seem to increase as the disease progresses (49). While these paraproteins are present in only small quantities, an occasional patient has been described with significant, even myeloma-like, levels (69). We have found that most of the paraproteins are IgG-κ. Ng et al. (69) have shown that most are IgG1 and that these are directed against antigens present in HIV. From these data, we believe that the oligoclonal and monoclonal immunoglobulins in HIV-infected subjects represent a rather brisk and somewhat unusual (and perhaps ineffective) antibody response to HIV. Whether the large quantities of one or few types of antibody are due to defects in immunoregulation, or the presence of continual antigen exposure, or both, is uncertain. Oligoclonal proteins have also been demonstrated in the CSF of HIV-infected subjects (73). The clinical significance of this finding is not certain.

Mono- or oligoclonal gammopathies can be found after HIV infection and before the development of AIDS. As with ALA, their presence indicates a pathologic state when compared with healthy controls, but they are neither sensitive nor specific enough to add predictive value to other markers. There is no evidence to suggest that paraproteins contribute to the various clinical pathological conditions associated with AIDS.

INHIBITORS

Sera from persons infected with HIV markedly inhibit the proliferation of lymphocytes from healthy individuals (49,74–78). The suppressive effect increases as HIV infection progresses (49). The cause and mechanism of inhibition are unclear. Suppressive sera have been described in other pathological conditions, but the methodologies of study vary sufficiently to make comparisons difficult.

Our assay, which is similar to those used by others examining HIV-infected individuals, is rather straightforward. We use 100,000–200,000 cells/well from a Ficoll-Hypaque gradient. Early on we discovered that the serum-to-cell ratio, as well as the amount of mitogen, were critical to obtain consistent results. Thus, our experiments usually involve 20% serum in a total volume of 200–250 μl and a suboptimal amount of mitogen, usually phytohemogglutinin (PHA). Sera from three healthy donors are studied and their mean net counts set as 100% proliferation. Sera from HIV-infected individuals are compared to this standard. Tritiated thymidine is added on day 3 of a 4-day culture and incorporation into DNA measured in a scintillation counter (74). Others have measured production of IL-2 as an endpoint (76,77).

In our system, almost all patients with the diagnosis of AIDS have serum inhibitors and the presence of inhibitors is a poor prognostic sign. We believe that there is more than one inhibitor since we found several patterns when we used cell lines as targets. Some sera inhibited all lines, some one set, others another set, and finally some sera inhibited no cell lines but still inhibited mitogen-driven peripheral blood lymphocytes. In addition, we had shown that some of the suppression of certain sera was reversed by cyclooxygenase inhibitors such as indomethacin or ibuprofen (79). Thus, we believe that there are at least three inhibitors, one of which releases prostaglandin from cells in culture.

The inhibitory activity is dilutable by sera from healthy subjects and the suppressive serum must be present within the first 48 hours of culture. IL-2, even in pharmacological doses, has no effect on reversing inhibition (1,79). It is likely that the inhibitors are cytokines and/or viral products, but their identity is not known at this time.

The role of suppressive factors is unknown. Potentially they have the effect of augmenting immune incompetence. Conceptually, it may be that these products reduce the viral load by suppressing cell activation and hence viral activation. Thus, investigators attempting to reverse inhibition must be aware of this potentially undesirable effect. In one set of experiments on a single subject, we were able to increase CD4 cell levels significantly with plasmapheresis. At the same time, serum suppressor levels decreased (1,80). Subsequently, we have determined that monkeys infected with simian immunodeficiency virus (SIV) also have serum inhibitors.

The incidence of serum inhibitors increases as HIV clinically progresses (49). Thus, their presence is a good guide for prognosis.

OTHER FACTORS

A number of other serum factors have been measured that may have some predictive value and/or provide insight into the pathogenesis of HIV infection. However, studies on these are so few in number that judgements on their ultimate clinical role cannot be made. Antibodies to collagen have an increased incidence, and IL-6 is present in larger quantities in HIV infection. The presence of anticollagen antibodies may be another example of immunological apoplexy leading to breakthrough of measurable concentrations of autoantibodies (81). The increase in IL-6 is provocative since so many functions have been ascribed to that interesting molecule (82). IL-6 may be at least partly involved in the paraproteinemia described earlier, since it stimulates the production of immunoglobulins and has been implicated as a trigger for overproduction of monoclonal proteins in multiple myeloma. One report has shown a direct correlation between serum levels of IL-6 and that of IL-2R in all stages of HIV infection (82a).

Tumor necrosis factor (TNF/cachectin) was increased in nine of nine AIDS patients (83). It is attractive to attribute the weight loss associated with AIDS to this cytokine. Serum levels of soluble CD4 and CD8 have been measured and shown to be elevated in HIV-infected individuals (84). In addition, infection with HIV seems to have effects on the serum concentrations of a number of trace elements (85). It is too early to judge the importance of these compounds in predicting the course of HIV infection; their role in the pathogenesis of HIV infection is also unknown.

CONCLUSIONS

Before HIV was determined to be the cause of AIDS, there was an active search to find some way of identifying those who had the disease. Measurement of both antibodies to HIV and HIV antigens or use of polymerase chain reaction (PCR) to find provirus or virus provide powerful tools to answer this question. Now the focus has shifted towards an attempt to predict when those infected with HIV will develop AIDS. In this chapter, we have discussed several possible analytes that may be examined in serum. Our own investigations suggest that elevation of sII-2 receptors is a sensitive indicator of HIV infection, but that the presence of measurable lymphocyte proliferation inhibitors is a better predictor for the development of AIDS. Antilymphocyte antibodies and paraproteins become abnormal in the time interval between the onset of elevation of sII-2R and the first detection of inhibitors.

Work done by others suggests that neopterin and β-2 microglobulin are even more sensitive than sII-2R for detecting those infected with HIV (15). Furthermore, the absolute amount of these analytes seems to be predictive of the appearance of AIDS, i.e., HIV-infected patients with higher levels are more likely to develop AIDS earlier than those with lower levels. The individual variations in time to development of AIDS may be remarkably wide. Both lower and higher levels appear to reflect therapeutic

responses to zidovudine therapy, and elevated β-2 microglobulin in the CSF has been associated with AIDS dementia.

Whether or not any one or a combination of several of these determinants are as predictive as the absolute CD4 lymphocyte count remains controversial and will not be resolved until several well-controlled prospective studies are completed. The existing data are promising enough to suggest that neopterin or β-2 microglobulin will prove to be as useful as CD4 cell counts. These assays are more easily performed and a good deal less costly. With the possible exception of sII-2R, it is unlikely that the other factors, as currently measured, will have much practical value in following patients infected with HIV. A significant exception might be the inhibitory factors, were they better understood and able to be assayed in a less cumbersome and less expensive manner.

Speculation on the role each of these factors might play in the pathogenesis of AIDS is beyond the scope of this chapter. Together they indicate the presence of an activated and deregulated immune system with secondary consequences of autoimmunity and immunodeficiency. A better understanding of these processes will add to our comprehension of the pathogenesis of AIDS and enhance efforts to treat this disease.

REFERENCES

1. Miller LE, Hennig AK, John PA, Kloster BE, Tomar RH. Serological factors in the pathogenesis of AIDS. In: Wormser GP, Stahl RE, Bottone EJ, eds. *AIDS and Other Manifestations of HIV Infection.* Park Ridge, NJ: Noyes Publications, 1987;380–97.
2. Williams AF, Barclay AN. The immunoglobulin superfamily-domains for cell surface recognition. *Annu Rev Immunol* 1988;6:381–405.
3. Perarnau B, Siegrist C, Gillet A, Vincent C, Kimura S, Lemonnier FA. Beta-2 microglobulin restriction of antigen presentation. *Nature* 1990;346:751–4.
3a.Kozlowski S, Takeshita T, Boehncke WH, et al. Excess β2 microglobulin promoting functional peptide association with purified soluble class I MHC molecules. *Nature* 1991;349:74–7.
4. Bethea M, Forman DT. Beta-2 microglobulin: its significance and clinical usefulness. *Ann Clin Lab Sci* 1990;20:163–8.
5. Crisp AJ, Coughlan RJ, Mackintosh D, Clark B, Panayi GS. β-2-microglobulin plasma levels reflect disease activity in rheumatoid arthritis. *J Rheumatol* 1983;10:954–6.
6. Weissel M, Scherak O, Fritzche H, Kolarz G. Serum β-2 microglobulin and SLE. *Arthritis Rheum* 1976;19:968.
7. Strom T, Evrin PK, Karlsson A. Serum beta-2-microglobulin Sjögren's syndrome. *Scand J Rheumatol* 1978;7:97–100.
8. Descos L, Andre C, Beorchia S, Vincent C, Revillard JP. Serum levels of β-2 microglobulin—A new marker of activity in Crohn's disease. *N Engl J Med* 1979;301:440.
9. Morell A, Riesen W. Serum β-2 microglobulin, serum creatinine and bone marrow plasma cells in benign and malignant monoclonal gammopathy. *Acta Haematol* 1980;64:87–93.
10. Bataille R, Durie BGM, Grenier J, Sany J. Prognostic factors and staging in multiple myeloma: a reappraisal. *J Clin Oncol* 1986;4:80–7.
11. Cassuto JP, Krebs BP, Viot G, Dujardin P, Masseyeff R. β-2 microglobulin, a tumour marker of lymphoproliferative disorder. *Lancet* 1978;2:950.
12. Simonsson B, Wibell L, Nilsson K. β-2 microglobulin in chronic lymphocytic leukaemia. *Scand J Haematol* 1980;24:174–80.

13. Zolla-Pazner S, Des Jarlais DC, Friedman SR, et al. Nonrandom development of immunologic abnormalities after infection with human immunodeficiency virus: implications for immunologic classification of the disease. *Proc Natl Acad Sci USA* 1987;84:5404–8.

14. Calabrese LH, Proffitt MR, Gupta MK, et al. Serum beta-2 microglobulin and interferon in homosexual males: relationship to clinical findings and serologic status to the human T lymphotropic virus (HTLV-III). *AIDS Res* 1984/5;1:423–38.

15. Fahey JL, Taylor JMG, Detels R, et al. The prognostic value of cellular and serologic markers in infection with human immunodeficiency virus type 1. *N Engl J Med* 1990;322:166–72.

16. Franzetti F, Cavalli G, Foppa CU, Amprino MC, Gaido P, Lazzarin A. Raised serum beta-2 microglobulin levels in different stages of human immunodeficiency virus infection. *J Clin Lab Immunol* 1988;27:133–7.

17. Howard MR, McVerry BA, Cooper EH. A longitudinal study of serum beta-2 microglobulin levels in haemophilia. *Clin Lab Haematol* 1988;10:427–34.

18. Morfeldt-Manson J, Julander I, von Stedingk LV, Wasserman J, Nilsson B. Elevated serum beta-2 microglobulin—a prognostic marker for development of AIDS among patients with persistent generalized lymphadenopathy. *Infection* 1988;16:109–10.

19. Anderson RE, Lang W, Shiboski S, Royce R, Jewell N, Winkelstein W, Jr. Use of beta-2 microglobulin level and CD4 lymphocyte count to predict development of acquired immunodeficiency syndrome in persons with human immunodeficiency virus infection. *Arch Intern Med* 1990;150:73–7.

20. Hofmann B, Wang YX, Cumberland WG, Detels R, Bozorgmehri M, Fahey JL. Serum beta-2 microglobulin level increases in HIV infection: relation to seroconversion CD4 T-cell fall and prognosis. *AIDS* 1990;4:207–14.

21. Moss AR, Bacchetti P, Osmond D, et al. Seropositivity for HIV and the development of AIDS or AIDS related condition: three year follow up of the San Francisco General Hospital cohort. *Br Med J [Clin Res]* 1988;296:745–50.

22. Jacobson MA, Abrams DI, Volberding PA, et al. Serum beta-2 microglobulin decreases in patients with AIDS or ARC treated with azidothymidine. *J Infect Dis* 1989;159:1029–36.

23. Elovaara I, Iivanainen M, Poutiainen E, Valle SL, Weber T, Suni J, Lahdevirta J. CSF and serum beta-2 microglobulin in HIV infection related to neurological dysfunction. *Acta Neurol Scand* 1989;79:81–7.

24. Brew BJ, Bhalla RB, Fleisher M, et al. Cerebrospinal fluid beta-2 microglobulin in patients infected with human immunodeficiency virus. *Neurology* 1989;39:830–4.

25. Sonnerborg AB, von Stedingk LV, Hansson LO, Strannegard O. Elevated neopterin and beta-2 microglobulin levels in blood and cerebrospinal fluid occur early in HIV-1 infection. *AIDS* 1989;3:277–83.

26. Werner ER, Werner-Felmayer G, Fuchs D, et al. Tetrahydrobiopterin biosynthetic activities in human macrophages, fibroblasts, THP-1 and T 24 cells. GTP-cyclohydrolase I is stimulated by interferon-gamma, and B-pyruvoyl tetrahydropterin synthase and sepiapterin reductase are constitutively present. *J Biol Chem* 1990;265:3189–92.

27. Wachter H, Fuchs D, Hausen A, Reibnegger G, Werner ER. Neopterin as a marker for activation of cellular immunity: immunological basis and clinical application. *Adv Clin Chem* 1989;27:81–141.

28. Fuchs D, Jaeger H, Popescu M, et al. Comparison of serum and urine neopterin concentrations in patients with HIV-1 infection. *Clin Chim Acta* 1990;187:125–30.

29. Reibnegger G, Fuchs D, Goedert JJ, et al. Urinary neopterin concentrations and T-cell subset data in HIV-1 infection. *Klin Wochenschr* 1990;68:43–8.

30. Fuchs D, Milstien S, Kramer A, et al. Urinary neopterin concentrations vs. total neopterins for clinical utility. *Clin Chem* 1989;35:2305–7.

31. Fuchs D, Spira TJ, Hausen A, et al. Neopterin as a predictive marker for disease progression in human immunodeficiency virus type 1 infection. *Clin Chem* 1989;35:1746–9.

32. Kramer A, Wiktor SZ, Fuchs D, et al. Neopterin: a predictive marker of acquired immune deficiency syndrome in human immunodeficiency virus infection. *J Acquired Immune Deficiency Syndrome* 1989;2:291–6.

33. Bogner JR, Matuschke A, Heinrich B, Eberle E, Goebel FD. Serum neopterin levels as predictor of AIDS. *Klin Wochenschr* 1988;66:1015–8.

34. Melmed RN, Taylor JM, Detels R, Bozorgmehri M, Fahey JL. Serum neopterin changes in HIV-infected subjects: indicator of significant pathology, CD4 T cell changes, and the development of AIDS. *J Acquired Immune Deficiency Syndrome* 1989;2:70–6.

35. Fuchs D, Banekovich M, Hausen A, et al. Neopterin estimation compared with the ratio of T-cell subpopulations in persons infected with human immunodeficiency virus-1. *Clin Chem* 1988;34:2415–7.

36. Fuchs D, Chiodi F, Albert J, et al. Neopterin concentrations in cerebrospinal fluid and serum of individuals infected with HIV-1. *AIDS* 1989;3:285–8.

37. Smith KA. The interleukin 2 receptor. *Annu Rev Cell Biol* 1989;5:397–425.

38. Waldmann TA. The multichain interleukin 2 receptor. A target for immunotherapy in lymphoma, autoimmune disorders and organ allografts. *JAMA* 1990;12:272–4.

39. Nelson DL, Kurman CC, Fritz ME, Boutin B, Rubin LA. The production of soluble and cellular interleukin-2 receptors by cord blood mononuclear cells following in vitro activation. *Pediatr Res* 1986;20:136–9.

40. Treiger BF, Leonard WJ, Svetlik P, Rubin LA, Nelson DL, Green WC. A secreted form of the human interleukin-2 receptor encoded by an "anchor minus" cDNA. *J Immunol* 1986;136:4099–105.

41. Nelson DL, Rubin LA, Kurman CC, Fritz ME, Boutin B. An analysis of the cellular requirements for the production of soluble interleukin-2 receptors in vitro. *J Clin Immunol* 1986;6:114–20.

42. Rubin LA, Kurman CC, Fritz ME, et al. Soluble interleukin 2 receptors are released from activated human lymphoid cells in vitro. *J Immunol* 1985;135:3172–7.

43. Manoussakis MN, Papadopoulos GK, Drosos AA, Moutsopoulos HM. Soluble interleukin-2 receptor molecules in the serum of patients with autoimmune diseases. *Clin Immunol Immunopathol* 1989;50:321–32.

44. Chilosi M, Semenzato G, Vinante F, et al. Increased levels of soluble interleukin-2 receptor in non-Hodgkin's lymphomas. *Am J Clin Pathol* 1989;92:186–91.

45. Symons JA, Wood NC, Di Giovine FS, Duff GW. Soluble IL-2 receptor in rheumatoid arthritis correlation with disease activity, IL-1 and IL-2 inhibition. *J Immunol* 1988;141:2612–8.

46. Kloster BE, John PA, Miller LE, et al. Soluble interleukin-2 receptors are elevated in patients with AIDS or at risk of developing AIDS. *Clin Immunol Immunopathol* 1987;45:440–6.

47. Honda M, Kitamura K, Matsuda K, et al. Soluble IL-2 receptor in AIDS correlation of its serum level with the classification of HIV-induced diseases and its characterization. *J Immunol* 1989;142:4248–55.

48. Prince HE, Kleinman S, Williams AE. Soluble IL-2 receptor levels in serum from blood donors seropositive for HIV. *J Immunol* 1988;140:1139–41.

49. Tomar RH, Hennig AK, Oates RP, Yuille MA, John PA. Serum factors in the progression of human immunodeficiency virus type 1 infection to AIDS. *J Clin Lab Anal* 1990;4:218–23.

50. Schulte C, Meurer M. Soluble IL-2 receptor serum levels—a marker for disease progression in patients with HIV-1 infection. *Arch Dermatol Res* 1989;281:299–303.

51. Prince HE, Kermani-Arab V, Fahey JL. Depressed interleukin-2 receptor expression in acquired immune deficiency and lymphadenopathy syndromes. *J Immunol* 1984;133:1313–7.

52. Lang JM, Coumaros G, Levy S, et al. Elevated serum levels of soluble interleukin-2 receptors in HIV infection: no correlation with activated T cells. *Nouv Rev Fr Hematol* 1989;31:9–11.

53. Allen JB, McCartney-Francis N, Smith PD, et al. Expression of interleukin-2 receptors by monocytes from patients with acquired immunodeficiency syndrome and induction of monocyte interleukin-2 receptors by human immunodeficiency virus in vitro. *J Clin Invest* 1990;85:192–9.

54. Tsunetsugu-Yokota Y, Honda M. Effect of cytokines on HIV release and IL-2 receptor alpha expression in monocytic cell lines. *J Acquired Immune Deficiency Syndrome* 1990;3:511–6.

55. Griffin DE, McArthur JC, Cornblath DR. Soluble interleukin-2 receptor and soluble CD8 in serum and cerebrospinal fluid during

human immunodeficiency virus-associated neurologic disease. *J Neuroimmunol* 1990;28:97–109.

56. Gallo P, Piccinno MG, Pagni S, et al. Immune activation in multiple sclerosis study of IL-2, sIL-2R, and gamma-IFN levels in serum and cerebrospinal fluid. *J Nerol Sci* 1989;92:9–15.

57. DeHoratius RJ. Lymphocytotoxic antibodies. *Prog Immunol* 1980;4:151–74.

58. Morimoto C, Reinherz EL, Distaso JA, Steinberg AD, Schlossman SF. Relationship between SLE T cell subsets, anti-T cell antibodies, and cell function. *J Clin Invest* 1984;73:689–700.

59. Schroeder TJ, Munda R, Pedersen SH, Hurtubise PE, Alexander JW, First MR. Failure of orthoclone OKT3 retreatment in a pancreas transplant recipient with anti-murine antibodies. *J Clin Lab Anal* 1990;4:99–101.

60. Tomar RH, John PA, Hennig AK, Kloster B. Cellular targets of antilymphocyte antibodies in AIDS and LAS. *Clin Immunol Immunopathol* 1985;37:37–47.

61. Kloster BE, Tomar RH, Spira TJ. Lymphocytotoxic antibodies in the acquired immune deficiency syndrome (AIDS). *Clin Immunol Immunopathol* 1984;30:330–5.

62. Dorsett BH, Cronin W, Ioachin HC. Presence and prognostic significance of antilymphocyte antibodies in symptomatic and asymptomatic human immunodeficiency virus infection. *Arch Intern Med* 1990;150:1025–8.

63. Daniel V, Weimer R, Schimpf K, Opelz G. Autoantibodies against CD4- and CD8-positive T lymphocytes in HIV-infected hemophilia patients. *Vox Sang* 1989;57:172–6.

64. Daniel V, Schimpf K, Opelz G. Lymphocyte autoantibodies and alloantibodies in HIV-positive hemophilia patients. *Clin Exp Immunol* 1989;75:178–83.

65. Pruzanski W, Jacobs H, Laing LR. Lymphocytotoxic antibodies against peripheral blood B and T lymphocytes in homosexuals with AIDS and ARC. *AIDS Res* 1984;1:211–20.

66. Ozturk GE, Kohler PE, Horsborgh CR Jr, Kirpatrick CH. The significance of antilymphocyte antibodies in patients with acquired immune deficiency syndrome (AIDS) and their sexual partners. *J Clin Immunol* 1987;7:130–9.

67. De La Barrera S, Fainboim L, Lugo S, Picchio GR, Muchinik GR, DeBracco MME. Anti-class II antibodies in AIDS patients and AIDS risk groups. *Immunology* 1987;62:599–604.

68. Heriot K, Hallquist AE, Tomar RH. Paraproteinemia in patients with acquired immunodeficiency syndrome (AIDS) or lymphadenopathy syndrome (LAS). *Clin Chem* 1985;31:1224–6.

69. Ng VL, Ohen KH, Hwang KM, Khayam-Bashi H, McGrath MS. The clinical significance of human immunodeficiency virus type 1-associated paraproteins. *Blood* 1989;74:2471–5.

70. Papadopoulos NM, Lane HC, Costello R, Moutsopoulos HM, Masur H, Gelmann EP. Oligoclonal immunoglobulins in patients with the acquired immunodeficiency syndrome. *Clin Immunol Immunopathol* 1985;35:43–6.

71. Kouns DM, Marty AM, Sharpe RW. Oligoclonal bands in serum protein electrophoretograms of individuals with human immunodeficiency virus antibodies. *JAMA* 1986;256:2343.

72. Crapper RM, Deam DR, Mackay IR. Paraproteinemias in homosexual men with HIV infection: lack of association with abnormal clinical or immunologic findings. *Am J Clin Pathol* 1987;88:348–51.

73. Grimaldi LME, Castagna A, Lazzorin A, et al. Oligoclonal IgG bands in cerebrospinal fluid and serum during asymptomatic human immunodeficiency virus infections. *Ann Neurol* 1988;24:277–9.

74. Hennig AK, Tomar RH. Inhibition of in vitro lymphocyte proliferation by serum from acquired immune deficiency syndrome patients depends on the ratio of cells to serum in culture. *Clin Immunol Immunopathol* 1984;33:258–67.

75. Donnelly RP, Tsang KY, Galbraith GMP, Wallace JI. Inhibition of interleukin-2-induced T-cell proliferation by sera from patients with acquired immune deficiency syndrome. *J Clin Immunol* 1986;6:92–101.

76. Farmer JL, Gottlieb AA, Nishihara T. Inhibition of interleukin-2 production and expression of the interleukin-2 receptors by plasma from acquired immune deficiency syndrome patients. *Clin Immunol Immunopathol* 1986;38:235–43.

77. Siegel JP, Djeu JY, Stocks NI, Masur H, Gelmann EP, Quinnan GV Jr. Sera from patients with the acquired immune deficiency syndrome inhibit production of interleukin-2 by normal lymphocytes. *J Clin Invest* 1985;75:1957–64.

78. Cunningham-Rundles S, Michelis MA, Masur H. Serum suppression of lymphocyte activation in vitro in acquired immunodeficiency disease. *J Clin Immunol* 1983;3:2.

79. Hennig AK, John PA, Blair DC, Tomar RH. Sera from AIDS patients contain multiple factors that suppress in vitro proliferation of lymphoid cells. *J Clin Anal* 1988;2:215–9.

80. Tomar RH, Kloster BE, Lamberson HV. Plasmapheresis increases T4 lymphocytes in a patient with AIDS. *Am J Clin Pathol* 1984;81:518–21.

81. Grant MD, Weaver MS, Tsoukas C, Hoffman GW. Distribution of antibodies against denatured collagen in AIDS risk groups and homosexual AIDS patients suggests a link between autoimmunity and the immunopathogenesis of AIDS. *J Immunol* 1990;144:1241–50.

82. Breen EC, Rezai AR, Nakajima K, et al. Infection with HIV is associated with elevated IL-6 levels and production. *J Immunol* 1990;144:480–4.

82a. Honda M, Kitamura K, Mizutani Y, et al. Quantitative analysis of serum IL-6 and its correlation with increased levels of serum IL-2R in HIV-induced diseases. *J Immunol* 1990;145:4059–64.

83. Lahdevirta J, Maury J, Teppo AM, Repo H. Elevated levels of circulating cachectin/tumor necrosis factor in patients with acquired immunodeficiency syndrome. *Am J Med* 1988;85:289–90.

84. Reddy MM, Vodian M, Grieco MH. Effect of azidothymidine on soluble CD4 levels in patients with AIDS or AIDS-related complex. *J Clin Lab Anal* 1990;4:396–8.

85. Beck KW, Schramel P, Hedl A, Jager H, Kaboth W. Trace element concentrations in HIV infected patients. *Oncology* 1989;12[Suppl 3]:43–7.

AIDS and Other Manifestations of HIV Infection,
Second Edition, Edited by Gary P. Wormser.
Raven Press, Ltd., New York © 1992.

CHAPTER 13

Care of the Adult Patient with HIV Infection

Gary P. Wormser and Harold Horowitz

Skillful management of the HIV-infected patient involves blending common sense and compassion with up-to-date knowledge of the latest pertinent scientific discoveries. Care of HIV-infected patients is constantly changing and improving, which is reflected by objective increases in patient survival (1–3). These rapid changes impose additional challenges on the clinician for whom "routine" management often requires the use of investigational as well as approved therapies. A partial list of drugs already widely used in the care of HIV-infected patients, but that were not Food and Drug Administration (FDA) approved until well after the epidemic began, are zidovudine (AZT), aerosol and parenteral pentamidine preparations, ganciclovir, fluconazole, clofazimine, foscarnet sodium, didanosine (ddI), and interferon α-2. Diagnostic procedures and methods are also in flux, continually being tailored to the specific needs of this patient population.

Recently acquired information on the natural history of HIV infection has indicated the necessity of, and proper timing for, beginning prophylaxis for prevention of *Pneumocystis carinii* pneumonia (4–8). This single intervention will in turn have far-reaching consequences on the natural history of HIV infection and on management approaches in the years to come.

INITIAL ASSESSMENT

Table 1 outlines the initial assessment procedures (9). Although the diagnostic term AIDS is rigorously defined (albeit with several revisions) (10–12) and has been immensely helpful for surveillance in following the epidemic (especially prior to the discovery of HIV), it is of limited value to clinicians in the care of individual patients. It is preferable to think in terms of HIV infection per se, and the clinical and immunologic consequences thereof. The definition of AIDS has been principally based on events that occur secondary to a state of advanced immunodeficiency. For example, the day after the diagnosis of *Pneumocystis carinii* pneumonia is made, the patient has AIDS; the day before the patient did not, despite the same degree of immunodeficiency. If that patient had received pneumocystis prophylaxis, the diagnosis of AIDS would likely have been postponed for several years, or perhaps never made at all, despite the likelihood of further progression of the immunodeficiency. A proposed revision of the surveillance definition (scheduled to become effective in 1992) will address this problem by incorporating the number of T-helper cells as a diagnostic criterion (13).

The most straightforward management approach for the HIV-infected patient is to focus attention on and monitor the course of HIV-induced immune deficiency. The most helpful, readily available laboratory tool to do this for adult patients is the number of helper T-cells (CD4+) in peripheral blood.

CD4+ Cell Count

CD4+ cells are expressed either as a percentage of the total lymphocyte count, or as an absolute number, which is a calculated value, derived from the percentage of CD4+ cells multiplied times the total lymphocyte count. For healthy non-HIV-infected adults, the average CD4+ cell count is approximately 1,000 cells/mm^3, but the values may range widely, from as low as approximately 500 to as high as 1,500 cells/mm^3 (14,15).

A CD4 cell count of 200/mm^3 marks an especially important point in the course of HIV-infected patients, since serious opportunistic infections infrequently occur before this level of immune deficiency is reached (5–7).

G. P. Wormser and H. Horowitz: Division of Infectious Diseases, Department of Medicine, Westchester County Medical Center, New York Medical College, Valhalla, New York 10595.

TABLE 1. *Initial assessment of HIV-infected patients[a]*

Strongly recommended for all patients
  History and complete physical examination
  Complete blood count with differential and platelet count
  Chemistry profile, including LDH, CPK, liver function tests
  CD4+ cell count and percentage
  Treponemal antibody test
  Hepatitis B surface antigen, surface antibody, and core antibody
  PPD with control skin tests
  Papanicolaou smear for female patients
  Chest roentgenogram
Tests to be considered
  Antibody titers for toxoplasma and hepatitis C virus
  Stool for ova and parasites (for homosexual men and for persons who have traveled to at-risk geographic areas)
  Serum amylase level
  Triglyceride level
  Vitamin B_{12} and folate levels
  Glucose-6-phosphate dehydrogenase enzyme level (if initiating dapsone)

[a] See ref. 9.
CPK, creatine phosphokinase; LDH, lactate dehydrogenase, PPD, purified protein derivative (of tuberculin).

A CD4 cell count of 500/mm³ is also an important juncture, since clinical benefit from the use of AZT has been demonstrated to date only for patients with counts at or below this level (16,17).

As vital as the CD4 count has become in the general management of the HIV-infected patient, there are several noteworthy limitations. First, any single determination may be aberrant (Table 2). The reasons why a particular count may be inconsistent from other values for a specific patient are not always apparent. Since the CD4 count is dependent on the total lymphocyte count, the fluctuations and variability in the total white blood cell or differential count determinations will greatly impact test results (18–20). Inappropriate storage conditions

TABLE 2. *Serial CD4+ lymphocyte counts on peripheral blood samples of two HIV-infected patients*

Patient A[a]			Patient B[b]		
Date	Count	Percentage	Date	Count	Percentage
3/88	591	30	11/88	500	24
10/88	277	15	4/89	406	23
12/88	724	35	8/89	301	21
4/89	445	24	11/89	604	24
7/89	554	31	4/90	332	28
12/89	402	26	8/90	237	22
4/90	426	22	10/90	342	19
8/90	166	22	2/91	244	19
9/90	349	27			
12/90	408	24			
3/91	297	28			
8/91	353	22			

[a] AZT begun 7/88.
[b] AZT begun 12/88.

and delayed transportation of blood samples to the laboratory may adversely affect CD4 lymphocyte determinations (21). In addition, factors such as test methodology, quality control, and type of laboratory equipment employed may influence the accuracy of the test (22).

Stress, exercise, season, use of exogenous glucocorticoids, serum cortisol level, and the presence of acute or chronic illnesses, have all been reported to affect CD4+ cell counts (18,23–27). In addition, there is a normal diurnal variation of approximately 60 CD4+ cells/mm³ in HIV-infected patients, with the highest values present in the evening (20,28), implying that specimen collection times should be standardized. The effect of diurnal variation is greatest for persons who have relatively high CD4 cell counts.

Splenectomy is associated with a large and prolonged increase in peripheral blood CD4+ lymphocyte count, often several hundred cells/mm³ in magnitude (29). In these patients, the CD4+ lymphocyte percentage presumably reflects the level of immunodeficiency more accurately. Falsely low CD4+ cell counts have been observed in up to 11% of blacks (and in lesser numbers of Asians and Caucasians) who lack or have a partial deficiency of the OKT4 epitope (30,31). Since the OKT4 monoclonal antibodies are widely used to identify T-helper cells, these individuals may appear to have no CD4+ cells when in fact they have normal numbers of T-helper cells if identified by other monoclonal antibody markers (e.g., Leu3a).

Thus, the initial CD4+ lymphocyte count for a patient, or counts significantly out of line with prior determinations, should be confirmed by repeat testing. During the first year of HIV infection the CD4 count falls approximately 400 cells/mm³ (14,32) and thereafter the average decline in CD4+ cells is approximately 60–100 cells/mm³ per year (33–35), except for those patients who, for unclear reasons, have entered into an accelerated phase, in which a decline of approximately 160 CD4+ cells/mm³ per year may be anticipated (36). Such patients are more likely to have detectable p24 antigen in serum and to have a more rapid progression to AIDS (36).

Caution should be exercised in overinterpreting small changes in CD4 test results. Patients often attach undue significance to minor rises or falls in these counts. They should be counseled that the overall trend of the CD4 count is more important than any single value (Fig. 1). In general, there is less test-to-test fluctuation in CD4 percentage compared with absolute number (37,38).

CD4 count enumerations are expensive tests ($100–200 per test in many commercial laboratories), and should not be done more frequently than is required for patient management. For patients with counts well above 600 cells/mm³, once or at most twice yearly tests are sufficient. As counts approach 500 cells/mm³, testing may be done every 3–4 months. When a level of 500

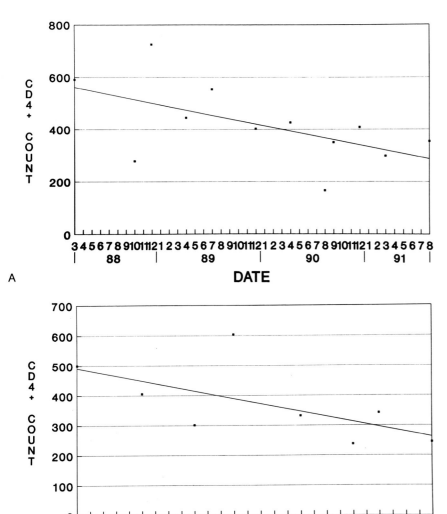

FIG. 1. a and b: Graphic display of the CD4+ lymphocyte counts of patients A (**a**) and B (**b**) shown in Table 2. A downward trend over time can be seen.

cells/mm³ is reached, testing frequency should be reduced to once or twice annually until the counts fall to around 300 cells/mm³, at which time they should be repeated every 3–4 months. At counts of 200 cells/mm³, there is no need, outside of a research protocol, to do additional testing, since further management changes are not directly dependent on these values.

Since low CD4 cell counts are associated with the development of the most serious opportunistic infections, understanding why some patients have a more rapid reduction in count, or why a sudden acceleration in the rate of fall occurs in the course of some HIV-infected patients, is an extremely important concern (39–45).

Other Laboratory Markers

Because of the variability (Table 2) and high cost of CD4 cell count determinations, other laboratory markers have been sought to assess prognosis and monitor the course of HIV-induced immunodeficiency. Two products of immune stimulation, neopterin and β-2 microglobulin, appear to be promising candidates (33,39,46,47). Neopterin is a metabolite of guanosine triphosphate produced by appropriately stimulated macrophages (48). β-2 Microglobulin is a subunit protein of the class I histocompatibility antigens, present on the surface of all nucleated cells. High baseline serum levels of either molecule are associated with an increased risk of progression to AIDS. The mechanisms for the increased levels of these cellular products are not fully understood. Furthermore, the proper timing of standard therapeutic interventions (AZT and *Pneumocystis carinii* pneumonia prophylaxis) based on either an absolute level or a change in level of these substances is unclear. Therefore, the role of these tests in the care of an individual HIV-infected patient remains experimental.

History and Physical Examination

A thorough history and physical examination is necessary to uncover symptoms and physical findings that may at the outset require further evaluation. Particular attention should be given to systemic complaints, visual disturbances, neurologic abnormalities, and gastroenterologic or respiratory problems. Physical examination should carefully document the patient's weight, cutaneous or oral mucosal abnormalities, and presence of enlarged lymph nodes.

LABORATORY TESTING

A complete blood count with a platelet count is essential (Table 3). Mild leukopenia and anemia may be seen and are especially common in the setting of advanced immunodeficiency (CD4+ cell count <200/mm³) (49). These hematologic abnormalities complicate the use of drugs that may further suppress the bone marrow, such as AZT or ganciclovir. Thrombocytopenia may occur at any level of CD4 cell count but is more common in advanced disease (49,50). In the absence of bleeding, no treatment is needed for patients with platelet counts above 20,000/mm³ (87). At levels below this, AZT is probably the treatment of choice for the nonbleeding patient, with reported efficacy rates of at least 50% (88,89). (Paradoxically, although AZT regularly causes anemia and leukopenia, it does not typically cause thrombocytopenia and indeed can reverse it.)

Blood chemistry testing is useful to pinpoint abnormalities of liver function, which may be due to a variety of

TABLE 3. *Selected test results in HIV-infected patients*

Test	Expected result (Ref.)
Hemoglobin	Progressive reduction over time; 10–20% of asymptomatic HIV+ persons are anemic vs. 70% of AIDS patients (49)
Leukocyte count	Progressive reduction over time from 10% of asymptomatic HIV+ persons to 65% of AIDS patients (49)
Platelet count	Reduced in approximately 10% of asymptomatic HIV+ persons and in up to 45% of AIDS patients (49,50)
Neutrophil count	Reduced in 20–50% of AIDS patients (49,50)
Lymphocyte count	Reduced in 70% of AIDS patients with opportunistic infections (49,50)
CD4+ lymphocyte count	Progressive reduction over time (51,52)
CD8+ lymphocyte count	Initially increased, falls later (52)
CD4/CD8 ratio	Progressive reduction over time (52)
Serum sodium	Hyponatremia present in ≥30% of AIDS patients, often attributed to renal salt wasting and (rarely) to hypoadrenalism (53–55)
Serum glucose	Pentamidine (especially by the IV/IM route) may cause hyper- or hypoglycemia and diabetes (56,57)
Creatinine	Increased in a small proportion of cases, especially among black men who are intravenous drug users (54,58)
Liver function tests	Abnormal in 90% but usually mildly i.e., ≤twofold, above upper limits of normal (59,60)
Creatine phosphokinase	Usually normal; when elevated may indicate the presence of myopathy due to either HIV or AZT (61–63)
Lactate dehydrogenase	Frequently mildly elevated; elevated in 90% of patients with *Pneumocystis carinii* pneumonia (64)
Serum globulins	Hypergammaglobulinemia is usual (51,65,66)
Amylase	Increased in 8% (67)
Triglycerides	Elevated in 50% of HIV-infected patients (68)
HBsAg	Present in approximately 10% (69,70)
HBcAb	Present in 90% (69,70)
Hepatitis C antibody	Positivity rates >50% among intravenous drug users and hemophiliacs (71,72)
PPD	Positivity rates highest in Haitians, intravenous drug users, prisoners, and the homeless (73–76)
Papanicolaou smear	Cervical dysplasia in one-third (77,78)
Treponemal antibody test (e.g., MHA-TP)	Positive in 45% of HIV-infected homosexual men (79)
Toxoplasma antibody	Present in 15–80% (80,81)
Cytomegalovirus antibody	Present in 70–100% (81,82)
Herpes simplex antibody	Present in 30–100% (81,82)
Vitamin B₁₂ level	Abnormally low levels in 7–15% of HIV-infected patients (83)
p24 antigen	Variably present (84–86); detectable immediately after HIV acquisition prior to seroconversion, and again in the later stages of immunodeficiency

PPO, purified protein derivative (of tuberculin).

causes including chronic viral hepatitis (59,60,69–72). Interferon-α-2 may be considered for therapy of selected patients with non-A, non-B hepatitis (90,91) or hepatitis B (92,93), although this usage should be regarded as investigational in the setting of HIV infection. Liver dysfunction may affect the pharmacokinetics of medications, which should be taken into account when any drug is prescribed. A baseline LDH (lactate dehydrogenase) is useful to serve as a basis for comparison during suspected bouts of *Pneumocystis carinii* pneumonia, since the LDH level is characteristically elevated in this form of pneumonia (64). A baseline CPK (creatine phosphokinase) may be helpful in detecting HIV-related myopathy or to serve as a basis for comparison should muscle pain or weakness develop during AZT therapy (AZT-induced myopathy) (61–63).

Syphilis Serology

It has been observed that the prevalence of a positive serologic test for syphilis is five times higher among HIV-infected homosexual men compared with those without HIV infection (79). HIV-infected individuals with latent syphilis based on the isolated finding of a positive serology, who have never been adequately treated or evaluated, should undergo a lumbar puncture (94–97). Cerebrospinal fluid abnormalities, even if nonspecific, warrant strong consideration for the parenteral administration of penicillin in doses adequate for the treatment of neurosyphilis (98,99). In the absence of cerebrospinal fluid abnormalities, benzathine penicillin G at a dose of 2.4 million units should be given intramuscularly weekly for 3 consecutive weeks to those patients judged to have late latent syphilis (98). However, benzathine penicillin can not be relied on in patients with neurosyphilis due to very low cerebrospinal fluid drug levels (99,100). HIV-infected patients with neurosyphilis should be treated with aqueous crystalline penicillin G at a dose of approximately 3 million units IV every 4 hours for 10–14 days (98). The serum Venereal Disease Research Laboratory (VDRL) or rapid plasma reagin (RPR) values should be closely followed after treatment in all patients, with particularly frequent testing done for patients with early syphilis (primary, secondary, or early latent, i.e., $\leq$1 year's duration) (96,98).

Tests for Hepatitis B

Hepatitis B (HB) surface antigen is present in approximately 10% of HIV-infected patients (69,70). This infection may be associated with chronic liver disease and may pose an additional occupational hazard for health care workers with parenteral blood exposures to these patients (101,102). Patients without prior hepatitis B infection (i.e., with a negative test for HBcAb) should be considered for hepatitis B vaccination (see below).

PPD with an Anergy Panel

The purified protein derivative (PPD) skin test-positive HIV-infected patient has a 5–10% risk per year of developing active tuberculosis (103) and consequently should receive chemoprophylaxis with isoniazid for 1 year (after active disease has been excluded) (104–107). Induration at the PPD skin test site of 5 mm (versus the usual 10 mm) is regarded as indicative of tuberculous infection for HIV-infected patients (108,109). Patients who are anergic but who have had a positive tuberculin skin test in the past and did not receive prior antituberculous treatment should also be given chemoprophylaxis (109). Presently, it is impossible to judge the need for prophylactic therapy in an anergic person whose skin test history is unknown. Some authorities would give isoniazid prophylaxis to such individuals if they are deemed to be at high risk for past exposure to tuberculosis (i.e., members of a group in which the prevalence of tuberculous infection is $\geq$10%) (109).

Papanicolaou Smear

Because of the high incidence of papillomavirus infection (31–67%) (110,111) and cervical dysplasia (32%) (77,112,113) among women with HIV infection, Papanicolaou smears should be performed at least annually (78).

Chest Roentgenogram

In asymptomatic HIV-infected patients the chest roentgenogram is typically normal. A baseline film is very useful for comparison with later studies done for the evaluation of respiratory tract symptoms.

Toxoplasma Antibody

The seroprevalence of toxoplasma antibody in adults varies widely according to geographic location (from 15% to 80%) (80,81). Since most cases of active toxoplasmosis among HIV-infected patients represent reactivation of latent infection, only those with a positive antibody test are, in general, at risk (114). This serologic result is helpful in the evaluation of neurologic abnormalities and may in the future be used to identify a subgroup of patients who would benefit from specific chemoprophylaxis for this infection, should a satisfactory regimen be established. Seronegative persons should be counseled on how toxoplasmosis is acquired (i.e., through ingestion of undercooked meat containing tissue cysts of *Toxoplasma gondii* or any food contaminated with oocysts that originate in cat feces) and on ways to reduce this occurrence (80).

Hepatitis C Antibody

Coinfection with hepatitis C is very common among HIV-infected intravenous drug users and hemophiliacs (>50%) (71,72). This form of hepatitis may explain abnormalities of liver function in these patients and, like hepatitis B, may pose an additional occupational risk for health care workers with needlestick accidents (115). Whether commercially available α-interferon preparations will ameliorate chronic hepatitis C infection in HIV-infected patients, as it does in approximately 50% of non-HIV-infected individuals (90,91), is unknown.

Stool Examination for Ova and Parasites

Homosexual men, or persons who have resided in areas endemic for *Strongyloides stercoralis* (most tropical and subtropical areas), should have stool examinations for ova and parasites. Patients who are infected with *Strongyloides* may be at risk for developing dissemination of this helminth as the immunodeficiency progresses (116). Consequently, all carriers should be treated, with thiabendazole being the treatment of choice (117). Homosexual men infected with *Giardia lamblia* or *Entamoeba histolytica* should also receive appropriate chemotherapy (117).

Serum Amylase

For unclear reasons, serum amylase levels are modestly elevated in approximately 8% of HIV-infected patients who have no clinical signs of pancreatic disease (67). In the few instances in which isoenzyme analysis has been done, approximately 75% of the serum amylase was of the salivary type, and in other cases the elevation was due to the presence of macroamylasemia (67). Results of a baseline amylase level may be helpful for use in comparison to subsequent testing in patients with abdominal pain, nausea, or vomiting, and in patients prior to treatment with ddI, which is associated with the development of pancreatitis in approximately 10% of patients receiving the drug (118).

Serum Triglyceride Level

The fasting serum triglyceride level is often elevated in HIV-infected patients (68) and may be one factor contributing to the increased incidence of pancreatitis in this patient population. The elevated triglyceride level directly correlates with the serum α-interferon level, implying a possible etiologic role for the cytokine in the disordered lipid metabolism (119).

Vitamin B$_{12}$ and Folate Levels

Vitamin B$_{12}$ levels are often modestly depressed in up to 15% of HIV-infected patients due to malabsorption, which may occur even in the absence of diarrhea or other clinical or laboratory abnormalities indicative of intestinal disease (83). Because low B$_{12}$ or folate levels may be associated with increased hematologic toxicity from trimethoprim–sulfamethoxazole, pyrimethamine, trimetrexate, or AZT, replacement therapy should be given.

Glucose-6-Phosphate Dehydrogenase Levels

Dapsone is being increasing utilized for patients intolerant of, or unable to take, both oral trimethoprim-sulfamethoxazole and aerosol pentamidine (120–123). Because of the risk of hemolysis in glucose-6-phosphate dehydrogenase (G-6-PD)-deficient patients, the enzyme should be assayed prior to administration of dapsone [doses of 50 mg or less per day, however, are not associated with G-6-PD-related hemolysis (124)].

INTERVENTIONS FOR HIV-INFECTED ADULTS

The standard interventions are listed in Table 4.

Counseling

Various counseling activities are an integral part of the care of HIV-infected persons (Table 5) (9). Counseling often first begins at the time that an individual requests or is advised to have HIV antibody testing. Because of the extraordinary psychosocial impact of a diagnosis of HIV infection, it is essential for the person being tested to have a clear understanding of the implications of the test results. The purpose and meaning of the test, the testing procedure itself, and the potential issues of discrimination should be explained to the patient. Informed consent is obtained prior to testing.

HIV test results should generally be communicated in person at which time posttest counseling is done. This

---

TABLE 4. *Standard interventions for HIV-infected adults*[a]

Counseling
Pneumococcal vaccine—once only
Influenza A and B vaccines yearly
Isoniazid for 1 year if PPD positive (now or in past)
Evaluation and treatment of syphilis (including asymptomatic seropositives)
Initiation of antiretroviral therapy: AZT for patients with CD4 counts ≤500 cells/mm^3
Initiation of *Pneumocystis carinii* pneumonia prophylaxis for patients with CD4 counts ≤200 cells/mm^3
Caloric dietary supplementation, as needed

[a] See ref. 9.
PPD, purified protein derivative (of tuberculin).

TABLE 5. *Topics to be considered in counseling HIV-infected adults*

Methods of transmission of HIV
Partner notification (needle-sharing and/or sexual partners)
Food safety issues to prevent toxoplasmosis and
salmonellosis
Nautral history of HIV infection, timing and nature of
interventions

should include a discussion of coping strategies after learning of a positive result, issues regarding potential discrimination, behavioral changes to reduce the risk of secondary transmission, available medical treatments, and the importance of notifying needle sharing and/or sexual contacts. Food safety issues to reduce transmission of *Toxoplasma gondii* (80) and enteric pathogens such as *Salmonella* sp. (125,126), should also be discussed. These discussions should not be limited to the first or second patient visit but should continue throughout the long-term care of the individual.

Vaccinations

HIV-infected adults respond less well than their HIV-uninfected counterparts to many vaccines. Response to hepatitis B vaccine, influenza A and B vaccines, and pneumococcal vaccines depends upon the degree of immunodeficiency present at the time of vaccination (127–135). Asymptomatic HIV-infected patients with CD4+ cell counts well in excess of 200/mm^3 respond the best. The theoretical argument that antigenic stimulation of the immune system will lead to increased HIV replication and progression of disease has not been substantiated in vaccine trials to date (132–138).

Since the inactivated preparations appear safe and potentially beneficial, they should be routinely administered to HIV-infected individuals. The pneumococcal vaccine is given once (139,140), while the latest preparation of the influenza A and B vaccine is given annually during the fall (141). Patients who are susceptible to hepatitis B (HBcAb-negative) who remain at risk of exposure to this virus should be vaccinated. An exception would be the patient with a recent exposure to hepatitis B who may be incubating the virus. For unclear reasons, hepatitis B vaccination of such individuals has been associated with an increased rate of chronic HBsAg carriage (142).

Patients should be informed that the extent and duration of protective efficacy of these vaccines are still uncertain. Whether there may be a role for booster doses of the pneumococcal or hepatitis B vaccines in this patient population is unknown.

Haemophilus influenzae is also a potential cause of infection in HIV-infected adults, although the serotypes most frequently causing disease have only been elucidated in a few instances (143). If *H. influenzae* type b is confirmed as the most important serotype, then use of the conjugate Hib vaccine may be considered. There are few data, however, regarding the efficacy of this vaccine in HIV-infected adults (144, 441).

Initiation of Antiretroviral Therapy—AZT

AZT at a dose of 500 mg/day (100 mg every 4 hours while awake) may be initiated at CD4 counts of 500/mm^3 and below. In placebo-controlled trials, AZT significantly delayed progression to an AIDS-defining diagnosis in such patients (16,17). Whether AZT is similarly beneficial for patients with CD4+ lymphocyte counts above 500/mm^3 is unknown. Typically, patients with CD4+ lymphocyte counts of 200–500/mm^3 are able to tolerate the 500-mg daily dose of AZT extremely well, although dose-limiting anemia and leukopenia may occur. Hematologic parameters should be carefully monitored in all AZT-treated patients (145–147). It is helpful to forewarn patients about headaches, insomnia, nausea, or vomiting that may complicate AZT usage during the first days of therapy, but that tend to abate spontaneously over time (Table 6). Long-term AZT administration may lead to darkening of the nails (148). We usually obtain a complete blood count and SMA profile with CPK at 2-week intervals during the first 4 weeks of AZT treatment and then monthly or bimonthly thereafter, depending on individual tolerance.

Patients with CD4+ lymphocyte counts below 200/mm^3 should also receive AZT (149,150). We use the same dosage of 500 mg/day although others may wish to give 1,200 mg/day for 1 month followed by 600 mg/day thereafter, as recommended by the drug manufacturer (145). Because AZT is generally less well tolerated in these more ill patients, they should be especially closely monitored. AZT may be continued despite severe anemia if blood transfusion support is given. Alternatively, in an attempt to reduce the need for red blood cell transfusions, the dose of AZT can be lowered. Preliminary data from one study have suggested equivalent efficacy

TABLE 6. *Selected potential adverse reactions associated with zidovudine (AZT) therapy*[a]

Anemia
Leukopenia
Headaches
Insomnia
Nausea
Vomiting
Rash
Myopathy
Hepatic dysfunction
Darkening of nails
Malaise

[a] For a complete list of adverse reactions to zidovudine please consult the *Physicians Desk Reference* or the package insert for the drug (145).

for a 300 mg daily dose of AZT (151). During AZT therapy the mean corpuscular volume of erythrocytes usually becomes elevated, and, curiously, when this does not occur, there is a much greater likelihood of developing severe anemia (147). Despite the macrocytosis, vitamin B_{12} or folate supplementation is not indicated, unless these vitamin levels are found to be deficient. Recombinant human erythropoietin at doses of 100 units/kg to 300 units/kg sc (or IV) three times per week has been shown to decrease erythrocyte transfusion requirements significantly in anemic patients with endogenous erythropoietin levels of less than 500 mU/ml (152,153). Erythropoietin may be considered an alternative approach to blood transfusion support, or AZT dosage reduction, although the high cost and the inconvenience of chronic subcutaneous injections are drawbacks to this modality.

AZT dosage should be decreased to approximately half the full dose if the neutrophil count falls below 1,000–1,250 cells/mm^3 and should be stopped in patients who develop severe granulocytopenia (<500–750 cells/mm^3). This effect of AZT on the bone marrow may be offset by the use of granulocyte or granulocyte-macrophage colony-stimulating factor (GCSF and GMCSF), but this is an expensive and impractical form of therapy for long-term use (154–157). Also, more data are needed on the effect of these agents on HIV replication in vivo, since under certain experimental conditions in vitro, GMCSF (but not GCSF) can markedly enhance the production of virus (158).

Other medications such as ganciclovir, cytotoxic chemotherapeutic agents, and high-dose trimethoprim-sulfamethoxazole, which are all myelosuppressive, are difficult to use in conjunction with AZT (159). As a general approach, we temporarily discontinue AZT during the acute therapy of intercurrent serious opportunistic infections. When discontinuing AZT, the physician must watch for the rapid progression of myelopathy or meningoencephalitis, but this appears to be extremely rare (160,161). Whenever possible, AZT is resumed following the completion of acute therapy of these infections.

Although there is a theoretical reason to believe that drugs such as acetaminophen or aspirin would increase AZT toxicity though competition for hepatic glucuronidization, when studied, enhanced rather than impaired clearance of AZT has actually been observed (162). Concomitant administration of probenecid, however, will increase AZT blood levels because of a reduction in AZT metabolism; probenecid also causes impaired renal excretion of the 5′ glucuronide metabolite of AZT (163,164).

AZT is not curative in HIV infection. Opportunistic infections and further reduction in CD4+ lymphocyte counts may still occur, even as early as within 6 months after drug initiation (165). Moreover, recent reports have

demonstrated decreased susceptibility to AZT of HIV isolates recovered from the blood of long-term AZT recipients (166,167). The development of new opportunistic infections or of unexplained weight loss warrants consideration of substituting other antiretroviral drugs for AZT, such as ddI (168). ddI should also be considered for patients unable to take AZT because of severe anemia or granulocytopenia (due to AZT or to other causes). It is likely that many changes in the approach to antiretroviral therapy will occur in the 1990s, representing perhaps the most dynamic area in clinical management (169–171).

Pneumocystis carinii Pneumonia Prophylaxis

HIV-infected patients are at risk for such serious opportunistic infections as *Pneumocystis carinii* pneumonia, cytomegalovirus retinitis, cryptococcosis, toxoplasmosis, or disseminated *Mycobacterium avium-intracellulare* infection, principally when the CD4+ lymphocyte count falls below 200 cells/mm^3 (5–7). Without specific chemoprophylaxis, it has been estimated that up to 75% of HIV-infected individuals with such low CD4+ lymphocyte counts will develop *Pneumocystis carinii* pneumonia (4), an infection that has a mortality rate of up to 30% per episode (172–176).

The discovery that this form of pneumonia can be largely prevented by chemoprophylaxis was a major achievement in the care of HIV-infected patients (8,177–183). The two forms of chemoprophylaxis that are most widely used are once monthly aerosol pentamidine, at a dose of 300 mg delivered by the Respirgard II jet nebulizer (Marquest, Englewood, CO) or trimethoprim–sulfamethoxazole given orally (8). The dose of pentamidine is diluted in 6 ml of sterile water and delivered at 6 L/min from a 50-pound/square inch (PSI) compressed air source until the reservoir is dry. Regimens of trimethoprim–sulfamethoxazole using as small a dose as one double-strength tablet (160 mg trimethoprim–800 mg sulfamethoxazole) every other day (183), or three times weekly (182), are highly effective. The advantages and disadvantages of aerosol pentamidine versus trimethoprim–sulfamethoxazole are displayed in Table 7 (183–189). We prefer trimethoprim–sulfamethoxazole using an every other day low-dose regimen, which is well tolerated by approximately 50% of patients during long-term administration (183–188). The most frequent cause of intolerance is hypersensitivity reactions, particularly rashes. Preliminary data from a direct comparison of trimethoprim–sulfamethoxazole with aerosol pentamidine have demonstrated significantly greater efficacy for trimethoprim–sulfamethoxazole in secondary prophylaxis of *Pneumocystis carinii* pneumonia (189).

For patients with CD4+ lymphocyte counts ≤200/mm^3 who are not already receiving AZT, we prefer to begin trimethoprim–sulfamethoxazole before AZT, and

TABLE 7. *Comparison of aerosol pentamidine vs. low-dose oral trimethoprim–sulfamethoxazole for prevention of* Pneumocystis carinii pneumonia in HIV-infected adults[a]

	Advantages	Disadvantages
Aerosol pentamidine	Minimal systemic absorption Tolerated by most patients	Expensive (>$100 per month) Requires special equipment 5–25% breakthrough rate Requires cooperative patients Unknown risk to health care personnel from exposure to pentamidine aerosol Unknown risk of long-term exposure on lung tissue Potential spread of other respiratory tract pathogens, e.g., *Mycobacterium tuberculosis* due to coughing Inactive against extrapulmonary pneumocystosis Significantly less effective than TMP-SMX in secondary prophylaxis of *Pneumonia carinii* pneumonia Inactive against potential pathogens other than pneumocystis
Trimethoprim–sulfamethoxazole (TMP-SMX)	Inexpensive (<5$ per month) <10% breakthrough rate No special equipment Likely to be effective against extrapulmonary pneumocystosis Possibly effective in preventing: salmonellosis, shigellosis, pneumococcal infection, *Haemophilus influenzae* infection, isospora infection, nocardiosis, listeriosis, toxoplasmosis	Limited data on tolerability of AZT Hypersensitivity reactions or other adverse reactions in 30–50% of patients

[a] See refs. 183–189.

if the hematologic parameters, liver chemistries, and renal function are stable at 2 weeks, then introduce AZT in standard doses.

It is important to emphasize that when patients who are compliant with trimethoprim–sulfamethoxazole prophylaxis develop respiratory tract symptoms and an abnormal chest roentgenogram, *Pneumocystis carinii* is unlikely to be the cause. In contrast, in our experience *Pneumocystis carinii* pneumonia remains the most common cause of this clinical picture in patients receiving aerosol pentamidine, although the roentgenographic findings may be atypical for this form of pneumonia [e.g., upper lobe infiltrates (190–192)]. Hypoglycemia (193) and pancreatitis (194–196) are much less common with aerosol pentamidine compared with intravenous administration, but may still rarely occur.

Although most HIV-infected patients with *Pneumocystis carinii* pneumonia have a CD4+ lymphocyte count of <200 cells/mm³, approximately 5% have higher counts (5). Identification of those HIV-infected patients with higher CD4+ lymphocyte counts who are at risk for pneumocystosis may be problematic. Patients with thrush, or those who have had a prior bout of *Pneumocystis carinii* pneumonia, should receive pneumocystis prophylaxis regardless of the CD4+ lymphocyte count

(6). Some authorities begin prophylaxis for all HIV-infected patients with a CD4 lymphocyte percentage ≤20%, regardless of the absolute CD4 count (8).

MANAGEMENT OF SPECIFIC COMPLICATIONS

Fever

The majority of HIV-infected patients will develop fever at some point in the course of their illness. Aside from primary HIV infection, sustained fevers are rarely, if ever, attributable to HIV infection itself and are usually due to serious but treatable superimposed infections (Table 8) (197). Management of the febrile HIV-infected patient is integrally related to establishing a specific etiology for the fever. Finding the source of fever, however, can at times be very challenging. Fever may be related to nonopportunistic infections presenting typically or atypically, opportunistic infections [sometimes multiple (198)], hypersensitivity reactions to medications, and malignancies, particularly lymphomas. Furthermore, nosocomial infections from intravascular catheters, decubitii, and urinary tract infections must not be overlooked in the hospitalized febrile HIV-infected patient (197).

TABLE 8. *General principles in the approach to the HIV-infected patient with fever* [a]

Except for primary HIV infection, sustained fevers are due to causes other than HIV infection itself
Serious opportunistic infections usually first occur in patients with CD4+ lymphocyte counts of less than 200 cells/mm³
Multiple opportunistic infections and/or neoplasia may occur simultaneously, even in the same organ or tissue
Serodiagnostic studies and tuberculin skin testing may be ambiguous
Growth of some opportunistic organisms, e.g., cytomegalovirus or *Mycobacterium avium-intracellulare,* from urine or sputum samples may not indicate active infection

[a] See ref. 197.

It is important at the outset to know whether the patient is highly immunocompromised (i.e., has a CD4+ lymphocyte count <200 cells/mm³) and is thus predisposed to serious opportunistic infections. If not, evaluation may be directed towards the discovery of less unusual microbial pathogens and conditions, for example sinusitis (199), herpes zoster infection (200), or tuberculosis (201).

It is also important to note epidemiologic clues that may help in identifying specific infectious risks (202). For example, Haitians, as well as intravenous drug users from major metropolitan areas, have an increased risk of tuberculosis (75,109). Patients from the southwestern United States (and occasionally those who have previously resided there) are at risk for disseminated *Coccidioides immitis* infection (203–205). Histoplasmosis may be a consideration in individuals who have resided in areas endemic for this fungus in the United States (206) or elsewhere, including certain areas of the Carribean such as Puerto Rico (207,208).

An approach to the evaluation of fever in the HIV-infected patient with advanced immunodeficiency is found in Table 9. If the source of fever has not been identified on routine diagnostic studies such as blood and urine culture or chest roentgenogram, then further

testing is necessary. Blood cultures for fungi and mycobacteria should be obtained (209) [two are sufficient (210)]. Mycobacterial blood cultures should include lysis of the cellular fraction of the specimen, followed by plating on a standard solid mycobacterial culture medium or by liquid culture with radiometric detection (211). Multiple cultures of stool, urine, and sputum for mycobacteria should also be considered. Stool acid-fast smears and cultures are helpful in the diagnosis of disseminated *Mycobacterium avium-intracellulare* infection, since the intestinal tract is often involved in the disease process (211–215). However, single positive cultures from stool and sputum for nontuberculous mycobacteria may represent contamination or colonization and not indicate true infection. Stool acid-fast cultures may also be useful in the diagnosis of *Mycobacterium tuberculosis* infection, although usually the sputum is culture positive in these instances (75).

Although cytomegalovirus infection may be a cause of fever in these patients, positive cultures for this virus from urine, pharynx, bronchial lavage fluid, or even blood are so frequent that they cannot be relied on to pinpoint the cause of fever (216,217). For the same reasons, serology for cytomegalovirus is also nondiagnostic (81,82,216). It is of utmost importance to attempt to

TABLE 9. *A diagnostic approach for evaluation of fever in HIV-infected patients* [a]

Evaluate if patient falls into a group at high risk for serious opportunistic infections, i.e., CD4 cell count less than 200 cells/mm³
Direct history to determine possible geographic, ethnic, or lifestyle risk factors for specific infections; pay particular attention to neurologic, respiratory, dermatologic, visual, and gastrointestinal complaints
Note medication list
Physical examination
Laboratory tests: CBC; chemistry profile, including liver function tests; urine analysis; cultures of blood, urine, and sputum for bacteria; chest roentgenogram; stool culture if diarrhea present.
If initial cultures are negative, culture blood, urine, sputum, and stool for mycobacteria and blood, urine, and sputum for fungi; do serum cryptococcal antigen, toxoplasma titer, and VDRL; do PPD with controls unless known to be anergic; sputum for IFA test for *Pneumocystis carinii*
If no source yet identified, consider:
  Gallium scan of lung
  Computed tomography of abdomen
  Examination by ophthalmologist for CMV retinitis
  Lymph node biopsy if enlarged node is accessible
  Bone marrow biopsy and aspiration (especially if anemic)
  Skin lesion biopsy (if present)
  Lumbar puncture if clinical signs warrant
  Bronchoscopy with bronchial alveolar lavage and/or biopsy (if respiratory tract signs or abnormalities are present)
  Liver biopsy (if liver function studies are abnormal)

CMV, cytomegalovirus; IFA, immunofluorescent antibody; PPD, purified protein derivative (of tuberculin).
[a] See ref. 197.

establish the pathogenicity of an organism that has been cultured, since specific treatment for microorganisms such as cytomegalovirus or *Mycobacterium avium-intracellulare* may be at best partially effective, potentially toxic, inconvenient (require multiple drugs or intravenous administration), or prolonged. Further, administration of ganciclovir for cytomegalovirus infection may preclude the use of AZT, due to potential additive bone marrow suppression (159).

Additional diagnostic studies should include a test for serum cryptococcal antigen, since it is positive in 75–95% of HIV-infected patients with cryptococcosis (218,219). Sputum should be obtained (induced if necessary) for detection of *Pneumocytsis carinii* using an immunofluorescent monoclonal antibody assay (220–222). This is especially important for patients with respiratory complaints, an abnormal chest roentgenogram, or gallium-67 uptake by the lung on scintography (223). If an induced sputum sample is nondiagnostic or unavailable, bronchoscopy for bronchial alveolar lavage and/or biopsy should be considered for patients with objective pulmonary signs or test abnormalities (224).

Serodiagnosis of *Histoplasma capsulatum* and *Coccidioides immitis* is helpful for selected patients (203–206). Also, Giemsa-stained preparations of the buffy coat of peripheral blood may be useful in the diagnosis of disseminated histoplasmosis (225). An experimental test for a histoplasma polysaccharide antigen was positive on urine and/or serum samples in more than 95% of AIDS patients with histoplasmosis, according to the test's originator (226).

A careful funduscopic examination by an ophthalmologist may help establish the diagnosis of disseminated cytomegalovirus infection. Although the patient with cytomegalovirus retinitis usually reports visual disturbances, this is not uniformly true, particularly in patients with an altered mental status (227).

Biopsies for culture, special stains, and histologic examination of sites such as bone marrow, lymph nodes, gastrointestinal tract, or skin lesions may be very helpful in the diagnosis of disseminated fungal, mycobacterial, or cytomegalovirus infection, bacillary epithelioid angiomatosis, lymphoma, and Kaposi's sarcoma, when other modalities of diagnosis are either nondiagnostic or negative. It is particularly helpful to perform a lymph node biopsy in patients who have a single group of lymph nodes that are disproportionately enlarged or that have rapidly increased in size (228).

Computed tomography may be used to locate intraabdominal masses or enlarged lymph nodes for biopsy. In patients with an elevated alkaline phosphatase level and fever, a liver biopsy for histologic examination and culture may be useful (209,229). This procedure is not often necessary, however, since other sources of culture material are usually diagnostic.

Before embarking on any biopsy procedure it is important to determine if the patient has a potential bleeding diathesis, such as thrombocytopenia. Platelet transfusions, intravenous infusions of immunoglobulin G preparations, or other measures to elevate the platelet count at least transiently may be required for patients with platelet counts below 50,000–100,000/mm^3, depending on the bleeding time and the type and urgency of the invasive procedure to be done. Partial thromboplastin times and (less often) prothombin times may be prolonged in HIV-infected patients. Usually this is due to the presence of a lupus-like anticoagulant, found in up to 70% of HIV-infected patients, particularly those with opportunistic infections (230–232). The "anticoagulants" are immunoglobulins that interfere with several in vitro coagulation assays. The presence of these anticoagulants can be confirmed by several diagnostic tests, such as the $\frac{1}{2} + \frac{1}{2}$ correction or the Russell's viper venom time (233). The majority of patients who have these factors are not predisposed to bleeding unless the level of coagulation factors is abnormal, or qualitative/quantitative platelet abnormalities coexist (230).

Empiric Treatment for Infection in the HIV-Infected Patient

The empiric use of broad-spectrum antibiotics is not routinely indicated for the febrile HIV-infected patient, since these drugs may be toxic, lead to increasingly resistant organisms, or confound the diagnostic evaluation. However, if the patient is clinically unstable or profoundly neutropenic (fewer than 500 neutrophils/mm^3), broad-spectrum antibiotics should be administered promptly. Certain other indications for empiric therapy are found in Table 10.

When an opportunistic infection (or infections) is diagnosed, specific therapy should be initiated (Table 11) (234–307). It is important to note that treatment of opportunistic infections in HIV-infected patients is rarely curative (308,309). More often, chronic maintenance therapy for an indefinite period is necessary after completion of the acute treatment.

Diarrhea

Diarrhea is a frequent complaint in HIV-infected patients occurring in at least 20–30% of patients at some point during their course (310,311). There is a large differential diagnosis ranging from common bacterial pathogens, such as *Campylobacter jejuni* (312) and *Salmonella* sp. (292–295), to previously rare protozoans, such as cryptosporidia (285,286) and microsporidia (282–284) (see Table 12 for a partial listing) (313–318). An infectious etiology has been found in up to 85% of cases (319). If diarrhea persists despite negative initial cultures and smears, colonoscopy and possibly gastroduodenos-

TABLE 10. *Clinical situations in which empiric therapy may be useful in HIV-infected adults prior to confirmation of diagnosis*[a]

Condition	Microorganism to which therapy is directed	Recommended therapy
Clinically unstable (septic appearing) or profoundly neutropenic (<500 PMNs/mm³)	*Staphylococcus aureus* *Streptococcus pneumoniae* *Haemophilus influenzae* *Salmonella* sp. Aerobic gram-negative rods	Third-generation cephalosporin with or without an aminoglycoside
Lobar pneumonia	*Streptococcus pneumoniae* *Haemophilus influenzae* *Moraxella catarrhalis* *Staphylococcus aureus* *Legionella* sp. *Klebsiella* sp. *Escherichia coli*	Third-generation cephalosporin plus erythromycin
Ring-enhancing mass lesion(s) on cranial MRI or CT, especially if serum toxoplasma titer is positive	*Toxoplasma gondii*	Pyrimethamine plus sulfadiazine plus folinic acid
Diffuse pulmonary infiltrates and hypoxia, especially if not on trimethoprim–sulfamethoxazole chemoprophylaxis	*Pneumocystis carinii*	Trimethoprim–sulfamethoxazole
Dysphagia or odynophagia	*Candida albicans*	Ketoconazole
PPD+ and ill-appearing, especially with abnormal chest roentgenogram (or if PPD− and anergic, but at high epidemiologic risk for tuberculosis)	*Mycobacterium tuberculosis*	Isoniazid, rifampin, pyrazinamide

[a] See ref. 197.
CT, computed tomography; MRI, magnetic resonance imaging; PPD, purified protein derivative (of tuberculin); PMN, polymorphonuclear (leukocytes).

copy are warranted for biopsy and cultures (Table 13) (320).

If an infectious agent is either not diagnosed, or not effectively treated with available antimicrobials, as for example with cryptosporidia or microsporidia, antiperistaltic agents such as loperamide may be tried (321). Somatostatin analog in doses of 100–300 μg three times daily sc or IM has been used successfully in anecdotal reports to reduce the diarrhea associated with cryptosporidia infection (286).

Stenotic Biliary Tract Disease

Stenotic biliary tract disease is being increasingly recognized in HIV-infected individuals (322,323). These patients typically have fever and epigastric or right upper quadrant pain (322). Blood chemistries reveal a markedly elevated alkaline phosphatase level, with relatively lower bilirubin and hepatocellular enzyme elevations. Dilated intra- or extrahepatobiliary ducts are frequently found on ultrasound examination or by computed tomography. Papillary stenosis and sclerosing cholangitis may be present together or individually on endoscopic evaluation. Cytomegalovirus and/or cryptosporidia are often present in bile or observed on histologic preparations of ampulla of Vater tissue, or papillary or peri-

papillary duodenal tissue. *Mycobacterium avium-intracellulare* infection, Kaposi's sarcoma, and lymphoma have also been demonstrated in periampullary or biliary ductal tissue (324). However, in 45% of cases, no opportunistic infection or neoplasm has been discovered (322). The role of HIV itself in the entity is unknown. Endoscopic sphincterotomy may be useful in relieving pain and reducing fever. However, the alkaline phosphatase level may continue to rise, suggesting progression of intrahepatic sclerosing cholangitis or the presence of diffuse hepatic parenchymal disease.

Renal Manifestations

Clinically apparent renal disease occurs in 10–30% of AIDS patients in certain geographic areas (54,58,325–328). In HIV-infected populations in which many patients are young black men who use intravenous drugs, proteinuria of greater than 0.5g/24 h has been reported to occur in more than 40% of AIDS patients, with nephrotic-range proteinuria in up to 10% (325,328). In other HIV-infected populations, the incidence of clinically apparent renal disease appears to be much lower.

AIDS patients with renal disease have been divided into three groups based upon the presentation of renal disease (326). Group 1 consists of patients who suddenly

TABLE 11. *Guide to therapy of opportunistic infections in HIV-infected patients*

Infection	Specific treatment	Alternative treatment	Maintenance therapy	References
Fungal infections				
Oral candidiasis (thrush)	Clotrimazole troches (10 mg) 5×/day	Nystatin oral suspension 100,000 units/cc 5 cc QID swish/swallow; or ketoconazole 200–400 mg/day; or fluconazole 100 mg/day	Same as initial therapy but may reduce frequency of administration	234–236
Candida esophagitis	Ketoconazole 200–400 mg/day	Fluconazole 100 mg/day; or amphotericin B 15–25 mg IV/day	Same as initial therapy	236–239
Histoplasmosis	Amphotericin B, ≥0.5 mg/kg/day; 2 g total dose	Ketoconazole 400 mg/day	Amphotericin B 50–80 mg biweekly	206,236,240
Cryptococcosis	Amphotericin B, ≥0.5 mg/kg/day; 1–2 g total dose	Fluconazole 200–400 mg/day	Fluconazole 200 mg/day	218,219,236,241–245
Coccidioidomycosis (without CNS involvement)	Amphotericin B, ≥0.5 mg/kg/day; ≥1 g total dose	Fluconazole 400 mg/day	Fluconazole 400 mg/day	203,205,236,246,248,249
Viral infections				
Localized herpes zoster	Acyclovir 800 mg PO 5×/day ×7–10 days	None	None	236,250,251
Disseminated varicella zoster	Acyclovir 10 mg/kg IV Q8H ×10 days	Foscarnet 40–60 mg IV Q8H ×10 days	Consider high-dose oral acyclovir if recurrences are seen	236,252,253
Localized, nonhealing herpes simplex infection, nasolabial, genital, or perianal areas	Acyclovir 200 mg PO 5×/day ≥10 days	Foscarnet 40–60 mg IV Q8H ≥10 days	Acyclovir 200 mg PO TID or 400 mg PO BID	236,254–261
Cytomegalovirus retinitis	Foscarnet 60 mg IV Q8H ×14–21 days	Ganciclovir 5 mg/kg IV Q12H ×14–21 days	Foscarnet 90 mg IV Q24H or ganciclovir 5 mg/kg IV Q24H	236,262–268
Progressive multifocal leukoencephalopathy (JC virus infection)	None	None	None	269,270
Parvo virus B19	Immunoglobulin G IV 0.4 g/kg ×5 days	None	If relapse occurs within 6 months after initial treatment, give single-day infusions of 0.4 g/kg IgG every 4 weeks	271
Protozoal infections				
Pneumocystis carinii[a] pneumonia	Trimethoprim (15–20 mg/kg/day) with Sulfamethoxazole (75–100 mg/kg/day) in 3–4 divided doses IV or PO × 21 days plus a tapering dose of corticosteroids if PaO₂ <70 or A-a gradient >35 mm Hg One possible regimen is: prednisone 40 mg PO BID ×days 1–5, prednisone 40 mg PO daily ×days 6–10, prednisone 20 mg daily ×days 11–21	Pentamidine 3–4 mg/kg IV daily × 21 days; or trimethoprim 20 mg/kg/day PO in 4 divided doses plus dapsone 100 mg PO daily × 21 days; or clindamycin 600 mg IV Q6H plus Primaquine 15 mg base PO QD × 21 days Plus steroids when indicated, for all of the above regimens	Trimethoprim–sulfamethoxazole 160 mg/800 mg PO TIW, or aerosol Pentamidine 300 mg once/month by the Respirgard II nebulizer, or dapsone 100 mg PO every other day	236,272–277

continued

TABLE 11. *Continued.*

Infection	Specific treatment	Alternative treatment	Maintenance therapy	References
Cerebral toxoplasmosis	Pyrimethamine 25–50 mg/day PO with sulfadiazine 1 g PO QID plus folinic acid 5 mg/day PO, until resolution or stabilization, with improvement of clinical signs and CT abnormalities	Clindamycin up to 1,200 mg IV Q8H with pyrimethamine 50 mg/day PO with folinic acid 5 mg PO/day	Pyrimethamine 25 mg/day Sulfadiazine 1 g/day Folinic 5 mg/day	227,236,278–281
Microsporidial enteric infection	None (metronidazole 500 mg PO TID—experimental)	None	None	282–284
Cryptosporidiosis	None	None	None	285–286
Isospora belli enteric infection	160 mg trimethoprim–800 mg sulfamethoxazole PO QID ×10 days	Pyrimethamine 75 gm PO, folinic acid 5 mg PO daily ×10 days	160 mg Trimethoprim–800 mg sulfamethoxazole TIW; or pyrimethamine 25 mg/day plus folinic acid 5 mg/day	287–289
Helminthic infection *Strongyloides stercoralis*	Thiabendazole 25 mg/kg Q12H × ≥5 days	Ivermectin 200 μg/kg × ≥1 dose (experimental)	None	117,290
Bacterial infections Nocardiosis	Sulfadiazine 1 g PO QID	None established (consider minocycline, primaxin, and other agents—see ref 291)	Sulfadiazine 1 g PO QID	291
Salmonella bacteremia	Ciprofloxacin 750 mg PO BID ×6 weeks	Amoxicillin 500 mg PO TID; trimethoprim 160 mg—sulfamethoxazole 800 mg PO TID	? None, if ciprofloxacin is used as primary therapy; otherwise, continue primary therapy	292–295
Mycobacterium tuberculosis	Isoniazid 300 mg PO daily with pyridoxine 50 mg PO daily, rifampin 600 mg PO daily, pyrazinamide 20–30 mg/kg per day PO once daily or in 3–4 divided doses (up to a daily maximum of 2 g) All ×2 months (if drug resistance suspected, use ≥4 drugs)	Isoniazid 300 mg PO daily with pyridoxine 50 mg PO daily, ethambutol 25 mg/kg/day, pyrazinamide 20–30 mg/kg/day	Isoniazid 300 mg PO daily with pyridoxine 50 mg PO daily, rifampin 600 mg PO daily—both ×9–18 months total course (including initial 2 months)	73,75,76,104–107
Mycobacterium avium-intracellulare	Rifampin 600 mg PO daily, ethambutol 15–25 mg/kg/day PO, ciprofloxacin 750 mg PO BID/day, clofazimine 100 mg PO daily	Add other antimycobacterial drugs e.g., amikacin 7.5 mg/kg IV Q12H–24H, or clarithromycin 500 mg PO BID (experimental therapy)	Continue initial therapy	236,296–302
Bacillary epitheliod angiomatosis	Erythromycin 250–500 mg PO QID ×2–4 weeks	None firmly established; see ref. 305	None	303–306

[a] Recent evidence suggests that *Pneumocystis carinii* is a fungus (306).

TABLE 12. *Microorganisms and/or conditions that have been associated with diarrhea in HIV-infected patients[a]*

Microorganisms
  Bacteria
    Campylobacter jejuni
    Shigella sp.
    Salmonella sp.
    Mycobacterium avium-intracellulare
  Protozoans
    Cryptosporidia
    Giardia lamblia
    Isospora belli
    Microsporidia
  Helminths
    Strongyloides stercoralis
  Viruses
    Cytomegalovirus
    Adenovirus
    Rotavirus
    HIV itself (? cause of AIDS enteropathy)
Tumors
  Lymphoma
  Kaposi's sarcoma (uncommon cause of diarrhea)
Miscellaneous
  Side effects of medications
  Clostridium difficile colitis

[a] Listing not meant to be exhaustive. See refs. 292–295 and 310–319.

develop renal failure because of an acute insult to the kidneys, such as dehydration, sepsis, hypotension, hypoxia, or nephrotoxic agents, including nonsteroidal antiinflammatory agents, pentamidine, foscarnet sodium, trimethoprim–sulfamethoxazole, or radiocontrast dye. In general, the clinical course of acute renal failure and response to treatment in AIDS patients is similar to that of nonimmunocompromised patients, and these patients benefit from dialysis when it is required (326,329). Both hemodialysis and peritoneal dialysis have been used successfully.

Group 2 consists of HIV-infected patients with renal disease due to HIV-associated nephropathy. For unclear reasons the majority of these patients (approximately 90%) are young black men, about half of whom have

TABLE 13. *Approach to the evaluation of the HIV-infected patient with diarrhea*

Standard evaluation
  Stool sample for
    Culture and sensitivity for routine enteric pathogens
    Ova and parasite examination[a]
    Cryptosporidia smear[a]
    Mycobacterial culture and smear
    Clostridium difficile (antigen, toxin, or culture assay)
Further evaluation if above negative or nondiagnostic
  Colonoscopy with biopsy
  Gastroduodenoscopy with biopsy[b]

[a] Examination of several stool samples will enhance yield.
[b] Electron microscopic examination necessary to detect microsporidia.

used intravenous drugs (54,58). [It is of interest that blacks also appear to develop idiopathic and heroin-associated variants of focal and segmental glomerulosclerosis much more commonly than other races (327,330–333)]. These patients have nephrotic syndrome and, even in the absence of ischemic or nephrotoxic injury, a rapidly progressive course to uremia over 6–12 months. An interesting clinical finding is the notable absence of hypertension during both early and late stages of disease, despite severe renal failure (58). The most common pathologic abnormality seen in these patients is a form of focal and segmental glomerulosclerosis, which is reminiscent of the glomerular lesions seen in patients using illicit drugs intravenously before the AIDS epidemic (334). The etiology of these lesions is unknown. CD4 receptors have been demonstrated on glomerular cell membranes, suggesting that direct infection of these cells by HIV may be involved (335). Proviral HIV DNA has been demonstrated in tubular and glomerular epithelial cells of patients with HIV-associated nephropathy using in vitro DNA hybridization techniques (336). Those patients with advanced HIV-induced immunodeficiency fare poorly on dialysis with complications of severe cachexia, malnutrition, and opportunistic infections, frequently leading to death within months. The therapeutic role of steroids or other immunosuppressive agents in this group is unclear. In anecdotal cases there have been beneficial effects from AZT (58,337).

Group 3 are patients who have end-stage renal disease of diverse causes unrelated to HIV infection (e.g., heroin-induced nephropathy or diabetic glomerulosclerosis). HIV infection may precede or follow the development of chronic renal failure. Seroprevalence surveys in chronic hemodialysis units have shown HIV seropositivity rates ranging from 0.77% in broad-based geographical studies (338) to 12–40% (339,340) in inner-city hemodialysis units. These patients usually have a progressive downhill course once the diagnosis of frank AIDS is made. The majority have died within 1 year with marked cachexia unresponsive to nutritional support by hyperalimentation (58). However, patients with asymptomatic HIV infection on chronic dialysis can live for years (339,341). The effect of chronic dialysis on the natural history of HIV infection per se remains to be defined.

Cardiac Manifestations

Cardiac abnormalities are common in AIDS patients, judging from an up to 77% prevalence at postmortem examination (342–346). However, they are much less often recognized antemortem, unless sensitive testing procedures are done specifically to identify them. Aside from electrocardiographic abnormalities, the cardiac conditions most likely to be appreciated clinically are cardiomyopathy (including myocarditis) and pericardial effusion (Table 14) (342). Cardiac disease is most common in HIV-infected individuals with advanced immunodeficiency (342) and reportedly directly contributes to the death of 1.1–6.3% of patients (347).

Electrocardiographic abnormalities occur in up to 44% of HIV-infected patients and may be due to myocarditis or pericarditis, or may reflect the presence of fever, sepsis, electrolyte disturbances, or drug toxicities (348–350). The findings are generally minor and consist of low-voltage, ST-T wave changes, bundle branch block, and intraventricular conduction delays (348,350). However, ventricular tachycardia has been reported, which may result in congestive heart failure or sudden death (349). Intravenous pentamidine (but not aerosol pentamidine) may cause QT interval prolongation and lead to *torsades de point,* a polymorphic ventricular tachycardia (351,352).

Symptoms and signs of congestive heart failure and/or embolic phenomena are the usual presenting manifestations of HIV-associated cardiomyopathy. Although most commonly felt to be due to active myocarditis, or to be postinfectious in origin, nutritional deficiencies of selenium or vitamin B_1 and abuse of ethanol or cocaine may play a role (342,353–355). Congestive heart failure has also been attributed to the use of AZT (442) and to high-dose α-interferon for the treatment of Kaposi's sarcoma (356). Doxorubicin hydrochloride, which is included in some combination chemotherapy protocols

TABLE 14. *Cardiac manifestations in HIV-infected patients*

Myocarditis
  Idiopathic
  Infectious—toxoplasmosis, cytomegalovirus infection,
    coxsackievirus infection, cryptococcosis, aspergillosis,
    candidiasis, mycobacterial infection, nocardiosis
  HIV-related (?)
Pericarditis
  Idiopathic
  Infectious—tuberculosis, *Mycobacterium avium-intracellulare* infection, cytomegalovirus infection,
    nocardiosis, toxoplasmosis, salmonellosis,
    cryptococcosis, herpes simplex infection
  Neoplastic—Kaposi's sarcoma, lymphoma
Endocarditis
  Infectious—*Staphylococcus aureus* and others
  Nonbacterial thrombotic endocarditis (marantic)
Cardiomyopathy
  Myocarditis
  Postinfectious (presumed)
  Nutritional deficiencies—selenium, vitamin B_1
  Toxins—alcohol, cocaine
  Drug-induced—Adriamycin, interferon, AZT
Primary pulmonary hypertension
Arrhythmias
  Underlying cardiac disease
  Fever/sepsis
  Electrolyte abnormalities
  Medications—IV pentamidine, interferon

for Kaposi's sarcoma, is a well-known cause of cardiomyopathy (357).

Myocarditis is a relatively common cardiac finding at postmortem examination in HIV-infected patients (342). Although infections such as toxoplasmosis (the most commonly recognized infectious cause) (346), cytomegalovirus infection (358), coxsackievirus infection (359), cryptococcosis (343,360), aspergillosis (361), candidiasis (344), mycobacterial infection (345), and nocardiosis (346) are potential etiologies, most often the cause is not identified.

The pathogenesis of myocarditis in the absence of an infectious agent is unclear. HIV can be demonstrated by a variety of techniques in the myocardium of certain cases implying a possible direct or indirect etiologic role for HIV itself (362–365). However, CD4 antigen has not been detected in normal human myocardium (364), and there has been no histologic evidence of HIV infection of the myocyte specifically. One group has hypothesized that an autoimmune process, as evidenced by the presence of serum antibodies to cardiac antigens, may play a role in pathogenesis (366).

Specific treatment for myocarditis is rarely possible except when caused by opportunistic infections, which are usually diagnosed based on cultures obtained from sites outside of the myocardium. In the absence of an alternative diagnosis, we empirically treat patients with a positive toxoplasma serology for toxoplasmosis. "Idiopathic" cases sometimes resolve spontaneously (367) or in one case (368) coincident with the introduction of antiretroviral therapy.

Pericardial effusions occur in up to 38% of AIDS patients and are the most common cause of clinical cardiovascular symptoms and signs (342,369–375). Although these effusions are often small, remain asymptomatic, and spontaneously resolve in 50% of cases (369), rarely cardiac tamponade may develop (370,376). Pericardial effusion may be "idiopathic" in origin or be caused by infection or neoplasms. In some instances, idiopathic effusions have been associated with chronic pulmonary disease and isolated right ventricular dilatation (346,347). *Mycobacterium tuberculosis* is the most commonly identified infectious cause, responsible for 22–50% of cases (370,377). Other infectious agents that have caused pericarditis in HIV-infected patients include *Mycobacterium avium-intracellulare* (377), cytomegalovirus (376), nocardia (378), *Toxoplasma gondii* (377), *Salmonella typhimurium* (377), and cryptococcus (379). Malignant effusions may be due to lymphoma (380) or Kaposi's sarcoma (344). Successful treatment of cases due to tuberculosis, toxoplasmosis, salmonellosis, and cryptococcosis has been possible (377). However, pericardial effusions due to *Mycobacterium avium-intracellulare* infection, lymphoma, or Kaposi's sarcoma are usually refractory to treatment. Drainage procedures such as pericardiotomy or pericardiocentesis have proved beneficial in selected patients with symptomatic disease (370,381).

Endocarditis in HIV-infected persons may be due to infection, but is more commonly due to nonbacterial thrombotic endocarditis (marantic endocarditis), which accompanies many wasting illnesses (344,346,382). Intravenous drug users who continue to inject drugs are at risk for infective endocarditis due principally to *Staphylococcus aureus,* but also to gram-negative organisms and fungi (383).

Primary pulmonary hypertension, with or without cor pulmonale, has been reported in a small number of HIV-infected patients (384–386). Echocardiograms have shown right atrial enlargement, right ventricular enlargement, or paradoxical septal motion. In several patients, underlying lung infections were also present (385). The etiology is unknown. However, a role for HIV has been speculated, either as the primary cause, or as an inciting agent for an immune response that leads to pulmonary vascular damage. Primary pulmonary hypertension should be suspected in an HIV-infected patient who presents with dyspnea on exertion in the presence of a normal chest roentgenogram.

Rheumatologic Manifestations

Arthralgia, arthritis, myopathies (which are mentioned elsewhere in this chapter and in other chapters), various forms of vasculitis, a sicca syndrome, and numerous autoimmune phenomena are the principal rheumatologic complications of HIV infection (387,388). Intermittent arthralgias without synovitis may occur during primary HIV infection and in up to one-third of patients at a later time (388–390). Although sometimes intensely painful (389), the cause is unknown and treatment is symptomatic.

Joint infections are surprisingly uncommon among HIV-infected adults. Anecdotally, we have seen a case due to *Staphylococcus aureus,* and other reported pathogens include *Sporothrix schenkii, Cryptococcus neoformans, Mycobacterium haemophilum, Salmonella* sp. and *Campylobacter fetus* (388,391–394). Microbiologic studies are an essential component in the evaluation of joint fluid in the HIV-infected patient with arthritis.

Reactive arthritides and Reiter's syndrome are the most frequently recognized forms of arthritis in HIV infection, occurring in 2–10% of adults depending on geographic area (387–389,395). The majority of North American patients with Reiter's syndrome have the HLA-B27 allele (387). Organisms known to trigger reactive arthritis are, however, rarely discovered (391,396). It should be noted that reactive arthritis or Reiter's syndrome may be the first clinical manifestation of HIV

infection. Psoriasis is also common in HIV infection occurring in 5–20% of patients and is complicated by a psoriatic-like arthritis in up to one-half of cases (389,397).

A less etiologically well-defined type of oligoarthritis termed "HIV-related arthritis" (387) has been described, which is characterized by subacute painful involvement of the knees and ankles with fewer than 10,000 leukocytes/mm^3 on synovial fluid analysis (398,390). Proposed pathophysiologic mechanisms include: direct HIV infection of joints (390,398–400); immune-complex deposition (390,401,402); and an atypical form of reactive arthritis occurring in the absence of HLA-B27, antecedent genitourinary or enteric infections, and inflammatory synovial fluid.

For patients with these forms of arthritis or with Reiter's syndrome, nonsteroidal antiinflammatory agents are the mainstay of treatment. A trial of sulfasalazine may be warranted in instances of sustained inflammation (388), but steroids and other immunosuppressive medications are potentially harmful and may increase the risk of developing opportunistic infections and Kaposi's sarcoma (391,403).

Several types of vasculitis have been reported in HIV-infected patients (404–413), including those of the polyarteritis nodosa type (405,406,414–416). The latter patients present primarily with a peripheral sensory or sensorimotor neuropathy. The etiology for the vasculitis is unknown in most cases, although cytomegalovirus infection is one recognized cause (417,418).

A syndrome characterized by massive parotid enlargement and xerostomia that superficially resembles Sjögren's syndrome is a well-reported but relatively infrequent complication (419,420). In adults the syndrome appears to have an immunogenetic basis and is found principally in blacks who have the DR5 allele (420). It is characterized by markedly elevated numbers of CD8+, CD29+ lymphocytes in blood that infiltrate various glandular and extraglandular tissues (388). Consequently, it has been designated as the "diffuse infiltrative lymphocytosis syndrome." Unlike classic Sjögren's syndrome, autoantibodies are usually absent. Extraglandular involvement may include the liver, lung, gastrointestinal tract, kidney, thymus, and nervous system (421). The possibility of HIV infection should always be considered in individuals with unexplained bilateral parotid enlargement. Anecdotally, we have observed striking resolution of parotid enlargement following irradiation of the gland.

Various autoimmune phenomena have been associated with HIV infection including the production of autoantibodies (387). Aside from antiplatelet antibodies that may be responsible for thrombocytopenia (422,423), antibodies directed at other targets, including red blood cells, leukocytes, and nuclear and cardiolipin antigens, are usually clinically silent (387). The same can probably be said for the presence of circulating immune complexes (401,402) and cryoglobulins (424).

Neurologic Manifestations

Nearly 50% of HIV-infected adults at some point will manifest a clinically apparent neurologic disorder (425–431) (Table 15). Direct HIV infection seems to play an important role in certain CNS manifestations. Complicating the primary neurologic disease process caused by HIV are various potential opportunistic infections, as well as lymphomas, both of which may cause diffuse or focal neurologic abnormalities.

The neurologic history and examination should attempt to ascertain the duration, course, and focality of the disease process. Frequently cerebrospinal fluid (CSF) analysis is required. CSF studies should include cell counts and cytology, protein and glucose determination, VDRL, cultures for bacteria, mycobacteria, and fungi, gram and acid-fast stains, India ink examination, and cryptococcal antigen determination. If there are no focal findings on physical examination, lumbar puncture can be performed prior to radiologic imaging. Computed tomography or magnetic resonance imaging frequently provide useful information. Neurologic consultation is helpful and should be a standard aspect of the care of these patients.

Diagnostic considerations (Table 15) and therapies are discussed in detail in several other chapters in this volume.

FUTURE PROSPECTS

Studies of novel chemo- and immunotherapeutic approaches to control HIV infection are likely to increase at an ever-expanding pace during the remainder of the 1990s and into the 21st century (432–438). Particular impetus will surely be given to the use of combination therapies. Such therapeutic strategies will be designed to take advantage of potential additive or synergistic antiviral effects, and to prevent or retard the emergence of resistant strains, a phenomenon regularly observed during long-term AZT therapy (166,167) and probably likely to occur with any of the nucleoside analogs (439). Putative benefits of any new therapy will continue to be judged against the efficacy and safety profile of AZT.

Because of the effectiveness of *Pneumocystis carinii* pneumonia prophylaxis, a reduction in the frequency of cases will occur, and other complications, particularly disseminated *Mycobacterium avium-intracellulare* infection and lymphoma, will become relatively more prominent (211,440). These conditions in turn will engender intensive efforts directed at improved diagnostic,

TABLE 15. *Common neurologic presentations in HIV-infected adults and usual etiologies*

Meningitis
  HIV
  Syphilis
  Cryptococcosis
  Tuberculosis
  Lymphoma (primary outside of CNS)
  Listeria (rare)
  Bacterial (e.g., pneumococcus, salmonella) (rare)
Encephalitis
  HIV
  Herpes simplex infection
  Cytomegalovirus infection
  Toxoplasmosis
Dementia
  HIV
  Progressive multifocal leukoencephalopathy
  Cytomegalovirus infection
  Toxoplasmosis
  Alcohol abuse
Focal CNS disease
  Toxoplasmosis
  Primary CNS lymphoma
  Progressive multifocal leukoencephalopathy
  Cryptococcosis (rare)
  Tuberculosis (rare)
  Aspergillosis (rare)
  Nocardiosis (rare)
Transient ischemic attacks/strokes
  Toxoplasmosis
  Syphilis
  Cryptococcosis
  Herpes zoster vasculitis
  Tuberculosis
  Aspergillosis
  Marantic endocarditis
  Embolus from mural thrombus (2° to cardiomyopathy)
  Vasculitis
  Idiopathic
  Coagulopathy and thrombocytopenia
Myelopathy/myelitis
  Vacuolar myelopathy
  Human T-cell lymphotropic virus type I
  Varicella-zoster infection
  Lymphoma/plasmacytoma
  Syphilis
  Cytomegalovirus infection
  Tuberculosis
  Epidural or intramedullary abscess
Peripheral neuropathy
  Autoimmunity
  HIV
  Drug toxicity
  Cytomegalovirus infection (polyradiculopathy)
Myopathy
  HIV
  AZT

therapeutic, and preventive measures. Advances that may come from these efforts will in turn further alter the natural history of HIV infection and lead to different research priorities.

ACKNOWLEDGMENTS

The authors thank Drs. R. Lerner, M. Weiss, B. Koppel, and M. Wolinsky for their helpful advice and Mrs. Shirley Gamble for typing the manuscript.

REFERENCES

1. Piette J, Mor V, Fleishman J. Patterns of survival with AIDS in the United States. *Health Services Res* 1991;26:75–95.
2. Moore RD, Hidalgo J, Sugland BW, Chaisson RE. Zidovudine and the natural history of the acquired immunodeficiency syndrome. *N Engl J Med* 1991;324:1412–6.
3. Lemp GF, Payne SF, Rutherford GW, et al. Projections of AIDS morbidity and mortality in San Francisco. *JAMA* 1990; 263:1497–501.
4. Hay JW, Osmond DH, Jacobson MA. Projecting the medical costs of AIDS and ARC in the United States. *J Acquired Immune Deficiency Syndrome* 1988;1:466–85.
5. Masur H, Ognibene FP, Yarchoan R, et al. CD4 counts as predictors of opportunistic pneumonias in human immunodeficiency virus (HIV) infection. *Ann Intern Med* 1989;111:223–31.
6. Phair JP, Munoz A, Detels R, et al. The risk of *Pneumocystis carinii* pneumonia among men infected with human immunodeficiency virus type 1. *N Engl J Med* 1990;322:161–5.
7. Crowe SM, Carlin JB, Stewart KI, Lucas R, Hoy JF. Predictive value of CD4 lymphocyte numbers for the development of opportunistic infections and malignancies in HIV-infected persons. *J Acquired Immune Deficiency Syndrome* 1991;4:770–6.
8. CDC. Guidelines for prophylaxis against *Pneumocystis carinii* pneumonia for persons infected with human immunodeficiency virus. *MMWR* 1989;39:[Suppl S-5]:1–9.
9. Horowitz H, Wormser GP. Human immunodeficiency virus (HIV)-infected patient. In: Taylor RB, ed. *Difficult medical management.* Philadelphia: WB Saunders, 1991;290–9.
10. CDC. Update on the acquired immune deficiency syndrome (AIDS)—United States. *MMWR* 1982;31:507–8, 513–4.
11. CDC. Revision of the case definition of acquired immunodeficiency syndrome for national reporting—United States. *MMWR* 1985;34:373–5.
12. CDC. Revision of the CDC surveillance case definition for acquired immunodeficiency syndrome. *MMWR* 1987;36 [Suppl-1]:1S–15S.
13. Zurawsky C. Revised AIDS definition draws fire. *Infectious Dis News* 1991;4:1,16.
14. Giorgi JV, Detels R. T-cell subset alterations in HIV-infected homosexual men: NIAID Multicenter AIDS Cohort Study. *Clin Immunol Immunopathol* 1989;52:10–8.
15. Wormser GP, Joline C, Sivak SL, Arlin ZA. Human immunodeficiency virus infections: considerations for health care workers. *Bull NY Acad Med* 1988;64:203–15.
16. Volberding PA, Lagakos SW, Koch MA, et al. Zidovudine in asymptomatic human immunodeficiency virus infection. A controlled trial in persons with fewer than 500 CD4-positive cells per cubic millimeter. *N Engl J Med* 1990;322:941–9.
17. Fischl MA, Richman DD, Hansen N, et al. The safety and efficacy of zidovudine (AZT) in the treatment of patients with mildly symptomatic human immunodeficiency virus type 1 (HIV) infection: a double-blind, placebo-controlled trial. *Ann Intern Med* 1990;112:727–37.
18. Signore A, Cugini P, Letizia C, Lucia P, Murano G, Possilli P. Study of the diurnal variation of human lymphocyte subsets. *J Clin Lab Immunol* 1985;17:25–8.
19. Saunders AM. Sources of physiological variation in differential leukocyte counting. *Blood Cells* 1985;11:31–48.
20. Malone JL, Simms TE, Gray GC, Wagner KF, Burge JR, Burke DS. Sources of variability in repeated T-helper lymphocyte counts from human immunodeficiency virus type 1-infected patients: total lymphocyte count fluctuations and diurnal cycle are

important. *J Acquired Immune Deficiency Syndrome* 1990; 3:144–51.
21. Miller CH, Levy NB. Effects of storage conditions on lymphocyte phenotypes from healthy and diseased persons. *J Clin Lab Anal* 1989;3:296–300.
22. Kidd PG, Vogt RF Jr. Report of the workshop on the evaluation of T-cell subsets during HIV infection and AIDS. *Clin Immunol Immunopathol* 1989;52:3–9.
23. Bertouch JV, Roberts-Thomson PJ, Bradley J. Diurnal variation of lymphocyte subsets identified by monoclonal antibodies. *Br Med J* 1983;286:1171–2.
24. Miyawaki T, Taga K, Nagaoki T, Seki H, Suzuki Y, Taniguchi N. Circadian changes of T lymphocyte subsets in human peripheral blood. *Clin Exp Immunol* 1984;55:618–22.
25. Fennerty AG, Jones KP, Davies BH. Lymphocytes are rhythmic: is this important? *Br Med J* 1985;290:152–3.
26. Hedfors E, Holm G, Ivansen M, Wahren J. Physiological variation of blood lymphocyte reactivity: T-cell subsets, immunoglobulin production, and mixed lymphocyte reactivity. *Clin Immunol Immunopathol* 1983;27:9–14.
27. Slade JD, Hepburn B. Prednisone-induced alterations of circulating human lymphocyte subsets. *J Lab Clin Med* 1983; 101:479–87.
28. Martini E, Muller J-Y, Doinel C, et al. Disappearance of CD4-lymphocyte circadian cycles in HIV-infected patients: early event during asymptomatic infection. *AIDS* 1988;2:133–4.
29. Tunkel AR, Rein MF, Kelsall B, Vollmer K, Wispelweg B. Marked increase in absolute CD4 lymphocyte counts following splenectomy in human immunodeficiency virus (HIV)-infected patients. 31st Interscience Conference on Antimicrobial Agents Chemotherapy, Chicago, October, 1991; 1385 (abst).
30. Bach M-A, Phan-Dinh-Tuy F, Bach J-F, et al. Unusual phenotypes of human inducer T-cells as measured by OKT4 and related monoclonal antibodies. *J Immunol* 1981;127:980–2.
31. Parker WA Jr, Hensley RE, Houk RA, Reid MJ. Heterogeneity of the epitopes of CD4 in patients infected with HIV. *N Engl J Med* 1988;319:581–1.
32. Lang W, Perkins H, Anderson RE, Royce R, Jewell N, Winkelstein NW Jr. Patterns of T lymphocyte changes with human immunodeficiency virus infection: from seroconversion to the development of AIDS. *J Acquired Immune Deficiency Syndrome* 1989;2:63–9.
33. Moss AR, Bachetti P. Natural history of HIV infection. *AIDS* 1989;3:55–61.
34. Phillips AN, Lee CA, Elford J, et al. Serial CD4 lymphocyte counts and development of AIDS. *Lancet* 1991;337:389–92.
35. Moss AR, Bacchetti P, Osmond D, et al. Seropositivity for HIV and the development of AIDS or AIDS related condition: three year follow-up of the San Francisco General Hospital Cohort. *Br Med J* 1988;296:745–50.
36. MacDonell KB, Chmiel JS, Poggensee L, Wu S, Phair JP. Predicting progression to AIDS: combined usefulness of CD4 lymphocyte counts and p24 antigenemia. *Am J Med* 1990; 89:706–12.
37. Taylor JM, Fahey JL, Detels R, Giorgi JV. CD4 percentage, CD4 number, and CD4:CD8 ratio in HIV infection: which to choose and how to use. *J Acquired Immune Deficiency Syndrome* 1989;2:114–24.
38. Kessler HA, Landay A, Pottage JC Jr, Benson CA. Absolute number versus percentage of T-helper lymphocytes in human immunodeficiency virus infection. *J Infect Dis* 1990;161:356–7.
39. Polis MA, Masur H. Predicting the progression to AIDS. *Am J Med* 1990;89:701–5.
40. Eyster ME, Gail MH, Ballard JO, Al-Mondhiry H, Goedert JJ. Natural history of human immunodeficiency virus infection in hemophiliacs: effects of T-cell subsets, platelet counts and age. *Ann Intern Med* 1987;107:1–6.
41. Pedersen C, Lindhardt BO, Jensen BL, et al. Clinical course of primary HIV infection: consequences for subsequent course of infection. *Br Med J* 1989;299:154–7.
42. Kaslow RA, Duqesnoy R, Van Raden M, et al. Al, CW7, B8, DR3 HLA antigen combination associated with rapid decline of

T-helper lymphocytes in HIV-1 infection. *Lancet* 1990; 335:927–30.

43. Fabio G, Scorza R, Smeraldi A, et al. Susceptibility to HIV infection and AIDS in Italian hemophiliacs is HLA associated. *Br J Haematol* 1990;75:531–6.

44. de Wolf F, Goudsmit J, Paul DA, et al. Risk of AIDS related complex and AIDS in homosexual men with persistent HIV antigenemia. *Br Med J* 1987;295:569–72.

45. Schnittman SM, Greenhouse JJ, Psallidopoulos MC, et al. Increasing viral burden CD4+ T-cells from patients with human immunodeficiency virus (HIV) infection reflects rapidly progressive immunosuppression and clinical disease. *Ann Intern Med* 1990;113:438–43.

46. Melmed RN, Taylor JM, Detels R, Bozorgmehri M, Fahey JL. Serum neopterin changes in HIV-infected subjects: indication of significant pathology, CD4 T cell change, and the development of AIDS. *J Acquired Immune Deficiency Syndrome* 1989;2:70–6.

47. Fahey JL, Taylor JMG, Detels R, et al. The prognostic value of cellular and serologic markers in infection with human immunodeficiency virus type 1. *N Engl J Med* 1990;322:166–72.

48. Huber C, Batchelor JR, Fuchs D, et al. Immune response-associated production of neopterin: release from macrophages primarily under control of interferon-gamma. *J Exp Med* 1984;160:310–6.

49. Zon L, Arkin C, Groopman JE. Haematologic manifestations of the human immune deficiency virus (HIV). *Br J Haematol* 1987;66:251–6.

50. Murphy MF, Metcalfe P, Waters AH, et al. Incidence and mechanism of neutropenia and thrombocytopenia in patients with human immunodeficiency virus infection. *Br J Haematol* 1987;66:337–40.

51. Gottlieb MS, Schroff R, Schanker HM, et al. *Pneumocystis carinii* pneumonia and mucosal candidiasis in previously healthy homosexual men: evidence of a new acquired cellular immunodeficiency. *N Engl J Med* 1981;305:1425–31.

52. Zolla-Pazner S, Des Jarlais DC, Friedman SR, et al. Non-random development of immunologic abnormalities after infection with human immunodeficiency virus: implications for immunologic classification of the disease. *Proc Natl Acad Sci USA* 1987;84:5404–8.

53. Cusano AJ, Thies HL, Siegal FP, Dreisbach AW, Maesaka JK. Hyponatremia in patients with acquired immune deficiency syndrome. *J Acquired Immune Deficiency Syndrome* 1990; 3:949–53.

54. Glassock RJ, Cohen AH, Danovitch G, Parsa KP. Human immunodeficiency virus (HIV) infection and the kidney. *Ann Intern Med* 1990;112:35–49.

55. Membreno L, Irony I, Dere W, et al. Adrenocortical function in acquired immunodeficiency syndrome. *J Clin Endocrinol* 1987;65:482–7.

56. Pearson RD, Hewlett EL. Pentamidine for the treatment of *Pneumocystis carinii* and other protozoal diseases. *Ann Intern Med* 1985;103:782–6.

57. Waskin H, Stehr-Green JK, Helmick CG, et al. Risk factors for hypoglycemia associated with pentamidine therapy for *Pneumocystis carinii* pneumonia. *JAMA* 1988;260:345–7.

58. Rao TKS. Human immunodeficiency virus (HIV) associated nephropathy. *Annu Rev Med* 1991;42:391–401.

59. Lebovics E, Thung SN, Schaffner F, et al. The liver in the acquired immunodeficiency syndrome: a clinical and histologic study. *Hepatology* 1985;5:293–8.

60. Dworkin BM, Stahl RE, Giardina MA, et al. The liver in acquired immune deficiency syndrome: emphasis on patients with intravenous drug abuse. *Am J Gastroenterol* 1987;82:231–6.

61. Till M, MacDonell KB. Myopathy with human immunodeficiency virus type 1 (HIV-1) infection: HIV-1 or zidovudine. *Ann Intern Med* 1990;113:492–4.

62. Delakas MC, Illa I, Pezeshkpour GH, Laukaitis JP, Cohen B, Griffin JL. Mitochondrial myopathy caused by long-term zidovudine therapy. *N Engl J Med* 1990;322:1098–105.

63. Arneudo E, Dalakas M, Shanske S, Moraes CT, DiMauro S, Schon EA. Depletion of muscle mitochondrial DNA in AIDS patients with zidovudine-induced myopathy. *Lancet* 1991; 337:508–10.

64. Zaman MZ, White DA. Serum lactate dehydrogenase levels and *Pneumocystis carinii* pneumonia. *Am Rev Respir Dis* 1988; 137:796–800.

65. Kekow J, Hobusch G, Gross WL. Predominance of IgG 1 subclass in the hypergammaglobulinemia observed in pre-AIDS and AIDS. *Cancer Detect Prev* 1988;12:211–6.

66. Jacobson DL, McCutchan JA, Spechko PL, et al. The evolution of lymphadenopathy and hypergammaglobulinemia are evidence for early and sustained polyclonal B lymphocyte activation during human immunodeficiency virus infection. *J Infect Dis* 1991;163:240–6.

67. Lambertus MW, Anderson RE. Hyperamylasemia in patients with human immunodeficiency virus infection. *N Engl J Med* 1990;323:1708–9.

68. Grunfeld C, Kotler DP, Hamadeh R, Tierney A, Wang J, Pierson RN Jr. Hypertriglyceridemia in the acquired immunodeficiency syndrome. *Am J Med* 1989;86:27–31.

69. Ravenholt RT. Role of hepatitis B virus in the acquired immune deficiency syndrome. *Lancet* 1983;2:885–6.

70. Rustgi VK, Hoofnagle JH, Gerin JC, et al. Hepatitis B virus infection in the acquired immunodeficiency syndrome. *Ann Intern Med* 1984;101:795–7.

71. Wormser GP, Forseter G, Joline C, Tupper B, O'Brien TA. Hepatitis C in HIV-infected intravenous drug users and homosexual men in suburban New York City. *JAMA* 1991;265:2958.

72. Esteban JI, Esteban R, Viladomio L, et al. Hepatitis C virus antibodies among risk groups in Spain. *Lancet* 1989;2:294–7.

73. CDC. Diagnosis and management of mycobacterial infection and disease in persons with human immunodeficiency virus infection. *Ann Intern Med* 1987;106:254–6.

74. Braun MM, Truman BI, Maguire B, et al. Increasing incidence of tuberculosis in a prison inmate population. *JAMA* 1989; 261:393–7.

75. Barnes PF, Bloch AB, Davidson PT, Snider DE Jr. Tuberculosis in patients with human immunodeficiency virus infection. *N Engl J Med* 1991;324:1644–50.

76. CDC. Tuberculosis and human immunodeficiency virus infection: recommendations of the Advisory Committee for the Elimination of Tuberculosis. *MMWR* 1989;38:236–50.

77. Marte C, Cohen M, Fruchter R, Kelly P. Pap test and STD finding in HIV+ women at ambulatory care sites. 6th International Conference on AIDS, San Francisco, June, 1990;211(abst).

78. Maiman M, Fruchter R, Klein R, Marte C, Shultz S. Risk for cervical disease in HIV-infected women—New York City. *MMWR* 1990;39:846–9.

79. Schultz S, Araneta MRG, Joseph SC. Neurosyphilis and HIV infection. *N Engl J Med* 1987;317:1474.

80. McCabe RE, Remington JS. Toxoplasmosis: the time has come. *N Engl J Med* 1988;318:313–5.

81. Maayan S, Wormser GP, Hewlett D, et al. Acquired immunodeficiency syndrome (AIDS) in an economically disadvantaged population. *Arch Intern Med* 1985;145:1607–12.

82. Rogers ME, Moren DM, Stewart JA, et al. National case-control study of Kaposi's sarcoma and *Pneumocystis carinii* pneumonia in homosexual men: Part 2. Laboratory results. *Ann Intern Med* 1983;99:151–8.

83. Harriman GR, Smith PD, Horne MK, et al. Vitamin B-12 malabsorption in patients with acquired immunodeficiency syndrome. *Arch Intern Med* 1989;149:2039–41.

84. Kessler HA, Bloauw B, Spear J, Paul PA, Falk LA, Landay A. Diagnosis of human immunodeficiency virus infection in seronegative homosexuals with an acute viral syndrome. *JAMA* 1987;258:1196–9.

85. Wittek AE, Phelan MA, Wells MA, et al. Detection of human immunodeficiency virus core protein in plasma by enzyme immunoassay. Association of antigenemia with symptomatic disease and T-helper cell depletion. *Ann Intern Med* 1987; 107:286–92.

86. Allain JP, Laurian Y, Paul DA, et al. Long-term evaluation of HIV antigen and antibodies to p24 and gp41 in patients with hemophilia. Potential clinical importance. *N Engl J Med* 1987;317:1114–21.

87. Finazzi G, Mannucci PM, Lazzarin A, et al. Low incidence of bleeding from HIV-related thrombocytopenia in drug addicts

and hemophiliacs: implication for therapeutic strategies. *Eur J Haematol* 1990;45:82–5.

88. The Swiss Group for Clinical Studies on the Acquired Immunodeficiency Syndrome (AIDS). Zidovudine for the treatment of thrombocytopenia associated with human immunodeficiency virus (HIV). A prospective study. *Ann Intern Med* 1988; 109:718–21.

89. Oksenhendler E, Bierling P, Ferchal F, Clauval J-P, Seligmann M. Zidovudine for thrombocytopenic purpura related to human immunodeficiency virus (HIV) infection. *Ann Intern Med* 1989;110:365–368.

90. Di Bisceglie AM, Martin P, Kassianides C, et al. Recombinant interferon alfa therapy for chronic hepatitis C. A randomized, double-blind, placebo-controlled trial. *N Engl J Med* 1989; 321:1506–10.

91. Davis GL, Balart LA, Schiff ER, et al. Treatment of chronic hepatitis C with recombinant interferon alfa. A multicenter randomized, controlled trial. *N Engl J Med* 1989;321:1501–6.

92. Perillo RP, Schiff ER, Davis GL, et al. A randomized controlled trial of interferon alpha-2b alone and after prednisone withdrawal for the treatment of chronic hepatitis B. *N Engl J Med* 1990;323:295–301.

93. Korenman J, Baker B, Waggoner J, Everhart JE, Di Bisceglie AM, Hoofnagle JH. Long-term remission of chronic hepatitis B after alpha-interferon therapy. *Ann Intern Med* 1991; 114:629–34.

94. Johns DR, Tierney M, Felsenstein D. Alteration in the natural history of neurosyphilis by concurrent infection with the human immunodeficiency virus. *N Engl J Med* 1987;316:1569–72.

95. Lukehart SA, Hook EW II, Baker-Zander SA, Collier AC, Critchlow CW, Handsfield HH. Invasion of the central nervous system by *Treponema pallidum*: implications for diagnosis and treatment. *Ann Intern Med* 1988;109:855–62.

96. CDC. Syphilis in HIV-infected patients. *MMWR* 1989;38:12–3.

97. Musher DM, Hamill RJ, Baughn RE. Effect of human immunodeficiency virus (HIV) infection on the course of syphilis and on the response to treatment. *Ann Intern Med* 1990;113:872–81.

98. CDC. 1989 Sexually Transmitted Diseases Treatment Guidelines. *MMWR* 1989;38:S-8:5–15.

99. Berry CD, Hooton TM, Collier AC, Lukehart SA. Neurologic relapse after benzathine penicillin therapy for secondary syphilis in a patient with HIV infection. *N Engl J Med* 1987; 316:1587–89.

100. Mohr JA, Griffiths W, Jackson R, Saadah H, Bird P, Riddle J. Neurosyphilis and penicillin levels in cerebrospinal fluid. *JAMA* 1976;236:2208–9.

101. Seef LB, Wright EC, Zimmerman HJ, et al. Type B hepatitis after needle-stick exposure. prevention with hepatitis B immune globulin. Final report of the Veterans Administration Cooperative Study. *Ann Intern Med* 1978;88:285–93.

102. Henderson DK, Saah AJ, Zak BJ, et al. Risk of nosocomial infection with human T-cell lymphotropic virus type III/lymphadenopathy-associated virus in a large cohort of intensively exposed health care workers. *Ann Intern Med* 1986;104:644–7.

103. Selwyn PA, Hartel D, Lewis VA, et al. A prospective study of the risk of tuberculosis among intravenous drug users with human immunodeficiency virus infection. *N Engl J Med* 1989; 320:545–30.

104. CDC. Diagnosis and management of mycobacterial infection and disease in persons with human T-lymphotropic virus type III/lymphadenopathy-associated virus infection. *MMWR* 1986; 35:448–52.

105. American Thoracic Society. Treatment of tuberculosis and tuberculosis infection in adults and children. *Am Rev Respir Dis* 1986;134:355–63.

106. American Thoracic Society. Mycobacterioses and the acquired immunodeficiency syndrome. *Am Rev Respir Dis* 1987; 136:492–6.

107. Small PM, Schecter GF, Goodman PC, Sande MA, Chaisson RE, Hopewell PC. Treatment of tuberculosis in patients with advanced human immunodeficiency virus infection. *N Engl J Med* 1991;324:289–94.

108. CDC. The use of preventive therapy for tuberculosis infection in the United States. Recommendations of the Advisory Committee for Elimination of Tuberculosis. *MMWR* 1990;39:9–12.

109. CDC. Purified protein derivative (PPD)-tuberculin anergy and HIV infection: guidelines for anergy testing and management of anergic persons at risk of tuberculosis. *MMWR* 1991;40:27–32.

110. Feingold AR, Vermund SH, Burk RD, et al. Cervical cytologic abnormalities and papilloma virus in women infected with human immunodeficiency virus. *J Acquired Immune Deficiency Syndrome* 1990;3:896–903.

111. Vermund S, Kelley KF, Burk RD, et al. Risk of human papilloma virus (HPV) and cervical squamous intraepithelial lesions (SIL) highest among women with advanced HIV disease. 6th International Conference on AIDS, San Francisco, June, 1990;215(abst).

112. Henry MJ, Stanley MW, Cruikshank S, Carson L. Association of human immunodeficiency virus-induced immunosuppression with human papilloma virus infection and cervical intraepithelial neoplasia. *Am J Obstet Gynecol* 1989;160:352–3.

113. Maiman M, Fruchter RG, Serur E, et al. Human immunodeficiency virus infection and cervical neoplasia. *Gynecol Oncol* 1990;38:377–82.

114. Cohn JA, McMeeking A, Cohen W, Jacobs J, Holzman RS. Evaluation of the policy of empiric treatment of suspected *Toxoplasma* encephalitis in patients with the acquired immunodeficiency syndrome. *Am J Med* 1989;86:521–7.

115. Kiyosawa K, Sodeyama T, Tanaka E, et al. Hepatitis C in hospital employees with needlestick injuries. *Ann Intern Med* 1991;115:367–9.

116. Maayan S, Wormser GP, Widerhorn J, Sy ER, Kim YH, Ernst JA. *Strongyloides stercoralis* hyperinfection in a patient with the acquired immune deficiency syndrome. *Am J Med* 1987; 83:945–8.

117. [Anonymous]. Drugs for parasitic infection. *Med Lett* 1990;32:23–30.

118. Videx (didanosine). Package insert. Bristol Laboratories; October, 1991.

119. Grunfeld C, Kotler DP, Shigenago JK, et al. Circulating interferon-α levels and hypertriglyceridemia in the acquired immunodeficiency syndrome. *Am J Med* 1991;90:154–62.

120. Kemper CA, Tucker RM, Lang OS, et al. Low-dose dapsone prophylaxis of *Pneumocystis carinii* pneumonia in AIDS and AIDS-related complex. *AIDS* 1990;4:1145–8.

121. Hughes WT, Kennedy W, Dugdale M, et al. Prevention of *Pneumocystis carinii* pneumonitis in AIDS patients with weekly dapsone. *Lancet* 1990;336:1066.

122. Metroka CE, Jacobus D, Lewis N. Successful chemoprophylaxis for pneumocystis with dapsone or bactrim. 5th International Conference on AIDS, Montreal, Canada, June, 1989.

123. Metroka CE, McMechan MF, Andrade R, Laubenstein LJ, Jacobus DP. Failure of prophylaxis with dapsone in patients taking dideoxyinosine. *N Engl J Med* 1991;325:737.

124. DeGowin RL. A review of therapeutic and hemolytic effects of dapsone. *Arch Intern Med* 1967;120:242–8.

125. Telzak EE, Budnick LD, Greenberg MSZ, et al. A nosocomial outbreak of *Salmonella enteritidis* infection due to the consumption of raw eggs. *N Engl J Med* 1990;323:394–7.

126. Mishu B, Griffin PM, Tauxe RV, Cameron DN, Hutcheson RH, Schaffner W. *Salmonella enteritidis* gastroenteritis transmitted by intact chicken eggs. *Ann Intern Med* 1991;115:190–4.

127. Collier AC, Corey L, Murphy VL, Handsfield HH. Antibody to human immunodeficiency virus and suboptimal response to hepatitis B vaccination. *Ann Intern Med* 1988;109:101–5.

128. Carne JA, Weller IVD, Waite J, et al. Impaired responsiveness of homosexual men with HIV antibodies to plasma derived hepatitis B vaccine. *Br Med J* 1987;294:866–8.

129. Odaka N, Elred L, Cohn S, et al. Comparative immunogenicity of plasma and recombinant hepatitis B vaccines in homosexual men. *JAMA* 1988;260:3635–7.

130. Geseman M, Scheiemann N, Brockmeyer N, et al. Clinical evaluation of a recombinant hepatitis B vaccine in HIV-infected vs. uninfected persons. In: Zuckerman AJ, ed. *Viral hepatitis and liver disease*. New York: Alan R. Liss, 1988;1076–8.

131. Loke RHT, Anderson MG, Tsiquaye KN, et al. Reduced immunogenicity of recombinant yeast-derived hepatitis B vaccine in HIV antibody positive male homosexuals. In: Zuckerman AJ, ed.

Viral hepatitis and liver disease. New York: Alan R. Liss 1988;1074–5.

132. Nelson KE, Clements ML, Miotti P, Cohn S, Polk BF. The influence of human immunodeficiency virus infection on antibody responses to influenza vaccines. *Ann Intern Med* 1988; 109:383–8.

133. Miotti PG, Nelson KE, Dallabetta GA, Farzadegan H, Margolick J, Clements ML. The influence of HIV infection on antibody responses to a two-dose regimen of influenza vaccine. *JAMA* 1989;262:779–83.

134. Huang K-L, Ruben FL, Rinaldo CR Jr, Kingsley L, Lyter DW, Ho M. Antibody responses after influenza and pneumococcal immunization in HIV-infected homosexual men. *JAMA* 1987;257:2047–50.

135. Klein RS, Selwyn PA, Maude D, Pollard C, Freeman K, Schiffman G. Response to pneumococcal vaccine among asymptomatic heterosexual partners of persons with human immunodeficiency virus. *J Infect Dis* 1989;160:826–31.

136. McLaughlin M, Thomas P, Onorato I, et al. Use of live virus vaccines in HIV-infected children: a retrospective survey. *Pediatrics* 1988;82:229–33.

137. Janoff EN, Douglas JM, Gabriel M, et al. Class specific antibody response to pneumococcal capsular polysaccharides in men infected with human immunodeficiency virus type 1. *J Infect Dis* 1988;158:983–90.

138. Buchbinder S, Hessol N, Lifson A, et al. Does infection with hepatitis B virus or vaccination with plasma-derived hepatitis B vaccine accelerate progression to AIDS? 6th International Conference on AIDS, San Francisco, June, 1990.

139. American College of Physicians. *Guide for adult immunization,* 2nd ed. Philadelphia, 1990.

140. Immunization Practices Advisory Committee. Pneumococcal polysaccharide vaccine. *MMWR* 1989;38:64–76.

141. [Anonymous]. Influenza vaccine, 1991–1992. *Med Lett* 1991; 33:86.

142. Hadler SC, Judson FN, O'Malley PM, et al. Outcome of hepatitis B virus infection in homosexual men and its relation to prior human immunodeficiency virus infection. *J Infect Dis* 1991;163:454–9.

143. Moreno S, Martinex R, Barros C, Gonzalez-Lahoz J, Garcia-Delgado E, Bouza E. Latent *Haemophilus influenzae* pneumonia in patients infected with HIV. *AIDS* 1991;5:967–70.

144. Janoff EN, Worel S, Douglas JM. Natural immunity and response to conjugate vaccine for *Haemophilus influenzae* type B in men with HIV. 30th Interscience Conference on Antimicrobial Agents and Chemotherapy, Atlanta, October, 1990.

145. Retrovir capsules (zidovudine). In: *Physicians Desk Reference,* 45th ed. Oradell, NJ: Medical Economics Data, 1991;788–92.

146. Richman DD, Fischl MA, Grieco MH, et al. The toxicity of azidothymidine (AZT) in the treatment of patients with AIDS and AIDS-related complex: a double-blind, placebo-controlled trial. *N Engl J Med* 1987;317:192–7.

147. Walker RE, Parker RJ, Kovacs JA, et al. Anemia and erythropoiesis in patients with the acquired immunodeficiency syndrome (AIDS) and Kaposi's sarcoma treated with zidovudine. *Ann Intern Med* 1988;108:372–6.

148. Dun PC, Fusco F, Fried P, et al. Nail dyschromia associated with zidovudine. *Ann Intern Med* 1990;112:145–6.

149. Fischl MA, Richman DD, Grieco MH, et al. The efficacy of azidothymidine (AZT) in the treatment of patients with AIDS and AIDS-related complex: a double-blind, placebo-controlled trial. *N Engl J Med* 1987;317:185–91.

150. Fischl MA, Parker CB, Pettinelli C, et al. A randomized controlled trial of a reduced daily dose of zidovudine in patients with the acquired immunodeficiency syndrome. *N Engl J Med* 1990;323:1009–14.

151. Collier AC, Bozzette S, Coombs R, et al. A pilot study of low-dose zidovudine in human immunodeficiency virus infection. *N Engl J Med* 1990;323:1015–21.

152. Fischl M, Galpin JE, Levine JD, et al. Recombinant human erythropoietin for patients with AIDS treated with zidovudine. *N Engl J Med* 1990;322:1488–93.

153. Phair JP, Abels RI. Recombinant human erythropoietin (R-HuEPO) treatment IND program for the anemia of AIDS—data from 1024 patients. 31st Interscience Conference on Antimicrobial Agents Chemotherapy, Chicago, October, 1991;1354(abst).

154. Groopman JE, Mitsuyasu RT, DeLeo MJ, Oette DH, Golde DW. Effect of recombinant human granulocyte-macrophage colony stimulating factor on myelopoiesis in the acquired immunodeficiency syndrome. *N Engl J Med* 1987;317:593–8.

155. Miles SA, Mitsuyasu RT, Moreno J, et al. Combined therapy with recombinant G-CSF and erythropoietin decreases hematologic toxicity from zidovudine. *Blood* 1991;77:2109–17.

156. Mitsuyasu R, Levine J, Miles SA, et al. Effects of long term subcutaneous administration of recombinant granulocyte-macrophage colony stimulating factor (GM-CSF) in patients with HIV-related leukopenia. *Blood* 1988;72[Suppl 1]:356(abst).

157. Mitsuyasu RT. Use of recombinant interferons and hematopoietic growth factors in patients infected with human immunodeficiency virus. *Rev Infect Dis* 1991;131:979–84.

158. Koyanagi Y, O'Brien WA, Zhau JQ, Golde DW, Gasson JC, Chen ISY. Cytokines alter production of HIV-1 from primary mononuclear phagocytes. *Science* 1988;241:1673–5.

159. Hochster H, Dieterich D, Bozzette S, et al. Toxicity of combined ganciclovir and zidovudine for cytomegalovirus disease associated with AIDS. An AIDS Clinical Trial Group Study. *Ann Intern Med* 1990;113:111–7.

160. Luke RHT, Wade JPH, Murray-Lyon IM. Myelopathy after stopping zidovudine. *Lancet* 1988;2:279.

161. Helbert M, Robinson D, Peddle B, et al. Acute meningoencephalitis on dose reduction of zidovudine. *Lancet* 1988; 1:1249–52.

162. Sattler FR, Ko R, Antoniskis D, et al. Acetaminophen does not impair clearance of zidovudine. *Ann Intern Med* 1991; 114:937–40.

163. Kornhauser DM, Petty BG, Hendrix CW, et al. Probenecid and zidovudine metabolism. *Lancet* 1989;2:473–5.

164. de Miranda P, Good SS, Yarchoan R, et al. Alteration of zidovudine pharmacokinetics by probenecid in patients with AIDS or AIDS-related complex. *Clin Pharm Ther* 1989;46:494–500.

165. Bach MC. Failure of zidovudine to maintain remission in patients with AIDS [Letter]. *N Engl J Med* 1989;320:594–5.

166. Larder BA, Darby G, Richman DD. HIV with reduced sensitivity to zidovudine (AZT) isolated during prolonged therapy. *Science* 1989;243:1731–4.

167. Larder BA, Kemp SD. Multiple mutations in HIV-1 reverse transcriptase confer high level resistance to zidovudine (AZT). *Science* 1989;246:1155–8.

168. Bach MC. Clinical response to dideoxyinosine in patients with HIV infection resistant to zidovudine. *N Engl J Med* 1990;323:275.

169. Vogt MW, Hirsch MS. Treatment of human immunodeficiency virus infection. *Infect Dis Clinic North Am* 1987;1:323–39.

170. Johnson RP, Schooley RT. Update on antiretroviral agents other than zidovudine. *AIDS* 1989;3[Suppl 1]:S145–S151.

171. Broder S, Mitsuya H, Yarchoan R, Pavlakis GN. Antiretroviral therapy in AIDS. *Ann Intern Med* 1990;113:604–18.

172. Haverkos HW. Assessment of therapy for *Pneumocystis carinii* pneumonia: PCP therapy project group. *Am J Med* 1984; 76:501–8.

173. Kales CP, Murren JR, Torres RA, Crocco JA. Early predictors of in-hospital mortality for *Pneumocystis carinii* pneumonia in the acquired immunodeficiency syndrome. *Arch Intern Med* 1987;147:1413–7.

174. Allen DW, Mc Avinue SM, Spahr HT, Chaisson RE. Organism load in *Pneumocystis carinii* pneumonia correlates with disease severity. 31st Interscience Conference on Antimicrobial Agents and Chemotherapy, Chicago, October, 1991;225(abst).

175. Kovacs JA, Masur H. *Pneumocystis carinii* pneumonia: therapy and prophylaxis. *J Infect Dis* 1988;158:254–9.

176. Klein NC, Duncanson FP, Lenox TH, et al. Trimethoprim-sulfamethoxazole vs pentamidine for *Pneumocystis carinii* pneumonia in AIDS patients. Results of a large, prospective, randomized treatment trial AIDS (in press).

177. Kovacs JA, Masur H. Prophylaxis of *Pneumocystis carinii* pneumonia: an update. *J Infect Dis* 1989;160:882–6.

178. Hirschel B, Lazzarin A, Chopard P, et al. A controlled trial for

primary prevention of *Pneumocystis carinii* pneumonia. *N Engl J Med* 1991;324:1079–83.

179. Montaner JSG, Lawson LM, Gervais A, et al. Aerosol pentamidine for secondary prophylaxis of AIDS-related *Pneumocystis carinii* pneumonia. A randomized, placebo-controlled trial. *Ann Intern Med* 1991;114:948–53.

180. Armstrong D, Bernard E. Aerosolized pentamidine for the prevention and treatment of pneumocystosis. *AIDS Updates* 1990;3:1–7.

181. Leoung GS, Feigal DW Jr, Montgomery AB, et al. Aerosolized pentamidine for prophylaxis against *Pneumocystis carinii* pneumonia. The San Francisco Community Prophylaxis Trial. *N Engl J Med* 1990;323:769–75.

182. Ruskin J, LaRiviere M. Low-dose co-trimoxazole for prevention of *Pneumocystis carinii* pneumonia in human immunodeficiency virus disease. *Lancet* 1991;337:468–71.

183. Wormser GP, Horowitz HW, Duncanson FP, et al. Low-dose intermittent trimethoprim-sulfamethoxazole for prevention of *Pneumocystis carinii* pneumonia in patients with human immunodeficiency virus infection. *Arch Intern Med* 1991;151:688–92.

184. Gordin F, Simon G, Wofsy C, Mills J. Adverse reactions to trimethoprim-sulfamethoxazole in patients with the acquired immunodeficiency syndrome. *Ann Intern Med* 1984;100:495–9.

185. CDC. *Mycobacterium tuberculosis* transmission in a health clinic —Florida 1988. *MMWR* 1989;38:256–64.

186. Smaldone GC, Vinciguerra C, Marchese J. Detection of inhaled pentamidine in health care workers. *N Engl J Med* 1991;325:891–2.

187. Raviglione MC. Extrapulmonary pneumocystosis: the first 50 cases. *Rev Infect Dis* 1990;12:1127–8.

188. Telzak EE, Cote RJ, Gold JWM, Campbell SW, Armstrong D. Extrapulmonary *Pneumocystis carinii* infection. *Rev Infect Dis* 1990;12:380–6.

189. NIAID, NIH. Important therapeutic information on prevention of recurrent *Pneumocystis carinii* pneumonia in persons with AIDS. Written communication, October 11, 1991.

190. Abel AG, Nierman DM, Ilowite JS, et al. Bilateral upper lobe *Pneumocystis carinii* pneumonia in a patient receiving inhaled pentamidine prophylaxis. *Chest* 1988;94:329–31.

191. Scannell KA. Atypical presentation of *Pneumocystis carinii* pneumonia in patients receiving inhalational pentamidine. *Am J Med* 1988;85:881–4.

192. Jules-Elysee K, Stover D, Zaman M, et al. Aerosolized pentamidine: effect on the diagnosis and presentation of *Pneumocystis carinii* pneumonia. *Ann Intern Med* 1990;112:750–7.

193. Karboski JA, Godley PJ. Inhaled pentamidine and hypoglycemia. *Ann Intern Med* 1988;108:490.

194. Herer B, Chinet T, Labrune L, et al. Pancreatitis associated with pentamidine by aerosol. *Br Med J* 1989;298:695.

195. Hart CC. Aerosolized pentamidine and pancreatitis. *Ann Intern Med* 1989;111:691.

196. Murphy RL, Noskin GA, Ehrenpreis ED. Acute pancreatitis associated with aerosolized pentamidine. *Am J Med* 1990; 88:5-53N–5-56N.

197. Horowitz H, Wormser GP. Human immunodeficiency virus-related disease. In: Taylor RB, ed. *Difficult medical management*. Philadelphia: WB Saunders 1991;300–12.

198. Wormser GP. Multiple opportunistic infections and neoplasms in the acquired immunodeficiency syndrome. *JAMA* 1985; 253:3441–2.

199. Meiteles LZ, Lucente FE. Sinus and nasal manifestations of the acquired immunodeficiency syndrome. *Ear Nose Throat J* 1990;69:454–9.

200. Melbye M, Grossman RJ, Goedert JJ, Eyster ME, Biggar RJ. Risk of AIDS after herpes zoster. *Lancet* 1987;1:728–30.

201. Theuer CP, Hopewell PC, Elias D, Schecter GF, Rutherford GW, Chaisson RE. Human immunodeficiency virus infection in tuberculosis patients. *J Infect Dis* 1990;162:8–12.

202. Selik RM, Starcher ET, Curran JW. Opportunistic diseases reported in AIDS patients: frequencies, associations, and trends. *AIDS* 1987;1:175–82.

203. Bronnimann DA, Adam RD, Galgiani JN, et al. Coccidioidomycosis in the acquired immunodeficiency syndrome. *Ann Intern Med* 1987;106:372–9.

204. Fish DG, Ampel NM, Galgiani JN, et al. Coccidioidomycosis during human immunodeficiency virus infection. A review of 77 patients. *Medicine* 1990;69:384–91.

205. Galgiani JN, Ampel NM. Coccidioidomycosis in human immunodeficiency virus-infected patients. *J Infect Dis* 1990; 162:1165–9.

206. Wheat LJ, Connolly-Stringfield PA, Baker RL, et al. Disseminated histoplasmosis in the acquired immune deficiency syndrome: clinical findings, diagnosis and treatment, and review of the literature. *Medicine* 1990;69:361–74.

207. Mandell W, Goldberg DM, Neu HC. Histoplasmosis in patients with the acquired immune deficiency syndrome. *Am J Med* 1986;81:974–8.

208. Ankobiah WA, Vaidya K, Powell S, et al. Disseminated histoplasmosis in AIDS. Clinicopathologic features in seven patients from a non-endemic area. *NY State J Med* 1990;90:234–8.

209. Prego V, Glatt AE, Roy V, Thelmo W, Dincsoy H, Raufman J-P. Comparative yield of blood culture for fungi and mycobacteria, liver biopsy, and bone marrow biopsy in the diagnosis of fever of undetermined origin in human immunodeficiency virus-infected patients. *Arch Intern Med* 1990;150:333–6.

210. Yagupsky P, Menegus MA. Cumulative positivity rates of multiple blood cultures for *Mycobacterium avium-intracellulare* and *Cryptococcus neoformans* in patients with the acquired immunodeficiency syndrome. *Arch Pathol Lab Med* 1990;114:923–5.

211. Horsburgh CR Jr. *Mycobacterium avium* complex infection in the acquired immunodeficiency syndrome. *N Engl J Med* 1991;324:1332–8.

212. Gillin JS, Urmacher C, West R, et al. Disseminated *Mycobacterium avium intracellulare* infection in acquired immunodeficiency syndrome mimicking Whipples' disease. *Gastroenterology* 1983;85:1187–91.

213. Gray JR, Rabeneck L. Atypical mycobacterial infection of the gastrointestinal tract in AIDS patients. *Am J Gastroenterol* 1989;84:1521–4.

214. Monsour HP Jr, Quigley EMM, Markin RS, Dalke PD, Goldsmith JC, Harty RF. Endoscopy in the diagnosis of gastrointestinal *Mycobacterium avium-intracellulare* infection. *J Clin Gastroenterol* 1991;13:20–4.

215. Greenson JK, Belitsos PC, Yardley JH, Bartlett JG. AIDS enteropathy: occult enteric infections and duodenal mucosal alterations in chronic diarrhea. *Ann Intern Med* 1991;114:366–72.

216. Quinnan GV, Masur H, Rook AH, et al. Herpesvirus infections in the acquired immune deficiency syndrome. *JAMA* 1984;252:72–7.

217. Salmon D, Lacassin F, Harzic M, et al. Predictive value of cytomegalovirus viraemia for the occurrence of CMV organ involvement in AIDS. *J Med Virol* 1990;32:160–3.

218. Kovacs JA, Kovacs AA, Polis M, et al. Cryptococcosis in the acquired immunodeficiency syndrome. *Ann Intern Med* 1985;103:533–8.

219. Zuger A, Louie E, Holzman RS, Simberkoff MS, Rahal JJ. Cryptococcal disease in patients with the acquired immunodeficiency syndrome. *Ann Intern Med* 1986;104:234–40.

220. Bigby TD, Margolskee D, Curtis JL, et al. The usefulness of induced sputum in the diagnosis of *Pneumocystis carinii* pneumonia in patients with the acquired immunodeficiency syndrome. *Am Rev Respir Dis* 1986;133:515–8.

221. Zaman MK, Wooten OJ, Suprahmanya B, Ankobiah W, Finch PJP, Kamholtz SL. Rapid non-invasive diagnosis of *Pneumocystis carinii* from induced liquified sputum. *Ann Intern Med* 1988;109:7–10.

222. Kovacs JA, Ng VS, Masur H, et al. Diagnosis of *Pneumocystis carinii* pneumonia: improved detection in sputum with use of monoclonal antibodies. *N Engl J Med* 1988;318:589–93.

223. Barron TF, Birnbaum NS, Shane LB, Goldsmith SJ, Rosen MJ. *Pneumocystis carinii* pneumonia studied by gallium-67 screening. *Radiology* 1985;154:791–3.

224. Stover DE, White DA, Romano PA, Gellene RA. Diagnosis of pulmonary disease in acquired immune deficiency syndrome (AIDS). Role of bronchoscopy and bronchoalveolar lavage. *Am Rev Respir Dis* 1984;130:659–62.

225. Henochowicz S, Sahovic E, Pistole M, et al. Histoplasmosis diag-

nosed on peripheral blood smear from a patient with AIDS. *JAMA* 1985;253:3148.

226. Wheat LJ, Connolly-Stringfield P, Kohler RB, Frame PT, Gupta MR. *Histoplasma capsulatum* polysaccharide antigen detection in diagnosis and management of disseminated histoplasmosis in patients with acquired immunodeficiency syndrome. *Am J Med* 1989;87:396–400.

227. Wormser GP. Unpublished observations, 1991.

228. Hewlett D Jr, Duncanson FP, Jagadha V, Lieberman J, Lenox TH, Wormser GP. Lymphadenopathy in an inner-city population consisting principally of intravenous drug abusers with suspected acquired immunodeficiency syndrome. *Am Rev Respir Dis* 1988;137:1275–9.

229. Cappell MS, Schwartz MS. Clinical utility of liver biopsy in patients with serum antibodies to the human immunodeficiency virus. *Am J Med* 1990;88:123–30.

230. Bloom EJ, Abrams DI, Rodgers G. Lupus anticoagulant in the acquired immunodeficiency syndrome. *JAMA* 1986;256:491–3.

231. Taillan B, Roul C, Fuzibet J-G, et al. Antiphospholipid antibodies associated with human immunodeficiency virus infection. *Arch Intern Med* 1990;150:1975.

232. Stimmler MM, Quismorio FP Jr, McGehee WG, Boylen T, Sharma OP. Anticardiolipin antibodies in acquired immunodeficiency syndrome. *Arch Intern Med* 1989;149:1833–5.

233. Thiagarajan P, Shapiro SS. Lupus anticoagulants. In: Coleman RW, ed. *Methods in hematology: disorders of thrombin formation.* New York: Churchill-Livingstone, 1983;101–8.

234. [Anonymous]. Oral candidosis in HIV infection. *Lancet* 1989;2:1491–2.

235. Blum RA, D'Andrea DT, Florentino BM, et al. Increased gastric pH and the bioavailability of fluconazole and ketoconazole. *Ann Intern Med* 1991;114:755–7.

236. [Anonymous]. Drugs for AIDS and associated infections *Med Lett* 1991;33:95–102.

237. Haulk AA, Sugar AM. Candida esophagitis. *Adv Intern Med* 1991;36:307–18.

238. Medoff G. Controversial areas in antifungal chemotherapy. Short-course and combination therapy with amphotericin B. *Rev Infect Dis* 1987;9:403–7.

239. Tavilian A, Rauffman JP, Rosenthal LE, et al. Ketoconazole resistant candida esophagitis in patients with acquired immunodeficiency syndrome. *Gastroenterology* 1986;90:443–5.

240. Mc Kinsey DS, Gupta MR, Riddler SA, Driks MR, Smith DL, Kurtin PJ. Long-term amphotericin B therapy for disseminated histoplasmosis in patients with the acquired immunodeficiency syndrome (AIDS). *Ann Intern Med* 1989;111:655–9.

241. Chuck SL, Sande MA. Infections with *Cryptococcus neoformans* in the acquired immunodeficiency syndrome. *N Engl J Med* 1989;321:794–9.

242. Stern JJ, Hartman BJ, Sharkey P, et al. Oral fluconazole therapy for patients with acquired immunodeficiency syndrome and cryptococcosis: experience with 22 patients. *Am J Med* 1988;85:477–80.

243. Zuger A, Schuster M, Simberkoff MS, Rahal JJ, Holzman RS. Maintenance amphotericin B for cryptococcal meningitis in the acquired immunodeficiency syndrome (AIDS). *Ann Intern Med* 1988;109:592–3.

244. Bozette SA, Larsen RA, Chiu J, et al. A placebo-controlled trial of maintenance therapy with fluconazole after treatment of cryptococcal meningitis, in the acquired immunodeficiency syndrome. *N Engl J Med* 1991;324:580–4.

245. Sugar AM, Saunders C. Oral fluconazole as suppressive therapy of disseminated cryptococcosis in patients with acquired immunodeficiency syndrome. *Am J Med* 1988;85:481–9.

246. P. Kelly MD, Personal communication, October, 1991.

247. Knoper SR, Galgiani JN. Coccidioidomycosis. *Infect Dis Clin North Am* 1988;2:861–75.

248. Tucker RM, Galgiani JN, Denning DW, et al. Treatment of coccidioidal meningitis with fluconazole. *Rev Infect Dis* 1990;12:S380–S389.

249. Zar FA, Fernandez M. Failure of ketoconazole maintenance therapy for disseminated coccidioidomycosis in AIDS. *J Infect Dis* 1991;164:824–5.

250. Huff JC, Bean B, Balfour HH, et al. Therapy of herpes zoster with oral acyclovir. *Am J Med* 1988;85:85–9.

251. Morton P, Thompson AN. Oral acyclovir in the treatment of herpes zoster in general practice. *NZ Med J* 1989;102:93–5.

252. Balfour HH Jr, Bean B, Laskin OL, et al. Acyclovir halts progression of herpes zoster in immunocompromised patients. *N Engl J Med* 1983;308:1448–53.

253. Safrin S, Berger TG, Gibson I, et al. Foscarnet therapy in five patients with AIDS and acyclovir-resistant varicella-zoster virus infection. *Ann Intern Med* 1991;115:19–21.

254. Bryson YJ, Dillon M, Lovett M, et al. Treatment of first episodes of genital herpes simplex virus infection with oral acyclovir. A randomized double-blind controlled trial in normal subjects. *N Engl J Med* 1983;308:916–21.

255. Mertz GJ, Crutchlow CW, Benedetti J, et al. Double-blind, placebo controlled trial of oral acyclovir in first-episode genital herpes simplex virus infections. *JAMA* 1984;252:1147–51.

256. Ehrlich KS, Jacobson MA, Koehler JE, et al. Foscarnet therapy for severe acyclovir-resistant herpes simplex virus type-2 infection in patients with the acquired immunodeficiency syndrome (AIDS): an uncontrolled trial. *Ann Intern Med* 1989;110:710–3.

257. Chatis PA, Miller CH, Schroager LE, Crumpacker CS. Successful treatment with foscarnet of an acyclovir-resistant mucocutaneous infection with herpes simplex virus in a patient with acquired immunodeficiency syndrome. *N Engl J Med* 1989;320:297–300.

258. Birch CJ, Tachedjian G, Doherty RR, Hayes K, Gust ID. Altered sensitivity to antiviral drugs of herpes simplex virus isolates from a patient with the acquired immunodeficiency syndrome. *J Infect Dis* 1990;162:731–4.

259. Safrin S, Assaykeen T, Follansbee S, Mills J. Foscarnet therapy for acyclovir-resistant mucocutaneous herpes simplex virus infection in 26 AIDS patients: preliminary data. *J Infect Dis* 1990;161:1078–84.

260. Safrin S, Crumpacker C, Chatis P, et al. A controlled trial comparing foscarnet with vidarabine for acyclovir-resistant mucocutaneous herpes simplex in the acquired immunodeficiency syndrome. *N Engl J Med* 1991;325:551–5.

261. Strauss SE, Croen KD, Sawyer MH, et al. Acyclovir suppression of frequently recurring genital herpes. *JAMA* 1988;260:2227–30.

262. Studies of Ocular Complications of AIDS Research Group, in Collaboration with the AIDS Clinical Trial Group. Mortality in patients with the acquired immunodeficiency syndrome treated with either foscarnet or ganciclovir for cytomegalovirus retinitis. *N Engl J Med* 1992;326:213–20.

263. Jacobson MA, O'Donnell JJ, Porteous D, Brodie HR, Feigal D, Mills J. Retinal and gastrointestinal disease due to cytomegalovirus in patients with the acquired immune deficiency syndrome: prevalence, natural history, and response to ganciclovir therapy. *Q J Med* 1988;67:473–86.

264. Jabs DA, Enger C, Bartlett JG. Cytomegalovirus retinitis and acquired immunodeficiency syndrome. *Arch Ophthalmol* 1989;107:75–80.

265. Drew WL. Cytomegalovirus infection in patients with AIDS. *J Infect Dis* 1988;158:449–56.

266. Chachoua A, Dieterich D, Krasinski K, et al. 9-(1,3, dihydroxy-2-propoxymethyl) guanine (ganciclovir) in the treatment of cytomegalovirus gastrointestinal disease with the acquired immunodeficiency syndrome. *Ann Intern Med* 1987;107:133–7.

267. Wilcox CM, Diehl DL, Cello JP, Margaretten W, Jacobson MA. Cytomegalovirus esophagitis in patients with AIDS. A clinical, endoscopic, and pathologic correlation. *Ann Intern Med* 1990;113:589–93.

268. Walmsley SL, Chew E, Read SE, et al. Treatment of cytomegalovirus retinitis with trisodium phosphonoformate hexahydrate (foscarnet) *J Infect Dis* 1988;157:569–72.

269. Krupp LB, Lipton RB, Swerdlow MD, Leeds NE, Llena J. Progressive multifocal leukoencephalopathy: clinical and radiographic features. *Ann Neurol* 1985;17:344–9.

270. Chaisson RE, Griffin DE. Progressive multifocal leukoencephalopathy in AIDS. *JAMA* 1990;264:79–82.

271. Frickhofen N, Abkowitz JL, Safford M, et al. Persistent B19 parvovirus infection in patients infected with human immunodeficiency virus type 1 (HIV-1): a treatable cause of anemia in AIDS. *Ann Intern Med* 1990;113:926–33.

272. Wharton JM, Coleman DL, Wofsey CB, et al. Trimethoprim-sulfamethoxazole or pentamidine for *Pneumocystis carinii* pneumonia in the acquired immunodeficiency syndrome. *Ann Intern Med* 1986;105:37–44.

273. Sattler FR, Cowan R, Nielsen DM, Ruskin J. Trimethoprim-sulfamethoxazole compared with pentamidine for treatment of *Pneumocystis carinii* pneumonia in the acquired immunodeficiency syndrome: a prospective, non-crossover study. *Ann Intern Med* 1988;109:280–7.

274. The National Institute of Health–University of California Expert Panel for Corticosteroids as Adjunctive Therapy for Pneumocystis Pneumonia. Consensus statement on the use of corticosteroids as adjunctive therapy for pneumocystis pneumonia in the acquired immunodeficiency syndrome. *N Engl J Med* 1990;323:1500–4.

275. Medina I, Mills J, Leoung G, et al. Oral therapy for *Pneumocystis carinii* pneumonia in the acquired immunodeficiency syndrome. A controlled trial of trimethoprim-sulfamethoxazole versus trimethoprim-dapsone. *N Engl J Med* 1990;323:776–82.

276. Toma E, Fournier S, Poisson M, Morisset R, Phaneuf D, Vega C. Clindamycin with primaquin for *Pneumocystis carinii* pneumonia. *Lancet* 1989;1:1046–8.

277. Ruf B, Pohle HD. Clindamycin/primaquin for *Pneumocystis carinii* pneumonia. *Lancet* 1989;2:626–7.

278. Leport C, Raffi F, Matheron S, et al. Treatment of central nervous system toxoplasmosis with pyrimethamine/sulfadiazine combination in 35 patients with the acquired immunodeficiency syndrome: efficacy of long-term continuous therapy. *Am J Med* 1988;84:94–100.

279. Rolston KVI, Hoy J. Role of clindamycin in the treatment of central nervous system toxoplasmosis. *Am J Med* 1987;83:551–4.

280. Dannermann BR, Israelski DM, Remington JS. Treatment of toxoplasmic encephalitis with intravenous clindamycin. *Arch Intern Med* 1988;148:2477–82.

281. Leport C, Bastuji-Garin S, Perronne C, et al. An open study of the pyrimethamine-clindamycin combination in AIDS patients with brain toxoplasmosis. *J Infect Dis* 1989;160:557–8.

282. Shadduck JA. Human microsporidiosis and AIDS. *Rev Infect Dis* 1989;11:203–7.

283. Orenstein JM, Chiang J, Steinberg W, Smith P, Rotterdam H, Kotler DP. Intestinal microsporidiosis as a cause of diarrhea in HIV-infected patients. A report of 20 cases. *Hum Pathol* 1990;21:475–81.

284. Schattenkerk JKM, Van Gool T, Van Ketel RJ, et al. Clinical significance of small-intestinal microsporidiosis in HIV-1 infected individuals. *Lancet* 1991;337:895–8.

285. Connolly GM, Dryden MS, Shanson D, Gazzard BG. Cryptosporidial diarrhea in AIDS and its treatment. *Gut* 1988;29:593–7.

286. Cook DJ, Kelton JG, Stanisz AM, Collins SM. Somatostatin treatment for cryptosporidial diarrhea in a patient with the acquired immunodeficiency syndrome (AIDS). *Ann Intern Med* 1988;108:708–9.

287. De Hovitz JA, Pape JW, Boncy M, et al. Clinical manifestations and therapy of *Isospora belli* infection in patients with the acquired immunodeficiency syndrome. *N Engl J Med* 1986;315:87–90.

288. Pape JW, Verdier R-I, Johnson WD Jr. Treatment and prophylaxis of *Isospora belli* infection in patients with the acquired immunodeficiency syndrome. *N Engl J Med* 1989;320:1044–7.

289. Weiss LM, Perlman DC, Sherman J, Tanowitz H, Wittner M. *Isospora belli* infection: treatment with pyrimethamine. *Ann Intern Med* 1988;109:474–5.

290. Datry A, Mayorga R, Lyagoubi M, et al. Treatment of *Strongyloides stercoralis* infection with ivermectin versus albendazole. Results of a 44 case study. 31st Interscience Conference on Antimicrobial Agents Chemotherapy, Chicago, October, 1991; 692(abst).

291. Kim J, Minamoto GY, Grieco MH. Nocardial infection as a complication of AIDS: report of six cases and review. *Rev Infect Dis* 1991;13:624–9.

292. Bottone EJ, Wormser GP, Duncanson FP. Nontyphoidal *Salmonella* bacteremia as an early infection in acquired immunodeficiency syndrome. *Diagn Microbiol Infect Dis* 1984;2:247–50.

293. Sperber SJ, Schleupner CJ. Salmonellosis during infection with human immunodeficiency virus. *Rev Infect Dis* 1987;9:925–34.

294. Jacobson MA, Hahn SM, Gerberding JL, Lee B, Sande MA. Ciprofloxacin for *Salmonella* bacteremia in the acquired immunodeficiency syndrome. *Ann Intern Med* 1989;110:1027–9.

295. Karabulut N, Porwancher R, Cherney C, Ricketti A, Friedland R. Clinical presentation and quinolone therapy of *Salmonella* in HIV infection. 5th International Conference on Acquired Immunodeficiency syndrome, Montreal, Canada, June, 1989.

296. Hawkins CH, Gold JWM, Whimbey E, et al. *Mycobacterium avium* complex infection in patients with the acquired immunodeficiency syndrome. *Ann Intern Med* 1986;105:184–8.

297. Young LS. *Mycobacterium avium* complex infection. *J Infect Dis* 1988;157:863–7.

298. Hoy J, Mijch A, Sandland M, Grayson L, Lucas R, Dwyer B. Quadruple-drug therapy for *Mycobacterium avium-intracellulare* bacteremia in AIDS patients. *J Infect Dis* 1990;161:801–5.

299. Agins BD, Berman DS, Spicehandler D, el Sadr W, Simberkoff MS, Rahal JJ. Effect of combined therapy with ansamycin, clofazimine, ethambutal, and isoniazid for *Mycobacterium avium* infection in patients with AIDS. *J Infect Dis* 1989;159:784–7.

300. Chiu J, Nussbaum J, Bozzette S, et al. Treatment of disseminated *Mycobacterium avium* complex infection in AIDS with amikacin, ethambutol, rifampin and ciprofloxacin. *Ann Intern Med* 1990;113:358–61.

301. Horsburgh CR, Havlik JA, Metchock BG, Thompson SE. Oral therapy of disseminated *Mycobacterium avium* complex infection in AIDS relieves symptoms and is well tolerated. *Am Rev Respir Dis* 1991;143:Suppl:A115. (Abstract).

302. Saint-Marc T, Touraine JL. Clinical experience with a combination of clarithromycin and clofazimine in the treatment of disseminated *M. avium* infection in AIDS. 31st Interscience Conference on Antimicrobial Agents Chemotherapy, Chicago, October, 1991;237(abst).

303. Le Boit PE, Berger TG, Egbert BM, et al. Epithelioid haemangioma-like vascular proliferation in AIDS: manifestation of cat scratch disease bacillus infection. *Lancet* 1988;1:960–3.

304. Relman DA, Loutit JS, Schmidt TM, et al. The agent of bacillary angiomatosis: an approach to the identification of uncultured pathogens. *N Engl J Med* 1990;323:1573–80.

305. Perkocha LA, Geaghan SM, Benedect Yen TS, et al. Clinical and pathological features of bacillary peliosis hepatis in association with human immunodeficiency virus infection. *N Engl J Med* 1990;323:1581–6.

306. Cockerill CJ, LeBoit PE. Bacillary angiomatosis: a newly characterized pseudoneoplastic, infectious, cutaneous vascular disorder. *J Am Acad Dermatol* 1990;22:501–12.

307. Edman JC, Kovacs JA, Masur H. Ribosomal RNA sequence shows *Pneumocystis carinii* to be a member of the fungi. *Nature* 1988;334:519–22.

308. Armstrong D, Gold JWM, Dryjanski J, et al. Treatment of infection in patients with the acquired immunodeficiency syndrome. *Ann Intern Med* 1985;103:738–43.

309. Glatt AE, Chirgwin K, Landesman SH. Treatment of infections associated with human immunodeficiency virus. *N Engl J Med* 1988;318:1439–48.

310. Rolston KV, Rodriguez S, Hernandez M, Bodey GP. Diarrhea in patients with the human immunodeficiency virus. *Am J Med* 1989;86:137–8.

311. Dworkin B, Wormser GP, Rosenthal WS, et al. Gastrointestinal manifestations of the acquired immunodeficiency syndrome: a review of 22 cases. *Am J Gastroenterol* 1985;80:774–8.

312. Dworkin B, Wormser GP, Abdoo RA, Cabello F, Aquero ME, Sivak SL. Persistence of multiply antibiotic-resistant *Campylobacter jejuni* in a patient with the acquired immune deficiency syndrome. *Am J Med* 1986;80:965–70.

313. Rene E, Marche C, Regnier B, et al. Intestinal infections in patients with acquired immunodeficiency syndrome. *Dig Dis Sci* 1989;34:773–80.

314. Janoff EN, Orenstein JM, Manischewitz JF, Smith PD. Adenovirus colitis in the acquired immunodeficiency syndrome. *Gastroenterology* 1991;100:976–9.

315. Friedman SL, Wright TL, Altman DF. Gastrointestinal Kaposi's sarcoma in patients with acquired immunodeficiency syndrome. *Gastroenterology* 1985;89:102–8.

316. Kotler DP, Gaetz HP, Lange M, Klein EB, Holt PR. Enteropathy

associated with the acquired immunodeficiency syndrome. *Ann Intern Med* 1989;101:421–8.

317. Ullrich R, Zeitz M, Heise W, L'age M, Hoffken G, Riecken EO. Small intestinal structure and function in patients infected with human immunodeficiency virus (HIV): evidence for HIV-induced enteropathy. *Ann Intern Med* 1989;111:15–21.

318. Fox CH, Kotler D, Tierney A, Wilson CS, Fauci AS. Detection of HIV-1 RNA in the lamina propria of patients with AIDS and gastrointestinal disease. *J Infect Dis* 1989;159:467–71.

319. Smith PD, Lane HC, Gill VJ, et al. Intestinal infections in patients with acquired immunodeficiency syndrome (AIDS). Etiology and response to therapy. *Ann Intern Med* 1988;108:328–33.

320. Gelb A, Miller S. AIDS and gastroenterology. *Am J Gastroenterol* 1986;81:619–22.

321. Johnson JF, Sonnenberg A. Efficient management of diarrhea in the acquired immunodeficiency syndrome. *Ann Intern Med* 1990;112:942–8.

322. Cello JP. Acquired immunodeficiency syndrome cholangiopathy: spectrum of disease. *Am J Med* 1989;86:539–46.

323. Cappell MS. Hepatobiliary manifestations of the acquired immune deficiency syndrome. *Am J Gastroenterol* 1991;86:1–15.

324. Kaplan LD, Kahn J, Jacobson M, Bottles K, Cello J. Primary bile duct lymphoma in the acquired immunodeficiency syndrome (AIDS). *Ann Intern Med* 1989;110:161–2.

325. Pardo V, Aldana M, Colton RM, et al. Glomerular lesions in the acquired immunodeficiency syndrome. *Ann Intern Med* 1984;101:429–34.

326. Rao TKS, Friedman EA, Nicastri AD. The types of renal disease in the acquired immunodeficiency syndrome (AIDS). *N Engl J Med* 1987;316:1062–8.

327. Seney FD Jr, Burns DK, Silva FG. Acquired immunodeficiency syndrome and the kidney. *Am J Kidney Dis* 1990;16:1–13.

328. Soni A, Agarwal A, Chander P, et al. Evidence for an HIV-related nephropathy: a clinico-pathological study. *Clin Nephrol* 1989; 31:12–7.

329. Bourgoignie JJ, Meneses R, Ortiz C, Jaffe D, Pardo V. The clinical spectrum of renal disease associated with human immunodeficiency virus. *Am J Kidney Dis* 1988;12:131–7.

330. Bakir AA, Bazilinski NG, Rhee HL, et al. Focal segmental glomerulosclerosis. A common entity in nephrotic black adults. *Arch Intern Med* 1989;149:1802–4.

331. Cunningham EE, Brentjens JR, Zielezny MA, et al. Heroin nephropathy: a clinicopathologic and epidemiologic study. *Am J Med* 1980;68:47–53.

332. Cunningham EE, Zielezny MA, Venuto RC. Heroin-associated nephropathy: a nationwide problem. *JAMA* 1983;250:2935–6.

333. Friedman EA, Rao TKS. Why does uremia in heroin abusers occur predominantly among blacks? *JAMA* 1983;250:2965–6.

334. Rao TK, Filippone EJ, Nicastri AD, et al. Associated focal and segmental glomerulosclerosis in the acquired immunodeficiency syndrome. *N Engl J Med* 1984;310:669–73.

335. Karlsson-Parra A, Dimeny E, Fellstrom B, Klareskog L. HIV receptors (CD4 antigen) in normal human glomerular cells. *N Engl J Med* 1989;320:741.

336. Cohen AH, Sun NC, Shapshak P, Imagawa DT. Demonstration of human immunodeficiency virus in renal epithelium in HIV-associated nephropathy. *Mod Pathol* 1989;2:125–8.

337. Babut-Gay M-L, Echard M, Kleinknecht D, Meyrier A. Zidovudine and nephropathy with human immunodeficiency virus (HIV) infection. *Ann Intern Med* 1989;111:856–7.

338. Marcus R, Solomon SL, Favero MSS, et al. Human immunodeficiency virus (HIV) antibody in patients undergoing chronic hemodialysis. *Kidney Int* 1988;35:255(abst).

339. Reiser IW, Shapiro WB, Porush JG. The incidence and epidemiology of human immunodeficiency virus infection in 320 patients treated in an inner-city hemodialysis center. *Am J Kidney Dis* 1990;16:26–31.

340. Chirgwin K, Rao TKS, Landesman SH, Friedman EA. Seroprevalence of antibody to human immunodeficiency virus (HIV) in patients treated by maintenance hemodialysis. *Kidney Int* 1988;35:242(abst).

341. Ortiz C, Meneses R, Jaffe D, et al. Outcome of patients with human immunodeficiency virus on maintenance hemodialysis. *Kidney Int* 1988;34:248–53.

342. Francis CK. Cardiac involvement in AIDS. *Curr Probl Cardiol* 1990;15:569–639.

343. Baroldi G, Corallo S, Moroni M, et al. Focal lymphocytic myocarditis in acquired immunodeficiency syndrome (AIDS): a correlative morphologic and clinical study in 26 consecutive fatal cases. *J Am Coll Cardiol* 1988;12:463–9.

344. Lewis W. AIDS: cardiac findings from 115 autopsies. *Prog Cardiovasc Dis* 1989;32:207–15.

345. Anderson DW, Virmani R, Reilly JM, et al. Prevalent myocarditis at necropsy in the acquired immunodeficiency syndrome. *J Am Coll Cardiol* 1988;11:792–9.

346. Roldan EO, Moskowitz L, Hensley GT. Pathology of the heart in acquired immunodeficiency syndrome. *Arch Pathol Lab Med* 1987;111:943–6.

347. Anderson DW, Renu V. Emerging patterns of heart disease in human immunodeficiency virus infection. *Hum Pathol* 1990;21:253–9.

348. Raffanti SP, Chiaramida AJ, Purnendu S, et al. Assessment of cardiac function in patients with the acquired immunodeficiency syndrome. *Chest* 1988;93:592–4.

349. Reilly JM, Cunnion RE, Anderson DW, et al. Frequency of myocarditis, left ventricular dysfunction and ventricular tachycardia in the acquired immune deficiency syndrome. *Am J Cardiol* 1988;62:789–93.

350. Levy WS, Simon GL, Rios JC, et al. Prevalence of cardiac abnormalities in human immunodeficiency virus infection. *Am J Cardiol* 1989;63:86–9.

351. Bibler MR, Chou TC, Toltzis RJ, et al. Recurrent ventricular tachycardia due to pentamidine-induced cardiotoxicity. *Chest* 1988;94:1303–6.

352. Thalhammer C, Bogner JR, Goegel F-D, et al. No arrhythmogenic QT-prolongation by pentamidine aerosol prophylaxis in 44 patients. 7th International Conference on Acquired Immunodeficiency Syndrome, Florence, Italy, June, 1991.

353. Dworkin BM, Rosenthal WS, Wormser GP, et al. Abnormalities of blood selenium and glutathione peroxidase activity in patients with acquired immunodeficiency syndrome and AIDS-related complex. *Biol Trace Element Res* 1988;15:167–77.

354. Dworkin BM, Antonecchia PP, Smith F, et al. Reduced cardiac selenium content in the acquired immunodeficiency syndrome. *J PEN* 1989;13:644–7.

355. Chokshi SK, Moore R, Pandian NG, Isner JM. Reversible cardiomyopathy associated with cocaine intoxication. *Ann Intern Med* 1989;111:1039–40.

356. Deyton LR, Walker RE, Kovacs JA, et al. Reversible cardiac dysfunction associated with interferon alfa therapy in AIDS patients with Kaposi's sarcoma. *N Engl J Med* 1989;321:1246–9.

357. Myers CE, Chabner BA. Anthracyclines. In: Chabner BA, Collins JM, eds. *Cancer chemotherapy, principles and practice.* Philadelphia: Lippincott, 1990;356–81.

358. Welch K, Finkbeiner W, Alpers CE, et al. Autopsy findings in the acquired immune deficiency syndrome. *JAMA* 1984;252:1152–9.

359. Elliott WJ. Human immunodeficiency virus, coxsackie virus, and cardiomyopathy. *Ann Intern Med* 1988;108:308–9.

360. Lewis W, Lipsick J, Cammarosano BS. Cryptococcal myocarditis in acquired immune deficiency syndrome. *Am J Cardiol* 1985;55:1240.

361. Henochowicz S, Mustafa M, Lawrinson WE, et al. Cardiac aspergillosis in acquired immune deficiency syndrome. *Am J Cardiol* 1985;55:1239–40.

362. Calabrese LH, Proffitt MF, Yen-Lieberman B, et al. Congestive cardiomyopathy and illness related to the acquired immunodeficiency syndrome (AIDS) associated with isolation of retrovirus from myocardium. *Ann Intern Med* 1987;107:691–2.

363. Flomenbaum M, Soeiro R, Udem SA, et al. Proliferative membranopathy and human immunodeficiency virus in AIDS hearts. *J AIDS* 1989;2:129–35.

364. Grody WW, Cheng L, Lewis W. Infections of the heart by the human immunodeficiency virus. *Am J Cardiol* 1990;66:203–6.

365. Wu AY-Y, Forouhar F, Cartun RW, et al. Identification of human immunodeficiency virus in the heart of a patient with acquired immunodeficiency syndrome. *Mod Pathol* 1990; 3:625–30.

366. Herskowitz A, Willoughby S, Oliveira M, et al. HIV-associated cardiomyopathy: evidence for autoimmunity. 7th International Conference on Acquired Immunodeficiency Syndrome, Florence, Italy, 1991.

367. Hakas JF Jr, Generalovich T. Spontaneous regression of cardiomyopathy in a patient with the acquired immunodeficiency syndrome. *Chest* 1991;99:770–2.

368. Wilkins CE, Sexton DJ, McAllister HA. HIV-associated myocarditis treated with zidovudine (AZT). *Tex Heart Inst J* 1989;16:44–5.

369. Blanchard DG, Hagenhoff C, Chow LC, et al. Reversibility of cardiac abnormalities in human immunodeficiency virus (HIV)-infected individuals: a serial echocardiographic study. *J Am Coll Cardiol* 1991;17:1270–6.

370. Monsuez JJ, Kinney EL, Vittecoq D, et al. Comparison among acquired immune deficiency syndrome patients with and without clinical evidence of cardiac disease. *J Am Coll Cardiol* 1988;62:1311–3.

371. Caggesi L, Mantero A, Schlacht I, et al. Cardiac involvement in HIV infection. 7th International Conference on Acquired Immunodeficiency Syndrome, Florence, Italy, 1991.

372. Himelman RB, Chung WS, Chernoff DN, et al. Cardiac manifestations of human immunodeficiency virus infection: a two-dimensional echocardiographic study. *J Am Coll Cardiol* 1989;13:1030–6.

373. Corrallo S, Mutinelli MR, Moroni M, et al. Echocardiography detects myocardial damage in AIDS: prospective study in 102 patients. *Eur Heart J* 1988;9:887–92.

374. Veloso VG, Xavier SS, Cavalcante S, et al. Echocardiographic study in patients with HIV infection. 7th International Conference on Acquired Immunodeficiency Syndrome, Florence, Italy, June, 1991.

375. Hecht SR, Berger M, Van Tosh A, et al. Unsuspected cardiac abnormalities in the acquired immune deficiency syndrome. *Chest* 1989;96:805–8.

376. Nathan PE, Arsura EL, Zappi M. Pericarditis with tamponade due to cytomegalovirus in the acquired immunodeficiency syndrome. *Chest* 1991;99:765–76.

377. Kinney EL, Monsuez JJ, Kitis M. Treatment of AIDS-associated heart disease. *Angiology* 1989;40:970–6.

378. Holtz HA, Lavery DP, Kapila R. Actinomycetales infection in the acquired immunodeficiency syndrome. *Ann Intern Med* 1985;102:203–5.

379. Schuster M, Valentine F, Holzman R. Cryptococcal pericarditis in an intravenous drug abuser. *J Infect Dis* 1985;152:842.

380. Gill PS, Chandraratna AN, Meyer PR, et al. Malignant lymphoma: cardiac involvement at initial presentation. *J Clin Oncol* 1987;5:216–24.

381. De Miguel J, Pedreira JD, Campos V, et al. Tuberculous pericarditis and AIDS. *Chest* 1990;97:1273.

382. Cammarosano C, Lewis W. Cardiac lesions in acquired immune deficiency syndrome (AIDS). *J Am Coll Cardiol* 1985;5:703–6.

383. Nahass RG, Weinstein MP, Bartels J, et al. Infective endocarditis in intravenous drug users: a comparison of human immunodeficiency virus type 1-negative and positive patients. *J Infect Dis* 1990;162:967–70.

384. Coplan NL, Shimony RY, Ioachim HL, et al. Primary pulmonary hypertension associated with human immunodeficiency viral infection. *Am J Med* 1990;89:96–9.

385. Himelman RB, Dohrmann M, Goodman P, et al. Severe pulmonary hypertension and cor pulmonale in the acquired immunodeficiency syndrome. *Am J Cardiol* 1989;64:1396–9.

386. Legoux B, Piette AM, Bouchet PF, et al. Pulmonary hypertension and HIV infection. *Am J Med* 1990;89:122.

387. Kaye BR. Rheumatologic manifestations of infection with human immunodeficiency virus (HIV). *Ann Intern Med* 1989;111:156–67.

388. Winchester R. AIDS and the rheumatic diseases. *Bull Rheum Dis* 1990;39:1–10.

389. Berman A, Espinoza LR, Aguillar JL, et al. Rheumatic manifestations of human immunodeficiency virus infection. *Am J Med* 1988;85:59–64.

390. Rynes RI, Goldenberg DL, DiGiacomo R, Olson R, Hussain M, Veazey J. Acquired immunodeficiency syndrome-associated arthritis. *Am J Med* 1988;84:810–6.

391. Winchester R, Bernstein DH, Fischer HD, Enlow R, Solomon G: The co-occurrence of Reiter's syndrome and acquired immunodeficiency. *Ann Intern Med* 1987;106:19–26.

392. Lipstein-Kresch E, Isenberg HD, Singer C, Cooke O, Greenwald RA. Disseminated *Sporothrix schenkii* infection with arthritis in a patient with acquired immunodeficiency syndrome. *J Rheumatol* 1985;12:805–8.

393. Ricciardi DD, Sepkowitz DV, Berkowitz LB, Bienenstock H, Maslow M. Cryptococcal arthritis in a patient with acquired immune deficiency syndrome. Case report and review of the literature. *J Rheumatol* 1986;13:455–8.

394. Rogers PL, Walker RE, Lane HC, et al. Disseminated *Mycobacterium haemophilum* infection in two patients with the acquired immunodeficiency syndrome. *Am J Med* 1988;84:640–2.

395. Winchester R, Brancato L, Itescu S, Skovron ML, Solomon G. Implications from the occurrence of Reiter's syndrome and related disorders in association with advanced HIV infection. *Scand J Rheumatol* 1988;74:89–93.

396. Oberlin F, Leblond V, Camus JP. Arthrites reactionnelles chez deux homosexuels à serologie HIV positive [Letter]. *Presse Med* 1987;16:355.

397. Solomon G, Brancato LJ, Itescu S, Skovorn ML, Mildvan D, Winchester RJ. Arthritis, psoriasis and related syndromes associated with HIV infection. *Arthritis Rheum.* 1988;31[Suppl 2]:S12.(abst).

398. Onerheim RM, Wang NS, Gilmore N, Jothy S. Ultrastructural markers of lymph nodes in patients with acquired immune deficiency syndrome and in homosexual males with unexplained persistent lymphadenopathy. A quantitative study. *Am J Clin Pathol* 1984;82:280–8.

399. Forster SM, Seifert MH, Keat AC, et al. Inflammatory joint disease and human immunodeficiency virus infection. *Br Med J* [Clin Res] 1988;296:1625–7.

400. Withrington RH, Cornes P, Harris JR, et al. Isolation of human immunodeficiency virus from synovial fluid of a patient with reactive arthritis. *Br Med J* [Clin Res] 1987;294:484.

401. Euler HH, Kern P, Loffler H, Dietrich M. Precipitable immune complexes in healthy homosexual men, acquired immune deficiency syndrome and the related lymphadenopathy syndrome. *Clin Exp Immunol* 1985;59:267–75.

402. McDougal JS, Hubbard M, Nicholson JK, et al. Immune complexes in the acquired immunodeficiency syndrome (AIDS): relationship to disease manifestation, risk group, and immunologic defect. *J Clin Immunol* 1985;5:130–8.

403. Duvic M, Johnson TM, Rapini RP, Freese T, Brewton G, Rios A. Acquired immunodeficiency syndrome-associated psoriasis and Reiter's syndrome. *Arch Dermatol* 1987;123:1622–32.

404. Rowe IF. AIDS and arthritis. *Br J Rheumatol* 1988;27:481–2.

405. Bardin T, Kuntz D, Gavdoven C, et al. Necrotizing vasculitis in human immunodeficiency virus (HIV) infection. *Arthritis Rheum* 1987;30:S105.

406. Calabrese LH, Yen-Lieberman B, Estes M, et al. Systemic necrotizing vasculitis and the human immunodeficiency virus (HIV). *Arthritis Rheum* 1988;31:S141.

407. Schwartz ND, So YT, Hollander H, Allen S, Fye KH. Eosinophilic vasculitis leading to amaurosis fugax in a patient with acquired immunodeficiency syndrome. *Arch Intern Med* 1986;146:2059–60.

408. Yanker BA, Skolnik PR, Shoukimas GM, Gabuzda DH, Sobel RA, Ho DD. Cerebral granulomatous angiitis associated with isolation of human T-lymphotropic virus type III from the central nervous system. *Ann Neurol* 1986;20:362–4.

409. Frank Y, Lim W, Kahn E, Farmer P, Gorey M, Pahwa S. Cerebral granulomatous angiitis causing multiple ischemic cerebrovascular accidents in a child with acquired immunodeficiency syndrome. *Ann Neurol* 1987;22:452–3(abst).

410. Velji AM. Leukocytoclastic vasculitis associated with positive HTLV-III serological findings [Letter]. *JAMA* 1986;256:2196–7.

411. Montilla P, Dronda F, Moreno S, Ezpeleta C, Bellas C, Buzon L. Lymphomatoid granulomatosis and the acquired immunodeficiency syndrome [Letter]. *Ann Intern Med* 1987;106:166–7.

412. Vinters HV, Anders KH. Lymphomatoid granulomatosis and

the acquired immunodeficiency syndrome (AIDS) [Letter]. *Ann Intern Med* 1987;107:945.

413. Guillon JM, Fouret P, Mayaud C, et al. Extensive T8-positive lymphocytic visceral infiltration in a homosexual man. *Am J Med* 1987;82:655–61.

414. Dalakas MC, Pezeshkpour GH. Neuromuscular complications of AIDS: diagnosis and management *Muscle Nerve* 1986;9 [Suppl]:92(abst).

415. Said G, Lacroix C, Andrieu JM, Gaudouen C, Leibowitch J. Necrotizing arteritis in patients with inflammatory neuropathy and human immunodeficiency virus infection. *Neurology* 1987; 37[Suppl 1]:176(abst).

416. Weber CA, Figueroa JP, Calabro JJ, Marcus EM, Gleckman RA. Co-occurrence of the Reiter syndrome and acquired immunodeficiency [Letter]. *Ann Intern Med* 1987;107:112–3.

417. Meiselman MS, Cello JP, Margaretten W. Cytomegalovirus colitis. Report of the clinical, endoscopic, and pathologic findings in two patients with the acquired immune deficiency syndrome. *Gastroenterology* 1985;88:171–5.

418. Burke G, Nichols L, Balogh K, et al. Perforation of the terminal ileum with cytomegalovirus vasculitis and Kaposi's sarcoma in a patient with acquired immunodeficiency syndrome. *Surgery* 1987;102:540–5.

419. Couderc LJ, D'Agay MF, Danon F, Harzic M, Brocheriou C, Clauvel JP. Sicca complex and infection with human immunodeficiency virus. *Arch Intern Med* 1987;147:898–901.

420. Itescu S, Brancato LJ, Buxbaum J, et al. A diffuse infiltrative CD8 lymphocytosis syndrome in human immunodeficiency virus (HIV) infection: a host immune response associated with HLA-DR5. *Ann Intern Med* 1990;112:3–10.

421. Itescu S, Brancato LJ, Buxbaum J, Solomon G, Winchester RJ. Sjögren's syndrome associated with HIV infection. *Clin Res* 1988;36:599A.

422. Stricker RB, Abrams DI, Corash L, Shuman MA. Target platelet antigen in homosexual men with immune thrombocytopenia. *N Engl J Med* 1985;313:1375–80.

423. Savona S, Nardi MA, Lennette ET, Karpatkin S. Thrombocytopenic purpura in narcotic addicts. *Ann Intern Med* 1985;102:737–41.

424. Kopelman RH, Zolla-Pazner S. Association of human immunodeficiency virus infection and autoimmune phenomenon. *Am J Med* 1988;84:82–8.

425. Gabuzda DH, Hirsch MS. Neurologic manifestations of infection with human immunodeficiency virus. *Ann Intern Med* 1987;107:383–91.

426. Petito CK, Navia BA, Cho ES, Jordon BD, George DC, Price RW. Vacuolar myelopathy pathologically resembling subacute combined degeneration in patients with the acquired immunodeficiency syndrome. *N Engl J Med* 1985;312:874–9.

427. Simpson DM, Wolfe DE. Neuromuscular complications of HIV infection and its treatment. *AIDS* 1991;5:917–26.

428. De La Monte SM, Gabuzda DH, Ho D, et al. Peripheral neuropathy in the acquired immunodeficiency syndrome. *Ann Neurol* 1988;23:485–92.

429. Engstrom JW, Lowenstein DH, Bredesen DE. Cerebral infarctions and transient neurologic deficits associated with acquired immunodeficiency syndrome. *Am J Med* 1989;86:528–32.

430. Price RW, Brew B. Management of the neurologic complications of HIV infection and AIDS. *Infect Dis Clin North Am* 1988;2:359–72.

431. Salloum E, Pella P, Horn D, Hewlett D. Stroke due to neurosyphilis: first manifestation of human immunodeficiency virus (HIV) infection in two homosexual men. *Infect Dis Clin Pract* 1992;1:43–5.

432. Skowron G, Merigan TC. Alternating and intermittent regimens of zidovudine (3'-azido-3'-deoxythymidine) and dideoxycytidine (2',3'-dideoxycytidine) in the treatment of patients with acquired immunodeficiency syndrome (AIDS) and AIDS-related complex. *Am J Med* 1990;88[Suppl 5B]:20S–23S.

433. Johnson VA, Merrill DP, Videler JA, et al. Two-drug combinations of zidovudine, didanosine, and recombinant interferon-α inhibit replication of zidovudine-resistant human immunodeficiency virus type 1 synergistically in vitro. *J Infect Dis* 1991;164:646–58.

434. Weinstein JN, Bunow B, Weislow S, et al. Synergistic drug combinations in AIDS therapy. *Ann NY Acad Sci* 1990;616:367–84.

435. Kovacs JA, Deyton L, Davey R, et al. Combined zidovudine and interferon-α therapy in patients with Kaposi sarcoma and the acquired immunodeficiency syndrome (AIDS). *Ann Intern Med* 1989;111:280–7.

436. Pedersen C, Sandstrom E, Petersen CS, et al. The efficacy of inosine pranobex in preventing the acquired immunodeficiency syndrome in patients with human immunodeficiency virus infection. *N Engl J Med* 1990;322:1757–63.

437. Lane HC. The role of immunomodulators in the treatment of patients with AIDS. *AIDS* 1989;3[Suppl 1]:S181–S185.

438. Redfield RR, Birx DL, Ketter N, et al. A phase I evaluation of the safety and immunogenicity of vaccination with recombinant gp 160 in patients with early human immunodeficiency virus infection. *N Engl J Med* 1991;324:1677–84.

439. St. Clair MH, Martin JL, Tudor-Williams G, et al. Resistance to ddI and sensitivity to AZT induced by a mutation in HIV-1 reverse transcriptase. *Science* 1991;253:1557–9.

440. Pluda JM, Yarchoan R, Jaffe ES, et al. Development of non-Hodgkin lymphoma in a cohort of patients with severe human immunodeficiency virus (HIV) infection on long-term antiretroviral therapy. *Ann Intern Med* 1990;113:276–82.

441. Steinhoff MC, Auerbach BS, Nelson KE, et al. Antibody responses to *Haemophilus influenzae* type B vaccines in men with human immunodeficiency virus infection. *N Engl J Med* 1991;325:1837–42.

442. Herskowitz A, Willoughby SB, Baughman KL, Schulman SP, Bartlett JD. Cardiomyopathy associated with antiretroviral therapy in patients with HIV infection: a report of six cases. *Ann Intern Med* 1992;116:311–3.

AIDS and Other Manifestations of HIV Infection,
Second Edition, Edited by Gary P. Wormser.
Raven Press, Ltd., New York © 1992.

CHAPTER 14

HIV Infection in Infants, Children, and Adolescents

Samuel Grubman, Richard Conviser, and James Oleske

We are guilty of many errors and many faults,
But our worst crime is abandoning the children,
Neglecting the fountain of life.
Many of the things we need can wait; the children
cannot.
Right now is the time his bones are being formed
His blood is being made and his senses are being
developed.
To him, we cannot answer "Tomorrow." His name is
"Today."

Gabriela Minstrel
Chilean Nobel Prize winning poet

In a discussion of human immunodeficiency virus (HIV) infection in infants, children, and adolescents, it is inevitable that comparisons should be made with HIV infection in adults. In the various age groups, there are differences in the disease's epidemiology and transmission, diagnosis, clinical manifestations, prognosis, and treatment. This chapter gives an overview of pediatric HIV infection, with an emphasis on those aspects of disease that differ between adults and younger people. It also addresses the question of developing standards of care for children with HIV infection and social issues complicating the delivery of care.

EPIDEMIOLOGY AND TRANSMISSION

In the United States, 2,903 cases of pediatric acquired immunodeficiency syndrome (AIDS) (birth to 13 years of age) had been reported through the end of February 1991 to the Centers for Disease Control (CDC), representing approximately 2% of all reported AIDS cases. Because AIDS is the most severe manifestation of HIV disease, this represents only a fraction of the total num-

ber of HIV-infected infants and children. The prevalence of pediatric HIV infection in the United States can best be estimated using the results of national surveys of HIV infection in childbearing women conducted between 1988 and 1990 (1). These results are based on anonymous HIV antibody screening of heelstick samples from all newborns in certain locations during intervals of several months; they suggest that approximately 1.5 newborns/1,000 in the United States are born to HIV-infected women. Seroprevalence rates varied by location, from 0.2/1,000 in the state of Minnesota (1/ 5,000 births) to 4.5/1,000 in Florida (1/222 births) to 15.8/1,000 in Essex County, New Jersey (1/63 births). A 1987 New York State study demonstrated a seroprevalence rate of 23.3/1,000 in the Bronx, New York (1/43 births) (2). Based on these statistics, an estimated 6,000 HIV-infected women will give birth annually in the United States (1). In conjunction with an estimated vertical transmission rate of 30%, these numbers translate to approximately 1,800 HIV-infected infants born annually in the United States. The estimated total number of HIV-infected children in the United States is currently between 10,000 and 20,000 (3).

The risk of being born with HIV infection in the United States varies significantly by race and ethnicity. Only 15% of all children in the United States are black (based on the 1980 census), but over 50% of those with AIDS are black; only 9% of all children are Hispanic, but over 20% of those with AIDS are. Of the 16,805 cases of AIDS among women over 13 years in the United States reported through March 1991, injecting drug use was the source of transmission for 51%; heterosexual transmission for 33%. Another 9% resulted from blood product transfusions, with other or unknown causes in 7%. The impact of heterosexual transmission is higher in mothers of HIV-infected children than in women taken as a

S. Grubman, R. Conviser, and J. Oleske: New Jersey Medical and Dental School, and Children's Hospital, Newark, New Jersey 07103.

whole. Heterosexual spread of HIV is an increasingly important mode of transmission for women, particularly in the black and Hispanic communities.

Although fewer than 1% of the reported cases of AIDS in the United States have been among adolescents, the impact of HIV disease in this age group is more serious than this figure might suggest. Of all reported AIDS cases in the country through early 1991, 20% were among those aged 20–29, with 4.2% of the total among those aged 20–24. The latency period from the acquisition of HIV infection to the development of AIDS in adults suggests that the majority of HIV-infected young adults under 25 acquired their infection as adolescents. The rising rates of other sexually transmitted diseases and unplanned pregnancies among adolescents are suggestive of a substantial risk for sexually transmitted HIV infection in this age group. Sexual exposure, including heterosexual, homosexual, bisexual, and sexual abuse, has been a prominent mode of HIV transmission among adolescent AIDS patients, with heterosexual transmission implicated in 43% of AIDS cases in adolescent females and homosexual transmission implicated in 43% of the cases in adolescent males. The impact of sexual spread is even higher in the group of young adult AIDS patients ages 20–24, with 67% of all cases reported as of December 31, 1989 involving sexual transmission. While intravenous drug use is relatively uncommon among adolescents, the disinhibiting effects of drug use—particularly alcohol, cocaine, and crack—as well as the cost of dependence result in increased sexual risk taking, including prostitution, and contribute to the further spread of HIV. In the United States, the cumulative male-to-female ratio of reported AIDS cases among adolescents is approximately 4:1, reflecting the influence of cases of AIDS among male patients with hemophilia.

Many of the earliest cases of pediatric HIV infection in the United States resulted from the presence of the virus in blood product transfusions used by children with hemophilia. Since universal screening of blood and treatment of blood products in the United States began in 1985, this vector of transmission has been all but eliminated. By early 1991, infection through blood and blood products accounted for approximately 7% of all reported pediatric HIV cases in the United States, while perinatal transmission accounted for 84%.

Transmission from mother to infant (vertical transmission) can occur both prenatally and at the time of delivery. Studies done with fetal tissue suggest that prenatal transmission of HIV can occur as early as the 8th week of gestation (4). HIV has been cultured as early as the 12th week of gestation from fetal brain, thymus, liver, spleen, and lung (5) and has been identified using other techniques in fetal brain tissue as early as 14 weeks gestation (6). Though the actual mixing of maternal and fetal circulation is prevented by the placenta, cellular ele-

ments and soluble factors can cross the placenta. CD4-positive cells have been demonstrated in the lining of the stroma of the chorionic villi (7), which is in close contact with maternal blood. HIV-specific IgA-containing immune complexes have been documented in amniotic fluid (8). The fact that infants often present with symptoms in the first months of life suggests prenatal infection. Serial serological evaluations of infants has documented the appearance of HIV-specific IgM, IgG3, and IgG1 antibodies in some who lacked HIV-specific IgM antibodies at birth (9), thereby providing evidence for HIV transmission around the time of delivery. This mode of transmission is also suggested by the documented perinatal transmission of other blood-borne viruses, such as hepatitis B virus. However, it is still unclear exactly when in relation to gestation and delivery the majority of transmission occurs and whether the timing of transmission correlates with the severity of disease. Studies evaluating the rate of transmission from mother to infant have yielded estimates ranging between 20% and 65%. The most recent studies, based upon larger numbers of cases, suggest a range of 25–35% (10–13).

Why some infants become infected and others do not is not yet known: ongoing research is investigating whether there are maternal factors that can predict the likelihood of perinatal transmission. It has been shown that levels of maternal antibody against gp120 correlate inversely with the transmission rate (14,15). In one retrospective study, the sera of 11 infected infants and their mothers had weak antibody reactivity to the principal neutralizing domain of gp120, whereas the sera of 4 uninfected infants and 3 of their mothers had strong reactivity (16). In another study, infants less than 6 months of age who were found to have antibody to the hypervariable loop of gp120 were proved to be uninfected more often than other infants (17). There is some evidence that women who are more immunocompromised at the time of pregnancy are more likely to transmit infection to their newborns (18,19). One study, however, showed that transmission is not correlated with the disease state of the mother (17). The presence of HIV antigenemia may also promote transmission. An explanation for the discordant transmission that has been described between both fraternal and identical twins is even more difficult to postulate. HIV transmission at the time of delivery is most likely associated with exposure to maternal body fluids, including blood and vaginal secretions. No differences have been found in transmission rates between women undergoing cesarean section and those having vaginal deliveries (12). Ongoing natural history studies of HIV infection in women and infants should help provide insight into these matters. Whether the antiretroviral drug zidovudine (AZT) can reduce the rate of vertical transmission is being addressed in an ongoing clinical trial through the AIDS Clinical Trial Group (ACTG).

Likewise, HIV-infected pregnant women should be considered as an appropriate group to be included in vaccine trials.

Postpartum transmission of HIV infection from mother to newborn via breastfeeding has been reported and documented in women who acquired HIV infection after delivery through sexual relations (13) and blood transfusion (20). The documented cases may be accounted for by the significant HIV antigenemia and presumed increased infectivity in the first 3–6 months after acquisition of HIV infection. Whether breastfeeding is a significant mode of transmission in women who are already HIV infected during pregnancy and clinically stable is unclear. One study suggests an increased rate of transmission in breastfed infants (12), but others do not support an increased incidence of vertical transmission in women who breastfeed (21). The risk–benefit ratio from breastfeeding in HIV-infected women is affected by the availability of sterile formula. Where it is readily available, infected women should use it rather than breastfeeding their infants. However, for Africa and most other Third-World areas, the World Health Organization has recommended that HIV-infected women breastfeed their infants since the likelihood of life-threatening disease secondary to ingestion of unsterile formula is significant.

Iatrogenic acquisition of HIV through transfusions and the use of unsterile needles is an ongoing problem in many countries in which blood products are not screened and disposable needles are not used. Recent reports of hospital-acquired HIV infection in Romania and the Soviet Union are examples of this continuing problem. Sexual abuse of infants, children, and adolescents is another documented mode of transmission of HIV infection (22). It is estimated that over 200,000 children are sexually abused each year in the United States. Among 15 sexually abused children and adolescents with a known HIV-infected attacker seen at Children's Hospital AIDS Program (CHAP) in Newark, New Jersey, three became infected.

DIAGNOSIS

In adolescents, children, and infants older than 15 months, definitive diagnosis of HIV infection is made in the same way as it is in adults, by using the enzyme-linked immunosorbent assay (ELISA) and confirmatory Western blot assays. These provide serological evidence of a humoral immune response to HIV by detecting HIV-specific IgG antibodies. However, since maternal IgG antibody is transferred to infants across the placenta, all infants born to HIV-infected women have a positive ELISA at birth. An IgG antibody response cannot be used to diagnose HIV infection definitively in

infants until they are 15 months of age, when maternal antibody is no longer present in their serum. Consequently, several other laboratory assays are being investigated to help diagnose infants less than 15 months of age. These include HIV viral culture, polymerase chain reaction (PCR), antigen capture assay, IgM and IgA ELISA assays, and in vitro antibody production assays.

Viral culture is performed on peripheral blood mononuclear cells cocultured with uninfected mononuclear cells that can support HIV growth and detect latent HIV infected cells by stimulating viral replication. Evidence of p24 antigen or reverse transcriptase activity indicates the presence of HIV in such samples. The sensitivity of this test is age dependent, exceeding 90% in infants greater than 4 months of age. The test is highly specific and is therefore useful if it is positive. It is probably the best test available at the current time to make a definitive laboratory diagnosis of HIV infection in children less than 15 months of age and should be done on at-risk infants at the age of 4–6 months. However, because the assay is not more sensitive, it cannot be used to rule out HIV infection.

The PCR assay facilitates the detection of minute amounts of HIV proviral DNA that have become incorporated into the DNA of infected cells. Neither its sensitivity nor its specificity has been standardized when it is performed on the lymphocytes of infants from different age groups. PCR may help determine the timing of HIV infection in infants and may have important implications for future investigational drug trials in newborns. Several recent studies have confirmed its diagnostic value (23). Research is ongoing to compare the effectiveness of PCR with that of HIV culture; one recent study suggested a 96% concordance between PCR and HIV coculture (24). At present, PCR cannot be used to rule out HIV infection.

While the ELISA assay tests for anti-HIV antibody, the antigen capture assay tests directly for the HIV p24 antigen levels in serum. There have been isolated false-positive antigen capture assay results reported in children (25) and the question remains whether it is possible that viral particles can be transferred from mother to infant without actual infection ensuing. Overall, though, this test is very specific and establishes the diagnosis if it is positive. Antigen capture is not at all sensitive, with only 30–50% of patients with AIDS having a positive p24 antigen. Thus, as with the other tests used in infants, it cannot be used to rule out HIV infection. More similar to standard IgG ELISA tests are ELISA assays for IgM (26) and IgA (27). These are capable of detecting infant antibody responses because these classes of antibody do not cross the placenta. IgM and IgA antibodies are present only in low concentrations in infants and are often transient; hence, serial testing needs to be done. There is also the concern of a cross-reactivity in the assay between

TABLE 1. *Definition of HIV infection in children*

Infants and children under 15 months of age are considered HIV infected if they meet one of the following criteria:
    Virus in blood or tissues
        or
    HIV antibody
        and
        Evidence of both cellular and humoral immune deficiency (i.e., increased immunoglobulin levels, depressed CD4 cell count, absolute lymphopenia, decreased CD4/CD8 ratio)
        and
        One or more symptoms of HIV infection included in class P-2[a]
        or
Symptoms meeting CDC case definition of AIDS

[a] See Table 3.

maternal IgG antibody and newborn IgM antibody. The sensitivity and specificity of these assays are yet to be determined; they are in the research stage of development and are not yet available commercially. Finally, in vitro antibody production is a functional assay that looks for anti-HIV antibody production by an infant's lymphocytes. Research on its development is under way and has met with some success (28–30).

Because these various tests are not always definitive and because they are not universally available to practitioners, diagnosis of HIV infection in infants frequently requires correlating clinical symptomatology with surrogate laboratory parameters. The 1987 CDC classification system for HIV infection for infants less than 15 months of age (31) defines an HIV-infected infant using clinical symptomatology in conjunction with laboratory parameters (Table 1). In infants and children as in adults, a depressed CD4 count or reversed CD4/CD8 ratio is indicative of immunocompromise. However, healthy infants and children normally have much higher counts than healthy adults. The median CD4 count for adults in a sample of uninfected subjects was 1,027, while the median CD4 count for infants 1–6 months of age in the same study was 3,211 and for those 7–12 months of age

3,128 (Table 2) (32). Whereas the absolute number of CD4 cells is higher in infants and children, the percentage of CD4 cells is relatively stable from infancy to adulthood, with a normal median value of approximately 50%. It is important to be familiar with the normal age-specific lymphocyte counts when evaluating the immune status of infants and children.

Most infants and children with HIV infection have hypergammaglobulinemia, which is indicative of polyclonal B-cell activation (33). Hypergammaglobulinemia has been described as the most common laboratory abnormality in HIV-infected children followed by a reversal of CD4/CD8 ratio (26). Normal immunoglobulin levels in infants and children are also age-specific and need to be considered when evaluating a child for hypergammaglobulinemia. Elevated β-2 microglobulin and neopterin levels have been reported in HIV-infected children. These two indicators correlate with disease progression in adults. Other laboratory abnormalities seen in pediatric HIV infection (some of them nonspecific) include: (1) hypogammaglobulinemia, seen in 3–5% of cases; (2) anemia, which is usually secondary to chronic disease and has been associated with disease progression; other causes such as iron deficiency, sickle cell, and lead toxicity must be ruled out; (3) thrombocytopenia, seen in about 10–20% of HIV-infected children (34) and documented to be associated with antiplatelet antibody in 80% of these (35); and (4) leukopenia. Other clinical manifestations possibly indicative of pediatric HIV infection are discussed below. The laboratory abnormalities seen in adolescent HIV infection are similar to those seen in adults and are discussed elsewhere in this volume.

Early definitive diagnosis of HIV in infants is important so that those infants who may benefit from antiretroviral treatment may be identified for enrollment into clinical trials of such therapy. Studies to assess the efficacy of early antiretroviral intervention with medications that have potentially adverse side effects would be more efficiently conducted if early definitive diagnosis could be made. In addition, early diagnosis helps to reduce the emotional strain currently experienced by care-

TABLE 2. *Normal CD4 lymphocyte counts for children*

	Age (months)				
	1–6	7–12	13–24	25–74	Adults
Absolute CD4 count					
Median	3,211	3,128	2,601	1,668	1,027
Range	1,153–5,285	967–5,289	739–4,463	505–2,831	237–1,817
Percent CD4					
Median	51.6	47.9	45.8	42.1	50.9
Range	36.3–67.1	32.8–63.0	31.2–60.4	32.2–52.0	34.7–67.1
CD4/CD8 ratio					
Median	2.2	2.1	2.0	1.4	1.7
Range	0.9–3.5	0.8–3.4	0.6–3.4	0.7–2.1	0.4–3.0

givers (natural or foster parents or extended family members) in waiting up to 15 months to learn whether their children are infected with HIV. Definitive diagnosis, however, is not needed to give appropriate care to at-risk infants, such as the initiation of *Pneumocystis carinii* pneumonia (PCP) prophylaxis or the administration of immunizations as detailed later in this chapter.

CLINICAL MANIFESTATIONS

HIV in infants and children is a chronic disease with multiorgan system involvement; indeed, there is probably not an organ system that is not affected by HIV. As in adults, HIV disease presents in infants and children with a broad spectrum of manifestations, some of them specific to young people. CDC has devised a classification system of HIV disease in children (31) with cases divided into three classes: (1) P-0 for indeterminate infection; (2) P-1 for asymptomatic infection with and without laboratory abnormalities; and (3) P-2 for symptomatic infection (see Table 3). Most of the symptomatic clinical manifestations of pediatric HIV disease are related to either direct HIV infection or the immunosuppression secondary to it. There is a wide range of clinical symptomatology from common nonspecific findings to severe manifestations of common childhood illnesses, AIDS-defining conditions, and end-organ dysfunction.

Common signs and symptoms seen in children with HIV that are not AIDS defining include lymphadenopathy, hepatomegaly, splenomegaly, parotitis, recurrent diarrhea, failure to thrive, and recurrent fevers. It is important to evaluate children for specific infectious etiologies for these conditions, although HIV or the ensuing immunodeficiency may be the sole cause. Common oropharyngeal signs include persistent thrush, severe painful gingivitis, recurrent aphthous stomatitis, and recurrent

herpetic gingivostomatitis. Some of these conditions are extremely common, and as with adults, lymphoproliferation manifesting as lymphadenopathy may be the first objective sign of disease.

As is true in other immunosuppressed conditions, children with HIV infection may have severe manifestations of otherwise relatively self-limited and usually non-life-threatening conditions common in childhood. Several common childhood illnesses that manifest more seriously in children with HIV infection include severe recurrent fungal skin and nail infections (tinea, candida), recalcitrant molluscum contagiosum, severe condylomata, recurrent and chronic otitis media and sinusitis, and recurrent upper respiratory tract infections.

Also included in this group are severe and life-threatening manifestations of varicella and measles. Prolonged disease with varicella is common in the immunocompromised child and includes progression to pneumonitis, hepatitis, pancreatitis, and encephalitis. In one study of HIV-infected children with varicella, seven of eight children had evidence suggestive of varicella pneumonitis (36). HIV-infected children with varicella should be treated aggressively with acyclovir as soon as there is evidence of disease. Varicella-exposed children should be given varicella-zoster immune globulin (VZIG) in an attempt to prevent or modify the course of the disease. Measles can also be life-threatening in the HIV-infected child (37). This is becoming a larger problem in the face of the current measles epidemic. Even with appropriate immunization, many HIV-infected children do not mount protective antibody responses against measles and continue to be susceptible because of their impaired humoral immune response. Any HIV-infected child who is exposed to measles should receive intramuscular serum immune globulin as prophylaxis. Some children with life-threatening manifestations of measles such as pneumonitis are being treated with IV ribavirin on an emergency IND compassionate use basis.

TABLE 3. *CDC classification system for HIV infection in children under 13 years of age*

Class	Symptom
P-0	Indeterminate infection
P-1	Asymptomatic infection
Subclass A	Normal immune function
Subclass B	Abnormal immune function
Subclass C	Immune function not tested
P-2	Symptomatic infection
Subclass A	Nonspecific findings
Subclass B	Progressive neurologic disease
Subclass C	Lymphoid interstitial pneumonitis
Subclass D	Secondary infectious diseases including opportunistic infections
Subclass E	Secondary cancers
Subclass F	Other diseases possibly due to HIV infection

OPPORTUNISTIC INFECTIONS

In both adults and children, the opportunistic infections related to the immunodeficiency caused by HIV are varied and frequently difficult to treat. AIDS-defining opportunistic infections in children often represent primary infection with the organism rather than the recrudescence that is typically the case in adults. This may be why PCP is a more severe illness in infants than in adults. Adult opportunistic infections that are rarely seen in children include toxoplasmosis, cryptococcal disease, and other disseminated fungal infections such as coccidioidomycosis and histoplasmosis. Their relative scarcity in children probably relates to a lack of exposure to the etiologic agents. These conditions are seen in adolescents, however. The types of opportunistic infections

TABLE 4. *Pharmacological treatment of HIV infection and its common sequela in children*

Condition	Treatment[a]
HIV infection	AZT (Retrovir, zidovudine), younger than 13 years: 180 mg/m²/dose orally Q6H, older than 13 years: 100 mg/dose orally Q4H, 5×/day ddI (Didanosine, Videx): 50–150 mg/m²/dose given orally 2×/day Investigational: ddI, ddC
Humoral immunodeficiency (with recurrent serious bacterial infections or documented functional antibody defect)	Immune globulin 400 mg/kg IV 1×/month
Pneumocystis carinii pneumonia	
Prophylaxis	Trimethoprim/sulfamethoxazole (TMP-SMX) 150 mg TMP/m²/day with 750 mg SMX/m²/day given orally divided BID 3×/week on consecutive days (e.g., M-T-W). Other dosing schedules include: (1) once daily dose 3×/week on consecutive days (e.g., M-T-W); (2) BID 7×/week; (3) BID dose given on alternate days (e.g., M-W-F) Alternate regimens: (1) dapsone 1 mg/kg/dose orally 1×/day not to exceed 100 mg/day; (2) aerosolized pentamidine (age 5 years or older) 300 mg/dose via Respirgard II 1×/month; (3) if above not tolerated: IV pentamidine 4 mg/kg/dose every 2 or 4 weeks
Treatment	Trimethoprim/sulfamethoxazole (TMP-SMX) 5 mg TMP/kg/dose with 25 mg SMX/kg/dose IV Q6H *or* Pentamidine isethionate 4 mg base/kg/day IV daily Investigational: steroids
Candida	
Thrush	Nystatin suspension 2–6 cc swish in cheeks 3–5×/day *or* Miconazole vaginal cream apply orally BID-QID *or* Terazol vaginal cream apply orally BID-QID *or* Clotrimazole troches, one troche in mouth 5×/day *or* Ketoconazole 5–10 mg/kg/day orally given once a day or BID *or* Fluconazole 2–8 mg/kg/day orally given once a day
Esophagitis	Ketoconazole 5–10 mg/kg/day orally given once a day or BID *or* Fluconazole loading dose of 10 mg/kg given orally then 3–8 mg/kg/day orally or IV given once a day *or* Amphotericin B 0.25–1.5 mg/kg/day IV
Disseminated cryptococcosis	Induction: amphotericin B 0.25–1.5 mg/kg/day IV Maintenance: amphotericin B 1 mg/kg 1–2×/week *or* Fluconazole 3–8 mg/kg/day orally 1×/day
Disseminated cytomegalovirus	Induction: ganciclovir 5 mg/kg/dose Q12H IV or 2–5 mg/kg/dose Q8H IV Alternative: foscarnet 60 mg/kg/dose Q8H IV Maintenance: ganciclovir 5 mg/kg/dose QD IV or 6 mg/kg/dose QD for 5 days/week Investigational: foscarnet 90–120 mg/kg QD IV (run over 2 hr)
Mycobacterium avium-intracellulare	No standard of therapy exists Investigational: (1) oral quadruple drug regimen: rifampin, ethambutol, ciprofloxacin, and clofazimine; (2) IV and oral quadruple drug regimen: oral ciprofloxacin, ethambutol and rifampin, and IV amikacin; (3) clarithromycin
Lymphoid interstital pneumonitis (LIP)	Steroids are indicated when LIP is associated with significant hypoxemia defined as a documented PaO₂ of less than 65 torr on three separate occasions over a 1-month period. Prednisone 2 mg/kg/day for 2–4 weeks or until there is an increase in PaO₂ of at least 20 torr, then gradually taper to 0.5 mg/kg every other day provided PaO₂ remains above 70. Duration of steroid therapy is not established.
Herpes simplex virus	Acyclovir 250 mg/m²/dose IV Q8H or 600 mg/m²/dose orally Q6H (in cases of visceral or disseminated infection use dose of 500 mg/m²/dose IV Q8H) Alternative for acyclovir resistant herpes: foscarnet

TABLE 4. *Continued.*

Condition	Treatment[a]
Varicella-zoster	Treatment: acyclovir 500 mg/m²/dose IV Q8H or 900 mg/m²/dose orally Q6H Exposure: varicella-zoster immune globulin (VZIG) 125 units (one vial) for each 10 kg of body weight (maximum of 625 units) IM within 96 hours of exposure to varicella
Measles	All children should be immunized with measles vaccine Exposure: immune globulin 0.5 ml/kg (maximum dose of 15 ml) IM within 6 days of exposure Investigational therapy: ribavirin

[a] The investigational therapies listed in this chart are available either by prescription, through enrollment in a treatment trial, or on a compassionate use basis through the pharmaceutical company.

children experience are likely to change as survival times increase and prophylaxis is initiated to prevent common infections like PCP. While space limitations preclude a comprehensive review of opportunistic infections in children, we will discuss some points that are particularly salient for pediatric HIV. The specific antimicrobial treatment of these infections is listed in Table 4 using weight-specific doses of drugs.

The most common opportunistic infection in infants and children is PCP, accounting for 45% of reported AIDS indicator diseases in children and up to 65% of opportunistic infections in the pediatric population (38,39). With the effective use of PCP prophylaxis, it is expected that there will be a drop in this statistic. Most cases occur in the first year of life, with the median age of presentation being 3–6 months. Prior to the use of PCP prophylaxis, among infants who developed AIDS in the first year of life, over half had PCP. Mortality is high even with effective therapy, and the median survival following an episode is 1–4 months (39). The clinical presentation of PCP varies, acute disease with rapid onset of respiratory failure being common in the first year of life. Diagnosis can be made using induced sputum, bronchoalveolar lavage, or lung biopsy. The use of gallium scans as a diagnostic modality is not standardized in children. Lymphoid interstitial pneumonitis (LIP) is an important part of the differential diagnosis in children. Because of the importance of aggressive management, it is not necessary to make a definitive diagnosis of PCP to initiate treatment. Based on adult recommendations, many clinicians are using steroids to treat PCP in children, even though the efficacy of this treatment has not been established for primary infection.

Candida esophagitis is the second most common opportunistic infection in pediatric AIDS. It may be seen with or without oral candidiasis. The symptoms of dysphagia, odynophagia, substernal pain, and fever are similar to those in adults. Infants and children who are either unable to verbalize or cannot localize pain frequently present with a decrease in oral intake, weight loss, and failure to thrive. Unusual neck movements may be seen

in a child who is attempting to relieve pain. The diagnosis is suggested by symptomatology and barium swallow, and is made definitively by endoscopy. Neurological causes of dysphagia are an important part of the differential diagnosis in children.

Mycobacterium avium-intracellulare (MAI) is associated with more severe immunocompromise. Among children seen with this condition at Children's Hospital AIDS Program in Newark, New Jersey, the CD4 count at the time of diagnosis has always been below 200/mm³ (40), regardless of the child's age. To date, MAI has been the AIDS-defining condition in about 3% of cases and has been seen at Children's Hospital in 14% of all children with AIDS; this percentage is likely to increase as children's survival times lengthen as a result of PCP prophylaxis and antiretroviral therapy. The most common clinical symptoms of MAI are fever, malaise, weight loss, diarrhea, and abdominal pain. All children followed at CHAP with MAI had the additional sign of a persistent failure to gain weight (40). Thus, all patients showing this sign should be evaluated for MAI. It is diagnosed chiefly by blood culture and also by means of bone marrow biopsy, liver biopsy, or stool culture.

Recurrent Bacterial Infections

HIV infection is associated with significant abnormalities in B-cell mediated immune responses. In infants, laboratory-documented B-cell dysfunction usually precedes T-cell abnormalities (41,42). This may be the result of an interference with normal B-cell maturation, as humoral immune responses are incomplete at birth. The normal maturation of B cells, including the ability to produce antigen-specific antibodies, requires lymphokines produced by functioning CD4 cells. Most adults with HIV infection were exposed to the common bacterial pathogens prior to becoming HIV infected; because of this, they tend to have circulating protective antibodies against them and circulating B cells with a retained anamnestic response to these pathogens. Thus, adults tend to get serious bacterial infections with common pathogens only late in the course of the disease, when they are severely immunocompromised. With improved survival in a more immunocompromised state, however, the problem of severe bacterial infections in adults is on the rise. In contrast, HIV-infected children have been shown to have defective primary and secondary antibody production to T cell-dependent and -independent antigens (41,43); when children are exposed to common bacterial pathogens for the first time, these abnormalities result in severe manifestations of infection early in the course of their HIV infection. Since 1987, multiple or recurrent serious bacterial infections have been a part of the CDC case definition of AIDS for children (44). The most common infections that meet the case definition are bacteremia and pneumonia. The most common organisms include *Streptococcus pnemoniae, Haemophilus influenzae, Salmonella* sp., and *Staphylococcus aureus* (45,46). Clinicians should be aggressive in treating less severe bacterial infections such as otitis or impetigo so as to prevent dissemination.

LYMPHOID INTERSTITIAL PNEUMONITIS

Lymphoid interstitial pneumonitis is a diffuse lymphocytic infiltration of the interstitium of the lung (47), which can interfere with gas exchange. It is an AIDS-defining condition only in children, and it has been the AIDS-defining condition in over 25% of cases of pediatric AIDS. It may result from dual infection with AIDS and Epstein-Barr virus (EBV) (48), but its etiology has not been definitively established. Hypoxemia, clubbing, and superimposed bacterial infections may be present, and long-standing LIP can progress to chronic bronchiectasis. PCP is rarely seen in patients who have LIP. Treatment is directed at the hypoxemia, which can be reversed with corticosteroids (49), the superimposed bacterial pneumonitis, and the chronic lung damage. Children with LIP often have other evidence of lymphoproliferative disease and tend to have significant lymphadenopathy, hepatomegaly, splenomegaly, and relatively frequently parotid enlargement.

CENTRAL NERVOUS SYSTEM INVOLVEMENT

Central nervous system (CNS) involvement is a more common manifestation of HIV infection in infants and children than in adults and is felt to occur in at least 60% of those infected. The severity of CNS dysfunction may relate to when in the course of pregnancy or delivery the infant became infected. HIV is believed to enter the CNS through HIV-infected macrophages, which can cross the blood–brain barrier. In infants, entry of HIV into the CNS may be facilitated by infection with HIV in utero prior to establishment of this barrier. It is unclear exactly how HIV causes neurological dysfunction; direct HIV effects and indirect effects through cells of the macrophage lineage and the elaboration of toxic cytokines have been postulated.

A broad clinical spectrum of neurological abnormalities is seen in pediatric HIV infection (50,51). Most children have some degree of developmental delay, whether subtle or blatant, affecting both motor and cognitive milestones. The presentation of developmental delay is variable. There may be relatively normal development suddenly followed by either a loss of milestones or a failure to attain new milestones. The onset of developmental delay may be followed by periods of relative stability in neurological function or a course of rapid neurodevelopmental deterioration. Pyramidal tract involvement may be seen, with resulting spastic paresis. Hypertonicity and hyperreflexia are common manifestations of motor involvement.

Static encephalopathy is seen in about one-quarter of children with HIV and is characterized by developmental delay of varying severity without loss of previously attained milestones. Children in this group can have improvement in neurological function with continued acquisition of developmental skills, but usually in a delayed fashion. Progressive encephalopathy, defined as a loss of previously attained cognitive or motor milestones, is often seen in patients who also have opportunistic infections (52). This accounts for its relatively low incidence as an AIDS indicator disease in pediatrics, despite its relative frequency. Progressive encephalopathy, which is associated with a very poor prognosis, can be characterized by a plateau course without continued loss of milestones, a subacute progressive course associated with slow continued losses in motor and nonmotor developmental milestones, or a rapidly progressive course. Radiological findings of HIV infection in children include cerebral atrophy and calcification of the basal ganglia. The possibility of a CNS lymphoma (53) must always be considered in the child who develops new neurological signs and symptoms.

Antiretroviral therapy has been shown to improve the neurodevelopmental functioning of infants and children with HIV (54). Children can regain lost motor and developmental milestones with therapy. In some this is dramatic, with the reversal of incontinence, gait abnormalities, or lost cognitive milestones after initiation of therapy. In pediatric trials, as opposed to those in adults, improvements in neurodevelopmental outcome is a primary goal of antiretroviral therapy.

PRESENTATION AND PROGNOSIS IN INFANTS AND CHILDREN

There are two general patterns of presentation of HIV in children (39,55). One of them, representing about one-third of all perinatally acquired infection, involves early onset of severe disease with rapid progression and poor prognosis (52). Infants in this group usually present with severe opportunistic infections (most often PCP) and/or encephalopathy, generally within the first 4–8 months of life. While these infants often have the manifestations of PCP or encephalopathy discussed above, they generally come to the attention of physicians and become identified as HIV infected because of severe illnesses that arise abruptly. PCP in this group is seldom insidious; infants may be seen by a physician one week with some mild general symptoms and have fulminant, life-threatening PCP the next. It is because of the presentation of illness in this group of patients that early PCP prophylaxis is required.

The second pattern of pediatric HIV infection involves later onset of disease symptomatology and is associated with a better prognosis. These children generally present after the first year of life with a more indolent disease course, consisting of a variety of the more general clinical manifestations discussed above. Relative to children diagnosed with AIDS in the first year of life, LIP is more common in this group, as are generalized lymphadenopathy and parotitis. It is not unusual for school-age children to be identified with perinatal HIV infection as a result of this type of presentation; there are children who are not diagnosed with AIDS or HIV infection until 10 or 11 years of age. One study has reported a median incubation period of over 6 years in this group, which is more comparable to the median reported for adults (56). Children who present relatively late may be clinically similar to asymptomatic adults or show only subtle HIV-related signs and symptoms before presenting with more obvious conditions such as thrush. Recurrent bacterial infections are likely to occur as AIDS-defining conditions in both early- and late-onset presentation of HIV. Renal and cardiac involvement usually occur as later manifestations of illness after other significant HIV-related disease is diagnosed.

It is unclear why some children present early with fulminant disease and others present later. One can speculate that this is related to the timing of infection—perinatal, early in gestation, or late in gestation. Initial reports of congenital cytomegalovirus (CMV) infection suggested that this was a uniformly fatal disease, but over time, it became obvious that these initial reports reflected the worst case scenarios and that other children who probably acquired their infection perinatally were less severely affected.

Although the median age of children at AIDS diagnosis is 12 months, this statistic is misleading in that it is heavily skewed toward those patients who present early with AIDS-defining conditions. Significant numbers of patients also present in the second to fifth year of life. In addition, many of the children in whom later onset will occur have yet to be identified. Thus it is likely that the actual median incubation period to AIDS for all perinatally infected children, including those in both early- and late-onset categories, will be in the range of 3–5 years. A statistical analysis of data from the New York State case registry of pediatric AIDS cases through 1987 by Auger et al. (56) revealed that approximately 20% developed AIDS in the first year of life with a rate of about 8% per year thereafter. Prospective studies of cohorts of infected and at-risk infants over time will answer the question of the true incubation period in children both to AIDS and to the development of clinical symptomatology. Though the actual incubation period to AIDS may be longer than initially thought, the incubation period to subtle HIV-attributable clinical symptomatology in children followed prospectively may be shorter. Scott et al. (39) reported that about 50% of children in her series had clinical symptoms suggestive of HIV infection, not AIDS, in the first year of life. With the current recommendations for early antimicrobial prophylaxis and antiretroviral therapy, and the inherent need for early identification of infected and at-risk infants, the true incubation periods will become clearer.

Two factors affect the prognosis of children with HIV infection: their specific HIV-related diseases and their age at presentation. A study of 172 perinatally infected children treated at a Miami hospital (39) showed median survival rates from diagnosis of 1 month for those with PCP, 5 months for those with nephropathy, 11 months for those with encephalopathy, 12 months for those with candida esophagitis, 50 months for those with recurrent bacterial infection, and 72 months for those with LIP. A study at the Children's Hospital of New Jersey (57) showed a median survival rate following PCP of 2 months. Another study of 94 children (52) showed 3-year survival rates of 48 ± 24% among those presenting with opportunistic infections or encephalopathy and 97 ± 3% among those presenting with LIP or recurrent bacterial infections. Opportunistic infections and encephalopathy appeared earlier than LIP, which did not present before the age of 16 months.

PCP has been the AIDS-defining condition in 53% of infants less than 1 year of age, and has had the worst prognosis in this group (55). In addition, a study at a New York hospital showed a mean survival time for perinatally infected children of 67 months, while the survival time from infection for children over 2 years of age infected by transfusion averaged 90 months (58). Thus both later presentation and later infection appear to be associated with longer survival.

It is important to note that an AIDS diagnosis, in and of itself, is not an accurate prognostic indicator for children. There is extreme variation in the prognosis that depends on the conditions responsible for the AIDS diagnosis. While opportunistic infections, encephalopathy, LIP, and recurrent bacterial infections are all AIDS-defining conditions, the first two of these are associated with a significantly worse prognosis than the last two. In addition, information about the average survival time for adults after an AIDS diagnosis is not valid for children. While an AIDS diagnosis may be of epidemiological interest and can be important in gaining access to care for children through eligibility for public entitlement programs, by itself it is of limited value in predicting survival time. Thus, contrary to the general impression held by many parents and caregivers, a diagnosis of AIDS does not mean that a child will die within a very short period of time; it is important for health care workers to discuss the prognosis for children in terms of specific conditions.

TREATMENT OF HIV AND RESULTING ILLNESSES IN CHILDREN

The medical management of children with HIV should begin with the identification of those who are at risk and their careful monitoring to determine the infection status. Once laboratory signs of immunosuppression or clinical symptoms of disease are evident, children should receive both HIV-specific treatment and general supportive management. Primary HIV-specific treatment centers on specific antimicrobial prophylaxis for opportunistic infections and antiretroviral therapy. General supportive management includes psychosocial support, pain management, nutritional supplementation, developmental intervention, patient education, and advocacy. In addition, medical management should encompass general pediatric care, including childhood immunizations.

HIV-Specific Treatment

PCP Prophylaxis

PCP in children with HIV infection is associated with a high rate of morbidity and mortality. It often presents acutely in the first 4–8 months of life. Because of the success of prophylaxis in adults with HIV infection and immunosuppressed children with cancer, a working group was sponsored by the National Pediatric HIV Resource Center to establish standards of care regarding PCP prophylaxis for children. The recommendations of the working group were endorsed by CDC and published in *MMWR* in March 1991 (59).

As with the adult recommendations for PCP prophylaxis, the recommendations for infants and children are based on CD4 lymphocyte counts. A recent retrospective review of children with PCP followed at the Children's Hospital AIDS Program in Newark, New Jersey (57) revealed that only 40% of the children had CD4 lymphocyte counts at or below 200/mm^3. In another study only 48% of perinatally infected children with PCP

had CD4 counts less than 500/mm^3 (60). Effective prophylaxis is recommended based on age-dependent CD4 values in infants and children; these differ from values in adults, as discussed earlier (see Table 2). Prophylaxis is recommended for children 1–11 months of age with CD4 counts under 1,500 cells/mm^3, for children 12–23 months of age with CD4 counts under 750, for those 24 months to 5 years of age with CD4 counts below 500, and for those greater than or equal to 6 years of age with CD4 counts below 200 (59). The normal percentage of CD4 lymphocytes does not vary with age, and regardless of age or CD4 counts, primary PCP prophylaxis is recommended for any child with a CD4 percent of less than 20 (Fig. 1). It is not necessary to make a definitive diagnosis of HIV infection in an infant to initiate PCP prophylaxis. For HIV-infected infants less than 15 months of age, it is not possible, given our current diagnostic capabilities, to make a definitive diagnosis prior to initiating prophylaxis in most cases. Infants who are at risk for HIV infection should have their CD4 lymphocyte counts determined at 1 month of age and have PCP prophylaxis initiated based on these results. The usual regimen is trimethoprim/sulfamethoxazole (TMP-SMX) in the dosage of 150 mg TMP/m^2/day given orally in divided doses twice a day, three times per week, on consecutive days. Refer to Table 4 for alternative drug and dosing schedules.

Effective PCP prophylaxis for adults has been a part of the standard of care in that community for several years. Despite this, the most common AIDS-defining condition in adults continues to be PCP. In the adult community taken as a whole there has been only a small drop in the impact of PCP, whereas for individuals followed in the MAC study, tumors (including Kaposi's sarcoma) and not PCP, is currently the most common AIDS-defining diagnosis. In order to have more of an impact on morbidity, the establishment of effective standards must be followed by their timely dissemination and implementation in the context of accessible health care.

Antiretroviral Therapy

AZT

AZT was FDA-approved for use in children three years after it was approved for adults. Its approval for children was based on the results of efficacy trials in adults, pharmacokinetic and toxicity trials in children, and some efficacy data that were deduced from phase I and phase II studies in children. It is important that drug development in children proceed in parallel with development in adults, and not following that development. This process is improving, with current research into promising antiretrovirals for children proceeding more in conjunction with adult research.

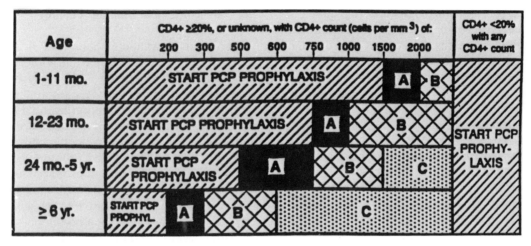

FIG. 1. Recommendations for initiation of *Pneumocystis carinii* pneumonia (PCP) prophylaxis for children ≥1 month old who are (1) HIV infected; (2) HIV seropositive; or (3) <12 months old and born to an HIV-infected mother. A CD4+ count and CD4+ % should be obtained for each child. Use test results and child's age as criteria for starting PCP prophylaxis. A, no prophylaxis recommended at this time; recheck CD4+ count in 1 month; B, no prophylaxis recommended at this time; recheck CD4+ count at least every 3–4 months; C, no prophylaxis recommended at this time; recheck CD4+ count at least every 6 months.

AZT is currently being used for children with symptomatic HIV infection (class P-2) and those with evidence of immunocompromise. However, because the pediatric guidelines were extrapolated from adult experience, they are not as clearly defined as the adult guidelines. With the recent advances in the knowledge of normal age-related CD4 cell counts in infants and children, it is probably appropriate to gear the beginning of antiretroviral therapy to age-specific CD4 counts, as is being done for PCP prophylaxis. At the Children's Hospital AIDS Program in Newark, New Jersey, AZT is being offered to all definitively diagnosed infants and children who meet criteria for PCP prophylaxis based on CD4 counts. Children older than 6 years of age are started on AZT using the adult guidelines of CD4 counts less than 500/mm³.

In adults, the use of AZT has been shown to prolong life, decrease the severity of opportunistic infections, and slow the progression of illness. No placebo-controlled efficacy studies have been completed in children, but other studies suggest similar results. Children with advanced HIV disease involved in ACTG protocol 043 (an open-label trial of AZT) experienced weight gains and improvements in cognitive function as measured by neuropsychological testing (61). The gains in cognitive function correlate with the results of phase I and II studies of AZT conducted by Pizzo et al. (54,62). The noted improvements in neurodevelopmental function is particularly important in pediatric HIV infection, as there are neurodevelopmental abnormalities in at least 60% of patients.

Children in ACTG protocol 043 had reductions in serum and cerebrospinal fluid (CSF) levels of p24 antigen. A further direct antiviral effect upon the central nervous system was seen in negative CSF viral cultures in the majority of children who had positive viral cultures at entry into the protocol. A positive CSF viral culture means that free virus is present in the CSF, so a negative culture in a patient who was previously positive implies a decrease in viral replication. Finally, changes in the CD4 cell counts of children in the protocol were consistent with those seen in adults: an increase during the first 12 weeks of therapy, followed by a subsequent decline by 24 weeks to counts at or above baseline.

The toxicity of AZT in children is similar to that in adults (63) and is primarily hematological. In protocol 043, one or more episodes of hematological toxicity occurred in 61% of the children, with anemia in 26% and neutropenia in 48% (61). Transfusions or dose modifications were required in 34% of the children because of hematological toxicity, while the remainder resolved spontaneously. As noted above, the children in the protocol had advanced disease: 57% of them were anemic at entry into the trial. Experience with AZT in adults has shown that those whose disease is less advanced when they begin taking the medication have a lower incidence of hematological toxicity. Thus, it is likely that the toxicity seen in protocol 043 represents the worst case scenario.

AZT is now available in a syrup formulation and is currently recommended for children in a dose of 180 mg/m² every 6 hours, comparable to the original high dose used in adults. A lower dose of AZT has become the standard of care in adults, and an ongoing pediatric trial is comparing the effects of the recommended dose with those of a dose half its size (90 mg/m²). Because of the significant improvement in neurodevelopmental outcome among children on the higher dose, investigators have been reluctant simply to extrapolate from adult experience and establish low-dose therapy as the standard of care for children. It remains to be seen whether the higher dose is necessary to reach appropriate concentrations in the central nervous system.

ddI

ddI is an antiretroviral whose mechanism of action is similar to that of AZT. It is FDA-approved for use in children who are intolerant of AZT or who have disease progression while on AZT. Currently there is an ongoing ACTG clinical trial comparing ddI with AZT and with a combination of ddI and AZT in children.

Evidence of the immunological efficacy of ddI in children was seen in the phase I and II trials (64), with a sustained increase in CD4 cell counts throughout the 24 weeks of the trials. A decrease in p24 antigen levels has also been demonstrated with ddI use. There is some indication of improvement in neurodevelopmental function of children on ddI; whether these preliminary observations are accurate will be determined with further pediatric experience with the drug. There appears to be variability of absorption of ddI in children, which may be related to gastric acidity. The improvements noted with ddI correlated with serum levels of ddI; those children with higher levels experienced more significant improvements.

In phase I and II pediatric trials with ddI, the main toxicity seen has been hyperamylasemia, with pancreatitis occurring in 2 of 43 patients studied (64). Pancreatitis appears to be dose related, having occurred in the patients receiving the two highest doses in the trial. Although peripheral neuropathy has been reported in adults on ddI, this symptom was not reported in any of the children in phase I and II trials. However, it is generally the patient who reports this symptom, which may account for its being underreported in children who cannot verbalize.

ddC

Another antiretroviral being used in clinical trials in children is ddC. Its mechanism of action is similar to that of AZT, but, like ddI, it does not cause significant hematological toxicity. In a small pilot study in HIV-infected children, ddC has been shown to decrease p24 antigen levels and raise CD4 counts (65). A dose-dependent toxicity of ddC seen in adults, painful peripheral neuropathy, has yet to appear in the limited-time trials at lower doses in children. Rashes and mouth sores have been the main side effects seen in children. An ongoing ACTG protocol is examining the effects of ddC in children who are intolerant of AZT or show evidence of disease progression while on AZT.

Intravenous Immune Globulin Therapy

Intravenous immune globulin (IVIG) is part of the standard treatment for children and adults with primary humoral immunodeficiency disorders such as Bruton's agammaglobulinemia. Passive immunotherapy in the form of IVIG provides protection against a wide range of bacterial and viral organisms. As discussed above, children with HIV infection often have functional abnormalities of their B-cell mediated immune system, which places them at risk for infections that require an intact humoral immune response. Though most children with HIV infection have elevated immunoglobulin levels, they are felt to represent nonspecific polyclonal B-cell activation. Many children fail to mount an antibody response to routine childhood immunizations (43), indicating a functional immunodeficiency.

Pediatric immunologists have been using IVIG on HIV-infected children with B-cell immunodeficiency since early in the epidemic (66). Uncontrolled studies have suggested that IVIG therapy is efficacious in reducing the frequency of sepsis (67) and other clinical symptomatology (68). Improvements in mitogen-induced lymphoproliferative responses and a decrease in the concentration of circulating immune complexes has also been shown to occur in some children on IVIG. Other researchers have been skeptical regarding the effectiveness of IVIG relative to other modalities such as prophylactic antibiotics. The National Institute of Child Health and Human Development (NICHD) recently completed a placebo-controlled trial using IVIG in HIV-infected children. The trial found that IVIG prolonged the time free from serious laboratory-proven bacterial or clinically diagnosed infections in symptomatic HIV-infected children with CD4 counts greater than 200/mm^3. This study suggests the value for using IVIG in some children with HIV infection. Unfortunately, this trial did not separately evaluate the efficacy in those children with documented B-cell defects but looked only at groups based on CD4 counts.

At Children's Hospital AIDS Program in Newark, New Jersey, IVIG is being used in HIV-infected children with documented humoral immunodeficiency based on either a history of recurrent serious bacterial infections or a documented lack of a specific antibody response to immunizations or infecting pathogens. IVIG is also useful in the treatment of HIV-related thrombocytopenia.

Childhood Immunizations

Immunizations represent the cornerstone of preventive medicine for children. The current measles epidemic is a result of the failure of the US health care system to provide access to health care for its citizens of lower socioeconomic status. Immunization schedules for HIV-infected children must take into account the potential for complications secondary to live or attenuated viral vaccines. Paralytic poliomyelitis is a potential complication of the oral polio vaccine (OPV) for both the immunocompromised patient and immunocompromised family members through excreted virus in stool. There is also a potential for serious complications from other attenuated viral vaccines such as measles. However, no serious side effects have been documented in immunized HIV-infected children. The use of inactivated polio vaccine (IPV) instead of OPV is recommended for these children. In the case of measles, for which no alternative is available, the use of MMR is recommended routinely for HIV-infected children. Despite immunization, many children may continue to be susceptible to the immunized organisms; inadequate antibody responses have been documented in some children (41,43). The current recommendations for immunization of HIV-infected children are listed in Table 5.

Early Identification of HIV-Infected and At-Risk Infants

Though there is currently no cure for HIV infection, there are several available interventions, as discussed above, that can reduce morbidity and delay progression of disease. New treatments directed at both HIV and the opportunistic infections secondary to HIV are increasingly being investigated. A delay in disease progression may eventually allow access to medication that will be life-saving. Because of this, adults are encouraged to have confidential and voluntary HIV testing with informed consent. Voluntary testing of newborns would be sensible from a medical standpoint so that those who are at risk can be identified for: (1) early initiation of PCP prophylaxis; (2) early initiation of antiretroviral therapy when appropriate; (3) change in immunization schedule from the use of OPV to IPV and the inclusion of pneumococcal and influenza vaccines; and (4) access

TABLE 5. *Recommendations for routine immunization of HIV-infected children—United States*

Vaccine	Known HIV infection	
	Asymptomatic	Symptomatic
DTP	Yes	Yes
OPV	No	No
IPV	Yes	Yes
MMR	Yes	Yes
HbCV	Yes	Yes
Pneumococcal	Yes	Yes
Influenza	No[a]	Yes

[a] Not contraindicated.

DTP, diphtheria and tetanus toxoids and pertussis vaccine, adsorbed. DTP may be used up to the seventh birthday. OPV, poliovirus vaccine live oral, trivalent; contains poliovirus types 1, 2, and 3; IPV, poliovirus vaccine inactivated: contains poliovirus types 1, 2, and 3; MMR, measles, mumps, and rubella virus vaccine, live; HbCV, vaccine composed of *Haemophilus influenzae* b polysaccharide antigen conjugated to a protein carrier.

to social service benefits to ensure better access to health care. Testing of newborns, however, by definition, includes testing of their mothers. Part of the informed consent surrounding voluntary newborn testing should clearly include, in addition to the benefits of such testing, information that the testing of the infant is in fact revealing the HIV status of the mother. Ideally maternal testing should be encouraged prenatally so that reproductive options and anticipatory health guidance can be thoroughly reviewed, and appropriate HIV-specific therapy initiated. Simultaneous with voluntary testing of infants and women, there must be assurance of confidentiality, protection against discrimination, and access to state of the art health care.

Pain Management

Pain management is an especially important but frequently undertreated clinical problem in HIV-infected infants. Children with AIDS suffer from two types of pain—the pain of the disease, both acute and chronic, and the pain of the multiple diagnostic and therapeutic procedures these children need. Physicians in general are poorly trained in the control of pain by medication, and many do not appreciate that newborns and infants experience pain. While many fear they will make their patients drug addicts, only 0.4% of patients given narcotics in hospitals ever have a problem with opiate dependence.

A much more aggressive approach must be taken to controlling pain in children; there is a lot of good literature, especially in the oncology field, to draw upon. Vigorous and proactive use of appropriate pain medication including aspirin, acetaminophen, codeine, ibuprofen, morphine, and methadone is essential to the overall quality of life for HIV-infected children. Both health care providers and families need to be educated as to the appropriate use of these medications. Specific barriers to the management of pain in HIV-infected children include: (1) the difficulty of assessing pain in young children; (2) the difficulty of assessing pain in children with neurological impairment; (3) parental denial of their children's disease; and (4) resistance to the use of narcotics by families who have a history of drug use (69). At the Children's Hospital AIDS Program, a combination of methadone and valium is used in children with chronic end-stage pain. Nonpharmacological approaches to pain management (including relaxation, hypnosis, play therapy, visualization, and distraction) should also be applied in the control of pain, especially when it is related to procedures.

SOCIAL ISSUES IN THE DELIVERY OF CARE

The epidemiological data on pediatric HIV disease make it clear that in the United States, there has been a disproportionate impact upon the poor and people of color, particularly those with histories of injecting drug use. The health care needs of these people have traditionally been underserved, and previous contact with public agencies may dispose them toward distrust and discourage them from seeking timely medical care (70). Often one of the first relationships of trust that affected families develop is with the health care providers who treat their children. Health care professionals should attempt to establish a partnership with the family rather than reinforcing the more traditional role of passivity and dependence (71).

The conditions of poverty, including inadequate housing, may interfere with the delivery of optimal health care. Mothers are typically the strongest advocates for their children, but this advocacy may be hindered by the fact that the mothers of HIV-infected children are often single parents and poor. In some cases, symptomatic HIV infection or drug use may interfere with a mother's ability to care properly for her child; more often, however, mothers are assertive in seeking care for their children while neglecting their own care needs. The general shortage of slots in drug treatment programs is especially severe for women who are HIV-infected or pregnant or who have children. All of these socioeconomic conditions have to be addressed in designing effective health care systems for families with HIV infection.

Families can also benefit from psychosocial support in dealing with many aspects of an HIV diagnosis in a child. The diagnosis may be the first evidence that a parent is infected and may give rise to guilt or anger leading to further disruption of the family unit. Apparently resolved emotional issues may require periodic reexamination, as for example when parents are confronted repeatedly by the differences between a child who is developmentally delayed and healthy peers (72). Decisions about the disclosure of an HIV diagnosis may arise repeatedly as different audiences are encountered such as family, friends, siblings of the infected child, the child himself, day care workers, school nurses, and teachers. Many parents choose to disclose the diagnosis on a need-to-know basis. However, children and their siblings often find it less stressful to know the diagnosis than to be left in the dark about something unnamed but apparent. Counseling may help parents to decide whether and how to disclose the diagnosis. Uninfected siblings often have mental health needs as well, especially when they face the eventual loss of siblings and one or both parents. A failure to deal successfully with psychosocial issues may impede families from seeking to obtain optimal medical care for their children.

DEVELOPING STANDARDS OF CARE FOR CHILDREN WITH HIV

Twenty years ago, 95% of the children with leukemia died; today, up to 85% are cured. The intensity of effort put into controlling childhood leukemia should serve as a template for our efforts to treat HIV-infected children. The effort to improve the quality of life while working toward a cure for HIV will require a multidisciplinary approach, calling on the skills of physicians, nurses, social workers, nutritionists, pharmacists, dentists, and developmental specialists. This effort must take the child's entire family into consideration, whether it be the family of birth or a foster family. At Children's Hospital AIDS Program in Newark, New Jersey, 40% of the children with HIV are in foster or adoptive care, often given by a member of the extended family. These families need supportive services, like any family caring for a multiply handicapped fragile baby.

The symptomatic care of HIV-infected children has been developed both to prolong survival and to improve the quality of life. The challenge to pediatric HIV treatment centers is to make investigational antiretroviral, immunomodulating, and antimicrobial therapies available rapidly. Potentially useful investigational drug studies for HIV-infected infants and children should be pursued in parallel to studies in adults. Programs using research and those providing clinical care should be linked synergistically.

This chapter began with a quote from Gabriela Minstrel. HIV-infected children truly can not wait for a tomorrow they may not have. Their name is today, and we must mobilize the necessary resources to ensure their access to investigational and state of the art medical care. It is just as important that their encounter with the health care system occur in an environment of compassion, hope, and kindness. Any less of a response is an abdication of our trust to nurture and care for our children.

REFERENCES

1. Gwinn M, Pappaionaou M, George JR et al. Prevalence of HIV infection in childbearing women in the United States: surveillance using newborn blood samples. *JAMA* 1991;265:1704–8.
2. Novick LF, Berns D, Strickoff R, Stevens R. HIV seroprevalence in newborn infants in New York State. 4th International Conference on AIDS, Stockholm, Sweden, 1987; 7221 (abst).
3. Oleske J. Natural history of HIV infection. In: *Report of the Surgeon General's workshop on children with HIV infection and their families.* Washington, DC: DHHS; 1987;24–5; DHHS publication no (HRS)-D-MC-87-1.
4. Lewis SH, Reynolds-Kohler C, Fox HE, Nelson JA. HIV-1 in trophoblastic and villous Hofbauer cells, and haematological precursors in eight-week fetuses. *Lancet* 1990;1:565–8.
5. Falloon J, Eddy J, Wiener L, Pizzo P. Human immunodeficiency virus in children. *J Pediatr* 1989;114:1–30.
6. Lyman WD, Kress Y, Rashbaum WK, et al. An AIDS virus-associated antigen localized in human fetal brain. *Adv Neuroimmunol* 1988;540:628–9.
7. Maury W, Potts BJ, Rabson AB. HIV-1 infection of first trimester and term human placental tissue: a possible mode of maternal-fetal transmission. *J Infect Dis* 1989;160:583–8.
8. Calvelli TA, Dubrovsky L, Freyman B, Lyman W, Soeiro R, Rubinstein A. IgA and IgM in amniotic fluid of HIV-positive women: anti-HIV reactivity and association with immune complexes. 7th International Conference on AIDS, Florence, Italy, 1991.

9. Pyun KH, Ochs HD, Dufford M, Wedgwood RJ. Perinatal infection with human immunodeficiency virus: specific antibody responses by the neonate. *N Engl J Med* 1987;317:611–4.
10. European Collaborative Study. Mother-to-child transmission of HIV infection. *Lancet* 1988;2:1039–42.
11. Italian Multicentre Study. Epidemiology, clinical features, and prognostic factors of paediatric HIV infection. *Lancet* 1988;2:1043–5.
12. Blanche S, Rouzioux C, Moscato M-LG, et al. A prospective study of infants born to women seropositive for human immunodeficiency virus type 1. *N Engl J Med* 1989;320:1643–8.
13. Ryder RW, Nsa E, Hassig SE, et al. Perinatal transmission of the human immunodeficiency virus type 1 to infants of seropositive women in Zaire. *N Engl J Med* 1989;320:1637–42.
14. Goedert JJ, Mendez H, Willoughby A, Landesman SH. High perinatal HIV rates with prematurity or low anti-gp120. 5th International Conference on AIDS, Montreal, Canada, 1989; ThAO6 (abst).
15. Goedert JJ, Mendez H, Drummond JE, et al. Mother-to-infant transmission of human immunodeficiency virus type 1: association with prematurity or low anti-gp 120. *Lancet* 1989;2:1351–4.
16. Devash Y, Calvelli TA, Wood DG, Reagan KJ, Rubinstein A. Vertical transmission of human immunodeficiency virus is correlated with the absence of high-affinity/avidity maternal antibodies to the gp120 principal neutralizing domain. *Proc Natl Acad Sci USA* 1990;87:3445–9.
17. Broliden PA, Moschese V, Ljunggren K, et al. Diagnostic implications of specific immunoglobulin G patterns of children born to HIV-infected mothers. *AIDS* 1989;9:577–82.
18. Mok JYQ, Hague RA, Yap PL, et al. Vertical transmission of HIV: a prospective study. *Arch Dis Child* 1989;64:1140–5.
19. Calvelli TA, Rubinstein A. Pediatric HIV infection: a review. *Immunodeficiency Rev* 1990;2:83–127.
20. Ziegler JB, Cooper DA, Johnson RO, Gold J. Post-natal transmission of AIDS-associated retrovirus from mother to infant. *Lancet* 1985;1:896–8.
21. Oxtoby MJ. Human immunodeficiency virus and other viruses in human milk: placing the issues in broader perspective. *Pediatr Infect Dis J* 1988;7:825–35.
22. Oleske JM. Human immunodeficiency virus testing of sexually abused children and their assistants. *Pediatr Infect Dis J* 1990;9:67.
23. Chadwick EG, Yogev R, Kwok S, Sninsky JJ, Kellogg KE, Wolinsky SM. Enzymatic amplification of the human immunodeficiency virus in peripheral blood mononuclear cells from pediatric patients. *J Infect Dis* 1989;160:954–9.
24. Krivine A, Yakudima A, Le May M, Pena-Cruz V, Huang AS, McIntoch K. A comparative study of virus isolation, polymerase chain reaction, and antigen detection in children of mothers infected with human immunodeficiency virus. *J Pediatr* 1990;116:372–6.
25. Borkowsky S, Krasinski K, Paul D, et al. Human immunodeficiency virus type 1 antigenemia in children. *J Pediatr* 1989;114:940–5.
26. Johnson JP, Nair P, Hines SE, et al. Natural history and serologic diagnosis of infants born to human immunodeficiency virus-infected women. *Am J Dis Child* 1989;143:1147–53.
27. Weiblen B, McIntosh K, Pelton S, Landesman S, Nahamias A, Hoff R. Detection of IgA HIV antibodies for diagnosis of HIV-infected infants. 6th International Conference on AIDS, San Francisco, June, 1990; SB206 (abst).
28. Amadori A, de Rossi A, Giaquinto C, Faulkner-Valle G, Zacchello F, Chieco-Bianchi L. In vitro production of HIV-specific antibody in children at risk of AIDS. *Lancet* 1988;1:852–4.
29. Pahwa S, Chirumale N, Leombruno C, et al. In vitro synthesis of human immunodeficiency virus-specific antibodies in peripheral blood lymphocytes of infants. *Proc Natl Acad Sci USA* 1989;86:7532–6.
30. Amadori A, deRossi A, Chieco-Bianchi L, Giaquinto C, de Maria A, Ades AE. Diagnosis of human immunodeficiency virus 1 infection in infants: in vitro production of virus-specific antibody in lymphocytes. *Pediatr Infect Dis J* 1990;9:26–30.
31. CDC. Classification system for human immunodeficiency virus (HIV) infection in children under 13 years of age. *MMWR* 1987;36:1–6.
32. Denny TN, Niven P, Skuza C, et al. Age-related changes of lymphocyte phenotypes in healthy children. *Pediatr Res* 1990;27:155A (abst).
33. Joshi V, Kaufman S, Olesde J, et al. Polyclonal polymorphic B-cell lymphoproliferative disorder with prominent involvement in children with AIDS. *Cancer* 1987;59:1455–62.
34. Wiznia A, Rubinstein A. Acquired immunodeficiency syndrome in infants and children. *Ann Nestle* 1988;46:154–75.
35. Ellaurie M, Burns ER, Bernstein LJ, Shah K, Rubinstein A. Thrombocytopenia and human immunodeficiency virus in childhood. *Pediatrics* 1988;82:905–8.
36. Jura E, Chadwick EG, Josephs SH, et al. Varicella-zoster virus infections in children infected with human immunodeficiency virus. *Pediatr Infect Dis J* 1989;8:586–90.
37. CDC. Measles in HIV infected children. *MMWR* 1988;37:183–6.
38. Rubinstein A, Morecki R, Silverman B, et al. Pulmonary disease in children with acquired immune deficiency syndrome and AIDS-related complex. *J Pediatr* 1986;108:498–503.
39. Scott GB, Hutto C, Makuch RW, et al. Survival in children with perinatally acquired HIV-1 infection. *N Engl J Med* 1990;321:1791–6.
40. Hoyt L, Conner E, Oleske J. Atypical mycobacterial infection (AM) in pediatric AIDS. 6th Annual National Pediatric AIDS Conference, Washington, 1991, session 09;13 (abst).
41. Bernstein LJ, Ochs HD, Wedgwood RJ, Rubinstein A. Defective humoral immunity in pediatric acquired immunodeficiency syndrome. *J Pediatr* 1985;107:352–7.
42. Pahwa S, Fikrig S, Menez R, Pahwa R. Pediatric acquired immunodeficiency syndrome: demonstration of B lymphocyte defects in vitro. *Diagn Immunol* 1986;4:24–30.
43. Borkowsky W, Steele CJ, Grubman S, Moore T, LaRussa P, Krasinski K. Antibody responses to bacterial toxoids in children infected with human immunodeficiency virus. *J Pediatr* 1987;110:563–6.
44. CDC. Revision of the CDC surveillance case definition for acquired immunodeficiency syndrome. *MMWR* 1987;36:1S.
45. Bernstein LJ, Krieger BZ, Novick B, Sicklick MJ, Rubinstein A. Bacterial infection in the acquired immunodeficiency syndrome of children. *Pediatr Infect Dis* 1985;4:472–5.
46. Krasinski K, Borkowsky W, Bonk S, Lawrence R, Chadwani S. Bacterial infections in human immunodeficiency virus infected children. *Pediatr Infect Dis J* 1988;7:323–8.
47. Joshi V, Oleske J, Minnefor AB, et al. Pathologic pulmonary findings in children with acquired immune deficiency syndrome: a study of ten cases. *Hum Pathol* 1985;16:241–6.
48. Chayt K, Harper M, Lewis E, et al. Detection of HTLV-III RNA in lungs of patients with the acquired immune deficiency syndrome and pulmonary involvement. *JAMA* 1986;256:2356–9.
49. Rubinstein A, Bernstein LJ, Charytan M, Krieger BZ, Ziprokowski M. Corticosteroid treatment for pulmonary lymphoid hyperplasia in children with the acquired immune deficiency syndrome. *Pediatri Pulmonol* 1988;4:13–7.
50. Epstein LG, Sharer LR, Oleske JM, et al. Neurologic manifestations of human immunodeficiency virus infection in children. *Pediatrics* 1986;78:678–87.
51. Belman AL, Diamond G, Dickson D, et al. Pediatric acquired immunodeficiency syndrome: neurologic syndromes. *Am J Dis Child* 1988;149:29–35.
52. Blanche S, Tardieu M, Duliege AM, et al. Longitudinal study of 94 symptomatic infants with perinatally acquired human immunodeficiency virus infection: evidence for a bimodal expression of clinical and biological symptoms. *Am J Dis Child* 1990;144:1210–5.
53. Epstein L, DiCarlo F, Joshi V, et al. Primary lymphoma of the central nervous system in children with acquired immunodeficiency syndrome. *Pediatrics* 1988;82:355–63.
54. Pizzo PA, Eddy J, Falloon J, et al. Effect of continuous infusion of zidovudine (AZT) in children with symptomatic HIV infection. *N Engl J Med* 1988;319:889–96.
55. Oxtoby MJ. Perinatally acquired human immunodeficiency virus infection. *Pediatr Infect Dis J* 1990;9:609–19.
56. Auger I, Thomas P, De Gruttola V, et al. Incubation periods for paediatric AIDS patients. *Nature* 1988;336:575–7.
57. Connor E, Bagarazzi M, McSherry G, et al. Clinical and laboratory correlates of *Pneumocystis carinii* pneumonia in children infected with HIV. *JAMA* 1991;265:1693–7.
58. Krasinski K, Borkowsky W, Holzman RS. Prognosis of human

immunodeficiency virus infection in children and adolescents. *Pediatr Infect Dis J* 1989;8:216–20.

59. CDC. Guidelines for prophylaxis against *Pneumocystis carinii* pneumonia for children infected with human immunodeficiency virus. *MMWR* 1991;40:RR-2.

60. Kovacs A, Frederick T, Church J, Eller A, Oxtoby M, Mascola L. CD4 T-lymphocyte counts and *Pneumocystis carinii* pneumonia in pediatric HIV infection. *JAMA* 1991;265:1698–703.

61. McKinney RE, Maha MA, Connor EM. A multicenter trial of oral zidovudine in children with advanced human immunodeficiency virus disease. *N Engl J Med* 1991;324:1018–25.

62. Brouwers P, Moss H, Wolters P, et al. Effect of continuous-infusion zidovudine therapy on neuropsychologic functioning in children with symptomatic human immunodeficiency virus infection. *J Pediatr* 1990;117:980–5.

63. McKinney RE, Pizzo PA, Scott GB, et al. Safety and tolerance of intermittent intravenous and oral zidovudine therapy in human immunodeficiency virus-infected pediatric patients. *J Pediatr* 1990;116:640–7.

64. Butler KM, Husson RN, Balis FM, et al. Dideoxyinosine in children with symptomatic human immunodeficiency virus infection. *N Engl J Med* 1991;324:137–44.

65. Pizzo PA, Butler K, Balis F, et al. Dideoxycytidine alone and in alternating schedule with zidovudine in children with symptomatic human immunodeficiency virus infection. *J Pediatr* 1990;117:799–808.

66. Oleske JM, Connor EM, Bobila R, et al. The use of IVIG in children with AIDS. In: Perrel BA, Baumgartra C, eds. *Workshop in immunoglobulin therapy of lymphoproliferative syndromes, mainly AIDS-related complex, and AIDS. VOX Sang* 1987;52:11.

67. Calvelli T, Rubinstein A. Intravenous gamma-globulin in infant acquired immunodeficiency syndrome. *Pediatr Infect Dis* 1986;5:S207–10.

68. Hague RA, Yap PL, Mok JYQ, et al. Intravenous immunoglobulin in HIV infection: evidence for the efficacy of treatment. *Arch Dis Child* 1989;64:1146–50.

69. Czarniecki L, Oleske J. Pain in children with HIV infection. *Journal Pain Symptom Management* 1991;6:177(abst).

70. Boyd-Franklin N, Aleman J. Black, inner-city families and multigenerational issues: the impact of AIDS. *Psychologist* 1990;40:14–7.

71. Boland MG, Mahan-Rudolph P, Evans P. Special issues in the care of the child with HIV infection/AIDS. In: Martin B, ed. *Pediatric hospice care: what helps.* Los Angeles: Los Angeles Children's Hospital, 1989;116–44.

72. Jessop DJ, Stein REK. Meeting the needs of individuals and families. In: Stein R, ed. *Caring for children with chronic illness.* New York: Springer, 1989;63–74.

AIDS and Other Manifestations of HIV Infection,
Second Edition, Edited by Gary P. Wormser.
Published by Raven Press, Ltd., New York 1992.

CHAPTER 15

AIDS-Related Complex and Persistent Generalized Lymphadenopathy Syndrome

Thomas R. O'Brien and Scott D. Holmberg

Infection with human immunodeficiency virus (HIV) results in an evolving clinical picture ranging from asymptomatic infection to the acquired immunodeficiency syndrome (AIDS). In this chapter we discuss some aspects of the early manifestations of HIV infection. We trace the origin, changing definitions, and limitations of the terms AIDS-related complex (ARC) and persistent generalized lymphadenopathy (PGL), and describe inclusive systems for classifying HIV infection. We then summarize current knowledge regarding the prognosis, evaluation, and treatment of persons with early symptoms of HIV infection.

HISTORY OF THE TERMS AIDS, ARC, AND PGL

The AIDS epidemic manifested as a major public health problem in the United States several years before the discovery of its etiologic agent, HIV-1. As a result, some terms used to describe manifestations of HIV infection, including AIDS, ARC, and PGL, were coined without full knowledge of the spectrum of HIV infection. As understanding of HIV infection has evolved over time, so have some of the definitions.

AIDS

The definition of AIDS has broadened over time to encompass conditions that were previously included in some definitions of ARC. Because definitions of ARC always exclude AIDS conditions, an understanding of

T. R. O'Brien and S. D. Holmberg: Division of HIV/AIDS, National Center for Infectious Diseases, Centers for Disease Control, Public Health Service, U.S. Department of Health and Human Services, Atlanta, Georgia 30333.

these changes is necessary to understand the evolution of the term ARC.

In 1981, the HIV epidemic was heralded by reports of *Pneumocystis carinii* pneumonia (PCP) among homosexual men with marked abnormalities of their cellular immune systems (1). The following year, the Centers for Disease Control (CDC) developed a formal AIDS case definition that included about a dozen opportunistic infections and Kaposi's sarcoma (KS) (Table 1). The purpose of the definition was to standardize epidemiologic surveillance of the AIDS epidemic geographically and over time (2).

Epidemiologic surveillance definitions often represent a compromise between conflicting desires for high predictive value, sensitivity, and specificity, as well as simplicity and completeness (3). As a result, surveillance definitions may not capture all cases of the disease under surveillance. To make the positive predictive value of the AIDS definition high, CDC epidemiologists excluded from the definition infections that occurred frequently in persons without impaired cellular immunodeficiency, such as pyogenic bacterial infections. To maintain a high level of completeness of reporting, the indicator diseases were limited to serious conditions that usually required hospitalization. Less serious conditions, such as oral candidiasis, were not included in the AIDS definition, even though such conditions might indicate impaired cellular immunity.

When the AIDS surveillance definition was originated in 1982, CDC epidemiologists recognized that the definition probably would not include all persons infected with (or exposed to) the then unknown etiologic agent of AIDS (2). With the advent of serologic tests for HIV-1 infection and a better understanding of the spectrum of HIV disease, CDC twice expanded the AIDS surveillance definition to include additional serious illnesses in

TABLE 1. *The 1982 CDC AIDS case surveillance definition*

A disease, at least moderately predictive of a defect in cell-mediated immunity, occurring in a person with no known cause for diminished resistance to that disease. Such diseases include Kaposi's sarcoma, *Pneumocystis carinii* pneumonia, and other serious opportunistic infections. These infections include pneumonia, meningitis, or encephalitis due to one or more of the following: aspergillosis, candidiasis, cryptococcosis, cytomegalovirus, nocardiosis, strongyloidosis, toxoplasmosis, zygomycosis, or atypical mycobacteriosis (species other than tuberculosis or lepra); esophagitis due to candidiasis, cytomegalovirus, or herpes simplex virus; progressive multifocal leukoencephalopathy; chronic enterocolitis (more than 4 weeks) due to cryptosporidiosis; or unusually extensive mucocutaneous herpes simplex of more than 5 weeks duration.

From CDC, ref. 2.

HIV antibody test-positive persons. In 1985, CDC added disseminated histoplasmosis, isosporiasis, bronchial or pulmonary candidiasis, and certain types of non-Hodgkin's lymphomas to the case definition (4). In late 1987, the definition of AIDS underwent a major expansion to include HIV encephalopathy, HIV wasting syndrome, extrapulmonary tuberculosis, and some other conditions in persons with a positive HIV antibody test (Table 2) (5).

Persistent Generalized Lymphadenopathy (PGL)

In 1982, even before AIDS was formally defined, clinicians reported cases of unexplained lymphadenopathy among homosexual men with evidence of cellular immune system abnormalities (6). The epidemiologic and clinical similarities between these persons with lymph-

TABLE 2. *Conditions included in the 1987 CDC AIDS case surveillance definition*

Candidiasis of bronchi, trachea, or lungs
Candidiasis, esophageal
Coccidioidomycosis, disseminated or extrapulmonary
Cryptococcosis, extrapulmonary
Cryptosporidiosis, chronic intestinal (>1 month duration)
Cytomegalovirus disease (other than liver, spleen, or nodes)
Cytomegalovirus retinitis (with loss of vision)
HIV encephalopathy
Herpes simplex: chronic ulcer(s) (>1 month duration); or bronchitis, pneumonitis, or esophagitis
Histoplasmosis, disseminated or extrapulmonary
Isosporiasis, chronic intestinal (>1 month duration)
Kaposi's sarcoma
Lymphoma, Burkitt's (or equivalent term)
Lymphoma, immunoblastic (or equivalent term)
Lymphoma, primary in brain
Mycobacterium avium complex or *M. kansasii,* disseminated or extrapulmonary
Mycobacterium tuberculosis, disseminated or extrapulmonary
Mycobacterium, other species or unidentified species, disseminated or extrapulmonary
Pneumocystis carinii pneumonia
Progressive multifocal leukoencephalopathy
Salmonella septicemia, recurrent
Toxoplasmosis of brain
Wasting syndrome due to HIV

From CDC, ref. 5.

adenopathy and persons with opportunistic infections led to speculation that these cases might be etiologically related. PGL, also referred to as lymphadenopathy syndrome or generalized lymphadenopathy syndrome, has been a term used to describe persons with lymphadenopathy of at least 3 months' duration that involves two or more extrainguinal sites for which no other explanation is apparent. The definition of PGL has generally remained unchanged from its original usage.

AIDS-Related Complex

In 1983, the NCI/NIAID Extramural AIDS Working Group first defined the term ARC to describe persons whose clinical condition did not meet the AIDS surveillance definition, but who exhibited at least two clinical and two laboratory abnormalities that appeared to be related to AIDS (R. Selik, personal communication, and ref. 7). The term was created to improve communication between researchers and to encourage uniformity in epidemiologic and clinical studies. PGL was included as a clinical manifestation of ARC, as was fever, weight loss, diarrhea, fatigue, and night sweats.

The isolation of HIV-1 and subsequent development of serologic tests for detection of antibody to that virus led to confirmation that PGL, ARC, AIDS, and some other clinical conditions were all manifestations of HIV infection (8). The original meaning of ARC was soon supplanted by a variety of definitions. A 1986 definition included oral candidiasis, hairy leukoplakia, herpes zoster, sinusitis, several dermatologic conditions, and certain constitutional symptoms among the ARC-defining clinical conditions (9). The San Francisco City Clinic Cohort Study investigators have used a definition of ARC that is limited to oral candidiasis, hairy leukoplakia, and specific constitutional symptoms (10). Moreover, the term ARC is used by some persons to indicate any symptomatic manifestation of HIV other than AIDS (11), a definition that is complicated by the changing definition of AIDS over time. Therefore, although still in use, the term ARC has varied over time and lacks specificity. In 1988, the Institute of Medicine's Committee for Oversight of AIDS Activities suggested that the term ARC was no longer useful and should be discarded (12). We discourage further use of the term and believe that

TABLE 3. *The 1986 CDC classification system for human immunodeficiency virus infection*

Group	Condition
I	Acute infection
II	Asymptomatic infection[a]
III	Persistent generalized lymphadenopathy[a]
IV	Other diseases
A	Constitutional disease
B	Neurologic disease
C	Secondary infectious disease
C-1	Specified secondary infectious diseases listed in the CDC surveillance definition for AIDS[b]
C-2	Other specified secondary infectious diseases
D	Secondary cancers[b]
E	Other conditions

From CDC, ref. 14.

[a] Patients in groups II and III may be subclassified on the basis of a laboratory evaluation.

[b] Includes those patients whose clinical presentation fulfills the definition of AIDS used by CDC for national reporting.

those who do use it should explicitly state their definition.

In this chapter we minimize use of the term ARC and, instead, whenever possible, discuss specific conditions that have been included in the ARC definition. The most common such conditions are oral candidiasis, oral hairy leukoplakia, herpes zoster, and constitutional symptoms that do not fulfill the criteria for the HIV-wasting syndrome.

HIV CLASSIFICATION SYSTEMS

Acute HIV infection can be accompanied by a mononucleosis-like syndrome with onset 1–8 weeks after initial infection (13). Chronic HIV infection results in an evolving clinical spectrum that ranges from asymptomatic infection to life-threatening opportunistic infections and cancers. The stage of HIV infection is also measured by the number of T-helper (CD4+) lymphocytes in the blood and other markers of immunological competence. Several systems for classifying HIV-infected adults are in use.

Under the 1986 CDC HIV classification system, HIV-infected persons were divided into four mutually exclusive groups based solely on clinical symptoms (14) (Table 3). The scheme was not meant to be a staging system (i.e., groups and subgroups were not meant to have explicit prognostic significance). Group I included persons with signs and symptoms of acute HIV infection, as confirmed by laboratory studies. Group II consisted of patients with no signs or symptoms of HIV infection. Group III included persons with PGL, but no findings that would place them in group IV. Group IV included all infected persons with signs and symptoms of HIV infection other than PGL. All persons who met the CDC AIDS surveillance definition were included in group IV; however, not all persons in group IV had AIDS.

CDC has recently proposed a classification system for HIV infection that is simpler and more prognostically oriented (15). The revised system consists of a matrix of mutually exclusive categories hierarchically arrayed along two axes: one axis has categories (A–C) of clinical conditions attributable to HIV infection and the other axis has categories of CD4+ lymphocyte measurements (Table 4).

Clinical category A includes acute HIV infection, asymptomatic HIV infection, and PGL. Included in category B are persons with symptomatic conditions that are attributed to or complicated by HIV infection, and that are *not* included in the 1987 AIDS surveillance case definition. Examples of clinical conditions in category B include bacterial pneumonia, oral candidiasis, oral hairy leukoplakia, and herpes zoster. Category C consists of any condition meeting the 1987 AIDS surveillance case definition (Table 2). HIV-infected persons are classified on the basis of the most severe clinical condition ever diagnosed and the lowest available CD4+ lymphocyte count. The CD4+ percent of total lymphocytes is the basis for laboratory categorization if the absolute count is unavailable.

The Walter Reed Classification staging system (Table 5) (16) employs clinical and laboratory measures of immune system deficiency to classify HIV-infected persons into one of six stages. The laboratory measures are skin testing for delayed hypersensitivity to four antigens and measurement of T-helper lymphocytes. Stage WR1 includes persons with acute HIV infection and HIV-

TABLE 4. *The proposed CDC HIV classification system for adolescents and adults*

	Clinical category		
CD4+ cell category	Asymptomatic (A)	Symptomatic, not AIDS (B)	AIDS (C)
0: Unavailable	A0	B0	C0
1: ≥500/mm³	A1	B1	C1
2: 200–499/mm³	A2	B2	C2
3: <200/mm³, or ≤10%	A3	B3	C3

From Mills, ref. 15.

TABLE 5. *The Walter Reed staging classification system for human immunodeficiency virus infection*

Stage	HIV antibody and/or virus	Chronic lymphadenopathy	T-helper cells/mm³	Delayed hypersensitivity	Thrush	Opportunistic infections
WR1	+	−	>400	Normal	−	−
WR2	+	+	>400	Normal	−	−
WR3	+	±	<400	Normal	−	−
WR4	+	±	<400	Partial energy	−	−
WR5	+	±	<400	Complete energy and/or thrush		−
WR6	+	±	<400	Partial or complete energy	±	+

Additional designations:
  B, fever (3 weeks), weight loss (10% of body weight over 3 months), night sweats (3 weeks), or diarrhea (1 month)
  K, Kaposi's sarcoma
  CNS, demyelinating disease, encephalopathy, or neuropathy
  N, neoplasms other than Kaposi's sarcoma

From Redfield et al., ref. 16, with permission.

infected persons without any clinical or laboratory manifestations of immune deficiency. WR2 includes persons with PGL, but no other manifestation of HIV infection. To be classified in stages WR3 or higher requires a T-helper count of 400 cells/mm³ or less. WR4 requires partial anergy on skin testing and WR5 requires complete anergy or the diagnosis of thrush. Persons with opportunistic infections are classified in category WR6. Other manifestations of HIV infection are designated with additional letters.

The World Health Organization has recently proposed "an interim staging system" for HIV infection that is primarily based on clinical markers and a performance scale (17). People are classified into four stages that range from asymptomatic/PGL (stage 1) to persons who have CDC-defined AIDS or who are bedridden for greater than 50% of the day (stage 4). In addition to the "clinical axis," a "laboratory axis" will further subdivide patients on the basis of the number of CD4+ lymphocytes per mm³ or absolute lymphocyte count.

EARLY MANIFESTATIONS OF HIV INFECTION AND DISEASE PROGRESSION

Lymphadenopathy develops soon after infection in many persons who have an acute HIV illness (13,18) and may be found at some time in a sizable percentage of all HIV-infected persons (19). In at least some studies, HIV-infected persons with generalized lymphadenopathy had no greater likelihood of developing AIDS than HIV-infected people without any signs or symptoms. In one prospective study of 75 homosexual men, the 5-year cumulative incidence of AIDS after onset of PGL was 29% (20), with an increased risk of developing AIDS after the third year of lymphadenopathy (21). Thus, lymphadenopathy in itself is not a reliable prognostic indicator for the development of AIDS. For this reason, persons with generalized lymphadenopathy and no other sign or symptom are often categorized as "asymptomatic" (15).

The resolution of PGL was found to be an ominous prognostic sign by some investigators (22), but not by others (23).

Because there are, as yet, no data on the incubation period from infection to onset of "ARC" conditions, that period may best be estimated indirectly, by considering the incubation period to AIDS and the time required to develop AIDS after the onset of these conditions. For some HIV-infected persons, however, an AIDS-defining illness will be the initial manifestation of HIV infection.

Studies of the natural history of HIV-1 infection have shown a variable incubation period from time of infection to the development of AIDS, with a median incubation period of 7–10 years (10,24). These studies have also demonstrated that the AIDS hazard (i.e., the risk of developing AIDS within a given time interval) is nonconstant, low during the early years of infection and increasing greatly thereafter (10). It is likely that the hazard for other HIV-associated conditions also follows a similar pattern, which may, in conjunction with the wide range of definitions of ARC by various investigators, explain the different rates of development of ARC observed among various HIV-seroprevalent cohorts.

In contrast to the limited prognostic value of PGL, data suggest that many "ARC" conditions are prognostic indicators of more severe HIV-related disease. Studies have shown that HIV-infected persons with oral candidiasis (thrush) are at increased risk of developing AIDS (25,26). Oral hairy leukoplakia (27), and herpes zoster (shingles) should also be considered poor prognostic indicators (20,28). After 6–40 months of observation of a group of heterosexual HIV-infected persons in Lusaka, Zambia, 62/212 (29.7%) of herpes zoster patients had progressed to AIDS, compared with 19/200 (9.5%) of persons with PGL (29). In a cohort of homosexual men, constitutional symptoms (i.e., fever, night sweats, or weight loss) presaged progression to AIDS (30), and these nonspecific symptoms were more powerful predictors of AIDS outcome than thrush, hairy leukoplakia, or shingles. In 49 intravenous drug users in Bologne, Italy, "ARC" (defined as CDC group IVA or IVC2) symptoms preceded the development of AIDS in 24 (49%) of them within 3 years (31).

The CD4+ lymphocyte count appears to be the strongest prognostic indicator for the development of AIDS (32,33). Constitutional symptoms—such as fever, weight loss, and diarrhea—and low T-helper cell count are substantially better predictors of the development of AIDS than is PGL. In one study of 18 men with ARC and a low CD4+ cell count, 9 (50%) developed AIDS, compared with only 5 (9%) of 57 patients without these clinical or laboratory parameters ($p < 0.001$) (21). Again, this risk was determined more by low CD4+ cell count than by the presence of enlarged lymph nodes at two or more extrainguinal sites; the 4-year cumulative incidence of AIDS was inversely related to observed CD4+ cell counts (21). Yet another study of 81 HIV-infected men with generalized lymphadenopathy showed that 77% of those with oral candidiasis (thrush) or constitutional symptoms and 80–88% of those with immunodeficiency as assessed by various indices, including <200 CD4+ cells/mm^3, developed AIDS (34).

Given that low or declining CD4+ cell counts best predict the development of AIDS, it would be useful if symptoms or signs could be correlated with CD4+ count. A recent study indicates that, excluding AIDS-defining conditions, the symptoms most significantly associated with a CD4+ cell count $< 200/mm^3$ were seborrheic dermatitis, oral candidiasis, hairy leukoplakia, unexplained weight loss (≥ 10 pounds/1 month), and diarrhea (≥ 1 month) (35).

PATHOLOGY AND PATHOGENESIS

Although manifestations of HIV infection such as thrush and shingles are well-known results of immunosuppression, the etiology of some other HIV-associated conditions is less obvious. Oral hairy leukoplakia, a lesion first described in HIV-infected men, is reviewed in detail by Greenspan and Greenspan (this volume). This condition appears to be associated with specific viral infections (36,37). Greenspan et al. (36) have demonstrated replication of Epstein-Barr virus within oral hairy leukoplakia tissue (36).

Recent research suggests that some cases of diarrhea in HIV-infected persons may result from direct effects of HIV. In situ DNA hybridization of intestinal biopsy specimens from AIDS patients has shown the presence of HIV in epithelial cells, suggesting that HIV directly causes some of the gastrointestinal disorders (38). Maturational defects in enterocytes (39) and detection of HIV-1 RNA in the lamina propria of HIV-infected persons (40) further suggest direct effects of HIV in persons with HIV-associated enteropathy. One group of researchers has demonstrated that tissue content of HIV (by p24 antigen quantitative assay) and interleukin-1 content correlate with diarrhea in HIV-infected patients (41). In a simian model that used eight monkeys, simian immunodeficiency virus (SIV) RNA was found in jejunal tissues of four monkeys with and two without malabsorptive diarrhea (42). Again, the pathogenic mechanism in this model may also involve direct SIV infection of enterocytes.

The reason that HIV-infected persons develop PGL is unclear. HIV is present in enlarged lymph nodes of infected persons and, in fact, lymph nodes were the tissue source for the first reported isolation of the virus. Lymph nodes from patients with PGL most commonly have reactive changes consistent with follicular hyperplasia (43,44), a pattern that is not specific for HIV infection. As HIV infection progresses, the enlarged lymph nodes may have fewer follicles and a depletion of lymphocytes (45). Enlarged lymph nodes in HIV-infected persons may, less commonly, be due to Kaposi's sarcoma, lymphoma, or opportunistic infections (46).

ISSUES IN CLINICAL EVALUATION AND MANAGEMENT

In addition to measurement of the CD4+ lymphocyte count and other relevant laboratory parameters, evaluation of the HIV-infected patient should be directed toward detecting unrecognized HIV-associated conditions (47). The rationale behind this is both prognostic and therapeutic. Some conditions, such as oral thrush or hairy leukoplakia, are poor prognostic signs; constitutional symptoms—weight loss, diarrhea, persistent fever —are also predictive of a rapid progression to AIDS. Yet other signs, such as generalized lymphadenopathy, are not associated with rapid development of opportunistic infections. In addition to counseling the patient as to what he or she may expect, the expanding indications for therapies earlier in HIV-associated disease necessitate good clinical evaluation.

Therapies for persons with early manifestations of HIV infection have concentrated on prophylaxis to prevent the development of opportunistic infections. Thus, zidovudine and other antiviral agents have been investigated more thoroughly than have therapies for the specific constitutional signs and symptoms, e.g. diarrhea.

A 1987 double-blinded, placebo-controlled study indicated that zidovudine (AZT) use delayed death and opportunistic infections over 24 weeks of observation in 122 men with ARC (defined as weight loss or thrush, plus one of the following: fever, PGL, oral hairy leukoplakia, night sweats, shingles, diarrhea) (48). A controlled trial with longer (median, 11 months) follow-up also showed the utility of AZT therapy in those with early HIV-associated symptoms (49); 36/351 in the placebo group had disease progression, compared with 15/360 in the AZT-treated group. A 1990 study has also shown that AZT therapy is beneficial to asymptomatic persons with less than 500 CD4+ lymphocytes/mm^3 (50). While there is substantial evidence that AZT therapy delays disease progression, studies with longer follow-up suggest that a substantial proportion of persons with symptomatic HIV infection will develop AIDS or die within 2 years of starting AZT therapy. In a study of 80 ARC patients who received AZT (1,200 mg or 600 mg/day) for an average of 102 weeks of follow-up (51), 26 (33%) died (mean, 66 weeks) and 26 developed AIDS (mean, 45 weeks) after starting the drug. Likewise, in a study of 301 AZT-treated men with ARC (undefined), 69 (23%) developed an AIDS-defining condition during a 15-month period (52). In sum, AZT therapy in persons with early manifestations of HIV infection delays onset of AIDS, but that delay may be of relatively short duration.

Antiretroviral therapies other than AZT are generally of unproven benefit in preventing HIV disease progression. Isoprinosine (inosine pranobex) reduced the likelihood of the development of AIDS in Scandinavian patients with CDC group II or III HIV infection, but not in 98 persons who had CDC group IV disease that did not meet the AIDS definition (53).

Various other antiretroviral therapies appear to be well tolerated when given to persons in initial, phase I studies. These include ribavirin (54), dideoxyinosine (ddI) (55), ampligen (56), and soluble recombinant human CD4 immunoglobulin (57,58). Some controversial therapies—such as dextran sulfate (59)—have also been given with apparent safety to patients with early manifestations of HIV infection. Studies of combinations of antiviral medications, such as the combination of AZT with acyclovir are also in progress (60,61). However, beyond their safety, the efficacies of these therapies in preventing AIDS in patients who already have symptoms of HIV infection are not clear.

One important issue that has received recent attention is the psychological well-being of persons who are symptomatic, but have not yet developed AIDS; many suffer from severe stress or psychiatric illness. Men with early manifestations of HIV infection appear to experience high levels of psychological stress, as well as suicidal ideation, delirium, dementia, and major affect or adjustment disorder (62–64). Thus, good clinical management of HIV-infected patients should extend beyond antiretroviral therapies and prophylaxis for opportunistic infections to the psychological well-being of the patient.

CONCLUSIONS

Infection with HIV can result in a wide range of disease. Our understanding of this spectrum is incomplete despite 10 years of clinical observation of HIV-infected patients. PGL describes HIV-infected persons with otherwise unexplained lymphadenopathy of at least 3 months' duration that involves two or more sites. The term ARC has several definitions and is sometimes used to describe any symptomatic manifestation of HIV infection that does not meet the CDC surveillance definition of AIDS. HIV-associated conditions included in many definitions of ARC are oral hairy leukoplakia, herpes zoster, oral candidiasis, and constitutional symptoms that do not fulfill the criteria for the HIV-wasting syndrome. Because ARC lacks a specific definition, the term is probably no longer useful. Persons with PGL do not appear to have a greater risk of developing AIDS than HIV-infected persons without any symptoms or signs. By contrast, oral hairy leukoplakia, herpes zoster, thrush, and constitutional symptoms are poor prognostic signs, often heralding development of AIDS. In the short term, AZT therapy is effective in preventing the development of AIDS in persons with these manifestations of HIV infection; the value of AZT therapy to improve long-term survival is yet to be determined.

REFERENCES

1. CDC. *Pneumocystis* pneumonia—Los Angeles. *MMWR* 1981;30:250–2.
2. CDC. Update on acquired immune deficiency syndrome (AIDS) United States. *MMWR* 1982;31:507–14.
3. Thacker SB, Berkelman RL. Public health surveillance in the United States. Epidemiol Rev 1988;164–90.
4. CDC. Revision of the case definition of acquired immunodeficiency syndrome for national reporting—United States. *MMWR* 1985;34:373–5.
5. CDC. Revision of the CDC surveillance case definition for acquired immunodeficiency syndrome. *MMWR* 1987;36[Suppl. 1S]:1S–15S.
6. CDC. Persistent generalized lymphadenopathy among homosexual males. *MMWR* 1982;31:249–52.
7. Abrams DI. Definition of ARC. In: Cohen PT, Sande MA, Volberding PA, eds. *The AIDS knowledge base—a textbook on HIV disease from the University of California, San Francisco and San Francisco General Hospital*. Waltham, MA: The Medical Publishing Group, 1990;4.1.3.
8. Groopman JE, Mayer KH, Sarnagadharan MG, et al. Seroepidemiology of human T-lymphotropic virus type III among homosexual men with the acquired immunodeficiency syndrome or generalized lymphadenopathy and among asymptomatic controls in Boston. *Ann Intern Med* 1985;102:334–7.
9. Nunes B, Frutchey C. *Coping with ARC*. San Francisco: San Francisco AIDS Foundation, 1986.
10. Rutherford GW, Lifson AR, Hessol NA, et al. Course of HIV-1 infection in a cohort of homosexual and bisexual men: an 11-year follow-up study. *Br Med J* 1990;301:1183–8.
11. Abrams DI. The Pre-AIDS syndromes. *Infect Dis Clin North Am* 1988;2:343–51.
12. Institute of Medicine/National Academy of Sciences. *Confronting AIDS: update 1988*. Washington, DC: National Academy Press, 1988;37.
13. Cooper DA, Gold J, Maclean P, et al. Acute AIDS retrovirus infection—definition of a clinical illness associated with seroconversion. *Lancet* 1985;1:537–40.
14. CDC. Classification system for human T-lymphotropic virus type III/lymphadenopathy-associated virus infections. *MMWR* 1986;35:334–9.

15. Mills J. Primary care for the HIV-positive patient: a manageable step-by-step strategy. *Modern Medicine* 1992;60:50–6.
16. Redfield RR, Wright DC, Tramont EC. The Walter Reed staging classification for HTLV-III/LAV Infection. *N Engl J Med* 1986;314:131–2.
17. World Health Organization. Acquired immunodeficiency syndrome. Interim proposal for a WHO staging system for HIV infection and disease. *Weekly Epidemiol Rec* 1990;65:221–8.
18. Tindall B, Barker S, Donovan B, et al. Characterizations of the acute clinical illness associated with human immunodeficiency virus infection. *Arch Intern Med* 1988;148:945–9.
19. Lang W, Anderson RE, Perkins H, et al. Clinical, immunologic, and serologic findings in men at risk for acquired immunodeficiency syndrome. *JAMA* 1987;257:326–30.
20. Kaplan JE, Spira TJ, Fishbein DB, et al. A six-year follow-up of HIV-infected homosexual men with lymphadenopathy. Evidence for an increased risk for developing AIDS after the third year of lymphadenopathy. *JAMA* 1988;260:2694–7.
21. Kaplan JE, Spira TJ, Fishbein DB, Pinsky PF, Schonberger LB. Lymphadenopathy syndrome in homosexual men. Evidence for continuing risk of developing the acquired immunodeficiency syndrome. *JAMA* 1987;257:335–7.
22. Mathur-Wagh MU, Enlow RW, Spigland I, et al. Longitudinal study of persistent generalised lymphadenopathy in homosexual men: relation to acquired immunodeficiency syndrome. *Lancet* 1984;1:1033–8.
23. El-Sadr W, Marmor M, Zoll-Pazner S, et al. Four-year prospective study of homosexual men: correlation of immunologic abnormalities, clinical status, and serology to human immunodeficiency virus. *J Infect Dis* 1987;155:789–93.
24. Ward JW, Bush TJ, Perkins HA, et al. The natural history of transfusion-associated HIV infection: factors influencing progression to disease. *N Engl J Med* 1989;321:947–52.
25. Klein RS, Harris CA, Small CB, Moll B, Lesser M, Friedland GH. Oral candidiasis in high risk patients as the initial manifestation of the acquired immunodeficiency syndrome. *N Engl J Med* 1984;311:354–8.
26. Phair J, Munoz A, Detels R, et al. The risk of *Pneumocystis carinii* pneumonia among men infected with human immunodeficiency virus type 1. *N Engl J Med* 1990;322:161–5.
27. Greenspan D, Greenspan DS, Hearst NG, et al. Relation of oral hairy leukoplakia to infection with human immunodeficiency virus and the risk of developing AIDS. *J Infect Dis* 1987;155:475–81.
28. Melbye M, Goedert JJ, Grossman JR, Eyster ME, Biggar RE. Risk of AIDS after herpes zoster. *Lancet* 1987;1:728–30.
29. Hira S, Tembo G, Wadhawan D, Kamanga J, Macuacua R, Perine P. Risk of AIDS in patients with herpes zoster, PGL or "other" features of ARC. 5th International Conference on AIDS, Montreal, Canada, June, 1989;128 (abst WAP54).
30. Moss AR, Bacchetti P, Osmond D, et al. Seropositivity for HIV and the development of AIDS or AIDS-related condition: three-year follow-up of the San Francisco General Hospital cohort. *Br Med J* 1988;296:745–50.
31. Raise E, Vannini V, Sabbatani S, et al. Progression of ARC to AIDS in a population of drug abusers and correlation with CD4 decrease and rise of HIV1 antigenemia. 5th International Conference on AIDS, Montreal, Canada, June, 1989;93 (abst MP94).
32. Fahey JL, Taylor JMG, Detels R, et al. The prognostic value of cellular and serologic markers in infection with human immunodeficiency virus type 1. *N Engl J Med* 1990;322:166–72.
33. Goedert JJ, Biggar RJ, Melbye M, et al. Effect of T4 count and cofactors on the incidence of AIDS in homosexual men infected with human immunodeficiency virus. *JAMA* 1987;257:331–4.
34. Murray HW, Godbold JH, Jurica KB, Roberts RB. Progression to AIDS in patients with lymphadenopathy or AIDS-related complex: reappraisal of risk and predictive factors. *Am J Med* 1989;86:533–8.
35. Lifson AR, Buchbinder SP, Hessol NA, Barnhart JL, Underwood R, Holmberg SD. Is clinical status a surrogate marker for low CD4 counts? In: *Program and Abstracts of the 30th Interscience Conference on Antimicrobial Agents and Chemotherapy.* Washington, DC; American Society for Microbiology, 1990:105 (abst 113).
36. Greenspan JS, Greenspan D, Lennette ET, et al. Replication of Epstein-Barr virus within the epithelial cells of oral "hairy" leuko-

plakia, an AIDS-associated lesion. *N Engl J Med* 1985;313:1564–71.
37. Greenspan D, Greenspan JS, Conant M, et al. Oral "hairy" leukoplakia in male homosexuals: evidence of association with papillomavirus and a herpes group virus. *Lancet* 1984;2:831–6.
38. Nelson JA, Wiley CA, Reynolds-Kohler C, Reese CE, Margaretten W, Levy JA. Human immunodeficiency virus detected in bowel epithelium from patients with gastrointestinal symptoms. *Lancet* 1988;1:259–62.
39. Ullrich R, Zeitz M, Heise W, L'age M, Höffken G, Rieken EO. Small intestinal structure and function in patients infected with human immunodeficiency virus (HIV): evidence for HIV-induced enteropathy. *Ann Intern Med* 1989;111:15–21.
40. Fox CH, Kotler D, Tierney A, Wilson CS, Fauci AS. Detection of HIV-1 RNA in the lamina propria of patients with AIDS and gastrointestinal disease. *J Infect Dis* 1989;159:467–71.
41. Reka S, Borcich A, Cronin W, Kotler DP. Intestinal HIV infection in AIDS and ARC: correlation with tissue content of p24 and interleukin-1 beta. 5th International Conference on AIDS, Montreal, Canada, June, 1989:514 (abst MCO27).
42. Dandekar S, Helse C, Martfeld D, et al. Pathogenesis of intestinal dysfunction in human and simian AIDS. 6th International Conference on AIDS, San Francisco, June, 1990;3:98 (abst SA11).
43. Biberfeld P, Porwit-Ksiazek A, Bottiger B, Morfeldt-Mansson L, Biberfeld G. Immunohistopathology of lymph nodes in HTLV-III infected homosexuals with persistent adenopathy or AIDS. Cancer Res 1985;45 [Suppl 9]:4665s–70s.
44. O'Murchadha MT, Wolf BC, Neiman RS. The histologic features of hyperplastic lymphadenopathy in AIDS-related complex are nonspecific. *Am J Surg Pathol* 1987;11:94–9.
45. Chadburn A, Metroka C, Mouradian J. Progressive lymph node histology and its prognostic value in patients with acquired immunodeficiency syndrome and AIDS-related complex. *Hum Pathol* 1989;20:579–87.
46. Levine AM, Meyer PR, Gill PS, et al. Results of initial lymph node biopsy in homosexual men with generalized lymphadenopathy. *J Clin Oncol* 1986;4:165–9.
47. Abrams DI. The pre-AIDS syndromes. Asymptomatic carriers, thrombocytopenic purpura, persistent generalized lymphadenopathy, and AIDS-related complex. *Infect Dis Clin North Am* 1988;2:343–51.
48. Fischl MA, Richman DD, Grieco MH, et al. The efficacy of azidothymidine (AZT) in the treatment of patients with AIDS and AIDS-related complex. A double-blind placebo-controlled trial. *N Engl J Med* 1987;317:185–91.
49. Fischl MA, Richman DD, Hansen N, et al. The safety and efficacy of zidovudine (AZT) in the treatment of subjects with mildly symptomatic human immunodeficiency virus type 1 (HIV) infection. *Ann Intern Med* 1990;112:727–37.
50. Volberding PA, Lagakos SW, Koch MA, et al. Zidovudine in asymptomatic human immunodeficiency virus infection. *N Engl J Med* 1990;322:941–9.
51. Dournon E, Matheron D, Michon C, et al. Long-term efficacy of zidovudine in ARC and AIDS patients. 6th International Conference on AIDS, San Francisco, June, 1990;3:197 (abst SB447).
52. Swanson CE, Cooper DA. Zidovudine therapy in homosexual/bisexual men with AIDS-related complex (ARC) in Australia. 5th International Conference on AIDS, Montreal, Canada, June, 1989:410 (abst WBP350).
53. Pedersen C, Sandström E, Pedersen CS, et al. The efficacy of inosine pranobex in preventing the acquired immunodeficiency syndrome in patients with human immunodeficiency virus infection. *N Engl J Med* 1990;322:1757–63.
54. Crumpacker C, Pearlstein G, van der Horst C, Valentine F, Spector S, Mills J. A phase one increasing dose trial of oral ribavirin (RBV) in patients with AIDS and ARC. 6th International Conference on AIDS, San Francisco, June, 1990;3:203 (abst SB468).
55. Connolly KJ, Allan JD, Fitch H, Jackson-Pope L, McLaren C, Groopman J. A phase 1 study of 2'-3'-dideoxyinosine (ddI) administered orally twice daily to patients with AIDS or ARC and hematologic intolerance to azidothymidine (AZT). 6th International Conference on AIDS, San Francisco, June, 1990;3:204 (abst SB473).
56. Strayer DR, Brodsky I, Pequignot E, et al. Improvement in T4 level and decrease in opportunistic infections and lymphomas (OI/

L) in ARC/pre-AIDS patients (T4 = 60–300) receiving ampligen compared to placebo. 6th International Conference on AIDS, San Francisco, June, 1990;3:205 (abst SB479).

57. Hodges TL, Kahn J, Kaplan L, et al. Phase I study of the safety and pharmacokinetics of recombinant human CD4 immunoglobulin (rCD4-IgG) administered by intramuscular (IM) injection in patients with AIDS and ARC. 6th International Conference on AIDS, San Francisco, June, 1990;3:205 (abst SB478).

58. Yarchoan R, Pluda JM, Adamo D, et al. Phase I study of rCD4-IgG administered by continuous intravenous (IV) infusion to patients with AIDS or ARC. 6th International Conference on AIDS, San Francisco, June, 1990;3:205 (abst SB479).

59. Abrams DI, Kuno S, Wong R, et al. Oral dextran sulfate (UA001) in the treatment of acquired immunodeficiency syndrome (AIDS) and AIDS-related complex. *Ann Intern Med* 1989;110:183–8.

60. Collier AC, Bozzette S, Coombs RW, et al. A pilot study of low-dose zidovudine in human immunodeficiency virus infection. *N Engl J Med* 1990;323:1015–21.

61. Surbone A, Yarchoan R, McAtee N, et al. Treatment of the acquired immunodeficiency syndrome (AIDS) and AIDS-related complex with a regimen of 3'-azido-2',3'-dideoxythymidine (azidothymidine or zidovudine) and acyclovir. A pilot study. *Ann Intern Med* 1988;108:534–40.

62. Schmidt RM, Castro FP Jr. The relationship between health status and psychological well-being among healthy men and men with ARC or AIDS. 5th International Conference on AIDS, Montreal, Canada, June, 1989:778 (abst D524).

63. O'Dowd MA, McKegney FP. Does AIDS reduce psychiatric illness? AIDS patients compared with other medically ill HIV+ patients seen in consultation. 6th International Conference on AIDS, San Francisco, June, 1990;2:355 (abst 2006).

64. Orr D, O'Dowd MA, McKegney FP, Natali C. A comparison of self reported suicidal behaviors in different stages of HIV infection. 6th International Conference on AIDS, San Francisco, June, 1990;1:141. (abst ThB30).

AIDS and Other Manifestations of HIV Infection,
Second Edition, Edited by Gary P. Wormser.
Published by Raven Press, Ltd., New York 1992.

CHAPTER 16

Pneumocystis carinii Disease in HIV-Infected Persons

Anthony Martinez, Anthony F. Suffredini, and Henry Masur

Pneumocystis pneumonia has achieved notoriety as the most important pulmonary pathogen associated with the acquired immunodeficiency syndrome (AIDS). Before the popular use of antipneumocystis prophylaxis, it was estimated that 80% of North American AIDS patients would develop one or more episodes of pneumocystis pneumonia during the course of their illness (1). With the advent of antiviral therapy and antipneumocystis prophylaxis, it is difficult to predict how many cases of AIDS-associated pneumocystis pneumonia will occur each year during the 1990s. Based on the expanding population of HIV-infected patients who are unaware of their retroviral infection, and the difficulties for many patients in gaining access to health care, it is likely that there will be tens of thousands of cases of AIDS-associated pneumocystis pneumonia per year through the 1990s (2).

With the tragic experience of AIDS has come the impetus and the opportunity to study the biology of human pneumocystis and its interactions with host defense mechanisms. The dramatic increase in the number of cases has allowed the development of novel therapeutic, preventive, and diagnostic modalities that can reduce the mortality and the incalculable physical, psychological, and socioeconomic disabilities that pneumocystis disease causes in this population.

Despite considerable progress, much is still unknown. Human pneumocystis is an enigmatic organism that still eludes successful cultivation, precise taxonomic classification, and extensive knowledge of its basic biology and life cycle. The presence of pneumocystis disease cannot be established by serologic assays. The diagnosis rests entirely on the demonstration of pneumocystis organisms in body fluids or tissue. Peculiar to AIDS patients with active pneumocystis pneumonia are the often subtle clinical presentations, the frequency of relapse, the frequency of adverse responses to medications, and the simultaneous occurrence of other pulmonary processes such as Kaposi's sarcoma or cytomegalovirus disease (3,4). This chapter will review the current status of knowledge about pneumocystis pneumonia as it relates to patients infected with HIV.

HISTORY

Several excellent reviews are available detailing the historical aspects of *Pneumocystis carinii* as a pulmonary pathogen (5–8). It was first described by Chagas (1909) and later Carini (1910), though both considered the cysts to be stages in the life cycle of the trypanosome. Subsequently Delanoes (1912) correctly identified the cysts in the lungs of Parisian sewer rats as a new protozoan species (7). The relationship of pneumocystis to human disease was not established until later, when in 1942, Van der Meer and Berg in Europe noted the association of pneumocystis and interstitial plasma cell pneumonitis (9). During the post-World War II era in Europe, epidemics of plasma cell pneumonitis occurred in nurseries and orphanages and carried a 50% mortality rate, using supportive rather than specific treatment (5,6). With improvement in living conditions and general nutrition in Europe, this devastating illness decreased in incidence, though the mortality rate per episode remained high. The first case in the United States was not described until 1956 (10). During the following decade, pathologists learned how to recognize the organism in lung tissue samples obtained by open lung biopsy or at autopsy. By 1967, 107 cases had been reported in the United States (11). From 1967 to 1970, 184 cases were reported to the

A. Martinez, A. F. Suffredini, and H. Masur: National Institutes of Health, Bethesda, Maryland 20892.

Centers for Disease Control. These occurred in immunocompromised children and adults with underlying malignancies, congenital immunodeficiency disorders, or organ transplants (12). No effective therapy was available until the introduction of pentamidine in Europe in 1958. This therapy dramatically decreased the mortality rate for infants with plasma cell pneumonitis from 50% to 3% (13).

After pentamidine became available in the United States in 1967, the fatality rate for pneumocystis pneumonia fell to 58% in the first 163 pentamidine-treated cases (12). The next major therapeutic advance occurred in the 1970s when Hughes showed that trimethoprim-sulfamethoxazole (TMP-SMX) was effective in treating pneumocystis pneumonia and was associated with a 75–80% response rate (14,15).

Successful endeavors in the prevention of pneumocystis pneumonia with biweekly doses of sulfadoxine and pyrimethamine in marasmic infants was reported in 1971 (16). Several years later, in a controlled study of children with malignancies, Hughes demonstrated that the trimethoprim–sulfamethoxazole combination was also highly effective in the prevention of pneumocystis pneumonia (17).

There were few other major diagnostic or therapeutic advances until the 1980s. The AIDS epidemic in the early 1980s was the catalyst for these innovations.

BIOLOGY

Some authorities refer to the pneumocystis organism derived from the rat as *Pneumocystis carinii,* and to the organism derived from humans as *Pneumocystis jiroveci* (18), but there is no consensus on nomenclature. In this chapter, pneumocystis will be the term used to refer to the organism that is derived from any host.

Based on morphologic studies, three stages in the life cycle of pneumocystis appear to exist: trophozoite, cyst, and sporozoite. The trophozoites vary in diameter from 2 μm to 5 μm, are pleomorphic in appearance, and tend to cluster together (19,20). Their nucleus is often eccentrically located, the cytoplasm is reticular, and the membrane is not well defined. Other internal structures in the trophozoites include endoplasmic reticulum, poorly developed mitochondria, ribosomes, and microtubules. No Golgi apparatus, flagellum, or cilium has been found in any stage of this organism (19,21,22).

Ultrastructurally, trophozoites are oval to spherical in shape. As development proceeds it would appear that they become pleomorphic. Based on transmission electron microscopy studies, the trophozoite has a pellicle (or wall) that consists of an electron-dense outer layer and inner plasma membrane (19,21,23).

Lobopodia (pseudopodia) are usually seen, but other features that would be characteristic of phagocytic activity have never been observed. Filopodia (tubular expansions) are characteristic structures of trophozoites (21,23,24). These structures increase in number as trophozoites develop and are arranged in clusters frequently facing another organism or host cell. The exact function and morphology of tubular expansions are not known. Some investigators have postulated that these organelles are used for anchoring and for nutritional uptake by the organism (21,25).

Cysts are the easiest form to recognize. They are 5–8 μm in diameter (19). Ultrastructurally, the pellicle of the cyst is very thick, and contains three layers: an electron-dense outer layer, an electron-lucent middle layer, and an innermost plasma layer (19,21,23,26). The pellicle of the cyst has a thickened portion that protrudes inward. This latter structure may be important for excystation and is also responsible for the so-called parentheses-like structures seen in the Gomori methenamine silver stain (21,27). The middle layer is only present in the cyst form and may be composed of β-1,3 glucan (28).

The mature cyst contains eight intracystic bodies. Each of these sporozoites contains a single nucleus, mitochondria, and abundant endoplasmic reticulum and ribosomes (19,26).

Thin-walled cysts, as well as precysts, are terms used in the literature to describe what appears to be the transition from trophozoite to cyst (23,26). Certain distinct differences have been described between the precyst and cyst: the presence of a synaptonemal complex is characteristic of the precyst stage (21,25). In other organisms this complex is known to conduct the precise alignment of homologous chromosomes and is visible only during meiotic division (21,25).

The sporozoite (also referred to as the intracystic body) is found only within the cyst (19). It is a small cell, 1–2 μm in diameter, surrounded by a very thin pellicle that contains a nucleus, a mitochondrion, and variably developed endoplasmic reticulum. Unlike the trophozoite, the sporozoite lacks surface projections and dense bodies in the cytoplasm (29). There may be up to eight of these crescent-shaped intracystic bodies found in one cyst (19).

Although a number of different versions have been proposed, the life cycle of this organism remains unknown. In 1916, Carini and Maciel first proposed that the eight intracystic merozoites escaped from the cyst and each small cell would then develop into one cyst (30). Other earlier investigators also recognized that the trophozoite could replicate itself by binary fission or a budding process (31,32). In a successful in vitro cultivation of pneumocystis organisms, trophozoites were reported to attach to the host cell (33). While attached to the host cell, convolutions were noted in the trophozoites, suggestive of the early development of the sporozoite form. Transformation to the cyst form was heralded by detachment of the organism from the host cell. Once detached, the cyst then became spherical. The cell wall thickened and contained as many as eight sporozoites. Excystment of sporozoites through one or more breaks in the cyst wall was observed. Upon leaving the cyst the sporozoite was referred to as a trophozoite. Cysts were observed completing the excystment process or enlarging to a dormant phase. The entire life cycle of pneumocystis occurred during a 4–6-hour period in this in vitro culture system (33). No phase of intracellular parasitism was noted in this study.

In addition to the asexual forms of multiplication, a sexual mode of multiplication has been postulated based on the discoveries by electron microscopy of synaptonemal complexes in the precyst stage of this organism (21,25). In eukaryotic cells this synaptonemal complex is visible only during prophase of the first meiotic division and has been used as evidence of a sexual cycle (21). Due to the number of developmental stages that have been identified, more complex life cycles have been postulated. Aside from the cyst-forming sexual cycle, multiplication could occur by binary fission as well as endogeny of haploid or diploid trophozoites (19,21,34).

TRANSMISSION AND EPIDEMIOLOGY

The pneumocystis organism appears to be acquired from the environment mainly by an air-borne route (19). Animal–animal transmission of pneumocystis clearly can occur in this way (19,35,36). Standard laboratory rats raised under conventional environmental conditions, treated with corticosteroids, and fed a low-protein diet as an adjunct to immunosuppression develop progressive pneumocystis pneumonia in a 6–12 week period. The pneumocystis pneumonia that develops is thought to represent reactivation of a latent focus of infection due to the immunosuppressive effect of corticosteroid treatment and protein deficiency (19,37). However, if germ-free rats are kept in a germ-free environment or raised in a protected environment and treated with the same immunosuppressive regimen, they do not develop pneumocystis pneumonia, even when exposed to pneumocystis-contaminated food or infective tissue, soil, or water (35,38). Germ-free rats will develop primary infection with pneumocystis when exposed to either unfiltered air or to other rats who have pneumocystis pneumonia (35,38).

Additional studies in athymic mice reveal that pneumocystis pneumonia can be successfully transmitted by intrapulmonary injection of lung homogenates or continued exposure to infected mice and rats (39). Transtracheal inoculation into germ-free, corticosteroid-treated rats also reliably produces heavy infections (40). No evidence of transplacental transmission was reported in murine studies.

In humans, the clusters of cases of infantile interstitial pneumonitis described in earlier case reports, as well as outbreaks in cancer patients, suggest that person-to-person transmission of pneumocystis may occur by the respiratory route (19,41,42). Epidemics of pneumocystis pneumonia occurring in nurseries have been well documented in the earlier literature (41,42). The most striking evidence of possible person-to-person transmission was a report of a cluster of 11 patients with predominantly hematologic malignancies that occurred in a 3-month period (43). An outbreak of 11 pediatric patients in an oncology ward was also reported at a different institution (44). Another report of pneumocystis pneumonia in ten pediatric patients with acute lymphoblastic leukemia could not be related to changes in chemotherapy (45). In this outbreak, no cases of pneumocystis pneumonia had been documented during the preceding 2 years, and in six of ten patients a direct association was noted between length of hospitalization and development of pneumocystis pneumonia, compared with uninfected controls matched by the date of initiation of chemotherapy (45).

Nonrespiratory routes of transmission in humans have rarely been reported. Case reports of pneumocystosis in a stillborn infant, a 2-day-old infant, and a 3-day-old infant suggest that in utero transmission is possible (19,46,47).

Thus, pneumocystis appears to be transmitted mainly by an air-borne route in both humans and rats. It is unknown whether pneumocystis from one animal species can infect another species. The infective form of this organism is also unknown. Based on recent immunologic studies it appears that the organisms that infect humans are antigenically different from those infecting rats, making transmission from one species to another less likely (48,49).

Pneumocystis has been isolated from numerous mammalian species including mice, rats, cats, dogs, horses, and cows, as well as from humans throughout the world (19). Except for one isolated case reported in birds, the hosts for this organism have been limited to mammals (50). Whether pneumocystis can survive outside of mammalian hosts in environmental sites, such as dust, dirt, or water, is unknown.

Based on numerous case reports and seroepidemiologic surveys, pneumocystis infection in animals and humans has a world-wide geographic distribution (19). The presence of antibodies to this organism in 70–80% of healthy humans over the age of 4 in North America and Europe indicates that most healthy adults have been infected with pneumocystis and that exposure to this organism occurs early in life (51,52).

TAXONOMY

Pneumocystis has been traditionally referred to as a protozoan based on its historical misidentification as a trypanosome, its morphology, its response to antiprotozoan drugs, and its failure to be cultivated on fungal media (23,31,53). The taxonomy of this organism has not been agreed upon by all authorities. The presumed airborne mode of spread, significant affinity for fungal stains, and ultrastructural features such as lack of organelles of motility suggest a fungal classification (26,54). Recent application of molecular biologic techniques has revealed significant homology between the ribosomal RNA of pneumocystis and the fungus *Saccharomyces cerevisae,* as compared with the ribosomal RNA of protozoa, such as the *Trypanosoma* species (55). Furthermore, in vitro assessment of enzyme structure and function of rat pneumocystis has revealed distinct differences when compared with protozoa (56). Unlike the protozoa, which usually have large, bifunctional enzymes mediating both dihydrofolate reductase and thymidylate synthetase activity, the isolated rat pneumocystis dihydrofolate reductase is of lower molecular weight and is lacking thymidylate synthetase activity (56–58).

Chemical properties of the cyst wall resemble those of fungi. It has been reported that the middle layer of the cyst wall contains β-1,3 glucan, which in *S. cerevisae* is thought to be responsible for the structural integrity of the yeast cell wall (28). In contrast, the organism's response to certain antibacterial agents and morphologic similarity to trypanosomes distinguish pneumocystis from known pathogenic fungi. Definitive classification of this unique organism is still uncertain.

HOST–ORGANISM INTERACTION

Humoral Immunity

Humoral immunity against pneumocystis has been difficult to assess because of the lack of a pure and well-defined antigen. The humoral response to, and antigenic characteristics of, pneumocystis have been evaluated by indirect immunofluorescence (IFA), ELISA (enzyme-linked immunosorbent assay), and immunoblot techniques.

Based on the specific immunoreactivity of monoclonal antibodies, it appears that rat pneumocystis has a large surface glycoprotein band that is approximately 110–120 kd in molecular weight, while the human pneumocystis has a surface glycoprotein of 95 kd molecular weight (49,59–61). Of six monoclonal antibodies developed against the rat pneumocystis organism, only one cross-reacted with human pneumocystis (62). The major surface protein bands of rat and human pneumocystis, however, have been found to be inconsistently immunoreactive when tested against sera of normal and infected hosts (62,48). Studies by Western blot technique have found IgG antibody responses to the 116-, 50-, and 45-kd antigen of rat pneumocystis and the 40-kd antigen of human pneumocystis by healthy persons and by patients with pneumocystis pneumonia (49,63–65). From the accumulated data, it appears that shared antigens exist between rat and human pneumocystis, but that species-specific antigenic determinants also exist (48,49).

Antibodies to pneumocystis are absent in young rats and mice but appear when they are exposed to other rodents with active or latent pneumocystis (63,66,67). This is presumed to reflect air-borne exposure and subclinical infection. IgG, IgA, and IgM anti-pneumocystis antibodies have been identified in serum and bronchoalveolar lavage fluid (51,59,67–69). It has been previously demonstrated that the addition of hyperimmune sera to freshly explanted alveolar macrophages of rats or mice enhances phagocytosis of pneumocystis (13). Additionally, infusion of monoclonal antibodies reactive against the 116-kd pneumocystis protein in ferrets appears to be partially protective (70).

The serologic response in humans parallels the experience noted in rodents. Antibodies against pneumocystis are rarely present before the age of 1 year. However, by age 4 years, more than 80% of children demonstrate such antibodies by IFA or ELISA (51,52,71). Using the more specific Western immunoblot analysis, a seropositivity rate of 80–90% was detected in older children and adults. The antibody response was primarily IgG and was directed against a 40-kd antigen (61,65). Patients with pneumocystis pneumonia generally have antibodies against pneumocystis that are not quantitatively or qualitatively different from patients without recent active disease (61).

Thus, extensive serologic studies in animals and humans have clearly demonstrated that there is a humoral response to pneumocystis. However, the presence of antibodies to this organism does not necessarily confer immunity or prevent the development of pneumocystis pneumonia in animals or humans.

Cell-Mediated Immunity

The vast majority of patients with pneumocystis pneumonia have severe cell-mediated immune defects. While pneumocystis pneumonia also occurs in patients with B-cell defects, it rarely, if ever, occurs in patients with pure defects in number or function of B lymphocytes (6,12,72,73). Macrophages play a crucial role in host defense against pneumocystis. Attachment of pneumocystis to macrophages has been reported to be fibronectin mediated (10,55). Pneumocystis are extracellular organisms that can be ingested and promptly digested by macrophages. They can also be damaged by soluble products secreted by macrophages. A previous in vitro study has demonstrated that freshly explanted alveolar macrophages will ingest or digest pneumocystis in the presence of hyperimmune sera (13). Further in vitro studies suggest that macrophages may contribute to the extracellular death of pneumocystis. When stimulated by interferon, macrophages separated from pneumocystis by a semiimpermeable membrane produce substances that are lethal to this organism (74). Tumor necrosis factor, a cytokine secreted by activated macrophages, has been reported to be directly lethal to pneumocystis in vitro (74).

The importance of T cells to host defense against

pneumocystis is supported by the observation that corticosteroids and, more importantly, cyclosporin, can induce pneumocystis pneumonia in experimental animals. Corticosteroids interfere with neutrophil, B-lymphocyte, and T-lymphocyte function, and also cause lymphopenia and reversal of the T-helper cell to T-suppressor cell ratio. Upon withdrawal of treatment, T-cell subpopulations return to normal, and pneumocystis pneumonia is cleared. Cyclosporin has a more selective effect on T-cell number and is also associated with the development of pneumocystis pneumonia (75).

T lymphocytes, in particular T-helper cells (CD4), have an active role in the control of pneumocystis in animals. Treatment of normal mice with monoclonal antibodies against circulating CD4 cells causes selective depletion of T-helper cells (76). Animals who are then exposed to pneumocystis by tracheal inoculation develop active pneumocystis pneumonia. Further, the importance of CD4 cells was demonstrated using severe combined immunodeficiency (SCID) mice, which are quite susceptible to pneumocystis pneumonia (54). Infusion of spleen cells from immunocompetent mice allows these SCID mice to reduce their pneumocystis burden significantly. Treatment with monoclonal anti-CD4 antibodies eliminates the ability of these spleen cell-infused mice to resolve their pneumocystis infection (54). In contrast, treatment with anti-CD8 monoclonal antibodies did not impair pneumocystis clearance (54). Thus, in this mouse model, CD4 cells clearly have an important role in host defense.

Evidence for the importance of cell-mediated immunity in humans is based mainly on the type of disease states that have a predilection for this form of pneumonia. In HIV-infected patients with circulating CD4 cells greater than 250/mm³, or 25% of total lymphocytes, pneumocystis pneumonia rarely occurs (77,78). Most cases develop in HIV-infected patients with CD4 lymphocyte counts of less than 100/mm³ (77). In a prospective study, HIV-infected patients with an initial CD4 count of less than 200/mm³ had a likelihood of developing pneumocystis at 6 months of 8.4%, at 12 months of 18.4%, and at 36 months of 33% (78). Thus, both experimental animal studies and human investigations support a central role for CD4-positive lymphocytes in host defense against pneumocystis.

Interaction of Pneumocystis and the Lung

Ultrastructural studies have demonstrated that there is selective attachment of pneumocystis trophozoites to type I alveolar epithelial cells. Adherence requires close apposition and interdigitation of cell membranes of pneumocystis and alveolar epithelial cells. Contrary to previous reports, fusion or filopodia attachment does not appear to occur (79–81). Although tubular extensions are seen, they are always separated from the target

cells by amorphous material that surrounds the trophozoite (79). Attachment of pneumocystis to its epithelial target cells is probably mediated at least in part by fibronectin (82). Such attachment to alveolar macrophages may allow the organism to be anchored within the alveolus and initiate infection (82). Intact cytoskeleton function is necessary for adherence to alveolar epithelial cells since antimotility agents interfere with adherence (83). It is of interest that adherence appears to impair lung cell replication (83).

Type II alveolar epithelial cells are responsible for the production of surfactant. In rats and humans with active pneumocystis pneumonia, surfactant levels in bronchoalveolar lavage fluid are reduced, apparently because of increased surfactant catabolism rather than decreased production (84).

In experimental pneumocystosis, rats treated with corticosteroids develop mild pneumocystis pneumonia within 4 weeks, reaching peak intensity by 7 or 8 weeks of corticosteroid treatment (37,85–88). Initially, the pneumonia is multifocal and, except for the presence of a few macrophages, an inflammatory response is absent (87). Focal necrosis of type I alveolar epithelial cells with regeneration of type II cells can also be seen (85,87). By week 8, greater than 75% of alveoli are involved with extensive degeneration of type I cells but no attachment of pneumocystis to type II cells. There is also alteration of alveolar–capillary permeability (86–88). By the late stages of experimentally induced pneumocystis pneumonia, frequently observed alterations in histology are: type I cell necrosis, type II cell hyperplasia, areas of pulmonary edema, interstitial fibrosis, and extensive pulmonary exudate (85–87). Macrophages are increased in number, but neutrophils are rare (85,87). The alveolar spaces are filled mostly by trophozoites, which may be responsible for the visualized eosinophilic honeycomb material (85,87).

Although clinical recovery in rats occurs when steroids are withdrawn, persistent attachment of pneumocystis to the type I cell is observed (85,87). Type II cell hyperplasia, along with progression of interstitial fibrosis, may continue despite clinical recovery (85–87).

Thus, pneumocystis organisms propagate slowly with selective attachment to type I cells and subsequent extensive degeneration of these target cells. Reduced surfactant levels, alteration of alveolar–capillary permeability, and pulmonary exudates occur with the progression of pneumocystis pneumonia.

CLINICAL MANIFESTATIONS OF PNEUMOCYSTIS PNEUMONIA

Predisposing Factors

The susceptibility of HIV-infected patients to develop pneumocystis pneumonia correlates best with their number or percentage of circulating CD4-positive lymphocytes (77,78). Those with fewer than 200/mm^3 are most susceptible, especially those who also have fever, weight loss, or thrush (78).

Symptoms

HIV-infected patients with pneumocystis pneumonia typically first note mild chest tightness. Subsequently, the chest tightness increases in severity, and exercise intolerance, cough, and fever develop (3,89,90). These symptoms may persist in mild form for months, or may accelerate abruptly until the diagnosis is established (3). As the disease progresses, dyspnea at rest may be noted. Cough is usually nonproductive: purulent or bloody sputum is quite unusual. Fever can be low grade (37–38°C) or high and spiking (greater than 40°C) (3,90). About 10–20% of patients never manifest a fever. In some patients, pneumocystis pneumonia is suspected on the basis of a chest x-ray or gallium scan done for other reasons before any pulmonary symptoms are present.

Physical Examination

Pneumocystis disease rarely causes striking abnormalities on physical examination except for vital sign abnormalities. The most common abnormalities seen are tachypnea and fever (3,90–92). Auscultation of the chest is abnormal in less than 50% of cases (3,90). Rales and rhonchi rather than signs of consolidation are the most common findings. Occasionally patients will present with manifestations that produce striking physical findings such as pneumothorax, or extrapulmonary manifestations, such as skin lesions, retinal lesions, or hepatomegaly (93–97).

Laboratory Evaluation

AIDS patients with pneumocystis pneumonia usually have a white blood count that is elevated over baseline. Since many of these patients are quite leukopenic at baseline, this relative leukocytosis might not be apparent unless a baseline value is known. For example, a patient with a baseline white blood cell count of 2,100/mm^3 may present with a white blood cell count of 5,500/mm^3. There also may be a modest rise in the percentage of granulocytes. Lymphopenia is characteristic. Serum chemistries are helpful only in terms of serum lactate dehydrogenase (LDH) which is elevated in 90% of patients, but this is a nonspecific abnormality (98,99). Arterial blood gases may be abnormal, depending on how advanced the pneumocystis pneumonia is, revealing a widening alveolar-to-arterial oxygen gradient (3,90).

Comparison of Presenting Features

Pneumocystis pneumonia is a more insidious disease in AIDS patients than in patients with other forms of immunosuppression (3). When compared with other immunosuppressed patients assessed at the time the pneumocystis pneumonia was diagnosed, AIDS patients had a longer median duration of symptoms (28 days versus 5 days), a lower respiratory rate (23 bpm versus 30 bpm), and a higher room air arterial oxygen tension (68 mm Hg versus 52 mm Hg) (3).

Extrapulmonary Pneumocystosis

Clinically apparent extrapulmonary pneumocystosis is an infrequent occurrence in HIV-infected patients. Patients may present with pulmonary complaints, or may have pain or other symptoms associated with other involved organs. Pneumocystosis has been reported in almost every organ including brain, retina, lymph nodes, liver, spleen, kidney, and skin (94,96,100–104).

In a retrospective analysis of 34 patients with extrapulmonary pneumocystosis, the most frequent sites of involvement were: spleen (12 patients), liver (12 patients), lymph nodes (12 patients), eyes (9 patients), bone marrow (8 patients), gastrointestinal tract (8 patients), and thyroid (7 patients). In 17 patients, only one extrapulmonary site was documented (103).

The diagnosis of extrapulmonary pneumocystosis has been established antemortem by needle aspirations or surgical biopsies of involved organs (97), but the majority of cases are discovered postmortem.

From a laboratory perspective, elevated liver enzymes, hypoalbuminemia, and coagulopathy have been reported in 9 of 14 cases of hepatic pneumocystosis. Less frequently, cytopenias have been noted in patients with bone marrow involvement (97). Characteristic radiographic and sonographic abnormalities have been associated with extrapulmonary pneumocystosis (97,105, 106). Findings of low-attenuation lesions and multiple small calcifications in lymph nodes and abdominal organs have been described by computed tomography. Clinical evidence of extrapulmonary pneumocystosis is still fairly unusual, but more aggressive diagnostic studies may demonstrate that this entity is more common then currently suspected (103,104,106).

Differential Diagnosis

There are no distinct clinical features that separate pneumocystis pneumonia from the many other possible causes of pneumonia that affect HIV-infected patients. Any HIV-infected patient with a CD4 lymphocyte count less than 200/mm^3 and any symptom or sign of chest disease should have pneumocystis pneumonia consid-

TABLE 1. *Differential diagnosis of respiratory failure in HIV-infected patients who fail to respond to anti-pneumocystis therapy*

Noninfectious causes
    Drug toxicity
    Pulmonary emboli
    Alveolar hemorrhage
    Pneumothorax
    Adult respiratory distress syndrome
    Congestive heart failure
    Nonspecific interstitial pneumonitis
    Lymphocytic interstitial pneumonitis
    Malignancies:
        Kaposi's sarcoma
        Non-Hodgkin's lymphoma
Infectious causes
    Refractory pneumocystis pneumonia
    Bacterial pneumonia
        Legionella
        Streptococcus pneumoniae
        Haemophilus influenzae
        Mycobacteria
            M. tuberculosis
            M. kansasii
            M. avium-intracellulare
    Fungal pneumonia
        Cryptococcus
        Histoplasma
        Coccidioides
        Aspergillus
    Viral pneumonia
        Cytomegalovirus pneumonia
        Influenza (uncommon)

ered in the differential diagnosis (Table 1). In virtually all situations a diagnostic procedure should be done to establish the etiology.

DIAGNOSTIC PROCEDURES

Diagnosis of pneumocystis disease is made by identification of the organism in pulmonary secretions, lung tissue, or extrapulmonary tissue specimens. Human pneumocystis has never been cultured in vitro, and reliable serologic assays have not been developed. Chest radiographs, CT scans, nuclear scans, and pulmonary function tests all lack the specificity to establish the diagnosis of pneumocystis pneumonia. Since a minority of HIV-infected patients with low CD4 lymphocyte counts and pulmonary symptoms will have pneumocystis pneumonia, it is important to make a specific diagnosis so that appropriate therapy can be given and unnecessary therapy avoided.

Chest Radiograph

The usual radiographic pattern of pneumocystis in HIV-infected patients is bilateral perihilar or diffuse interstitial infiltrates (Fig. 1A and B) (107). Documented pneumocystis pneumonia has also been recognized in

association with: an asymmetric distribution, lobar consolidation, pseudonodular infiltrates, cavities, granulomas, or cystic-appearing infiltrates (Fig. 1C) (6,108–111). Patients with histologically severe disease can also have a normal-appearing radiograph, particularly early in the clinical course. If patients are receiving aerosolized pentamidine, "atypical" radiographic findings seem to be more common, including: focal or upper lobe infiltrates, pulmonary cavities, and pneumothoraces (112–117). In one study, diffuse infiltrates were present in only 52% of patients who received aerosolized pentamidine chemoprophylaxis compared with 90% of patients not receiving chemoprophylaxis (116). Apical or upper lobe infiltrates were seen in 38% who received aerosolized pentamidine compared with 7% in patients receiving no aerosol prophylaxis (116).

Nuclear Medicine Procedures

Gallium-67 citrate scans represent a sensitive, expensive, and nonspecific screening test for active pulmonary disease in AIDS patients. The scan is conventionally performed 48–72 hours after injection of the isotope. The sensitivity for pneumocystis pneumonia approaches 90–98%, although its specificity ranges only from 40% to 47% (118–120). Pneumocystis pneumonia has been reported with normal or minimally abnormal scans, but typically the lung fields show diffuse symmetric pulmonary uptake that is at least equal to bone marrow uptake (91,121). Thus, the utility of gallium scanning seems marginal given the ease and safety of bronchoscopic procedures.

Serology

Currently serologic tests for pneumocystis serve no role in clinical practice. Their utility is primarily for epidemiologic research.

Pulmonary Function Testing

Pulmonary function tests in patients with pneumocystis pneumonia typically show a decrease in lung volumes (vital capacity and total lung capacity), an increase in flow rates (forced expired volume in 1 second to forced vital capacity ratio), and a decreased diffusing capacity. Although statistically significant differences occur in these measurements between AIDS patients with and without pneumocystis pneumonia, there is substantial overlap between both groups (122,123). In addition, a decrease in diffusing capacity with a normal chest radiograph has been noted to occur with other conditions such as, for example, intravenous drug use (123,124). Thus, there is little diagnostic utility in obtaining pulmonary function tests.

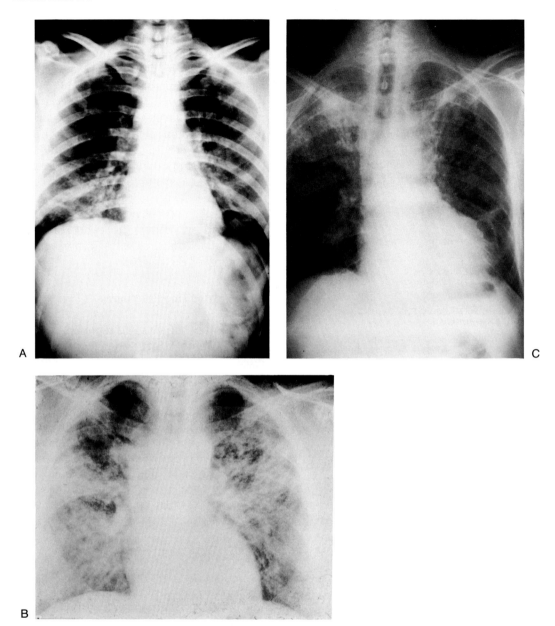

FIG. 1. PA chest radiographs of lavage-documented pneumocystis pneumonia in HIV-infected patients. **A:** Bilateral diffuse interstial infiltrates in a patient with mild disease. **B:** Extensive air-space disease in a patient with respiratory failure. **C:** Atypical findings with predominant right upper lobe involvement.

Microscopic Identification

Definitive diagnosis of pneumocystis disease is dependent on demonstration of pneumocystis cysts or trophozoites in samples of secretions or tissue (Table 2). The toluidine blue O, the Gram Weigert, and the methenamine silver stains can be used to identify the cyst form of pneumocystis (20,125,126). These staining techniques also identify fungi, which can be confused with pneumocystis cysts by inexperienced observers. Pneumocystis cysts are distinguished from fungal forms by the absence of budding, the intraalveolar location, and the more oval shape (125). Stains for trophozoites and

sporozoites used on tissue imprints or pulmonary secretions include the Giemsa, Diff Quik, and Gram stain. These stains take considerable expertise to read accurately (90,127).

The Papanicolaou stain has been used on bronchial washings and lavage fluid to identify pneumocystis. Pneumocystis cysts appear as an amphophilic amorphous granular mass (128). A modification of the Papanicolaou smear views the material under ultraviolet light. Cysts emit bright fluorescence, permitting localization and identification. This procedure may complement the use of other conventional stains, although most reference laboratories do not rely on cytologic techniques (129).

TABLE 2. *Demonstration of forms of pneumocystis in pulmonary specimens using brightfield or fluorescent microscopy and various staining techniques*

Pulmonary specimen and staining technique	Ability to stain pneumocystis		
	Cyst wall	Sporozoite	Trophozoite
Bronchoalveolar lavage and induced sputum			
Hematoxylin and eosin	−	−	−
Methenamine silver	+	−	−
Toluidine blue O	+	−	−
Gram Weigert	+	−	−
Cresyl echt violet	+	−	−
Glemsa	−	+	+
Monoclonal immunofluorescence	+	−	+
Lung imprint			
Hematoxylin and eosin	−	−	−
Methenamine silver	+	−	−
Toluidine blue O	+	−	−
Gram Weigert	+	−	−
Cresyl echt violet	+	−	−
Giemsa	−	+	+
Monoclonal immunofluorescence	+	−	+
Lung histology-Paraffin sections			
Hematoxylin and eosin	−	−	−
Methenamine silver	+	−	−
Toluidine blue O	+	−	−
Gram Weigert	+	−	−
Cresyl echt violet	+	−	−
Giemsa	−	−	−

Sputum Examination

Sputum analysis should be the first test performed to diagnose pneumocystis pneumonia. AIDS patients with pneumocystis pneumonia characteristically have a nonproductive cough. Thus, expectorated sputum is difficult to obtain. One of the advances in the management of pneumocystis pneumonia in AIDS patients has been the ability to establish the diagnosis on induced sputum samples (130–132). Sputum can be induced in almost every patient by having the patient inhale 3% hypertonic saline mist via an ultrasonic nebulizer for up to 30 minutes. The technique used to obtain the specimen is crucial to the success of this approach and is outlined in Table 3. Specimens should be processed regardless of their apparent quality.

The technique of processing the specimen is also crucial to the yield of this approach. Dithiothreitol dissolves the mucous in the sputum and allows better concentration of cellular elements (133). Conventional staining of specimens can yield the diagnosis in up to 70–85% of cases (131). Immunofluorescent staining techniques (using three different monoclonal antibodies directed at human pneumocystis) improves the diagnostic yield to 90–95% (131,134). The immunofluorescent stains can be read rapidly. Their specificity should approach 100% (131,134).

Patients receiving aerosol pentamidine prophylaxis represent a special diagnostic problem. The yield in this patient population is only 60%, and organisms may be particularly scant in number (135).

Since induced sputum samples are often not assessed for pathogens other than pneumocystis, the possibility that other etiologic agents are also present must be considered, especially for patients not responding promptly to antipneumocystis therapy.

Fiberoptic Bronchoscopy

When evaluated prospectively, bronchoalveolar lavage has been demonstrated to have an 87–89% sensitivity for the diagnosis of pneumocystis pneumonia (92,136,137). Lavage combined with transbronchial biopsies increased the sensitivity rate to 94–100%, unless more than 1–2 weeks of empiric antipneumocystis therapy had been given (136,138). The negative predictive value of bronchoscopy for pneumocystis pneumonia when both bronchoalveolar lavage and transbronchial biopsy are performed and no pneumocystis is found is greater than 92% (137). In patients with adequate lavage and transbronchial biopsy specimens, this degree of reliability of a negative result strongly suggests an alternative diagnosis.

In most HIV-infected patients in whom the diagnosis of pneumocystis pneumonia is strongly suspected but testing of induced sputum is negative, it is reasonable to proceed to bronchoalveolar lavage without transbron-

TABLE 3. *Induction and processing of sputum for the diagnosis of pneumocystis pneumonia*

1. Procedure should be explained to the patient. Cooperation, effort and deep coughing by the patient, as well as adequate time, are necessary to produce a good specimen.
2. In order to minimize contamination of specimens with mouth flora and debris, have the patient gargle with 10–15 ml aliquots of 3% saline three times before the procedure.
3. Fill the reservoir of an ultrasonic nebulizer with 150 ml of 3% saline. Adjust to mist that is tolerable to the patient. Have patient breathe normally with occasional deep breaths. Continue for up to 30 minutes if necessary.
4. Process any specimen produced if the patient is coughing, regardless of its appearance. Specimens resembling saliva are often positive. Quantity of the specimen does not correlate with diagnostic yield.
5. Dilute the specimen 1:1 with sterile water to minimize hypertonicity-induced morphologic distortion. Mix the specimen with 2 volumes of dithiothreitol (sputolysin Stat-Pak, Behring Diagnostics, San Diego, CA), vortex briefly, incubate 3 minutes at 37°C, add 10 ml phosphate-buffered saline, and centrifuge at 2,500 × *g* for 5 minutes.
6. To the pellet and 1.5 ml of remaining supernatant add 0.15 ml of a solution containing 1% Rhozyme P11 (Genencor, Inc., South San Francisco, CA) and 10% Tween 20 (Sigma Chemical Co., St. Louis, MO), vortex briefly, and incubate at 37°C for 3 minutes.
7. Several direct smears or cytospin slides may be prepared using 0.2–0.3 ml of processed specimen per slide and stained for pneumocystis by toluidine blue-O, Giemsa, or immunofluorescence.

chial biopsy. However, the diagnostic approach should be modified in HIV-infected patients who have received prophylactic aerosolized pentamidine. Peculiar to this subset of patients is apical and upper lobe involvement of pneumocystis (112,114–117). Furthermore, the overall organism burden may be appreciably less (116). A diminished sensitivity of bronchoalveolar lavage to 62% in these patients has been reported (116). In patients receiving aerosol pentamidine selective lavage of the upper lobes is recommended, especially if that is the location of the infiltrate. At some institutions the yield of directed lavage is close to 100% if the specimen is stained by the immunofluorescent technique. At other institutions, transbronchial biopsy is necessary in order to obtain satisfactory sensitivity (116).

Although the overall mortality and morbidity associated with fiberoptic bronchoscopy is low, a significant occurrence of transient atrial arrhythmias (32%) and ventricular arrhythmias (20%) has been reported (139). In most patients, transient abnormalities in pulmonary function occur during and after the procedure, with associated decreased arterial oxygen tension, but these usually have little clinical significance (140). Major complications associated with bronchoalveolar lavage and transbronchial biopsy include hemoptysis, which occurs in 1–4% of patients, and pneumothorax, which has been reported in 5% of patients (141,142). Fever with chills, or transient new pulmonary infiltrates, can be experienced after the procedure (143). The frequencies of these complications vary as a function of the skill of the bronchoscopist, the patient population, and the condition under which the procedure is done. The likelihood of pneumothorax can be minimized by performance of biopsies under fluoroscopic guidance. Contraindications to transbronchial biopsy include a significant bleeding diathesis (platelet count less than 50,000/mm³, prothrombin time greater than 3 seconds above control values, or uremia), severe hypoxemia, positive end expiratory pressures greater than 5 cm H_2O while on mechanical ventilation, and pulmonary hypertension. In many of these patients bronchoalveolar lavage alone can be a useful diagnostic procedure.

Nonbronchoscopic Lavage

Variations in the technique of bronchoalveolar lavage have been described using: (1) a control (movable) tipped catheter placed into the lung segments fluoroscopically (138); (2) lung lavage by catheters passed blindly into lung segments of intubated patients (144); or (3) endobronchial lavage using conventional endotracheal suctioning techniques (145). The use of blindly placed tracheal catheters in unintubated patients has also been reported. Tracheobronchial lavage obtained by this procedure detected 35 of 40 cases of pneumocystis pneumonia that were diagnosed by bronchoalveolar lavage (146).

Currently, nonbronchoscopic techniques cannot be routinely recommended and appear to offer no advantage over induced sputum analysis. When sputum induction is not available or obtainable and bronchoscopy is unavailable, they may be a valuable means of evaluating a patient who is deteriorating rapidly.

Transthoracic Needle Aspiration

Percutaneous needle aspiration of the lung has been used to diagnose pneumocystis pneumonia, but its use as a routine diagnostic procedure in adults is made undesirable by the high rate of associated pneumothoraces (147). As currently performed percutaneous needle aspiration of the lung cannot be recommended as a routine procedure in AIDS patients with pulmonary disease.

Open Lung Biopsy

It is unusual for properly performed bronchoalveolar lavage and transbronchial biopsies to fail to detect disease due to pneumocystis. Open lung biopsy may be necessary, however, in patients whose respiratory status is deteriorating such that fiberoptic bronchoscopy is contraindicated, when bronchoalveolar and transbronchial biopsies are otherwise contraindicated or nondiagnostic, and when certain other diagnoses such as cytomegalovirus infection or Kaposi's sarcoma are suspected.

Summary of Diagnostic Approaches

An algorithm for diagnosing pneumocystis pneumonia is shown in Fig. 2.

In the absence of active pneumocystis pneumonia, it is extremely unusual to detect pneumocystis organisms in respiratory tract specimens in previously untreated HIV-infected patients (148). Therefore, antipneumocystis therapy, should be initiated for untreated patients in whom the organism has been observed.

If pneumocystis pneumonia is suspected on the basis of clinical signs, symptoms, or radiographic abnormalities, empiric therapy should be started in all but extremely mild cases. An induced sputum is the initial diagnostic procedure of choice. If results of induced sputum are negative, fiberoptic bronchoalveolar lavage should be performed so that the toxicity of unnecessary

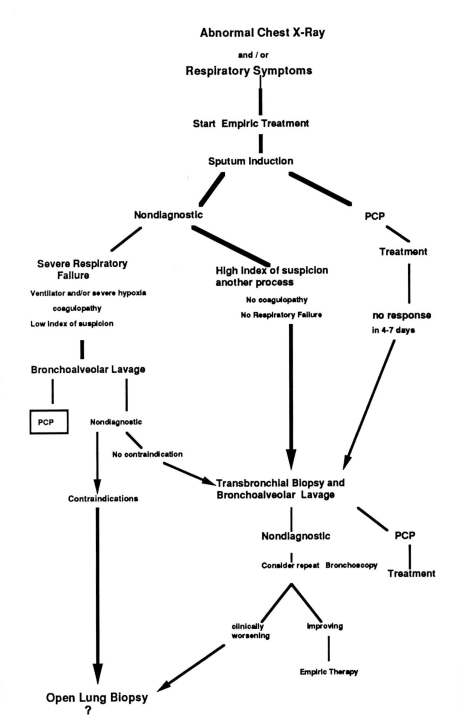

FIG. 2. Algorithm for evaluation of pneumocystis pneumonia *(PCP)* in an HIV-infected person with an abnormal chest x-ray or with respiratory symptoms.

drugs can be avoided, and other appropriate specific therapies promptly instituted. A transbronchial biopsy should be considered in patients if the bronchoalveolar lavage is nondiagnostic and the respiratory status continues to deteriorate.

Patients with the diagnosis of pneumocystis pneumonia established by induced sputum or bronchoalveolar lavage, who have worsening clinical signs or lack of clinical improvement after 5–7 days of therapy, should undergo fiberoptic bronchoscopy with bronchoalveolar lavage and biopsy. If these results are nondiagnostic, and the severity of the patient's clinical status warrants an aggressive evaluation, an open lung biopsy should then be performed.

THERAPY

Background

The development of drugs active against pneumocystis has been hampered by the inability to grow this organism in an axenic culture system and by the limited understanding of the physiology of this organism. The experimental animal model has been the mainstay of drug development (19,149).

Dihydrofolate Reductase Inhibitors

Dihydrofolate reductase inhibitors (DHFR) are a class of compounds that inhibit several metabolic pathways essential for nucleotide synthesis. The ideal dihydrofolate reductase inhibitor is one that is extremely selective for pneumocystis dihydrofolate reductase rather than the mammalian enzyme. This may be achieved by differential enzyme affinity or by differential ability to be transported into microbial as opposed to mammalian cells. Trimethoprim, pyrimethamine, and trimetrexate are all examples of dihydrofolate reductase inhibitors.

Dihydropteroate Synthetase Inhibitors

Critical to pneumocystis are intracellular enzymes such as dihydropteroate synthetase, which permit the utilization of paraaminobenzoic acid (PABA) (150). Many paraaminobenzoate analogs have been developed to inhibit this reaction, which include the sulfonamide (such as sulfamethoxazole) and sulfone (such as dapsone) compounds (150).

Conventional Therapy

Trimethoprim–sulfamethoxazole, a fixed combination inhibitor, is the drug of choice for pneumocystis pneumonia.

Trimethoprim is a dihydrofolate reductase inhibitor. It is eliminated by the kidney with only 20% of the drug dose metabolized to inactive metabolites (151,152). Levels at 5–10 μg/ml have been associated with a favorable outcome in the treatment of *P. carinii* pneumonia (14,153,154). Sulfamethoxazole, an inhibitor of dihydropteroate synthetase, is metabolized in the liver with less than 20% of the drug eliminated by the kidney (151,152). Concurrent administration of leucovorin has been used in an attempt to reduce hematologic toxicity, but there is little evidence that this is necessary or useful (155).

Trimethoprim and sulfamethoxazole are well absorbed from the gastrointestinal tract (152). The half-lives of trimethoprim and sulfamethoxazole are 9 and 14 hours, respectively, and they are believed to accumulate. Recommended dosing schedules are trimethoprim (20 mg/kg) and sulfamethoxazole (100 mg/kg) per day in three or four divided doses. Peak levels of 5–10 μg/ml of trimethoprim and 100–150 μg/ml of sulfamethoxazole (drawn 1.5–2 hours after administration) have been associated with successful outcome (14,153). Lower doses with lower serum levels have not been directly compared with this regimen, but doses of 15 mg/kg/day of trimethoprim and 75 mg/kg/day of sulfamethoxazole have been used successfully (154). Adverse effects of trimethoprim–sulfamethoxazole include nausea, vomiting, erythroderma, fever, tremors, hepatotoxicity, bone marrow suppression with leukopenia, thrombocytopenia, and megaloblastic anemia (3,4,89,151,154,156–159). These adverse effects occur in 50–80% of HIV-infected patients, but are rarely life-threatening; in a few cases severe blistering skin lesions have been described.

Pentamidine Isethionate

Pentamidine isethionate, an aromatic diamidine, was the first agent found to be effective against pneumocystis. The principal mechanism of action may be inhibition of DNA synthesis (160).

Initially, pentamidine was only given by the intramuscular route because of early reports of seizures, hypotension, and sudden death associated with rapid intravenous infusion (160). Intramuscular injections were not easy to tolerate: local discomfort at the injection site and sterile abscess formation occurred in at least 18% of cases. The intravenous route was reevaluated and has been shown to be well tolerated without significant hypotension when given as a slow infusion in 150 ml of 5% dextrose in water over a 1-hour period (12,161,162). Aerosol pentamidine has been tried for acute therapy, but unsatisfactory efficacy and a high relapse rate have been observed (163,164).

Pentamidine has a large volume of distribution. Less than 5% of the drug is cleared by the kidneys (151,165).

Toxicities include nephrotoxicity, dysglycemia, torsade de pointes arrhythmias, leukopenia, and a metallic taste (160,166,167). Hypoglycemia can be severe and usually occurs during the second or third week of therapy, but may be encountered at any point during therapy, and even days or weeks after pentamidine has been discontinued (167). Acute, and rapidly progressive renal failure has been reported, especially in association with concomitant amphotericin B treatment (168). Renal failure is usually reversible when pentamidine is discontinued.

These toxicities are probably related to the accumulated dose of pentamidine. A reduced daily dose of 3 mg/kg/day has been used to improve patient tolerance without compromising overall clinical efficacy (154). Whether this lower dose produces efficacy comparable to 4 mg/kg/day dose is uncertain.

Dapsone

Dapsone is a paraaminobenzoic acid analog. In vitro it has been found to be a potent inhibitor of the dihydropteroate synthetase of pneumocystis. Dapsone can only be administered orally. The plasma half-life ranges from 10 hours to 83 hours (169,170). Only 5–15% of the drug dose is renally excreted (151). Dapsone is eliminated from the body primarily by acetylation and oxidative metabolism. Half the dose of dapsone is hydroxylated to dapsone hydroxylamine. It is believed that this metabolite is primarily responsible for the methemoglobinemia that is commonly seen (151,171). Mean peak levels of 2.1 μg/ml measured after 6 hours of administration of dapsone–trimethoprim have been reported in successfully treated AIDS patients (151). Steady state is usually achieved after 7 days. When dapsone is given concurrently with trimethoprim, higher levels of both dapsone and trimethoprim are achieved (151). The increased dapsone levels may contribute to the toxicity, as well as the efficacy, of this combination (151,172).

As with most sulfones, hypersensitivity reactions occur frequently. Anemia and methemoglobinemia (>60%) have been reported in AIDS patients treated with the combination of dapsone and trimethoprim (151,172,173). It is advised that patients be screened for possible glucose 6-phosphate dehydrogenase deficiency (G6PD) before instituting therapy. Regular monitoring for methemoglobinemia and for anemia is equally important (151,172,173).

EXPERIMENTAL THERAPIES

Clindamycin–Primaquine

The combination of clindamycin and primaquine is effective in the prophylaxis and treatment of pneumocystis in an experimental animal model (174). The mech-

anism of action against pneumocystis is unknown. When used alone, each of these drugs is ineffective against pneumocystis in vitro and in the immunosuppressed rat model (175,176). Initial studies in AIDS patients with mild-to-moderate pneumocystis pneumonia are encouraging (177,178). This regimen is relatively well tolerated, although cutaneous reactions and reversible methemoglobinemia are common.

Treatment regimens used to date have included oral primaquine base (15 mg/day) and oral or intravenous clindamycin (600 mg four times daily); primaquine base (30 mg orally) and intravenous or oral clindamycin (900 mg four times daily). Both treatment regimens appear to have efficacy (177,178).

Dihydrofolate Reductase Inhibitors

Trimetrexate and piritrexim are lipid-soluble analogs of methotrexate that are very potent inhibitors of DHFR (150,179,180). These lipid-soluble compounds readily diffuse into pneumocystis as well as host cells. Cytotoxicity to host cells is minimized by the concurrent administration of leucovorin (150,179,181,182). Studies of trimetrexate have shown that this drug has considerable efficacy, but efficacy is not as high as that for trimethoprim–sulfamethoxazole, and the relapse rate is unacceptably high (183). Thus, this drug has little current role in management except as an alternative agent for patients who have either failed or manifested serious intolerance to both pentamidine and trimethoprim–sulfamethoxazole.

Piritrexim, another lipid-soluble methotrexate analog, is structurally similar to trimetrexate but has better oral bioavailability (150,180). Results of a small clinical trial suggest that its efficacy and relapse rate are comparable to trimetrexate (184).

BW566C80

The hydroxynapthoquinone BW566C80 has in vitro and animal model activity against plasmodium, toxoplasma, and pneumocystis (185). Hydroxynapthoquinones block protozoal respiratory chain electron transport and probably function as analogs of ubiquinone (185).

Activity against pneumocystis has been demonstrated in vitro and in the experimental murine model. In a pilot study of 34 AIDS patients with mild to moderately severe pneumocystis pneumonia who were treated with 566C80 750 mg po BID to QID, efficacy was 79% (186). Therapy was discontinued in four patients, all in the high-dose cohort group, due to the development of rash (two patients) or drug fever (two patients). An additional four patients developed rash and three patients had elevated transaminase levels but completed therapy. Pharmacokinetic studies show somewhat erratic absorption (186). There is currently no intravenous preparation.

Thus, preliminary clinical studies suggest that BW566C80 is an effective and well-tolerated therapy in HIV-infected patients with pneumocystis pneumonia. A phase III study comparing oral BW566C80 to oral trimethoprim–sulfamethoxazole was completed in October 1991. Patients with mild or moderate pneumocystis pneumonia were assessed in a blinded fashion. Preliminary analysis of data suggests that BW566C80 was almost as effective as trimethoprim–sulfamethoxazole, but was much better tolerated (186a).

Other Experimental Therapeutics

A number of drugs have been shown to have activity in vitro or in animal models, but not in clinical trials.

Antifungals, specifically β-1,3 glucan synthesis inhibitors, have been observed to cause rapid clearing of pneumocystis cysts in immunosuppressed rats with active pneumocystis (187). The specificity of this novel therapeutic approach is based on the presence of β-1,3 glucan in the cyst wall, since there is no known counterpart of β-1,3 glucan synthesis in mammalian cells (28,187).

Sulfonylureas, such as carbutamide, have been shown in a rat model to be effective (188).

Novel pentamidine analogs, some with good oral bioavailability, have been developed and some appear to be effective in preliminary studies in the experimental induced pneumocystis animal model (189). An inosine analog, 9-deazonainozine, has also been reported to be effective against pneumocystis in vitro and in the immunosuppressed animal model (190).

WR6026 and WR238 are primaquine analogues with excellent activity in vitro and in animal models (191). Trials with these compounds are expected to be initiated in 1992.

Adjuvant Therapy

Three trials have demonstrated unequivocal clinical benefit when corticosteroids are administered with specific therapy as the initial regimen for patients with moderate or severe pneumocystis pneumonia (192–194). When corticosteroids were started during the initial 72 hours of therapy in patients whose initial arterial oxygen pressure on room air was less than 70 mm Hg, oxygenation deterioration, respiratory failure, and death were all reduced in frequency (192,194). Adverse effects of the corticosteroids were not life-threatening: oral thrush and mucocutaneous herpes simplex virus infection did occur with increased frequency (194). The recommended regimen is: days 1–5, 40 mg of oral prednisone twice daily; days 6–10, 40 mg daily; and days 11–21, 20 mg daily (195). Whether corticosteroids benefit patients with mild pneumocystis pneumonia (i.e., arterial oxygen pressure on room air of more than 70 mm Hg) has not been shown; these patients have such a good prognosis in general that it would take a very large trial to prove benefit, and such a trial has not been done.

Therapeutics: An Overview

Over the past decade a variety of novel therapeutic approaches have been developed (Table 4). Thus far, none has been proved to surpass the clinical efficacy of trimethoprim–sulfamethoxazole or parenteral pentamidine. Trimethoprim–sulfamethoxazole (15–20 mg/kg/day trimethoprim and 75–100 mg/kg/day sulfamethoxazole administered intravenously or orally in divided doses at 6–8-hour intervals) is the agent of choice due to high efficacy, low frequency of life-threatening side effects, and ease of administration. Trimethoprim-dapsone (trimethoprim 20 mg/kg/day at 8-hour intervals and dapsone 100 mg once/day) is a suitable alterna-

TABLE 4. *Drugs for therapy of pneumocystis pneumonia*

Drug	Total daily dose	Route	Interval	Duration (days)	Adverse effects
Trimethoprim and sulfamethoxazole	15–20 mg/kg 75–100 mg/kg	IV or PO	Q6–8 H Q6–8 H	21	Fever, rash, leukopenia, thrombocytopenia, and hepatic disturbances
Pentamidine isethionate	3–4 mg/kg	IV	Q24 H	21	Hypotension with rapid IV administration Cardiac arrythmias, hypocalcemia, pancreatitis, dysglycemias, nephrotoxicity
Trimethoprim and dapsone	20 mg/kg 100 mg	PO	Q8 H Q24 H	21	Anemia, hyperkalemia, and methemoglobinemia Screen for G6PD deficiency in selected patients
Trimetrexate with leucovorin	45 mg/m² 20 mg/m²	IV IV or PO	Q24 H	21	Elevated transaminases, leukopenia, and thrombocytopenia
Clindamycin and primaquine	2.4–3.6 g 15–30 mg	IV, PO PO	Q8 H Q24 H	21	Rash and methemoglobinemia Screen for G6PD deficiency
BW566C80	2,250 mg	PO	Q8 H	21	? Rash and elevated transaminases

tive for mild-to-moderate disease, since efficacy is probably comparable and toxicity appears to be less frequent than with trimethoprim–sulfamethoxazole (172).

In patients with severe pneumocystis pneumonia who have serious allergies to trimethoprim–sulfamethoxazole, intravenous pentamidine (4 mg/kg IV once a day) should be used.

In cases of moderate-to-severe pneumocystis as defined by an arterial oxygen pressure of less than 70 mm Hg or an alveolar–arterial gradient of greater than 35, during the initial 72 hours after the institution of therapy, corticosteroids (oral prednisone 40 mg orally twice daily for 5 days before tapering) should be started (195).

Patients with mild disease and those already incorporated into the health care system can receive oral trimethoprim–sulfamethoxazole or trimethoprim–dapsone therapy and be followed carefully as outpatients. They should be educated about the adverse effects of the medication and the disease process.

Severely ill patients should receive intravenous therapy until substantial clinical improvement is observed. After therapy is initiated, the clinician should anticipate worsening of pulmonary function during the initial 3–4 days of therapy. This worsening does not imply a poor prognosis. The cause of this transient worsening is not clear, but may be related to the release of antigen or activation of immunologic mediators by dying organisms. Generally the initial therapy should be continued for a minimum of 5–10 days before poor response would warrant changing the regimen.

Many clinicians prefer to treat for 21 days rather than the customary 14-day duration of therapy for non-AIDS patients. While this is the standard of practice, there is no evidence that a 21-day course of therapy, compared with a 14-day course, lowers the relapse rate or improves overall survival. Once definitive therapy is completed, prophylaxis should be immediately initiated (2).

Patients whose conditions do not improve or, as determined by symptoms, signs, arterial blood gas values, or chest radiographs after 5–10 days of therapy should be considered treatment failures. A bronchoscopic evaluation, preferably with transbronchial biopsies, should be considered, especially if the initial diagnosis was established by sputum evaluation. Pneumocystis organisms are almost invariably present after 5–10 days of therapy even in patients who are responding well. Thus, the goal of the procedure is to look for other treatable processes such as cytomegalovirus, mycobacteria or fungal infection.

If pneumocystis is the only pathogen identifiable, the options after 5–10 days of initial therapy include: switching from trimethoprim–sulfamethoxazole to pentamidine (or vice versa); switching to trimetrexate; or switching to primaquine–clindamycin. In addition to these maneuvers, adjunctive corticosteroids can be added to any of these regimens. There are no data defining the best approach: each has been used successfully in anecdotal cases.

PROGNOSIS

Based on early experience in the treatment of HIV-infected patients with pneumocystis pneumonia, the clinical or laboratory features at presentation that suggest a favorable prognosis include: a low respiratory rate (<25 bpm); higher room air arterial oxygen tension (>70 mm Hg); low alveolar–arterial oxygen tension gradient (<25 mm Hg); high lymphocyte counts (900/mm^3); high albumin levels (>3.3 g/L); low serum LDH levels (<388 units/L); and a normal chest radiograph (3,90,99,197). Patients with their first episode of pneumocystis pneumonia and mild disease have a greater than 90% chance of survival (90,157). HIV-infected patients with pneumocystis pneumonia and respiratory failure who require mechanical ventilation have been reported to have a survival prognosis of 0–50% depending on patient selection criteria (3,90,196,198,199).

Early recognition and treatment of concurrent pulmonary infection may also impact on survival. It has been noted that 10% of HIV-infected patients with biopsy-proven pneumocystis pneumonia have concurrent pulmonary pathogens. The pulmonary infections found in this retrospective report included bacterial pneumonia (four), cytomegalovirus pneumonitis (three), cryptococcosis (two), pulmonary tuberculosis (two), *Mycobacterium avium-intracellulare* infection, and one case of pulmonary toxoplasmosis. The mortality rate for patients with pneumocystis pneumonia and one of the above-mentioned coexistent infections was 50% compared with 18% for patients with pneumocystis alone (90). Thus, early recognition and treatment of other potential pulmonary pathogens may play a role in improved survival. The clinical significance of finding *Mycobacterium avium-intracellulare* in bronchoalveolar lavage fluid is unknown but has been detected more frequently in nonsurvivors (90,196).

In contrast, one retrospective review from an institution that recently experienced an improved in-hospital survival of 40% (previously reported 14%) in AIDS patients with pneumocystis pneumonia and respiratory failure found no differences in coexisting opportunistic infections or patient characteristics that could account for the improved outcome (198). Improved survival may be related to the overall accumulated experience or familiarity of particular institutions with AIDS-related diseases (198,200). A lower in-hospital mortality of 12% has been observed in AIDS patients treated for pneumocystis pneumonia at hospitals with a high level of experience with AIDS patients (greater than 30 HIV-related discharges per 10,000 hospital discharges) compared with a 33% mortality rate at hospitals with less experience (less than 30 HIV-related discharges per 10,000 hospital discharges) (200).

PROPHYLAXIS

Chemoprophylaxis against pneumocystis pneumonia is termed primary if the goal is to prevent an initial episode. The risk of an HIV-infected person developing pneumocystis pneumonia is directly related to the degree and duration of suppression of CD4 counts (2). In a prospective study of 1,665 HIV-infected homosexual or bisexual adult males who did not have AIDS and had not received antipneumocystis prophylaxis, the risk of developing pneumocystis pneumonia within 6 months, based on the initial CD4 count/mm^3, was: greater than 350/mm^3, 0%; between 201 and 350/mm^3, 0.5%; and less than 200/mm^3, 8.4%. Fever and thrush were additional independent risk factors that directly correlated with an increased likelihood of developing pneumocystis pneumonia (78). Thus, prospective data have defined the period of highest susceptibility for HIV-infected patients.

The risk of an initial episode of pneumocystis pneumonia in HIV-infected patients has been assessed in a retrospective study of 119 episodes of pulmonary dysfunction in HIV-infected patients. Of the 49 cases of pneumocystis pneumonia that were reported, CD4 cells below 200/mm^3 were documented prior to the diagnosis of pneumocystis in 46 of 49 episodes (77). This finding substantiates the utility of using a CD4 count of approximately 200/mm^3 as a reasonable indicator of susceptibility to pneumocystis pneumonia among adults. Similar data substantiate the appropriateness of using a CD4 percent of 20 as a reasonable indicator of susceptibility. Generally, either when a patient's total CD4 count falls below 200/mm^3 *or* the percent falls below 20, the patient is considered susceptible.

While CD4 counts are important for indicating when primary prophylaxis is most useful, it is also important to note the limitations of CD4 counts. Splenectomized patients will have falsely elevated absolute CD4 counts, and thus the percentage of CD4 cells reflects the degree of immunosuppression more accurately than the absolute count (2). By contrast, some black and Hispanic patients may lack the OKT4 epitope. Since OKT4 monoclonal antibodies are used in many laboratories to identify T-helper cells, some blacks and Hispanics may appear to have no CD4 cells when, in fact, they have normal numbers of T-helper cells that can be identified by other monoclonal antibody markers such as Leu3 (201).

Prophylaxis is referred to as secondary prophylaxis if the objective is to prevent an episode of pneumocystis pneumonia in an AIDS patient who has already had at least one occurrence of pneumocystis pneumonia. Following an episode of pneumocystis pneumonia, AIDS patients who are given zidovudine without specific antipneumocystis prophylaxis have a likelihood of recurrence of 65% after 1 year (202). Based on the defined risk, antipneumocystis prophylaxis should be given to all patients who either have a CD4 cell count of less than 200/mm^3, or have had an episode of pneumocystis pneumonia, even if they are receiving zidovudine.

Trimethoprim–Sulfamethoxazole

In children with acute lymphoblastic leukemia, the clinical efficacy of chemoprophylaxis using trimethoprim (5 mg/kg/day)–sulfamethoxazole (25 mg/kg/day) orally in two divided doses every day, or 3 consecutive days per week, has been well established in controlled studies (17,203).

In the only published study assessing AIDS patients that was controlled, 30 patients with Kaposi's sarcoma were given trimethoprim (160 mg) and sulfamethoxazole (800 mg) twice daily as primary prophylaxis. None of the 30 patients in the treatment arm developed pneumocystis pneumonia compared with 16 of 30 patients in the untreated group (204). Prophylaxis had to be discontinued in 17% of patients in the treatment group due to adverse effects, which included severe erythroderma and fever (four patients) and persistent neutropenia (one patient). An additional 50% of treated patients suffered minor toxicities, the most common of which was erythroderma, but prophylaxis was able to be continued.

Recently a trial involving 310 patients who had no known severe intolerance to trimethoprim–sulfamethoxazole, and a history of recently completing therapy for pneumocystis pneumonia was completed (204a). Patients were randomly assigned to oral trimethoprim–sulfamethoxazole (one double-strength tablet daily) or aerosol pentamidine (300 mg once monthly by Respirgard nebulizer) in a nonblinded fashion. Relapse rates, based on intent-to-treat analysis and computed as 1-year actual rates, were 4.5% for oral trimethoprim–sulfamethoxazole and 18.5% for aerosol pentamidine. The frequencies of toxicities were, surprisingly, similar for the two groups, although significantly more patients had trimethoprim–sulfamethoxazole discontinued because of toxicity (27%) than had aerosol pentamidine discontinued (4%). Thus, trimethoprim–sulfamethoxazole was shown to be more effective but also more toxic as secondary prophylaxis for this group of patients.

The clinical efficacy and safety of trimethoprim–sulfamethoxazole as a secondary prophylaxis agent has also been assessed in less rigorous studies. In an open prospective clinical trial with a median follow-up of 8 months, only 3/50 (6%) who received trimethoprim 160 mg and sulfamethoxazole 800 mg daily had recurrence of pneumocystis compared with 11/16 (69%) patients who did not receive secondary prophylaxis (205). This dosing regimen was well tolerated; none of the patients discontinued prophylaxis due to adverse effects. The efficacy of trimethoprim–sulfamethoxazole has been suggested by several trials that did not have concurrent controls. In a small, open, uncontrolled clinical trial, AIDS patients received an intermittent dosing regimen of trimethoprim 160 mg and sulfamethoxazole 800 mg twice daily for 3 consecutive days as primary or secondary prophylaxis (206). No episodes of pneumocystis pneumonia were reported in the 34 patients receiving primary prophylaxis (mean follow-up of 10.9 months). One episode occurred (after 10 months) among the 19 patients who received secondary prophylaxis. No major toxicities were reported in the primary prophylaxis group, but secondary prophylaxis was discontinued in 3 of the 19 patients due to the development of rash (2 patients) and a threefold elevation of transaminase (1 patient). No significant bone marrow suppression was reported in any patient. Thus, trimethoprim–sulfamethoxazole appears to have a high degree of efficacy in those patients who can tolerate this drug. It is currently unclear, however, which dosing schedule is optimal to maximize efficacy and minimize intolerance.

Aerosol Pentamidine

Aerosol pentamidine has been a very popular antipneumocystis prophylactic regimen. Selective delivery of pentamidine to the lungs by the aerosolized route offers a number of potential advantages as a prophylactic agent. The overall clinical efficacy of aerosolized pentamidine is dependent on the particle size (described by mass median aerodynamic diameter, MMAD) produced by the delivery device; the amount of drug deposited in the intra-alveolar spaces; the patient's breathing pattern and position. Particle sizes of 1 to 2 μ (MMAD) result in more peripheral deposition and less airway deposition (207–210). Larger particle sizes have been associated with more airway deposition and bronchospasm (207).

In an unblinded, controlled community based trial, aerosolized pentamidine was administered by the Respirgard II nebulizer to 408 HIV-infected patients for both primary and secondary prophylaxis (211). These patients were randomly assigned to one of three dosage arms of inhaled pentamidine. Rates of occurrence of pneumocystis, with a median follow up of 10 months, were: 24% (33 of 135 patients) of the patients who received pentamidine 30 mg every two weeks; 19% (25 of 135 patients) of the patients who received 150 mg every two weeks, and 13% (18 of 139 patients) who received 300 mg every 4 weeks. The efficacy of 300 mg of aerosolized pentamidine administered once a month by the Respirgard nebulizer was statistically superior to the low-

est dosage regimen of 30 mg in preventing secondary pneumocystis pneumonia (211). Therapy was well tolerated; only 5.6% of the participants had to discontinue prophylaxis due to bronchospasm or cough. Overall, coughing and bronchospasm occurred in 36% and 11%, respectively, of patients.

Other studies have assessed aerosolized pentamidine using different delivery systems. The Fisoneb ultrasonic nebulizer has been assessed in a double-blinded, placebo-controlled study of 162 Canadian AIDS patients with previous episodes of pneumocystis pneumonia (212). Patients were randomized to either aerosolized pentamidine (60 mg every 2 weeks after initial loading) or placebo, and patients were followed prospectively for a mean of 6 months. Of the 78 patients in the placebo arm, 27 cases (35%) had recurrences compared with 5 of 84 (5.9%) in the treatment arm. Aerosol pentamidine delivered by this system was well tolerated: cough or bronchospasm was reported in 25% of pentamidine-treated patients. In no case did toxicities preclude continued administration of inhaled pentamidine. Pretreatment with albuterol (salbutamol) reduced the incidence of bronchospasm but not cough (105). A controlled trial in the United States that did not have a placebo arm provided confirmatory results for the efficacy of aerosol pentamidine delivered by the Fisoneb system (213).

An additional trial carried out in Europe has assessed the Ultraneb ultrasonic nebulizer for primary prophylaxis (214). Fifty-one patients were randomized to receive 4 mg/kg of pentamidine mesylate monthly (after initial loading) or placebo. Recurrences of pneumocystis pneumonia occurred in 9% of the treated group and 66% of the placebo group, after a mean follow-up of 10 and 8.7 months, respectively. The delivery system was also well tolerated.

In a trial of 223 patients randomized to either aerosol pentamidine delivered by Respirgard nebulizer or placebo for primary prophylaxis, the pneumocystis pneumonia rate was 6% in the former and 33% in the latter. This finding confirms the efficacy of aerosol pentamidine as primary prophylaxis (215).

Thus, several controlled trials and extensive uncontrolled experiences have demonstrated that aerosol pentamidine can be a safe and effective method of prophylaxis. Which delivery technique and dosing schedule are optimal in terms of efficacy, toxicity, and convenience has not as yet been clearly delineated. Both the Respirgard system and the Fisoneb system can be recommended based on extensive clinical experience.

It is important to reiterate that aerosolized pentamidine can have a dramatic influence on the clinical manifestations and diagnosis of pneumocystis pneumonia. Focal or upper lobe radiographic infiltrates, pulmonary cysts, and pneumothoraces have been reported and probably occur more often in association with aerosolized pentamidine than in patients on other forms of prophy-

TABLE 5. *Potential antipneumocystis prophylaxis regimens for HIV-infected patients*

Drug	Route	Dose	Interval	
Trimethoprim–	Oral	160 mg/800 mg	BID	(2, 3, or 7 days/week)
sulfamethoxazole	Oral	160 mg/800 mg	Qday	(2, 3, or 7 days/week)
Dapsone	Oral	25-50 mg	Q12	
Pyrimethamine–dapsone	Oral	25–50 mg/100–200 mg	Qweek	
Pentamidine (isethionate)				
Respigard	Aerosol	300 mg	QMonth	
Fisoneb	Aerosol	60 mg	Q2Weeks	

laxis or on no prophylaxis (112,114–116). For example, in one study, upper lobe infiltrates were noted radiographically in 38% of patients receiving aerosolized pentamidine compared with 7% not receiving aerosolized pentamidine (116). Extrapulmonary pneumocystosis also appears to occur with increased frequency in patients receiving aerosol pentamidine. In a retrospective analysis of 34 AIDS patients with extrapulmonary involvement, the organs affected included spleen, liver, lymph nodes, eyes, gastrointestinal tract, bone marrow, and thyroid (103). The diagnosis of pneumocystis pneumonia may be more difficult in patients receiving aerosol pentamidine. A significantly lower diagnostic yield of bronchoalveolar lavage (62%) was found in 21 patients receiving aerosol pentamidine prophylaxis compared with a 100% yield in 30 patients not receiving aerosol pentamidine (116). Similarly, sputum examinations have a significantly lower diagnostic yield (60%) in patients receiving aerosolized pentamidine compared with those (90%) on no chemoprophylaxis (135).

Other Investigational Agents

Most clinicians currently use either trimethoprim–sulfamethoxazole or aerosolized pentamidine for prophylaxis. Other prophylactic agents being assessed include dapsone (administered weekly at doses of 100 mg, 200 mg, or 300 mg orally). In one study that assessed dapsone 100–300 mg weekly, after a mean prospective follow-up of 9 months only 1 of 60 patients had a breakthrough episode of pneumocystis pneumonia (216). Adverse effects occurred in 13% (eight patients). Its long half-life and low cost makes dapsone a promising agent although its efficacy and toxicity need to be compared with trimethoprim–sulfamethoxazole. Fansidar (pyrimethamine 25 mg plus sulfadoxine 500 mg) has been assessed, but its toxicity appears high compared with its efficacy (217,218). Trials are currently being considered with BW566C80 and with clindamycin–primaquine.

Thus, there is an expanding list of potential regimens for antipneumocystis prophylaxis (Table 5). Many of these regimens clearly have some efficacy, although their efficacy and toxicity relative to trimethoprim–sulfa-

methoxazole or aerosol pentamidine are difficult to determine without additional data.

Currently, it is reasonable to initiate trimethoprim–sulfamethoxazole at a dose of one double-strength tablet (trimethoprim 320 mg and sulfamethoxazole 1,600 mg) once daily 7 days per week (or twice daily, three times a week, i.e., Monday-Wednesday-Friday) and to reserve aerosol pentamidine (300 mg once monthly by Respirgard nebulizer) for those who are intolerant of trimethoprim–sulfamethoxazole. For those few individuals who are intolerant of both trimethoprim–sulfamethoxazole and aerosol pentamidine, there are few well-studied alternatives, although a dapsone-containing regimen or oral BW566C80 might be tried.

REFERENCES

1. Murray JF, Garay SM, Hopewell PC, Mills J, Snider GL, Stover DG. NHLBI workshop summary: pulmonary complications of the acquired immune deficiency syndrome: an update. *Am Rev Respir Dis* 1987;135:504–9.
2. CDC. Guidelines for prophylaxis against *Pneumocystis carinii* pneumonia for persons infected with human immunodeficiency virus. *MMWR* 1989;38[S-5]:1–9.
3. Kovacs JA, Hiemenz JW, Macher AM, et al. *Pneumocystis carinii* pneumonia: a comparison between patients with the acquired immunodeficiency syndrome and patients with other immunodeficiencies. *Ann Intern Med* 1984;100:663–71.
4. Gordin FM, Simon GL, Mills J, Wofsy CB. Adverse reactions to trimethoprim–sulfamethoxazole in patients with acquired immune deficiency syndrome. *Ann Intern Med* 1984;100:495–9.
5. Gajdusek DC. *Pneumocystis carinii* as the cause of human disease: historical perspective and magnitude of the problem. In: Robbins JB, DeVita VT, Dutz W, eds. *Symposium on* Pneumocystis carinii *infection.* NCI Monograph 43. Washington, DC: National Cancer Institute, 1973:1–10.
6. Burke BA, Good RA. *Pneumocystis carinii* infection. *Medicine (Baltimore)* 1973;52:23–51.
7. Hughes WT. Pneumocystis pneumonia: a plague of the immunosuppressed. *Johns Hopkins Med J* 1978;143:184–92.
8. Young LS (ed). Pneumocystis carinii *pneumonia: pathology, diagnosis, treatment.* New York: Marcel Dekker, 1984.
9. Van der Meer G, Brug SC. Infection par pneumocystis chez l'homme et chez les animaux. *Ann Soc Belge Med Trop* 1942;22:301–7.
10. Duazier G, Willis T, Barnett RN. *Pneumocystis carinii* in an infant. *Am J Clin Pathol* 1956;26:787–93.
11. LeClair RA. Descriptive epidemiology of interstitial pneumocystic pneumonia: an analysis of 107 cases from the United States, 1955–1967. *Am Rev Respir Dis* 1969;99:542–7.
12. Walzer PD, Krogstad DJ, Rawson PG, Schultz MG. *Pneumocys-*

tis carinii pneumonia in the United States: epidemiologic, diagnostic, and clinical features. *Ann Intern Med* 1974;80:83–93.

13. Masur H, Jones TC. The interaction in vitro of *Pneumocystis carinii* with macrophages and L-cells. *J Exp Med* 1978; 147:157–70.

14. Hughes WT, Feldman S, Sanyal SK. Treatment of *Pneumocystis carinii* pneumonitis with trimethoprim–sulfamethoxazole. *Can Med Assoc J* 1975;112:47–50.

15. Hughes WT, Feldman S, Chaudhary SC, Ossi MJ, Cox F, Sanyal SK. Comparison of pentamidine isethionate and trimethoprim-sulfamethoxazole in the treatment of *Pneumocystis carinii* pneumonia. *J Pediatr* 1978;92:285–91.

16. Post C, Fakouhi T, Dutz W, Bandarizadeh B, Kohout EE. Prophylaxis of epidemic infantile pneumocystosis with a 20:1 sulfadoxine+pyrimethamine combination. *Curr Ther Res* 1971; 13:273–9.

17. Hughes WT, Kuhn S, Chaudhary S, et al. Successful chemoprophylaxis for *Pneumocystis carinii* pneumonitis. *N Engl J Med* 1977;297:1419–26.

18. Frenkel JK. *Pneumocystis jiroveci n. sp.* from man: morphology, physiology, and immunology in relation to pathology. *Natl Cancer Inst Monogr* 1976;43:13–30.

19. Hughes WT. Pneumocystis carinii *pneumonitis.* Boca Raton: CRC Press, 1987.

20. Ruffolo JJ, Cushion MT, Walzer PD. Techniques for examining *Pneumocystis carinii* in fresh specimens. *J Clin Microbiol* 1986;23:17–21.

21. Yoshida Y. Ultrastructural studies of *Pneumocystis carinii. J Protozool* 1989;36:53–60.

22. Barton EG Jr, Campbell WG Jr. Further observations on the ultrastructure of pneumocystis. *Arch Pathol* 1967;83:527–34.

23. Yoneda K, Walzer PD, Richey CS, Birk MG. *Pneumocystis carinii* freeze-fracture study of stages of the organism. *Exp Parasitol* 1982;53:68–76.

24. Grimes MM, LaPook JD, Bar MH, Wasserman HS, Dwork A. Disseminated *Pneumocystis carinii* infection in a patient with acquired immunodeficiency syndrome. *Hum Pathol* 1987; 18:307–8.

25. Matsumoto Y, Yoshida Y. Sporogony in *Pneumocystis carinii* synaptonemal complexes and meiotic nuclear divisions observed in precysts. *J Protozool* 1984;31:420–8.

26. Vavra J, Kucera K. *Pneumocystis carinii* delanoe, its ultrastructure and ultrastructural affinities. *J Protozool* 1970;17:463–83.

27. Yoshikawa H, Yoshida Y. Localization of silver deposits on *Pneumocystis carinii* treated with Gomori's methanamine silver nitrate stain. *Zentralbl Bakteriol Mikrobiol Hyg* [A] 1987; 264:363–72.

28. Matsumoto Y, Matsuda S, Tegoshi T. Yeast glucan in the cell wall of *Pneumocystis carinii. J Protozool* 1990;36:21S–22S.

29. Bedrossian CW. Ultrastructure of *Pneumocystis carinii.* A review of internal and surface characteristics. *Semin Diagn Pathol* 1989;6:212–37.

30. Carinii A, Maciel J. Ueber *Pneumocystis carinii. Zentralbl Bakteriol* [Orig A] 1916;77:46–50.

31. Campbell WG Jr. Ultrastructure of *Pneumocystis* in human lung. Life cycle in human pneumocystosis. *Arch Pathol* 1972; 93:312–24.

32. Vanek J, Jirovec O. Paritare Pneumonie. "Interstitile" Plasmazellenpneumonie der Fruhgeborenen, verursacht durch *Pneumocystis carinii. Zentralbl Bakteriol* [Orig A] 1952;158:120–7.

33. Pifer LL, Hughes WT, Murphy MJ Jr. Propagation of *Pneumocystis carinii* in vitro. *Pediatr Res* 1977;11:305–16.

34. Richardson JD, Queener SF, Bartlett M. Binary fission of *Pneumocystis carinii* trophozoites grown in vitro. *J Protozool* 1989;36:27S–29S.

35. Hughes WT, Bartley DL, Smith BM. A natural source of infection due to *Pneumocystis carinii. J Infect Dis* 1983;147:595–9.

36. Hendley JO, Weller TH. Activation and transmission in rats of infection with *Pneumocystis. Proc Soc Exp Biol Med* 1971;137:1401–4.

37. Frenkel JK, Good JT, Schultz JA. Latent *Pneumocystis* infection of rats, relapse and chemotherapy. *Lab Invest* 1966;15:1559–77.

38. Hughes WT. Natural mode of acquisition for de novo infection with *Pneumocystis carinii. J Infect Dis* 1982;145:842–8.

39. Walzer PD, Schnelle V, Armstrong D, Rosen PP. Nude mouse: a new experimental model for *Pneumocystis carinii* infection. *Science* 1977;197:177–9.

40. Bartlett MS, Queener SF, Jay MA, Durkin MM, Smith JW. Improved rat model for studying *Pneumocystis carinii* pneumonia. *J Clin Microbiol* 1987;25:480–4.

41. Gajdusek DC. *Pneumocystis carinii* etiologic agent of interstitial plasma cell pneumonia of premature and young infants. *Pediatrics* 1957;19:543.

42. Ivady G, Paldy L, Koltay M, Toth G, Kovacs Z. *Pneumocystis carinii* pneumonia. *Lancet* 1967;1:616–7.

43. Singer C, Armstrong D, Rosen PP, Schottenfeld D. *Pneumocystis carinii* pneumonia: a cluster of eleven cases. *Ann Intern Med* 1975;82:772–7.

44. Chusid MJ, Heyrman KA. An outbreak of *Pneumocystis carinii* pneumonia at a pediatric hospital. *Pediatrics* 1978;62:1031–5.

45. Ruebush TK, Weinstein RA, Baehner RL, et al. An outbreak of pneumocystis pneumonia in children with acute lymphocytic leukemia. *Am J Dis Child* 1978;132:143–8.

46. Baaz GR, Manfredi OL, Howard RG, Claps AA. *Pneumocystis carinii* pneumonia in three full-term siblings. *J Pediatr* 1970;76:767.

47. Post C, Dutz W, Nasarian I. Endemic *Pneumocystis carinii* pneumonia in South Iran. *Arch Dis Child* 1964;39:35–5.

48. Kovacs JA, Halpern JL, Lundgren B, Swan JC, Parrillo JE, Masur H. Monoclonal antibodies to *Pneumocystis carinii:* identification of specific antigens and characterization of antigenic differences between rat and human isolates. *J Infect Dis* 1989;159:1–2.

49. Walzer PD, Linke MJ. A comparison of the antigenic characteristics of rat and human *Pneumocystis carinii* by immunoblotting. *J Immunol* 1987;138:2257–65.

50. Shimizu A, Kimura F, Kimura S. Occurrence of *Pneumocystis carinii* in animals in Japan. *Jpn J Vet Sci* 1985;47:309–11.

51. Meuwissen JH, Tauber I, Leeuwenberg AD, Beckers PJ, Sieben M. Parasitologic and serologic observations of infection with *Pneumocystis* in humans. *J Infect Dis* 1977;136:43–9.

52. Pifer LL, Hughes WT, Stagno S, Woods D. *Pneumocystis carinii* infection: evidence for high prevalence in normal and immunosuppressed children. *Pediatrics* 1978;61:35–41.

53. Carinii A. Formas de eschizogonia de *Trypanosoma lewisii. Arch Soc Med Ci Sao Paulo* August 16, 1910;204.

54. Harmsen AG, Stankiewicz M. Requirement for CD4[+] cells in resistance to *Pneumocystis carinii* pneumonia in mice. *J Exp Med* 1990;172:937–45.

55. Edman JC, Kovacs JA, Masur H, Santi DV, Elwood HJ, Sogin ML. Ribosomal RNA sequence shows *Pneumocystis carinii* to be a member of the fungi. *Nature* 1988;334:519–22.

56. Allegra CJ, Kovacs JA, Drake JC, Swan JC, Chabner BA, Masur H. Activity of antifolates against *Pneumocystis carinii* dihydrofolate reductase and identification of a potent new agent. *J Exp Med* 1987;165:926–31.

57. Beverley SM, Ellenberger TE, Cordingley JS. Primary structure of the gene encoding the bifunctional dihydrofolate reductasethymidilate synthase of *Leishmania major. Proc Natl Acad Sci USA* 1986;83:2584–8.

58. Garrett CE, Coderre CE, Meek TD, et al. A bifunctional thymidilate synthetase-dihydrofolate reductase in protozoa. *Mol Biochem Parasitol* 1984;11:257–65.

59. Graves DC. Immunological studies of *Pneumocystis carinii. J Protozool* 1989;36:60–9.

60. Kovacs JA, Halpern JL, Swan JC, Moss J, Parrillo JE, Masur H. Identification of antigens and antibodies specific for *Pneumocystis carinii. J Immunol* 1988;140:2023–31.

61. Lundgren B, Lipschik GY, Kovacs JA. Purification and characterization of a major human *Pneumocystis carinii* surface antigen. *J Clin Invest* 1991;87:163–70.

62. Gigliotti F, Stokes DC, Cheatham AB, Davis DS, Hughes WT. Development of murine monoclonal antibodies to *Pneumocystis carinii. J Infect Dis* 1986;154:315–21.

63. Walzer PD, Stanforth D, Linke MJ, Cushion MT. *Pneumocystis carinii* immunoblotting and immunofluorescent analyses of serum antibodies during experimental rat infection and recovery. *Exp Parasitol* 1987;63:319–28.

64. Graves DC, McNabb SJ, Worley MA, Downs TD, Ivey MH.

Analyses of rat *Pneumocystis carinii* antigens recognized by human and rat antibodies by using western immunoblotting. *Infect Immun* 1986;54:96–103.

65. Peglow SL, Smulian AG, Linke MJ, et al. Serologic responses to *Pneumocystis carinii* antigens in health and disease. *J Infect Dis* 1990;161:296–306.

66. Walzer PD, Rutledge ME. Serum antibody responses to *Pneumocystis carinii* among different strains of normal and athymic mice. *Infect Immun* 1982;35:620–6.

67. Walzer PD, Rutledge ME. Humoral immunity in experimental *Pneumocystis carinii* infection. I. Serum and bronchial lavage fluid antibody responses in rats. *J Lab Clin Med* 1981;97:820–33.

68. Hofmann B, Odum N, Platz P, et al. Humoral responses to *Pneumocystis carinii* in patients with acquired immunodeficiency syndrome and in immunocompromised homosexual men. *J Infect Dis* 1985;152:838–40.

69. Blumenfeld W, Mandrell RE, Jarvis GA, Griffiss JM. Localization of host immunoglobulin G to the surface of *Pneumocystis carinii*. *Infect Immun* 1990;58:456–63.

70. Gigliotti F, Hughes WT. Passive immunoprophylaxis with specific monoclonal antibody confers partial protection against *Pneumocystis carinii* pneumonitis in animal models. *J Clin Invest* 1988;81:1666–8.

71. Pifer LL, Niell HB, Langdon SB, et al. Evidence for depressed humoral immunity to *Pneumocystis carinii* in homosexual males, commercial plasma donors, and patients with acquired immunodeficiency syndrome. *J Clin Microbiol* 1987;25:991–5.

72. Leggiadro RJ, Winkelstein JA, Hughes WT. Prevalence of *Pneumocystis carinii* pneumonitis in severe combined immunodeficiency. *J Pediatr* 1981;99:96–8.

73. Saulsbury FT, Bernstein MT, Winkelstein JA. *Pneumocystis carinii* pneumonia as the presenting infection in congenital hypogammaglobulinemia. *J Pediatr* 1979;95:559–61.

74. Pesanti EL. Interaction of cytokines and alveolar cells with *Pneumocystis carinii* in vitro. *J Infect Dis* 1991;163:611–6.

75. Hardy AM, Wajszczuk CP, Suffredini AF, Hakala TR, Ho M. *Pneumocystis carinii* pneumonia in renal-transplant recipients treated with cyclosporine and steroids. *J Infect Dis* 1984; 149:143–7.

76. Shelito J, Suzara V, Blumenfeld W, et al. A new model of Pneumocystis carinii infection in mice selectively depleted of helper T lymphocytes. *J Clin Invest* 1990;85:1686–92.

77. Masur H, Ognibene FP, Yarchoan R, et al. CD4 counts as predictors of opportunistic pneumonias in human immunodeficiency virus (HIV) infection. *Ann Intern Med* 1989;111:223–31.

78. Phair J, Muñoz A, Detels R, et al. The risk of *Pneumocystis carinii* pneumonia among men infected with human immunodeficiency virus type 1. *N Engl J Med* 1990;322:161–5.

79. Yoneda K, Walzer PD. Attachment of *Pneumocystis carinii* to type I alveolar cells studied by freeze-fracture electron microscopy. *Infect Immun* 1983;40:812–5.

80. Henshaw NG, Carson JL, Collier AM. Ultrastructural observations of *Pneumocystis carinii* attachment to rat lung. *J Infect Dis* 1985;151:181–6.

81. Long EG, Smith JS, Meier JL. Attachment of *Pneumocystis carinii* to rat pneumocytes. *Lab Invest* 1986;54:609–15.

82. Pottratz ST, Martin WJ II. Role of fibronectin in *Pneumocystis carinii* attachment to cultured lung cells. *J Clin Invest* 1990;85:351–6.

83. Limper AH, Martin WJ II. *Pneumocystis carinii*: inhibition of lung cell growth mediated by parasite attachment. *J Clin Invest* 1990;85:391–6.

84. Kernbaum S, Masliah J, Alcindor LG, Bouton C, Christol D. Phospholipase activities of bronchoalveolar lavage fluid in rat *Pneumocystis carinii* pneumonia. *Br J Exp Pathol* 1983; 64:75–80.

85. Walzer PD, Powell RD Jr, Yoneda K, Rutledge ME, Milder JE. Growth characteristics and pathogenesis of experimental *Pneumocystis carinii* pneumonia. *Infect Immun* 1980;27:928–37.

86. Yoneda K, Walzer PD. Interaction of *Pneumocystis carinii* with host lungs: an ultrastructural study. *Infect Immun* 1980; 29:692–703.

87. Lanken PN, Minda M, Pietra GG, Fishman AP. Alveolar response to experimental *Pneumocystis carinii* pneumonia in the rat. *Am J Pathol* 1980;99:561–88.

88. Yoneda K, Walzer PD. The effect of corticosteroid treatment on the cell surface glycocalyx of the rat pulmonary alveolus: relevance to the host-parasite relationship in *Pneumocystis carinii* infection. *Br J Exp Pathol* 1984;65:347–54.

89. Engelberg LA, Lerner CW, Tapper ML. Clinical features of *Pneumocystis* pneumonia in the acquired immune deficiency syndrome. *Am Rev Respir Dis* 1984;130:689–94.

90. Kales CP, Murren JR, Torres RA, Crocco JA. Early predictors of in-hospital mortality for *Pneumocystis carinii* pneumonia in the acquired immunodeficiency syndrome. *Arch Intern Med* 1987;147:1413–17.

91. Tuazon CU, Delaney MD, Simon GL, Witorsch P, Varma VM. Utility of gallium 67 scintigraphy and bronchial washings in the diagnosis and treatment of *Pneumocystis carinii* pneumonia in patients with the acquired immune deficiency syndrome. *Am Rev Respir Dis* 1985;132:1087–92.

92. Ognibene FP, Shelhamer J, Gill V, et al. The diagnosis of *Pneumocystis carinii* pneumonia in patients with the acquired immunodeficiency syndrome using subsegmental bronchoalveolar lavage. *Am Rev Respir Dis* 1984;129:929–32.

93. Sherman M, Levin D, Breidbart D. *Pneumocystis carinii* pneumonia with spontaneous pneumothorax. A report of three cases. *Chest* 1986;90:609–10.

94. Coulman CU, Greene I, Archibald RW. Cutaneous pneumocystosis. *Ann Intern Med* 1987;106:396–8.

95. Eng RH, Bishburg E, Smith SM. Evidence for destruction of lung tissues during *Pneumocystis carinii* infection. *Arch Intern Med* 1987;147:746–9.

96. Macher AM, Bardenstein DS, Zimmerman LE, et al. *Pneumocystis carinii* choroiditis in a male homosexual with AIDS and disseminated pulmonary and extrapulmonary *P. carinii* infection [Letter]. *N Engl J Med* 1987;316:1092–9.

97. Northfelt DW, Clement MJ, Safrin S. Extrapulmonary pneumocystosis: clinical features in human immunodeficiency virus infection. *Medicine* 1990;69:392–8.

98. Zaman MK, White DA. Serum lactate dehydrogenase levels and *Pneumocystis carinii* pneumonia. Diagnostic and prognostic significance. *Am Rev Respir Dis* 1988;137:796–800.

99. Garay SM, Greene J. Prognostic indicators in the initial presentation of *Pneumocystis carinii* pneumonia. *Chest* 1989;95:769–72.

100. Gallant JE, Enriquez RE, Cohen KL, Hammers LW. *Pneumocystis carinii* thyroiditis. *Am J Med* 1988;84:303–6.

101. Gherman CR, Ward RR, Bassis ML. *Pneumocystis carinii* otitis media and mastoiditis as the initial manifestation of the acquired immunodeficiency syndrome. *Am J Med* 1988;85:250–2.

102. Schinella RA, Breda SD, Hammerschlag PE. Otic infection due to *Pneumocystis carinii* in an apparently healthy man with antibody to the human immunodeficiency virus. *Ann Intern Med* 1987;106:399–400.

103. Raviglione MC. Exrapulmonary pneumocystosis: the first 50 cases. *Rev Infect Dis* 1990;12:1127–38.

104. Telzak EE, Cote RJ, Gold JWM, et al. Extrapulmonary *Pneumocystis carinii* infections. *Rev Infect Dis* 1990;12:380–6.

105. Montaner JS, Lawson LM, Gervais A, et al. Aerosol pentamidine for secondary prophylaxis of AIDS-related *Pneumocystis carinii* pneumonia. *Ann Intern Med* 1991;114:948–53.

106. Radin DR, Baker EL, Klatt EC, et al. Visceral and nodal calcification in patients with AIDS-related *Pneumocystis carinii* infection. *AJR* 1990;154:27–31.

107. DeLorenzo LJ, Huang CT, Maguire GP, Stone DJ. Roentgenographic patterns of *Pneumocystis carinii* pneumonia in 104 patients with AIDS. *Chest* 1987;91:323–7.

108. Israel HL, Gottlieb JE, Schulman ES. Hypoxemia with normal chest roentgenogram due to *Pneumocystis carinii* pneumonia. Diagnostic errors due to low suspicion of AIDS. *Chest* 1987;92:857–9.

109. Doppman JL, Geelhoed GW, De Vita VT. Atypical radiographic features in *Pneumocystis carinii* pneumonia. *Radiology* 1975;114:39–44.

110. Sirotzky L, Memoli V, Roberts J. Recurrent pneumocystis pneumonia with normal chest roentgenograms. *JAMA* 1978; 240:1513–5.

111. Smith DE, McLuckie A, Wyatt J, Gazzard B. Severe exercise hypoxaemia with normal or near-normal x-rays: a feature of *Pneumocystis carinii* infection. *Lancet* 1988;2:1049–52.

112. Abd AG, Nierman DM, Ilowite JS, Pierson RNJr, Bell AL Jr. Bilateral upper lobe *Pneumocystis carinii* pneumonia in a patient receiving inhaled pentamidine prophylaxis. *Chest* 1988; 94:329–31.

113. Hardy WD, Northfelt DW, Drake TA. Fatal, disseminated pneumocystosis in a patient with acquired immunodeficiency syndrome receiving prophylactic aerosolized pentamidine. *Am J Med* 1989;87:329–31.

114. Sepkowitz KA, Telzak EE, Gold WM, et al. Pneumothorax in AIDS. *Ann Intern Med* 1991;114:455–9.

115. Scannell KA. Pneumothoraces and *Pneumocystis carinii* pneumonia in two AIDS patients receiving aerosolized pentamidine. *Chest* 1990;97:479–80.

116. Jules-Elysee K, Stover D, Zaman M, et al. Aerosolized pentamidine: effect on the diagnosis and presentation of *Pneumocystis carinii* pneumonia. *Ann Intern Med* 1990;112:750–7.

117. Lowery S, Fallat R, Feigal DW, Montgomery AB, Berge J. Changing patterns of *Pneumocystis carinii* pneumonia on pentamidine aerosol prophylaxis. 4th International Conference on AIDS, Montreal, Canada, 1989;7167 (abst).

118. Murray JF, Felton CP, Garay SM, et al. Pulmonary complications of the acquired immunodeficiency syndrome. Report of a National Heart, Lung, and Blood Institute workshop. *N Engl J Med* 1984;310:1682–8.

119. Curtis J, Goodman P, Hopewell P. Noninvasive tests in the diagnostic evaluation for *P. carinii* pneumonia in patients with or suspected of having AIDS. *Am Rev Respir Dis* 1986; 133:A182(abst).

120. Barron TF, Birnbaum NS, Shane LB, Goldsmith SJ, Rosen MJ. *Pneumocystis carinii* pneumonia studied by gallium-67 scanning. *Radiology* 1985;154:791–3.

121. Coleman DL, Hattner RS, Luce JM, Dodek PM, Golden JA, Murray JF. Correlation between gallium lung scans and fiberoptic bronchoscopy in patients with suspected *Pneumocystis carinii* pneumonia and the acquired immune deficiency syndrome. *Am Rev Respir Dis* 1984;130:1166–9.

122. Stover DE, White DA, Romano PA, Gellene RA, Robeson WA. Spectrum of pulmonary diseases associated with the acquired immune deficiency syndrome. *Am J Med* 1985;78:429–37.

123. Hopewell PC, Luce JM. Pulmonary involvement in the acquired immunodeficiency syndrome. *Chest* 1985;87:104–12.

124. Cohen BA, Pomeranz S, Rabinowitz JG, et al. Pulmonary complications of AIDS: radiologic features. *AJR* 1984;143:115–22.

125. Gosey LL, Howard RM, Witebsky FG, et al. Advantages of a modified toluidine blue-O stain and bronchoalveolar lavage for the diagnosis of *Pneumocystis carinii* pneumonia. *J Clin Microbiol* 1985;22:803–7.

126. Hasleton PS, Curry A, Rankin EM. *Pneumocystis carinii* pneumonia: a light microscopical and ultrastructural study. *J Clin Pathol* 1981;34:1138–46.

127. Macher AM, Shelhamer J, MacLowry J, Parker M, Masur H. *Pneumocystis carinii* identified by gram stain of lung imprints. *Ann Intern Med* 1983;99:484–5.

128. Rorat E, Garcia RL, Skolom J. Diagnosis of *Pneumocystis carinii* pneumonia by cytologic examination of bronchial washings. *JAMA* 1985;254:1950–1.

129. Ghali VS, Garcia RL, Skolom J. Fluorescence of *Pneumocystis carinii* in Papanicolaou smears. *Hum Pathol* 1984;15:907–9.

130. Bigby TD, Margolskee D, Curtis JL, et al. The usefulness of induced sputum in the diagnosis of *Pneumocystis carinii* pneumonia in patients with the acquired immunodeficiency syndrome. *Am Rev Respir Dis* 1986;133:515–8.

131. Kovacs JA, Ng VL, Masur H, et al. Diagnosis of *Pneumocystis carinii* pneumonia: improved detection in sputum with use of monoclonal antibodies. *N Engl J Med* 1988;318:589–93.

132. Weiss LM, Udem SA, Salgo M, Tanowitz HB, Wittner M. Sensitive and specific detection of toxoplasma DNA in an experimental murine model: use of *Toxoplasma gondii*-specific cDNA and the polymerase chain reaction. *J Infect Dis* 1991;163:180–6.

133. Zaman MK, Wooten OJ, Suprahmanya B, Ankobiah W, Finch PJ, Kamholz SL. Rapid noninvasive diagnosis of *Pneumocystis carinii* from induced liquefied sputum. *Ann Intern Med* 1988;109:7–10.

134. Gill VJ, Evans G, Stock F, Parrillo JE, Masur H, Kovacs JA. Detection of *Pneumocystis carinii* by fluorescent-antibody stain using a combination of three monoclonal antibodies. *J Clin Microbiol* 1987;25:1837–40.

135. Levine SJ, Masur H, Gill VJ, et al. The effects of aerosolized pentamidine prophylaxis on the diagnosis of *Pneumocystis carinii* pneumonia by induced sputum examination in patients infected with the human immunodeficiency virus. *Am Rev Respir Dis* 1991;144:760–4.

136. Stover DE, White DA, Romano PA, Gellene RA. Diagnosis of pulmonary disease in acquired immune deficiency syndrome (AIDS). Role of bronchoscopy and bronchoalveolar lavage. *Am Rev Respir Dis* 1984;130:659–62.

137. Broaddus C, Dake MD, Stulbarg MS, et al. Bronchoalveolar lavage and transbronchial biopsy for the diagnosis of pulmonary infections in the acquired immunodeficiency syndrome. *Ann Intern Med* 1985;102:747–52.

138. Caughey G, Wong H, Gamsu G, Golden J. Nonbronchoscopic bronchoalveolar lavage for the diagnosis for *Pneumocystis carinii* pneumonia in the acquired immunodeficiency syndrome. *Chest* 1985;88:659–62.

139. Katz AS, Michelson EL, Stawick J, et al. Cardiac arrythmias: frequency during fiberoptic bronchoscopy and correlation with hypoxia. *Arch Intern Med* 1981;141:603–6.

140. Albertini RE, Harell JH, Kurihara N, et al. Arterial hypoxemia induced by fiberoptic bronchoscopy. *JAMA* 1974;230:1666–7.

141. Herf SM, Suratt PM, Arora NS. Deaths and complications associated with transbronchial lung biopsy. *Am Rev Respir Dis* 1977;115:708–11.

142. Zavala DC. Pulmonary hemorrhage in fiberoptic transbronchial biopsy. *Chest* 1976;70:584–8.

143. Pereira W, Kovnat DM, Khan MA, et al. Fever and pneumonia after flexible fiberoptic bronchoscopy. *Am Rev Respir Dis* 1975;112:59–64.

144. Mann JM, Altus CS, Webber CA, Smith PR, Muto R, Heurich AE. Nonbronchoscopic lung lavage for diagnosis of opportunistic infection in AIDS. *Chest* 1987;91:319–22.

145. Karpel JP, Prezant D, Appel D, Bezahler G. Endotracheal lavage for the diagnosis of *Pneumocystis carinii* pneumonia in intubated patients with acquired immune deficiency syndrome. *Crit Care Med* 1986;14:741–74.

146. Martin WR, Albertson TE, Siegel B. Tracheal catheters in patients with acquired immunodeficiency syndrome for the diagnosis of *Pneumocystis carinii* pneumonia. *Chest* 1990;98:29–32.

147. Schilling PJ, Vadhan-Raj S. Concurrent cytomegalovirus and pneumocystis pneumonia after fludarabine therapy for chronic lymphocytic leukemia. *N Engl J Med* 1990;323:833–4.

148. Ognibene FP, Masur H, Rogers P, et al. Nonspecific interstitial pneumonitis without evidence of *Pneumocystis carinii* in asymptomatic patients infected with human immunodeficiency virus (HIV). *Ann Intern Med* 1988;109:874–9.

149. Frenkel JK, Good JT, Shultz JA. Latent pneumocystis infection of rats, relapse, and chemotherapy. *Lab Invest* 1966;15:1559–77.

150. Kovacs JA, Allegra CJ, Swan JC, et al. Potent antipneumocystis and antitoxoplasma activities of piritrexim, a lipid-soluble antifolate. *Antimicrob Agents Chemother* 1988;32:430–3.

151. Lee BL, Medina I, Benowitz NL, Jacob P III, Wofsy CB, Mills J. Dapsone, trimethoprim, and sulfamethoxazole plasma levels during treatment of pneumocystis pneumonia in patients with the acquired immunodeficiency syndrome (AIDS): Evidence of drug interactions. *Ann Intern Med* 1989;110:606–11.

152. Rubin R, Swartz M. Trimethoprim-sulfamethoxazole. *N Engl J Med* 1980;303:426–31.

153. Lau WK, Young LS. Trimethoprim-sulfamethoxazole treatment of *Pneumocystis carinii* pneumonia in adults. *N Engl J Med* 1976;295:716–8.

154. Sattler FR, Cowan R, Nielsen DM, Ruskin J. Trimethoprim-sulfamethoxazole compared with pentamidine for treatment of *Pneumocystis carinii* pneumonia in the acquired immunodeficiency syndrome. A prospective, noncrossover study. *Ann Intern Med* 1988;109:280–7.

155. Dantonio RG, Johnson DB, Winn RE, van Dellen AF, Evans

ME. Effect of folinic acid on the capacity of trimethoprim-sulfamethoxazole to prevent and treat *Pneumocystis carinii* pneumonia in rats. *Antimicrob Agents Chemother* 1986;29:327–9.

156. Wharton JM, Coleman DL, Wofsy CB, et al. Trimethoprim-sulfamethoxazole or pentamidine for *Pneumocystis carinii* pneumonia in the acquired immunodeficiency syndrome. *Ann Intern Med* 1986;105:37–44.

157. Haverkos HW. Assessment of therapy for *Pneumocystis carinii* pneumonia: PCP therapy project group. *Am J Med* 1984; 76:501–8.

158. Small CB, Harris CA, Friedland GH, Klein RS. The treatment of *Pneumocystis carinii* pneumonia in the acquired immunodeficiency syndrome. *Arch Intern Med* 1985;145:837–40.

159. Jaffe HS, Abrams DI, Ammann AJ, Lewis BJ, Golden JA. Complications of co-trimoxazole in treatment of AIDS-associated *Pneumocystis carinii* pneumonia in homosexual men. *Lancet* 1983;2:1109–11.

160. Pearson RD, Hewlett EL. Pentamidine for the treatment of *Pneumocystis carinii* and other protozoal diseases. *Ann Intern Med* 1985;103:782–6.

161. Navin TR, Fontaine RE. Intravenous versus intramuscular administration of pentamidine [Letter]. *N Engl J Med* 1984;311:1701–2.

162. Mallory DL, Parrillo JE, Bailey KR, et al. Cardiovascular effects and safety of intravenous and intramuscular pentamidine isethionate. *Crit Care Med* 1987;15:503–5.

163. Conte JE, Chernoff D, Feigal DW, Joseph P, McDonald C, Golden JA. Intravenous or inhaled pentamidine for treating *Pneumocystis carinii* pneumonia in AIDS. *Ann Intern Med* 1990;113:203–9.

164. Soo Hoo GW, Mohsenifar Z, Meyer RD. Inhaled or intravenous pentamidine therapy for *Pneumocystis carinii* pneumonia in AIDS. *Ann Intern Med* 1990;113:195–202.

165. Conte JE Jr, Upton RA, Phelps RT, Wofsy CB, Zurlinden E, Lin ET. Use of a specific and sensitive assay to determine pentamidine pharmacokinetics in patients with AIDS. *J Infect Dis* 1986;154:923–9.

166. Bibler M, Chou T, Toltzis R, et al. Recurrent ventricular tachycardia due to pentamidine-induced cardiotoxicity. *Chest* 1988; 94:1302–6.

167. Waskin H, Stehr Green JK, Helmick CG, Sattler FR. Risk factors for hypoglycemia associated with pentamidine therapy for *Pneumocystis* pneumonia. *JAMA* 1988;260:345–7.

168. Antoniskis D, Larsen RA. Acute, rapidly progressive renal failure with simultaneous use of amphotericin B and pentamidine. *Antimicrob Agents Chemother* 1990;34:470–2.

169. Hughes WT. Comparison of dosages, intervals, and drugs in the prevention of *Pneumocystis carinii* pneumonia. *Antimicrob Agents Chemother* 1988;32:623–5.

170. Hughes WT, Smith BL. Efficacy of diaminodiphenylsulfone and other drugs in murine *Pneumocystis carinii* pneumonitis. *Antimicrob Agents Chemother* 1984;26:436–40.

171. Kramer P, Glader B, Li T. Mechanism of methemoglobin formation by diphenylsulfones. *Biochem Pharmacol* 1972;21:1265–75.

172. Medina I, Mills J, Leoung G, et al. Oral therapy for *Pneumocystis carinii* pneumonia in the acquired immunodeficiency syndrome—a controlled trial of trimethoprim-sulfamethoxazole versus trimethoprim-dapsone. *N Engl J Med* 1990;323:776–82.

173. Leoung GS, Mills J, Hopewell PC, Hughes W, Wofsy C. Dapsone-trimethoprim for treatment of *Pneumocystis carinii* pneumonia in the acquired immunodeficiency syndrome. *Ann Intern Med* 1986;105:45–8.

174. Queener SF, Bartlett MS, Richardson JD, Durkin MM, Jay MA, Smith JW. Activity of clindamycin with primaquine against *Pneumocystis carinii* in vitro and in vivo. *Antimicrob Agents Chemother* 1988;32:807–13.

175. Brzosko W, Madalinski K, Nowoslawski A. Immunofluorescent and immunoelectrophoretic reactions in children with pneumonia caused by *Pneumocystis carinii*. *Med Dosw Mikrobiol* 1967;19:373–80.

176. Hughes WT, McNabb PC, Makres TD. Efficacy of trimethoprim and sulfamethoxazole in the prevention and treatment of *Pneumocystis carinii* pneumonitis. *Antimicrob Agents Chemother* 1974;5:289–93.

177. Toma E, Fournier S, Poisson M, Morisset R, Phaneuf D, Vega C. Clindamycin with primaquine for *Pneumocystis carinii* pneumonia. *Lancet* 1989;1:1046–8.

178. Ruf B, Pohle HD. Clindamycin/primaquine for *Pneumocystis carinii* pneumonia. *Lancet* 1989;2:626–7.

179. Allegra CJ, Kovacs JA, Drake JC, Swan JC, Chabner BA, Masur H. Activity of antifolates against *Pneumocystis carinii* dihydrofolate reductase and identification of a potent new agent. *J Exp Med* 1987;165:926–31.

180. Queener SF, Bartlett MS, Jay MA, Durkin MM, Smith JW. Activity of lipid-soluble inhibitors of dihydrofolate reductase against *Pneumocystis carinii* in culture and in a rat model of infection. *Antimicrob Agents Chemother* 1987;31:1323–7.

181. Allegra CJ, Chabner BA, Tuazon CU, et al. Trimetrexate for the treatment of *Pneumocystis carinii* pneumonia in patients with the acquired immunodeficiency syndrome. *N Engl J Med* 1987;317:978–85.

182. Kovacs JA, Allegra CJ, Kennedy S, et al. Efficacy of trimetrexate, a potent lipid-soluble antifolate in the treatment of rodent *Pneumocystis carinii* pneumonia. *Am J Trop Med Hyg* 1988; 39:491–6.

183. Sattler FR, Allegra CJ, Verdegem TD, et al. Trimetrexate-leucovorin dosage evaluation study for treatment of *Pneumocystis carinii* pneumonia. *J Infect Dis* 1990;161:91–6.

184. Fallon J, Kovacs J, Allegra C, et al. A pilot study of piritrexim (PTX) with leucovorin (LCV) for the treatment of pneumocystis pneumonia. 6th International Conference on AIDS, San Francisco, June, 1990; ThB399(abst).

185. Hughes WT, Gray VL, Gutteridge WE, Latter VS, Pudney M. Efficacy of a hydroxynaphthoquinone, 566C80, in experimental *Pneumocystis carinii* pneumonitis. *Antimicrob Agents Chemother* 1990;34:225–8.

186. Fallon J, Kouacs J, Hughes W, et al. A preliminary evaluation of 566C80 for the treatment of *pneumocystis* pneumonia in patients with AIDS. *N Eng J Med* 1991;325:1534–8.

186a. Hughes W, Leung G, Kramer F, et al. Comparison of JGGC80 and trimethoprim sulfamethoxazole (TMP-SME) for treatment of p. carinii pneumonitis (PCP). Submitted to the 8th International Conference on AIDS.

187. Schmatz DM, Romancheck MA, Pittarelli LA, et al. Treatment of *Pneumocystis carinii* pneumonia with 1,3-β-glucan synthesis inhibitors. *Proc Natl Acad Sci USA* 1990;87:5950–4.

188. Hughes WT, Smith McCain BL. Effects of sulfonylurea compounds on *Pneumocystis carinii*. *J Infect Dis* 1986;153:944–7.

189. Jones SK, Hall JE, Allen MA, et al. Novel pentamidine analogs in the treatment of experimental *Pneumocystis carinii* pneumonia. *Antimicrob Agents Chemother* 1990;34:1026–30.

190. Smith JW, Bartlett MS, Queener SF, et al. *Pneumocystis carinii* pneumonia therapy with 9-deazainosine in rats. *Diagn Microbiol Infect Dis* 1987;7:113–8.

191. Bartlett MS, Queener SF, Tidwell RR, et al. 8-Aminoquinolones from the Walter Reed Army Institute for Research for treatment and prophylaxis of pneumocystis pneumonia in the rat models. *Antimicrob Agents Chemother* 1991;35:277–82.

192. Gagnon S, Boota AM, Fischl MA, Baier H, Kirksey OW, La Voie L. Corticosteroids as adjunctive therapy for severe *Pneumocystis carinii* pneumonia in the acquired immunodeficiency syndrome—double-blind, placebo-controlled trial. *N Engl J Med* 1990;323:1444–50.

193. Montaner JSG, Lawson LM, Levitt N, Belzberg A, Schechter MT, Ruedy J. Oral corticosteroids prevent early deterioration in patients with moderately severe AIDS-related *Pneumocystis carinii* pneumonia. *Ann Intern Med* 1990;113:14–20.

194. Bozzette SA, Sattler FR, Chiu J, et al. A controlled trial of early adjunctive treatment with corticosteroids for *Pneumocystis carinii* pneumonia in the acquired immunodeficiency syndrome. *N Engl J Med* 1990;323:1451–7.

195. Masur H (chairman). Consensus statement on the use of corticosteroids as adjunctive therapy for pneumocystis pneumonia in the acquired immunodeficiency syndrome. *N Engl J Med* 1990;323:1500–4.

196. el Sadr WM, Simberkoff MS. Survival and prognostic factors in severe *Pneumocystis carinii* pneumonia requiring mechanical ventilation. *Am Rev Respir Dis* 1988;137:1264–7.

197. Wachter RM, Russi MB, Bloch DA, Hopewell PC, Luce JM. *Pneumocystis carinii* pneumonia and respiratory failure in AIDS. *Am Rev Respir Dis* 1991;143:251-6.

198. Smith RL, Levine SM, Lewis ML. Prognosis of patients with AIDS requiring intensive care. *Chest* 1989;96:857-61.

199. Wachter RM, Luce JM, Turner J, Volberding P, Hopewell PC. Intensive care of patients with the acquired immunodeficiency syndrome. Outcome and changing patterns of utilization. *Am Rev Respir Dis* 1986;134:891-6.

200. Bennett CL, Garfinkle JB, Greenfield S, et al. The relation between hospital experience and in-hospital mortality for patients with AIDS-related PCP. *JAMA* 1989;261:2975-9.

201. Bach M, Phan-Dinh-Tuy F, Bach J, et al. Unusual phenotypes of human inducer T cells as measured by OKT4 and related monoclonal antibodies. *J Immunol* 1981;127:980-2.

202. Fischl MA, Parker CB, Pettielli C, et al. A randomized controlled trial of reduced daily dose of zidovudine in patients with the acquired immunodeficiency syndrome. *N Engl J Med* 1990;323:1010-25.

203. Hughes WT, Rivera GK, Schell MJ, Thornton D, Lott L. Successful intermittent chemoprophylaxis for *Pneumocystis carinii* pneumonitis. *N Engl J Med* 1987;316:1627-32.

204. Fischl MA, Dickinson GM, La Voie L. Safety and efficacy of sulfamethoxazole and trimethoprim chemoprophylaxis for *Pneumocystis carinii* pneumonia in AIDS. *JAMA* 1988;259:1185-9.

204a.Hardy WD, Feinberg J, Finkelstein D, et al. Trimethoprim sulfamethoxazole versus pentamidine for secondary prophylaxis of pneumocystis carinii pneumonia in AIDS patients. Submitted for publication.

205. Pedersen C, Lungren J, Nielsen T, Andersen W. The outcome of *Pneumocystis carinii* pneumonia in Danish patients with AIDS. *Scand J Infect Dis* 1989;21:375-80.

206. Raviglione M, Nash E, Cortes H, et al. Intermittent co-trimoxazole prophylaxis against *Pneumocystis carinii* pneumonia. *Lancet* 1990;336:180.

207. O'Doherty MJ, Thomas S, Page C, et al. Differences in relative efficacy of nebulizers for pentamidine administration. *Lancet* 1988;2:1283-6.

208. O'Doherty MJ, Thomas SH, Page CJ, Bradbeer C, Nunan TO, Bateman NT. Does inhalation of pentamidine in the supine position increase deposition in the upper part of the lung. *Chest* 1990;97:1343-8.

209. Baskin M, Abd G, Ilowite J. Regional deposition of aerosolized pentamidine. *Ann Intern Med* 1990;113:677-83.

210. Monk J, Benfield P. Inhaled pentamidine. An overview of its pharmacological properties and review of its therapeutic use in *Pneumocystis carinii* pneumonia. *Drugs* 1990;39:741-56.

211. Leoung GS, Feigal DW Jr, Montgomery AB, et al. Aerosolized pentamidine for prophylaxis against *Pneumocystis carinii* pneumonia—the San Francisco Community Prophylaxis Trial. *N Engl J Med* 1990;323:769-75.

212. Montaner JSG, Lawson LM, Gervais A. Aerosol pentamidine for secondary prophylaxis of AIDS-related *Pneumocystis carinii* pneumonia. *Ann of Intern Med* 1991;114:948-53.

213. Murphy R, Lavelle J, Allan J, et al. Aerosol pentamidine prophylaxis following *Pneumocystis carinii* pneumonia in AIDS patients. *Am J Med* 1991;90:418-26.

214. Girard PM, Landman R, Gaudebout C, et al. Prevention of pneumocystis carinii pneumonia relapse by pentamidine aerosol in zidovudine-treated AIDS patients. *Lancet* 1989;1:1348-52.

215. Hirschel B, Lazzanin A, Chopard P, et al. A controlled study of inhaled pentamidine for primary prevention of *Pneumocystis carinii* pneumonia. *N Eng J Med* 1991;324:1079-83.

216. Hughes WT, Kennedy W, Dugdale M, et al. Prevention of *Pneumocystis carinii* pneumonitis in AIDS patients with weekly dapsone. *Lancet* 1990;336:1066.

217. Hardy D, Wolfe PR, Gottlieb MS. Long term follow-up of fansidar prophylaxis for *Pneumocystis carinii* pneumonia in patients with AIDS. 1st International Conference on AIDS, Atlanta, Georgia, 1985.

218. Fischl MA, Dickinson GM. Fansidar prophylaxis of *Pneumocystis* pneumonia in the acquired immunodeficiency syndrome [Letter]. *Ann Intern Med* 1986;105:629-62.

AIDS and Other Manifestations of HIV Infection,
Second Edition, Edited by Gary P. Wormser.
Raven Press, Ltd., New York © 1992.

CHAPTER 17

Cytomegalovirus Infections in AIDS

Robert L. Yarrish

Some of the earliest reports of the acquired immune deficiency syndrome noted a remarkable frequency and severity of cytomegalovirus (CMV) infection among affected patients (1–5). Along with the already known "immunosuppressive" properties of CMV (6,7) and the extremely high prevalence of CMV infection among homosexual men (8), this led to speculation that CMV might even be the cause of the new syndrome. Discovery of the human immunodeficiency virus (HIV) soon put an end to such speculation, but as the epidemic has unfolded, CMV infection has clearly established itself as one of the most common and devastating complications of AIDS (9–14). At the same time, AIDS, more than any other condition, has allowed us to view the full pathogenic potential of CMV in the adult patient, and it constantly reminds us of the deficiencies in our diagnostic and therapeutic approaches to this virus. This has fortunately proved to be a strong impetus for research on CMV infection, and it is probably no coincidence that the greatest strides in anti-CMV chemotherapy have been made only since the appearance of AIDS.

THE VIRUS

Human CMV belongs taxonomically to the *Herpesviridae* and has the same basic structure as the other members of this family. The complete enveloped virus ranges from 180 to 250 nm in diameter, making it second in size only to the poxviruses among human viral pathogens. The large CMV genome—approximately 150×10^6 daltons—is sufficient to code for over 30 proteins and imparts great genetic and antigenic complexity to the virus. One consequence of this is the variability found among CMV strains. Although all appear to share at least 80% DNA homology (15), it is uncommon to

find two strains with identical nucleic acid composition except when they can be linked epidemiologically (16). Strains also seem to vary in their antigenicity (17,18) and in their cytopathic effects in tissue culture (19); but these differences have been difficult to classify, and there are still no widely accepted serotyping or biotyping systems for CMV.

Although it is morphologically indistinguishable from other herpesviruses, human CMV shares no cross-reactive antigens with any of them and has enough biological peculiarities to set it apart as the prototype of its own subfamily, the *Betaherpesvirinae*. Other members of this group include the cytomegaloviruses of mice, guinea pigs, and swine; and all share properties of slow focal growth in culture and narrow host range. Human CMV, in fact, causes in vivo infection only in humans and productive in vitro infection only in human fibroblasts. Infected cells typically show enlargement, or *cytomegaly*, and both nuclear and cytoplasmic inclusion bodies. Although these inclusions consist mainly of virions and viral proteins (20), it is likely that much of the cytomegaly stems from the stimulation of host cell nucleic acid and protein synthesis that accompanies CMV infection (21,22).

An important property that CMV shares with other herpesviruses is *latency;* that is, the ability of the virus to persist indefinitely in the infected host in a quiescent state, subject to reactivation by appropriate stimuli. Unlike the other human herpesviruses, CMV has no clearly identified site of latency; but CMV antigens have been detected in several types of cells—including pulmonary alveolar and renal tubular epithelium, hepatocytes and Kupffer cells, splenic lymphocytes and macrophages, cerebral astrocytes, and endothelial cells in several organs—in apparently normal tissues of patients dying of trauma or acute illnesses not related to CMV (23). Transmission of CMV via transfused blood components (24) and renal allografts (25,26) also suggests that at least some white blood cells and some cells in the kidney may

R. L. Yarrish: St. Vincent's Hospital and Medical Center of New York, New York, New York 10011.

harbor latent virus. Spontaneous reactivation of CMV infection in healthy individuals, such as commonly occurs with herpes simplex and varicella-zoster infections, is not well documented; but reactivation does occur reliably when cytotoxic immunosuppressive therapy is instituted after organ transplantation (25,27,28). This, along with the observation that fulminant CMV infections almost always occur in settings of profoundly depressed cell-mediated immunity (e.g., AIDS, bone marrow transplantation), is generally felt to indicate that cell-mediated immunity is the host's main defense against the virus. That such infections run a malignant course despite the presence of neutralizing antibody has been cited as evidence that humoral immunity plays little role in CMV infection; but antibodies may in fact benefit the host in certain situations. One study of premature infants who acquired CMV via blood transfusions strongly suggests that although maternal antibodies may not prevent infection, they almost certainly diminish its severity (29). Similar conclusions about the role of humoral immunity may be drawn from studies showing that administration of CMV hyperimmune plasma or globulin, or even commercially available intravenous immunoglobulin, may substantially decrease morbidity from CMV infection when given prophylactically to bone marrow and kidney transplant recipients (30–33).

EPIDEMIOLOGY

Since CMV infection persists for the life of the host, the presence of antibody to the virus is considered a reliable indicator of infection. The prevalence of CMV infection in a population can therefore be assessed by seroepidemiologic means. One of the most comprehensive studies of this kind found that the frequency of CMV complement-fixing antibodies among healthy blood donors ranged from 40 to 60% in Europe, North America, and Australia, and from 80 to 100% in South America, Asia, and Africa (34). While clearly demonstrating the widespread occurrence of CMV infection among inhabitants of developing nations, this study probably underestimates the eventual probability of infection for residents of the industrialized world. It is well known that children in developing countries tend to acquire their CMV infections early in life (35), with almost universal infection, and hence a flat age-specific prevalence curve, by the end of childhood. In the developed countries, however, the age-specific prevalence of CMV infection appears to increase throughout life, with periods of rapid acquisition during early adulthood in white, middle-class populations and during adolescence among nonwhite individuals (36,37). It should also be noted that the complement fixation test used in most of the earlier studies of CMV prevalence is not highly sensitive (38). For example, when we recently tested sera from over 400 middle-aged and elderly adults (mean age 60 yr) in Philadelphia, the

complement fixation test showed a CMV seroprevalence of 66%, while the more sensitive indirect immunofluorescence test showed a prevalence of 95% (unpublished data). In any case, it seems likely that CMV infection is an almost inescapable fact of life for people throughout the world.

As might be expected for a virus of such ubiquity, there are many ways in which CMV transmission is known or suspected to occur. Transmission via blood transfusions (24) and renal allografts (25,26) is well documented but obviously accounts for a very small proportion of infections. Vertical transmission—that is from mother to child—is certainly much more common, especially in the Third World, where the prevalence of infection among young mothers is very high. Transplacental transmission leading to congenital infection occurs in approximately 0.5 to 2.5% of live births, varying little from study to study and region to region (39). Intrapartum transmission via infected cervical secretions (40,41) and postpartum transmission via breast milk (42) are probably much more common routes of infection, however. For the infant who avoids vertical CMV transmission, opportunities for horizontal transmission abound, especially for children cared for in group settings. Unusually high rates of infection have been observed in day care centers and Israeli kibbutz nurseries (43–45), and although the route of transmission is not certain, transfer of virus via saliva on toys and hands seems most likely (43–46).

Acquisition of CMV by older children and adults is common in the developed countries but more difficult to explain than infection in early childhood. The acceleration in the rate of CMV infection seen in adolescence and early adulthood has two likely explanations. One is transmission via urine and saliva from young children to their parents (47). The other likely mode of CMV acquisition in this age group, and the one that is more relevant to the majority of AIDS patients, is venereal transmission. CMV has been cultured from cervical secretions of up to 13% of women attending venereal disease clinics in England and the United States (48,49). Likewise, CMV may be present in semen in large quantities, but this appears to be uncommon in the general population. In two studies from the United States and Canada, semen specimens from several hundred men, including college students, prison inmates, professional blood donors, venereal disease patients, and fertility clinic patients, were cultured for CMV, and between 0.6 and 10% of specimens from the different groups were positive (50,51). Excretion of CMV in the semen of homosexual men may be much more common, however, as suggested by several studies in which over one-third of specimens from a total of 227 individuals were culture-positive (51–54).

Evidence that such virus-laden fluids actually transmit CMV during sexual intercourse is circumstantial but highly suggestive. In developed nations, the age at which people most commonly contract CMV infection seems to coincide with the age of peak sexual activity, and several studies have noted a strong correlation between CMV infection and other sexually transmitted diseases (48,49,55). There is also a report of an outbreak of CMV mononucleosis in a group of college students in which sex partners were involved while roommates were spared (56). The best evidence for venereal transmission probably comes from a study of women attending a venereal disease clinic in Seattle and their sex partners (57). CMV was cultured from the cervix in 46 (13.3%) of 347 women, and 64% of the women were seropositive for CMV. Testing of 58 male sex partners showed that 74% of partners of CMV-seropositive women were seropositive themselves, as opposed to only 31% of partners of seronegative women. In addition, restriction endonuclease analysis of CMV isolates from three pairs of sex partners showed that, in two pairs, both partners were infected by the same CMV strain, almost certainly a result of transmission of the virus from one partner to the other.

Venereal transmission probably accounts for the unusual epidemiology of CMV infection in homosexual men. Studies of this group typically show CMV seropositivity rates of 90% or more, which is significantly higher than the 40–70% seen in age-matched controls (8,54,58). In addition, uninfected but sexually active homosexual men seem to acquire CMV infection rapidly. One study of such men found that 71% of those who were originally seronegative became infected during 9 months of follow-up (53), suggesting an extraordinary intensity of CMV transmission among the study population. This would be consistent with observations that homosexual men are much more likely than controls to have anti-CMV IgM antibody (58,59), which is most commonly found in recent infections (60) and might be expected to occur more often in a setting of frequent infection and reinfection. It is also of note that the first instances of active infection with more than one strain of CMV were documented in homosexual men with AIDS (61,62); and more recent data suggest that multiple CMV infections in homosexual men, regardless of HIV status, may be relatively common (63). Two studies suggest that the major route of CMV transmission in this group is anal receptive intercourse (52,54), a finding consistent with the high rate of seminal CMV excretion observed in homosexual men.

Epidemiologic data on CMV infection in other AIDS risk groups are less abundant. One small study of AIDS patients who were intravenous drug users or of Haitian origin showed them to be 80 and 100% seropositive for CMV, respectively, but with antibody titers significantly lower than those of homosexual men (64). This finding would be consistent with infection early in life but without primary infection or reinfections during adulthood. Differences in recentness and intensity of infection may explain why homosexual men seem to suffer more mor-

bidity from CMV infections than do patients from other risk groups (65; R. E. Stahl, *unpublished data*).

The epidemiology of CMV in hemophiliacs, a much smaller AIDS risk group, is also not well documented. Two studies involving over 170 American hemophiliacs found an age-specific prevalence of CMV infection similar to that of the general population (66,67), and another smaller study found no significant differences between hemophiliacs and controls in terms of CMV seropositivity and antibody titers (68). These data indicate that, unlike hepatitis B and HIV, CMV is not transmitted efficiently by factor VII concentrate or cryoprecipitate. One might also infer that because of a lower prevalence of infection, hemophiliac AIDS patients would suffer less morbidity from CMV than would members of other AIDS risk groups, and this may, in fact, be the case (65).

MANIFESTATIONS OF CMV INFECTION

The most common manifestation of CMV infection is no disease at all. There is no syndrome associated with the latent infections that prevail among most people, and the primary infections that precede them appear, in the vast majority of cases, either to be asymptomatic or to pass unrecognized in the succession of "benign viral illnesses" that punctuate everyone's medical history. The only indication that such infections have occurred is the presence of anti-CMV antibody. The syndromes associated with the minority of cases that are symptomatic have been well described in several excellent reviews (69–72) and include cytomegalic inclusion disease of the newborn and CMV mononucleosis. The latter is similar in many ways to the more common infectious mononucleosis caused by Epstein-Barr virus, but it usually occurs in young adults and features lymphadenopathy and exudative pharyngitis in only a minority of cases (71).

An illness similar to CMV mononucleosis has been described in patients 1–2 months after cardiac surgery and labeled the "postperfusion syndrome" (73). It has since been observed in other types of multiply transfused patients and is felt to result from CMV transmission by blood. The exact cell that carries the virus is unknown but is probably some type of leukocyte. Transfusion of leukocytes from CMV-seropositive donors appears to transmit CMV infection to bone marrow transplant recipients (74,75), and, conversely, use of only frozen deglycerolized red cells seems to carry less risk of transmission than the use of whole blood (76). Although the postperfusion syndrome, like CMV mononucleosis, is a benign, self-limited illness in most cases, certain patients, such as heavily immunosuppressed transplant recipients (70), may suffer severe morbidity or even death from transfusion-related CMV infections. One study of bone marrow transplant recipients suggests that such problems can be avoided in CMV-seronegative patients by using only blood products from seronegative donors (77). Whether this practice might also benefit the small number of CMV-seronegative AIDS patients is not known.

Primary CMV infection in the immunocompetent host, when symptomatic at all, usually features poorly localized symptoms such as fever, fatigue, and malaise. Clinical involvement of specific organs is not uncommon, however. Some degree of hepatitis is seen in the majority of cases of CMV mononucleosis, but it also occurs independently of the rest of the syndrome. Hepatitis caused by CMV is usually accompanied by selective elevation of the serum alkaline phosphatase and may show granulomata on histopathology, both unusual findings for a viral hepatitis (78,79). Liver failure and significant jaundice fortunately are rare. Skin rashes occur in approximately one-third of CMV mononucleosis cases and are usually described as maculopapular (71). A wide variety of other lesions, including erythema nodosum (80), have been described, however. Most other types of organ-specific involvement—for example, encephalitis, myo- and pericarditis, pneumonia, gastrointestinal ulceration, and retinitis—are very uncommon in the normal host (71). One condition that deserves special mention is the Guillain-Barré syndrome, a type of polyneuritis that occurs sporadically and is usually idiopathic. Various studies have used viral cultures and serology to implicate CMV in 10–25% of cases, making this virus one of the best documented etiologies of this poorly understood disease (81,82). One patient, in fact, experienced two cases of CMV-related Guillain-Barré syndrome—one after vaccination with an attenuated CMV strain and the second after infection transmitted via a kidney transplant (83).

Despite its benign behavior in most infected individuals, CMV is a well-established cause of serious and frequently lethal disease in persons with impaired cell-mediated immunity. The pathology of CMV infection in AIDS patients exemplifies this perfectly, but AIDS has certainly not provided our first opportunity to observe the pathogenic potential of the virus. By the early 1960s it was known that CMV-induced lesions could be found at autopsy in patients with various types of malignancies (84,85). Both localized and disseminated disease were seen, with the former most commonly involving the gastrointestinal tract with ulceration, diarrhea, and hemorrhage, and the latter most often affecting the lungs, adrenals, and liver. The spleen, pancreas, kidneys, and myocardium were also occasionally involved, suggesting that in an appropriately compromised host, CMV was capable of causing disease in almost any organ. CMV infections superimposed on malignancy initially appeared to be rare (86,87) but subsequently seem to be increasing in frequency, perhaps coincident with the use of more immunosuppressive chemotherapy regimens, especially in the treatment of lymphomas (88).

Since the late 1960s, CMV has also emerged as one of the major problems of renal transplant patients, and this group in particular has taught us many important lessons about the biology of CMV infection. CMV latency and its propensity to reactivate during immunosuppression were first convincingly demonstrated in renal transplant patients (89). In this setting it also became clear that the virus could be transmitted even in its latent phase, as is the case when a renal allograft from a healthy donor is followed by active infection in the graft recipient (25). Most infections in this group are asymptomatic, and the most common CMV-related illness is a nonspecific febrile syndrome sharing many clinical features with CMV mononucleosis (70). Unfortunately, this is sometimes accompanied by severe neutropenia, which may lead to serious bacterial and fungal superinfections (90,91). Next most common is an often fatal interstitial pneumonia. A problem peculiar to this group is a form of glomerulopathy, which affects the allograft and is characterized by necrosis and enlargement of endothelial cells and accumulation of mononuclear cells in glomerular capillaries (92). Clinically, it is difficult to distinguish from allograft rejection; but unlike rejection, it responds to decreased immunosuppression.

In renal transplant patients, primary CMV infections —that is, those occurring in individuals with no evidence of previous infection—are much more likely to cause symptoms and serious disease than are reinfections or reactivated latent infections (93,94). This strongly suggests that preexisting immunity may help to moderate infection, even during immunosuppression. However, after allogeneic bone marrow transplantation, where ablation of the patient's immune response is a necessary part of the procedure, CMV immunity prior to transplantation does not appear to affect the course of post-transplant CMV infection (75,95). Bone marrow transplant recipients, in fact, appear to be more vulnerable to severe morbidity from CMV infection than are other transplant patients, and CMV is the most common cause of infectious death following allogeneic marrow transplantation (96). Most of the mortality results from CMV pneumonia, which occurs in approximately 15% of patients and until recently had a case fatality rate approaching 90%. The strong correlation between this condition and graft-versus-host disease, along with its relative rarity in AIDS patients, has led to suggestions that CMV pneumonia in bone marrow transplant recipients results mainly from a cytotoxic T-cell response to viral antigens being expressed on cells in the lung, and not from direct viral damage to those cells (97).

Other CMV-associated problems in transplant recipients include ulcerative disease of the gastrointestinal tract, hepatitis, arthritis, retinitis, leukopenia, and prolonged fevers. It is interesting to note that many of these problems, which were previously viewed mainly as complications of transplantation, are now encountered relatively commonly in AIDS patients and that these two groups of patients show striking similarities in their responses to CMV infection.

CMV AS A CAUSE OF IMMUNOSUPPRESSION

As the above discussion is meant to suggest, the most serious forms of CMV infection occur almost exclusively in patients with impaired cell-mediated immunity. That CMV itself may cause significant immunosuppression, and thereby render some of these already vulnerable individuals even more susceptible to opportunistic infections, is a more recent idea and one that remains somewhat speculative. The first investigations into CMV immunosuppression were to some extent prompted by earlier studies, which found impairment of cell-mediated immunity in mice infected with murine cytomegalovirus (98). Hirsch and co-workers subsequently showed that lymphocytes from patients with CMV mononucleosis showed decreased responsiveness to mitogens (99) and various herpesvirus antigens. This phenomenon correlated with increased suppressor activity, which appeared to be mediated by monocytes and T lymphocytes (7,100). The same group later demonstrated that, in the acute phase of CMV mononucleosis, patients show a reversal of the normal helper/suppressor T-cell ratio, with both decreased numbers of helper cells and increased numbers of suppressor cells (101).

The basis for the changes in lymphocyte function observed during CMV mononucleosis is still poorly understood, but the excessive numbers of suppressor cells generated are probably at least partly responsible. Carney et al. found that when cultures of mononuclear cells from CMV mononucleosis patients were depleted of OKT8+ lymphocytes, proliferative and cytotoxic functions of the remaining cells increased significantly (102). A direct effect of CMV on lymphocyte function is also possible, however. Human lymphocytes and monocytes can be infected with CMV in vitro (103) and in vivo (104), apparently resulting in expression of some viral proteins but without production of whole virus. Monocytes that are infected appear to be normal in terms of their ability to activate lymphocytes by presenting CMV antigens to them, while infected lymphocytes are less responsive to mitogens than are uninfected cells (105).

As provocative as these studies are, evidence that CMV causes clinically significant immunosuppression has been difficult to find. Despite the abnormal performance of their lymphocytes in vitro, CMV mononucleosis patients seem to have no special susceptibility to opportunistic infections. Patients with more serious forms of CMV infection, on the other hand, are usually already immunosuppressed, and it has been difficult to show that the virus makes their immune function any worse. In an attempt to do so, Chatterjee et al. followed 35 renal

allograft recipients and found that mortality and severe morbidity from opportunistic infections were limited to those patients who were CMV-seronegative prior to transplantation (106). Of the four patients who died of fungal infections, three had documented active CMV infections. The authors concluded that primary CMV infections in the post-transplant period render patients more susceptible to opportunistic fungal infections, while reactivated CMV infections appear to have no such effect. In another study, Schooley et al. found that among 18 recipients of cadaveric kidney grafts, both primary and reactivated CMV infections occurring in the first 3 months after transplantation were invariably followed by inversions of the helper/suppressor ratio similar to those seen in CMV mononucleosis patients (107). Among ten patients who received kidneys from living related donors, and were therefore less heavily immunosuppressed than the cadaver graft recipients, T-cell subset inversions also occurred, but only in the presence of symptomatic CMV infection. In both groups, CMV-related inversions of the helper/suppressor ratio were associated with an increased frequency of opportunistic infections.

Although they involve relatively small numbers of patients, these two prospective studies provide some evidence that CMV infection leads to clinically significant immunosuppression in patients who are receiving immunosuppressive therapy after organ transplantation. Might a similar scenario occur in patients who are immunosuppressed as a result of HIV infection? If so, the presence or absence of active CMV infection could to some extent account for the differences in susceptibility to various opportunistic infections observed among AIDS patients.

Assessing the possible role of CMV as a cofactor in the development of AIDS has been complicated by the fact that the vast majority of individuals infected with HIV also show serologic or virologic evidence of CMV infection. A prospective study of HIV-positive homosexual men found that CMV antibody titers greater than 300 mg/dl showed a significant correlation with progression to AIDS (108), but this finding may well reflect reactivation of latent CMV infection due to HIV-induced immunosuppression rather than a more rapid progression of HIV infection somehow mediated by CMV. Somewhat more suggestive is a recent study of HIV-seropositive hemophiliacs, which included substantial numbers of CMV-seronegative patients (109). In this study, the patients with CMV infection appeared to have a 2.5-fold greater risk of progression to AIDS than did patients without CMV infection during 1.3–9 years of follow-up. Survival curves also showed that the CMV-seropositive patients progressed to AIDS more rapidly than did the seronegative patients.

If CMV really does act as a cofactor in the development of AIDS, it may be a result of the "immunosuppressive" properties of the virus described above. These may weaken host defenses against both HIV itself and the opportunistic infections that define most cases of AIDS. In addition, in vitro data suggest that CMV and HIV enhance each other's replication when they coinfect the same cell (110). A possible in vivo correlate of this phenomenon may be found in two recently reported cases of simultaneous primary infection with both CMV and HIV in intravenous drug users. The clinical disease experienced by both patients was more severe than would be expected from acute infection with either virus, and both showed unusually early and severe declines in their CD4 cell counts (111). In any case, the role of a CMV as a cofactor in AIDS remains to be established with certainty; but it also remains quite plausible and now enjoys some support from laboratory, epidemiologic, and clinical observations.

CMV INFECTIONS IN AIDS PATIENTS

Whether or not CMV has any role in the pathogenesis of AIDS, its significance as a major cause of morbidity and mortality among AIDS patients is undeniable. Defining the frequency of CMV infections and their complications during the course of AIDS, however, is extremely difficult. Signs and symptoms of CMV infection are often nonspecific and subtle, and most infections go undiagnosed during the life of the patient (10,11,13). As a result, data based on clinical case reporting may severely underestimate the importance of CMV in AIDS. A 1986 update from the Centers for Disease Control, for instance, reported CMV infection in only 7% of AIDS cases (112); and that same year, serious CMV infection was diagnosed in 7.4% of 761 patients attending the AIDS clinic at San Francisco General Hospital (113). In contrast, postmortem studies typically find evidence of CMV infection in well over 50% of patients dying with AIDS, making CMV by far the most common opportunistic pathogen associated with AIDS at autopsy (10–14,114). These studies also reveal that AIDS-related CMV infections tend to be disseminated and may at times involve almost every organ.

Pathology caused by CMV in AIDS ranges from occasional scattered cytomegalic cells with little or no surrounding inflammation to large areas of necrosis with a prominent neutrophilic or mononuclear cell response. The pattern and severity of involvement vary widely from patient to patient, and even from organ to organ in the same patient (12). Clinical manifestations of these infections do not always correlate well with histopathology and range from no apparent disease to life-threatening dysfunction of major organ systems. It is quite likely that CMV is also a frequent cause of nonspecific febrile illness in AIDS, but this has been difficult to document since these patients so commonly have several different active infections at once.

Table 1 presents a list of manifestations of CMV infection, which have been described in connection with AIDS. Although the virus may attack virtually any organ, not all the lesions observed have definite clinical significance. The most important ones will be discussed below.

Retinitis

CMV retinitis is both the most common intraocular infection and the most important cause of visual impairment in AIDS. Although this condition is familiar to most clinicians who care for AIDS patients, its precise frequency is difficult to deduce from published data. It was diagnosed in 5.7% of AIDS clinic patients seen at San Francisco General Hospital in 1986 (113), and Klatt and Shibata found it in approximately 5% of 164 autopsies of AIDS patients (14). Two smaller autopsy series, which were concerned specifically with ocular pathology, found it in 20 and 26% of AIDS cases (115,116). Thus CMV retinitis is probably much less common than CMV-related pathology at many other sites, such as the adrenals, gastrointestinal tract, and brain. Because its cardinal symptom—loss of vision—is so distressing and its physical findings are so distinctive, however, CMV retinitis is the manifestation of CMV infection most likely to be diagnosed during life in AIDS patients. It may present as the patient's first opportunistic infection, but it more

TABLE 1. *Sites of CMV infection in AIDS patients*

Established clinical significance
    Disseminated infection
    Retina
    Colon
    Esophagus
    Stomach
    Small bowel
    Gallbladder and bile ducts
    Brain
    Spinal cord
    Peripheral nerves and nerve roots
    Skin
    Epididymis
Probable clinical significance
    Lungs
    Adrenal glands
Questionable clinical significance
    Liver
    Pancreas (islets and acini)
    Kidneys
    Spleen
    Lymph nodes
    Heart
    Testes
    Prostate
    Thyroid gland
    Parathyroid glands
    Pituitary gland

typically occurs in the later stages of HIV infection. Holland et al. found a median interval of 9 months from the diagnosis of AIDS to the diagnosis of CMV retinitis, and the median survival after diagnosis of retinitis was 5 months for all patients and 7 months for those treated with ganciclovir (117).

The clinical findings and course of CMV retinitis are treated in detail elsewhere in this volume and in two recent reviews (118,119), and they need not be repeated here. The primary pathologic process involves one or more foci of retinal necrosis with varying degrees of associated inflammation. Depending on the location of these foci, visual loss may range from clinically inapparent to profound. Involved areas of the retina remain atrophic and functionless even after the disease is arrested by antiviral therapy. Most patients will nonetheless experience substantial improvement in their vision during treatment, probably due to resolution of vitreous inflammation and macular edema. Retinal detachment originating in atrophic areas is a serious late complication that may occur despite complete control of active disease.

Of all CMV-related lesions, retinitis is probably the most responsive to antiviral therapy. Making the correct diagnosis is therefore extremely important; and this can be done without invasive procedures. Clinicians should routinely perform ophthalmoscopy on all AIDS patients, and patients with abnormal findings or visual symptoms should be immediately referred to an ophthalmologist. If findings suggest CMV retinitis, induction therapy with ganciclovir or foscarnet should be initiated, followed by a lower maintenance dose to be continued indefinitely. Regular ophthalmoscopic examinations should continue for patients on maintenance therapy since a high percentage will show breakthrough after initial stabilization or slowly progressive "smoldering" disease (120,121). Most of these patients, fortunately, appear to benefit from a repeat course of induction therapy (121).

Gastrointestinal Ulceration

After retinitis, ulcerative disease of the gastrointestinal tract is the next most commonly diagnosed complication of CMV infection in AIDS, probably due to the accessibility of lesions for biopsy. It has been reported from 2.2% of AIDS patients at San Francisco General Hospital (113), but autopsy series suggest a higher frequency between 5 and 50% (10,12,14).

The colon and terminal ileum seem to be the gastrointestinal sites most commonly affected by CMV. In the mildest form of the disease, viral inclusions are found in the endothelial, epithelial, or mesenchymal cells of the gut with little or no necrosis or inflammation. Such lesions are often found in patients with no history of gastrointestinal symptoms, and it is difficult to determine if they are ever clinically significant. More advanced disease involves mucosal ulceration, which may be extensive and often shows bacterial or fungal superinfection (12,122). This stage is often severely symptomatic, with chronic, watery diarrhea that is difficult to distinguish from the other types of diarrhea that so commonly affect AIDS patients. One helpful differential feature may be abdominal pain, which tends to be more prominent with CMV than with the other causes of diarrhea (123). Weight loss and wasting may be profound, and some patients eventually die from refractory diarrhea (12,124). In its most severe form, CMV infection may lead to focal or extensive hemorrhagic necrosis in the terminal ileum, colon, or rectum. The underlying lesion in such cases appears to be a vasculitis of the bowel wall caused by CMV infection of endothelial cells (12,125), and reported outcomes include bowel perforation, peritonitis, and massive hemorrhage necessitating emergency colectomy (10,126).

Both roentgenographic and endoscopic findings in CMV enterocolitis are quite nonspecific. Barium enema usually shows mucosal granularity, superficial erosions, and effacement of haustral markings resembling, to some extent, ulcerative colitis (127); but terminal ileitis resembling Crohn's disease has also been reported (128). Lesions seen endoscopically may also be confused with inflammatory bowel disease (124), pseudomembranous colitis (125), or even Kaposi's sarcoma (127). Diagnosis therefore rests on histopathology of biopsies taken from suspicious lesions.

CMV involvement of the upper gastrointestinal tract also occurs in AIDS, but it appears to be less common than colonic disease. Patients with CMV esophagitis typically present with some combination of odynophagia, dysphagia, and substernal chest pain (129–131). Discrete, shallow ulcers involving the mid-to-distal esophagus are the usual endoscopic findings; but diffuse mucosal erosion may be seen, and one case even featured a large exophytic mass resembling a tumor (132). The underlying pathology is once again vasculitis (129, 131,132). CMV-related ulcerations have also been reported in the gastric fundus and antrum and in the duodenum (124,131). Such lesions are usually clinically silent, but postprandial vomiting and epigastric pain have been reported with antral disease (131). CMV lesions of the upper gastrointestinal tract, like those of the colon, have no specific radiographic or endoscopic features; and biopsy with microscopic examination is required to distinguish them from similar lesions caused by candida, herpes simplex, gastroesophageal reflux, and peptic ulcer disease.

The experience with ganciclovir therapy in CMV gastrointestinal disease in AIDS is still somewhat limited, but two series comprising a total of over 100 patients suggest that clinical response rates of 75% or better can be expected (133,134). Relapse is likely if chronic maintenance therapy is not given (134), however, and median survival is around 6 months even for patients who respond to therapy (132,134).

Hepatobiliary Disease

Although hepatitis is a common feature of CMV mononucleosis in normal hosts, it is rarely reported in AIDS-related CMV infections. In one autopsy series, which concentrated specifically on hepatic pathology, over 80% of cases had systemic CMV infection, but only 6% showed liver involvement (134). This was limited to scattered viral inclusions present mainly in Kupffer cells, but also in some hepatocytes, endothelial cells, and biliary epithelial cells. Several other series describe similar findings in between 2 and 20% of cases, but in none of them does CMV hepatitis appear to be a clinically important entity (9,12–14,122).

One of the most surprising lesions associated with CMV infection in AIDS is acalculous cholecystitis (135,136). The first three patients reported with this complication all underwent laparotomy for severe, progressive abdominal pain, which had been present for several months in two patients. Gallbladder disease was suspected preoperatively in each case because of findings such as right upper quadrant tenderness, abnormal oral cholecystogram, and elevated alkaline phosphatase; and in one case each, ultrasonography and computed tomography strongly suggested a diagnosis of acalculous cholecystitis. Cholecystectomy was performed on all three; and gallbladder pathology showed extensive mucosal ulceration and, in one case, areas of transmural necrosis. Numerous CMV inclusions were found in epithelial cells in all three gallbladders, and two also showed endothelial involvement. In one case, CMV appeared to be the cause of all pathology, and postmortem examination several months later showed a necrotizing cholangitis due to CMV in the common bile duct and major intrahepatic ducts. Simultaneous infections with *Candida albicans* and cryptosporidium in the other cases make the role of CMV difficult to determine. In any case, it is important for clinicians to be aware of the syndrome of acalculous cholecystitis in AIDS since timely surgery may relieve the patient's pain and avoid rupture of the gallbladder.

An additional biliary syndrome—papillary stenosis with sclerosing cholangitis—has been linked to CMV in five cases on the basis of histopathology of the ampulla of Vater or adjacent tissue (137). In other cases, however, cryptosporidium was the only pathogen identified. These patients generally seemed to benefit from endoscopic sphincterotomy, but low-grade fever and pain persisted in many. A trial of ganciclovir might therefore be warranted in such patients if an ampullary biopsy suggests CMV.

Infections of the Nervous System

Central nervous system (CNS) infection with CMV is relatively common in AIDS patients. Autopsy studies report it in between 6 and 33% of cases (10,12,14,138), and, in one such study, CMV encephalitis was ranked as the third most common cause of death, after CMV pneumonia and *Pneumocystis carinii* pneumonia (12).

The microscopic lesion most commonly described in CMV encephalitis is the microglial nodule, a focal, dense collection of glial cells that may or may not include a few cytomegalic cells (138–140). Even in the absence of diagnostic cytopathology, CMV antigens and DNA can be detected in neurons and glial cells of most nodules using immunocytochemical or *in situ* hybridization techniques (138,140). These lesions are most abundant in the cerebral and spinal gray matter but may be found in white matter as well. The next most common lesions are microscopic infarctions, which are presumed to result from occlusion of microvasculature by enlarged, CMV-infected cells (138). Infection appears to progress by direct extension from both types of lesion, and foci up to several centimeters in diameter may eventually develop (138). Other lesions attributed to CMV include areas of demyelination in the brain and spinal cord (141), vasculitis of larger vessels (142), leptomeningitis (140), and choroid plexitis (140). In many cases, CMV infection appears to show an affinity for the ventricular ependyma and to spread centrifugally from there (138,140).

Relating the histopathologic lesions of CMV encephalitis and myelitis to signs and symptoms is difficult for several reasons. There is no characteristic cerebrospinal fluid profile; and imaging studies such as CT and MRI typically show nonspecific findings or no abnormalities, despite florid microscopic pathology (140,143). Consequently, nearly all cases are diagnosed at autopsy, and reports rarely detail the clinical signs and symptoms. In addition, the majority of cases of CMV encephalitis occur along with other CNS infections (138,140), of which HIV encephalopathy is the most common. An early study of the neurologic complications of AIDS described a syndrome of "subacute encephalitis" characterized by slowly progressive cognitive changes, lethargy, and psychomotor retardation, and terminating in severe dementia (144). Microglial nodules were found in the brains of most patients dying with this syndrome, and the disease was attributed to CMV. This attribution probably deserves reexamination, however, in light of the more recently recognized neuropathic properties of HIV itself. Striking focal neurologic abnormalities, including hemi- and quadraparesis, gaze palsies, and sensory deficits, have been described in connection with necrotizing lesions of CMV encephalitis involving critical areas of the brain and internal capsule, but such cases appear to be rare (145–147). Clinical and radiographic findings are usually not diagnostic, although the uncommon finding of diffuse periventricular enhancement on CT scanning should strongly suggest CMV encephalitis (143). Viral cultures of the cerebrospinal fluid are not helpful since they appear to be neither sensitive nor specific for histopathologically verifiable infection (140,148). Rigorous attempts at tissue diagnosis of accessible lesions are probably justified, however, since patients with CMV encephalitis may show clinical improvement when treated with ganciclovir (140,145).

In addition to its role as a CNS pathogen, CMV is probably an important cause of inflammatory radiculopathy and neuropathy in AIDS patients. Characteristic inclusions of CMV, with associated inflammation and necrosis, have been found in both ventral and dorsal nerve roots and in cranial and peripheral nerves (148–151). CMV infection of Schwann cells appears to cause much of the pathology in these lesions (149), which present clinically as either focal or extensive motor and sensory deficits. The association of CMV with dorsal root ganglionitis makes it possible that the virus may be involved in the painful peripheral neuropathy of AIDS patients. One study found a close temporal relationship between the onset of painful symptoms and the appearance of CMV infection at other sites in 9 of 12 patients, but histopathologic confirmation of CMV neuropathy was not obtained (152). Nerve roots, of course, are not available for biopsy, and the focality of the lesions in CMV neuropathy probably renders a single peripheral nerve biopsy unsatisfactory as a diagnostic procedure (150). Cerebrospinal fluid culture for CMV is also not reliably positive (148,149). Thus CMV radiculopathy and neuropathy are likely to remain important syndromes that are rarely diagnosed during life, and a trial of antiviral therapy should probably be considered in patients with suggestive signs and symptoms and any evidence of active CMV infection. Unfortunately, the early experience with such an approach in advanced disease has not been encouraging (153).

Pneumonitis

Pulmonary infection caused by CMV is extremely common in AIDS patients, but its clinical importance is not at all clear. Several AIDS autopsy studies rank CMV pneumonitis as a major cause of death, and giant cells typical of CMV infection are found postmortem in the lungs of 50–90% of AIDS patients (10,11,13,14,122, 154). The frequency with which CMV pneumonitis is reported during life, however, is somewhat lower and is highly dependent on the diagnostic criteria that are used. Early clinical series, which based their diagnoses on either histopathology *or* positive viral cultures of lung tissue, found CMV pneumonitis in between 17 and 56% of AIDS patients with symptomatic pulmonary disease (155–157); but in over two-thirds of these cases, CMV was found along with *Pneumocystis carinii* or some other pathogen. A more recent study from the National Institutes of Health, which required both the presence of cytomegalic cells in a biopsy specimen and the absence of any concurrent pathogen or neoplasm as diagnostic criteria, found CMV pneumonitis in only 8 (7%) of 119 episodes of AIDS-related pulmonary disease (158).

Whatever its true incidence, the significance of CMV pneumonitis as a clinical syndrome in AIDS patients is now being critically reappraised. Behind this reappraisal lies the hypothesis, derived mainly from experience in bone marrow transplantation, that assigns a major role in the pathogenesis of CMV pneumonitis to cell-mediated immunity (97,159). If this hypothesis is correct, it is quite possible that most AIDS patients are simply unable to mount the sort of immune response that so commonly produces CMV pneumonitis in bone marrow transplant recipients. Observational support for the relative lack of importance of CMV as a pulmonary pathogen in AIDS comes from three recent studies, all of which found CMV in a high percentage of bronchoalveolar lavage (BAL) fluids from AIDS patients, but none of which found any association between the presence of the virus and the clinical findings or outcome of the pulmonary disease (160–162). In one of these studies, some patients with positive viral cultures were treated with ganciclovir, but they showed no survival advantage over patients who received no antiviral therapy (160). In another, none of 31 patients with positive cultures received antiviral therapy, yet all but 2 of these recovered, including 6 in whom CMV was the only pathogen identified (162).

These studies strongly suggest that CMV is not a major pulmonary pathogen in AIDS and that viral cultures for CMV have little or no utility in AIDS patients with pneumonia. It remains possible, however, that in a subset of profoundly immunosuppressed individuals, CMV may cause disease in the lungs by direct cytopathic effect and vascular compromise, much as it does in other organs. This would be consistent with the NIH group's finding that rigorously diagnosed CMV pneumonitis is essentially limited to patients whose CD4 cells constitute less than 5% of their total circulating lymphocytes (158).

The lack of generally accepted diagnostic criteria and the high frequency of concurrent infections make it difficult to ascribe a set of "typical" pathologic findings to CMV pneumonitis in AIDS. CMV inclusions have been observed in pulmonary endothelial and epithelial cells and in pulmonary macrophages, however, sometimes in association with alveolar neutrophilic exudates and interstitial lymphocytic infiltrates (12,14). One report also describes diffuse alveolar damage in connection with most cases (154). The clinical syndrome of CMV pneumonitis also awaits precise definition, but it is likely to resemble that of the other interstitial pneumonitides, with dyspnea, nonproductive cough, hypoxemia, and diffuse infiltrates on chest x-ray as cardinal findings (156).

For the time being, CMV pneumonitis should probably be diagnosed only in patients who have suggestive clinical illness, histopathologic findings of CMV infection in lung tissue, and no evidence of other pulmonary infection. The value of ganciclovir therapy in such patients has yet to be established, but there is little rationale for withholding it in the face of severe illness. In bone marrow transplant recipients, whose disease probably has a somewhat different pathogenesis, ganciclovir alone has not been effective in the treatment of CMV pneumonitis, but most patients seem to respond to a combination of ganciclovir and high-dose immune globulin (163).

Adrenalitis

After the lungs, the organ most commonly affected by CMV in AIDS patients is the adrenal gland. CMV adrenalitis has been reported in 40–90% of AIDS patients coming to autopsy (10,12,14,122,164), and some suggest that it is a special feature of AIDS since it occurs much more frequently in this condition than in other immunodeficiency states (165). It has also been noted that adrenal necrosis caused by CMV in AIDS patients is often disproportionate to damage caused by the virus in other organs (122), suggesting that the adrenals are especially vulnerable to attack by CMV in AIDS.

The pathology of CMV adrenalitis in AIDS has been well described. Nuclear and cytoplasmic inclusions may be seen in endothelial, medullary, and cortical epithelial cells; but disease tends to be worst in the medulla and in many cases is entirely limited to this part of the gland (122,164). Involvement varies from focal, single-cell necrosis in the medulla to hemorrhagic infarction of the entire gland (166). In most cases, however, cortical destruction is less than 50% (164). Cellular infiltration appears to differ according to the extent of the necrosis, with lymphocytes and plasma cells in areas of sparse involvement, but with neutrophils predominating in zones of confluent necrosis.

The clinical significance of CMV adrenalitis in AIDS has not yet been convincingly established. Hypoadrenalism occurs in AIDS patients but has not been definitely linked to any well-defined adrenal pathology (167). Conversely, other studies note that patients in whom subtotal adrenal necrosis was found at autopsy showed no obvious findings of hypoadrenalism during life (12,164). It is likely that in most cases of adrenalitis, enough functional cortex remains to avoid frank adrenal insufficiency; but this is obviously not the case in pa-tients with bilateral total adrenal necrosis. Especially in the terminal phases of AIDS, many patients exhibit fever, hypotension, hyponatremia, and other abnormalities that are consistent with hypoadrenalism, but corticotrophin stimulation tests, which would allow a definitive diagnosis, are rarely performed. When eight patients with documented cytomegalovirus end-organ disease along with postural hypotension, low-grade fevers, and fatigue were subjected to such testing at San Francisco General Hospital, three had subnormal responses (113). Physicians caring for AIDS patients should thus be alert to the possibility of hypoadrenalism and perhaps be more aggressive in testing adrenal function so that steroid replacement can be undertaken on a more timely and rational basis.

Other Sites

CMV disease of the thyroid, parathyroid, and pituitary glands has been found at autopsy in up to 25% of AIDS patients. Involvement is generally limited to scattered inclusion-bearing cells, however, without the prominent necrosis seen in the adrenals (10,12). Thus far, endocrine dysfunction secondary to CMV, other than hypoadrenalism, has not been reported in AIDS. Cytomegalic cells are also commonly found in the pancreas at autopsy, but symptomatic pancreatitis due to CMV seems to be rare, even in the face of diffuse involvement of the gland (168,169).

CMV-related lesions of the kidneys are mentioned in several autopsy series and are probably not uncommon (10,11,122). In one study, it was further noted that the glomeruli seem to be most affected, raising the question of whether a clinically significant CMV glomerulopathy, perhaps analogous to that described in renal transplant recipients (92), may eventually be recognized in AIDS. Elsewhere in the urinary tract, symptomatic epididymitis due to CMV has been reported in an AIDS patient (122), and this diagnosis is worth considering when clinical epididymitis appears in this setting with negative urine cultures and no apparent benefit from antibiotic therapy.

One study noted four AIDS cases in which CMV caused focal necrosis in the myocardium (12). Although congestive heart failure, arrhythmias, and electrocardiographic changes were not detected in these patients, there is no reason to doubt that clinically significant cardiomyopathy will occur in more severe cases, and physicians should remain alert to this possibility.

Finally, unusual CMV-related skin lesions have recently been described in AIDS patients. In one case, violaceous skin lesions were presumed to be Kaposi's sarcoma until biopsy showed a cutaneous vasculitis due mainly to CMV (170). In two others, verrucous skin lesions were found to be caused by CMV infection of keratinocytes (171). The lesson is clear: skin lesions in AIDS patients may have many etiologies and must be biopsied to avoid serious diagnostic errors.

IMPACT ON MORTALITY

The manifestations of CMV infection in AIDS are many, and their consequences for patients may be grave. Perhaps the ultimate measure of the importance of any pathogen in AIDS, however, is its impact on mortality. Because several severe infections often present simultaneously in the later stages of AIDS, the cause of a patient's death cannot always be determined unequivocally. Several autopsy studies have attempted to do so (10–14,122), however, and their findings with respect to CMV are summarized in Table 2. Some caution must be exercised in generalizing from these data since they are based on only a tiny fraction of the AIDS patients who have died in the United States to date. All these studies also deal mainly with homosexual men, who may have a higher frequency of CMV-related complications than do members of other AIDS risk groups. Even with these caveats in mind, however, the data are impressive. CMV was the most common pathogen in all but one series, being found in 49–90% of all patients. Either alone or in combination with some other process, CMV infection was also determined to be the most frequent immediate cause of death in all series except those of Moskowitz et al. (11) and Klatt and Shibata (14), where *Pneumocystis carinii* pneumonia was responsible for more deaths. The most lethal form of CMV infection reported in these studies is pneumonitis, with colitis and encephalitis also contributing significantly to mortality.

CMV AND KAPOSI'S SARCOMA

In 1972, Giraldo and colleagues at the Memorial Sloan–Kettering Cancer Center noted herpesvirus-like particles in several cell lines derived from African cases of Kaposi's sarcoma (KS) (172). A strain of CMV was eventually isolated from one of those cell lines (173), and in the meantime, another group had demonstrated CMV's potential for oncogenic transformation of human cells in vitro (174). This combination of findings

led to a hypothesis that CMV might be the cause of Kaposi's sarcoma, or at least an important cofactor in its pathogenesis. What followed were two studies showing that American and European patients with KS tend to have higher titers of anti-CMV antibodies than do appropriately matched controls (175,176) and two others in which CMV antigens and nucleic acids were detected in small numbers of biopsy specimens of KS lesions (177,178). Notably, no single marker of CMV infection was found in more than half of the specimens, and most were found in considerably less than half.

When AIDS was first recognized among homosexual men, there seemed to be additional circumstantial evidence linking CMV to KS in the sudden appearance of large numbers of KS cases in a group known to have an extremely high prevalence of CMV infection. Drew et al. were the first to look for CMV in KS tissue from AIDS patients, and they found CMV antigens and/or RNA in most, but not all, of the ten specimens they studied (179). Over the next several years, despite improvements in the sensitivity and specificity of techniques for detecting viral markers, other groups obtained similar results; that is, CMV proteins and nucleic acids were found frequently, but not consistently, in KS cells (180,181). The one study that compared levels of anti-CMV antibodies in AIDS patients with and without KS found no significant difference between the two groups (182). Taken together then, the evidence to date does not support an essential role for CMV in the pathogenesis of KS; but the virus is probably able to infect KS cells and may in some way affect their behavior.

In the meantime, the percentage of AIDS patients reported to have KS has been declining steadily (183), and theories about its pathogenesis and biology have changed markedly. It now seems likely that KS is a multicentric proliferative process rather than a true neoplasm (184) and that malignant transformation by CMV or any other virus is not part of its etiology. The proliferative stimulus in KS has yet to be identified, but the epidemiology of the disease suggests a sexually transmitted pathogen other than HIV itself (183,185). A role for CMV, or perhaps one or more specialized strains of the virus, has not been definitively ruled out but does not enjoy great support at present.

TABLE 2. *CMV infection as the immediate cause of death (ICOD) in AIDS patients*

Autopsy study (ref. no.)	Total number of cases	Number with CMV infections (%)	Number with CMV as ICOD (%)
Reichert et al., 1983 (122)	10	9 (90%)	4 (40%)
Welch et al., 1984 (10)	36	25 (69%)	18 (40%)
Mobley et al., 1985 (13)	12	10 (83%)	6 (50%)
Moskowitz et al., 1985 (11)	54	30 (56%)	10 (19%)
Niedt and Schinella, 1985 (12)	56	43 (77%)	30 (54%)
Klatt and Shibata, 1988 (14)	164	81 (49%)	17 (10%)

DIAGNOSIS OF CMV INFECTION

The past decade has seen many significant advances in our ability to diagnose CMV infection. Unfortunately, most of these have been of little help in the setting of AIDS, where the usual problem is not simply to demonstrate the presence of CMV infection, but rather to identify those patients who have clinically significant CMV-related disease that warrants antiviral therapy.

IgG antibodies to CMV can be detected in serum by a wide variety of tests, including complement fixation, indirect immunofluorescence, enzyme immunoassay, indirect hemagglutination, latex agglutination, and the new dot immunobinding "cube" assay. When performed with commercially available reagents, they all show good sensitivity and specificity, but the recently developed latex agglutination and dot immunobinding assays require the least specialized equipment and may be the easiest to perform in most laboratories (38,186,187). None of these tests can distinguish latent from active infection with a single specimen; but when performed quantitatively on serial specimens, they can be used to demonstrate a rise in antibody titer, which generally indicates active infection. The presence of IgM antibody, which can be detected by indirect immunofluorescence or enzyme immunoassay, is also considered a marker of active infection in most cases (60,188,189). Serologic tests such as these are rarely useful in AIDS patients since nearly all of them have IgG anti-CMV antibodies, frequently at high titers; and fourfold increases in titer may occur even in the absence of clinical disease (190,191). Likewise, IgM anti-CMV antibody is often present even in asymptomatic individuals with HIV infection or absent in those with serious CMV-related disease (190,192).

Isolation of CMV, using human fibroblasts in tissue culture, is much more expensive and technically demanding than serodiagnosis but is a better indicator of active infection (193). Because of the slow development of CMV's characteristic cytopathic effect in cultured fibroblasts, virologic confirmation of CMV infection has traditionally required up to 3 weeks. It has recently become possible to detect CMV in cultures of body fluids between 16 and 48 h after inoculation, however, by first centrifuging specimens onto the fibroblast monolayer and later staining with a monoclonal antibody directed against an early viral protein after a short incubation. Infected cells can then be visualized using immunofluorescence or immunoperoxidase techniques, with both a sensitivity and a specificity of over 90% when compared with standard culture techniques (194,195). Specimens typically used for CMV isolation include urine, saliva, peripheral blood leukocytes, and BAL fluid, but virus can also be cultured from homogenized tissues and even from mucolysed induced sputum (196). Although excellent for documenting active CMV infection, these culture techniques are rarely helpful in diagnosing clinically significant infections in AIDS patients since such a high proportion of these patients persistently shed CMV in body fluids. Many, in fact, are persistently viremic, even when no apparent CMV-related disease is present (190,197).

Alternative methods for rapid diagnosis use nucleic acid hybridization to detect CMV DNA in urine specimens (198–200) and either *in situ* hybridization or monoclonal antibody staining to detect viral markers in cells separated from peripheral blood (201–203) or BAL fluid (204–206). The hybridization techniques appear to be somewhat less sensitive than virus isolation for demonstrating active infection, while the monoclonal antibody staining techniques show comparable sensitivity. When used qualitatively, however, these techniques offer no advantage over isolation in terms of specificity for clinically significant CMV infection.

In the setting of AIDS, the diagnosis of CMV-related disease—with the notable exception of CMV retinitis—currently requires finding typical CMV cytopathology in some organ. The characteristic "owl's eye" cell of CMV infection is markedly enlarged with a large, ovoid, eosinophilic inclusion, surrounded by a clear halo, occupying most of the nucleus. Cells may also contain large, globular cytoplasmic inclusions or dense cytoplasmic granules. Such cells can usually be found in tissue sections stained with hematoxylin and eosin or in Giemsa-stained touch preparations of biopsy specimens. The sensitivity of the latter is only around 50% when compared with standard histologic diagnosis, however (207). Another rapid diagnostic procedure involves the immunofluorescent staining of frozen sections of biopsy specimens with anti-CMV monoclonal antibodies (208). Although it has excellent sensitivity, the specificity of this procedure with regard to CMV infections in AIDS has not been determined.

The disadvantages of biopsy-dependent diagnosis, of course, include the requirement for an invasive procedure, with its attendant risk to the patient, and the need to identify a diseased organ that is both accessible for biopsy and likely to show diagnostic cytopathology. This latter requirement is not always easily met in disseminated CMV infection, which may have nonspecific symptoms and clinical findings. Sampling error is an additional problem in organs where typical cytomegalic cells may be few in number and difficult to detect. The result is that, at our current level of diagnostic sophistication, the only manifestations of CMV infection commonly diagnosed during life in AIDS patients are retinitis, for which presumptive ophthalmoscopic diagnosis is considered adequate, and ulcerative gastrointestinal tract disease, where lesions can easily be biopsied endoscopically.

Clearly, there is a need for more noninvasive means that will allow clinicians to recognize a broader range of significant CMV infections, and this need may some day be met by quantitative virologic techniques. In congenital CMV infection, there is a strong correlation between the amount of virus shed in the urine and the degree of clinical illness (209). The standard quantitative techniques used to make this observation are extremely cumbersome, but recent work suggests that the time required for quantitative CMV cultures can be reduced from 2 weeks to 20 h by using a monoclonal antibody coupled with a biotin–avidin–peroxidase staining system (210). This technique has not yet been applied to body fluids from AIDS patients, but it offers diagnostic possibilities worthy of study.

An even simpler approach might involve the quantitation of infected polymorphonuclear cells in the blood of patients. This can be done using cytospin centrifugation followed by monoclonal antibody staining for CMV immediate-early antigens, and such a technique has already been used on small numbers of samples from AIDS patients. Although rigorous correlation with biopsy-proven disease is still lacking, symptoms compatible with CMV infection appear to occur with numbers of infected polymorphonuclear cells greater than 50–80 per 2×10^5 cells (211,212). In two instances, investigators were also able to demonstrate simultaneous regression of symptoms and the disappearance of infected cells from the blood in response to antiviral therapy (211).

ANTIVIRAL CHEMOTHERAPY

The 1970s and early 1980s were a time of unprecedented progress in the therapy of herpesvirus infections. Throughout most of this period, however, it appeared that CMV possessed an exceptional resistance to inhibition by antiviral drugs as first vidarabine (213,214) and then acyclovir (215–217) failed decisively in clinical trials against CMV infection in transplant recipients. In retrospect, these results could have been anticipated on the basis of in vitro studies, which have shown that both agents are active against CMV only at concentrations that would be toxic to patients (218,219). In the case of acyclovir, these findings are easily understandable as well since this drug depends on activation by a viral thymidine kinase for its activity. Both herpes simplex and varicella-zoster virus have genes that code for such an enzyme; CMV does not.

Prospects for anti-CMV chemotherapy began to improve in 1983 when two groups demonstrated significant in vitro activity against the virus by a new purine analog then known as 9-(1,3-dihydroxy-2-propoxymethyl)guanine, or DHPG, but now called by its official generic name *ganciclovir* (220,221). Despite close structural similarity to acyclovir, this agent does not depend on thymidine kinase for phosphorylation and presumably is activated by one or more of the cellular kinases induced by

CMV infection. In any case, levels of the active ganciclovir triphosphate are approximately ten times higher in infected cells than in uninfected cells, imparting some measure of selectivity to the drug (222,223). In its active form, ganciclovir appears to block viral DNA synthesis by inhibiting the binding of deoxyguanosine triphosphate to DNA polymerase. Unlike acyclovir, it does not have the additional action of DNA chain termination, probably because of the presence of a hydroxymethyl substituent at the 3′ position on its acyclic side chain.

Human studies with ganciclovir were begun in 1984, and initial results were mixed. At doses of 7.5 and 15 mg/kg/day, the drug was effective at eliminating CMV from blood, urine, and sputum of bone marrow recipients with CMV pneumonia, but nine of the 10 patients so treated died of respiratory failure (224). In addition, therapy had to be discontinued in three cases because of severe neutropenia. At the same time, two other groups reported much better results in the treatment of several AIDS patients with retinitis (225,226). Patients received 7.5 or 15 mg/kg/day of ganciclovir for 20–30 days, and all had dramatic improvements in visual acuity and fundoscopic examination. When the drug was stopped, all patients experienced worsening of retinitis within weeks but responded to the institution of daily maintenance therapy. Serious toxicity was not noted in these patients.

Since then, ganciclovir has been given to thousands of AIDS patients, mostly for treatment of CMV retinitis and colitis, and, in 1989, it was approved in the United States by the Food and Drug Administration for the treatment of CMV retinitis in immunocompromised patients. Reported response rates for retinitis in AIDS patients have for the most part been favorable. When doses of ganciclovir between 7.5 and 10 mg/kg/day are used, visual acuity and retinal findings can be expected to improve initially in over 80% of patients (133,227,228). Earlier observations of the need for long-term maintenance to prevent relapse have been confirmed, however, and, even when such therapy is given, most patients will eventually "break through" and show progression of disease at intervals varying from 3 to 46 weeks (medians of 7.5–21 weeks in various studies) (121,133,227). Approximately 10% of patients who initially appear to respond may also show slowly progressive "smoldering" retinitis (121). In an attempt to enhance these results, one group used CMV hyperimmune globulin as adjunctive therapy to ganciclovir for CMV retinitis, but no benefit was found (229).

The experience with ganciclovir in CMV-related gastrointestinal disease is much more limited, but either symptomatic improvement or complete resolution can be expected in over 70% of patients treated (132–134,227). As with retinitis, early relapse is likely to occur if maintenance therapy is not given. Experience with ganciclovir therapy for less common complications of CMV infection is limited to sporadic reports, some of which were mentioned earlier (140,145). The experience in CMV pneumonia in AIDS patients suggests a beneficial effect but cannot be interpreted with confidence due to imprecise diagnostic criteria (133). In addition to its specific affects on identified CMV-related diseases, ganciclovir may also effect nonspecific improvements in the health of treated patients, including weight gain, repletion of body cell mass and fat, and increased serum albumin concentration (230). The effect of the drug on mortality has not yet been investigated rigorously, but at least two studies suggest that patients who are treated may experience a survival advantage when compared with untreated patients (117,231).

Although ganciclovir therapy of CMV infections in AIDS represents a major improvement over the hopeless situation that prevailed in the early years of the epidemic, its use entails many serious problems. Since the drug is not currently available for oral administration, patients being treated can anticipate a lifetime of intravenous therapy, which usually requires insertion of an indwelling central venous access device. Drug-related toxicity is also considerable. Over 40% of patients treated will experience neutropenia (granulocyte count <1000/mm^3), and nearly half of these will develop granulocyte counts less than 500/mm^3 (133). This usually responds to discontinuation of the drug but may be irreversible. Thrombocytopenia occurs in approximately 20% of patients, with rashes, nausea, vomiting, fever, anemia, diarrhea, and seizures each being reported in 3–6% of patients (133). With the exception of neutropenia and thrombocytopenia, the relation of the drug to these adverse effects is uncertain. The hematologic toxicity of ganciclovir is greatly augmented by zidovudine, and the two drugs should probably not be used concurrently (232). An additional concern about ganciclovir is the development of resistance among CMV strains, and this has already been documented in several patients in association with secondary treatment failure (233).

Current regimens for the use of ganciclovir usually involve an induction period of 14–21 days, during which the drug is given at a dose of 5 mg/kg every 12 h, followed by an indefinite maintenance period with doses of 5 mg/kg daily or 6 mg/kg five days a week. All infusions should be given over a 1-hr period to avoid excessive serum levels and increased toxicity. Since ganciclovir is excreted almost entirely by the kidneys, patients whose creatinine clearance is less than 80 ml/min require a reduction in dosage. Some authorities also use a reduced dose when neutropenia and thrombocytopenia are encountered (113).

After ganciclovir, the agent that has been most extensively studied for therapy of CMV infections in AIDS patients is foscarnet, also known as trisodium phosphonoformate. This drug is a pyrophosphate analog that, like ganciclovir, reversibly inhibits CMV DNA polymerase (234). Unlike ganciclovir, it is also active against re-troviral reverse transcriptases (235); and it appears to have some in vivo activity against HIV, as manifested by decreased levels of serum p24 antigen in treated patients (236,237). Several small clinical trials suggest that foscarnet's efficacy in the treatment of CMV retinitis is comparable to that of ganciclovir in terms of both initial response and ability to sustain remission (237–239). Results of a multicenter trial directly comparing the two drugs have recently been published and show that while both agents have equal efficacy against CMV retinitis, patients treated with foscarnet have a longer median survival (239a). The toxicity profile of foscarnet differs from that of ganciclovir in that it causes a reversible decline in renal function in 20–50% of patients. Other common side effects include proteinuria, hypomagnesemia, hypocalcemia, hypokalemia, hypophosphatemia, and diabetes insipidus, all presumably due to renal tubular damage (237–240). Foscarnet has also been associated with anemia, paresthesias, seizures, and genital ulcers. By itself, foscarnet rarely causes significant neutropenia, but a decline in granulocyte count may be anticipated in patients treated concurrently with zidovudine (237). Given its formidable toxicity, it seems unlikely that foscarnet will represent a major therapeutic advance over ganciclovir unless the early findings of increased patient survival are confirmed. It may also have a role in the treatment of resistant infections since it is active against some ganciclovir-resistant strains of CMV (241).

Like ganciclovir, foscarnet must be administered intravenously. Therapy is usually begun with a dose of 60 mg/kg given over 1 hr every 8 h for 14–21 days, followed by chronic maintenance with 90–120 mg/kg given over 2 h once daily. Maintaining adequate hydration with 1 liter of normal saline prior to each dose of foscarnet may help to limit nephrotoxicity; and serum creatinine, calcium, magnesium, potassium, and phosphorus should be monitored two to three times per week during induction and every 1–2 weeks during maintenance. Dose adjustment is required for patients with abnormal renal function.

If nothing else, our early experience with antiviral therapy for CMV infection in AIDS makes it clear that we need more and better drugs for this indication. A variety of agents, including both nucleoside analogs (242,243) and anthraquinones (unpublished data) have shown promising activity in vitro, and it is certain that the development of these and other agents will continue at a rapid pace to meet the urgent demand of CMV infection in the AIDS epidemic.

SUMMARY

Infection with human cytomegalovirus is extremely common in all populations, but transmission of infection seems to be particularly intense among sexually active homosexual men. In immunocompetent individuals, CMV may cause a form of mononucleosis but is most often asymptomatic. In patients with impaired cell-mediated immunity, however, CMV causes severe and even life-threatening disease. There are also data that suggest that CMV infection itself may have an immunosuppressive effect and adversely modify the course of HIV infection.

CMV infection is the most common opportunistic infection and one of the most frequent causes of death in AIDS patients. Manifestations include retinitis, ulcerative gastrointestinal tract disease, encephalomyelitis, peripheral neuritis and radiculitis, pneumonitis, adrenalitis, and disease at numerous other sites. Diagnosis of clinically significant CMV infection in AIDS may be extremely difficult and currently rests on the demonstration of characteristic histopathology. Ganciclovir, a new antiviral agent, has produced good results in the treatment of CMV retinitis and gastrointestinal disease in AIDS patients, but prolonged maintenance therapy is required to sustain remission.

REFERENCES

1. Gottlieb MS, Schroff R, Schanker HM, et al. *Pneumocystis carinii* pneumonia and mucosal candidiasis in previously healthy homosexual men. *N Engl J Med* 1981;305:1425–31.
2. Masur H, Michelis MA, Greene JB, et al. An outbreak of community-acquired *Pneumocystis carinii* pneumonia: initial manifestation of cellular immune dysfunction. *N Engl J Med* 1981;305:1431–8.
3. Siegal FP, Lopez C, Hammer GS, et al. Severe acquired immunodeficiency in male homosexuals manifested by chronic perianal ulcerative herpes simplex lesions. *N Engl J Med* 1981;305:1439–44.
4. Urmacher C, Myskowski P, Ochoa M, Kris M, Safai B. Outbreak of Kaposi's sarcoma and cytomegalovirus infection in young homosexual men. *Am J Med* 1982;72:569–75.
5. Mildvan D, Mathur U, Enlow RW, et al. Opportunistic infections and immune deficiency in homosexual men. *Ann Intern Med* 1982;96:700–4.
6. Levin MJ, Rinaldo CR, Leary PL, Zaia JA, Hirsch MS. Immune response to herpesvirus antigens in adults with acute cytomegalovirus mononucleosis. *J Infect Dis* 1979;140:851–7.
7. Rinaldo CR, Carney WP, Richter BS, Black PH, Hirsch MS. Mechanisms of immunosuppression in cytomegaloviral mononucleosis. *J Infect Dis* 1980;141:488–95.
8. Drew LW, Mintz L, Miner RC, Sands M, Ketterer B. Prevalence of cytomegalovirus infection in homosexual men. *J Infect Dis* 1981;143:188–92.
9. Guarda LA, Luna MA, Smith JL, Mansell PW, Gyorkey F, Roca AN. Acquired immune deficiency syndrome: postmortem findings. *Am J Clin Pathol* 1984;81:549–57.
10. Welch K, Finkbeiner W, Alpers CE, et al. Autopsy findings in the acquired immune deficiency syndrome. *JAMA* 1984;252:1152–9.
11. Moskowitz L, Hensley GT, Chan JC, Adams K. Immediate cause of death in acquired immunodeficiency syndrome. *Arch Pathol Lab Med* 1985;109:735–8.
12. Niedt GW, Schinella RA. Acquired immunodeficiency syndrome: clinicopathologic study of 56 autopsies. *Arch Pathol Lab Med* 1985;109:727–34.
13. Mobley K, Rotterdam HZ, Lerner CW, Tapper M. Autopsy findings in the acquired immune deficiency syndrome. *Pathol Annu* 1985;20:45–65.
14. Klatt EC, Shibata D. Cytomegalovirus infection in the acquired immunodeficiency syndrome. *Arch Pathol Lab Med* 1988;112:540–4.
15. Huang E-S, Kilpatrick BA, Huang Y-T, Pagano JS. Detection of human cytomegalovirus and analysis of strain variation. *Yale J Biol Med* 1976;49:29–43.
16. Huang E-S, Huang S-M, Tegtmeier GE, Alford C. Cytomegalovirus: genetic variation of viral genomes. *Ann NY Acad Sci* 1980;354:332–46.
17. Beutner KR, Morag A, Deibel R, Morag B, Raiken D, Ogra P. Strain-specific local and systemic cell-mediated immune responses to cytomegalovirus in humans. *Infect Immun* 1978;20:82–7.
18. Waner JL, Weller TH. Analysis of antigenic diversity among human cytomegaloviruses by kinetic neutralization tests with high-titered rabbit antisera. *Infect Immun* 1978;21:151–7.
19. Albrecht T, Weller TH. Heterogeneous morphologic features of plaques induced by five strains of human cytomegalovirus. *Am J Clin Pathol* 1980;73:648–54.
20. Kanich RE, Craighead JE. Human cytomegalovirus infection of cultured fibroblasts. I. Cytopathologic effects induced by an adapted and a wild strain. *Lab Invest* 1972;27:263–72.
21. St. Jeor SC, Albrecht TB, Funk RD, Rapp F. Stimulation of cellular DNA synthesis by human cytomegalovirus. *J Virol* 1974;13:353–62.
22. Stinski MF. Sequence of protein synthesis in cells infected by human cytomegalovirus: early and late virus-induced polypeptides. *J Virol* 1978;26:686–701.
23. Toorkey CB, Carrigan DR. Immunohistochemical detection of an immediate early antigen of human cytomegalovirus in normal tissues. *J Infect Dis* 1989;160:741–51.
24. Adler SP. Transfusion-associated cytomegalovirus infections. *Rev Infect Dis* 1985;6:979–93.
25. Betts RF, Freeman RB, Douglas RG, Talley TE, Rundell B. Transmission of cytomegalovirus infection with renal allograft. *Kidney Int* 1975;8:387–94.
26. Chou S. Acquisition of donor strains of cytomegalovirus by renal transplant recipients. *N Engl J Med* 1986;314:1418–23.
27. Marker SC, Howard RJ, Simmons RL, et al. Cytomegalovirus infection: a quantitative prospective study of 320 consecutive renal transplants. *Surgery* 1981;89:660–71.
28. Pollard RB, Rand KH, Arvin AM, Merigan TC. Cell-mediated immunity to cytomegalovirus infection in normal subjects and cardiac transplant patients. *J Infect Dis* 1978;137:541–9.
29. Yeager AS, Grumet FC, Hafleigh EB, Arvin AM, Bradley JS, Prober CG. Prevention of transfusion-acquired cytomegalovirus infections in newborn infants. *J Pediatr* 1981;98:281–7.
30. Winston DJ, Pollard RB, Ho WG, et al. Cytomegalovirus immune plasma in bone marrow transplant recipients. *Ann Intern Med* 1982;97:11–8.
31. O'Reilly RJ, Reich L, Gold J, et al. A randomized trial of intravenous hyperimmune globulin for the prevention of cytomegalovirus (CMV) infections following bone marrow transplantation: preliminary results. *Transplant Proc* 1983;15:1405–11.
32. Winston DJ, Ho WG, Lin C-H, Budinger MD, Champlin RE, Gale RP. Intravenous immunoglobulin for modification of cytomegalovirus infections associated with bone marrow transplantation. *Am J Med* 1984;76(3A):128–33.
33. Snydman DR, Werner BG, Heinze-Lacey B, et al. Use of cytomegalovirus immune globulin to prevent cytomegalovirus disease in renal-transplant recipients. *N Engl J Med* 1987;317:1049–54.
34. Krech U. Complement-fixing antibodies against cytomegalovirus in different parts of the world. *Bull WHO* 1973;49:103–6.
35. Krech U, Tobin J. A collaborative study of cytomegalovirus antibodies in mothers of young children in 19 countries. *Bull WHO* 1981;59:605–10.
36. Wentworth BB, Alexander ER. Seroepidemiology of infections due to members of the herpesvirus group. *Am J Epidemiol* 1971;94:496–507.
37. White NH, Yow MD, Demmler GJ, et al. Prevalence of cytomeg-

alovirus antibody in subjects between the ages of 6 and 22 years. *J Infect Dis* 1989;159:1013–7.

38. Horodniceanu F, Michelson S. Assessment of cytomegalovirus antibody detection techniques. *Arch Virol* 1980;64:287–301.

39. Hanshaw JB, Dudgeon JA, Marshall WC. *Viral diseases of the fetus and newborn.* Philadelphia: Saunders; 1985.

40. Reynolds DW, Stagno S, Hosty TS, Tiller M, Alford CA. Maternal cytomegalovirus excretion and perinatal infection. *N Engl J Med* 1973;289:1–5.

41. Montgomery R, Youngblood L, Medearis DN. Recovery of cytomegalovirus from the cervix in pregnancy. *Pediatrics* 1972; 49:524–31.

42. Stagno S, Reynolds DW, Pass RF, Alford CA. Breast milk and the risk of cytomegalovirus infection. *N Engl J Med* 1980; 302:1073–6.

43. Pass RF, August AM, Dworsky M, Reynolds DW. Cytomegalovirus infection in a day-care center. *N Engl J Med* 1982;307:477–9.

44. Hutto C, Ricks R, Garvie M, Pass RF. Epidemiology of cytomegalovirus infection in young children: day care vs. home care. *Pediatr Infect Dis* 1985;4:149–152.

45. Sarov B, Naggan L, Rosenzveig R, Katz S, Haikin H, Sarov I. Prevalence of antibodies to human cytomegalovirus in urban, kibbutz, and Bedouin children in southern Israel. *J Med Virol* 1982;10:195–201.

46. Faix RG. Survival of cytomegalovirus on environmental surfaces. *J Pediatr* 1985;106:649–52.

47. Yeager AS. Transmission of cytomegalovirus to mothers by infected infants: another reason to prevent transfusion-acquired infections. *Pediatr Infect Dis* 1983;2:295–7.

48. Jordan MC, Rousseau WE, Noble GR, Steward JA, Chin TD. Association of cervical cytomegalovirus with venereal disease. *N Engl J Med* 1973;288:932–4.

49. Wilmott FE. Cytomegalovirus in female patients attending a VD clinic. *Br J Vener Dis* 1975;51:278–80.

50. Lang DJ, Kummer JF. Cytomegalovirus in semen: observations in selected populations. *J Infect Dis* 1975;132:472–3.

51. Embil JA, Manuel FR, Garner JB, Coveney L. Cytomegalovirus in the semen. *Can Med Assoc J* 1982;126:391–2.

52. Mintz L, Drew WL, Miner RC, Braff EH. Cytomegalovirus infections in homosexual men: an epidemiological study. *Ann Intern Med* 1983;99:326–9.

53. Lange M, Klein EB, Kornfield H, Cooper LZ, Grieco MH. Cytomegalovirus isolation from healthy homosexual men. *JAMA* 1984;252:1908–10.

54. Collier AC, Meyers JD, Corey L, Murphy VL, Roberts PL, Handsfield HH. Cytomegalovirus infection in homosexual men: relationship to sexual practices, antibody to human immunodeficiency virus, and cell-mediated immunity. *Am J Med* 1987;82:593–601.

55. Chandler SH, Alexander ER, Holmes KK. Epidemiology of cytomegaloviral infection in a heterogeneous population of pregnant women. *J Infect Dis* 1985;152:249–56.

56. Chretien JH, McGinniss CG, Muller A. Venereal causes of cytomegalovirus mononucleosis. *JAMA* 1977;238:1644–5.

57. Handsfield HH, Chandler SH, Caine VA, et al. Cytomegalovirus infection in sex partners: evidence for sexual transmission. *J Infect Dis* 1985;151:344–8.

58. Kryger P, Gerstoft J, Pedersen NS, Nielsen JO. Increased prevalence of cytomegalovirus antibodies in homosexual men with syphilis: relation to sexual behavior. *Scand J Infect Dis* 1984;16:381–4.

59. Buimovici-Klein E, Tinker MK, O'Beirne AJ, Lange M, Cooper Z. IgM detection by ELISA in the diagnosis of cytomegalovirus infections in homosexual and heterosexual immunosuppressed patients. *Arch Virol* 1983;78:203–12.

60. Langenhuysen MMAC, The TH, Nieweg HO, Kapsenberg JG. Demonstration of cytomegalovirus antibodies as an aid to early diagnosis in adults. *Clin Exp Immunol* 1970;6:387–93.

61. Drew WL, Sweet ES, Miner RC, Mocarski ES. Multiple infections by cytomegalovirus in patients with acquired immunodeficiency syndrome: documentation by Southern blot hybridization. *J Infect Dis* 1984;150:952–3.

62. Spector SA, Hirata KK, Neuman TR. Identification of multiple cytomegalovirus strains in homosexual men with acquired immunodeficiency syndrome. *J Infect Dis* 1984;150:953–5.

63. Collier AC, Chandler SH, Handsfield HH, Corey L, McDougall JK. Identification of multiple strains of cytomegalovirus in homosexual men. *J Infect Dis* 1989;159:123–6.

64. Guinan ME, Thomas PA, Pinsky PF, et al. Heterosexual and homosexual patients with the acquired immunodeficiency syndrome. A comparison of surveillance, interview, and laboratory data. *Ann Intern Med* 1984;100:213–8.

65. Blaser MJ, Cohen DL. Opportunistic infections in patients with AIDS: clues to the epidemiology of AIDS and the relative virulence of pathogens. *Rev Infect Dis* 1986;8:21–30.

66. Enck RE, Betts RF, Brown MR, Miller G. Viral serology (hepatitis B virus, cytomegalovirus, Epstein-Barr virus) and abnormal liver function tests in transfused patients with hereditary hemorrhagic diseases. *Transfusion* 1979;19:32–8.

67. Cheeseman SH, Sullivan JL, Brettler DB, Levine PH. Analysis of cytomegalovirus and Epstein-Barr virus antibody responses in treated hemophiliacs: implications for the study of acquired immune deficiency syndrome. *JAMA* 1984;252:83–5.

68. Landay A, Poon M-C, Abo T, Stagno S, Lurie A, Cooper MD. Immunologic studies in asymptomatic hemophilia patients: relationship to acquired immune deficiency syndrome (AIDS). *J Clin Invest* 1983;71:1500–4.

69. Betts RF. Syndromes of cytomegalovirus infection. *Adv Intern Med* 1980;26:447–66.

70. Ho M, Dowling JN. Cytomegalovirus infections in transplant and cancer patients. *Curr Clin Topics Infect Dis* 1980;1:45–67.

71. Cohen JI, Corey GR. Cytomegalovirus infection in the normal host. *Medicine* 1985;64:100–114.

72. Alford CA, Stagno S, Pass RF, Britt WJ. Congenital and perinatal cytomegalovirus infections. *Rev Infect Dis* 1990;12:S745–53.

73. Lang DJ, Scolnik EM, Willerson JT. Association of cytomegalovirus infection with the postperfusion syndrome. *N Engl J Med* 1968;278:1147–9.

74. Winston DJ, Ho WG, Howell CL, et al. Cytomegalovirus infections associated with leukocyte transfusions. *Ann Intern Med* 1980;93:671–5.

75. Hersman J, Meyers JD, Thomas ED, Buckner CD, Clift R. The effect of granulocyte transfusions on the incidence of cytomegalovirus infection after allogeneic marrow transplantation. *Ann Intern Med* 1982;96:149–52.

76. Bayer WE. The effect of frozen blood on the relationship of cytomegalovirus and hepatitis virus to infection and disease. In: Dawson RB, Barnes A, eds. *Clinical and practical aspects of the use of frozen blood.* Washington, DC: American Association of Blood Banks; 1977:133–47.

77. Mackinnon S, Burnett AK, Crawford RJ, Cameron S, Leask BGS, Sommerville RG. Seronegative blood products prevent primary cytomegalovirus infection after bone marrow transplantation. *J Clin Pathol* 1988;41:948–50.

78. Bonkowski HL, Lee RV, Klatskin G. Acute granulomatous hepatitis: occurrence in cytomegalovirus mononucleosis. *JAMA* 1975;233:1284–8.

79. Clarke J, Craig RM, Saffro R, Murphy P, Yokoo H. Cytomegalovirus granulomatous hepatitis. *Am J Med* 1979;66:264–9.

80. Spear JB, Kessler HA, Dworin A, Semel J. Erythema nodosum associated with acute cytomegalovirus mononucleosis in an adult. *Arch Intern Med* 1988;148:323–4.

81. Leonard JC, Tobin JO. A report from various centers: polyneuritis associated with cytomegalovirus infection. *Q J Med* 1971;40:435–42.

82. Dowling P, Menonna J, Cook S. Cytomegalovirus complement fixation antibody in Guillain-Barré syndrome. *Neurology* 1977;27:1153–6.

83. Donaghy M, Gray JA, Squier W, et al. Recurrent Guillain-Barré syndrome after multiple exposures to cytomegalovirus. *Am J Med* 1989;87:339–41.

84. Wong TW, Warner NE. Cytomegalic inclusion disease in adults. Report of 14 cases with review of literature. *Arch Pathol* 1962;74:403–21.

85. Gottman AW, Beatty EC. Cytomegalic inclusion disease in children with leukemia or lymphosarcoma. *Am J Dis Child* 1962;21:415–25.

86. Bodey GP, Wertlake PT, Douglas G, et al. Cytomegalic inclusion disease in patients with acute leukemia. *Ann Intern Med* 1965;62:899–906.

87. Rosen P, Hadju S. Cytomegalovirus inclusion disease at autopsy of patients with cancer. *Am J Clin Pathol* 1971;55:749–56.
88. Armstrong D, Rosen P. Cytomegalovirus and herpes simplex pneumonia complicating neoplastic disease. In: von Graevenitz A, Sall A, eds. *Pathogenic microorganisms from atypical sources.* New York: Marcel Dekker; 1975:89–99.
89. Craighead JE, Hanshaw JB, Carpenter CB. Cytomegalovirus infection after renal allotransplantation. *JAMA* 1967;201:725–8.
90. Peterson PK, Balfour HH, Marker SC, Fryd DS, Howard RJ, Simmons RL. Cytomegalovirus disease in renal allograft recipients: a prospective study of the clinical features, risk factors, and impact on renal transplantation. *Medicine* 1980;59:283–300.
91. Glenn J. Cytomegalovirus infections following renal transplantation. *Rev Infect Dis* 1981;3:1151–78.
92. Richardson WP, Colvin RB, Cheeseman SH, et al. Glomerulopathy associated with cytomegalovirus viremia in renal allografts. *N Engl J Med* 1981;305:57–63.
93. Suwansirikul S, Rao N, Dowling JN, Ho M. Primary and secondary cytomegalovirus infection: clinical manifestations after renal transplantation. *Arch Intern Med* 1977;137:1026–29.
94. Betts RF, Freeman RB, Douglas RG, Talley TE. Clinical manifestations of renal allograft derived primary cytomegalovirus infection. *Am J Dis Child* 1977;131:759–63.
95. Peterson PK, McGlave P, Ramsay NKC, et al. A prospective study of infectious diseases following bone marrow transplantation: emergence of aspergillus and cytomegalovirus as the major causes of mortality. *Infect Control* 1983;4:81–9.
96. Meyers JD, Flournoy N, Thomas ED. Risk factors for cytomegalovirus infection after human marrow transplantation. *J Infect Dis* 1986;153:478–88.
97. Grundy JE, Shanley JD, Griffiths PD. Is cytomegalovirus interstitial pneumonitis in transplant recipients an immunopathological condition? *Lancet* 1987;2:996–9.
98. Howard RJ, Miller J, Najarian JS. Cytomegalovirus induced immune suppression. II. Cell-mediated immunity. *Clin Exp Immunol* 1974;18:119–26.
99. Rinaldo CR, Black PH, Hirsch MS. Interaction of cytomegalovirus with leukocytes from patients with mononucleosis due to cytomegalovirus. *J Infect Dis* 1977;136:667–77.
100. Carney WP, Hirsch MS. Mechanisms of immunosuppression in cytomegalovirus mononucleosis. II. Virus–monocyte interactions. *J Infect Dis* 1981;144:47–54.
101. Carney WP, Rubin RH, Hoffman RA, Hansen WP, Healey K, Hirsch MS. Analysis of T lymphocyte subsets in cytomegalovirus mononucleosis. *J Immunol* 1981;126:2114–6.
102. Carney WP, Iacoviello V, Hirsch MS. Functional properties of T lymphocytes and their subsets in cytomegalovirus mononucleosis. *J Immunol* 1983;130:390–3.
103. Rice GPA, Schrier RD, Oldstone MBA. Cytomegalovirus infects human lymphocytes and monocytes: virus expression is limited to immediate-early gene products. *Proc Natl Acad Sci USA* 1984;81:6134–8.
104. Schrier RD, Nelson JA, Oldstone MBA. Detection of human cytomegalovirus in peripheral blood lymphocytes in a natural infection. *Science* 1985;230:1048–51.
105. Wahren B, Ljungman P, Paulin T, Ringdén O. Enhancive and suppressive effects of cytomegalovirus on human lymphocyte responses *in vitro. J Virol* 1986;58:909–13.
106. Chatterjee SN, Fiala M, Weiner J, Stewart JA, Stacey B, Warmer N. Primary cytomegalovirus and opportunistic infections. Incidence in renal transplant recipients. *JAMA* 1978;240:2446–9.
107. Schooley RT, Hirsch MS, Colvin RB, et al. Association of herpesvirus infections with T-lymphocyte subset alterations, glomerulopathy, and opportunistic infections after renal transplantation. *N Engl J Med* 1983;308:307–13.
108. Polk BF, Fox R, Brookmeyer R, et al. Predictors of the acquired immunodeficiency developing in a cohort of seropositive homosexual men. *N Engl J Med* 1987;316:61–6.
109. Webster A, Cook DG, Emery VC, et al. Cytomegalovirus infection and progression towards AIDS in hemophiliacs with human immunodeficiency virus infection. *Lancet* 1989;2:63–6.
110. Skolnik PR, Kosloff BR, Hirsch MS. Bidirectional interactions between human immunodeficiency virus type 1 and cytomegalovirus. *J Infect Dis* 1988;157:508–13.
111. Bonetti A, Weber R, Vogt M, Wunderli W, Siegenthaler W, Lüthy R. Co-infection with human immunodeficiency virus-type 1 (HIV-1) and cytomegalovirus in two intravenous drug users. *Ann Intern Med* 1989;111:293–6.
112. Centers for Disease Control. Update: acquired immunodeficiency syndrome—United States. *MMWR* 1986;35:17–21.
113. Jacobson MA, Mills J. Serious cytomegalovirus disease in the acquired immunodeficiency syndrome (AIDS): clinical findings, diagnosis, and treatment. *Ann Intern Med* 1988;108:585–94.
114. Jessurun J, Angeles-Angeles A, Gasman N. Comparative autopsy and demographic findings in acquired immune deficiency syndrome in two Mexican populations. *J Acquired Immune Deficiency Syndrome* 1990;3:579–83.
115. Holland GN, Pepose JS, Pettit TH, Gottlieb MS, Yee RD. Acquired immune deficiency syndrome: ocular manifestations. *Ophthalmology* 1983;90:859–73.
116. Palestine AG, Rodrigues MM, Macher AM, et al. Ophthalmic involvement in acquired immunodeficiency syndrome. *Ophthalmology* 1984;91:1092–9.
117. Holland GN, Sison RF, Jatulis DE, Haslop MG, Sakamoto MJ, Wheeler NC. Survival of patients with the acquired immune deficiency syndrome after development of cytomegalovirus retinopathy. *Ophthalmology* 1990;97:204–11.
118. Bloom JN, Palestine AG. The diagnosis of cytomegalovirus retinitis. *Ann Intern Med* 1988;109:963–9.
119. Palestine AG. Clinical aspects of cytomegalovirus retinitis. *Rev Infect Dis* 1988;10:S515–9.
120. Jacobson MA, O'Donnell JJ, Brodie HR, Wofsy C, Mills J. Randomized prospective trial of ganciclovir maintenance therapy for cytomegalovirus retinitis. *J Med Virol* 1988;25:339–49.
121. Gross JG, Bozzette SA, Mathews WC, et al. Longitudinal study of cytomegalovirus retinitis in acquired immune deficiency syndrome. *Ophthalmology* 1990;97:681–6.
122. Reichert CM, O'Leary TJ, Levens DL, Simrell CR, Macher AM. Autopsy pathology in the acquired immune deficiency syndrome. *Am J Pathol* 1983;112:357–82.
123. Connolly GM, Shanson D, Hawkins DA, Harcourt Webster JN, Gazzard BG. Non-cryptosporidial diarrhoea in human immunodeficiency virus (HIV) infected patients. *Gut* 1989;30:195–200.
124. Knapp AB, Horst DA, Eliopoulos G, et al. Widespread cytomegalovirus gastroenterocolitis in a patient with acquired immunodeficiency syndrome. *Gastroenterology* 1983;85:1399–1402.
125. Frank D, Raicht RF. Intestinal perforation associated with cytomegalovirus infection in patients with acquired immunodeficiency syndrome. *Am J Gastroenterol* 1984;79:201–5.
126. Meiselman MS, Cello JP, Margareten W. Cytomegalovirus colitis: report of clinical, endoscopic, and pathologic findings in two patients with the acquired immune deficiency syndrome. *Gastroenterology* 1985;88:171–5.
127. Balthazar EJ, Megibow AJ, Frazzini E, Opulencia JF, Engel I. Cytomegalovirus colitis in AIDS: radiographic findings in 11 patients. *Radiology* 1985;155:585–9.
128. Wajsman R, Cappell MS, Biempica L, Cho KC. Terminal ileitis associated with cytomegalovirus and the acquired immune deficiency syndrome. *Am J Gastroenterol* 1989;84:790–3.
129. St. Onge G, Bezahler GH. Giant esophageal ulcer associated with cytomegalovirus. *Gastroenterology* 1982;83:127–30.
130. Gertler SL, Pressman J, Price B, Brezinsky S, Katsumi M. Gastrointestinal cytomegalovirus infection in a homosexual man with severe acquired immunodeficiency syndrome. *Gastroenterology* 1983;85:1403–6.
131. Balthazar EJ, Megibow AJ, Hulnick DH. Cytomegalovirus esophagitis and gastritis in AIDS. *Am J Radiol* 1985;144:1201–4.
132. Wilcox CM, Diehl DL, Cello JP, Margareten W, Jacobson MA. Cytomegalovirus esophagitis in patients with AIDS: a clinical, endoscopic, and pathologic correlation. *Ann Intern Med* 1990;113:589–93.
133. Buhles WC, Mastre BJ, Tinker AJ, et al. Ganciclovir treatment of life- and sight-threatening cytomegalovirus infection: experience in 314 immunocompromised patients. *Rev Infect Dis* 1988;10:S495–505.
134. Dieterich DT, Chachoua A, Lafleur F, Worrell C. Ganciclovir treatment of gastrointestinal infections caused by cytomegalovirus in patients with AIDS. *Rev Infect Dis* 1988;10:S532–7.
135. Blumberg RS, Kelsey P, Perrone T, Dickersin R, Laquaglia M,

Ferruci J. Cytomegalovirus- and cryptosporidium-associated acalculous cholecystitis. *Am J Med* 1984;76:1118–23.

136. Kavin H, Jonas RB, Chowdhury L, Kabins S. Acalculous cholecystitis in cytomegalovirus infection in the acquired immunodeficiency syndrome. *Ann Intern Med* 1986;104:53–54.

137. Cello JP. Acquired immunodeficiency syndrome cholangiopathy: spectrum of disease. *Am J Med* 1989;86:539–46.

138. Wiley CA, Nelson JA. Role of human immunodeficiency virus and cytomegalovirus in AIDS encephalitis. *Am J Pathol* 1988;133:73–81.

139. Bale JF. Human cytomegalovirus infection and disorders of the nervous system. *Arch Neurol* 1984;41:310–20.

140. Vinters HV, Kwok MK, Ho HW, et al. Cytomegalovirus in the nervous system of patients with the acquired immune deficiency syndrome. *Brain* 1989;112:245–68.

141. Moskowitz LB, Gregorios JB, Hensley GT, Berger JR. Cytomegalovirus induced demyelination associated with acquired immune deficiency syndrome. *Arch Pathol Lab Med* 1984;180:873–7.

142. Hawley DA, Schaefer JF, Schulz DM, Muller J. Cytomegalovirus encephalitis in acquired immunodeficiency syndrome. *Am J Clin Pathol* 1983;80:874–7.

143. Post MJD, Hensley GT, Moskowitz LB, Fischl M. Cytomegalic inclusion virus encephalitis in patients with AIDS: CT, clinical, and pathologic correlation. *Am J Radiol* 1986;146:1229–34.

144. Snider WD, Simpson DM, Nielsen S, Gold JW, Metroka CE, Posner JB. Neurological complications of acquired immune deficiency syndrome. *Ann Neurol* 1983;14:403–18.

145. Masdeu JC, Small CB, Weiss L, Elkin CM, Llena J, Mesa-Tejada R. Multifocal cytomegalovirus encephalitis in AIDS. *Ann Neurol* 1988;23:97–9.

146. Reyes MG. Cytomegalovirus encephalitis in acquired immunodeficiency syndrome. *Ann Neurol* 1988;24:98.

147. Fuller GN, Guiloff RF, Scaravilli F, Harcourt Webster JN. Combined HIV–CMV encephalitis presenting with brainstem signs. *J Neurol Neurosurg Psychiatry* 1989;52:975–9.

148. Singh BM, Levine S, Yarrish RL, Hyland MJ, Jeanty D, Wormser GP. Spinal cord syndromes in the acquired immune deficiency syndrome. *Acta Neurol Scand* 1986;73:590–98.

149. Behar R, Wiley C, McCutchan JA. Cytomegalovirus polyradiculopathy in acquired immune deficiency syndrome. *Neurology* 1987;37:557–61.

150. Grafe MR, Wiley CA. Spinal cord and peripheral nerve pathology in AIDS: the roles of cytomegalovirus and human immunodeficiency virus. *Ann Neurol* 1989;25:561–6.

151. Small PM, McPhaul LW, Sooy CD, Wofsy CB, Jacobson MA. Cytomegalovirus infection of the laryngeal nerve presenting as hoarseness in patients with acquired immunodeficiency syndrome. *Am J Med* 1989;86:108–10.

152. Fuller GN, Jacobs JM, Guiloff RJ. Association of painful peripheral neuropathy in AIDS with cytomegalovirus infection. *Lancet* 1989;2:937–40.

153. de Gans J, Portegies P, Tiessens G, et al. Therapy for cytomegalovirus polyradiculitis in patients with AIDS: treatment with ganciclovir. *AIDS* 1990;4:421–5.

154. Nash G, Fligiel S. Pathologic features of the lung in the acquired immune deficiency syndrome (AIDS): an autopsy study of seventeen homosexual males. *Am J Clin Pathol* 1984;81:6–12.

155. Murray JF, Felton CP, Garay SM, et al. Pulmonary complications of the acquired immunodeficiency syndrome: report of a National Heart, Lung, and Blood Institute Workshop. *N Engl J Med* 1984;310:1682–8.

156. Blumenfeld W, Wagar E, Hadley K. Use of the transbronchial biopsy for diagnosis of opportunistic pulmonary infections in acquired immunodeficiency syndrome (AIDS). *Am J Clin Pathol* 1984;81:1–5.

157. Stover DE, White DA, Romano PA, Gellene RA, Robeson WA. Spectrum of pulmonary diseases associated with the acquired immune deficiency syndrome. *Am J Med* 1985;78:429–37.

158. Masur H, Ognibene FP, Yarchoan R, et al. CD4 counts as predictors of opportunistic pneumonias in human immunodeficiency virus (HIV) infection. *Ann Intern Med* 1989;111:223–31.

159. Zaia JA. Epidemiology and pathogenesis of cytomegalovirus disease. *Semin Hematol* 1990;27(2 suppl 1):1–5.

160. Bower M, Barton SE, Nelson MR, et al. The significance of the detection of cytomegalovirus in the bronchoalveolar fluid in AIDS patients with pneumonia. *AIDS* 1990;4:317–20.

161. Miles PR, Baughman RP, Linnemann CC. Cytomegalovirus in the brochoalveolar lavage fluid of patients with AIDS. *Chest* 1990;97:1072–6.

162. Millar AB, Patou G, Miller RF, et al. Cytomegalovirus in the lungs of patients with AIDS. Respiratory pathogen or passenger. *Am Rev Respir Dis* 1990;141:1474–7.

163. Emanuel D, Cunningham I, Jules-Elysee K, et al. Cytomegalovirus pneumonia after bone marrow transplantation successfully treated with the combination of ganciclovir and high-dose intravenous immune globulin. *Ann Intern Med* 1988;109:777–82.

164. Glasgow BJ, Steinsapir KD, Anders K, Layfield J. Adrenal pathology in the acquired immune deficiency syndrome. *Am J Clin Pathol* 1985;84:594–7.

165. Tapper ML, Rotterdam HZ, Lerner CW, Al'Khafaji K, Seitzman PA. Adrenal necrosis in the acquired immunodeficiency syndrome. *Ann Intern Med* 1984;100:239–41.

166. Macher AM, Reichert CM, Straus SE, et al. Death in the AIDS patient. *N Engl J Med* 1983;309:1454.

167. Greene LW, Cole W, Greene JB, et al. Adrenal insufficiency as a complication of the acquired immunodeficiency syndrome. *Ann Intern Med* 1984;101:497–8.

168. Brivet F, Coffin B, Bedossa P, et al. Pancreatic lesions in AIDS. *Lancet* 1987;2:570–1.

169. Schwartz MS, Brandt LJ. The spectrum of pancreatic disorders in patients with the acquired immune deficiency syndrome. *Am J Gastroenterol* 1989;84:459–62.

170. Kwan TH, Kaufman HW. Acid-fast bacilli with cytomegalovirus and herpesvirus inclusions in the skin of an AIDS patient. *Am J Clin Pathol* 1986;85:236–8.

171. Bournérias I, Boisnic S, Patey O, et al. Unusual cutaneous cytomegalovirus involvement in patients with acquired immunodeficiency syndrome. *Arch Dermatol* 1989;125:1243–6.

172. Giraldo G, Beth E, Haguenau F. Herpes-type virus particles in tissue culture of Kaposi's sarcoma from different geographic regions. *J Natl Cancer Inst* 1972;49:1509–26.

173. Glaser R, Geder L, St. Jeor S, Michelson-Fiske S, Haguenau F. Partial characterization of a herpes-type virus (K9V) derived from Kaposi's sarcoma. *J Natl Cancer Inst* 1977;59:55–60.

174. Geder L, Lausch R, O'Neill F, Rapp F. Oncogenic transformation of human embryo lung cells by human cytomegalovirus. *Science* 1976;192:1134–7.

175. Giraldo G, Beth E, Kourilsky FM, et al. Antibody patterns to herpesviruses in Kaposi's sarcoma: serological association of European Kaposi's sarcoma with cytomegalovirus. *Int J Cancer* 1975;15:839–48.

176. Giraldo G, Beth E, Henle W, et al. Antibody patterns to herpesviruses in Kaposi's sarcoma. II. Serological association of American Kaposi's sarcoma with cytomegalovirus. *Int J Cancer* 1978;22:126–31.

177. Giraldo G, Beth E, Huang E-S. Kaposi's sarcoma and its relationship to cytomegalovirus (CMV). III. CMV DNA and CMV early antigens in Kaposi's sarcoma. *Int J Cancer* 1980;26:23–9.

178. Boldogh I, Beth E, Huang E-S, Kyalwaszi SK, Giraldo G. Kaposi's sarcoma. IV. Detection of CMV DNA, CMV RNA, and CMNA in tumor biopsies. *Int J Cancer* 1981;28:469–74.

179. Drew WL, Miner RC, Ziegler JL, et al. Cytomegalovirus and Kaposi's sarcoma in young homosexual men. *Lancet* 1982;2:125–7.

180. Delli Bovi P, Donti E, Knowles DM, et al. Presence of chromosomal abnormalities and lack of AIDS retrovirus DNA sequences in AIDS-associated Kaposi's sarcoma. *Cancer Res* 1986;46:6333–8.

181. van den Berg F, Schipper M, Jiwa M, Rook R, van de Rijke F, Tigges B. Implausibility of an aetiological association between cytomegalovirus and Kaposi's sarcoma shown by four techniques. *J Clin Pathol* 1989;42:128–31.

182. Johnston GS, Jockusch J, McMurty LC, Shandera WX. Cytomegalovirus (CMV) titers among acquired immunodeficiency syndrome (AIDS) patients with and without a history of Kaposi's sarcoma. *Cancer Detect Prev* 1990;14:337–42.

183. Beral V, Peterman TA, Berkelman RL, Jaffe HW. Kaposi's sar-

coma among persons with AIDS: a sexually transmitted infection? *Lancet* 1990;335:123–8.

184. Fukunaga M, Silverberg SG. Kaposi's sarcoma in patients with acquired immune deficiency syndrome: a flow cytometric DNA analysis of 26 lesions in 21 patients. *Cancer* 1990;66:758–64.

185. Friedman-Kien AE, Saltzman BR, Cao Y, et al. Kaposi's sarcoma in HIV-negative homosexual men. *Lancet* 1990; 335:168–9.

186. McHugh TM, Casavant C, Wilber JC, Stites DP. Comparison of six methods for the detection of antibody to cytomegalovirus. *J Clin Microbiol* 1985;22:1014–9.

187. Gleaves CA, Wendt SF, Dobbs DR, Meyers JD. Evaluation of the CMV-CUBE assay for detection of cytomegalovirus serologic status in marrow transplant patients and marrow donors. *J Clin Microbiol* 1990;28:841–2.

188. Rasmussen L, Kelsall D, Nelson R, et al. Virus-specific IgG and IgM antibodies in normal and immunocompromised subjects infected with cytomegalovirus. *J Infect Dis* 1982;145:191–9.

189. Schaefer L, Cesario A, Demmler G, et al. Evaluation of Abbott CMV-M enzyme immunoassay for detection of cytomegalovirus immunoglobulin M antibody. *J Clin Microbiol* 1988;26:2041–3.

190. Quinnan GV, Masur H, Rook AH, et al. Herpesvirus infections in the acquired immune deficiency syndrome. *JAMA* 1984;252:72–7.

191. Halbert SP, Kiefer DJ, Friedman-Kien AE, Poiesz B. Antibody levels for cytomegalovirus, herpes simplex virus, and rubella in patients with acquired immune deficiency syndrome. *J Clin Microbiol* 1986;23:318–21.

192. Landini MP, Mirolo G, Re MC, Ripalti A, La Placa M. Antibody reactivity to cytomegalovirus structural polypeptides in subclinical and clinical human immunodeficiency virus infections. *Eur J Clin Microbiol Infect Dis* 1989;8:159–63.

193. Marsano L, Perillo RP, Flye MW, et al. Comparison of culture and serology for the diagnosis of cytomegalovirus infection in kidney and liver transplant recipients. *J Infect Dis* 1990; 161:454–61.

194. Shuster EA, Beneke JS, Tegtmeier GE, et al. Monoclonal antibody for rapid laboratory detection of cytomegalovirus infections: characterization and diagnostic application. *Mayo Clinic Proc* 1985;60:577–85.

195. Swenson PD, Kaplan MH. Rapid detection of cytomegalovirus in cell culture by indirect immunoperoxidase staining with monoclonal antibody to an early nuclear antigen. *J Clin Microbiol* 1985;21:669–73.

196. Rush JD, Ng VL, Hopewell PC, Hadley WK, Mills J. Comparative recovery of cytomegalovirus from saliva, mucolysed induced sputum, and bronchoalveolar lavage fluid from patients at risk for or with acquired immunodeficiency syndrome. *J Clin Microbiol* 1989;27:2864–5.

197. Epstein JS, Frederich WR, Rook AH, et al. Selective defects in cytomegalovirus- and mitogen-induced lymphocyte proliferation and interferon release in patients with acquired immunodeficiency syndrome. *J Infect Dis* 1985;152:727–33.

198. Chou S, Merigan TC. Rapid detection and quantitation of human cytomegalovirus in urine through DNA hybridization. *N Engl J Med* 1983;308:921–5.

199. Schuster V, Matz B, Wiegand H, Traub B, Kampa D, Neumann-Haefelin D. Detection of human cytomegalovirus in urine by DNA–DNA and RNA–DNA hybridization. *J Infect Dis* 1986;154:309–14.

200. Musiani M, Zerbini M, Gentilomi G, et al. Rapid detection of cytomegalovirus DNA in urine samples with a dot blot hybridization immunoenzymatic assay. *J Clin Microbiol* 1990;28:2101–3.

201. van der Bij W, Torensma R, van Son WJ, et al. Rapid diagnosis of active cytomegalovirus infection by monoclonal antibody staining of blood leukocytes. *J Med Virol* 1988;25:179–88.

202. van der Bij W, Schirm J, Torensma R, van Son WJ, Tegzess AM, The TH. Comparison between viremia and antigenemia for detection of cytomegalovirus in blood. *J Clin Microbiol* 1988;26:2531–5.

203. Danker WM, McCutchan JA, Richman DD, Hirata K, Spector SA. Localization of human cytomegalovirus in peripheral blood leukocytes by *in situ* hybridization. *J Infect Dis* 1990;161:31–6.

204. Martin WJ, Smith TF. Rapid detection of cytomegalovirus in

205. Emanuel D, Peppard J, Stover D, Gold J, Armstrong D, Hammerling U. Rapid diagnosis of cytomegalovirus pneumonia by bronchoalveolar lavage using human and murine monoclonal antibodies. *Ann Intern Med* 1986;104:476–81.

206. Gleaves CA, Myerson D, Bowden RA, Hackman RC, Meyers JD. Direct detection of cytomegalovirus from bronchoalveolar lavage samples by using a rapid *in situ* DNA hybridization assay. *J Clin Microbiol* 1989;27:2429–32.

207. Schulman HM, Hackman RC, Sale GE, Meyers JD. Rapid cytologic diagnosis of cytomegalovirus interstitial pneumonia on touch imprints from open lung biopsy. *Am J Clin Pathol* 1982;77:90–4.

208. Hackman RC, Myerson D, Meyers JD, et al. Rapid diagnosis of cytomegaloviral pneumonia by tissue immunofluorescence with a murine monoclonal antibody. *J Infect Dis* 1985;151:325–9.

209. Stagno S, Reynolds DW, Tsiantos A, Fucillo DA, Long W, Alford CA. Comparative serial virologic and serologic studies of symptomatic and subclinical congenitally and natally acquired cytomegalovirus infections. *J Infect Dis* 1975;132:568–77.

210. Chou S, Scott KM. Rapid quantitation of cytomegalovirus and assay of neutralizing antibody by using monoclonal antibody to the major immediate-early viral protein. *J Clin Microbiol* 1988;26:504–7.

211. Gerna G, Parea M, Percivalle E, et al. Human cytomegalovirus viremia in HIV-1-seropositive patients at various clinical stages of infection. *AIDS* 1990;4:1027–31.

212. Gerna G, Revello MG, Percivalle E, Zavattoni M, Parea M, Battaglia M. Quantification of human cytomegalovirus viremia by using monoclonal antibodies to different viral proteins. *J Clin Microbiol* 1990;28:2681–8.

213. Marker SC, Howard RJ, Groth KE, Mastri AR, Simmons RL, Balfour HH. A trial of vidarabine for cytomegalovirus infection in renal transplant patients. *Arch Intern Med* 1980;140:1441–4.

214. Meyers JD, McGuffin RW, Bryson YJ, Cantell K, Thomas ED. Treatment of cytomegalovirus pneumonia after marrow transplantation with combined vidarabine and human leukocyte interferon. *J Infect Dis* 1982;146:80–4.

215. Wade JC, Hintz M, McGuffin RW, Springmeyer SC, Connor JD, Meyers JD. Treatment of cytomegalovirus pneumonia with high-dose acyclovir. *Am J Med* 1982;73:249–56.

216. Wade JC, McGuffin RW, Springmeyer SC, Newton B, Singer JW, Meyers JD. Treatment of cytomegaloviral pneumonia with high-dose acyclovir and human leukocyte interferon. *J Infect Dis* 1983;148:557–62.

217. Shepp DH, Newton BA, Meyers JD. Intravenous lymphoblastoid interferon and acyclovir for treatment of cytomegaloviral pneumonia. *J Infect Dis* 1984;150:776–7.

218. Tyms AS, Seamans EM, Naim HM. The *in vitro* activity of acyclovir and related compounds against cytomegalovirus infections. *J Antimicrob Chemother* 1981;6:65–72.

219. Spector SA, Kelley E. Inhibition of human cytomegalovirus by combined acyclovir and vidarabine. *Antimicrob Agents Chemother* 1985;27:600–4.

220. Smee DF, Martin JC, Verheyden JPH, Matthews TR. Anti-herpesvirus activity of the acyclic nucleoside 9-(1,3-dihydroxypropoxymethyl)guanine. *Antimicrob Agents Chemother* 1983; 23:676–82.

221. Mar EC, Cheng YC, Huang E-S. Effect of 9-(1,3-dihydroxy-2-propoxymethyl)guanine on human cytomegalovirus replication *in vitro*. *Antimicrob Agents Chemother* 1983;24:518–21.

222. Freitas VR, Smee DF, Chernow M, Boehme R, Matthews TR. Activity of 9-(1,3-dihydroxy-2-propoxymethyl)guanine compared with that of acyclovir against human, monkey, and rodent cytomegaloviruses. *Antimicrob Agents Chemother* 1985;28: 240–5.

223. Matthews T, Boehme R. Antiviral activity and mechanism of action of ganciclovir. *Rev Infect Dis* 1988;10:S490–4.

224. Shepp DH, Dandliker PS, de Miranda P, et al. Activity of 9-[2-hydroxy-1-(hydroxymethyl)ethoxymethyl]guanine in the treatment of cytomegalovirus pneumonia. *Ann Intern Med* 1985;103: 368–73.

225. Felsenstein D, D'Amico DJ, Hirsch MS, et al. Treatment of cyto-

megalovirus retinitis with 9-[2-hydroxy-1-(hydroxymethyl)eth-oxymethyl]guanine. *Ann Intern Med* 1985;103:377–80.

226. Bach MC, Bagwell SP, Knapp NP, Davis KM, Hedstrom PS. 9-(1,3-dihydroxy-2-propoxymethyl)guanine for cytomegalovirus infections in patients with the acquired immunodeficiency syndrome. *Ann Intern Med* 1985;103:381–2.

227. Jacobson MA, O'Donnell JJ, Porteous D, et al. Retinal and gastrointestinal disease due to cytomegalovirus in patients with the acquired immune deficiency syndrome: prevalence, natural history, and response to ganciclovir therapy. *Q J Med* 1988;67:473–86.

228. Mills J, Jacobson MA, O'Donnell JJ, Cederberg D, Holland GN. Treatment of cytomegalovirus retinitis in patients with AIDS. *Rev Infect Dis* 1988;10:S522–7.

229. Jacobson MA, O'Donnell JJ, Rousell R, Dionian B, Mills J. Failure of adjunctive cytomegalovirus intravenous immune globulin to improve efficacy of ganciclovir in patients with acquired immunodeficiency syndrome and cytomegalovirus retinitis. *Antimicrob Agents Chemother* 1990;34:176–8.

230. Kotler DP, Tierney AR, Altilio D, Wang J, Pierson RN. Body mass repletion during ganciclovir treatment of cytomegalovirus infections in patients with acquired immunodeficiency syndrome. *Arch Intern Med* 1989;149:901–5.

231. Kotler DP, Culpepper-Morgan JA, Tierney AR, Klein EB. Treatment of disseminated cytomegalovirus with 9-(1,3-dihydroxy-2-propoxymethyl)guanine: evidence of prolonged survival in patients with the acquired immunodeficiency syndrome. *AIDS Res* 1986;2:299–308.

232. Hochster H, Dieterich D, Bozzette S, et al. Toxicity of combined ganciclovir and zidovudine for cytomegalovirus disease associated with AIDS: an AIDS Clinical Trials Group study. *Ann Intern Med* 1990;113:111–7.

233. Erice A, Chou S, Biron K, Stanat SC, Balfour HH, Jordan MC. Progressive disease due to ganciclovir-resistant cytomegalovirus in immunocompromised patients. *N Engl J Med* 1989; 320:289–93.

234. Eriksson B, Oberg B, Wahren B. Pyrophosphate analogues as inhibitors of DNA polymerases of cytomegalovirus, herpes simplex virus and cellular origin. *Biochim Biophys Acta* 1982;696:115–23.

235. Oberg B. Antiviral effects of phosphonoformate (PFA, foscarnet sodium). *Pharmacol Ther* 1983;19:387–415.

236. Jacobson MA, Crowe S, Levy J, et al. Effect of foscarnet therapy on infection with human immunodeficiency virus in patients with AIDS. *J Infect Dis* 1988;158:862–5.

237. Palestine AG, Polis MA, De Smet MD, et al. A randomized, controlled trial of foscarnet in the treatment of cytomegalovirus retinitis in patients with AIDS. *Ann Intern Med* 1991; 115:665–73.

238. Jacobson MA, O'Donnell JJ, Mills JF. Foscarnet treatment of cytomegalovirus retinitis in patients with the acquired immunodeficiency syndrome. *Antimicrob Agents Chemother* 1989; 33:736–41.

239. Fanning MM, Read SE, Benson M, et al. Foscarnet therapy of cytomegalovirus retinitis in AIDS. *J Acquired Immune Deficiency Syndrome* 1990;3:472–9.

239a. Studies of ocular complications of AIDS research group in collaboration with the AIDS clinical trials group. *N Engl J Med* 1992;326:213–20.

240. Farese RV, Schambelan M, Hollander H, Stringari S, Jacobson MA. Nephrogenic diabetes insipidus associated with foscarnet treatment of cytomegalovirus retinitis. *Ann Intern Med* 1990;112:955–6.

241. Biron KK, Fyfe JA, Stanat SC, et al. A human cytomegalovirus mutant resistant to the nucleoside analog 9-{[2-hydroxy-1-(hydroxymethyl)ethoxyl]methyl}guanine (BW B759U) induces reduced levels of BW B759U triphosphate. *Proc Natl Acad Sci USA* 1986;83:8769–73.

242. Colacino JM, Lopez C. Efficacy and selectivity of some nucleoside analogs as anti-human cytomegalovirus agents. *Antimicrob Agents Chemother* 1983;24:505–8.

243. Colacino JM, Lopez C. Antiviral activity of 2'-deoxy-2'-fluoro-β-D-arabinofuranosyl-5-iodocytosine against human cytomegalovirus in human skin fibroblasts. *Antimicrob Agents Chemother* 1985;28:252–8.

AIDS and Other Manifestations of HIV Infection,
Second Edition, Edited by Gary P. Wormser.
Raven Press, Ltd., New York © 1992.

CHAPTER 18

Bacterial Infections in Patients with HIV Infection

Michael S. Simberkoff and Howard L. Leaf

ABNORMALITIES OF HOST DEFENSES AGAINST BACTERIAL INFECTION

A variety of specific and nonspecific host defense mechanisms are essential for the prevention of bacterial infection. These include elaboration of specific immunoglobulins, phagocytic cell activity, and the integrity of the skin and mucous membranes. Each of these defenses may be compromised in patients with human immunodeficiency virus (HIV) infection, predisposing them to infections with pyogenic bacteria.

Early in the HIV epidemic, immunoglobulin abnormalities were recognized as very common among patients with HIV/AIDS. Although concentrations of serum immunoglobulins are usually elevated, patients have been found to have paradoxically hypoactive B-cell function. B cells from patients with AIDS respond poorly to new antigenic stimuli, including protein (key-hole-limpet hemocyanin) and polysaccharide (pneumococcal) antigens in vitro and in vivo (1,2). In addition, their lymphocytes respond poorly to a variety of mitogens in vitro including phytohemagglutinin (T cell), pokeweed (T and B cell), and formalinized *Staphylococcus aureus* Cowan (B cell) (2,3). Depression of IgG$_2$ subclass levels in patients with AIDS or ARC with pyogenic infections has been noted, when compared to levels in comparable groups without bacterial infections (4). Beyond the fact that such dysgammaglobulinemias predispose to bacterial infection, a further difficulty is encountered in attempting to immunize patients, in whom adequate antibody responses may not occur against common bacterial pathogens.

Disordered phagocyte function is also seen in HIV infection. Granulocyte function may be affected due both to qualitative defects and as a result of granulocytopenia caused by various drug therapies. Decreased neutrophil chemotaxis to leukotriene B4 and the chemotactic peptide fMLP has been reported in HIV-infected patients who nevertheless exhibited normal spontaneous neutrophil migration (5). Others have reported decreased chemotactic responses to casein (6). Similar findings have been noted in children with HIV infection, who manifest more frequent episodes of bacterial infection than do adults (7). Interestingly, this chemotactic defect has been more pronounced in patients with earlier clinical stages of HIV infection (6,7). This surprising observation was also made by Ellis and colleagues (8), who demonstrated significantly less neutrophil chemotaxis in patients with AIDS-related complex (ARC) than in patients with AIDS (with Kaposi's sarcoma—KS) or in healthy heterosexual controls.

Decreased phagocytosis and killing of *Candida albicans* by polymorphonuclear leukocytes (9) and decreased killing of *S. aureus* (8) have also been reported. These defects in killing, as well as the observed chemotactic defects, may be due, in some degree, to serum abnormalities. Ras and colleagues (10) reported that serum from AIDS patients decreased the number of fMLP receptors on normal neutrophils. Moreover, opsonization of *S. aureus* by complement containing serum restored bacterial killing by neutrophils from patients with AIDS. It appears that defects in specific humoral immunity in patients with HIV infection contribute to deficient neutrophil phagocytosis and killing, and that other less well-defined serum factors, such as immune complexes (11), may also play a role in causing abnormal neutrophil

M. S. Simberkoff and H. L. Leaf: Infectious Diseases Section, New York Veterans Administration Medical Center, New York, New York 10010; and the Department of Medicine, New York University School of Medicine, New York, New York 10016.

function. GM-CSF has been noted to improve the defective bactericidal activity of neutrophils in HIV-infected children (7).

Bone marrow dysfunction is commonly observed in HIV-infected patients (12). Though anemia and thrombocytopenia predominate, granulocytopenia also may occur. In addition, granulocytopenia can result from use of anti-retroviral agents, such as zidovudine (13–15), to treat the HIV infection, cytotoxic agents to treat the malignancies associated with AIDS, or antimicrobial agents such as trimethoprim-sulfamethoxazole (16) or ganciclovir (17), which are used in the treatment of opportunistic infections.

Finally, the skin and mucous membranes of patients with AIDS are often affected by disease processes or therapeutic interventions that may lead to secondary pyogenic infections. Kaposi's sarcoma (KS) is one such disease process. The tumor may be confined to the skin, it may involve mucous membranes with or without lymph node involvement, or it may disseminate viscerally (18,19). The lesions on the skin and in the oral and gastrointestinal mucosa may be very numerous and coalesce (20). They can erode or bleed and serve as foci of infection by the microbial flora of the surface involved. The gingival mucosa is most frequently the site of superinfected KS lesions. However, bacterial pneumonia has also been reported as a complication of pulmonary Kaposi's sarcoma (21,22), and *Clostridium perfringens* (19) and *Streptococcus bovis* (see below) bacteremia have occurred in patients with gastrointestinal lesions.

Similarly, certain opportunistic infections, which may involve the skin or mucous membranes of patients with AIDS, can in turn become superinfected with pyogenic organisms. Cytomegalovirus infections of the lung, esophagus, colon, or gallbladder may lead to secondary bacterial infections; intestinal perforation with fecal peritonitis and/or bacteremia may occur (23) and secondary bacterial infection of cytomegalovirus cholecystitis has also been reported (24). Chronic oral and perianal infections due to herpes simplex, and seborrheic dermatitis, tinea faciale, and a variety of other dermatophyte infections, which are common in these patients (25,26), can become secondarily infected by bacterial pathogens. Furunculosis and impetigo have been described in patients with HIV infection and may serve as sources of persistent infection and bacteremia. Finally, *Candida* species are a common cause of pharyngitis and esophagitis in HIV-infected patients (27,28), although to our knowledge bacterial superinfection of these lesions and resultant bacteremias have not been reported.

Iatrogenic intervention also frequently impairs the integrity of the mucocutaneous barrier in AIDS. Cytotoxic agents may cause mucosal ulcerations in patients with malignancies. Hospitalized AIDS patients frequently require intravenous catheters, which can serve as conduits for bacterial invasion of the vascular system. Catheter-related infections have been documented to be a prominent source of the *Staphylococcus aureus* and gram-negative bacillary bacteremias seen in these patients (22). Patients with AIDS seem to be at higher risk for infection of indwelling central venous catheters. The infection rate per catheter day was tenfold higher in AIDS patients than in immunocompetent patients in one study (29). In another hospital survey, a fivefold higher rate was seen (30). Infections were largely due to *S. aureus,* in contrast to the usually higher percentage due to coagulase-negative staphylococci in patients with malignancies. Whether this relates to the aforementioned defects in neutrophil phagocytosis of *S. aureus* or to factors favoring colonization with *S. aureus* in this patient population is unclear. A higher prevalence of *S. aureus* colonization in HIV-infected patients has been noted (31).

BACTERIAL PNEUMONIA

It is now widely recognized that a significant proportion of pulmonary infections in HIV-infected patients are due to "classic" respiratory tract pathogens, particularly the encapsulated bacteria.

Estimates of the incidence of pyogenic pneumonia among AIDS patients have varied considerably. In one of the first descriptions of *Pneumocystis carinii* pneumonia (PCP) in the HIV epidemic, 3 of 11 patients developed a nosocomial gram-negative pneumonia during or after treatment for PCP (32). Two other patients in this group had bacterial sepsis. At the other extreme was the report of the first National Heart, Lung and Blood Institute Workshop on pulmonary complications of AIDS, which pooled data from six institutions (33). Of the reported 1067 patients with AIDS, 441 developed pulmonary infections or malignancies; 11 of these infections were caused by pyogenic bacteria and an additional 10 by *Legionella,* an incidence of less than 2%.

Several other reports cite figures somewhere between these two extremes. Of 100 patients with AIDS seen by Stover and colleagues during a 4-year period, nine cases of bacterial pneumonia were seen in four patients (34). *Haemophilus influenzae* or *Streptococcus pneumoniae* was recovered from sputum cultures in five of these cases; in the remainder, Gram stains suggested bacterial pneumonia but pathogens were not recovered. In 336 patients seen over 6 years by Polsky and colleagues, 18 episodes of community-acquired bacterial pneumonia occurred in 13 patients (21). Selwyn and colleagues have reported on the increased incidence of bacterial pneumonias associated with HIV infection in a cohort of intravenous drug users without AIDS (35). Ten percent developed bacterial pneumonias, 4% due to *S. pneumoniae.* These figures contrasted with the rate of 2% for bacterial pneumonias among HIV-seronegative intravenous drug users (IVDUs), with less than 1% due to *S. pneumoniae.*

In fact, the number of pyogenic organisms that have been associated with significant pulmonary disease in HIV-infected patients is fairly small. *Streptococcus pneumoniae* (21,34,36) and *H. influenzae* (21,34,37) have been responsible for the majority of community-acquired bacterial pneumonias, with occasional case reports of infection due to *Klebsiella* species (32,38), group B streptococcus, or *Moraxella catarrhalis* (21). A clustering of *Legionella* infections was noted early in the epidemic in New York City (33), although details of these cases, their clinical manifestations, and their responses to therapy have not been published.

Pneumococcal bacteremia is increasingly being recognized as an important cause of morbidity in HIV-infected patients. Through a review of microbiology records at ten San Francisco hospitals, Redd and colleagues identified 294 patients with pneumococcal bacteremia, 11% of whom had AIDS at the time of presentation, and 15% of whom were HIV-infected but without AIDS (39). From these and other data, a rate of pneumococcal bacteremia in AIDS patients was estimated at 9.4/ 1000 patient-years. Importantly, 82% of pneumococcal isolates in HIV-infected patients were of serotypes included in the current 23-valent pneumococcal vaccine (see below).

Excess rates of pneumococcal disease have therefore come to be used as effective epidemiologic markers for HIV infection within populations, at the hospital-wide (40), city-wide (41), or state-wide (42) levels.

Variable data on the clinical presentation and outcome of pneumococcal disease have been reported. It has been our observation (unpublished data) and that of others (39), that pneumococcal disease may present prior to the development of AIDS, suggesting that significant abnormalities in humoral immunity may develop prior to cellular immune deficits severe enough to predispose to opportunistic infections. One study (43) reported a high frequency of atypical presentations of pneumococcal disease in HIV-infected patients, with fever and leukocytosis present in only 57% and 59%, respectively, and a mortality rate of 33%. Others, however, have described more typical findings (39,40,44) of focal infiltrates, fever, leukocytosis, and a lower mortality rate. A recent review of radiologic findings in pyogenic bacterial pneumonias in HIV-infected patients supported the latter finding (45). Of 34 episodes of pyogenic pneumonias reviewed, 17 (50%) were associated with lobar consolidation on CXR. Pulmonary nodules and pleural effusions were also seen in this group but were absent in another group of 30 patients in whom PCP was diagnosed. Twelve of the 34 episodes were due to *Streptococcus pneumoniae* and 11 were due to *Staphylococcus aureus*. A 9% mortality rate was noted.

The presence of purulent sputum, which is microscopically consistent with a bacterial infection, is probably the most important indicator of a bacterial infection of the respiratory tract. However, polymicrobial infections are the rule rather than the exception in patients with AIDS, and the presence of a bacterial infection does not exclude the simultaneous occurrence of one or more opportunistic pulmonary infections. While there are no statistics regarding the frequency with which bacterial respiratory infections in patients with AIDS are associated with underlying, perhaps more chronic, opportunistic infections, the phenomenon is not uncommon. Following one memorable case in which a bacteremic pneumococcal pneumonia, PCP, and *Legionella* pneumonia were found simultaneously in a single patient (36), we usually presume the coexistence of PCP until diagnostic maneuvers or a favorable response to antibacterial therapy satisfy us that only the bacterial infection is present.

When treated promptly and appropriately, pyogenic respiratory infections among patients with AIDS frequently respond well to therapy. In Polsky's series of 18 episodes of community-acquired bacterial pneumonias in 13 patients, 16 of 18 episodes were cured (21). It would appear that the higher mortality rates have been reported from those series in which the patients had the most severely compromised immune systems (43). Thus it appears that the best indicator of immediate prognosis of severe bacterial pulmonary infection is the individual's overall clinical condition. Patients who have not been weakened by long hospitalizations or bouts with other infections tend to respond well.

An issue that has been repeatedly raised in discussions of pyogenic pneumonias in patients with AIDS has been the utility of prophylaxis of pneumococcal infections with the pneumococcal vaccine. Results of immunization in this population, however, have been extremely variable. Some have documented adequate antibody responses, with the suggestion that active immunization against pneumococcal disease in this population is a feasible proposition. Huang and colleagues (46) found no difference in antibody titers to 12 pneumococcal polysaccharide antigens in asymptomatic HIV-seropositive patients when compared to healthy controls. Patients with HIV infection and persistent generalized lymphadenopathy syndrome (PGL) showed mild impairment in their response. Others (47–50) have documented a wholly inadequate antibody response, citing the now well-recognized phenomenon of B-cell dysfunction among these patients. Ballet and colleagues (47) noted significantly lower antibody titers after pneumococcal vaccination in HIV-infected patients regardless of their clinical stage of disease; others have noted similarly disappointing results in asymptomatic or mildly symptomatic HIV-infected homosexual men (48,49). In one study of HIV-infected hemophiliacs, disappointing increases in antibody titer following vaccination were attributed to higher preimmunization titers than in seronegative controls (50). Finally, antibody responses to the 23-valent pneumococcal polysaccharide vaccine in HIV-seropositive asymptomatic heterosexual partners of IVDUs were lower than those seen in controls, although a majority of patients with low baseline type-specific antibodies to one or more antigens showed a rise in titer to at least one antigen (51). We have reported one frank clinical failure of the pneumococcal vaccine, in which bacteremia with a vaccine-type pneumococcus occurred 6 months after the vaccine was administered to an HIV-infected individual (36). Prospective evaluation of the efficacy of the 23-valent vaccine in our hospital's HIV-infected population is ongoing.

Despite the lack of clear demonstration of efficacy, the Advisory Committee on Immunization Practices now recommends vaccination for all adults with asymptomatic or symptomatic HIV infection (52). It would seem advisable to administer vaccine to patients as early in their course as possible. Whether or not there may be benefit from long-term oral penicillin prophylaxis in this patient population is unknown.

BACTEREMIA

Not surprisingly, given the higher incidences of bacteremic pneumococcal pneumonia and catheter-associated staphylococcal sepsis, the incidence of bacteremia in general is high among patients with AIDS (22,43,53). In epidemiologic surveys, increases in sepsis mortality among young populations have been correlated with high cumulative AIDS incidence (54).

Whimbey and colleagues reviewed 38 episodes of bacteremia occurring among 336 patients with AIDS followed at Memorial Sloan–Kettering Cancer Center in New York City (22). Nine of these were nosocomial infections, and seven were associated with vascular catheters. In addition, there were four episodes of candidemia associated with vascular catheters. Two cases of Pseudomonas aeruginosa bacteremia were observed. Both of these were associated with pneumonia and one of the patients was neutropenic. Two other episodes of bacteremia occurred in neutropenic patients. One was caused by Staphylococcus epidermidis and the other by Enterococcus faecalis. There were ten episodes of S. aureus bacteremia, nine community acquired and one nosocomial. The latter was associated with a vascular catheter and a mixed bacteremia (with group G streptococcus).

A survey of 35 bacteremic episodes from another institution with a largely IVDU population showed a similar distribution of pathogens (53). Outcomes were not reported. A San Francisco General Hospital series (43) reported on 44 episodes of community-acquired bacteremia in 38 AIDS patients, which accounted for 5% of all AIDS admissions. Of interest, fever occurred in only 57% of the episodes. The most common sources for the bacteremia were pneumonia, central venous line infections, and cellulitis. There was a 9% fatality rate.

In our own series of 817 patients with CDC-defined AIDS seen at the New York VA Medical Center, we observed bacteremias in 135 patients. There were 66 patients with S. aureus bacteremia, 42 with Pseudomonas aeruginosa bacteremia, 20 with S. pneumoniae bacteremia, 14 with Salmonella bacteremia, 10 with enterococcal bacteremia, and 8 with H. influenzae bacteremia. In addition, there were 12 episodes of Candida albicans or Torulopsis glabrata fungemia.

A high incidence of Pseudomonas infections was also seen in a survey from the M. D. Anderson Hospital (54), in which 76 episodes of bacterial infections during 304 admissions of HIV-infected patients were surveyed. Nine were due to enteric gram-negative bacilli, of which P. aeruginosa was the most frequent isolate.

Outside the United States and England (55), the proportion of bacteremias in HIV-infected patients due to Salmonella is higher. Non-typhi Salmonella accounted for 40% of 24 bacteremic episodes in AIDS patients seen in Pavia, Italy (56), and 10.3% of bacteremias in Barcelona (57).

Other organisms have caused bacteremia in patients with AIDS. There are reports of Listeria monocytogenes bacteremia in several patients with AIDS (58,59). Kales and Holzman (60) reported on listeriosis in seven patients with HIV infection and in four at risk for HIV infection seen at three New York City hospitals from 1981 to 1988. Three of the 11 had meningitis. Seven had bacteremia without an identified source of infection and one had endocarditis. All responded well to penicillin or ampicillin, with or without an aminoglycoside, and no relapses were observed. Why listeriosis, against which the host defense is largely cell-mediated, is not seen more frequently in AIDS, is an unsettled issue. One fatal case of Listeria bacteremia occurred in a postpartum 27-year-old Haitian immigrant (61), in whom AIDS was diagnosed when skin lesions noted on admission proved to be an inflammatory variant of Kaposi's sarcoma (62).

Other miscellaneous bacteremias have also been reported, including infections due to Campylobacter fetus in a patient with cholecystitis (63), Yersinia enterocolitica (64), and Shigella species (65), among the non-salmonella gastrointestinal pathogens. Group G streptococcus endocarditis (66) has been reported, and Streptococcus bovis bacteremia was observed in a 33-year-old Haitian male with gastrointestinal Kaposi's sarcoma (KS) (67). Clostridium perfringens bacteremia has also been observed in a patient with gastrointestinal KS (19). Cases of Rhodococcus equi infection (68) and reports of severe group A beta-hemolytic streptococcal cellulitis have also appeared (69,70).

We have found that response to treatment for bacteremia, as for pneumonia, directly correlates with the patient's overall clinical condition. Patients not weakened by chronic infections or malignancies respond well, while bacteremia is frequently the modus exitus of terminal individuals.

Two qualifications to these generalizations should be noted. First, a high rate of late metastatic infectious complications of treated *S. aureus* bacteremia has been observed (71). In 17 AIDS or ARC patients who survived at least 1 month after their initial bacteremia, a 35% rate of late metastatic complications was observed, with only one of the six affected patients initially receiving less than 2 weeks of appropriate therapy.

The second exception involves patients with *Salmonella* bacteremia. Although the topic of gastrointestinal infections in HIV infection is dealt with more fully elsewhere in this volume, the unique problem of non-typhi *Salmonella* bacteremia deserves mention here, as the majority of these patients present without gastrointestinal complaints (72). The increased incidence of bacteremic *Salmonella* infections, which may at times precede the diagnosis of AIDS, was recognized early in the epidemic (73–75), and recurrence after appropriate therapy, an AIDS-defining event (76), has been problematic. The increased incidence of bacteremic *Salmonella* infections is due largely to *S.* serotype *typhimurium* and *S.* serotype *enteritidis,* although *S. arizonae* infections in AIDS patients ingesting rattlesnake meat along the U.S.–Mexican border have been recently reported (77). Suppressive therapy with ampicillin or trimethoprim-sulfamethoxazole has been advocated (72), while ciprofloxacin appears to be a safe and effective alternative (78).

PEDIATRIC INFECTIONS

As the number of HIV-infected pediatric patients has risen, it has become evident that frequent and severe bacterial infections are a recognized feature of their illness (79). As in adult patients, cell-mediated immunity is depressed in children with AIDS, T-helper cell numbers are reduced, and T-cell ratios are reversed (80). Humoral immunity also is affected in these children. Bernstein and colleagues showed that the primary and secondary responses to bacteriophage antigens, tetanus toxoid, and pneumococcal vaccine were profoundly depressed in pediatric AIDS patients (81).

The clinical manifestations of AIDS in children and adults also have many similarities. Like adults, children become cachectic and may suffer from chronic diarrhea. Opportunistic infections are common, as is lymphoid interstitial pneumonia, which is less commonly seen in adults (82).

The high incidence of bacterial infections in children, including bacteremia, however, is so striking that recurrent severe bacterial infection has been included as an "indicator disease" in the case definition of AIDS in the pediatric population (76). Among the earliest series of pediatric AIDS, 5 of 7 patients reported by Rubinstein and colleagues (80), 5 of 8 cases reported by Oleske and colleagues (82), and 10 of 14 reported by Scott and colleagues (83) had infections with classic pyogenic organisms, including *S. aureus, S. pneumoniae,* and *E. coli* or other gram-negative bacilli. Recurrent infections with the same bacterial pathogen are very common among these patients. For example, we observed a child with four episodes of type 6A *S. pneumoniae* bacteremia at Bellevue Hospital.

Krasinski and colleagues (79) reviewed the records of 71 children infected with HIV. Thirty-seven percent of the children had a bacteriologically documented infection. Of the 125 episodes observed, 19% were pneumonias, 19% upper respiratory tract infections, 19% urinary tract infections, and 10% wound infections. Twenty-eight percent of episodes were bacteremic, with *S. pneumoniae* and *Salmonella* species the most common blood isolates. A generally prompt response to therapy was noted.

CONCLUSIONS

Bacterial infections, although less common than opportunistic infections among patients with HIV infection, cause a significant amount of morbidity and mortality in this population. HIV-infected children are particularly at risk for bacterial infections. HIV-infected adults are also at risk, both early in the course of HIV infection with relatively well-preserved cell-mediated immunity and much later, after long hospitalizations or bouts with other AIDS-related infections or malignancies. Predisposing factors for pyogenic infection include physical alterations in cutaneous and mucosal barriers, B-cell dysfunction, and reductions in phagocytic cell number and function. The clinician must be aware of the increased risk of these infections, consider prophylactic strategies where appropriate, and be prepared to initiate diagnostic studies and appropriate therapies promptly.

REFERENCES

1. Ammann AJ, Schiffman G, Abrams D, Volberding P, Ziegler J, Conant M. B-cell immunodeficiency in acquired immunodeficiency syndrome. *JAMA* 1984;251:1947–9.
2. Lane HC, Masur H, Edgar LC, Whalen G, Rook AH, Fauci AS. Abnormalities of B-cell activation in patients with the acquired immunodeficiency syndrome. *N Engl J Med* 1983;309:453–8.
3. Stahl RE, Friedman-Kien A, Dubin R, Marmor M, Zolla-Pazner S. Immunologic abnormalities in homosexual men; relationship to Kaposi's sarcoma. *Am J Med* 1982;73:171–8.
4. Parkin JM, Helbert M, Hughes CL, Pinching AJ. Immunoglobulin G subclass deficiency and susceptibility to pyogenic infections in patients with AIDS-related complex and AIDS. *AIDS* 1989; 3(1):37–9.
5. Valone FH, Payan DG, Abrams DI, Goetzl EJ. Defective polymorphonuclear leukocyte chemotaxis in homosexual men with persistent lymph node syndrome. *J Infect Dis* 1984;150:267–71.
6. Nielsen H, Kharazmi A, Faber V. Blood monocyte and neutrophil functions in the acquired immunodeficiency syndrome. *Scand J Immunol* 1986;24:291–6.
7. Roilides E, Mertins S, Eddy J, Walsh TJ, Pizzo PA, Rubin M. Impairment of neutrophil chemotactic and bactericidal function in children infected with human immunodeficiency virus type 1

and partial reversal after *in vitro* exposure to granulocyte–macrophage colony-stimulating factor. *J Pediatr* 1990;117:531–40.

8. Ellis M, Gupta S, Galant S, Hakim S, VandeVen C, Toy C, Cairo MS. Impaired neutrophil function in patients with AIDS or AIDS-related complex: a comprehensive evaluation. *J Infect Dis* 1988;158(6):1268–76.

9. Lazzarin A, Uberti Foppa C, Galli M, Montavani A, Poli G, Franzetti F, Novati R. Impairment of polymorphonuclear leukocyte function in patients with acquired immunodeficiency syndrome and with lymphadenopathy syndrome. *Clin Exp Immunol* 1986;65:105–11.

10. Ras GJ, Anderson R, Lukey PT. Defective polymorphonuclear leucocyte migration in AIDS. *S African Med J* 1985;68:292–3.

11. Cohen HJ, Takahashi K, Whitin JC, Chovaniec ME. Human neutrophil (PMN) interactions with human immune complexes (IC). *Pediatr Res* 1987;21:297A.

12. Spivak JL, Bender BS, Quinn TC. Hematologic abnormalities in the acquired immune deficiency syndrome. *Am J Med* 1984;77:224–8.

13. Richman DD, Fischl MA, Grieco MH, et al. The toxicity of azidothymidine (AZT) in the treatment of patients with AIDS and AIDS-related complex: a double-blind, placebo-controlled trial. *N Engl J Med* 1987;317:192–7.

14. Fischl MA, Richman DD, Hansen N, et al. The safety and efficacy of zidovudine (AZT) in the treatment of mildly symptomatic human immunodeficiency virus type 1 (HIV) infection: a double-blind, placebo-controlled trial. *Ann Intern Med* 1990;112:727–37.

15. Volberding PA, Lagakos SW, Koch MA, et al. Zidovudine in asymptomatic human immunodeficiency virus infection: a controlled trial in persons with fewer than 500 CD4-positive cells per cubic millimeter. *N Engl J Med* 1990;322:941–9.

16. Gordin FM, Simon GL, Wofsy CB, Mills J. Adverse reactions to trimethoprim-sulfamethoxazole in patients with the acquired immunodeficiency syndrome. *Ann Intern Med* 1984;100:495–9.

17. Masur HH, Lane C, Palestine A, et al. Effect of 9-(1,3-dihydroxy-2-propoxymethyl)guanine on serious cytomegalovirus disease in eight immunosuppressed homosexual men. *Ann Intern Med* 1986;104:41–4.

18. Krigel RL, Laubenstein LJ, Muggia FM. Kaposi's sarcoma: a new staging classification. *Cancer Treat Rep* 1983;67:531–4.

19. Laubenstein LJ. Staging and treatment of Kaposi's sarcoma in patients with AIDS. In: Friedman-Kien AE, Laubenstein LJ, eds. *AIDS: the epidemic of Kaposi's sarcoma and opportunistic infection.* New York: Masson Publishing; 1984:51–5.

20. Friedman-Kien AE, Ostreicher R. Overview of classical and epidemic Kaposi's sarcoma. In: Friedman-Kien AE, Laubenstein LJ, eds. *AIDS: the epidemic of Kaposi's sarcoma and opportunistic infection.* New York: Masson Publishing; 1984:23–4.

21. Polsky B, Gold JWM, Whimbey E, et al. Bacterial pneumonia in patients with the acquired immunodeficiency syndrome. *Ann Intern Med* 1986;104:38–41.

22. Whimbey E, Gold JWM, Polsky B, et al. Bacteremia and fungemia in patients with the acquired immunodeficiency syndrome. *Ann Intern Med* 1986;164:511–4.

23. Horowitz L, Stern JO, Sefarra S. Gastrointestinal manifestations of Kaposi's sarcoma and AIDS. In: Friedman-Kien AE, Laubenstein LJ, eds. *AIDS: the epidemic of Kaposi's sarcoma and opportunistic infection.* New York: Masson Publishing; 1984:235–40.

24. Kavin H, Jonas RB, Chowdhury L, Kabins S. Acalculous cholecystitis and cytomegalovirus in the acquired immunodeficiency syndrome. *Ann Intern Med* 1986;104:53–4.

25. Eisenstat BA, Wormser GF. Seborrheic dermatitis and butterfly rash in AIDS. *N Engl J Med* 1984;311:189.

26. Hatcher VA. Mucocutaneous infections in acquired immune deficiency syndrome. In: Friedman-Kien AE, Laubenstein LJ, eds. *AIDS: the epidemic of Kaposi's sarcoma and opportunistic infection.* New York: Masson Publishing; 1984:245–51.

27. Klein RS, Harris CA, Small CB, et al. Oral candidiasis in high-risk patients as the initial manifestation of the acquired immunodeficiency syndrome. *N Engl J Med* 1984;311:354–8.

28. Tavitian A, Raufman JP, Rosenthal LE. Oral candidiasis as a marker for esophageal candidiasis in the acquired immunodeficiency syndrome. *Ann Intern Med* 1986;104:54–5.

29. Skoutelis AT, Murphy RL, McDonnell KB, Von Roenn JH, Ster-

kel CD, Phair JP. Indwelling central venous catheter infections in patients with acquired immunodeficiency syndrome. *J AIDS* 1990;3(4):335–42.

30. Raviglione MC, Battan R, Pablos-Mendez A, Aceves-Cassillas P, Mullen MP, Taranta A. Infections associated with Hickman catheters in patients with acquired immunodeficiency syndrome. *Am J Med* 1989;86:780–6.

31. Weinke T, Scherer W, Rohde I, Schiller R, Fehrenbach FJ, Pohle HD. Increased carriage rate of *Staphylococcus aureus* among HIV patients. In: 6th International Conference on AIDS, San Francisco, June 1990.

32. Masur H, Michelis MA, Greene JB, et al. An outbreak of community-acquired *Pneumocystis carinii* pneumonia. Initial manifestation of cellular immune dysfunction. *N Engl J Med* 1981;305:1431–8.

33. Murray JF, Felton CP, Garay SM, et al. Pulmonary complications of acquired immunodeficiency syndrome; report of a National Heart, Lung and Blood Institute Workshop. *N Engl J Med* 1984;310:1682–6.

34. Stover DE, White DA, Romano PA, et al. Spectrum of pulmonary diseases associated with the acquired immune deficiency syndrome. *Am J Med* 1985;78:429–37.

35. Selwyn PA, Feingold AR, Hartel D, Schoenbaum EE, Alderman MH, Klein RS, Friedland GH. Increased risk of bacterial pneumonia in HIV-infected intravenous drug users without acquired immunodeficiency syndrome. *AIDS* 1988;2:267–72.

36. Simberkoff MS, El-Sad W, Schiffman G, Rahal JJ. *Streptococcus pneumoniae* infections and bacteremia in patients with the acquired immune deficiency syndrome, with report of a pneumococcal vaccine failure. *Am Rev Respir Dis* 1984;130:1174–6.

37. Schlamm HT, Yancovitz SR. *Hemophilus influenza* pneumonia in young adults with AIDS, ARC, or risk of AIDS. *Am J Med* 1989;86:11–4.

38. Hollschlanger CM, Khan FA, Chitkara RK, Shivaram U. Pulmonary manifestations of the acquired immunodeficiency syndrome (AIDS). *Chest* 1984;85:197–202.

39. Redd SC, Rutherford GW, Sande MA, Lifson AR, Hadley WK, Facklam RR, Spika JS. The role of human immunodeficiency virus infection in pneumococcal bacteremia in San Francisco residents. *J Infect Dis* 1990;162:1012–7.

40. Chirurgi VA, Edelstein H, McCabe R. Pneumococcal bacteremia as a marker for human immunodeficiency virus infection in patients without AIDS. *South Med J* 1990;83(8):895–9.

41. Stoneburner RL, Laussucq S, Benezra D. Increase in pneumonia mortality among young adults and the HIV epidemic—New York City, United States. *JAMA* 1988;260:2181–5.

42. Schuchat A, Stehr-Green J, Parkin W, Berkelman R, Broome CV. Use of pneumococcal disease surveillance to estimate the HIV-infected population (281). In: Twenty-ninth Interscience Conference on Antimicrobial Agents and Chemotherapy, Houston, 1989.

43. Krumholtz HM, Sande MA, Lo B. Community-acquired bacteremia in patients with acquired immunodeficiency syndrome: clinical presentation, bacteriology, and outcome. *Am J Med* 1989;86:776–9.

44. Witt DJ, Craven DE, McCabe WR. Bacterial infections in adult patients with the acquired immune deficiency syndrome (AIDS) and AIDS-related complex. *Am J Med* 1987;82:900–6.

45. Amorosa JK, Nahass RG, Nosher JL, Gocke DJ. Radiologic distinction of pyogenic pulmonary infection from *Pneumocystis carinii* pneumonia in AIDS patients. *Radiology* 1990;175:721–4.

46. Huang KL, Ruben FL, Rinaldo CR, Kingsley L, Lyter DW, Ho M. Antibody responses after influenza and pneumococcal immunization in HIV-infected homosexual men. *JAMA* 1987;257:2047–50.

47. Ballet JJ, Sulcebe G, Couderc LJ, et al. Impaired anti-pneumococcal antibody response in patients with AIDS-related persistent generalized lymphadenopathy. *Clin Exp Immunol* 1987;68:479–87.

48. Janoff EN, Douglas JM, Gabriel M, Blaser MJ, Davidson AJ, Cohn DL, Judson FN. Class-specific antibody response to pneumococcal capsular polysaccharides in men infected with human immunodeficiency virus type 1. *J Infect Dis* 1988;158:983–90.

49. Ochs HD, Junker AK, Collier AC, Virant FS, Handsfield HH, Wedgwood RJ. Abnormal antibody responses in patients with persistent generalized lymphadenopathy. *J Clin Immunol* 1988;8:57–63.

50. Ragni MV, Ruben FL, Winkelstein A, Spero JA, Bontempo FA, Lewis JH. Antibody responses to immunization of patients with hemophilia with and without evidence of human immunodeficiency virus (human T-lymphotropic virus type III) infection. *J Lab Clin Med* 1987;109:545–9.

51. Klein RS, Selwyn PA, Maude D, Pollard C, Freeman K, Schiffman G. Response to pneumococcal vaccine among asymptomatic heterosexual partners of persons with AIDS and intravenous drug users infected with human immunodeficiency virus. *J Infect Dis* 1989;160:826–31.

52. Centers for Disease Control. Recommendations of the Immunization Practices Advisory Committee. Pneumococcal polysaccharide vaccine. *MMWR* 1989;38:64–76.

53. Eng RHK, Bishburg E, Smith SM, Geller H, Kapila R. Bacteremia and fungemia in patients with acquired immune deficiency syndrome. *Am J Clin Pathol* 1986;86:105–7.

54. Rolston KVI, Uribe-Botero G, Mansell PWA. Bacterial infections in adult patients with the acquired immune deficiency syndrome (AIDS) and AIDS-related complex (letter). *Am J Med* 1987;83:604–5.

55. Shanson DC. Septicemia in patients with AIDS. *Trans R Soc Trop Med Hyg* 1990;84(suppl 1):14–6.

56. Marone P, Sacchi P, Grosi P, Gatti G. Severe bacterial infections in AIDS patients (MBP75). In: 5th International Conference on AIDS, Montreal, Canada, June 1989.

57. Ocana I, DeLuis A, Planes A, Plakissa A, Serra E, Martinez-Vazquez JM. *Salmonella* bacteremia and HIV infection (MBP67). In: 5th International Conference on AIDS, Montreal, Canada, June 1989.

58. Real FX, Gold JWM, Krown SE, Armstrong D. *Listeria monocytogenes* bacteremia in the acquired immunodeficiency syndrome. *Ann Intern Med* 1984;101:883–4.

59. Read EJ, Orenstein JM, Chorba TL, et al. *Listeria monocytogenes* sepsis and small cell carcinoma of the rectum: an unusual presentation of the acquired immunodeficiency syndrome. *Am J Clin Pathol* 1985;83:385–9.

60. Kales CP, Holzman RS. Listeriosis in patients with HIV infection: clinical manifestations and response to therapy. *J AIDS* 1990;3:139–43.

61. Wetli CV, Roldan EO, Fojaco RM. Listeriosis as a cause of maternal death: an obstetric complication of the acquired immunodeficiency syndrome (AIDS). *Am J Obstet Gynecol* 1983;147:7–9.

62. Wetli CV, Roldan EO, Fojaco RM. Reply to letter. *Am J Obstet Gynecol* 1983;147:805–6.

63. Wheeler AP, Gregg CR. Campylobacter bacteremia, cholecystitis, and the acquired immunodeficiency syndrome. *Ann Intern Med* 1986;105:804.

64. Cohen JI, Rodday P. *Yersinia enterocolitica* bacteremia in a patient with the acquired immunodeficiency syndrome. *Am J Med* 1989;86:254–5.

65. Lieb L, Tormey M, Ewert D, Wakamatsu P, Run G, Kerndt P. *Shigella* enteritis among AIDS cases in Los Angeles (MBP67). In: 5th International Conference on AIDS, Montreal, Canada, June 1989.

66. Kaplan JD, Musher DM, Hamill RJ. Group G streptococcal bacteremia with presumed endocarditis in a patient with AIDS (letter). *West J Med* 1988;149:344.

67. Glaser JB, Landesman SH. *Streptococcus bovis* bacteremia and acquired immunodeficiency syndrome. *Ann Intern Med* 1985;99:878.

68. Fierer J, Wolf P, Seed L, Gay T, Noonan K, Haghighi P. Nonpulmonary *Rhodococcus equi* in patients with acquired immunodeficiency syndrome (AIDS). *J Clin Pathol* 1987;40:556–8.

69. Hewitt WD, Farrar WE. Case report: bacteremia and ecthyma caused by *Streptococcus pyogenes* in a patient with acquired immunodeficiency syndrome. *Am J Med Sci* 1988;295:52–4.

70. Johnson MP, Rand KH. Group A beta-hemolytic streptococcal bacteremia and HIV infection. *South Med J* 1990;83:146–9.

71. Jacobson MA, Gellermann H, Chambers H. *Staphylococcus aureus* bacteremia and recurrent staphylococcal infection in patients with acquired immunodeficiency syndrome and AIDS-related complex. *Am J Med* 1988;85:172–6.

72. Sperber SJ, Schleupner CJ. Salmonellosis during infection with human immunodeficiency virus. *Rev Infect Dis* 1987;9:925–34.

73. Smith PD, Macher AM, Bookman MA, et al. *Salmonella typhimurium* enteritis and bacteremia in the acquired immunodeficiency syndrome. *Ann Intern Med* 1985;102:207–9.

74. Jacobs JL, Gold JWM, Murray HW, et al. *Salmonella* infections in patients with the acquired immunodeficiency syndrome. *Ann Intern Med* 1985;102:186–8.

75. Glaser JB, Morton-Kute L, Berger SR, et al. Recurrent *Salmonella typhimurium* bacteremia associated with the acquired immunodeficiency syndrome. *Ann Intern Med* 1985;102:189–93.

76. Centers for Disease Control. Revision of the CDC surveillance case definition for acquired immunodeficiency syndrome. *MMWR* 1987;36:1(S)–15(S).

77. Casner PR, Zuckerman MJ. *Salmonella arizonae* in patients with AIDS along the U.S.–Mexican border (letter). *N Engl J Med* 1990;323:198–9.

78. Jacobson MA, Hahn SM, Gerberding JL, Lee B, Sande SA. Ciprofloxacin for *Salmonella* bacteremia in the acquired immunodeficiency syndrome. *Ann Intern Med* 1989;110:1027–9.

79. Krasinski K, Borkowsky W, Bonk S, Lawrence R, Chadwani S. Bacterial infections in human immunodeficiency virus-infected children. *Pediatr Infect Dis J* 1988;7:323–8.

80. Rubinstein A, Sicklick M, Gupta A, et al. Acquired immunodeficiency with reversed T4/T8 ratios in infants born to promiscuous and drug-addicted mothers. *JAMA* 1983;249:2350–6.

81. Bernstein LJ, Ochs HD, Wedgewood RJ, Rubinstein A. Defective humoral immunity in pediatric acquired immune deficiency syndrome. *J Pediatr* 1985;107:352–7.

82. Oleske J, Minnefor A, Cooper R, et al. Immune deficiency in children. *JAMA* 1983;249:2345–9.

83. Scott GB, Buck BE, Leterman JG, Grederick LB, Parks WP. Acquired immunodeficiency in infants. *N Engl J Med* 1984;310:76–81.

AIDS and Other Manifestations of HIV Infection,
Second Edition, Edited by Gary P. Wormser.
Raven Press, Ltd., New York © 1992.

CHAPTER 19

Mycobacterial Disease in Patients with HIV Infection

Arthur E. Pitchenik and Debra Fertel

TUBERCULOSIS AND HIV INFECTION

Understanding tuberculosis (TB) in patients infected with human immunodeficiency virus (HIV) is important from many standpoints. First, among tuberculous-infected individuals, HIV immunosuppression is the greatest known single risk factor for contracting reactivation TB (1–3). Predictably, the incidence of TB is rising significantly in those populations and areas where dual HIV and tuberculous infection are prevalent [i.e., sub-Saharan Africa, parts of tropical America, and many urban areas of the United States with large populations of intravenous (IV) drug users and socioeconomically deprived ethnic minority groups] (1–7). Second, TB differs from other HIV-related infections in that it is spread by the respiratory route from human to human to both normal and immunocompromised hosts. The potential for an aerosol transmitted disease such as TB to spread rapidly among HIV-infected persons exposed to each other and from them to non-HIV-infected contacts (e.g., household members, health care personnel) is evident. Third, mycobacterial disease in HIV-infected patients often presents with an atypical clinical picture. Tuberculin skin anergy is common, the chest radiograph is often atypical, and there is a high incidence of extrapulmonary and disseminated disease that confounds diagnosis (1,8–17). The diagnosis may easily be missed unless these features are appreciated. Thus there must be a high index of suspicion for TB among persons who are HIV infected or in AIDS risk groups. Fourth, and most importantly, TB is preventable and curable even in an HIV immunosuppressed population (13,18,19).

A. E. Pitchenik and D. Fertel: Pulmonary Division, University of Miami; and Veterans Affairs Medical Centers, Miami, Florida 33125.

Controlling TB among HIV-infected populations demands: (a) early recognition and preventive isoniazid treatment of those persons who are dually HIV and tuberculous infected (i.e., widespread tuberculin skin testing and preventive therapy programs among AIDS risk groups), (b) early recognition and treatment of those HIV-infected patients who already have active TB (i.e., effective TB case finding), and (c) compulsive attention that patients comply with anti-TB therapy (which often includes fully supervised therapy). It also requires the institution and maintenance of strict environmental control measures in AIDS clinics and wards where HIV immunosuppressed patients, who are at high risk of contracting TB, are recurrently exposed to each other (20,21). Controlling TB among HIV-infected populations requires dealing with the HIV component as well. Efforts must be aimed at prevention of HIV infection through public education and screening the blood supply (which still may not be universal in some developing countries) (6,7), and at treatment of HIV infection itself.

PATHOGENESIS OF TUBERCULOSIS

The risk of acquiring TB is related to two separate stages: the risk of acquiring tuberculous infection (as identified by the development of a significant tuberculin skin reaction) and the risk of tuberculous infection progressing to tuberculous disease. The risk of acquiring tuberculous infection is primarily related to the frequency and density of TB bacilli in a person's environment (i.e., the risk of inhaling a tubercle bacillus) and to a lesser extent the natural resistance against primary tuberculous infection. (For example, if alveolar macrophages kill the tubercle bacilli on first exposure, infection is not established, a specific T-cell immune response is obviated, and the tuberculin skin test remains negative.) The risk of established tuberculous infection progressing to disease is related to a patient's T-cell immune response. Table 1 reveals the relative prevalences of TB among populations with low and high rates of tuberculous infection and with or without HIV immunosuppression. As seen, Haitian entrants with AIDS, who have both a very high prevalence of tuberculous infection (i.e., 79–90%) (22) and a severe state of immunosuppression, have an extremely high prevalence of active TB compared to the other groups. Such comparative data demonstrate the extreme risk for contracting active TB when a tuberculous-infected individual becomes HIV immunosuppressed.

Response to Inhaled Tubercle Bacilli

Inhaled tubercle bacilli that reach the alveolar space are usually ingested by alveolar macrophages where they may be killed immediately (natural immunity) (23). If not killed, they may persist or replicate within macrophages or lyse them and then infect other alveolar macrophages. The tubercle bacilli are then transported within macrophages to the regional lymph nodes and from there may be widely disseminated hematogenously throughout the body. Most primary pulmonary and disseminated lesions remain asymptomatic and heal with the development of T-cell immunity (granulomatous reaction) during a 2–8-week period after primary infection. During this time the tuberculin skin test becomes positive, documenting the occurrence of tuberculous infection. In general, only 5% of persons contract TB within the first two years following primary infection and an additional 5% contract TB at some later time during their life. If a tuberculous-infected person becomes HIV infected, there is a much greater likelihood for reactivation TB to occur at some critical point during the slow but inexorable progression of HIV-induced immunosuppression (24). If a patient is severely HIV immunosuppressed (e.g., has AIDS) at the time of initial tuberculous infection, then rapid progression to TB within weeks to months is expected (20,21,25).

Macrophages are pivotal in the generation of an immune response against mycobacteria (23,26,27). Macrophages phagocytose and process mycobacterial antigens, which are then presented to antigen-specific T-helper lymphocytes within lymph nodes. These T-helper lymphocytes with specific receptors recognize the mycobacterial antigens as well as HLA-DR ("self") proteins on the macrophage membranes and become activated. T-cell activation also requires the synthesis and release of interleukin-1 (IL-1), a soluble cytokine, from macrophages. Once T-helper cells are activated, they produce soluble factors (lymphokines) that promote both further clonal T-cell proliferation (IL-2) and increased macrophage antigen presentation, recruitment, and effector reactivity (γ-interferon, macrophage activating factor, macrophage chemotactic factor, macrophage migration inhibition factor).

In response to immunologically competent T lymphocytes that enter the areas of tuberculous infection, monocytes enter the area, undergo transformation into activated macrophages and subsequently into specialized histiocytic cells, which are organized into granulomas (tubercles). These lymphokine-activated macrophages exhibit increased metabolic and enzymatic activities and have an enhanced ability to ingest tubercle bacilli and inhibit their growth. Further multiplication and spread of mycobacteria are usually then arrested within the microscopic granulomas at the initial pulmonary site of infection, in regional lymph nodes and at distant sites. A small number of living organisms persist in dormant foci often for the life of the patient and may reactivate at anytime if host defenses decline. This cellular immune response not only confers protection against mycobacterial disease but is also intimately linked with cellular hypersensitivity as expressed by a positive tuberculin skin test reaction, formation of tissue granulomas, caseation necrosis, and liquefaction and cavity formation. Although activated macrophages limit replication of mycobacteria, they are also responsible through their liberated enzymes for much of the tissue damage. Paradoxically, if the immune-mediated tissue damage is too extensive (i.e., caseous necrosis and cavity formation), a favorable environment for multiplication of mycobacteria may result, leading to classic fibrocavitary TB in a relatively immune competent host.

TABLE 1. *Prevalence of TB among different populations by risk of acquiring tuberculous infection and risk of developing active disease*

Population (ref.)	Prevalence of TB	Risk of acquiring tuberculous infection	Risk of developing TB after infection
United States population (2)	0.01%	Low	Low
Haitian entrants (Florida) (22)	0.65%	High	Low
United States born homosexual men with AIDS (Florida) (66)	3.2%	Low	High
Haitian entrants with AIDS (Florida) (14, 32, 62, 66)	27.3–60%	High	High

From Pitchenik AE, Fertel D. Tuberculosis and non-tuberculous mycobacterial disease in HIV infected patients. *Med Clin North Am* 1992;76:121–71, with permission.

Role of HIV

The HIV virus causes a profound immune defect by producing a qualitative and progressive quantitative deficiency of the CD4+ T-lymphocyte population, which in turn results in the impairment of B-cell function, cytotoxic T-cell function, natural killer (NK) cell function, and macrophage function including macrophage antigen presenting capabilities, recruitment, and activation (28–31). It is the immune defect involving macrophages that is most crucial in the defense against mycobacterial disease. Without the recruitment and activation of macrophages by T-cell secreted lymphokines, there is poor granuloma formation, poor containment of mycobacteria, frequent reactivation of mycobacterial disease with large organism loads, spread to regional lymph nodes, and wide hematogenous dissemination with mycobacteremia. In this setting, caseation necrosis and cavity formation (e.g., in the lung) is less prominent or absent and tuberculin skin tests are often falsely negative. Among individuals with mycobacterial disease, the frequency and severity of these features are directly related to the CD4+ peripheral blood count. Since *M. tuberculosis* is more virulent than nontuberculous mycobacteria or other opportunistic pathogens such as *Pneumocystis carinii,* reactivation TB tends to occur relatively early in the course of HIV immunosuppression and at higher peripheral blood CD4+ lymphocyte counts (e.g., often >200/mm^3) (13,14,32,33). There is some evidence in animals and humans that the ability to generate an immune response to TB has a genetic basis (23,34). Therefore even among tuberculous–HIV-infected populations, there might be variabilities in the time of onset and severity of TB.

HIV also infects monocytes and macrophages that bear the CD4 surface molecule. These cells are resistant to both the cytolytic and syncytium forming effects that HIV has on CD4+ lymphocytes. Although not destroyed, the HIV-infected monocyte and macrophage are defective in chemotaxis and other functions, serve as important reservoirs of persistent HIV infection, and probably transport HIV to the central nervous system (31,35,36). Alveolar macrophages may also be infected with HIV in vitro and in vivo. Furthermore, cytomegalovirus is frequently isolated from lung secretions of patients with AIDS, and in guinea pig models this virus markedly decreases metabolic functions of alveolar macrophages (37). Therefore it is possible that relatively small inocula of tubercle bacilli could primarily infect patients with AIDS because of impaired alveolar macrophage function (i.e., impaired natural immunity against inhaled mycobacteria) (28,35,36). If this is true, AIDS patients could be at relatively high risk for becoming tuberculous infected following exposure to a contagious patient, in addition to being at high risk for contracting tuberculous disease after infection is established.

EPIDEMIOLOGY OF TUBERCULOSIS AND AIDS

Developing Countries

The World Health Organization (WHO) estimates that 1 billion people are tuberculous infected, at least 5 million people are already HIV infected, and over 400,000 have AIDS worldwide (38,39). In countries where HIV infection has become prevalent and where tuberculous infection has long been endemic (e.g., sub-Saharan Africa, parts of Latin America and the Caribbean), a rise in the incidence of TB is almost inevitable (7,22,38,40–42). This has already been documented in Tanzania, Burundi, Uganda, Zaire, Abidjan, and Malawi (7,43,44).

TB has long been an important worldwide health problem with an estimated 8–10 million cases and 2–3 million deaths occurring each year. Over 75% of these cases of TB occur in the tropics; the highest rates occurring in Africa followed by Asia and Latin America (38). Overcrowding, poverty, and inadequate TB control programs create conditions favorable for the spread of TB within these areas. The WHO estimates that 30–60% of adults in developing countries are infected with *M. tuberculosis.* In some developing countries, over half the population become tuberculous infected by the time they reach adulthood (7,22,38,45). Due to underreporting, underdiagnosing, and delays in notification, accurate numbers of HIV-infected individuals in these areas are difficult to assess. Nevertheless, in parts of sub-Saharan Africa, 5–15% of the general urban population and 10–25% of sexually active urban young adults are thought to be infected with HIV. Fortunately, HIV infection has not yet become prevalent in Asia and the Middle East, areas where tuberculous infection is endemic—WHO pattern III areas (7). However, this may well change and worsen an already serious TB problem. When cell-mediated immunity declines due to HIV infection, populations coinfected with *M. tuberculosis* contract reactivation TB at an extremely high and rapid rate.

In developing countries, TB is one of the most common opportunistic infections among HIV-seropositive patients (38,41). The proportion of patients with AIDS who also had TB was 24% (171 of 718) in Rio de Janeiro, 21% (1068 of 5219) in Brazil, 21% (17 of 81) in Buenos Aires, 14% (13 of 93) in Mexico City (41), and 7% (234 of 3512) in Mexico (38,41,46). In Zimbabwe and Ethiopia, approximately one-third of patients infected with HIV present with TB as their initial manifestation (38). In several central and east African countries (Burundi, Uganda, Zaire, Malawi, Zambia), 27–61% of patients with TB have positive serologies for HIV; among three TB patient populations in Haiti, 21.7% (36/166), 24% (67/274), and 39% (56/143) were HIV seropositive (38,41,44,45,47–49). These HIV seroprevalence rates are 3 to more than 20 times the rates found in the general population in these countries. In two university hospitals in Rio de Janeiro, 41% (45/110) of HIV-positive and only 3% (4/135) of randomly selected HIV-negative patients had TB (50). The most likely explanation for these findings is an accelerated progression to TB among persons who are coinfected with *M. tuberculosis* and HIV (45). These findings also point out the large proportion of TB cases that may be related to HIV-1 infection in many developing countries. In addition, it is possible that the antigenic stimulation of CD4+ cells by *M. tuberculosis* or other mycobacteria could activate latent HIV infection and thereby speed the immunosuppression (29,31).

HIV-2 infection may also be a risk factor for TB in some developing countries. In certain areas of West Africa, HIV-2 seropositivity has been found in approximately 15% of TB patients, which was significantly greater than the prevalence of HIV-2 seropositivity among control blood donors (51–53). The likelihood of detecting serum antibodies against HIV-2, by U.S. licensed enzyme immunoassay kits designed to detect antibodies against HIV-1, varies among different manufacturers from 60 to 91% (54). Therefore some HIV-2-infected patients would be missed by conventional HIV-1 serologic testing.

HTLV-1, another human retrovirus, is endemic in discrete locales of Japan, the Caribbean, tropical America, and southeast United States and is associated with acute T-cell leukemia and tropical spastic paraparesis (55). In certain areas of Brazil, HTLV-1 seropositivity has recently been found to occur in 10.9% of TB patients (non-HIV infected) and only in 2–3% of healthy blood donors or hospital workers residing in the same locale (E. Duarte and W. Harrington Jr., *personal communication,* 1991). Although these three populations (approximately 100 in the TB group and 400 in the two control groups) may or may not be comparable, the possibility is at least raised that HTLV-1 infection may constitute a risk factor for contracting TB. Conversely, the antigenic stimulation of CD4+ cells by *M. tuberculosis* might result in recrudescence of latent HTLV-1 infection, which then becomes more easily detectable serologically.

United States

In the United States, there has recently been an unprecedented increase in the incidence of TB and this correlates directly with the AIDS epidemic. Between 1953, when national reporting was instituted, and 1984, there was a constant decline of TB case rates of approximately 5% per year. From 1984 to 1985, that decline had decreased to 0.2% (or 54 cases). In 1986, for the first time in over three decades since national TB reporting was implemented, there was an increase in the number of new TB cases (up 2.6%) from the previous year (567 case increase from 22,201 to 22,768). Since 1986, the yearly incidence of TB cases has either leveled off (1987 and 1988) or continued to rise. In 1989, 23,495 cases of TB were reported, up 5% compared with 1988 and preliminary 1990 statistics are running 6% ahead of 1989 (1–3,5,56–59). The TB control division of the Centers for Disease Control (CDC) estimates that in 1984–1990 there were 22,494 excess cases of TB over the number of cases expected, had the rate of decline seen in 1980–1984 continued (Fig. 1).

Evidence that AIDS Is Causing the Rising Incidence of TB

Several lines of evidence support the hypothesis that the AIDS epidemic is responsible for the unprecedented increase in the incidence of TB in the United States (1–5,8,14,24,60–66). Nationwide, there has been a disproportionate rise in the incidence of extrapulmonary versus pulmonary TB (20% versus 3% increase from 1984 to 1989) (3). Nationwide, the states and cities with the largest number of AIDS cases have had the largest increases in reported TB cases (including extrapulmonary TB cases) (i.e., New York City, Miami/Dade County, New Jersey, California, Florida, Texas). Furthermore, the increases in TB largely occurred among those demographic groups that have a relatively high prevalence of AIDS (i.e., blacks and Hispanics, 24–44 years of age).

In New York City, which has the largest number of AIDS cases, there was a 56% increase in TB cases over a

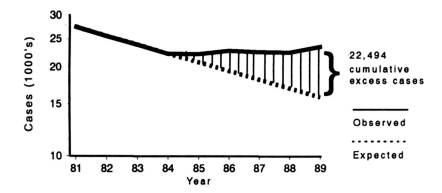

FIG. 1. Reported tuberculosis cases, observed and expected, in the United States, 1981–1989. Courtesy of CDC.

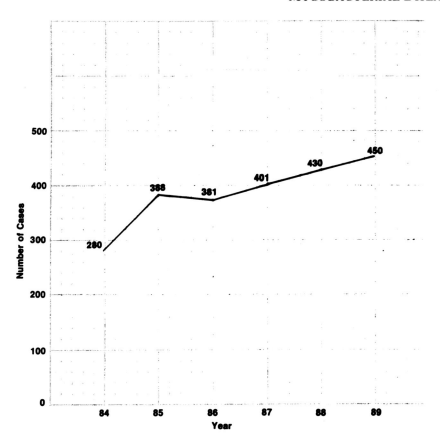

FIG. 2. Registered tuberculosis cases in Dade County, Florida, 1984–1989. Courtesy of Janice Burr, M.D.

6-year period (from 1630 in 1984 to 2223 in 1986 to 2545 in 1989). Furthermore, the greatest increases in TB cases occurred among young adult to middle-aged black and Hispanic males and in those areas of the city with a high incidence of AIDS (1,3,61). Figures 2 and 3 show similar data for Dade County, Florida (65). Figure 2 shows the rising incidence in TB cases in Dade County from 1984 to 1989. (Most of the cases were concentrated in the inner city—Miami.) Figure 3 shows that the increases of TB cases from 1985 to 1989 were most prominent among blacks and Hispanics 30–50 years of age. The excess in TB cases in young to middle-aged adults without a corresponding increase in young children suggests increased endogenous reactivation rather than increased transmission. Among the 443 reported TB cases in Dade County, Florida in 1990, the largest age group was, by far, 25–44 years, and well over half of the patients within this age group were HIV infected (Fig. 4).

Studies that have linked TB to AIDS in New York, Florida, Newark, Connecticut, and San Francisco have shown an extremely high incidence of TB among patients with AIDS ranging from 2 to 27%. This is scores to several hundred-fold higher than the incidence of TB in the general population, even after adjustment for age, race, and sex (1,13,22,61–64,66,67).

Perhaps the most compelling evidence linking TB to HIV infection comes from a study of 520 IV drug users

in New York City who were enrolled in a methadone maintenance program (24). In this study, 23% of the 217 HIV-seropositive subjects and 20% of the 303 HIV-seronegative subjects had positive tuberculin skin tests before entry into the study (P = NS). The rates of conversion from a negative to a positive PPD test were similar for seropositive (11%) and seronegative (13%) subjects

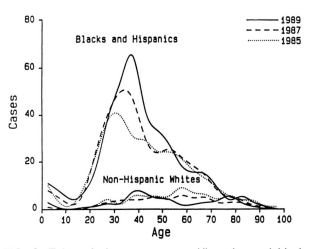

FIG. 3. Tuberculosis cases among Hispanics and blacks compared to non-Hispanic whites, Dade County, Florida, 1985, 1987, and 1989. Courtesy of Janice Burr, M.D.

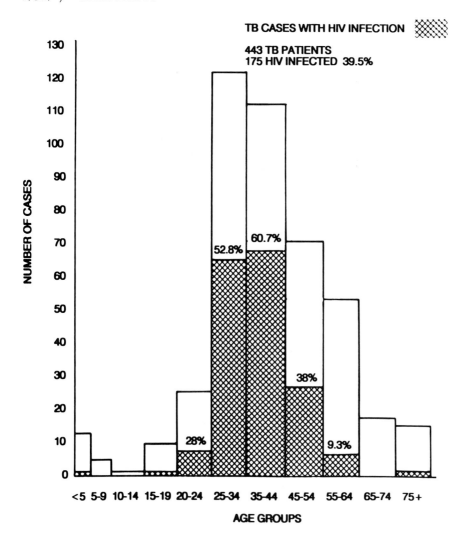

FIG. 4. Tuberculosis cases by age group showing those who are also HIV seropositive, Dade County, Florida, 1990. Courtesy of Janice Burr, M.D.

who were retested during the follow-up period (*P* = NS). Eight of the seropositive individuals (seven of whom were initially PPD positive) subsequently developed active TB while no seronegative subjects developed active TB during the follow-up period of 3–30 months (*P* < 0.002). The authors concluded that the prevalence and incidence of tuberculous infection detectable by a positive skin test (≥10-mm induration) was similar for both HIV-seropositive and HIV-seronegative IV drug users; however, the risk of active TB was increased only for seropositive subjects (approximately 8% per year). It is noteworthy that among HIV/tuberculous-infected subjects followed during the study period, none of 13 who received prophylactic isoniazid (INH) developed active TB whereas 7 of 36 who did not receive chemoprophylaxis did so. This emphasizes the importance of performing tuberculin skin tests *early* in persons who are proved or suspected to be HIV infected (while they can still react to tuberculin), and promptly instituting isoniazid prophylaxis among those who are found to be tuberculous infected.

Demographic Characteristics of AIDS/TB Cases by Geographic Area

Although AIDS/TB cases are disproportionately reported from urban areas, among minority groups and IV drug users, there are still marked variations in demographic characteristics of AIDS/TB cases depending on the geographic areas studied (1). An analysis of the characteristics of AIDS/TB patients in New York City (261 patients), Florida (109 patients), Newark (29 patients), and San Francisco (31 patients) revealed the following: the proportion of AIDS/TB patients who were black or Hispanic (minority groups) ranged from 35% in San Francisco to 81% in New York City to 90% in Florida to 100% in Newark. The proportion of AIDS/TB patients who were homosexual or bisexual ranged from 14% in Newark to 93% in San Francisco, whereas the proportion who were IV drug users with no other risk factors ranged from 7% in San Francisco to 69% in Newark. The proportion of AIDS/TB patients who were foreign born ranged from 14% in Newark to 22% in San Francisco to

31% in New York City to 60% in Florida. (In Florida 51% were from Haiti.) In all four areas, the mean and median ages of AIDS/TB patients were similar (33–37 years and 30–36 years, respectively).

Since 1987, extrapulmonary TB among HIV-infected patients has been counted as an AIDS defining condition (68). Through September 1990, 3110 cases of extrapulmonary TB were reported in patients with AIDS and the distributions by race/ethnicity and risk factors for HIV infection varied considerably throughout the country similar to that described above (i.e., in New York and New Jersey, there were many more cases in blacks, Hispanics, and IV drug users compared to California, where there were relatively more cases in non-Hispanic whites and homosexual men) (3).

Prevalence of TB Among Patients with AIDS

The prevalence of TB among patients with AIDS varies by race/ethnicity and AIDS risk group and is directly proportional to the prevalence of tuberculous infection within these groups (1,2,5). The prevalence of significant tuberculin skin test reactions was 79–91% among Haitian immigrants in Florida (22), 22.5% among drug addicts in New York City (69), and only 1.5% among predominantly white American-born Louisiana State University medical students in a similar age range (70). Predictably, the prevalence of TB among various groups of patients with AIDS in Florida varied widely from 27.3–60% in Haitians, to 11.7% in non-Haitian blacks, to 10.1% in IV drug users, to 5.8% in Hispanics, to 3.2% in homosexual/bisexual men, to only 1.8% in non-Hispanic whites (14,32,62,66). Nationally, among 74,880 AIDS patients reported to CDC from October 1987 through December 1989, extrapulmonary TB was documented in 14% of those born in a pattern II country, 5% of the blacks, 4.5% of the IV drug users, 2.8% of the Hispanics, and only 1.7% of the homosexual/bisexual men and 1.5% of the non-Hispanic whites (71).

In contrast to patients with AIDS in Miami and New York City, where a relatively high proportion are black, Haitian, Hispanic, and/or IV drug users, the majority of patients with AIDS in San Francisco are American-born white homosexuals, a group with a comparatively low rate of tuberculous infection. Not surprisingly, the proportion of AIDS cases in which TB is reported is only 2% in San Francisco (19) compared to 5% in New York City (61), 7% in Dade County, Florida, and 6% in the State of Florida (W. Bigler, *personal communication*, 1991).

Prevalence of HIV Infection or AIDS Among Patients with TB

HIV serologic data indicates that TB among patients with overt AIDS is only the tip of the iceberg. Of 408 consecutive TB patients presenting to the Dade County Florida Health Department from October 1, 1985 through October 31, 1987, 90 (22%) were HIV seropositive; only 11 (12%) met nontuberculous criteria for AIDS at the time of TB diagnosis. An additional 30 patients (33%) could be classified as having AIDS on the basis of the 1987 revised CDC criteria for AIDS, which include a positive HIV serology with extrapulmonary TB (13,68). As shown in Fig. 4, the proportion of TB cases that were associated with HIV infection in Dade County, Florida in 1990 rose to 39.5%. In San Francisco, prospective seroprevalence studies revealed that 28% of patients with TB were also HIV infected. This figure is considerably higher than the proportion of TB patients retrospectively reported as having AIDS (5.3% of TB patients reported in San Francisco from 1981 through 1988 had AIDS) (19,72). Similar high HIV seroprevalence rates among TB patients have been reported from clinics in New York (46%), Newark (34%), and Boston (27%) (3). HIV seroprevalence rates among TB patients, however, vary widely from 0 to 46% among different metropolitan areas and among different clinics within individual cities (3).

CLINICAL FEATURES

History and Physical Examination

Symptoms of TB in HIV-seropositive patients are non-specific, commonly occur with other conditions associated with AIDS, and are often present for many weeks before the diagnosis of TB is made or even considered. In contrast to pyogenic pneumonias in which the onset is abrupt over 1–2 days, the onset of TB is frequently insidious. Patients often present with constitutional symptoms of fever, night sweats, fatigue, malaise, and weight loss. Patients with pulmonary TB may have cough, sputum production, hemoptysis, pleuritic chest pain, and/or dyspnea. Signs and symptoms of extrapulmonary or disseminated TB depend on the organ and/or tissue affected (e.g., regional or generalized lymphadenopathy, hepatosplenomegaly, or CNS abnormalities).

Although TB may occur concomitantly with or after other AIDS-defining infections, it usually precedes these by 1 month to 2 years or more. Of 109 TB cases reported from Florida in patients with confirmed AIDS (by non-tuberculous criteria), the report of TB preceded the diagnosis of AIDS by more than 1 month in 62 cases (57%), occurred within 1 month of the diagnosis of AIDS in 30 cases (28%), and followed the diagnosis of AIDS by more than 1 month in only 17 cases (16%). Overall, TB was reported a median interval of 3 months before AIDS diagnosis (62). Other studies from other cities, states, and countries have yielded similar findings (8,14,17,32, 61,63,64,73–76) (Table 2). This is predictable since *M.*

TABLE 2. *Clinical presentation of TB in HIV-infected patients (retrospective versus prospective studies)*

Presentation of TB	AIDS/TB patients, 7 retrospective studies (8,14,19,63,73–75)	HIV+/TB patients, prospective study (13,17)	HIV−/TB patients, prospective study (13,17)
Number of patients	292	90	318
Time of TB diagnosis			
Before AIDS[a]	170/292 (58%) (46–79%)	79/90 (88%)	
At AIDS[a]	56/292 (19%) (11–45%)	11/90 (12%)	
After AIDS[a]	66/292 (23%) (0–38%)		
Site of TB			
Any pulmonary	216/292 (74%) (70–93%)	68/90 (76%)	293/318 (92%)
Any extrapulmonary	181/292 (62%) (50–72%)	31/90 (34%)	27/318 (8%)
Chest x-ray pattern			
Diffuse infiltrate	18/60 (30%) (14–60%)	15/68 (22%)	
Focal infiltrate	16/60 (27%) (21–35%)	42/68 (62%)	
Cavitation	7/60 (12%) (5–17%)	19/68 (28%)	33/43 (77%)
Intrathoracic lymphadenopathy	20/60 (33%) (20–45%)	10/68 (15%)	1/43 (2%)
Tuberculin skin reaction			
Significant[b]	61/191 (32%) (7–40%)	31/55 (56%)	183/202 (91%)
Not significant	130/191 (68%) (60–89%)	24/55 (44%)	19/202 (9%)

From Pitchenik AE, Fertel D. Tuberculosis and non-tuberculous mycobacterial disease in HIV infected patients. *Med Clin North Am* (in press), with permission.
[a] AIDS-defining disease other than TB.
[b] Induration of ≥ 10 mm.

tuberculosis is a more virulent organism than the other opportunistic infections that define AIDS, and among tuberculous-infected individuals, reactivation TB would be expected to occur at an earlier stage of HIV-induced immunosuppression. Thus TB is often a sentinel infection among patients with HIV immunosuppression and a HIV serology should always be obtained when TB is diagnosed or suspected.

Although most cases (90%) of TB in the United States, HIV related or not, are believed to represent activation of latent infection (77), HIV immunosuppressed patients are also vulnerable to exogenous tuberculous infection with rapid progression to active TB. Some cases of TB that follow diseases caused by less virulent pathogens may be the result of recent exposure to the tubercle bacillus. This should be suspected particularly when there are outbreaks of TB among AIDS patients (20,21,25).

Pulmonary Tuberculosis

Pulmonary involvement occurs in 70–93% of HIV-infected patients with TB (Table 2). The radiographic picture is often atypical (8,13,15,17,63,73,78). Hilar and mediastinal lymphadenopathy, lower lobe infiltrates, and diffuse alveolar, linear, or miliary infiltrates are relatively common among the more severely immunosuppressed patients with HIV infection. Although the severe immune defect often leads to a chest radiographic pattern resembling primary TB (i.e., hilar or mediastinal lymphadenopathy with or without noncavitating pulmonary infiltrates) (Figs. 5 and 6), epidemiologic evidence suggests that most patients have reactivation TB (15). Unilateral or bilateral pleural effusions may occur. An enlarged cardiac silhouette should raise the possibility of tuberculous pericarditis. Patients may also present with another pulmonary infection such as *Pneumocystis carinii* pneumonia with diffuse linear interstitial lung infiltrates, which confounds the radiographic diagnosis of concurrent pulmonary TB (15). Occasionally, sputum cultures are positive for *M. tuberculosis* despite the presence of a normal chest x-ray. Intrathoracic lymphadenopathy, diffuse miliary infiltrates, and pleural effusions are chest radiographic features that are diagnostically helpful when they occur in the setting of HIV-induced immunosuppression since they are typical of TB and

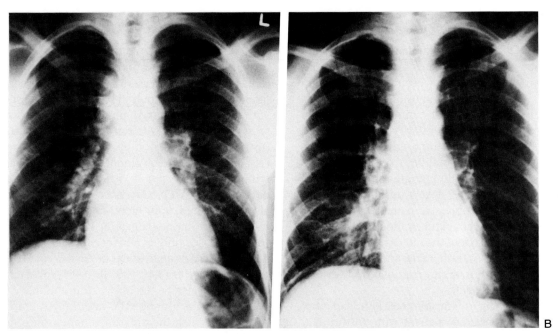

FIG. 5. A: Chest radiograph in a patient with tuberculosis and HIV infection. There is right paratracheal adenopathy (*arrow*) with clear lung fields. Sputum culture was positive for *M. tuberculosis*. **B:** The radiographic abnormality resolved (as did the patient's symptoms) following several months of anti-tuberculous drug treatment. (From ref. 1, with permission.)

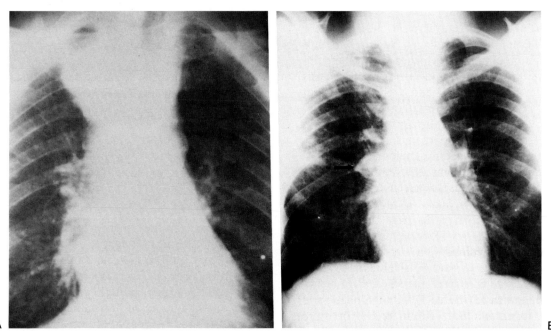

FIG. 6. A: Chest radiograph in a patient with tuberculosis and HIV infection. There is right paratracheal adenopathy with clear lung fields. The patient complained of dysphagia. Esophagoscopy with biopsy revealed granulomatous esophagitis with a positive tissue culture for *M. tuberculosis.* A CT scan (not shown) revealed air in the mediastinum; an esophagram (not shown) revealed extravasation of barium, consistent with a tuberculous mediastinal lymph node–esophageal fistula. The patient's symptoms and radiographic abnormalities resolved following anti-tuberculous drug treatment. [The CT scan and eso-phagram were previously reproduced elsewhere (1).] **B:** Chest radiograph in a patient with tuberculosis and HIV infection. Right paratracheal adenopathy (*arrow*) and a right upper lobe infiltrate are present. Sputum culture was positive for *M. tuberculosis* and the patient responded to anti-tuberculous drug treatment. Although the chest radiograph resembles primary tuberculosis (i.e., noncavitary pulmonary infiltrate with ipsilateral hilar lymphadenopathy), the patient was documented to have a strongly positive PPD-tuberculin skin reaction several years previously. (He never received INH preventive therapy.) The chest radiograph therefore probably represents an atypical pattern of reactivation TB due to HIV-induced immunosuppression. [Part (A) from ref. 1, with permission; part (B) from Pitchenik AE, Fertel D. Tuberculosis and non-tuberculous mycobacterial disease in HIV infected patients. *Med Clin North Am* 1992;76:121–71, with permission.]

highly atypical of *P. carinii* pneumonia. Classic tuberculous upper lobe infiltrates and cavitary lesions are also diagnostically helpful when they occur but are uncommon among severely HIV immunosuppressed patients. They are seen more commonly among patients who have contracted TB in the earlier stages of HIV infection (17,72). Even among HIV immunosuppressed patients, the chest radiographic abnormalities related to TB tend to clear, without scarring, within months of anti-TB drug therapy (15,19). The poor T-cell immune response among HIV immunosuppressed patients readily explains the reduced frequency of tuberculous-induced cavity formation and fibrosis and the increased frequency of miliary infiltrates and intrathoracic and extrathoracic lymphadenopathy representing regional and distant spread of the tubercle bacilli.

Radiographic evidence of intrathoracic lymphadenopathy in an HIV-seronegative patient with postprimary TB is rare even on computerized tomography (CT) scanning of the chest (79). We have found that radiographic evidence of intrathoracic lymphadenopathy among HIV-infected patients with pulmonary TB predicts a poor prognosis compared to that of HIV-infected pulmonary TB patients who do not have this radiographic finding (13). Furthermore, an atypical chest x-ray for reactivation TB among HIV-infected patients with culture-proven pulmonary TB correlates with tuberculin skin anergy (80). An HIV-seropositive patient who has culture-proven pulmonary TB and a chest x-ray that shows otherwise unexplained intrathoracic lymphadenopathy should therefore meet the current CDC criteria for AIDS (i.e., HIV seropositivity plus extrapulmonary TB) (68). The lymphadenopathy, although intrathoracic, is still extrapulmonary, and in this setting it is almost certainly tuberculous and predicts a relatively poor prognosis (13).

Extrapulmonary Tuberculosis

Extrapulmonary TB occurs in 34–72% of HIV-infected patients with TB (Table 2), with lymphatic and disseminated forms (miliary TB and/or two or more noncontiguous tuberculous sites) predominating. Involvement of bone marrow, genitourinary tract, and central nervous system are also common among HIV immunosuppressed patients. Furthermore, unusual clinical presentations of TB occur frequently in this setting (8,13,14,32,63,73–75). Tuberculous meningitis (81), brain abscesses (14,63,81–83), vertebral abscess (84), spinal cord abscess (85), meningomyelitis (86), choroiditis (87), pericarditis and pericardial effusion (88,89), pericardial–cutaneous fistula (90), mediastinal lymph node–esophageal fistula (1), esophago-bronchial and esophago-esophageal fistulas (91), mediastinal lymph node–endobronchial fistulas and endobronchial masses

(92,93), empyema (94), retrogastric mass with a gastric ulcer (95), small intestinal fistula (96), rectal abscess (63,97), prostatic abscess (98), testicular abscess (99), cutaneous ulcers or papules (100,101), soft tissue abscess with rib destruction (63), peritonitis with pancreatic abscess (1), peritonitis with retroperitoneal lymphadenopathy (presenting as abdominal masses) (102), liver abscess (98), ileocecal involvement (103), and generalized lymphadenopathy (14,17) have all been reported among patients with AIDS. *Mycobacterium tuberculosis* may also be cultured from blood and stool in the setting of HIV immunosuppression (104,105). With new lysis centrifugation techniques, mycobacterial blood cultures have yielded *M. tuberculosis* in 26–42% of HIV-infected patients with TB (3,12,106–108). Mycobacterial blood culture may also be the only extrapulmonary source of *M. tuberculosis* among HIV-infected patients and may therefore furnish the only documentation of an AIDS-defining illness (3,108).

Because of a high rate of dissemination of TB in AIDS, it should be noted that pulmonary and extrapulmonary TB commonly coexist, occurring in approximately 36% (Table 2) and as high as 55% of AIDS/TB cases (1). Even if a diagnosis of pulmonary TB is already established (and treatment wouldn't change), documentation of coexisting extrapulmonary TB is of importance in HIV-infected patients since it establishes criteria for AIDS with attendant medical, social, and economic benefits.

Concomitant Tuberculous and Nontuberculous Disease in AIDS

TB may present concomitantly with a nontuberculous opportunistic infection or tumor and both diseases may occur in the same tissue or organ. For example, pulmonary TB and *Pneumocystis carinii* pneumonia (PCP) have occurred together, in which case the chest x-ray revealed diffuse linear interstitial infiltrates suggestive of PCP alone (15); tuberculous and toxoplasma brain abscesses have occurred concomitantly in which a CT scan of the brain revealed multiple ring-enhancing lesions (the toxoplasma infection was initially missed) (83); *M. tuberculosis* and MAC have been isolated from the same sputum specimen and from the same skin lesions in AIDS (109; *unpublished data*); TB, Kaposi's sarcoma, and Hodgkin's disease have been identified in a single lymph node (110). Therefore clinical specimens from HIV-infected patients should be stained and cultured for mycobacteria regardless of other findings.

The Spectrum of TB Among HIV-Infected Patients: Retrospective Versus Prospective Studies

Retrospective studies from hospitals and health departments in Florida, New York, New Jersey, Connecticut, and California, in which AIDS and TB registries were matched, have revealed similar information regarding the clinical features of TB when it is associated with HIV infection and AIDS (8,14,15,19,61–64,73–75). Extrapulmonary and disseminated TB are very common, pulmonary TB is often manifested by atypical chest x-ray patterns, falsely negative tuberculin skin reactions are frequent, and the fatality rate from nontuberculous AIDS-related diseases is high. However, retrospective study designs select patients with TB who were all proved to have met nontuberculous AIDS-defining conditions during the study period (i.e., usually within a few years) (8,14,15,19,63,73–75). In contrast, prospective study designs select HIV-infected TB patients who may or may not meet nontuberculous criteria for AIDS during the study period (13,17,33,72). Therefore prospective studies include more HIV-associated cases of TB occurring earlier in the course of immunosuppression. They demonstrate that there is a much higher proportion of TB cases and a wider clinical spectrum of TB associated with HIV infection than was previously appreciated. Compared to retrospective studies, prospective studies not surprisingly encompass a higher proportion of patients who have classic fibrocavitary, upper lobe pulmonary TB, significant tuberculin skin reactions, less disseminated and extrapulmonary TB, and a longer time interval before progressing to nontuberculous AIDS-defining conditions and death. This is shown in Table 2 in which the clinical presentation of TB among 160 AIDS/TB patients compiled from seven retrospective studies (8,14,19,63,73–75) is compared with that of 90 HIV-seropositive TB patients and 318 HIV-seronegative TB patients consecutively diagnosed and studied prospectively (13,17). In our prospective study, we found that the subset of HIV-infected TB patients who presented (at the time of TB diagnosis) with reactive tuberculin skin tests and classic fibrocavitary upper lobe pulmonary infiltrates (without intrathoracic lymphadenopathy) were less likely to develop nontuberculous AIDS-defining illnesses and were more likely to survive during the study period (13).

DIAGNOSIS

As stated, in the setting of HIV-induced immunosuppression, the chest radiographic picture of pulmonary TB is atypical, and extrapulmonary, "unusual," and disseminated forms of TB are common. A high index of suspicion for TB and an aggressive diagnostic approach are required to avoid missing a contagious and highly treatable disease.

The generalized symptoms of TB such as fatigue, malaise, weight loss, fever, and night sweats, and the local symptoms of TB such as cough (or other local symptoms depending on the particular organ affected) are nonspe-cific and commonly occur with other conditions associated with HIV infection. Among patients with known or suspected HIV infection, there should be a particularly high index of suspicion for TB in IV drug users, Haitians, other immigrant and ethnic minority groups in whom tuberculous infection is highly prevalent, persons with a known past history of a significant tuberculin skin reaction, patients with chest radiographs suggestive of old TB (e.g., apical scarring), and persons with a history of recent TB exposure (8,14,63).

Conversely, in patients with proven TB, the physician should have a high index of suspicion for concomitant HIV infection if the patient is in an AIDS risk group, has "unusual" or extrapulmonary TB (especially disseminated and lymphatic), or has any symptoms or signs that are common in HIV infection but uncommon in TB (e.g., unexplained persistent diarrhea, thrush, hairy leukoplakia of the tongue, dysphagia, or generalized lymphadenopathy). In high-risk areas for AIDS, physicians, nurse practitioners, and public health nurses who care for patients with TB should routinely and periodically include an extended review of systems and physical examination to search for "nontuberculous" signs and symptoms consistent with an underlying HIV infection.

Pulmonary Tuberculosis

The medical evaluation of a patient suspected or proved to have HIV infection should include a baseline chest x-ray and a tuberculin skin test. If the patient has evidence of pulmonary disease, he/she should be placed in respiratory isolation and a workup begun to exclude pulmonary TB. At least three sputum samples should be sent for mycobacterial smear and culture. If adequate specimens cannot be obtained, sputum should be induced with aerosolized hypertonic saline. If the sputum smears are nondiagnostic, and there is evidence of unexplained pulmonary parenchymal disease either by an abnormal chest x-ray, increased alveolar–arterial pO_2 gradient at rest or with exercise, decreased diffusing capacity of the lung for carbon monoxide, and/or abnormal gallium scan, then a fiberoptic bronchoscopy with bronchoalveolar lavage and transbronchial lung biopsy is indicated. The specimens obtained should be stained and cultured for mycobacteria and other pathogens. This is especially true if the chest x-ray, gallium scan, or clinical presentation is atypical for PCP, making a diagnosis of "presumptive PCP" unlikely. We have noted that bronchoalveolar lavage results in a higher diagnostic yield for *M. tuberculosis* organisms than does transbronchial lung biopsy (13). It should be emphasized that smears and cultures of sputum and bronchoalveolar lavage fluid may be positive for tubercle bacilli when the chest x-ray reveals only lymphadenopathy and may even be positive when the chest x-ray appears normal

(10,15,17). Enlarged mediastinal lymph nodes may be sampled for study by an endobronchial needle aspiration during bronchoscopy, or at mediastinoscopy. Gallium scans may show uptake in hilar nodes even though chest x-rays appear normal. Among HIV-infected patients, such uptake is typical in pulmonary TB but atypical in PCP (111). Mediastinal gas may be seen on chest CT scans as the result of fistulas between tuberculous mediastinal lymph nodes and the esophagus or tracheobronchial tree (1,93).

Extrapulmonary Tuberculosis

The frequency of diagnosing extrapulmonary TB is related not only to the degree of the patient's immunosuppression but also to the extent of the diagnostic evaluation of extrapulmonary sites. If disseminated or extrapulmonary TB is suspected, then specimens can be obtained from extrapulmonary sites depending on clinical presentation. If the patient presents with fever of unknown origin and/or another unexplained systemic symptom, laboratory investigations should include a search for mycobacteria in blood, urine, stool, bone marrow, and/or liver biopsy specimens. If there is clinical, radiographic, or laboratory evidence of local disease, specimens should be obtained from these sites (e.g., urine, stool, pleural fluid, cerebrospinal fluid, bone marrow, liver, superficial, intrathoracic, and/or intra-abdominal lymph nodes, pericardium, brain, skin, and soft tissue) and studied for the presence of mycobacteria. Gallium scans, abdominal sonograms, and CT scans of the head, chest, and abdomen may all be helpful in localizing and defining the extent of tuberculous disease and in directing biopsies (1,82,83,89,95,102,111–114). Tuberculomas and tuberculous brain abscesses appear as ring-enhancing or hypodense mass lesions on CT scans. The chest x-ray is normal in 70% of cases and brain biopsy is often needed for definitive diagnosis. Acid-fast bacilli are seen on smear in most instances. The cerebrospinal fluid may show changes typical of tuberculous meningitis or may be normal (3,82). On abdominal CT scanning, the presence of focal lesions in the liver, spleen, kidneys, pancreas, gastrointestinal tract, or other viscera and enlarged lymph nodes with central or diffuse low attenuation suggest disseminated mycobacterial disease, particularly TB (115).

Although widespread lymphatic TB is frequent in AIDS patients, generalized lymphadenopathy occurs even more commonly with HIV-related lymphoid hyperplasia and also occurs with Kaposi's sarcoma and B-cell lymphoma. The likelihood that lymphadenopathy represents mycobacterial or another specific disease (as opposed to nonspecific lymphoid hyperplasia) increases markedly when chest x-ray abnormalities are present, fever is present, or when lymph nodes are tender, fluc-

tuant, matted, disproportionately large, and/or growing in a regional area (e.g., the neck or the abdomen). In these settings, we usually perform a lymph node aspiration, followed, if necessary, by an excisional lymph node biopsy. In cases of culture-proven tuberculous lymphadenitis, granulomas are usually evident and acid fast smears are positive in 67–90%, permitting an early presumptive diagnosis (12,13,108,116, and *unpublished data*) (Fig. 7). Interestingly, hilar and mediastinal lymphadenopathy are uncommon among HIV-infected patients with generalized peripheral lymphadenopathy secondary to nonspecific lymphoid hyperplasia. If it occurs, neoplastic, fungal, and especially mycobacterial disease should be suspected. Anemia and abnormal liver function tests are common among AIDS patients with TB but are nonspecific findings. However, an elevated alkaline phosphatase out of proportion to other liver function parameters suggests that granulomatous liver disease might be present. Quantification of adenosine deaminase activity in cerebrospinal fluid has been reported as a useful test for the early diagnosis of tuberculous meningitis in patients with and without AIDS (117,118). The test may also be useful in the diagnosis of tuberculous pleural effusions.

Bacteriology

The diagnosis of TB is confirmed by culture of body fluids or tissue specimens. There are conflicting reports whether HIV-infected patients with culture-proven pulmonary TB are less likely to have positive sputum smears than non-HIV-infected patients with pulmonary TB. Nevertheless, the smear is still positive in 44–65% of HIV-infected patients (13,19,72,119). The sensitivity of acid-fast sputum smears tends to be greater in those HIV-infected TB patients who are less immunosuppressed and have chest x-rays typical of reactivation TB compared to those who are more severely immunocompromised and have chest x-rays typical of primary or miliary TB (3,72,119). Although not common practice prior to the AIDS epidemic, laboratories should now routinely receive blood for culture for the diagnosis of mycobacterial disease in HIV-infected patients (104). In one report, 7 (26%) of 27 HIV-infected patients with TB had positive blood cultures for *M. tuberculosis,* and in several other studies this proportion was even higher (up to 42%) (3,12,106,108). Mycobacterial blood cultures should be obtained in HIV-infected patients whenever they have unexplained fever. The diagnostic yield is highest in patients with a temperature higher than 39.5°C, a miliary pattern on chest x-ray, and an elevated serum alkaline phosphatase or lactate dehydrogenase value (106). Acid-fast smears of stool are positive in 40% of patients with HIV infection and TB, probably representing organisms in swallowed sputum. Patients with

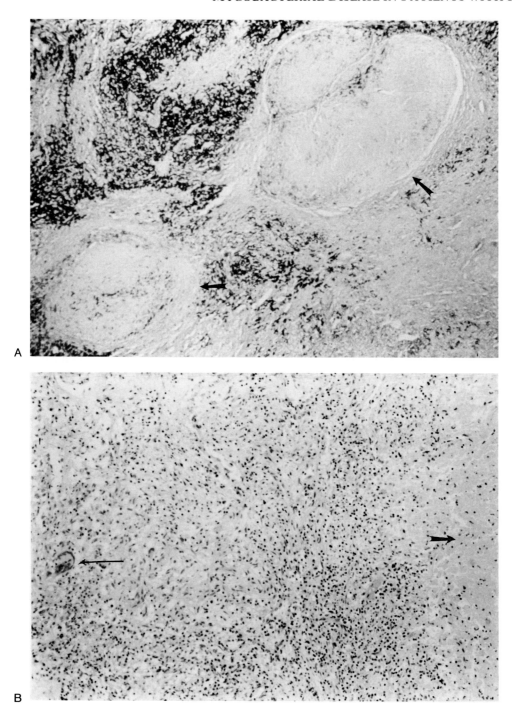

FIG. 7. Tuberculosis. **A:** Lymph node section (hematoxylin and eosin, ×50) from a patient with tuberculous lympadenitis presenting as his first AIDS-related infection. Well-formed tuberculous granulomas are seen (*arrows*). **B:** Bone marrow section (hematoxylin and eosin, ×700) from a patient with disseminated tuberculosis, revealing a multinucleated giant cell (*thin arrow*) and caseation necrosis (*thick arrow*). This is in contrast to the MAC-infected tissue seen in Fig. 8 in which granulomas and necrosis are absent. [Part (A) from ref. 1, with permission; part (B) from Pitchenik AE, Fertel D. Tuberculosis and nontuberculous mycobacterial disease in HIV infected patients. *Med Clin North Am* 1992;76:121–71, with permission.]

this finding almost invariably have pulmonary TB with positive acid-fast smears of sputum and rarely have clinical features of gastrointestinal TB (3,12,108). Therefore positive stool cultures for *M. tuberculosis* are usually not indicative of extrapulmonary TB. (This is in contrast to MAC disease in AIDS where primary gastrointestinal involvement is the rule.)

Recovery and identification of mycobacteria from clinical specimens and the availability of drug susceptibility results are significantly speeded by the use of Bactec radiometric broth (Johnston Laboratories, Inc., Towson, MD) (104,120). A combination of Bactec broth and conventional agar medium (i.e., Lowenstein Jensen or 7H11), in addition to acid-fast stains, provides a rapid and sensitive method of detecting mycobacteria. An isolation lysis centrifugation system (DuPont Co, Wilmington, DE) is used for mycobacterial blood cultures to enhance the isolation of mycobacteria in the culture media. The degree of mycobacteremia can be quantitated when the sediment from the isolator is cultured on 7H11 agar (121). A nucleic acid probe (Gen-Probe, San Diego, CA) can be used for rapid speciation of *M. tuberculosis* and *M. avium-intracellulare* (growing in culture media) (122). A method for detection of mycobacteria based on DNA amplification and hybridization has recently been reported (123). It appears to be a rapid, sensitive, and specific method for detecting *M. tuberculosis* directly from *noncultured* clinical specimens. The amplification procedure has significant advantages over existing methods for diagnosis of mycobacterial infections. It is much more sensitive and specific than direct examination for acid-fast bacilli and it is much more rapid (i.e., 1 day) than culture (even in Bactec broth, which still takes 1–2 weeks). Although this method is still a research tool, it has great potential for clinical practice worldwide (including developing countries).

Pathology

All tissue and fluid specimens from HIV-infected patients should routinely be stained and cultured for mycobacteria, regardless of histologic or other microbiologic findings. Specimens from HIV immunosuppressed patients may reveal mycobacteria on culture even though there are no acid-fast bacilli (AFB) on smear, no granulomas are seen, and/or coexisting nonmycobacterial infections or neoplasms are evident. The pathologist must therefore also have a high index of suspicion for mycobacterial disease when examining tissue from HIV-infected patients. The extent of granulomatous tissue reaction among HIV-infected patients with mycobacterial disease depends on their state of immune reactivity. Although some HIV-infected patients with TB have no granulomas in infected tissue, the majority do (Fig. 7A,B). This is in contrast to the more severely immunosuppressed patients with disseminated MAC in whom granuloma formation in infected tissues is usually poor to nonexistent (1) (Fig. 8A–E). Even among patients with TB, the frequency of detectable granulomas may vary by the site and type of biopsy. Among 11 HIV-seropositive patients who had culture-proven extrapulmonary TB (lymphatic, pleural, bone marrow, liver, and skin), biopsy from the tuberculous site revealed well-formed granulomas in ten (91%). In contrast, granulomas were found in the tissue specimens of only three (33%) of nine patients with culture-proven pulmonary TB who had transbronchial lung biopsies performed by fiberoptic bronchoscopy (13). Similar findings were reported by Sunderam et al. (63). This might be explained by the relatively small (millimeter) specimen size obtained by transbronchial lung biopsy. Among HIV-infected patients with disseminated TB presenting as fever of unknown origin, liver and bone marrow biopsies often furnish the most rapid clues to diagnosis because of the presence of AFB and/or granulomas in the specimens. Although blood culture also represents a good diagnostic source, is less invasive, and certainly should be done, blood smears for AFB have a much lower yield and culture takes weeks to detect growth (124).

Reasons for Delayed or Missed Diagnosis

Kramer et al. found that delayed or no treatment of TB in HIV-infected patients was common (48% of 52 patients) and was related more to errors in management (84% of times) than to atypical manifestations of TB (108). Of those in whom diagnosis was delayed, 45% died of TB. In most cases, delays could have been avoided if at least three sputum samples for acid-fast smear and mycobacterial culture had been obtained, and if empiric therapy for TB had been given to symptomatic patients in whom chest x-ray findings were suggestive of mycobacterial disease. Among HIV-infected patients with TB, acid-fast smears of sputum and bronchoscopic specimens are often negative and granulomatous reaction is frequently missed in the small transbronchial lung biopsy specimens (13,63,108). Therefore, after appropriate specimens have been obtained for mycobacterial culture, empiric anti-TB therapy should be instituted in all HIV-infected patients in whom chest x-ray abnormalities suggestive of TB are not explained by other causes (3,108). The tuberculin skin test is also seriously underutilized among symptomatic HIV-infected patients (125). Although anergy is common among HIV-infected patients with TB (44–89%), a significant number (up to 56%) still have a significant tuberculin skin reaction, which may be very useful in directing care (Table 2). For example, if an HIV-infected tuberculin-reactive patient is symptomatic (e.g., fever of unknown origin) and active TB cannot be excluded initially, full (multidrug) anti-TB therapy should be instituted.

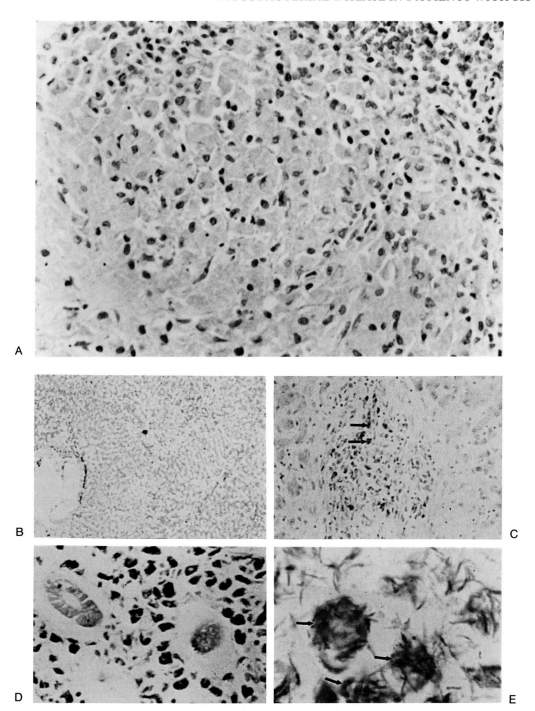

FIG. 8. MAC disease. **A:** Lymph node section (hematoxylin and eosin, ×700) from a patient with disseminated MAC presenting late in AIDS. Large histiocytes are present with abundant foamy cytoplasm. There are no formed granulomas or tissue necrosis, indicative of severe T-cell immunodeficiency. **B–E:** Liver, intestine, and lymph node from another patient with disseminated MAC disease and AIDS. (B) Liver section (hematoxylin and eosin ×200) reveals no granulomas and appears essentially within normal limits. (C) Liver section (Ziehl–Neelsen, ×200) reveals numerous acid-fast bacilli (*arrows*) proved on culture to be MAC. (D) Intestine section (Ziehl–Neelsen, ×800) and (E) lymph node section (Ziehl–Neelsen, ×1500) also reveal numerous acid-fast bacilli without granulomatous reaction. In (E), the acid-fast bacilli are seen, literally packing several macrophages (*arrows*). [Such macrophages appear large and foamy on hematoxylin and eosin staining as shown in (A).] [Parts (A) and (E) from Pitchenik AE, Fertel D. Tuberculosis and non-tuberculous mycobacterial disease in HIV infected patients. *Med Clin North Am* 1992;76:121–71, with permission; parts (B–D) from ref. 1, with permission.]

TREATMENT

Despite their immunosuppressed state, HIV-infected patients with TB who comply with a regimen of standard anti-TB drugs (including both isoniazid and rifampin) have rapid sterilization of sputum, radiographic and clinical improvement, and reasonably low rates of relapse (8,9,13–15,17,19,33,63,72,75,126). Treatment for TB should promptly be initiated whenever a positive AFB smear is found in a patient with proven or suspected HIV infection. It should not be withheld on the presumption that the AFB may represent nontuberculous mycobacteria such as *M. avium-intracellulare*. Initial treatment must be directed against the more virulent, contagious, and treatable *M. tuberculosis* until TB has been ruled out. If the culture later reveals a nontuberculous mycobacteria, treatment can then be changed or discontinued at the physician's discretion (10, 127,128).

Guidelines for the treatment of TB in the setting of HIV infection have been published by the American Thoracic Society, Centers for Disease Control, and others (3,127,129,130). Recommended treatment for adults is isoniazid (INH) 300 mg/day, rifampin (RIF) 600 mg/day (450 mg for persons weighing less than 50 kg), and pyrazinamide (PZA) 20–30 mg/kg daily. PZA is administered during the first 2 months of therapy and then discontinued. If INH resistance is suspected, ethambutol (EMB) 25 mg/kg daily should be included in the initial treatment regimen. (In Miami, we add EMB to the initial drug regimen routinely.) Treatment with INH and RIF should be continued for a total of 9 months or for 6 months after documented culture conversion, whichever is longer (3). Drug susceptibility tests should be performed routinely and the treatment regimen revised if there is resistance to any of the drugs being used. If either INH or RIF is not included in the treatment regimen because of resistance or intolerance, therapy should be continued with RIF and EMB for a total of 18 months (if INH cannot be used) or with INH and EMB for a total of 18–24 months (if RIF cannot be used). Both drug regimens should include PZA for at least the first 2 months and should be continued for 12 months after culture conversion. Some authorities would extend the use of PZA from the first 2 months to the full 18–24 months when drug regimens are used that do not include both INH and RIF (3). In this case, the dosage of EMB may be reduced from 25 to 15 mg/kg after the first 2 months of therapy. Although likely to be effective and well tolerated, it should be noted that the efficacy and toxicity of these recommended 18–24-month drug regimens (without INH or without RIF) are unknown in the setting of HIV immunosuppression. Noncompliance with therapy may be common among subgroups of AIDS patients, and, if suspected or anticipated, fully supervised directly administered ambulatory therapy should be initiated (130). If public health resources are strained (e.g., in developing countries or rural communities) and insufficient to provide for fully supervised therapy when needed, responsible family members or other laypersons (e.g., former TB patients known to be responsible) might be recruited for this purpose, perhaps on a paid, "per patient cured" basis.

Anti-TB drug toxicity (e.g., fever or hepatic, hematologic, or dermatologic reactions) may be difficult to monitor among HIV-infected patients because multiple and recurrent nontuberculous infections, non-TB drugs used concurrently, and/or TB itself may produce similar abnormalities. However, with some exceptions (8,19), most studies show that anti-TB drugs are reasonably well tolerated, and since they are vital, they should not be discontinued because of mild symptoms or mild laboratory abnormalities (14,17,63,72). It has been suggested, and it has been our experience as well, that significant adverse reactions to anti-TB drugs (especially to RIF) are more frequent among the more immunosuppressed patients with TB (i.e., those who contract TB in the later stages of AIDS) (9). In one retrospective study, 90% of adverse reactions (mostly to RIF) were seen during the first 2 months of treatment (19). Concurrent therapy with zidovudine and anti-TB medications seems to be well tolerated (131). Ketoconazole inhibits the absorption of RIF and can result in failure of TB treatment if the drugs are taken together (132). INH and/or RIF can reduce serum ketoconazole and fluconazole concentrations, resulting in ineffective antifungal therapy in some patients (132,133).

Although HIV-infected patients rarely die from TB when it's treated appropriately, subsequent fatal nontuberculous infections usually occur within 1–2 years (8,13,14,19,32,63,75). Furthermore, although TB in HIV-infected patients usually responds to therapy, the optimal duration of therapy to prevent relapse after anti-TB drugs are stopped is still unknown. Relapses, although uncommon, occasionally occur (13,19,99). Therefore HIV-infected patients with TB should have frequent follow-ups for life, and mycobacterial examinations should be repeated as clinically indicated. In addition, some consultants recommend indefinite continuation of isoniazid after completion of a course of anti-TB therapy.

Primary Drug-Resistant TB Acquired Late in AIDS

We recently encountered a large and serious nosocomial outbreak of primary multidrug-resistant TB among severely immunosuppressed HIV-infected patients attending an AIDS center (20,21). The typical patient was attending the center for a nontuberculous AIDS-defining condition at the time of contracting TB, which was resistant to INH and RIF and sometimes to EMB. In this subset of severely immunosuppressed patients, TB was widely disseminated, associated with atypical chest x-rays (e.g., diffuse pulmonary infiltrates), poorly responsive to anti-TB drug therapy, associated with a relatively high rate of drug toxicity (especially to RIF), and directly responsible for a high mortality rate. A few patients may have had a clinical and bacteriologic response (at least temporarily) to a drug regimen that included streptomycin, pyrazinamide, and ciprofloxacin. Since many of the cases occurred within months of each other, the time from TB exposure to tuberculous disease was probably very short. Although a few patients had a past history of previously treated TB, the documentation of the same unusual pattern of multidrug resistance in their isolates suggested another new primary infection rather than reactivation of old infection. It is not unexpected that immunosuppressed patients exposed to TB can be newly reinfected and contract TB despite old tuberculous infection and/or disease that was adequately treated in the past (20,21). This makes them that much more vulnerable to TB exposure.

The Value of HIV Serologic Testing in Patients with TB

All persons with TB should be questioned about risk factors for HIV infection and, whether or not risk factors are elicited, urged to have a HIV serology (129). The finding that a person with TB is HIV infected (a) alters plans for management of the TB (6-month chemotherapy is not recommended and lifetime follow-up is indicated), (b) forewarns the physician of imminent, multiple, and recurrent, nontuberculous opportunistic infections that require treatment in their own right and that also confound the evaluation of anti-TB therapy, (c) alerts the physician to the possible need for anti-HIV therapy (zidovudine) and PCP chemoprophylaxis, (d) establishes the diagnosis of AIDS if extrapulmonary TB is present (an AIDS diagnosis often establishes eligibility for certain social, medical, and economic benefits), and (e) often affords the earliest opportunity to counsel the patient about notification of sexual partners and risk of transmitting HIV infection to others.

Results of Treatment and Long-Term Outcome

Small et al., in a retrospective study, reviewed the course and outcome in 132 patients who were registered as having both AIDS and TB in San Francisco between January 1981 and December 1988 (19). Of 60 patients with pulmonary involvement, in whom follow-up sputum cultures were available, all showed clearance of acid-fast organisms from the sputum within 1–20 weeks from the start of treatment (median clearance time, 10 weeks). The delayed instances of clearance mainly represented late collection of sputum rather than delayed response. Of 58 patients with TB (all forms) who com-

pleted conventional therapy, only three (5%) relapsed over 82.3 patient years of follow-up. All three patients had been noncompliant with therapy. Only one treatment failure occurred in a patient with multiple drug-resistant organisms who was also noncompliant with therapy. Twenty-three patients (18%) required a change in anti-TB drug therapy (almost all within the first 2 months) because of adverse effects (mainly rashes and hepatitis). In two-thirds of these cases, the drug reaction was attributed to rifampin. One hundred three (78%) of the 132 AIDS/TB patients died during the study period. For 125 patients who were treated for TB, median survival was 16 months from the time of diagnosis of TB; however, TB was the major cause of death in only eight (6%) of these patients. Furthermore, in six of these eight patients, death occurred within the first month of TB therapy.

In another retrospective study of 1452 AIDS/TB cases, the crude mortality ratio was 62% (818/1452) and the median probability of survival from TB diagnosis was 20 months and from AIDS diagnosis was 18 months. Although patients with pulmonary and extrapulmonary TB had equally poor prognoses, it is unclear how patients with pulmonary TB and intrathoracic lymphadenopathy and/or pleural effusions were classified or how vigorously a diagnosis of extrapulmonary TB was sought after a diagnosis of pulmonary TB was made (134).

In a prospective study, Pitchenik et al. evaluated 90 patients with TB and HIV infection attending a public health TB clinic in Dade County, Florida (13). Between October 1985 and October 1987, 408 consecutive patients with TB were tested for HIV at TB diagnosis; the 90 who were seropositive constituted the study group who were treated and followed in the clinic. Final data regarding the efficacy of anti-TB therapy and the overall outcome were tabulated in October 1989. With respect to these parameters, the findings were similar to that of the retrospective studies described above (except for patient mortality rate, which was lower). Efficacy of TB therapy was good; 52 (96%) of 54 assessable patients with pulmonary TB converted sputum cultures to negative within 3 months post-therapy. Relapse rates were low for those who were compliant with therapy; only 11 (19%) of 59 assessable patients relapsed during the study period (10/85–10/89) and nine of the 11 were noncompliant with therapy. Case fatality rate, although lower than that of the retrospective studies, was still high; 36 (51%) of 70 assessable patients died during the study period (median duration from TB diagnosis to death was 20 months) and the cause of death was nontuberculous in the great majority (>90%). A report that included the first 34 of these HIV-seropositive patients with TB documented that less than 10% had adverse drug reactions severe enough to require change of the standard anti-TB chemotherapy regimen (17).

PREVENTION

All persons in risk groups for HIV infection must be made aware of three basic principles of TB control that are especially relevant to them (127,129,130,135). (a) Persons with tuberculous infection must be found and treated to prevent reactivation TB. (b) Persons with active TB must be found and treated before they infect others. (c) Persons exposed to patients with pulmonary TB (contacts) must be found and treated to prevent tuberculous infection from occurring and to prevent the progression of recent infection to active disease. Health care workers must also be aware of these principles and must apply them if the alarming rise in HIV-related TB is to be controlled.

Finding and Treating HIV/Tuberculous-Infected Persons to Prevent Reactivation TB

All persons in risk groups for HIV infection should be educated through all possible media to seek a tuberculin skin test within the health care system. Tuberculin testing (Mantoux test with five units of PPD tuberculin) should routinely be conducted at TB and chest disease clinics, substance abuse treatment centers, AIDS clinics, HIV counseling and testing sites, and other facilities where HIV testing is offered (136). In addition, tuberculin skin testing should routinely be offered within general medical offices, clinics, and hospitals whenever patients with proven or suspected HIV infection are encountered. Tuberculin skin testing and preventive therapy programs (including outreach efforts) should be a high priority for drug users, the homeless, and prison inmates since they have an extremely high incidence of HIV and tuberculous infection (129,136,137). Better definition is needed of subgroups among the foreign born (e.g., specific subgroups among Haitians) who are at high risk of dual HIV/tuberculous infection so they can also be included as a high priority in outreach tuberculin skin testing and preventive therapy programs (138). In addition, patients found to be tuberculous infected should be questioned for risk factors for HIV infection and should receive HIV serologic testing if a history of risk factors is elicited; the criteria for administering INH preventive therapy differs for patients with and without HIV infection.

Tuberculin skin testing should include the intradermal administration of five tuberculin units of PPD-tuberculin and at least two other recall antigens such as candida, mumps, or tetanus toxoid (3,139). Tuberculin reactive persons who are HIV infected, or whose HIV infection status is unknown but are suspected of being HIV infected, should have INH preventive therapy administered for 12 months regardless of age, after active TB has been excluded by clinical evaluation and chest x-ray (127,129,130,136,140). For HIV-infected persons or those suspected to be HIV infected, a significant tuberculin skin reaction is considered to be ≥5 mm of induration (140). HIV-infected persons who are anergic, but who have a history of a positive tuberculin skin test and never received treatment, have x-ray evidence of old untreated TB (e.g., apical scarring), are close contacts to patients with TB, or are members of indigenous or immigrant populations in whom tuberculous infection is highly prevalent (e.g., Haitians), should also receive 12 months of INH preventive therapy regardless of age, after active TB is excluded. Tuberculin reactive persons in high risk groups but who are HIV seronegative should be managed according to ATS/CDC preventive therapy guidelines for the general population (130). IV drug abuse may in itself be a risk factor for TB (69). Therefore IV drug users who have a significant tuberculin skin reaction should receive INH preventive therapy regardless of HIV status and regardless of age. If they are known to be HIV seronegative, a significant tuberculin skin reaction is considered to be 10 mm rather than 5 mm of induration, and preventive therapy is continued for 6 rather than 12 months (136). It should be emphasized that preventive therapy should be started only after a chest x-ray and clinical evaluation have excluded active pulmonary or extrapulmonary TB. If an HIV-infected tuberculin reactive patient is symptomatic and active TB cannot initially be excluded, full anti-TB therapy should be started as discussed above. If TB is subsequently excluded, preventive isoniazid and rifampin can be continued for a total of 6 months or, alternatively, isoniazid alone can be continued for a total of 12 months (127,130).

For the past $2\frac{1}{2}$ years, patients found to be HIV seropositive at the Dade County Florida Public Health Sexually Transmitted Disease Clinic have been referred for tuberculin skin testing (Mantoux test with five units PPD-tuberculin) at the adjacent TB clinic. Of 769 HIV-seropositive patients who had skin tests placed and read, 430 (56%) had negative tests (<5-mm induration to PPD-tuberculin and a significant skin reaction to one or more of three recall antigens), 175 (23%) were anergic (no significant skin reaction to PPD-tuberculin and three recall antigens), and 164 (21%) had a significant skin reaction of ≥5-mm induration to PPD-tuberculin (the majority had a reaction ≥ 10-mm induration). All the patients with significant tuberculin skin reactions and some anergic patients from populations likely to be tuberculous infected (e.g., Haitians) were placed on INH preventive therapy. To date, there has only been one known case of TB among these patients, and isoniazid drug toxicity has not been a problem (J. Burr, *personal communication,* 1991). It is of interest that 23% of the HIV-infected patients, many of whom were asymptomatic, had skin anergy.

Several additional studies have shown that asymptomatic adults with HIV infection may have an impaired response to PPD, and that skin anergy among certain populations is a strong predictor for contracting TB. Among HIV-infected patients, this supports the criteria of a 5-mm induration tuberculin skin reaction as indicating tuberculous infection, routine testing for skin anergy with multiple antigens (including tetanus toxoid), and instituting preventive therapy for certain subgroups who are anergic (139,141–144). Among HIV-infected patients with low CD4 counts (<200 mm³) and/or clinical AIDS, whose initial tuberculin skin test is negative, a second (booster) test has been reported to be of little value (145). However, if the patient is started on zidovudine, the skin test should be repeated in 2 months on the possibility that a falsely negative skin reaction to tuberculin might be restored back to positive following (even transient) zidovudine-induced immune restoration.

Since patients with both tuberculous and HIV infection have an extremely high rate of contracting TB, early tuberculin skin test screening and chemoprophylaxis are likely to be highly cost effective in the prevention and control of TB. In Africa and the United States, isoniazid has been shown to prevent TB among HIV/tuberculous-infected persons (24,146).

Finding and Treating Patients with Active TB Before They Infect Others

Persons who are HIV infected or at risk for HIV infection must be taught to recognize symptoms of TB and to seek medical care when these symptoms occur and persist. Physicians and nurses who evaluate the health problems of these patients should have a very high index of suspicion for TB and isolate patients as needed. When TB is diagnosed, every effort should be made to assure continuity of treatment and completion of the prescribed drug regimen. This includes scheduling clinic visits, at least monthly, to dispense medication, monitor response to treatment (bacteriologic response is most important), check for drug toxicity, detect noncompliance, and promote compliance. Certain risk groups for HIV infection are frequently noncompliant with TB therapy (13,19,147). Full compliance is probably the major obstacle in controlling the HIV-associated TB outbreak. If noncompliance is anticipated or is already suspected, fully supervised, intermittent, directly administered ambulatory therapy should be initiated promptly (130). Those few with active pulmonary TB who are still not compliant may require incarceration in a TB facility until completion of therapy.

Preventive Treatment of HIV-Infected Persons Exposed to TB (Contacts)

Although TB is not as contagious as communicable diseases of childhood, such as measles, where secondary attack rates among susceptibles range from 80 to 90%, at least 20% of household contacts of patients with pulmonary TB convert their skin tests (148). Close contacts who are HIV infected should receive isoniazid prophylaxis (after active TB is excluded) regardless of their tuberculin skin test status and regardless of previous therapy for tuberculous infection or disease.

Environmental Control

There have been TB outbreaks among HIV-infected inmates within a prison (149) and at least three reports of M. tuberculosis transmission to health care workers and HIV immunosuppressed patients within AIDS clinics and wards (20,21,25,150). The most serious outbreak involved 29 patients with INH- and rifampin-resistant organisms (20,21). Although both health care workers and AIDS patients became tuberculous infected, the AIDS patients (not surprisingly) progressed rapidly to active (multidrug-resistant) TB and transmitted TB to other HIV immunosuppressed patients within the AIDS facility and within their homes. The outbreak was related to delays in recognition and delays in adequate treatment of TB. The patients were admitted to the AIDS wards, followed in AIDS clinics (sharing a common waiting room), and/or received multiple aerosolized pentamidine treatments in clinic while still infectious. Additional problems included inadequate AFB isolation precautions on the HIV ward for some patients known to have active TB and improperly balanced ventilation in HIV wards and clinics. Air from pentamidine treatment and sputum induction rooms were improperly balanced and probably circulated into central treatment and waiting areas of the AIDS clinic.

These outbreaks of TB raise concern about the organization and management of hospital wards and clinics for patients with HIV infection. All HIV-infected patients admitted to the hospital with an undiagnosed pulmonary infiltrate and/or cough should be suspected of having TB, and appropriate precautions to prevent airborne transmission should be taken until TB is diagnosed and treated or ruled out (135,151,152). Early diagnosis is facilitated with radiometric culture techniques and DNA probes (120). Patients with positive sputum smears for acid-fast bacilli (AFB) should remain in isolation, on therapy, until clinically improved with substantial reduction in cough, and until the numbers of organisms in three sequential sputum AFB smears are decreasing (this usually takes at least 2 weeks). If infection with drug-resistant organisms is likely, isolation should be continued until AFB smears are negative (21,129,150,152,153). Patients with suspected pulmonary TB (pending culture results), who have three initial negative sputum smears for AFB, should remain isolated until they have had at least 3 days of effective anti-TB chemotherapy.

When TB patients are discharged, continued bacteriologic response to therapy must be insured and verified, fully supervised therapy must be promptly instituted when noncompliance is anticipated or suspected, and provisions should be made to prevent TB transmission in the outpatient setting, particularly in the AIDS clinics (21,150,152). We have designated a separate, appropriately ventilated facility (trailer) for AIDS/TB patients until they have successfully completed anti-TB treatment. If fully supervised anti-TB drug therapy is not instituted for noncompliant HIV-infected TB patients, they are likely to relapse rapidly, again become contagious, often with resistant organisms, and expose a large population of HIV immunosuppressed copatients within the AIDS clinic (20,21). Drug-resistant TB seriously compounds the problem since it may not be detected for months until drug susceptibility test results become available, it is much harder to treat, and patients may remain infectious despite therapy (which the physician thinks is adequate) (20,21). In addition to AIDS wards and clinics, AIDS hospices, prisons, and shelters for the homeless also represent risk areas for the rapid spread of TB among HIV-infected persons (137,149).

TB within an immunosuppressed population of patients frequently exposed to each other and to health care personnel is of vital concern and demands comprehensive control measures. Especially important are (a) the early identification and treatment of tuberculous infection and active disease, (b) isolation [rooms with negative pressure, ≥6 air exchanges per hour, nonrecirculated ventilation vented to the outside, very efficient particulate air (HEPA) filters, and ultraviolet lights] in both inpatient and outpatient AIDS facilities and during cough-inducing procedures, and (c) fully supervised therapy (129,130,135,150,152–155). The recent outbreaks of TB in AIDS facilities (20,21,25,150) support the use of strict environmental control, not only in rooms specifically designated for TB patient isolation and cough-inducing procedures (sputum induction, aerosol pentamidine therapy, bronchoscopy, pulmonary function testing), but also in waiting rooms, other clinic areas, and entire wards designated for HIV immunosuppressed patients. Specialized booths, occupied only by the patient, can be utilized for sputum induction and aerosol pentamidine therapy (154). Health care workers who are exposed to patients during cough-inducing procedures should wear properly fitted face masks that can filter out droplet nuclei. Candidates for aerosolized pentamidine therapy should be evaluated for the possibility of TB prior to therapy and before each treatment (3). In addition, if HIV-infected TB patients are to be treated in the AIDS clinics of general hospitals (rather than in public health TB clinics), then hospital health care nurses should be designated who have the specific responsibility for closely following these patients as a safeguard for public health. At each scheduled appointment, it should be documented that the appointment is kept, that patients are compliant with therapy, and that they are re-

ceiving fully supervised therapy as required. Surveillance of employees, working in AIDS areas, for tuberculin skin test conversions (e.g., every 6 months) will identify those who need preventive therapy and also identify possible lapses in TB control.

BCG Vaccination

BCG (a live attenuated bacterial vaccine) should not be given to any patient who is immunosuppressed (156–159). After BCG vaccination, three infants with symptomatic HIV infection developed BCG adenitis, and two infants with apparent asymptomatic HIV infection and two patients with AIDS developed disseminated BCG (156,160–163). Although the World Health Organization has recommended the use of BCG vaccine at birth (or as soon as possible thereafter) for HIV-infected children who are asymptomatic and residing in areas where the risk of TB is high, the risk versus benefit of this recommendation is still unknown and requires study (157,159,161). All agree that BCG should not be given to any HIV-infected child or adult who is symptomatic. Among populations where the risk of newly acquired tuberculous infection is low (e.g., most areas of the United States), BCG is withheld from any person known or suspected to be HIV infected, even if that person is asymptomatic (60,156,157). In the United States, with few exceptions, BCG is also not recommended for the general population (156).

FUTURE PROSPECTS

An estimated 1–1.5 million people in the United States are infected with HIV, and over the next decade the majority will develop varying degrees of immunosuppression and clinical disease (164,165). If, even by conservative estimate, 10% of these HIV immunosuppressed patients are also tuberculous infected (10 million people in the United States are estimated to be tuberculous infected) (166), a very large increase in the number of TB cases can be projected. Furthermore, the need for fully supervised therapy will increase as the numbers of noncompliant TB patients increase (e.g., IV drug users) (147). The situation is even more serious in developing countries where both HIV and tuberculous infection are more common, TB control is poorer, and the proportion of patients with HIV and tuberculous coinfection is higher. Unless worldwide TB control efforts are greatly expanded to meet this problem now, the incidence of TB will continue to rise, even more steeply (2,6,41,42, 45,167). Studies of INH preventive therapy for HIV/tuberculous-infected persons and studies of short course, supervised, intermittent chemotherapy for HIV-infected

TB patients are being conducted in developing countries with encouraging preliminary results (146,168). The "less expensive," longer course anti-TB drug regimens (which do not contain rifampin and do include thiacetazone, a sulfur-containing compound) are currently being used in many developing countries but are more toxic (in the setting of HIV infection), less effective, and less complied with. They should therefore be replaced (41,169,170). Streptomycin, an injectable, also carries the risk of HIV transmission if needles are reused without proper sterilization.

The Department of Health and Human Services Advisory Committee for the Elimination of TB (ACET) has set forth a comprehensive and ambitious plan with the goal of eradicating TB from the United States by the year 2010, and with an interim target goal of reducing the incidence of TB to 3.5 cases per 100,000 population by the year 2000 (171). (The incidence of TB in the United States at the present time is approximately 9.5 per 100,000 population.) A three-step plan of action was proposed: (a) more effective use of existing prevention and control methods, especially in high-risk populations (e.g., HIV/tuberculous-infected persons); (b) the development and evaluation of new technologies for diagnosis, treatment, and prevention of TB; and (c) the rapid assessment and transfer of newly developed technologies into clinical and public health practice.

Better methods to prevent, detect, and treat tuberculous infection and disease are badly needed. Priorities for new (breakthrough) technology development include: finding a vaccine that is much more effective than BCG; finding a sensitive serologic test that detects antibody to *M. tuberculosis* among anergic persons with tuberculous infection or disease; developing DNA amplification and hybridization techniques and/or monoclonal antibodies that are sensitive and specific enough to detect (within hours) *M. tuberculosis* at the species level from uncultured clinical specimens; and developing new immunotherapies, new drug delivery systems, and/or an intensive multidrug regimen that markedly simplify and shorten the current 6–12-month preventive and treatment regimens for patients with tuberculous infection and disease (171).

TB is life-threatening, transmissible, and pandemic, especially among the estimated 5–10 million HIV-infected persons worldwide (42). Fortunately, it is also treatable and preventable, but lack of compliance with therapy is a major obstacle to success. Better tests for identifying tuberculous infection and methods that simplify and shorten existing treatment and preventive drug regimens must be found. To be even moderately successful, the ACET plan to eradicate TB in the United States must heavily target the very large HIV/tuberculous-infected population. Furthermore, the plan must be adopted and implemented for developing countries where the problem is catastrophic (6,7,38,41,42,45,167).

MYCOBACTERIUM AVIUM INTRACELLULARE AND HIV INFECTION

Mycobacterium avium and *Mycobacterium intracellulare* are two closely related, slowly growing, nonchromogenic mycobacteria that cannot be distinguished in most laboratories. Therefore they are conventionally grouped together in the presently used term *Mycobacterium avium-intracellulare complex (MAC)*.

Prior to the AIDS epidemic, MAC disease classically presented as a slowly progressive chronic fibrocavitary pulmonary disease in middle-age persons (men > women, rual > urban) with underlying predisposing lung conditions that are characterized by poor lung drainage (e.g., chronic bronchitis and emphysema, bronchiectasis, pneumoconiosis). Extrapulmonary disease occurred primarily in the form of lymphadenitis in preschool children and disseminated disease was very rare (172,173). From 1940 to 1984, only 37 cases of disseminated MAC were described in non-AIDS patients, most of whom had other underlying immunosuppressive diseases (172). Therefore, even among immunosuppressed patients, disseminated MAC was rare prior to the AIDS epidemic.

With the advent of AIDS, MAC disease (particularly the disseminated form) has become very common, being diagnosed in 14–30% of HIV-infected patients during life (174–179) and in up to 50% or more of autopsy cases (175,176,178,180–182). In the United States and other developed countries, MAC is by far the most common mycobacteria isolated from patients with AIDS and is one of the most frequent opportunistic infections reported in these patients (174,178,183–185). [In Africa and other developing countries, *M. tuberculosis* is more frequently isolated (186–188).] Even if HIV status is unknown, culture-proven MAC (or *M. kansasii*) disease, at a site other than the lungs, skin, or cervical or hilar lymph nodes, meets the CDC surveillance case definition for AIDS (providing there is no other obvious cause for immunosuppression) (68). In contrast to TB, MAC disease is not believed to be transmitted from person to person, occurs uniformly among the AIDS risk groups, occurs late among the AIDS-related infections, and, in the setting of AIDS, is manifested histologically by poorly formed granulomas and macrophages that teem with acid-fast bacilli (1) (Figures 7 and 8). Among HIV-infected patients with MAC disease (in contrast to those with TB), chest x-rays are less specific for mycobacterial disease, pleuritis is uncommon, and positive stool cultures usually represent primary gastrointestinal invasion rather than infected sputum that is swallowed (3,12). Compared to TB, the efficacy of therapy for MAC disease is poor (1).

There is still much to learn about MAC infection and disease in both AIDS and non-AIDS patients. What is the primary route of infection (pulmonary and/or gastrointestinal)? Do the infecting strains of MAC and the route of infection differ in AIDS and non-AIDS patients, and if so, why? Why is the geographic distribution of MAC disease among AIDS patients different from that of non-AIDS patients? Is MAC disease usually the result of reactivation of a persistent latent infection (as in TB) or the result of direct progression of primary infection following recent exposure? What is the normal immune response to MAC infection? Why is MAC disease so common in AIDS, and why, in this setting, does it occur so much more frequently than other nontuberculous mycobacterial disease? Even in midwestern United States, where *M. kansasii* infection was thought to be more prevalent (pre-AIDS epidemic), disseminated MAC is tenfold more common than disseminated *M. kansasii* among patients with AIDS (189,190). Similar findings have been reported from England and Wales (191). Furthermore, among HIV-infected persons, colonization of stool or sputum with MAC appears much more likely to predispose to dissemination than does colonization of stool or sputum with other nontuberculous mycobacteria (192). What is the specific immune defect in AIDS that specifically favors disease from MAC (possibly even favoring only a few MAC serotypes) and can the selective immune defect be altered? Does disseminated MAC in AIDS patients contribute to their morbidity and mortality and does treatment make a difference? What are the best drugs, drug combinations, and dosages to use in treatment? Is drug susceptibility testing helpful in selecting drug regimens?

EPIDEMIOLOGY AND PATHOGENESIS

MAC Infection in Patients Without AIDS

The true prevalence of MAC disease in the United States (among AIDS and non-AIDS patients) is unknown since positive MAC cultures are not routinely reported to public health departments and isolation of MAC (especially from sputum) may represent colonization rather than disease. Nevertheless, prior to the AIDS epidemic, large nationwide skin test surveys (utilizing PPD-S and PPD-Battey) conducted by the U.S. Navy and Public Health Service suggested that MAC infection was common (10–70% prevalence depending on region), occurred most frequently in the southeast United States (≥70% prevalence), was more frequent in rural areas, and (in contrast to tuberculous infection) was more common at younger ages (190,193,194). A skin test survey conducted on medical students and hospital employees in New Orleans revealed similar findings (i.e., PPD-Battey skin reactivity was common in this area, and, among young adults, was much more common than PPD-S reactivity) (70). A nationwide survey of nontuberculous mycobacterial isolates in 1979 and 1980 re-

vealed that MAC accounted for 60% and that MAC isolation rates were highest in the Southeast, supporting the skin test survey results (195).

In contrast to TB, MAC is not transmitted from person to person but is acquired from the environment by means not well understood. MAC is the most ubiquitous nontuberculous mycobacteria in the environment. It is found in domestic animals, soil, dust, dried plants, and water (especially in fresh and brackish water in warmer climates such as estuaries and rivers along the southeast coast of the United States) (173,190,195–197). There is evidence that MAC-infected aerosols are produced from these waters and that those MAC strains that are preferentially aerosolized are the ones more commonly isolated from persons with disease (198). Plasmid containing MAC strains are associated with increased virulence in animal models of disease, are usually present in isolates associated with human disease, and are much more common in aerosols than in soil or dust (190,199). These studies, considered together, and the fact that MAC disease prior to the AIDS epidemic was most common in the southeast United States and was predominantly pulmonary, support the hypothesis of airborne transmission of infection from the environment to humans, at least among non-AIDS patients.

MAC Infection in Patients with AIDS

Among AIDS patients with disseminated MAC disease, autopsies have shown massive involvement of the small and large intestinal mucosa and submucosa and adjacent lymph nodes out of proportion to pulmonary involvement (200,201). During life, these patients tend to have more gastrointestinal symptoms than pulmonary symptoms and their chest x-rays are often normal (202,203). This strongly suggests that among AIDS patients, at least in part, infection is acquired from environmental sources via the oral route (i.e., primary gastrointestinal infection from ingesting food or water) (183,200,201). Furthermore, among AIDS patients, the prevalence of MAC disease is similar in most areas of the United States, in all AIDS risk groups regardless of socioeconomic status, in males and females, and in non-Hispanic whites and blacks (only Hispanics with AIDS have a lower prevalence) (189). This also supports the hypothesis that MAC infection is not spread from person to person but from the environment where the organism is ubiquitous (e.g., in water) and exposure is unavoidable and common to most if not all groups. The similar rate of disseminated MAC among all AIDS risk groups does not support homosexual intercourse as a means of transmission as has been proposed (200).

Although the prevalence of MAC disease among AIDS patients does not seem to vary by location, race, sex, or AIDS risk group, it does vary significantly by age, with higher rates occurring among younger age groups (189). This suggests that MAC frequently infects young persons, including infants and young children, and that disease results from recent infection rather than reactivation of latent infection (189,204). The lack of antibody response to MAC in patients with AIDS and disseminated MAC also suggests recent primary infection since AIDS patients lack the ability to mount antibody responses to other primary infections, but not to reactivation infections (185,205,206). A third line of evidence suggesting primary disease from recent environmental exposure is that asymptomatic MAC colonization of respiratory secretions and stool commonly precedes MAC bacteremia among patients with AIDS (175,185, 192,207,208). [Asymptomatic MAC colonization may also occur in the normal host but without dissemination (185).]

Differences in MAC Isolates from AIDS and Non-AIDS Patients

In addition to biochemical methods used to speciate MAC, one can recognize 28 types of MAC by seroagglutination. This has been helpful in epidemiologic studies since only a few serotypes predominate in human disease. A predominance of serotypes 1, 4, and 8 is seen among patients with AIDS (179). MAC isolates from patients with and without AIDS differ in various ways. The MAC isolates from AIDS patients (compared to isolates from non-AIDS patients) are more likely to be: serotype 4, plasmid containing, more virulent *in vitro* and in animal models, identical on DNA probe analysis, *M. avium* rather than *M. intracellulare* on DNA probe analysis, susceptible to ethionamide and cycloserine and resistant to kanamycin and rifampin (180,185,209–212). Interestingly, the most frequent MAC serotype found among AIDS patients in Germany was 8/21, in contrast to that found among AIDS patients in the United States where it was serotype 4 (213). Nevertheless, in both countries, the most common MAC serotypes isolated from AIDS and non-AIDS patients still differed. Whether these differences in MAC isolates from AIDS and non-AIDS patients are due to different virulence factors relative to different host susceptibilities, different routes of infection, and/or distinct geographical preponderances of different MAC serotypes remains to be determined (213).

Prevalence of Disseminated MAC in AIDS

From 1981 to 1987, 41,349 cases of AIDS were reported to the CDC and disseminated nontuberculous mycobacteria was seen in 2269 (5.5%) (189). Of the 2269 cases of disseminated nontuberculous mycobacteria, 21 (1.2%) were either *M. gordonae, M. fortuitum, or M. che-*

lonei, 57 (2.9%) were *M. kansasii,* and the overwhelming majority, 1906 (96.1%), were MAC. By December 31, 1990, 161,073 cases of AIDS were reported to the CDC and disseminated nontuberculous mycobacterial infection was seen in 12,202 (7.6%). Again, MAC represented the vast majority of the nontuberculous mycobacteria (185). This is markedly different from the distribution of disseminated nontuberculous mycobacteria before the AIDS epidemic (38% MAC, 33% *M. kansasii,* 14% *M. fortuitum-chelonei,* 13% scotochromogens) (173,189). Even in areas of midwestern United States where *M. kansasii* disease was relatively high prior to the AIDS epidemic, disseminated MAC accounted for more than 90% of disseminated nontuberculous mycobacteria (189).

The cumulative incidence of disseminated MAC and AIDS reported to the CDC, representing approximately 7% of all reported AIDS cases, is certainly an underestimate (185). This is so because disseminated MAC tends to occur in the late stages of HIV immunosuppression [a mean of 7–15 months after other AIDS defining conditions (e.g., PCP) have been diagnosed and reported to CDC as index AIDS cases]. In clinical studies, between 76 and 90% of MAC infections follow the AIDS diagnosis (185). In North America, clinical studies have shown disseminated MAC in 14–30% of AIDS patients and even these may be underestimates since autopsy series of AIDS patients have shown disseminated MAC in as high as 50% (174–182). In Europe, disseminated MAC is also common among patients with AIDS. In one study from Berlin, 29% of 102 autopsies performed on AIDS patients revealed a postmortem diagnosis of MAC infection; the diagnosis of MAC disease was made premortem in 25 (9%) of 281 AIDS patients (214). Since disseminated MAC is insidious in onset and presents late in the course of AIDS, the diagnosis is often missed during life and clinical studies can underestimate its true prevalence. On the other hand, autopsy data can overestimate the proportion of AIDS patients who develop disseminated MAC at sometime between AIDS diagnosis and death because of a bias toward patients who die with unexplained clinical syndromes (185). Even though a high proportion of AIDS patients are shown on autopsy to have died with disseminated MAC, the contribution of MAC to morbidity and mortality in AIDS is still unclear.

In summary, MAC disease among patients with AIDS appears markedly different from MAC disease among patients without AIDS (180,189,190,200,201,209–212). (a) It is much more common. (b) It constitutes a much higher proportion of all nontuberculous mycobacterial cases. (c) It is much more likely to be disseminated rather than a chronic fibrocavitary pulmonary disease superimposed on other chronic pulmonary diseases, which are characterized by poor lung drainage. (d) The route of infection seems to be mainly gastrointestinal rather than respiratory; dissemination appears to originate predominantly from the GI source. (e) It is commonest in the young age groups and appears to decrease with increasing age rather than occurring predominantly in persons who are middle aged or older. (f) The geographic distribution is fairly uniform throughout the United States rather than predominantly in the Southeast. (g) The serotypes, DNA sequence, prevalence of plasmids, virulence, and drug susceptibility patterns of AIDS MAC isolates have been found to be different from that of non-AIDS MAC isolates. Although the precise reasons for these differences are unclear, it is likely that AIDS patients have an immune defect that makes them uniquely susceptible to MAC infection and disease, especially via the gastrointestinal route. The ability to enter intestinal epithelial cells has been demonstrated with some MAC *in vitro,* a property that may contribute to the relative virulence of MAC for AIDS patients via the gastrointestinal tract (215). It is likely that once invasion of the gut epithelium has occurred, the profound immune defect of AIDS permits widespread dissemination. It is also possible that specific strains of MAC are uniquely virulent in this setting.

CLINICAL FEATURES

Unlike TB, MAC disease usually occurs in the late stages of HIV immunosuppression when malnutrition and multiple concurrent AIDS-related infections and/or advanced malignancies are present (175). At this time, patients are often on multiple medications, each having its own toxicity. The clinical signs and symptoms of MAC infection are nonspecific and therefore difficult to distinguish from other AIDS-related conditions or drug toxicities. Nevertheless, multiple studies have revealed fairly consistent information regarding the clinical picture of MAC disease among patients with AIDS (1,12,175–179,186,202,203,216–228). Common symptoms include fever, night sweats, fatigue, anorexia, malaise, and weight loss, all of which are often present for several months before the diagnosis is made (i.e., patients present with a chronic wasting syndrome). Abdominal pain and diarrhea may be prominent symptoms in patients with MAC infection of the bowel. Involvement of the small bowel can produce an illness mimicking Whipple's disease, with malabsorption and similar intestinal histologic findings (175,201,228–230). Enlarged infected periportal lymph nodes may cause extrahepatic biliary obstructive jaundice (175). Despite frequent pulmonary involvement, pulmonary symptoms are uncommon and should suggest another diagnosis (202,203).

On physical examination, patients are often febrile, cachectic, and may or may not have chest findings, peripheral and/or bulky intra-abdominal lymphadenopathy, and/or hepatosplenomegaly. Subclinical hepatitis,

thrombocytopenia, marked leukopenia, and progressive anemia (including red cell hypoplasia) (231) may occur, suggesting involvement of bone marrow and liver.

MAC disease among patients with AIDS has also presented as localized pneumonia (208), mediastinal–endobronchial fistulas presenting as endobronchial mass lesions on bronchoscopy (232,233), mediastinal-esophageal fistulas with esophagitis (234), terminal ileitis mimicking Crohn's disease (235), pericarditis (236), meningitis (204), endophthalmitis (237), septic arthritis and osteomyelitis (238), cutaneous abscesses (239), and infections of skin, lymph node, and rectal mucosa in association with Kaposi's sarcoma (175,240).

DIAGNOSIS

Disseminated MAC infection should be suspected in any HIV immunosuppressed patient who presents with unexplained systemic symptoms. The great majority of patients will have fever, debilitation, and weight loss with a peripheral blood CD4 count of less than $100/mm^3$ and/or an AIDS diagnosis already established by criteria other than MAC infection (12,175,176,241). Of 55 patients with MAC infection, Modilevsky et al. found that 48 (87%) had another AIDS-defining illness diagnosed 2–37 months (mean 7.8 months) before MAC infection was diagnosed (12). Of 50 patients with MAC infection diagnosed before death, Hawkins et al. found that 48 (96%) had an AIDS-defining illness 1–24 months (mean 9.3 months) before MAC infection was diagnosed (175). In one study of 21 HIV-infected patients with disseminated MAC, all had systemic signs and symptoms; of the 14 who had peripheral blood CD4 cell counts performed, all had counts of less than 100 cells/mm³ (242). In two other studies of AIDS patients with MAC infection, the concentration of peripheral blood CD4 lymphocytes averaged $52/mm^3$ and $70/mm^3$ (12,176). This is in contrast to HIV-infected patients with TB in whom the mean or median peripheral blood CD4 lymphocyte concentration was $170/mm^3$ in one study and $326/mm^3$ in another (12,72). In the study by Hawkins et al. (175), involving 67 patients with disseminated MAC, almost every patient had fever, malaise, and weight loss, 11 (16%) had chronic diarrhea and abdominal pain, 6 (9%) had a chronic malabsorption resembling Whipple's syndrome, and 2 (3%) presented with extrahepatic biliary obstruction secondary to enlarged intra-abdominal lymph nodes. Although PCP is the most common AIDS-defining infection, Pierone et al. found that the most frequent cause of fever of unknown origin (FUO) in AIDS was disseminated MAC infection (31.9%), followed by TB (26.2%) and PCP (9.5%) (243).

Although pulmonary involvement with MAC is frequent in AIDS patients, the chest x-ray is nonspecific and prominent pulmonary symptoms are rare (12,202,

203). Chest x-rays may show a nodular, diffuse, or patchy infiltrate with or without hilar or mediastinal adenopathy or, commonly, may be normal (despite the presence of disseminated disease) (219). Cavitary disease, pleural effusions, and a miliary pattern are uncommon (219). Although the radiographic findings are nonspecific, they lead to study of sputum, bronchoscopic washings, or lung biopsy specimens.

Abdominal CT scans may show marked hepatosplenomegaly, diffuse jejunal wall thickening, and large retroperitoneal and mesenteric lymph nodes of homogeneous soft tissue density, which are quite suggestive of disseminated MAC in this setting (115,244). Lymph nodes with central or diffuse low attenuation may also be seen in AIDS patients with disseminated MAC on CT scanning but are less common and more typical of TB (in which caseation necrosis is more frequent) (115). Gallium scans may also be useful to locate infected sites (e.g., lung, lymph node, bone marrow, skin) and to direct biopsies (114,239,245,246).

Bacteriology

Among patients with disseminated MAC, the organism has been cultured from almost every body fluid and tissue including blood, stool, urine, sputum, cerebrospinal fluid, lung, bone marrow, liver, lymph node, spleen, pancreas, tongue, esophagus, stomach, intestine, heart, adrenals, kidney, eye, and skin (2,12,14,104,121,175–177,180,196,200,207,247–252). The culture yield for MAC from various sites in AIDS patients with disseminated disease is shown in Table 3. A positive culture from a normally sterile site such as blood, bone marrow, liver, or lymph node (the most commonly involved and accessible sterile sites) is diagnostic of invasive and (usually) disseminated disease. False positive cultures of MAC and other mycobacteria due to contaminated laboratory reagents and/or other technical laboratory problems have occurred (253; and *unpublished data*).

Blood culture is a particularly good noninvasive test for disseminated MAC among HIV immunosuppressed patients and is the diagnostic procedure of choice in this setting. MAC bacteremia tends to be persistent and blood cultures, utilizing a lysis–centrifugation technique (Dupont Co., Wilmington, DE), are positive in the great majority of cases (e.g., 70–98%) (Table 3) (12,104,121, 175–177,179,180,248,251). One retrospective study suggested that two blood cultures will detect most cases (95%) of disseminated MAC infection (254). Since the MAC are usually not found free in plasma (255), a lysis–centrifugation technique is employed to increase the sensitivity of mycobacterial blood culture. This is accomplished by lysis of peripheral blood leukocytes with saponin, which releases viable intracellular mycobacteria, which are then concentrated by centrifugation. The concentrate can then be plated on conventional media (i.e., Lowenstein Jensen or 7H11 agar and Bactec radiometric broth). The radiometric Bactec system will allow rapid diagnosis by detecting growth of mycobacteria within 6–12 days; culture on 7H11 or Lowenstein Jensen agar takes 15–20 days. Plating on the solid agar, however, allows quantitative colony counts in blood, which are a useful means of determining both the magnitude of infection and the response to treatment (104,121,179,180). DNA probes for MAC can offer a rapid 2-hr species identification once mycobacterial growth in Bactec broth and/or on solid culture media is achieved (122,256). [As mentioned in the TB section, techniques of DNA augmentation are currently under study to increase the sensitivity of DNA probes so that species identification would be possible on raw, uncultured clinical specimens within one day (123).] Auramine fluorochrome staining of uncultured peripheral blood concentrate for AFB is insensitive for detecting mycobacteremia and is generally not done (as it is for all other specimens). Buffy coat smears for AFB are also insensitive but have been reported to detect mycobacteremia in patients with AIDS (250,257,258).

AFB smear and culture of stool are simple noninva-

TABLE 3. *Diagnostic yield of specimens in AIDS patients with disseminated MAC infection: a compilation of multiple studies*

References (patient series)	Specimen	Total number of patients cultured (all studies)	Average percent yield	Range
12, 175–177, 251	Blood	173	94%	70–98%
12, 175, 176, 180, 200	Stool	79	61%	36–100%
12, 175, 176	Sputum	85	59%	29–92%
12, 175	BAL	35	60%	41–78%
175	Urine	28	43%	—
12, 175, 176	Bone marrow	36	72%	40–100%
12, 175	Lymph node	5	80%	50–100%
175, 200	Bowel	7	86%	75–100%
251	CSF	19	11%	—

From Pitchenik AE, Fertel D. Tuberculosis and non-tuberculous mycobacterial disease in HIV infected patients. *Med Clin North Am* 1992;76:121–71, with permission.

sive tests that often correlate with invasive disease if the patient has constitutional symptoms (175). Positive MAC cultures from sputum or bronchial washings are common and raise suspicion for, but are not diagnostic of, invasive or disseminated disease (175,182,207,219). If MAC is found in pulmonary or stool specimens, other specimens from sterile sites (e.g., blood, bone marrow) should be cultured for MAC to search for proof of disseminated disease. Positive cultures from respiratory secretions and stool commonly precede bacteremia; therefore close clinical follow-up of patients with these findings is necessary (175,192,207,208). Horsburg et al. found that 8 (33%) of 24 patients colonized with MAC (in sputum or stool) progressed to disseminated disease with the same species they were colonized with, while none of 16 colonized with other nontuberculous mycobacterial species progressed to dissemination with the colonizing species ($P = 0.01$). [Mean follow-up was 5.2 months for patients colonized with MAC and 7.3 months for patients colonized with other mycobacteria (192).] Disseminated MAC can also occur, occasionally, in the absence of prior detectable respiratory or gastrointestinal colonization (259).

Pathology

The distinctive pathologic feature of MAC disease in patients with AIDS (on hematoxylin and eosin staining of tissue specimens) is a poorly defined granuloma consisting of pale blue striated histiocytes filled with mycobacteria (221,227,249,260–262). The striations within the histiocytes represent large numbers of acid-fast bacilli as demonstrated on Ziehl–Neelsen staining (Figures 8A–E). The features often described in typical granulomatous inflammation, such as lymphocytic infiltrates, caseation necrosis, epithelioid histiocytes, and Langhans' giant cells, are present only in a minority of cases. Occasionally, there is no suggestive tissue reaction at all, despite positive AFB smears and positive cultures for MAC (1,12) (Figures 8B,C). Culture of tissue may also be positive when the AFB smear is negative. Therefore all specimens from HIV immunosuppressed patients must be stained for AFB and cultured for mycobacteria regardless of tissue reaction, AFB smear results, or concomitant nonmycobacterial pathology. Bone marrow is easily biopsied and frequently yields diagnostic specimens, as do biopsies from lung, lymph node, liver, and GI tract. On gross inspection, involved organs may appear yellow because of the pigmentation of the organisms (185).

When disseminated MAC is suspected, the best specimens for culture are blood, stool, bone marrow, and, if necessary, liver. Taken together, the yield should be almost 100% (Table 3)(175). Cultures of respiratory, stool, and sterile site specimens are frequently positive when the smear of the specimen is negative (104).

TREATMENT

Assessment of Morbidity and Mortality from MAC Disease in AIDS

MAC infection among patients with AIDS disseminates widely and densely involves many tissues and organs (e.g., blood, bone marrow, liver, spleen, lymph node, and GI tract), but the organism has relatively low virulence. Autopsy series suggest that it does not usually cause significant tissue damage or organ failure (181,263). Among AIDS patients with PCP, who also have MAC in their respiratory secretions, it has been noted that anti-pneumocystis therapy alone usually results in recovery (264). Nevertheless, the bacterial load in disseminated MAC is formidable (as high as 10^4–10^5 colony forming units of MAC/ml blood within circulating monocytes and 10^9–10^{10} bacilli/g of tissue within fixed macrophages of the reticulo-endothelial system) and clinical studies suggest that disseminated infection contributes significantly to fever and debilitation among patients in the late stages of AIDS (202,248,265,266).

It is uncertain whether patients with disseminated MAC die from this disease or from multiple other coexisting infections (e.g., due to P. carinii or cytomegalovirus) (218,264). In one study involving AIDS patients with PCP, patient survival did not differ whether they were MAC infected or not (267). In another large national study, the median survival for AIDS patients with disseminated nontuberculous mycobacteria (almost all MAC) was 7.4 months, whereas the median survival for AIDS patients without MAC was 13.3 months ($P < 0.0001$) (189). The survival analyses for patients in this study, however, was challenged (264). In a third, subsequent study that controlled for CD4+ cell counts and antiviral therapy, the estimated survival of patients with AIDS and disseminated MAC infection was 4.1 months whereas the survival in comparable AIDS patients without disseminated MAC was 11.1 months (268). In a fourth study, involving 1044 patients with AIDS or ARC who were started on zidovudine, 12.4% developed MAC disease during 2 years of follow-up and this was found to be a strong independent predictor of death (241). It has been suggested that the shortened survival among AIDS patients with MAC disease (which frequently involves the intestine) results from inanition (176,185,249). Although the preponderance of evidence suggests that MAC disease does contribute (directly or indirectly) to the morbidity and mortality of AIDS in its late stages, the efficacy of therapy for MAC in improving quality of life (considering drug toxicity) and in improving survival is unclear.

Problems with Treatment for MAC Disease in AIDS

Pulmonary or disseminated MAC disease is very hard to treat in patients without AIDS because of relative drug resistance of the organism; MAC disease in patients with AIDS responds even less well to anti-mycobacterial chemotherapy (172,269,270). This is primarily due to the severe immune defect of AIDS, and possibly because AIDS MAC isolates have more virulence and/or different drug susceptibility patterns from that of non-AIDS isolates (180,209–212). Unlike the treatment for TB, it is unclear whether or not various drug regimens for disseminated MAC among AIDS patients have a significant impact on morbidity and mortality, which drug regimens and what drug doses are most effective, and whether or not *in vitro* drug susceptibility results (i.e., testing single drugs or drug combinations) predict bacteriologic and clinical response to therapy (265,271). *In vitro* drug concentrations that are easily achievable as serum levels *in vivo* and that predict clinical usefulness of the drug are well established for TB but are not well defined to guide treatment for MAC disease (especially in AIDS). In MAC disease, clinical response or lack of response to a drug is often poorly predicted by the results of standard qualitative drug susceptibility tests. The *in vitro* critical drug concentrations used in these qualitative tests were originally developed and standardized for *M. tuberculosis* and not for MAC (272).

Despite these reservations, Horsburgh et al. have documented improved responses among *non-AIDS* patients with MAC pulmonary disease, when several drugs were used to which the organism was susceptible, singly, *in vitro,* suggesting that the *in vitro* qualitative test results are sometimes clinically relevant in this setting (273). They found that the more drugs included in the regimen to which the MAC strain was susceptible *in vitro,* the more likely there was to be bacteriologic clearance in sputum. Although the same principle may also apply to AIDS patients with disseminated MAC, this has not yet been proved. To date, there have been no studies in patients with AIDS that relate successful treatment of MAC infections to *in vitro* drug susceptibility (265). Even if susceptibility is demonstrated to some drugs, it usually represents inhibition rather than killing of the organism at attainable plasma concentrations. Ciprofloxacin and amikacin offer some advantage in this regard, because they may kill (rather than inhibit) MAC at achievable levels in serum (unlike rifabutin and clofazimine) (274). Low bactericidal activities of drugs against MAC *in vitro,* however, do not exclude their therapeutic usefulness, because they may produce a synergistic effect in combination with other drugs. Drug combinations may therefore be therapeutically promising for patients whose isolates are susceptible on the basis of the minimal inhibitory concentration (MIC)(275,276).

Quantitative and Combination Drug Susceptibility Testing

Heifets and Iseman have described a radiometric method to determine minimal inhibitory concentrations

(MICs) of anti-mycobacterial drugs in 7H12 broth and proposed the use of MICs to quantitate the degree of susceptibility of *M. avium* isolates. Susceptible strains were those for which the MIC of an agent was below the drug concentrations achievable in humans and equal to or lower than the MIC of susceptible strains of *M. tuberculosis* (277,278). Such quantitative tests of drug susceptibility may prove to be superior to conventional single concentration qualitative tests in indicating the best drugs and doses for treatment of disseminated MAC in patients with AIDS. In contrast to standard qualitative drug susceptibility testing, the quantitative test has the advantage of being able to determine the proportion of resistant organisms (degree of resistance) at a wide range of drug concentrations and thereby possibly yields drug susceptibility data that correlate better with clinical response to treatment. Quantitative drug susceptibility testing is also the only practical way to evaluate the potential of new anti-MAC drugs (e.g., rifamycins, quinalones, clofazimine) for which clinically relevant *in vitro* drug concentrations have not been established. A MIC and MBC of the drug are determined and then compared with achievable serum-tissue concentrations (272).

Susceptibility testing to combinations of two to five drugs can also be performed on conventional agar plates or Bactec broth (272,278). The test is designed to determine if a mycobacterial isolate is susceptible to a certain combination of drugs to which it was found resistant in single drug tests. Such drug synergy has been demonstrated with MAC isolates (276,279). The technique may be especially applicable in selecting drug regimens for treatment of MAC disease due to isolates that are relatively resistant to most conventional anti-mycobacterial drugs. Quantitative and combination drug susceptibility testing represent state-of-the-art technology aimed to better evaluate, *in vitro,* existing and new drug regimens. Currently, these tests are only available in a few laboratories but may become increasingly used if they prove to be cost effective.

Results of Treatment

MAC is often resistant to most standard first-line anti-TB drugs (e.g., isoniazid, rifampin, pyrazinamide, and streptomycin) but shows variable susceptibilities *in vitro* to rifabutin, clofazimine, ciprofloxacin, ofloxacin, imipenem/cilastatin, rifapentine, cycloserine, amikacin, ethambutol, roxithromycin, clarithromycin, and azithromycin (179,265,271,272,274,280–283). The effects of drugs in combination are often additive and occasionally synergistic and bactericidal (276,279). Nevertheless, there have been conflicting reports on the clinical efficacy of regimens that include drugs to which MAC shows some susceptibility (127,175,176,179,183, 220,224,265,280,284–292). Initial reports indicated a lack of success using drug regimens that included rifabutin and clofazimine (175,285). Subsequently, several reports have shown that similar drug regimens, including rifabutin and clofazimine, with or without amikacin, have resulted in defervescence, resolution of night sweats, malaise, and (less frequently) diarrhea, decline in mycobacteremia, and, in some cases, sterilization of blood without bacteremic relapses (185,248,289–293). Symptomatic and bacteriologic responses have also been shown using a drug regimen without rifabutin (i.e., ethambutol, clofazimine, ciprofloxacin, and rifampin) (294) and without rifabutin and clofazimine (i.e., ethambutol, rifampin, ciprofloxacin, and amikacin) (295). The more favorable results in the more recent therapeutic studies may be explained by the use of more drugs to which MAC is susceptible (i.e., four or five), started earlier after the onset of symptoms (i.e., within 4 weeks) and continued for a longer time (i.e., ≥3 months) before assessment of response to therapy (185). To date, there have been no controlled studies evaluating which, if any, drug regimens increase overall survival, reduce bacteremia, and/or induce amelioration of symptoms. Although recent evidence suggests some clinical improvement with aggressive therapy, controlled studies are still needed (128). Because AIDS patients with disseminated MAC usually have continuous high-grade bacteremia, serial quantitative blood cultures provide at least one objective means for evaluating treatment (248).

Clinical Approach to Treatment

In contrast to TB, there is no evidence that MAC is communicable to the general population, and the efficacies of current drug regimens are modest (128,179,241, 289). Furthermore, MAC disease is less often fatal than TB when left untreated (12,108,125). Therefore when acid-fast bacilli are found in any specimen from a patient with AIDS or suspected AIDS, our approach, pending culture results, is to institute promptly standard anti-TB drugs as outlined in the section on TB. With new radiometric rapid culture methods (Bactec, Johnston Laboratories, Towson, MD) and specific DNA probes (Gen-Probe), mycobacteria are now routinely identified within 1–3 weeks (104,122,179,256,265). If culture reveals *invasive* MAC that accounts (or probably accounts) for significant symptoms (i.e., no other treatable opportunistic infections), the patient has reasonably intact renal and liver function, and the patient is willing to cooperate in a multidrug treatment plan, we may then initiate an anti-MAC drug regimen on a trial (e.g., 3-month) basis (128,265).

The following regimen includes the most promising drugs (based on susceptibility testing) that are currently available for clinical use in the treatment of MAC disease: rifampin (600 mg/day), clofazimine (100 mg/day), ethambutol (15–25 mg/kg/day), ciprofloxacin (750 mg twice a day), and amikacin (7.5 mg/kg im or iv every 12

hr or 10 mg/kg iv daily) (128,185,247,265,280). All drugs in this regimen are administered orally (except for amikacin) and are available commercially (296). If a clinical response is induced (usually within 2–8 weeks when it occurs), suppressive therapy should be continued for life with oral drugs and for as long as practical (e.g., 4–8 weeks) with amikacin (185,265). Amikacin (an injectible) can be administered intravenously once (instead of twice) daily, to facilitate its use on an outpatient basis. If the outpatient use of amikacin is still impractical, it can be withheld from the initial drug regimen or withdrawn on hospital discharge and added later if there is no response or if drug toxicity requires discontinuing one of the oral drugs (185). If, because of epidemiologic considerations, it is elected to initiate therapy for MAC prior to speciation of an acid-fast isolate, isoniazid should be added to the regimen described above until TB is excluded by culture. The aim of treatment is to reduce the bacterial load and thereby ameliorate symptoms and improve quality of life. These objectives, even if achievable, must be weighed against the significant toxicity of the multidrug regimen.

Drug Toxicity

Clofazimine, ciprofloxacin, and amikacin, although relatively active against MAC *in vitro,* have only recently been used for the treatment of MAC disease. The most common adverse effects of clofazimine are pink to brownish black discoloration of various tissues and fluids, skin dryness, rash, and gastrointestinal symptoms including nausea, vomiting, abdominal pain, diarrhea, and anorexia (271,296). The adverse effects of ciprofloxacin include occasional nausea, vomiting, abdominal pain, rash, headache, and lightheadedness. The adverse effects of amikacin are nephrotoxicity and ototoxicity; ototoxicity is frequent after 8 weeks of therapy and is sometimes irreversible (185,293). The toxicities of the conventional anti-mycobacterial drugs have been well described (130).

Rifabutin, which shows relatively good in vitro activity against MAC, may soon become available. It is generally well tolerated (at least as well as rifampin), and the types of adverse reactions from it have been similar to those reported for rifampin. The most common adverse effects are mild elevations of liver enzymes, gastrointestinal distress (nausea, vomiting, diarrhea), and hypersensitivity reactions such as rash and fever. Reversible bone marrow suppression with leukopenia and thrombocytopenia has also been observed (297). It has been shown that 80–100% of MAC strains are susceptible to rifabutin at concentrations of ≥1.0 μg/ml (271). Although plasma levels of rifabutin do not reach this concentration at conventional doses, high tissue distribution does occur (298). Compared to rifampin, rifabutin is a weaker enzyme inducer and may be less likely to interfere with the action of multiple drugs (e.g., coumarin, oral contraceptives, methadone, oral hypoglycemics, digitoxin, quinidine, disopyramide, dapsone, ketoconazole, and corticosteroids) (132,296). Rifabutin is excreted partly through the biliary route and partly through the kidney. In contrast to rifampin, the dose must be lowered in renal insufficiency (297). Interestingly, rifabutin has been shown to inhibit the replication of HIV although this is not of clinical significance (299).

Monitoring for toxicity of anti-mycobacterial drugs in patients with AIDS is often confounded by the occurrence of hepatic, hematologic, and dermatologic abnormalities from other drugs, nonmycobacterial disease, or the mycobacterial disease itself that has disseminated to the liver and bone marrow. The presence of such abnormalities is therefore not an absolute contraindication to the use of anti-mycobacterial agents. It has been shown that patients can tolerate concurrent therapy with zidovudine and conventional anti-mycobacterial drugs without unacceptable toxicity (131).

Experimental Considerations in Treatment and Prevention

The drug regimens rifabutin–clofazimine; amikacin; amikacin–clofazimine; amikacin–ciprofloxacin-imipenem/cilastatin; amikacin–rifapentine; and azithromycin have particularly good *in vitro* activity against MAC and have been effective in the treatment of disseminated MAC in immunocompromised (beige) mouse models (179,265,271,281). However, it is hard to extrapolate from animal data to humans. Rifabutin and clarithromycin are currently under clinical trials by Adria (rifabutin) and Abbott (clarithromycin) Laboratories and may become available for future use. Other variables such as drug–tissue concentrations and activity of agents within macrophages influence the relevance of serum drug concentration and *in vivo* drug efficacy (265). [For example, some β-lactam antibiotics, such as ampicillin, have promising *in vitro* activity against MAC but are not effective against intracellular organisms, thus limiting their clinical effectiveness (271).] Liposome encapsulation of drugs or other carrier technology might be used in the future to enhance delivery of drugs to intracellular sites and thereby increase drug activity against intracellular mycobacteria (265). Liposome encapsulation of amikacin improves its activity compared with free amikacin in the beige mouse model of MAC infection (271). Whether or not these newer anti-mycobacterial drugs, drug combinations, and/or drug delivery systems will improve survival in patients with AIDS remains to be determined. As new anti-HIV and immune stimulating drugs are developed, new and existing chemotherapy regimens for MAC may become more effective in the setting of AIDS and should be reevaluated.

Prevention

MAC is ubiquitous within the environment and it therefore seems impossible to prevent exposure. Measures to prevent MAC disease among HIV-infected patients might include the early use of zidovudine (e.g., when the T-helper-cell count falls below $500/mm^3$) (300) and the early preventive use of rifabutin (e.g., when the T-helper-cell count falls below $200/mm^3$) (301). The efficacy of rifabutin in preventing MAC disease in patients with AIDS has not yet been proved but is currently under study in a large prospective, multicenter, randomized trial conducted by Adria Laboratories.

Immune Regulation and Modulation in MAC Disease

The abnormal susceptibility of AIDS patients to mycobacteria has been attributed to deficiencies in T-lymphocyte-produced lymphokines that activate macrophages. Facilitating anti-mycobacterial macrophage activity and delivering effective drugs into the macrophage seem critical since tissue macrophages from AIDS patients with disseminated MAC are literally packed with these bacilli (271) (Figure 8C–E). Nevertheless, the precise mechanism by which the macrophage defends against MAC is unknown.

Recombinant granulocyte–macrophage colony-stimulating factor has been shown to inhibit growth of or kill MAC (302). Tumor necrosis factor has also been shown to enhance *in vitro* killing of MAC in human macrophages and the bactericidal effect was augmented when used in combination with antimicrobial agents (293,303). Tumor necrosis factor with interleukin-2 has also been demonstrated to reduce colony counts in MAC-infected mice (304). This raises the question of whether these cytokines play some role in enhancing macrophage defense against MAC infection *in vivo*.

Bermudez and Young and Toba et al. found that γ-interferon does not have macrophage activating factor activity for *M. avium* infection of human monocytes (305,306). This suggests that γ-interferon might not enhance the efficacy of chemotherapy for MAC disease. Schnittman et al. have shown that peripheral blood monocytes from both AIDS patients and normal controls can phagocytose and initially kill 50–99% of infecting MAC; however, surviving bacilli always multiplied rapidly in later phases of infection in both types of monocytes. Pretreatment of monocytes with γ-interferon, *in vitro*, only modestly enhanced initial MAC killing by normal monocytes and not at all by patient's monocytes, and outgrowth of MAC was still always observed in both. Persistent killing of MAC by normal monocytes also did not occur in the presence of tumor necrosis factor-α or even autologous lymphocytes primed with IL-2 (266). This *in vitro* study further dampens enthusiasm for the clinical use of lymphokines such as γ-interferon and IL-

2 in the treatment of disseminated MAC in AIDS. In the same study, however, high titered anti-MAC immune serum significantly enhanced the killing of MAC by monocytes from both AIDS patients and healthy controls and also prevented the outgrowth of surviving MAC. One way microorganisms may survive intracellular killing is by inhibition of fusion of lysosomes with the phagosomes containing the organisms, thus avoiding exposure to hydrolytic enzymes (307). Schnittman et al. hypothesized that the anti-MAC antibody may alter the outer capsule of the MAC bacillus, thereby overcoming the inhibition of fusion of the phagosome with the lysosome (266).

Winter et al. found that patients with AIDS and disseminated MAC infection had anti-MAC antibody levels similar to uninfected AIDS patients and normal controls, suggesting the inability to mount an anti-MAC antibody response in AIDS (206). Crowle et al. found that normal human serum inhibits the growth of *M. avium* in normal human macrophages and that sera from AIDS patients were deficient in this inhibitory property. Furthermore, macrophages from AIDS patients were unresponsive to the inhibitor in normal serum (308). Further studies on how normal macrophages respond to the serum inhibiter to suppress *M. avium* infection and studies on the clinical efficacy of hyperimmune (anti-MAC) gamma globulin in AIDS patients with disseminated MAC would be of interest.

The precise roles of monocyte–T-cell interactions and various cytokines, lymphokines, and antibody-dependent mechanisms in enhancing macrophage killing of MAC and other mycobacteria are still unknown. Even though MAC and *M. tuberculosis* are both intracellular pathogens, reside in monocytes and macrophages, and are presumably controlled by cellular immune responses, they may present different challenges to the immune system and may therefore be handled differently.

For example, as stated above, AIDS patients with disseminated MAC do not produce antibodies in response to infection and there is some evidence that humoral immunity may play a role in the defense against this organism (206,266,308). In contrast, AIDS patients with reactivation TB commonly have antibodies against *M. tuberculosis,* but humoral immunity seems unimportant in controlling the disease (205). Understanding the normal immune defense against MAC infection and understanding the basis of the specific vulnerability of AIDS patients to MAC will provide insight to the development of new preventive and therapeutic strategies. In the final analysis, prevention of immunosuppression and/or restoration of overall immune function will have the most impact on the overall morbidity and mortality of HIV-infected patients and remains the ultimate goal of therapy in AIDS.

OTHER NONTUBERCULOUS MYCOBACTERIAL INFECTIONS IN AIDS

Other mycobacteria have been isolated much less frequently from patients with AIDS and include *M. fortuitum, M. kansasii, M. gordonae, M. xenopi, M. chelonei, M. simiae, M. haemophilum, M. bovis* (from BCG vaccine), *M. malmoense, M. scrofulaceum, M. szulgai, M. marinum, M. flavescens,* and *M. asiaticum* (127,160, 162,189,247,309–316). The first eight mycobacteria listed have caused disseminated disease in patients with AIDS. Although all these organisms are potentially pathogenic in AIDS patients, with the exception of *M. kansasii,* there are no established guidelines for their treatment. Ciprofloxacin shows excellent in vitro activity against *M. fortuitum* and *M. xenopi* (282,283).

A retrospective review of 19 HIV-infected patients with *M. kansasii* disease has recently been published (317). Fourteen patients (74%) had pulmonary disease exclusively with either focal upper lobe infiltrates or diffuse interstitial infiltrates; thin-walled cavitary lung lesions occurred in nine patients. The disease occurred late in the course of HIV immunosuppression; the majority of patients (84%) had a previous diagnosis of AIDS and the median CD4+ lymphocyte count was 49 cells/mm^3 (range 0–198 cells/mm^3). Treatment with conventional therapy resulted in resolution of fever, symptoms, and radiographic infiltrates and in bacteriologic response without relapse while patients were on therapy. Recommended treatment consists of isoniazid, rifampin, and ethambutol for a minimum of 18 months and for at least 15 months after culture conversion (127).

REFERENCES

1. Pitchenik AE, Fertel D, Bloch AB. Mycobacterial disease: epidemiology, diagnosis, treatment and prevention. *Clin Chest Med* 1988;9:425–441.
2. Bloch AB, Rieder HL, Kelly GD, et al. The epidemiology of tuberculosis in the United States: implications for diagnosis and treatment. *Clin Chest Med* 1989;10:297–313.
3. Barnes PF, Bloch AB, Davidson PT, Snider DE Jr. Tuberculosis in patients with human immunodeficiency virus infection. *N Engl J Med* 1991;324:1644–50.
4. CDC. Tuberculosis—United States, 1985. *MMWR* 1986; 35:699–703.
5. Bloch AB, Rieder HL, Kelly GD, et al. The epidemiology of tuberculosis in the United States. *Semin Respir Infect* 1989; 4:157–70.
6. Murray JF. The J. Burns Amberson Lecture. The white plague: down and out or up and coming? *Am Rev Respir Dis* 1989;140:1788–95.
7. WHO Epidemiologic Record. *Global programme on AIDS and tuberculosis programmes.* Geneva: WHO, April 28, 1989.
8. Chaisson RE, Schecter GF, Theuer CP, Rutherford GW, Echenberg DF, Hopewell PC. Tuberculosis in patients with the acquired immunodeficiency syndrome. Clinical features, response to therapy, and survival. *Am Rev Respir Dis* 1987;136:570–4.
9. Chaisson RE, Slutkin G. Tuberculosis and human immunodeficiency virus infection. *J Infect Dis* 1989;159:96–100.

10. Fertel D, Pitchenik AE. Tuberculosis in acquired immune deficiency syndrome. *Semin Respir Infect* 1989;4:198–205.
11. Hopewell PC. Tuberculosis and the human immunodeficiency virus infection. *Semin Respir Infect* 1989;4:111–22.
12. Modilevsky T, Sattler FR, Barnes PF. Mycobacterial disease in patients with human immunodeficiency virus infection. *Arch Intern Med* 1989;149:2201–5.
13. Pitchenik A, Burr J, Fertel D, et al. Tuberculosis in HIV infected patients: epidemiology, infectivity, clinical features, response to treatment, prognostic factors and long term outcome. *International Congress for Infectious Disease,* Montreal, Canada, July 15–19, 1990:152(abst 426).
14. Pitchenik AE, Cole C, Russell BW, et al. Tuberculosis, atypical mycobacteriosis, and the acquired immunodeficiency syndrome among Haitian and non-Haitian patients in south Florida. *Ann Intern Med* 1984;101:641–5.
15. Pitchenik AE, Rubinson A. The radiographic appearance of tuberculosis in patients with the acquired immune deficiency syndrome (AIDS) and pre-AIDS. *Am Rev Respir Dis* 1985;31:393–6.
16. Theuer CP. Tuberculosis in patients with human immunodeficiency virus infection. *West J Med* 1989;150:700–4.
17. Pitchenik AE, Burr J, Suarez M, Fertel D, Gonzalez G, Moas C. Human T-cell lymphotropic virus-III (HTLV-III) seropositivity and related disease among 71 consecutive patients in whom tuberculosis was diagnosed. A prospective study. *Am Rev Respir Dis* 1987;135:875–9.
18. CDC. Diagnosis and management of mycobacterial infection and disease in persons with human T-lymphotropic virus type III/lymphadenopathy-associated virus infection. *MMWR* 1986;35:448–52.
19. Small PM, Schecter GF, Goodman PC, et al. Treatment of tuberculosis in patients with advanced human immunodeficiency virus infection. *N Engl J Med* 1991;324:289–94.
20. Pitchenik AE, Burr J, Laufer M, et al. Outbreaks of drug-resistant tuberculosis at an AIDS centre. *Lancet* 1990;336:440–1.
21. CDC. Nosocomial transmission of multidrug-resistant TB to health care workers and HIV-infected patients in an urban hospital—Florida. *MMWR* 1990;39:718–22.
22. Pitchenik AE, Russell BW, Cleary T, et al. The prevalence of tuberculosis and drug resistance among Haitians. *N Engl J Med* 1982;307:162–5.
23. Edwards D, Kirkpatrick CH. The immunology of mycobacterial diseases. *Am Rev Respir Dis* 1986;134:1062–71.
24. Selwyn PA, Hartel D, Lewis VA, et al. A prospective study of the risk of tuberculosis among intravenous drug users with human immunodeficiency virus infection. *N Engl J Med* 1989;320:545–50.
25. Di Perri G, Cruciani M, Danzi MC, et al. Nosocomial epidemic of active tuberculosis among HIV-infected patients. *Lancet* 1989;2:1502–4.
26. Collins FM. The immunology of tuberculosis. *Am Rev Respir Dis* 1982;125:42–9.
27. Dannenberg AM Jr. Pathogenesis of pulmonary tuberculosis. *Am Rev Respir Dis* 1982;125:25–30.
28. Rankin JA, Collman R, Daniele RP. Acquired immune deficiency syndrome and the lung. *Chest* 1988;94:155–64.
29. Seligmann M, Pinching AJ, Rosen FS, et al. Immunology of human immunodeficiency virus infection and the acquired immunodeficiency syndrome. An update. *Ann Intern Med* 1987;107:234–42.
30. Fauci AS. Immunologic abnormalities in the acquired immunodeficiency syndrome (AIDS). *Clin Res* 1985;32:491–9.
31. Fauci AS, Schnittman SM, Poli G, Koenig S, Pantaleo G. Immunopathogenic mechanisms in human immunodeficiency virus (HIV) infection. *Ann Intern Med* 1991;114:678–93.
32. Pitchenik AE, Fischl M, Dickinson G, et al. Opportunistic infections and Kaposi's sarcoma among Haitians: evidence of a new acquired immunodeficiency state. *Ann Intern Med* 1983;98:277–84.
33. Theuer CP, Chaisson RE, Schecter GF, et al. Human immunodeficiency virus in tuberculosis patients in San Francisco (abstract). *Am Rev Respir Dis* 1988;137:121.
34. Bothamley G, Beck JS, Gibbs J, et al. HLA phenotype and the

35. immune response to *Mycobacterium tuberculosis. Am Rev Respir Dis* 1991;143:A286(abst).
35. Prince HE, Moody DJ, Shubin BI, et al. Defective monocyte function in the acquired immune deficiency syndrome (AIDS): evidence for a monocyte T-cell proliferative system. *J Clin Immunol* 1985;5:21–5.
36. Smith PD, Ohura K, Masur H, et al. Monocyte function in the acquired immune deficiency syndrome. *J Clin Invest* 1984;74:2121–8.
37. Miller SA, Bia FJ, Coleman DL, Lucia HL, Young K Jr, Root RK. Pulmonary macrophage function during experimental cytomegalovirus interstitial pneumonia. *Infect Immun* 1985;47:211–6.
38. Harries AD. Tuberculosis and human immunodeficiency virus infection in developing countries. *Lancet* 1990;335:387–90.
39. WHO. *Weekly epidemiological record.* Geneva: WHO, January 5, 1990.
40. Lamoureux G, Davignon L, Turcotte R, Laverdière M, Mankiewicz E, Walker MC. Is prior mycobacterial infection a common predisposing factor to AIDS in Haitians and Africans? *Ann Inst Pasteur/Immunol* 1987;138:521–9.
41. Pitchenik AE. Tuberculosis control and the AIDS epidemic in developing countries. *Ann Intern Med* 1990;113:89–91.
42. Styblo K. The potential impact of AIDS on the tuberculosis situation in developed and developing countries. *Bull Int Union Tuberc Lung Dis* 1988;63:25–8.
43. Yesso G, Bretton R, Bretton G, et al. HIV infection and tuberculosis: tuberculosis trends in Abidjan, Côte d'Ivoire, 1985–1989. 6th International Conference on AIDS, San Francisco, June 1990, p 308; ThC732 (abst).
44. Kelly P, Burnham G, Radford C. HIV seropositivity and tuberculosis in a rural Malawi Hospital. *Trans R Soc Trop Med Hyg* 1990;84:725–7.
45. Slutkin G, Leowski J, Mann J. The effects of the AIDS epidemic on the tuberculosis problem and tuberculosis programmes. *Bull Int Union Tuberc Lung Dis* 1988;63:21–4.
46. Garcia ML, Valdespino JL, Salcedo A, Mora JL, Bravo E, Sepulveda JA. AIDS and tuberculosis. Encounter between two epidemics in a Latin American country. 6th International Conference on AIDS, San Francisco, June 1990, p 245; ThB492 (abst).
47. Clermont HC, Chaisson RE, Davis H, et al. HIV-1 infection in adult tuberculosis patients in Cite Soleil, Haiti. 6th International Conference on AIDS, San Francisco, June 1990, p 244; ThB490 (abst).
48. Long R, Scalcini M, Manfreda J, et al. Impact of human immunodeficiency virus type 1 on tuberculosis in rural Haiti. *Am Rev Respir Dis* 1991;143:69–73.
49. Elliott AM, Luo N, Tembo G, et al. Impact of HIV on tuberculosis in Zambia: a cross sectional study. *BMJ* 1990;301:412–15.
50. Quinões EP, Morais de sá CA, Ferreira Ramos Filho C, Weniger BG, Rodrigues LGM, Heyward WL. Comparison of tuberculosis in HIV-positive and HIV-negative inpatients in Rio de Janeiro, Brazil. 6th International Conference on AIDS, San Francisco, June 1990, p 245; ThB493 (abst).
51. Ekpini E, Gnaore E, Adjorlolo G, et al. Evaluation of clinical features and AIDS case definition in tuberculosis patients in Abidjan. 6th International Conference on AIDS, San Francisco, June 1990, p 439 (abst 3148).
52. Sabbatani S, Mangiarotti V, Fabbri A, et al. Fraction of excess tuberculosis morbidity attributable to HIV-2 infection in the population of Bissau district. 6th International Conference on AIDS, San Francisco, June 1990, p 434 (abst 3129).
53. Gnaore E, Adjorlolo G, Bretton G, et al. HIV-2 infection is associated with tuberculosis. 6th International Conference on AIDS, San Francisco, June 1990, p 246; FC663 (abst).
54. George JR, Rayfield MA, Phillips S, et al. Efficacies of U.S. Food and Drug Administration—licensed HIV-1-screening enzyme immunoassays for detecting antibodies to HIV-2. *AIDS* 1990;4:321–6.
55. Hammer SM, Feinberg M. Slow virus infections and retrovirus infections. In: Rubenstein E, Federman DD, eds. *Scientific American Medicine,* vol 2. 7, XXXII. New York: Scientific American Inc., 1989:1–30.

56. CDC. Cases of specified notifiable diseases, United States, weeks ending December 29, 1990 and December 30, 1989 (52nd week). *MMWR* 1991;39:944.

57. CDC. Update: tuberculosis elimination—United States. *MMWR* 1990;39:153–6.

58. Rieder HL, Cauthen GM, Kelly GD, Bloch AB, Snider DE Jr. Tuberculosis in the United States. *JAMA* 1989;262:385–9.

59. Rieder HL, Cauthen GM, Comstock GW, Snider DE Jr. Epidemiology of tuberculosis in the United States. *Epidemiol Rev* 1989;11:79–98.

60. CDC. Tuberculosis—United States, 1985—and the possible impact of human T-lymphotropic virus type III/lymphadenopathy-associated virus infection. *MMWR* 1986;35:74–6.

61. CDC. Tuberculosis and acquired immunodeficiency syndrome—New York City. *MMWR* 1987;36:785–90,795.

62. CDC. Tuberculosis and acquired immunodeficiency syndrome—Florida. *MMWR* 1986;35:587–90.

63. Sunderam G, McDonald RJ, Maniatis T, Oleske J, Kapila R, Reichman LB. Tuberculosis as a manifestation of the acquired immunodeficiency syndrome (AIDS). *JAMA* 1986;256:362–6.

64. CDC. Tuberculosis and AIDS—Connecticut. *MMWR* 1987;36:133–5.

65. Burr JM. Tuberculosis update in Dade County. *Miami Med* 1990;27–33.

66. Rieder HL, Cauthen GM, Bloch AB, et al. Tuberculosis and acquired immunodeficiency syndrome—Florida. *Arch Intern Med* 1989;149:1268–73.

67. CDC. Tuberculosis, final data—United States, 1986. *MMWR* 1987;36:817–20.

68. CDC. Revision of the CDC surveillance case definition for acquired immunodeficiency syndrome. *MMWR* 1987;36:3S–15S (suppl).

69. Reichman LB, Felton CP, Edsall JR. Drug dependence: a possible new risk factor for tuberculous disease. *Arch Intern Med* 1979;139:337–9.

70. Pitchenik AE. PPD-tuberculin and PPD-Battey dual skin testing of hospital employees and medical students. *South Med J* 1978;71:917–22.

71. Bloch AB, Snider DE Jr. Reported AIDS patients with extrapulmonary tuberculosis in the United States. 6th International Conference on AIDS, San Francisco, June 1990, p 437(abst 3140).

72. Theuer CP, Hopewell PC, Elias D, Schecter GF, Rutherford GW, Chaisson RE. Human immunodeficiency virus infection in tuberculosis patients. *J Infect Dis* 1990;162:8–12.

73. Duncanson FP, Hewlett D Jr, Maayan S, et al. *Mycobacterium tuberculosis* infection in the acquired immunodeficiency syndrome. A review of 14 patients. *Tubercle* 1986;67:295–302.

74. Handwerger S, Mildvan D, Senie R, et al. Tuberculosis and the acquired immunodeficiency syndrome at a New York City Hospital: 1978–1985. *Chest* 1987;91:176–80.

75. Louie E, Rice LB, Holzman RS. Tuberculosis in non-Haitian patients with acquired immunodeficiency syndrome. *Chest* 1986;90:542–5.

76. Pape JW, Liautaud B, Thomas F, et al. Characteristics of the acquired immunodeficiency syndrome (AIDS) in Haiti. *N Engl J Med* 1983;309:945–50.

77. Sbarbaro JA. Tuberculosis: the new challenge to the practicing clinician. *Chest* 1975;68:436–43(suppl).

78. Long R, Maycher B, Scalcini M, Manfreda J. The chest roentgenogram in pulmonary tuberculosis patients seropositive for human immunodeficiency virus type 1. *Chest* 1991;99:123–7.

79. Long R, Maycher B, Rigby M, Manfreda J, Hershfield E, Mendella L. Intrathoracic adenopathy (IA) in postprimary tuberculosis: a computed tomographic study. *Am Rev Respir Dis* 1991;143:A285(abst).

80. Silva VMC, Werneck E, Kritski AL, et al. Pulmonary tuberculosis (PT) and AIDS: chest radiographic (CR) features. 6th International Conference on AIDS, San Francisco, June 1990, p 248; ThB506 (abst).

81. Laguna F, Polo R, Saenz E, et al. Central nervous system tuberculosis in AIDS. 6th International Conference on AIDS, San Francisco, June 1990; ThB502(abst).

82. Bishburg E, Sunderam G, Reichman LB, Kapila R. Central nervous system tuberculosis with the acquired immunodeficiency syndrome and its related complex. *Ann Intern Med* 1986;105:210–13.

83. Fischl MA, Pitchenik AE, Spira TJ. Tuberculous brain abscess and toxoplasma encephalitis in a patient with the acquired immunodeficiency syndrome. *JAMA* 1985;253:3428–30.

84. Reichman LB. HIV infection: a new face of tuberculosis. *Bull Int Union Tuberc Lung Dis* 1988;63:19–26.

85. Doll DC, Yarbro JW, Phillips K, Klott C. Mycobacterial spinal cord abscess with an ascending polyneuropathy (letter) (published erratum appears in *Ann Intern Med* 1987;106:784). *Ann Intern Med* 1987;106:333–4.

86. Woolsey RM, Chambers TJ, Chung HD, McGarry JD. Mycobacterial meningomyelitis associated with human immunodeficiency virus infection. *Arch Neurol* 1988;45:691–3.

87. Croxatto JO, Mestre C, Puente S, Gonzalez G. Nonreactive tuberculosis in a patient with acquired immune deficiency syndrome. *Am J Ophthalmol* 1986;102:659–90.

88. Dalli E, Quesada A, Juan G, Navarro R, Payá R, Tormo V. Tuberculous pericarditis as the first manifestation of acquired immunodeficiency syndrome. *Am Heart J* 1987;114:905–6.

89. D'Cruz IA, Sengupta EE, Abrahams C, Reddy HK, Turlapati RV. Cardiac involvement, including tuberculosis pericardial effusion, complicating acquired immune deficiency syndrome. *Am Heart J* 1986;112:1100–2.

90. Lin RY, Schwartz RA, Lambert WC. Cutaneous–pericardial tuberculous fistula in an immunocompromised host. *Int J Dermatol* 1986;25:456–8.

91. de Silva R, Stoopack PM, Raufman JP. Esophageal fistulas associated with mycobacterial infection in patients at risk for AIDS. *Radiology* 1990;175:449–53.

92. Maguire GP, Delorenzo LJ, Brown RB, Davidian MM. Case report: endobronchial tuberculosis simulating bronchogenic carcinoma in a patient with the acquired immunodeficiency syndrome. *Am J Med Sci* 1987;294:42–4.

93. Wasser LS, Shaw GW, Talavera W. Endobronchial tuberculosis in the acquired immunodeficiency syndrome. *Chest* 1988;94:1240–4.

94. Cendan I, Talavera W, Busillo C, Garner G, Mullen M. Empyema thoracis: a complication of disseminated *Mycobacterium tuberculosis* (MTB) in AIDS. *Am Rev Respir Dis* 1991;143:A281(abst).

95. Brody JM, Miller DK, Zeman RK, et al. Gastric tuberculosis: a manifestation of acquired immunodeficiency syndrome. *Radiology* 1986;159:347–8.

96. Duncanson F, Prabakaran J, Selvaraj S, et al. Intestinal fistula formation in a man with mycobacterial disease and AIDS. *NY State J Med* 1985;85:702–4.

97. Lax JD, Haroutiounian G, Attia A, Rodriguez R, Thayaparan R, Bashist B. Tuberculosis of the rectum in a patient with acquired immune deficiency syndrome. Report of a case. *Dis Colon Rectum* 1988;31:394–7.

98. Moreno S, Pacho E, Lopez-Herce JA, Rodriguez-Creixems M, Martin-Scapa C, Bourza E. *Mycobacterium tuberculosis* visceral abscesses in the acquired immunodeficiency syndrome (AIDS). *Ann Intern Med* 1988;109:437.

99. Sunderam G, Mongura BT, Lombardo JM, et al. Failure of "optimal" four drug short course tuberculosis chemotherapy in a compliant patient with HIV. *Am Rev Respir Dis* 1987;136:1475–8.

100. Freed JA, Pervez NK, Chen V, Damsker B. Cutaneous mycobacteriosis: occurrence and significance in two patients with the acquired immunodeficiency syndrome. *Arch Dermatol* 1987;123:1601–3.

101. Stack RJ, Bickley LK, Coppel IG. Miliary tuberculosis presenting as skin lesions in a patient with acquired immunodeficiency syndrome. *J Am Acad Dermatol* 1990;23:1031–35.

102. Barnes P, Leedom JM, Radin DR, Chandrasoma P. An unusual case of tuberculous peritonitis in a man with AIDS. *West J Med* 1986;144:467–9.

103. Dickerman SA, Sherman A, Balthazar EJ, Hazzi C. Ileocecal tuberculosis in a patient with the acquired immune deficiency syndrome. *Am J Med* 1987;83:1010–11.

104. Kiehn TE, Cammarata R. Laboratory diagnosis of mycobacterial infections in patients with acquired immunodeficiency syndrome. *J Clin Microbiol* 1986;24:708–11.

105. Saltzman BR, Motyl MR, Friedland GH, McKitrick JC, Klein RS. *Mycobacterium tuberculosis* bacteremia in the acquired immunodeficiency syndrome. *JAMA* 1986;256:390–1.

106. Shafer RW, Goldberg R, Sierra M, Glatt AE. Frequency of *Mycobacterium tuberculosis* bacteremia in patients with tuberculosis in an area endemic for AIDS. *Am Rev Respir Dis* 1989;140:1611–3.

107. Barber TW, Craven DE, McCabe WR. Bacteremia due to *Mycobacterium tuberculosis* in patients with human immunodeficiency virus infection. A report of 9 cases and a review of the literature. *Medicine* 1990;69:375–83.

108. Kramer F, Modilevsky T, Waliany AR, Leedom JM, Barnes PF. Delayed diagnosis of tuberculosis in patients with human immunodeficiency virus infection. *Am J Med* 1990;89:451–56.

109. Lombardo PC, Weitzman I. Isolation of *Mycobacterium tuberculosis* and *M. avium* complex from the same skin lesions in AIDS. *N Engl J Med* 1990;323:916–17(lett).

110. Hayes MM, Coghlan PJ, King H, et al. Kaposi's sarcoma, tuberculosis and Hodgkin's lymphoma in a lymph node—possible acquired immunodeficiency syndrome. *S Afr Med J* 1984;66:226–29.

111. Ganz WI, Serafini AN. The diagnostic role of nuclear medicine in the acquired immunodeficiency syndrome. *J Nucl Med* 1989;30:1935–45.

112. Abiri MM, Kirpekar M, Abiri S. The role of ultrasonography in the detection of extrapulmonary tuberculosis in patients with acquired immunodeficiency syndrome (AIDS). *J Ultrasound Med* 1985;4:471–3.

113. Golden JA, Sollitto RA. The radiology of pulmonary disease: chest radiography, computed tomography and gallium scanning. *Clin Chest Med* 1988;9:481–95.

114. Skarzynski JJ, Sherman W, Lee HK, Berger H. Patchy uptake of gallium in the lungs of AIDS patients with atypical mycobacterial infection. *Clin Nucl Med* 1987;12:507–9.

115. Radin DR. Intraabdominal *Mycobacterium tuberculosis* vs. *Mycobacterium avium-intracellulare* infections in patients with AIDS: distinction based on CT findings. *Am J Roentgenol* 1991;156:487–91.

116. Hewlett D Jr, Duncanson FP, Jagadha V, Lieberman J, Lenox TH, Wormser GP. Lymphadenopathy in an inner-city population consisting principally of intravenous drug abusers with suspected acquired immunodeficiency syndrome. *Am Rev Respir Dis* 1988;137:1275–9.

117. Ena J, Crespo MJ, Valls V, De Salamanca RE. Adenosine deaminase activity in cerebrospinal fluid: a useful test for meningeal tuberculosis, even in patients with AIDS. *J Infect Dis* 1988;158:896.

118. Ribera E, Martinez-Vazquez JM, Ocana I, Segura RM, Pascual C. Activity of adenosine deaminase in cerebrospinal fluid for the diagnosis and follow-up of tuberculous meningitis in adults. *J Infect Dis* 1987;155:603–7.

119. Klein NC, Duncanson FP, Lenox TH III, Pitta A, Cohen SC, Wormser GP. Use of mycobacterial smears in the diagnosis of pulmonary tuberculosis in AIDS/ARC patients. *Chest* 1989;95:1190–2.

120. Saddiqi S, Libonati J, Middlebrook G. Evaluation of a rapid radiometric method for drug susceptibility testing of *Mycobacterium tuberculosis*. *J Clin Microbiol* 1981;13:908–12.

121. Kiehn TE, Cammarata R. Comparative recoveries of *Mycobacterium avium-M. intracellulare* from isolator lysis–centrifugation and BACTEC 13A blood culture systems. *J Clin Microbiol* 1988;26:760–1.

122. Kiehn TE, Edwards FF. Rapid identification using a specific DNA probe of *Mycobacterium avium* complex from patients with the acquired immunodeficiency syndrome. *J Clin Microbiol* 1987;25:1551–2.

123. Brisson-Noel A, Gicquel B, Lecossier D, Lévy-Frébault V, Nassif X, Hance AJ. Rapid diagnosis of tuberculosis by amplification of mycobacterial DNA in clinical samples. *Lancet* 1989;2:1069–71.

124. Prego V, Glatt AE, Roy V, Thelmo W, Dincsoy H, Raufman JP. Comparative yield of blood culture for fungi and mycobacteria, liver biopsy, and bone marrow biopsy in the diagnosis of fever of undetermined origin in human immunodeficiency virus-infected patients. *Arch Intern Med* 1990;150:333–6.

125. Flora GS, Modilevsky T, Antoniskis D, Barnes PF. Undiagnosed tuberculosis in patients with human immunodeficiency virus infection. *Chest* 1990;98:1056–9.

126. Ankobiah W. Treatment of tuberculosis in the acquired immunodeficiency syndrome. *Ann Intern Med* 1987;106:772–3.

127. American Thoracic Society/Centers for Disease Control. Mycobacterioses and the acquired immunodeficiency syndrome. *Am Rev Respir Dis* 1987;136:492–96.

128. Pitchenik AE. The treatment and prevention of mycobacterial disease in patients with HIV infection. *AIDS* 1988;2:S177–82.

129. CDC. Tuberculosis and human immunodeficiency virus infection: recommendations of the advisory committee for the elimination of tuberculosis ACET. *MMWR* 1989;38:236–238,243–50.

130. American Thoracic Society/Centers for Disease Control. Treatment of tuberculosis and tuberculosis infection in adults and children. *Am Rev Respir Dis* 1986;134:355–63.

131. Kavesh NG, Holzman RS, Seidlin M. The combined toxicity of azidothymidine and antimycobacterial agents. A retrospective study. *Am Rev Respir Dis* 1989;139:1094–7.

132. Engelhard D, Stutman HR, Marks MI. Interaction of ketoconazole with rifampin and isoniazid. *N Engl J Med* 1984;311:1681–3.

133. Lazar JD, Wilner KD. Drug interactions with fluconazole. *Rev Infect Dis* 1990;12(Suppl 3):S327–33.

134. Laroche E, Stoneburner R, Araneta M, Adler J. Survival experience after TB diagnosis in 1,452 AIDS cases: implications for the expansion of the AIDS case definition. 6th International Conference on AIDS, San Francisco, June 1990, p 298; ThC694(abst).

135. American Thoracic Society/Centers for Disease Control. Control of tuberculosis. *Am Rev Respir Dis* 1983;128:336–42.

136. CDC. Screening for tuberculosis and tuberculous infection in high-risk populations and the use of preventive therapy for tuberculous infection in the United States: recommendations of the Advisory Committee for the elimination of tuberculosis. *MMWR* 1990;39(RR-8):1–7.

137. Torres RA, Mani S, Altholz J, Brickner PW. Human immunodeficiency virus infection among homeless men in a New York City shelter. Association with *Mycobacterium tuberculosis* infection. *Arch Int Med* 1990;150:2030–6.

138. Nardell E, Salter J, Boutotte J, et al. HIV seroprevalence in an asymptomatic, PPD-positive (class II), predominantly nonwhite, foreign born, inner city, TB clinic population. *Am Rev Respir Dis* 1991;143:A278(abst).

139. CDC. Purified protein derivitive (PPD)–tuberculin anergy and HIV infection: guidelines for anergy testing and management of anergic persons at risk of tuberculosis. *MMWR* 1991;40:27–32.

140. CDC. The use of preventive therapy for tuberculous infection in the United States. Recommendations of the Advisory Committee for Elimination of Tuberculosis. *MMWR* 1990;39:9–12.

141. Johnson M, Clermont HC, Coberly J, et al. Impact of HIV infection on response to tuberculin skin tests in Haitian adults. *Am Rev Respir Dis* 1991;143:A280(abst).

142. Barry MA, Murray C, Foley K, et al. Skin test reactivity in various populations—Boston, 1988–90. *Am Rev Respir Dis* 1991;143:A282(abst).

143. Barry MA, Taylor J, King G, Murray C, McInnis B, Bernardo J. Development of active tuberculosis (TB) in homeless persons: risk based on skin test results. *Am Rev Respir Dis* 1991;143:A282(abst).

144. Cohen J, Nardell E. Anergy in intravenous drug users (IVDUs); prevalence, influence of HIV status, sex. 6th International Conference on AIDS, San Francisco, June 1990, p 203; FB502(abst).

145. Menzies R, Vissandjee B, Mannix S, Rocher I. The booster effect in two step tuberculin testing among those with HIV infection. *Am Rev Respir Dis* 1991;143:A280(abst).

146. Wadhawan D, Hira S, Mwansa N, Tembo G, Perine PL. Isoniazid prophylaxis among patients with HIV-1 infection. 6th International Conference on AIDS San Francisco, June 1990, p 249; ThB510(abst).

147. Brudney K, Dobkin J. Poor compliance is the major obstacle in controlling the HIV-associated tuberculosis (TB) outbreak. 5th International Conference on AIDS, Montréal, Québec, Canada, June 1989, p 427; ThB68(abst).

148. Riley RL. Disease transmission and contagion control. *Am Rev Respir Dis* 1982;125:16–9.

149. Braun MM, Truman BI, Morse DL, Maguire B, Broaddus R. Tuberculosis and the acquired immunodeficiency syndrome in prisoners. *JAMA* 1987;257:1471–2.

150. CDC. Mycobacterium and tuberculosis transmission in a health clinic—Florida, 1988. *MMWR* 1989;38:256–258,263–4.

151. CDC. Guidelines for preventing the transmission of tuberculosis in health care settings, with special focus on HIV related issues. *MMWR* 1990;39:1–29.

152. Garner JS, Simmons BP. Guidelines for isolation precautions in hospitals. *Infect Control* 1983;4:245–325.

153. CDC. *Guidelines for the prevention of TB transmission in hospitals.* Atlanta: U.S. Department of Health and Human Services; 1982: HSS Publication No. (CDC)82-8371.

154. Nardell EA. Dodging droplet nuclei: reducing the probability of nosocomial tuberculosis transmission in the AIDS era. *Am Rev Respir Dis* 1990;142:501–3.

155. Riley RL, Nardell EA. State of the art: clearing the air, the theory and application of ultraviolet air disinfection. *Am Rev Respir Dis* 1989;139:1286–94.

156. CDC. ACIP: Use of BCG vaccines in the control of tuberculosis. A joint statement by the ACIP and the Advisory Committe for Elimination of Tuberculosis. *MMWR* 1988;37:663–664,669–75.

157. WHO. Special programme on AIDS and expanded programme on immunization—joint statement: consultation on human immunodeficiency virus (HIV) and routine childhood immunization. *Wkly Epidemiol Rec* 1987;62:297–9.

158. Bregere P. BCG vaccination and AIDS. *Bull Int Union Tuberc Lung Dis* 1988;63:40–1.

159. Reichman LB. Why hasn't BCG proved dangerous in HIV infected patients? *JAMA* 1989;261:3246.

160. CDC. Disseminated *Mycobacterium bovis* infection from BCG vaccination of a patient with acquired immunodeficiency syndrome. *MMWR* 1985;34:227–8.

161. Ninane J, Grymonprez A, Burtonboy G, Francois A, Cornu G. Disseminated BCG in HIV infection. *Arch Dis Child* 1988; 63:1268–9.

162. Boudes P, Sobel A, Deforges L, Leblic E. Disseminated *Mycobacterium bovis* infection from BCG vaccination and HIV infection (letter). *JAMA* 1989;262:2386.

163. Houde D, Dery P. *Mycobacterium bovis* sepsis in an infant with human immunodeficiency virus infection. *Pediatr Infect Dis J* 1988;7:810–2.

164. Piot P. The natural history and clinical manifestations of HIV infection. 3rd International Conference on Acquired Immunodeficiency Syndrome (AIDS), Washington, DC, June 1987.

165. CDC. Human immunodeficiency virus infection in the United States. *MMWR* 1987;36:801–4.

166. Rieder HL, Snider DE Jr. Tuberculosis and the acquired immunodeficiency syndrome. *Chest* 1986;90:469–70.

167. WHO/IUATLD. Tuberculosis and AIDS. Statement on AIDS and tuberculosis, Geneva, March 1989. *Bull Int Union Tuberc Lung Dis* 1989;64:8–11.

168. Mukadi Y, Perriëns J, Willame JC, et al. Short course antituberculous therapy for pulmonary tuberculosis in HIV seropositive patients: a prospective controlled study. 6th International Conference on AIDS, San Francisco, June 1990, p 248; ThB507(abst).

169. Sugarman J, Cegielski P, Lallinger G, Mwakyusa D. Stevens-Johnson syndrome associated with treatment of tuberculosis in patients with HIV infection in Tanzania. 6th International Conference on AIDS, San Francisco, June 1990, p 249; ThB509(abst).

170. Eriki PP, Okwera A, Aisu T, et al. The influence of human immunodeficiency virus infection on tuberculosis in Kampala, Uganda. *Am Rev Respir Dis* 1991;143:185–7.

171. CDC. A strategic plan for the elimination of tuberculosis in the United States. *MMWR* 1989;38:269–72.

172. Horsburgh CR Jr, Mason UG III, Farhi DC, Iseman MD. Disseminated infection with *Mycobacterium avium-intracellulare:* a report of 13 cases and a review of the literature. *Medicine* 1985;64:36–48.

173. Wolinsky E. Nontuberculous mycobacteria and associated diseases. *Am Rev Respir Dis* 1979;119:107–59.

174. Murray JF, Felton CP, Garay S, et al. Pulmonary complications of the acquired immunodeficiency syndrome. Report of a National Heart, Lung and Blood Institute Workshop. *N Engl J Med* 1984;310:1682–8.

175. Hawkins CC, Gold JW, Whimbey E, et al. *Mycobacterium avium* complex infections in patients with the acquired immunodeficiency syndrome. *Ann Intern Med* 1986;105:184–8.

176. Wallace JM, Hannah JB. *Mycobacterium avium* complex infection in patients with the acquired immunodeficiency syndrome. *Chest* 1988;93:926–32.

177. Macher AM, Kovacs JA, Gill V, et al. Bacteremia due to *Mycobacterium avium-intracellulare* in the acquired immunodeficiency syndrome. *Ann Intern Med* 1983;99:782–5.

178. Fauci AS, Macher AM, Longo DL, et al. Acquired immunodeficiency syndrome: epidemiologic, immunologic and therapeutic considerations. *Ann Intern Med* 1984;110:92–106.

179. Young LS, Inderlied CB, Berlin OG, Gottlieb MS. Mycobacterial infections in AIDS patients, with an emphasis on the *Mycobacterium avium* complex. *Rev Infect Dis* 1986;8:1024–33.

180. Kiehn TE, Edwards FF, Brannan P, et al. Infections caused by *Mycobacterium avium* complex in immunocompromised patients: diagnosis by blood culture and fecal examination, antimicrobial susceptibility tests, and morphological and seroagglutination characteristics. *J Clin Microbiol* 1985;21:168–73.

181. Welch K, Finkbeiner W, Alpers CE, et al. Autopsy findings in the acquired immune deficiency syndrome. *JAMA* 1984;252: 1152–9.

182. Reichert CM, O'Leary TJ, Levens DL, Simrell CR, Macher AM. Autopsy pathology in the acquired immunodeficiency syndrome. *Am J Pathol* 1983;112:357–82.

183. Armstrong D, Gold JWM, Dryjanski J, et al. Treatment of infection in patients with the acquired immunodeficiency syndrome. *Ann Intern Med* 1985;103:738–43.

184. Horsburgh CR Jr, Cohn DL. *Mycobacterium avium* complex and the acquired immunodeficiency syndrome. *Ann Intern Med* 1986;105:968–9.

185. Horsburgh CR Jr. Current concepts: *Mycobactrium avium* complex infection in the acquired immunodeficiency syndrome. *N Engl J Med* 1991;324:1332–8.

186. Murray JF, Mills J. State of the art: pulmonary infectious complications of human immunodeficiency virus infection (part 1). *Am Rev Respir Dis* 1990;141:1356–72.

187. Gilks CF, Brindle RJ, Otieno LS, et al. Extrapulmonary and disseminated tuberculosis in HIV-1–seropositive patients presenting to the acute medical services in Nairobi. *AIDS* 1990;4:981–5.

188. Okello DO, Sewankambo N, Goodgame R, et al. Absence of bacteremia with *Mycobacterium avium-intracellulare* in Ugandan patients with AIDS. *J Infect Dis* 1990;162:208–10.

189. Horsburgh CR Jr, Selik RM. The epidemiology of disseminated nontuberculous mycobacterial infection in the acquired immunodeficiency syndrome (AIDS). *Am Rev Respir Dis* 1989;139:4–7.

190. O'Brien RJ. The epidemiology of nontuberculous mycobacterial disease. *Clin Chest Med* 1989;10:407–18.

191. Jenkins PA. AIDS and the lung. *Br Med J* 1987;295:331.

192. Horsburg CR Jr, Metchock BG, McGowan JE Jr, Thompson ST. Progression to disseminated infection in HIV-infected persons colonized with mycobacteria other than tuberculosis. *Am Rev Respir Dis* 1991;143(suppl):A279 (abst).

193. Edwards LB, Acquaviva FA, Livesay VT, Cross FW, Palmer CE. An atlas of sensitivity to tuberculin, PPD-B, and histoplasmin in the United States. *Am Rev Respir Dis* 1969;99:1.

194. Wijsmuller G, Erickson P. The reaction to PPD-Battey: a new look. *Am Rev Respir Dis* 1974;109:29.

195. Good RC, Snider DE Jr. Isolation of nontuberculous mycobacteria in the United States, 1980. *J Infect Dis* 1982;146:829–33.

196. Iseman MD, Corpe RF, O'Brien RJ, et al. Disease due to *Mycobacterium avium-intracellulare. Chest* 1985;87:1395–495.

197. Falkinham JO III, Parker BC, Gruft H. Epidemiology of infection by nontuberculous mycobacteria I. Geographic distribution in the eastern United States. *Am Rev Respir Dis* 1980;121:931–7.

198. Parker BC, Ford MA, Gruft H, Falkinham JO III. Epidemiology of infection by nontuberculous mycobacteria IV. Preferential aerosolization of *Mycobacterium intracellulare* from natural waters. *Am Rev Respir Dis* 1983;128:652–6.

199. Meissner PS, Falkinham JO III. Plasmid DNA profiles as epidemiologic markers for clinical and environmental isolates of *Mycobacterium avium, Mycobacterium intracellulare,* and *Mycobacterium scrofulaceum. J Infect Dis* 1986;153:325–31.

200. Damsker B, Bottone FJ. *Mycobacterium avium-intracellulare* in intestinal tracts of patients with the acquired immune deficiency syndrome: concepts regarding acquisition and pathogenesis. *J Infect Dis* 1985;151:179–81.

201. Roth RI, Owen RL, Keren DF, Volberding PA. Intestinal infection with *Mycobacterium avium* in acquired immune deficiency syndrome (AIDS). Histological and clinical comparison with Whipple's disease. *Dig Dis Sci* 1985;30:497–504.

202. Jacobson MA. Mycobacterial diseases. Tuberculosis and *Mycobacterium avium* complex. *Infect Dis Clin North Am* 1988;2:465–74.

203. MacDonnell KB, Glassroth J. *Mycobacterium avium* complex and other nontuberculous mycobacteria in patients with HIV infection. *Semin Respir Infect* 1989;4:123–32.

204. Hoyt L, Connor E, Oleske J. Atypical mycobacterial infection (AM) in pediatric AIDS. 6th International Conference on AIDS, San Francisco, June 1990, p 369(abst 2060).

205. Farber CM, Yernault JC, Legros F, Debruyn J, Van Vooren JP. Detection of anti-P32 mycobacterial IgG antibodies in patients with AIDS. *J Infect Dis* 1990;162:279–80.

206. Winter SM, Bernard EM, Gold JWH, Armstrong D. Humoral response to disseminated infection by *Mycobacterium avium-Mycobacterium intracellulare* in acquired immunodeficiency syndrome and hairy cell leukemia. *J Infect Dis* 1985;151:523–7.

207. Poropatich CO, Labriola AM, Tuazon CU. Acid-fast smear and culture of respiratory secretions, bone marrow, and stools as predictors of disseminated *Mycobacterium avium* complex infection. *J Clin Microbiol* 1987;25:929–30.

208. Tenholder MF, Moser RJ III, Tellis CJ. Mycobacteria other than tuberculosis: pulmonary involvement in patients with acquired immunodeficiency syndrome. *Arch Intern Med* 1988;148:953–5.

209. Horsburgh CR Jr, Cohn DL, Roberts RB, et al. *Mycobacterium avium-intracellulare* isolates from patients with or without acquired immunodeficiency syndrome. *Antimicrob Agents Chemother* 1986;30:955–7.

210. Crawford JT, Bates JH. Analysis of plasmids in *Mycobacterium avium-intracellulare* isolates from persons with acquired immunodeficiency syndrome. *Am Rev Respir Dis* 1986;134:659–61.

211. Guthertz LS, Damsker B, Bottone EJ, Ford EG, Midura TF, Janda JM. *Mycobacterium avium* and *Mycobacterium intracellulare* infections in patients with and without AIDS. *J Infect Dis* 1989;160:1037–41.

212. Hampson SJ, Portaels F, Thompson J, et al. DNA probes demonstrate a single highly conserved strain of *Mycobacterium avium* infecting AIDS patients. *Lancet* 1989;1:65–8.

213. Peters M, Schürmann D, Rüsch-Gerdes S, Schröder HJ, Ruf B. Serotype pattern of *Mycobacterium avium-intracellulare* isolates from German AIDS patients. *Am Rev Respir Dis* 1991; 143:A281(abst).

214. Schurmann D, Jantzke G, Thalmann U, et al. Prevalence and diagnosis of infection due to *Mycobacterium avium-intracellulare* in HIV infected patients. Results from a prospective study. *Am Rev Respir Dis* 1991;143:A279(abst).

215. Mapother ME, Singer JG. *In vitro* interaction of *Mycobacterium avium* with intestinal epithelial cells. *Infect Immun* 1984; 45:67–73.

216. Green JB, Sidhu GS, Lewin S, et al. *Mycobacterium avium-intracellulare.* A cause of disseminated life threatening infection in homosexuals and drug abusers. *Ann Intern Med* 1982;97:539–46.

217. Masur H, Michelis MA, Wormser GP, et al. Opportunistic infection in previously healthy women. *Ann Intern Med* 1982; 97:533–9.

218. Zakowski P, Fligiel S, Berlin GW, Johnson BL Jr. Disseminated *Mycobacterium avium-intracellulare* infection in homosexual men dying of acquired immunodeficiency. *JAMA* 1982;248: 2980–2.

219. Marinelli DL, Albelda SM, Williams TM, Kern JA, Iozzo RV, Miller WT. Nontuberculous mycobacterial infection in AIDS: clinical, pathologic and radiographic features. *Radiology* 1986;160:77–82.

220. Sathe SS, Reichman LB. Mycobacterial disease in patients infected with the human immunodeficiency virus. *Clin Chest Med* 1989;10:445–63.

221. Chester AU, Winn WC Jr. Unusual and newly recognized patterns of nontuberculous mycobacterial infection with emphasis on the immunocompromised host. *Pathol Annu* 1986;21: 251–70.

222. Horsburgh CR Jr. Mycobacterial infections in the immunocompromised host. *Semin Respir Med* 1989;10:61–7.

223. Nunn PP, McAdam KPWJ. Mycobacterial infections and AIDS. *Br Med Bull* 1988;44:801–13.

224. Spencer PM, Jackson GG. Fungal and mycobacterial infections in patients infected with human immunodeficiency virus. *J Antimicrob Chemother* 1989;23:107–25.

225. Shelhamer JH, Ognibene FP, Kovacs JA, et al. Infections due to *Pneumocystis carinii* and *Mycobacterium avium-intracellulare* in patients with acquired immunodeficiency syndrome. *Ann NY Acad Sci* 1984;437:394–9.

226. Elliott JL, Hoppes WL, Platt MS, Thomas JG, Patel IP, Gansar A. The acquired immunodeficiency syndrome and *Mycobacterium avium-intracellulare* bacteremia in a patient with hemophilia. *Ann Intern Med* 1983;98:290–3.

227. Sohn CC, Schroff RW, Kliewer KE, Lebel DM, Fligiel S. Disseminated *Mycobacterium avium-intracellulare* infection in homosexual men with acquired cell-mediated immunodeficiency: a histologic and immunologic study of two cases. *Am J Clin Pathol* 1983;79:247–52.

228. Gray JR, Rabeneck L. Atypical mycobacterial infection of the gastrointestinal tract in AIDS patients. *Am J Gastroenterol* 1989;84:1521–4.

229. Gillin JS, Urmacher C, West R, et al. Disseminated *Mycobacterium avium-intracellulare* infection in acquired immunodeficiency syndrome mimicking Whipple's disease. *Gastroenterology* 1983;85:1187–91.

230. Vazquez-Iglesia JL, Yañez J, Durana J, Arnal F. Infection by *Mycobacterium avium-intracellulare* in AIDS: endoscopic duodenal appearance mimicking Whipple's disease. *Endoscopy* 1988;20:279–80.

231. Gardener TD, Flanagan P, Dryden MS, Costello C, Shanson DC, Gazzard BG. Disseminated *Mycobacterium avium-intracellulare* infection and red cell hypoplasia in patients with the acquired immune deficiency syndrome. *J Infect* 1988;16:135–40.

232. Mehle ME, Adamo JP, Mehta AC, Weideman HP, Keys T, Longworth DL. Endobronchial *Mycobacterium avium-intracellulare* infection in a patient with AIDS. *Chest* 1989;96:199–201.

233. Packer SJ, Cesario T, Williams JH Jr. *Mycobacterium avium* complex infection presenting as endobronchial lesions in immunosuppressed patients. *Ann Intern Med* 1988;109:389–93.

234. Goodman P, Pinero SS, Rance RM, et al. Mycobacterial esophagitis in AIDS. *Gastrointest Radiol* 1989;14:103–5.

235. Schneebaum CW, Novick DM, Chabon AB, Strutynsky N, Yancovitz SR, Freund S. Terminal ileitis associated with *Mycobacterium avium-intracellulare* infection in a homosexual man with acquired immune deficiency syndrome. *Gastroenterology* 1987; 92:1127–32.

236. Woods GL, Goldsmith JC. Fatal pericarditis due to *Mycobacterium avium-intracellulare* in acquired immunodeficiency syndrome. *Chest* 1989;95:1355–7.

237. Cohen JI, Saragas SJ. Endophthalmitis due to *Mycobacterium avium* in a patient with AIDS. *Ann Ophthalmol* 1990;22:47–51.

238. Blumenthal DR, Zucker JR, Hawkins CC. *Mycobacterium avium* complex-induced septic arthritis and osteomyelitis in a patient with the acquired immunodeficiency syndrome. *Arthritis Rheum* 1990;33:757–8 (lett).

239. Barbaro DJ, Orcutt VL, Coldiron BM. *Mycobacterium avium-Mycobacterium intracellulare* infection limited to the skin and lymph nodes in patients with AIDS. *Rev Infect Dis* 1989;11: 625–8.

240. DeCoste SD, Dover JS. Kaposi's sarcoma and *Mycobacterium avium-intracellulare* with cellulitis in patient with acquired immunodeficiency syndrome. *J Am Acad Dermatol* 1989;21:574–6.

241. Chaisson RE, Keruly J, Richman DD, et al. Incidence and natural history of *Mycobacterium avium*-complex infection in ad-

vanced HIV disease treated with zidovudine. *Am Rev Respir Dis* 1991;143:A278(abst).

242. Havlik JA, Horsburgh CR Jr, Metchock B, Williams P, Thompson SE. Clinical risk factors for disseminated *Mycobacterium avium* complex infection (DMAC) in persons with HIV infection. 6th International Conference on AIDS, San Francisco, June 1990, p 250; ThB515(abst).

243. Pierone G, Lin J, Masci J, Nicholas P. Fever of unknown origin in AIDS. 6th International Conference on AIDS, San Francisco, June 1990, p 257; ThB540(abst).

244. Nyberg DA, Federle MP, Jeffrey RB, et al. Abdominal CT findings of disseminated *Mycobacterium avium-intracellulare* in AIDS. *AJR* 1985;145:297–99.

245. Bach MC, Bagwell SP, Masur H. Utility of gallium imaging in the diagnosis of *Mycobacterium avium-intracellulare* infection in patients with the acquired immunodeficiency syndrome. *Clin Nucl Med* 1986;11:175–7.

246. Allwright SJ, Chapman PR, Antico VF, Gruenewald SM. Cutaneous gallium uptake in patients with AIDS with *Mycobacterium avium-intracellulare* septicemia. *Clin Nucl Med* 1988;13:506–8.

247. CDC. Diagnosis and management of mycobacterial infection and disease in persons with human immunodeficiency virus infection. *Ann Intern Med* 1987;106:254–6.

248. Wong B, Edwards FF, Kiehn TE, et al. Continuous high grade *Mycobacterium avium-intracellulare* bacteremia in patients with the acquired immunodeficiency syndrome. *Am J Med* 1985;78:35–40.

249. Klatt EC, Jensen DF, Meyer PR. Pathology of *Mycobacterium avium-intracellulare* infection in acquired immunodeficiency syndrome. *Hum Pathol* 1987;18:709–14.

250. Truffot-Pernot C, Lecoeur HF, Maury L, Dautzenberg B, Grosset J. Results of blood cultures for detection of mycobacteria in AIDS patients. *Tubercle* 1989;70:187–91.

251. Whimbey E, Kiehn TE, Armstrong D. Disseminated *Mycobacterium avium-intracellulare* disease: diagnosis and therapy. In: Remington JS, Swartz MN, eds. *Current clinical topics in infectious diseases,* vol 9. New York: McGraw-Hill; 1986:112–33.

252. Jacob C, Henein S, Heurich A, Kamholz S. Nontuberculous mycobacterial meningitis in patients with AIDS. *Am Rev Respir Dis* 1991;143:A279(abst).

253. Graham L Jr, Warren NG, Tsang AY, Dalton HP. *Mycobacterium avium* complex pseudobacteriuria from a hospital water supply. *J Clin Microbiol* 1988;26:1034–6.

254. Barnes PF, Arevalo C. Blood culture positivity patterns in bacteremia due to *Mycobacterium avium-intracellulare*. *South Med J* 1988;81:1059–60.

255. Meylan PR, Richman DD, Kornbluth RS. Characterization and growth in human macrophages of *Mycobacterium avium* complex strains isolated from the blood of patients with acquired immunodeficiency syndrome. *Infect Immun* 1990;58:2564–8.

256. Drake TA, Hindler JA, Berlin GW, Bruckner DA. Rapid identification of *Mycobacterium avium* complex in culture using DNA probes. *J Clin Microbiol* 1987;25:1442–5.

257. Graham BS, Hinson MV, Bennett SR, et al. Acid-fast bacilli on buffy coat smears in the acquired immunodeficiency syndrome: a lesson from Hansen's bacillus. *South Med J* 1984;77:246–8.

258. Eng RH, Bishburg E, Smith SM, Mangia A. Diagnosis of *Mycobacterium* bacteremia in patients with acquired immunodeficiency syndrome by direct examination of blood films. *J Clin Microbiol* 1989;4:768–9.

259. Benson C, Kerns E, Sha B, Glick E, Harris A, Kessler H. Relationship of respiratory and GI tract colonization with *Mycobacterium avium* complex (MAC) to disseminated MAC disease in HIV infected (+) patients. 6th International Conference on AIDS, San Francisco, June 1990, p 250; ThB514(abst).

260. Solis OG, Belmonte AH, Ramaswamy G, Tchertkoff V. Pseudogaucher cells in *Mycobacterium avium-intracellulare* infections in acquired immune deficiency syndrome (AIDS). *Am J Clin Pathol* 1986;85:233–5.

261. Bottles K, McPhaul LW, Volberding P. Fine needle aspiration biopsy of patients with acquired immunodeficiency syndrome (AIDS): experience in an outpatient clinic. *Ann Intern Med* 1988;108:42–5.

262. Nash G, Fligiel S. Pathologic features of the lung in the acquired immunodeficiency syndrome (AIDS): an autopsy study of seventeen homosexual males. *Am J Clin Pathol* 1984;81:6–12.

263. Wilkes MS, Fortin AH, Felix JC, et al. Value of necropsy in acquired immunodeficiency syndrome. *Lancet* 1988;2:85–8.

264. Chaisson RE, Hopewell PC. Mycobacteria and AIDS morbidity (editorial). *Am Rev Respir Dis* 1989;139:1–3.

265. Young LS. *Mycobacterium avium* complex infection. *J Infect Dis* 1988;157:863–7.

266. Schnittman S, Lane HC, Witebsky FG, et al. Host defense against *Mycobacterium avium* complex. *J Clin Immunol* 1988;8:234–43.

267. Demopulos P, Sande MA, Bryant C, Wofsy C, Brodie H, Hopewell P. Influence of *Mycobacterium avium-intracellulare* (MAI) infection on morbidity and survival in patients with *Pneumocystis carinii* pneumonia (PCP) and the acquired immunodeficiency syndrome (AIDS). In: *25th Interscience Conference on Antimicrobial Agents and Chemotherapy.* Washington, DC: American Society for Microbiology; 1985:230(abst 745).

268. Horsburgh CR Jr, Havlik JA, Thompson SE. Survival of AIDS patients with disseminated *Mycobacterium avium* complex infection (DMAC): a case control study. 6th International Conference on AIDS, San Francisco, June 1990; ThB516(abst).

269. Bass JB. *Mycobacterium avium-intracellulare*—rational therapy of chronic pulmonary infection? *Am Rev Respir Dis* 1986;134:431–2.

270. Davidson PT. The diagnosis and management of disease caused by *M. avium* complex, *M. kansasii,* and other mycobacteria. *Clin Chest Med* 1989;10:431–43.

271. Cynamon MH, Klemens SP. New antimycobacterial agents. *Clin Chest Med* 1989;10:355–64.

272. Heifets L. Qualitative and quantitative drug–susceptibility tests in mycobacteriology. *Am Rev Respir Dis* 1988;137:1217–22.

273. Horsburgh CR Jr, Mason UG III, Heifets LB, Southwick K, Labrecque J, Iseman MD. Response to therapy of pulmonary *Mycobacterium avium-intracellulare* infection correlates with the results of *in vitro* susceptibility testing. *Am Rev Respir Dis* 1987;135:418–21.

274. Yajko DM, Nassos PS, Hadley WK. Therapeutic implications of inhibition versus killing of *Mycobacterium avium* complex by antimicrobial agents. *Antimicrob Agents Chemother* 1987;31:117–20.

275. Heifets L, Lindholm-Levy P. Comparison of bactericidal activities of streptomycin, amikacin, kanamycin, and capreomycin against *Mycobacterium avium* and *M. tuberculosis*. *Antimicrob Agents Chemother* 1989;33:1298–301.

276. Heifets LB, Iseman MD, Lindholm-Levy PJ. Combinations of rifampin or rifabutine plus ethambutol against *Mycobacterium avium* complex: bactericidal synergistic, and bacteriostatic additive or synergistic effects. *Am Rev Respir Dis* 1988;137:711–5.

277. Heifets LB, Iseman MD. Choice of antimicrobial agents for *M. avium* disease based on quantitative tests of drug susceptibility. *N Engl J Med* 1990;323:419–20.

278. National Jewish Centers for Immunology and Respiratory Medicine. *Resource guide: tuberculosis and non-TB mycobacterial disease.* Denver, CO: 1989.

279. Yajko DM, Kirihara J, Sanders C, Nassos P, Hadley WK. Antimicrobial synergism against *Mycobacterium avium* complex strains isolated from patients with acquired immune deficiency syndrome. *Antimicrob Agents Chemother* 1988;32:1392–5.

280. O'Brien RJ, Miller D, Pitchenik AE, et al. In highlights ATS symposia summaries and topics. *Am Rev Respir Dis* 1987;136:127–30.

281. Inderlied CB, Kolonoski PT, Wu M, Young LS. Azithromycin (AZ) is an effective therapeutic agent for disseminated *Mycobacterium avium* complex (MAC) infection in the beige mouse. 6th International Conference on AIDS, Stockholm, Sweden, June 1988, p 307(abst 7531).

282. Saito H, Watanabe T, Tomioka H, Sato K. Susceptibility of various mycobacteria to quinolones. *Rev Infect Dis* 1988;10:552.

283. Young LS, Berlin OG, Inderlied CB. Activity of ciprofloxacin and other fluorinated quinolones against mycobacteria. *Am J Med* 1987;82:23–6.

284. Ahn CH, Anderson RA, Murphy DT, et al. A four-drug regimen for initial treatment of cavitary disease caused by *Mycobacterium avium* complex. *Am Rev Respir Dis* 1986;134:438–41.

285. Masur H, Tuazon C, Gill V, et al. Effect of combined clofazimine and ansamycin therapy on *Mycobacterium avium–Mycobacterium intracellulare* bacteremia in patients with AIDS. *J Infect Dis* 1987;155:127–9.

286. Lucas CR, Mijch AM, Sandland AM, Grayson ML, Dwyer BW. Evidence that drug therapy may be effective in *Mycobacterium avium-intracellulare* (MAI) bacteraemia. 4th International Conference on AIDS, Stockholm, Sweden, June 1988, p 308(abst 7534).

287. Valenti W, Portmore A. Treatment of *M. avium-intracellulare* infections. 4th International Conference on AIDS, Stockholm, Sweden, June 1988, p 311(abst 7547).

288. O'Brien RJ, Lyle MA, Snider DE Jr. Rifabutin (ansamycin LM427): a new rifamycin-S derivative for the treatment of mycobacterial diseases. *Rev Infect Dis* 1987;9:519–30.

289. Polis MA, Tuazon CU. Clues to the early diagnosis of *Mycobacterium avium* infection in patients with acquired immunodeficiency syndrome. *Arch Pathol Lab Med* 1985;109:465–6.

290. Bach MC. Treating disseminated *Mycobacterium avium-intracellulare* infection. *Ann Intern Med* 1989;110:169–70.

291. Agins BD, Berman DS, Spicehandler D, Sadr W, Simberkoff MS, Rahal JJ. Effect of combined therapy with ansamycin, clofazimine, ethambutol, and isoniazid for *Mycobacterium avium* infection in patients with AIDS. *J Infect Dis* 1989;159:784–87.

292. Hoy J, Mijch A, Sandland M, Grayson L, Lucus R, Dwyer B. Quadruple drug therapy for *Mycobacterium avium-intracellulare* bacteremia in AIDS patients. *J Infect Dis* 1990;161:801–5.

293. Benson C, Pottage J, Kessler H. Treatment of AIDS-related disseminated *Mycobacterium avium*-complex disease (D-MAC) with a multiple drug regimen including amikacin. 6th International Conference on AIDS, San Francisco, June 1990; ThB517(abst).

294. Horsburgh CR Jr, Havlik JA, Metchock BG, Thompson SE. Oral therapy of disseminated *Mycobacterium avium* complex infection in AIDS relieves symptoms and is well tolerated. *Am Rev Respir Dis* 1991;413(suppl):A115(abst).

295. Chiu J, Nussbaum J, Bozzette S, et al. Treatment of disseminated *Mycobacterium avium* complex infection in AIDS with amikacin, ethambutol, rifampin and ciprofloxacin. *Ann Intern Med* 1990;113:358–61.

296. *Physicians Desk Reference,* 45th ed. Oradell, NJ: Medical Economics Co, 1991.

297. CDC: Rifabutin (ansamycin LM 427). *Informational material for physicians.* Washington, DC: CDC; 1986.

298. Skinner MH, Hsieh M, Torseth J, et al. Pharmacokinetics of rifabutin. *Antimicrob Agents Chemother* 1989;33:1237–41.

299. Anand R, Moore J, Curran J, Srinivasan A. Interaction between rifabutin and human immunodeficiency virus type 1: inhibition of replication, cytopathic effect, and reverse transcriptase *in vitro*. *Antimicrob Agents Chemother* 1988;32:684–8.

300. Volberding PA, Lagakos SW, Koch MA, et al. Zidovudine in asymptomatic human immunodeficiency virus infection. A controlled trial in persons with fewer than 500 CD4-positive cells per cubic millimeter. *N Engl J Med* 1990;322:941–9.

301. Siegal FP, Borenstein M, Gehan K, et al. Rifabutin may delay the onset of *Mycobacterium avium* complex infection (MAC) in patients with AIDS. 6th International Conference on AIDS, San Francisco, June 1990, p 251; ThB518(abst).

302. Bermudez LE, Young LS. Recombinant granulocyte–macrophage colony-stimulating factor activates human macrophages to inhibit growth or kill *Mycobacterium avium* complex. *J Leukocyte Biol* 1990;48:67–73.

303. Bermudez LE, Young LS. Activities of amikacin, roxithromycin, and azithromycin alone or in combination with tumor necrosis factor against *Mycobacterium avium* complex. *Antimicrob Agents Chemother* 1988;32:1149.

304. Bermudez LE, Stevens P, Kolonoski P, et al. Treatment of *Mycobacterium avium* complex (MAC) infection in mice with recombinant human interleukin-2 (IL-2) and tumor necrosis factor. In: 27th Interscience Conference on Antimicrobial Agents and Chemotherapy. Washington, DC: American Society for Microbiology 1987:104.

305. Bermudez LEM, Young LS. Tumor necrosis factor, alone or in combination with IL-2, but not IFN-γ, is associated with macrophage killing of *Mycobacterium avium* complex. *J Immunol* 1988;140:3006–31.

306. Toba H, Crawford JT, Ellner JJ. Pathogenicity of *Mycobacterium avium* for human monocytes: absence of macrophage-activating factor activity of gamma interferon. *Infect Immun* 1989;57:239–44.

307. Armstrong JA, Hart PD. Response of cultured macrophages to *Mycobacterium tuberculosis,* with observations on fusion of lysosomes with phagosomes. *J Exp Med* 1971;134:713–40.

308. Crowle AJ, Cohn DL, Poche P. Defects in sera from acquired immunodeficiency syndrome (AIDS) patients and from non-AIDS patients with *Mycobacterium avium* infection which decrease macrophage resistance to *M. avium. Infect Immun* 1989;57:1445–51.

309. Ausina V, Barrio J, Luquin M, et al. *Mycobacterium xenopi* infections in the acquired immunodeficiency syndrome. *Ann Intern Med* 1988;109:927–928.

310. Brady MT, Marcon MJ, Maddux H. Broviac catheter-related infection due to *Mycobacterium fortuitum* in a patient with acquired immunodeficiency syndrome. *Pediatr Infect Dis J* 1987;6:492–4.

311. Eng RHK, Forrester C, Smith SM, Sobel H. *Mycobacterium xenopi* infection in a patient with acquired immunodeficiency syndrome. *Chest* 1984;86:145–7.

312. Males BM, West TE, Bartholomew WR. *Mycobacterium haemophilum* infection in a patient with acquired immune deficiency syndrome. *J Clin Micro* 1987;25:186–90.

313. Sherer R, Sable R, Sonnenberg M, et al. Disseminated infection with *Mycobacterium kansasii* in the acquired immunodeficiency syndrome. *Ann Intern Med* 1986;105:710–2.

314. Rogers PL, Walker RE, Lane HC, et al. Disseminated *Mycobacterium haemophilum* infection in two patients with the acquired immunodeficiency syndrome. *Am J Med* 1988;84:640–2.

315. Lévy-Frébault V, Pangon B, Buré A, Katlama C, Marche C, David HL. *Mycobacterium simiae* and *Mycobacterium avium–M. intracellulare* mixed infection in acquired immune deficiency syndrome. *J Clin Microbiol* 1987;25:154–7.

316. Tecson-Tumang FT, Bright JL. *Mycobacterium xenopi* and the acquired immunodeficiency syndrome. *Ann Intern Med* 1984;100:461–2.

317. Levine B, Chaisson RE. *Mycobacterium kansasii:* a cause of treatable pulmonary disease associated with advanced human immunodeficiency virus (HIV) infection. *Ann Intern Med* 1991;114:861–8.

AIDS and Other Manifestations of HIV Infection,
Second Edition, Edited by Gary P. Wormser.
Raven Press, Ltd., New York © 1992.

CHAPTER 20

Neurological Complications of AIDS and HIV Infection

An Overview

Barbara S. Koppel

Neurological complications are common in HIV infection. At least 10% of cases of AIDS present with neurological symptoms, and over the course of the illness symptomatic involvement of the central or peripheral nervous system has been found in 30–63% of patients (1–5). Impressively, one prospective study found that neurologic findings were present in 90% of AIDS patients if they were examined by a neurologist (6). Postmortem examination of brains from patients dying of AIDS has revealed abnormalities in up to 88% of cases (7–10), and more than one disease process was frequently present (7) (Table 1). Some patients develop a mononucleosis-like syndrome with aseptic meningitis or cranial neuropathies as early as 2 weeks after primary HIV infection (1,2,5,11,12). Rarely, encephalopathy (13), brachial plexus neuritis (14), ganglioneuronitis (15), myelitis (16,17), peripheral neuropathy (18), stroke (19), or muscle necrosis with myoglobinuria (20) also occur at, or shortly after, HIV infection and seroconversion.

An asymptomatic period of variable duration follows primary infection, even if early neurological symptoms had occurred. During this "silent interval," special tests of nervous system function such as EEG and polysomnography (21,22), brainstem auditory evoked potentials (21,23,24), long latency evoked potentials (25,26), brain magnetic resonance imaging (MRI) (27–32), cerebrospinal fluid analysis (33–37), cerebral blood flow (38), and neuropsychological assessment (32,39–41) may detect

subclinical evidence of central nervous system (CNS) involvement or dysfunction by HIV.

Autoimmune disorders with neurological consequences may occur during the course of HIV infection as the body's immune system becomes dysfunctional. These include polyradiculopathy (42–45), peripheral polyneuropathy (46), mononeuritis multiplex (47–49), Bell's palsy (11,50), polymyositis (51,52), myasthenia gravis (53), thrombocytopenia leading to brain hemorrhage (54–57), and anticardiolipin antibodies causing cerebral infarction (58).

The brain may be devastated by a bland encephalitis, so-called AIDS–dementia complex (ADC), caused by HIV itself, even in patients whose immune function is relatively normal (59,60). ADC is clinically evident in 30% of cases, although there is pathological evidence of the encephalitis in many more (61–64). In about half the patients with ADC, myelopathy or peripheral neuropathy also develop.

Once the immune system is no longer capable of effective defense, the nervous system also becomes vulnerable to opportunistic infections, neoplasms, and infarction (65–67). Standard therapies often fail to control viral, treponemal, fungal, or mycobacterial disease in such immunosuppressed patients, and the course of these infections may be fulminant (68–72).

Drugs used to treat patients with AIDS may have neurotoxic side effects. Dideoxycytidine (DDC) causes neuropathy (73); didanosine (DDI) causes neuropathy and rarely seizures (74,75); zidovudine (AZT) causes a mitochondrial myopathy (76–78), Wernicke's encephalopathy (79), seizures (80), headache (81), and rarely delir-

B. S. Koppel: Department of Neurology, New York Medical College, Valhalla, New York 10595; and Metropolitan Hospital Center, New York, New York 10029.

TABLE 1. *Frequency (%) of neurologic complications in AIDS patients*

Reference	1, 10[a]	5, 9[a]	8[a]	4	6	2	3
Main risk[b]	HS	HS	HS	IVDU	IVDU	MIX	MIX
Site[c]	SF	NY	LA	NY	NY	BAL	Miami
Patient numbers	390	104	66	28	172	186	83
HIV							
Aseptic Meningitis	4	4	—	—	—	7	—
Encephalitis	25	66	85	25	39	16	14
Infection							
Toxoplasma	14	14	9	32	8	8	40
Cryptococcus	17	2	17	25	20	6	14
CMV[d]	3	27	21	—	<1	6	10
PML[e]	2	2	9	4	<1	<1	4
Mycobacteria	<1	3	6	4	6	—	2
Bacteria	<1	—	—	4	2	—	2
Herpes zoster	1	1	—	4	4	<1	—
Candida	<1	2	1	4	—	<1	1
Fungi[f]	<1	—	1	—	—	—	1
Tumor							
1° Lymphoma	6	5	4	11	<1	4	2
2° Lymphoma	<1	5	1	—	—	<1	—
Kaposi sarcoma, plasmacytoma	<1	2	—	—	—	—	—
Cerebrovascular							
Infarction	<1	3	20	—	3	<1	5
Hemorrhage	<1	3	20	—	2	—	—
Metabolic	—	—	9	—	—	3	6
Nerve	6	10	—	—	13	21	11
Muscle	<1	1	—	—	—	—	4

[a] Pathologic series.
[b] HS, homosexual men; IVDU, intravenous drug users; MIX, mixed group.
[c] SF, San Francisco; NY, New York; LA, Los Angeles; BAL, Baltimore.
[d] CMV, cytomegalovirus, including retinitis and encephalitis.
[e] PML, progressive multifocal leukoencephalopathy.
[f] Fungi include *Aspergillus, Coccidioides, Rhizopus,* and *Histoplasma.*

ium (81,82); 2'-fluoro-5-iodo-aracytosine (FIAC) causes myoclonus and delirium (83); compound Q causes aphasia and coma (84); trimethoprim-sulfamethoxazole causes aseptic meningitis (85); and pentamidine causes hypotension (86) and hypoglycemia (87). Antiepileptic drugs seem to have an unusually high incidence of toxicity (26%) (88,89), including orofacial dyskinesias from phenytoin (4), and neuroleptic agents often produce severe extrapyramidal effects (90,91) and sometimes neuroleptic malignant syndrome as well (92).

This chapter offers an approach to the neurologically impaired patient and provides descriptions of the more commonly encountered syndromes.

DIAGNOSTIC STUDIES

Neuroimaging

Structural lesions of the brain and spinal cord are defined and serially assessed by computerized tomography (CT) or magnetic resonance imaging (MRI). Because of the importance of early detection of opportunistic brain infection and tumor, some investigators have recommended routine CT scans at regular intervals even in asymptomatic patients (93), although this is generally not standard practice. CT findings of HIV-related conditions are summarized in Table 2.

The most common CT finding in cerebral HIV infection is diffuse atrophy with sulcal and ventricular enlargement (Fig. 1). The white matter changes associated with HIV infection, which are visible with MRI, are usually not evident with CT (94). If the amount of ventricular dilation is out of proportion to the degree of cortical atrophy, communicating obstructive hydrocephalus caused by chronic meningitis should be suspected (Fig. 2). Focal atrophy may be the result of infarction, previous trauma, or healed infection. Intracerebral calcification, especially of the basal ganglia, was previously thought to occur only in children with congenital HIV infection (95). However, as adults with opportunistic infections survive longer, parenchymal calcification may develop, especially in those with cytomegalovirus (CMV) infection (3,4,96) (Fig. 3). Thus calcification of lesions generally reflects chronicity, as in immunocompetent hosts, and should never be taken as evidence of

TABLE 2. *CT scan findings in HIV-infected patients*

Pathology	Typical location	Enhancement	Atrophy	Hydrocephalus	Edema or mass effect	Multiple sites
HIV encephalitis	White matter, especially frontal	Rarely	++ Progressive	+	−	−
Toxoplasma abscesses	Periventricular (basal ganglia, thalamus) corticomedullary	Variable: ring, homogeneous, or none	After treatment	Rare, with meningitis	Usually	Usually
Fungal[a] brain lesion	Cortical or near sinuses	+	−	−	+	Occasionally
Mycobacterial infection	Cortical	++ Ring or solid	−	++, after meningitis	+	Rarely
PML[b]	White matter, 10% posterior fossa	−	−	−	−	Occasionally (increased number over time)
Chronic meningitis[c]	−	Meninges, ependyma of ventricles	Generalized and focal	+	−	−
Lymphoma and other tumors	Periventricular, rarely cortical	++	−	−	++	+

Scale: −, absent; +, present; ++, prominent.
[a] *Candida, Asperigillus* (may be hemorrhagic), mucor.
[b] Progressive multifocal leukoencephalopathy due to JC papovavirus.
[c] Due to toxoplasma, cryptococcus, mycobacterial species, or tumor. May see infarctions as well.

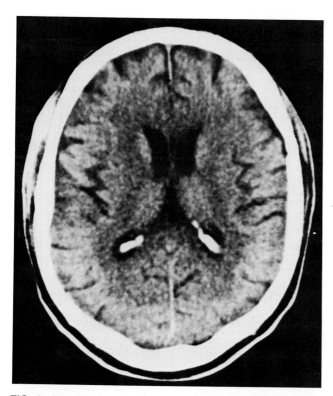

FIG. 1. Brain CT in a 34-year-old woman with ADC showing sulcal and ventricular dilation resulting from diffuse cerebral atrophy. There is hypodensity of the cerebral white matter adjacent to the ventricles, another common finding in patients with HIV infection of the brain.

inactive disease. Both lymphoma and toxoplasmosis favor periventricular and gray–white matter junction locations (Fig. 4), although they can occur almost anywhere. If a lesion has hemorrhagic elements on the nonenhanced scan, fungal infection, especially aspergillosis, should be considered.

Although parenchymal lesions can often be seen on unenhanced CT as hypodense lesions, with or without evidence of mass effect, contrast infusion greatly facilitates detection of lymphoma and abscesses due to bacterial or toxoplasma infection. Double-dose contrast injection with delayed imaging improves visualization of less intensely enhancing lesions (96–100), but use of this technique is often limited by the patient's renal function (96,97). When serial studies are performed in the same patient, it is important to use consistent amounts of contrast on each occasion to facilitate meaningful comparisons. Even with optimal use of current CT technology, however, the extent of brain pathology is almost always underrepresented (98). Ring enhancement correlates with better prognosis (101), because poor fibroblast recruitment limits capsule formation in many AIDS patients (102). Thus, in some patients, disappearance of enhancement may represent deterioration rather than response to treatment.

If a presumptive diagnosis of toxoplasmosis is made, an empiric trial of appropriate anti-infective agents can be instituted and the patient rescanned after 10–14 days.

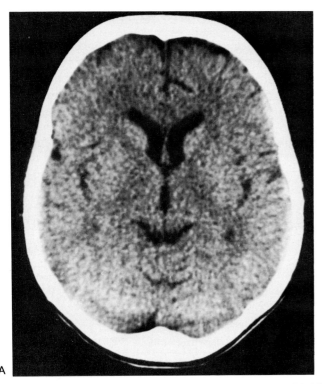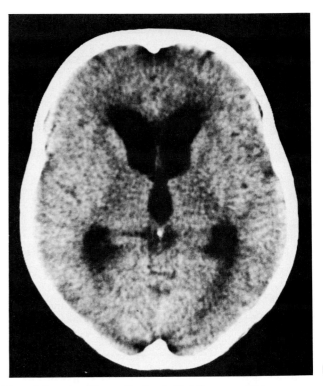

A   B

FIG. 2. A: Brain CT in a 30-year-old woman with AIDS and chronic otitis media due to *H. influenzae.* The only finding is mild atrophy. **B:** CT of same patient 1 month later during treatment for *H. influenzae* meningitis showing enlargement of third and lateral ventricles with absent cortical sulci, reflecting increased intracranial pressure and hydrocephalus.

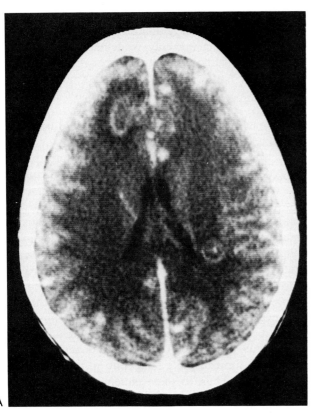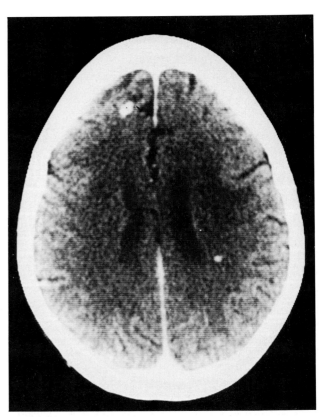

A   B

FIG. 3. A: Contrast-enhanced CT and brain scan in a 34-year-old HIV-infected man with seizures, showing right frontal and left parietal ring enhancing lesions surrounded by edema as well as multiple small lesions in the left frontal lobe adjacent to the falx, consistent with toxoplasmosis. (Courtesy of Dr. Michael Daras.) **B:** Noncontrast scan in the same patient after 8 weeks of empiric anti-toxoplasma therapy, showing a decrease in size and number of lesions and increased density of the right frontal and left parietal lesions representing calcification.

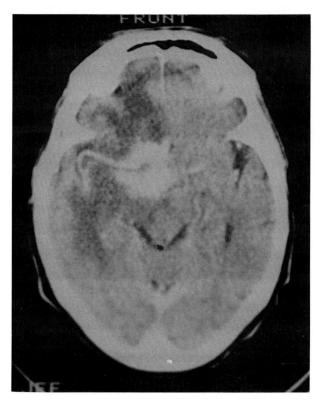

FIG. 4. Contrast-enhanced CT of the brain in a 57-year-old woman with AIDS who presented with headache and left hemiparesis, showing a densely homogeneously enhancing mass with extensive surrounding edema in the right suprasellar region, which proved to be lymphoma on biopsy. (Courtesy of Dr. John Mangiardi.)

To assess response to treatment most meaningfully, the size and number of lesions must be carefully determined, as well as the extent to which each enhances (103,104), while attempting to control for nonspecific beneficial effects of corticosteroids and technical aspects of the imaging procedure.

MRI is complementary to CT, especially in detecting white matter degeneration caused by HIV (28,98, 105,106) or by progressive multifocal leukoencephalopathy (107,108). It is more sensitive than CT in detecting lesions and in reflecting the extent of the pathological process, but findings are generally less specific and margins of lesions are not easily distinguishable from surrounding edema (105). Unlike iodine-based contrast agents used with CT, gadolinium DTPA, the contrast agent used with MRI, almost never evokes an allergic response. Furthermore, the small volume required, about 10 ml, allows gadolinium to be used in patients with renal failure. Like contrast-enhanced CT, gadolinium-enhanced MRI reveals alterations in blood–brain barrier and abnormal perfusion (98,109). In general, statements about the effect of contrast enhancement on CT-detected lesions apply to gadolinium and MRI. Pa-

tients with claustrophobia need prior conditioning or sedation to tolerate the procedure.

Similar MRI or CT abnormalities may be seen with different infections (94,97,100,102,105), or with infections and tumors (Fig. 4) (5,94,102). Even viral infections may rarely present as a focally enhancing lesion (1,98,106). Both CT and MRI can facilitate brain biopsy, and immediate postoperative scanning allows early detection of bleeding and confirmation that the lesion was accurately sampled (1,98,108,110,111).

MRI or CT accompanied by myelography is necessary to diagnose spinal cord compression from tumor or abscess.

Cerebrospinal Fluid (CSF) Examination

CSF examination is required when meningitis is suspected, but findings are frequently atypical in immunocompromised hosts compared to immunocompetent ones. For example, there may be a paucity of white cells in cryptococcal or other infectious meningitides due to the patients' inability to generate an inflammatory response; conversely, pleocytosis can be seen in the Guillain-Barré-like syndrome associated with HIV infection (45). Low CSF glucose is a reliable indicator of infection, but hypoglycorrachia can be seen with sarcoid or meningeal tumor as well. A serum glucose level should always be obtained simultaneously for comparison with CSF glucose measurements. Tests for antigen in CSF have been developed for cryptococcus (112), mycobacteria (113), and HIV (35,37,114,115), and for antibody in mycobacterial (tuberculosis) (116,117), bacterial (syphilis) (118–120), and viral (HIV, herpes simplex) infections (121–124). These are discussed in later sections dealing with specific infections. Amplification by polymerase chain reaction will likely assist in detecting minute quantities of pathogens in the future (115). Serological tests that rely on antibody production can be falsely negative (99). To detect tumor cells adequately, at least 3 ml of fluid should be preserved with an equal amount of alcohol and studied by millipore filtration or cytometry. Sometimes cytologic examination must be repeated several times before a positive sample is obtained. Measurement of myelin basic protein may be of interest in quantifying the extent of ongoing demyelination. Atypical oligoclonal band patterns occur as a nonspecific consequence of viral infection (125) or acute destructive processes and thus are usually not helpful. HIV can be cultured from CSF, so appropriate precautions in handling must be observed (59,126,127).

Clinical Neurophysiology

A wide variety of electroencephalographic (EEG) changes have been described in patients with HIV infection or AIDS. EEG is rarely of specific help, but diffuse abnormalities of background rhythms may assist in documenting organic cerebral dysfunction in patients with equivocal mental or psychological symptoms. Conversely, a normal EEG in an apparently demented patient should raise suspicion of a psychiatric disorder such as severe depression.

Early EEG findings in ADC include slowing of mean alpha rhythm frequency, loss of alpha rhythm, and increased diffuse slow frequency activity (89). Later, EEG activity becomes low voltage, and there is loss of faster frequency components (128) (Fig. 5). Quantitative computer-assisted methods of EEG analysis may increase the sensitivity for detecting abnormalities in asymptomatic patients with HIV encephalitis and predict progressive dementia (129,130). One study has claimed that electrophysiologic tests are the most sensitive indicators of subclinical CNS disease (21).

Patients with focal lesions usually show focal slowing over the appropriate regions. Herpes simplex encephalitis may be accompanied by a characteristic periodic sharp-wave pattern. Triphasic waves suggest metabolic encephalopathy. In patients with seizures, epileptiform discharges may be focal, multifocal, or generalized (88,89). Nonconvulsive status epilepticus may present

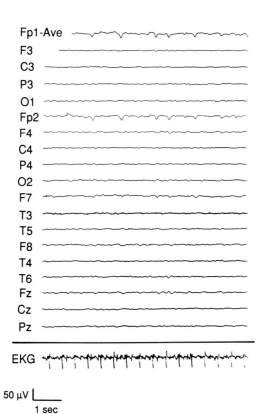

FIG. 5. Electroencephalogram of a 41-year-old HIV-infected man with dementia showing diffuse low-voltage slowing with reduction in faster frequency activity. (Courtesy of Dr. Cynthia Harden.)

as altered mental status and is diagnosable only by EEG (88).

Emerson et al. (131) have provided preliminary data that some neurologically asymptomatic HIV-infected individuals, as well as patients with early ADC, have a characteristic attenuation or loss of subcortical components (P14, N18) of the somatosensory evoked potential. Polysomnography has demonstrated disruption of stage IV sleep in some patients early in the course of HIV infection (22). Nerve conduction studies and electromyography are useful in quantifying neuropathy and in detecting myopathy and radiculopathy.

Brain Biopsy

Because of the similarity in clinical and neuroimaging presentations of etiologically different neurological complications, brain biopsy is often crucial for definitive diagnosis (111,132,133). This is especially important when empiric therapy, based on the most reasonable presumptive diagnosis, fails or new lesions develop. Tissue diagnosis is mandatory in such cases. Brain biopsy is also indicated in patients who are deteriorating too quickly for a therapeutic trial (103,104). Having said this, it is important to acknowledge that definitions of treatment failure and timing of biopsy are often disputed.

Brain biopsy has an increased incidence of complications in patients with AIDS, including infection (2,7) (Fig. 6) and hemorrhage (98,103). Although a bleeding diathesis is frequently present that may predispose to hemorrhage, such as thrombocytopenia, liver dysfunction with clotting abnormalities, or disseminated intravascular coagulopathy (4,5,96,133), AIDS patients seem to have increased bleeding even in the absence of these. Awareness of these problems can reduce their influence on surgical morbidity. Chance of hemorrhage can be minimized by replacing deficient clotting factors and platelets. Stereotactic-guided biopsy using either CT or MRI guidance and only a small burr hole or limited craniotomy allows safer access to deep lesions (98,110,111). The disadvantage of this is that only a small tissue sample is obtained, which is sometimes inadequate for diagnosis. An ultrasound probe, used with a small craniotomy, can help define the perimeter of a lesion, which maximizes detection of organisms in patients with brain abscess (Fig. 7). Ultrasonography is also helpful in detecting hemorrhagic complications.

Even with tissue obtained by biopsy, it is sometimes not possible to make an unambiguous diagnosis. This is usually because the amount of tissue is inadequate or because the sample is obtained from a part of the lesion that does not contain diagnostic pathology (1,99,100, 102,132,133). Review of frozen sections is helpful in confirming that an adequate sample has been obtained

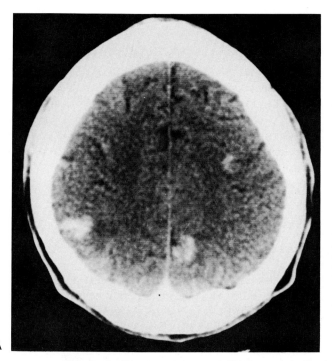
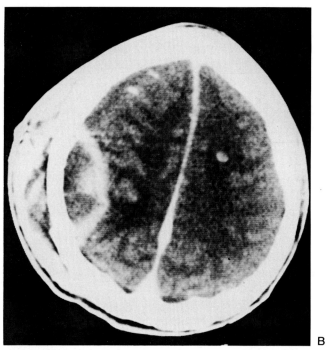

A   B

FIG. 6. A: Contrast-enhanced CT scan of the brain in a 38-year-old HIV-infected man with fever and seizures, revealing multiple enhancing nodular lesions. Biopsy revealed toxoplasmosis. **B:** Contrast-enhanced scan of same patient 10 days after open biopsy of right frontal lesion, showing dural enhancement and subgaleal swelling due to bacterial empyema.

(133). An additional problem is that sections stained with hematoxylin and eosin may appear normal even in the presence of infection (134). Thus special stains and cultures are always necessary and must not be overlooked. It is also important to recognize that multiple infectious agents may be present simultaneously (1,9,133,135–138), or that different pathological processes may coexist, such as toxoplasmosis with lymphoma (1,96,100,135). Finally, the histopathology may be atypical in the immunodeficient host, causing problems for the unwary. For example, toxoplasma tachyzoites may be round rather than crescentic (133); micro-

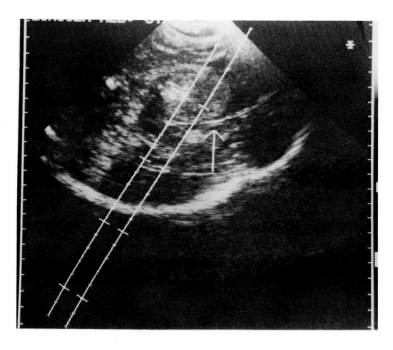

FIG. 7. Real-time ultrasonography performed during the biopsy of the patient described in Fig. 4, showing needle trajectory in center of lesion (lymphoma). (Courtesy of Dr. John Mangiardi.)

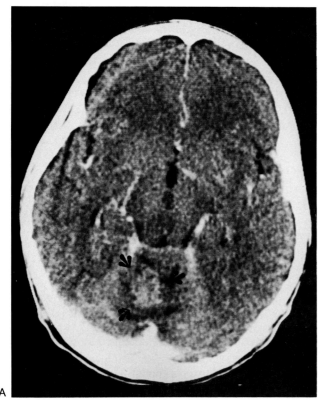
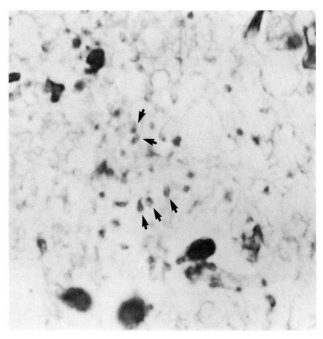

FIG. 8. A: Contrast-enhanced brain CT in a 32-year-old man with cryptococcal meningitis who developed gait ataxia on treatment. The scan shows a round, fairly homogeneously enhancing lesion in the cerebellar vermis. Biopsy revealed a cryptococcoma. **B:** Biopsy specimen of lesion shown in (A), demonstrating cryptococcal yeast forms surrounded by a blank space containing nonstaining capsular material (hematoxylin and eosin stain, ×800). (Courtesy of Dr. Tung Pui Poon.)

glial nodules may be seen with infections other than CMV and HIV; and capsules of cryptococcal yeast organisms may appear unusually small (139) (Fig. 8).

SYNDROMES DUE TO HIV INFECTION

HIV Encephalitis (AIDS–Dementia Complex)

Clinical and Laboratory Features

Early in the course of HIV infection, in some patients as early as 2 weeks after exposure to the virus, a flu-like syndrome occurs with muscle and joint aches, macular trunk rash, lymphadenopathy, and aseptic meningitis. Symptoms referable to the meningitis include headache, irritability, mild confusion, photophobia, and excessive sleepiness (11,140). Seizures are rare (13,88,89,140). Transient cranial neuropathies (1,2,5,141), especially facial (1,3,5,11,50), may appear. CSF shows a mild lymphocytic pleocytosis (36,142) with slight elevation in protein content but a normal sugar level (142). HIV-1 can be detected by polymerase chain reaction (PCR) (37,115) or other techniques (35,114). The aseptic men-

ingitis that occurs early is usually symptomatic for only a few days or sometimes weeks, but some patients continue to show a cellular reaction in CSF even after they become asymptomatic (2). Rarely chronic meningitis develops with persistent headache and confusion (142). Treatment with corticosteroids has been beneficial, but if required, these should be used only for short periods because of the undesirable immunosuppressive properties (143).

As brain infection evolves, several nonspecific markers appear in CSF in both patients and experimental animals infected with HIV. Concentrations of quinolinic acid, an excitotoxin, increase proportionally to the degree of neurological involvement (144,145) and correlate with the severity of neuropsychological and motor deficits (145). The ratio of quinolinic acid to kynurenic acid, an antagonist of the excitotoxic effects of quinolinic acid, also increases (146). CSF levels of neopterin, a putative marker of activated macrophages, also rise in parallel with the severity of neurological disease (147,148) and decrease in conjunction with clinical improvement associated with zidovudine therapy (147). Intrathecal production of α-tumor necrosis factor, one of the cytokines proposed to contribute to neurotoxicity

(149), also occurs with HIV brain infection, and CSF levels may correlate with ongoing active CNS disease (150). Measurable antibodies to HIV develop (122,123), and the virus may be cultured relatively easily (126,127).

For the next months to years the patient usually has no neurological symptoms, although aseptic meningitis can recur. Nonetheless, evidence of latent CNS infection can be demonstrated, including the presence of HIV-Ag (114) and β_2-microglobulin (151,152) in CSF, and intrathecal synthesis of anti-HIV IgG (123), which may precede other serologic markers of infection (33). The ratio of HIV antibody in CSF to that in serum is highest early in infection (34), and in acute cases, antibody may be found only in CSF (33). Although disputed (152–155), there is some evidence that careful neuropsychological assessment reveals increased abnormalities in at least a small percentage of neurologically asymptomatic HIV-seropositive individuals compared to controls (32,39–41). However, selection bias may play a role in the controversy regarding psychological findings, because studies other than one in military recruits (152) and another in a small group of intravenous drug users (IVDUs) (41) have all been of homosexual men. Members of nonhomosexual risk groups, especially IVDUs, tend to seek medical attention only when opportunistic infection occurs. It has thus been extremely difficult to correlate neuropsychological findings with HIV encephalitis in this group of patients. Furthermore, abnormal neuropsychological findings have been mostly observed in timed trials, which may reflect slowed motor ability rather than impaired cognitive function. Thus the clinical significance of the neuropsychological abnormalities reported to date early in HIV infection is unclear.

Other functional abnormalities in clinically asymptomatic patients have been reported using routine (128,129) and quantitative (130) electroencephalography, brainstem auditory evoked potentials (21,23,24), somatosensory evoked potentials (131), long-latency event-related potentials (25,26), and oculography (23, 156). ^{31}P magnetic resonance spectroscopy (157), positron emission tomography (158–160), and single photon emission computed tomography (SPECT) (38,161,162) (Fig. 9) have demonstrated *increased* metabolism within the thalamus and basal ganglia in patients with early symptoms and signs of ADC, and *decreasing* cortical metabolism as the disease progresses. Early changes in the central white matter fornices and corpus callosum have been reported using high-resolution magnetic resonance imaging (MRI) (23,27,28), and MRI abnormalities have been correlated with results of neuropsychological testing (27,32).

Eventually, clinical symptoms referable to HIV encephalitis emerge in approximately 85% of those with AIDS (155). Neurological abnormalities correlate well with the areas of the brain found to be most involved pathologically by the virus (163,164). Computed tomography shows atrophy (155,165), the degree of which parallels the stage of disease.

Children who are infected with HIV *in utero* or perinatally may be developmentally delayed and then, at about 2–3 years of age, develop a progressive syndrome characterized by loss of milestones, pyramidal tract signs, acquired microcephaly, seizures, and a behavioral and cognitive decline (95,166–168). Computed tomography (CT) in these children reveals diffuse brain atrophy with calcifications in the basal ganglia that correspond to min-

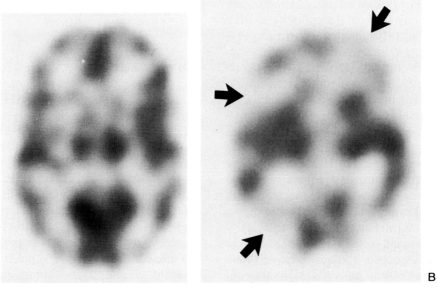

FIG. 9. A: Normal SPECT brain scan in a healthy control subject in the axial plane at the midthalamic level. **B:** Multifocal perfusion defects (*arrows*) are present in the SPECT scan from a patient with HIV encephalopathy. (Courtesy of Dr. Joseph Masdeu.)

eral deposits in blood vessels. MRI demonstrates delayed myelination (169).

Adults with HIV encephalitis develop apathy and depression and have trouble concentrating and organizing tasks (23,155,156), difficulties that are probably due to neuron loss within frontal lobes (170). Memory loss, language impairment, and occasional hallucinations can be attributed to involvement of the limbic system and temporal lobe (165). Bradykinesia, impaired eye movements, and involuntary movements such as myoclonus, tremor (6,61,171,172), asterixis, and posturing (173) result from abnormalities of basal ganglia and other subcortical nuclei (159). Ataxia reflects brainstem involvement (6,61). Loss of myelin within fiber tracts leads to delayed information processing, slow responses, impaired fine motor skills, and loss of bladder control. Pathologic reflexes such as grasp, snout and root responses appear as the disease progresses. Terminally, patients are mute, incontinent, quadriplegic and contracted.

Demyelination precedes inflammatory changes and frank atrophy (64). Once dementia is evident, the patient's average life span is less than 6 months (2). Sporadic generalized seizures occur in 25%–30% of patients, possibly reflecting increased levels of excitotoxins such as quinolinic acid (89,145).

Pathophysiology

Pathological evidence of HIV encephalitis, including microglial nodules and multinucleated giant cells, are found in up to 90 percent of patients with AIDS (62,174). Viral entry into brain is by HIV-infected monocytes and macrophages (175,176) or directly across capillary endothelium (155,177,178). Monocytes and microglial cells probably vary in their susceptibility to HIV infection (176). Although HIV rarely seems to infect neurons directly (178), it can cause release of excitatory substances that activate N-methyl-D-aspartate (NMDA) receptors (179). The gp 120 portion of the viral envelope is capable of increasing calcium influx into cultured rodent retinal ganglion and hippocampal cells with toxic consequences for the neurons (180). Blocking the calcium influx improves cell survival in this experimental situation (180). The Tat protein produced by HIV can depolarize cell membranes causing neuronal dysfunction and, at high concentrations, lead to pore formation with ion leakage and eventual cytotoxicity (181). Because a section of the viral envelope shares some amino acid sequences with neurotrophic factors such as neuroleukin (175,182,183) and vasoactive intestinal peptide (184–186), the virus may also block processes essential to ongoing required cell maintenance (59,155,185). Studies now indicate that HIV strains associated with prominent neurological disease differ biologically from those linked

to immune deficiency (59,63,149,187,188). Although the presence of opportunistic infection or tumor may obscure signs of ADC in nonhomosexual patients (190), differences in neurotropism of viral strains may explain the occasional occurrence of neurological symptoms due to HIV encephalitis without major changes in immune status and may partially account for the disparate frequency of ADC among the different risk behavior groups (8,59,63,126,149,187,191–195). Alcohol or other drug abuse has synergistic deleterious effects on the nervous system (189).

Prospective studies have not yet linked early episodes of aseptic meningitis or facial nerve palsy to the development of HIV encephalitis (142), but the ability of the virus to mutate may explain the high incidence of encephalitis in patients with prolonged (>3 years) infection (193–195). That is, even if the virus were not neurotropic at the time infection occurred, it may become so over time.

Therapy

Only zidovudine (AZT) has been studied to date as treatment for neurologic disease caused directly by HIV infection. It penetrates the blood–brain barrier and has possibly resulted in short-term clinical benefit (82,158, 160,196–200). Apparent remission of encephalopathy in children, however, may have been due to improved overall well being (199). Zidovudine has also been reported to restore CSF neopterin (147), cortisol, and biogenic amine levels to normal levels (200). In the future, liposomes may be used to facilitate drug delivery across the blood–brain barrier (203). Calcium channel blockers including nimodipine, nifedipine (180), and flunarizine (201) can prevent cell injury and death in experimental preparations, as can antibodies to the HIV envelope protein, gp120 (202).

HIV Myelopathy

Up to 40% of patients with ADC develop progressive spastic paraparesis that is usually accompanied by loss of bladder and bowel control (2,61–63,204). Eventually the arms may become weak as well, but a sensory level is rarely found.

Myelopathy is associated with a characteristic pathological picture mainly involving the lateral and posterior columns of the thoracic spinal cord, which resembles subacute combined degeneration seen in vitamin B_{12} deficiency (204,205) (Fig. 10). Although B_{12} levels are low in some of these patients, supplementation with B_{12} has not led to neurological improvement (206). No other primary nutritional or metabolic abnormality has been identified. Furthermore, unlike the brain in which there is evidence of inflammation and where HIV can readily

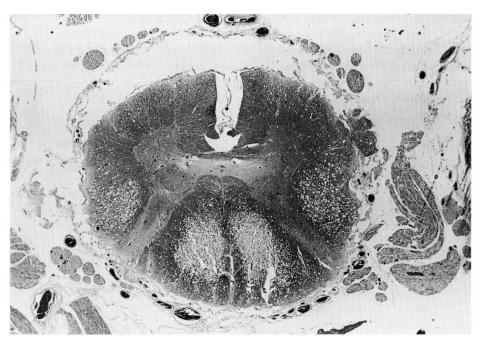

FIG. 10. Cross section of spinal cord stained with hematoxylin and eosin and luxol fast blue for myelin showing vacuolar changes in the posterior and lateral columns. (Courtesy of Dr. Seymour Levine.)

be demonstrated by appropriate probes, HIV-associated myelopathy is not associated with inflammatory changes (206–208), and HIV has been directly demonstrated only in regions of vacuolar change (209). Some investigators have proposed that these spinal cord changes may be secondary to Wallerian degeneration resulting from a primary process in the brain (174,206,210,211) or dorsal root ganglia (15,212). In children, the spinal cord may fail to myelinate fully (210). Other possible but unlikely causes for the vacuolar myelopathy include toxic effects from chemicals used in wound cleaning (213); nutritional deficiency or toxicity from therapeutic drugs such as isoniazid (2); and coinfection with other agents (214,215), most often the related retroviruses human T-lymphotropic virus type I (HTLV-I) (216–218) and HTLV-II (216). In most cases, however, HTLV-I, the causative agent of tropical spastic paraparesis, cannot be demonstrated (207,219,220). Whether other agents, acting alone or in synergy with HIV, cause myelopathy in AIDS patients is unknown.

There is no proved treatment for HIV myelopathy. Steroids may have helped in one case in which an inflammatory component attributed to coinfection with HTLV-I may have played a pathogenic role (218). Spasticity may be relieved by baclofen (although often at the expense of loss of strength), and urinary urgency is improved by oxybutynin or imipramine.

At least one case of amyotrophic lateral sclerosis (ALS) has occurred in a patient with AIDS (221), but another patient with a syndrome resembling motor neuron disease actually had severe, extensive peripheral neuropathy and myopathy (222).

HIV Peripheral Neuropathy

In up to 35% of AIDS patients a clinical sensory neuropathy occurs manifested by stocking/glove numbness, painful dysesthesias (mainly burning feet), and, uncommonly, weakness or autonomic dysfunction (223–228). Electrophysiological studies are consistent with axonal degeneration (44,227,229) or, rarely, segmental demyelination; these findings have been confirmed by nerve biopsy (227). Unlike the chronic inflammatory demyelinating polyneuropathy that resembles Guillain-Barré syndrome (142–148), inflammatory changes are generally absent in HIV sensory neuropathy, and the virus has not been demonstrated directly (227,228). However, viral antigen has been found within monocytes infiltrating the vasa nervorum of peripheral nerves (49), and viral-like particles have been seen with electron microscopy in the axoplasm of peripheral nerve (229). Although the pathological changes are consistent with direct viral invasion of the nerve (229,230) or "dying back" consequent to dorsal root ganglia infection (212), circulating immune complexes, toxins, or nutritional deficiency (2) may be contributing factors in some patients. This sensory neuropathy must be distinguished from the inflammatory polyneuritis, which occurs as a manifestation of immune dysregulation (see below).

Symptoms and signs of peripheral neuropathy usually stabilize (227,229) but may improve with zidovudine (160,231,232). Tricyclic antidepressants (amitriptyline, imipramine) or antiepileptic drugs (carbamazepine, phenytoin) can alleviate neuritic pain in some patients (223). Substance P releasing creams, such as capsaicin, can also be useful in suppressing neuralgic pain.

Muscle Disease

Most patients suffer from myalgias and weakness preterminally (233), and some patients have an inflammatory syndrome mimicking polymyositis (51,52,234–236). Affected patients have had myalgias, especially of the thighs (236,237), slowly worsening proximal weakness, and mild elevations of creatine phosphokinase. The electromyogram shows fibrillations, positive sharp waves, and polyphasic motor units. Muscle biopsy has revealed lymphocyte and macrophage infiltrates that stain for HIV gp41 antigen (238). Myoglobinuria not accompanied by inflammatory changes on muscle biopsy was reported in one HIV-infected patient before other symptoms of muscle disease (228), and myoglobinuria has also been reported rarely at the time of HIV seroconversion (20). Treatment with steroids (52,78), antiretroviral drugs (52), nonsteroidal anti-inflammatory drugs (78), or, rarely, plasmapheresis (234) leads to improvement in the majority of patients.

HIV wasting syndrome, which accounts for 15% of new cases of AIDS reported to the CDC, may rarely be due to a steroid-responsive myopathy in patients without signs of malabsorption (52).

Syndromes of Immune Dysregulation

In intermediate stages of HIV infection, autoimmune diseases can appear, probably because the virus has adversely affected lymphocyte function without yet causing complete immunosuppression. The most common of these is a subacute or chronic inflammatory demyelinating polyneuropathy (CIDP) or polyradiculopathy (42–48,227,239,240). Acute forms more typical of Guillain-Barré syndrome have been described, which may occur even at the time of HIV seroconversion (12). Clinical features include symmetric weakness of the arms and legs, which is most marked distally, and relatively milder sensory abnormalities, mainly of the hands and feet, with the ability to sense vibration being especially affected. Involvement of the autonomic nervous system is rare (225,226). Occasionally the disease is severe enough that respiratory insufficiency develops (42,227). Although this is mainly a disorder of adults, at least one child has been affected (239). Isolated facial palsy may be a restricted variant of the more widespread disorder (10,50). Nerve biopsies reveal inflammatory segmental demyelination with a variable amount of axonal degeneration (42,45,227,231). CSF protein is generally elevated to two to three times normal, and there may be a slight pleocytosis (<50 WBCs/mm^3) (42,227).

Polymyositis (51,52), vasculitis (234,241), and mononeuritis multiplex (47–49,242) also probably represent autoimmune phenomena, as does thrombocytopenia. Thrombocytopenia may lead to cerebral hemorrhage (57,66). Anticardiolipin antibodies or lupus anticoagulant (58,242) are found in some AIDS patients with cerebral infarction (234,237), as is vasculitis (241,243).

Despite the concern about accelerating immunosuppression (143), corticosteroids and plasmapheresis have been used with apparent benefit in some patients (42,43,46,48) with immune dysregulation disorders. However, it is also clear that symptoms subside spontaneously in some patients. In one of three refractory patients with HIV-related CIDP, intravenous immunoglobulin therapy was associated with improvement (240).

NEUROLOGIC SYNDROMES DUE TO OPPORTUNISTIC INFECTION, TUMOR, AND VASCULAR DISEASE

The clinical manifestations of opportunistic infections, tumors, and vascular disease affecting the nervous system in patients with AIDS can be conveniently grouped into syndromes that reflect predominantly focal cerebral, meningeal, spinal cord, or neuromuscular involvement.

Focal Cerebral Syndromes

A neurological picture marked by headache and focal signs is most often due to opportunistic infection or tumor affecting the brain parenchyma. Other causes of focal brain disease such as infarction or hemorrhage (244) are much less common. The particular manifestations of a cerebral lesion are a function of its location, acuity, and size. Focal hemispheric lesions commonly cause aphasia, spatial neglect or denial, lateralized changes in tone or strength, hemisensory loss, gaze preference, visual field defect, reflex asymmetry, and unilateral extensor plantar response. Focal or secondarily generalized seizures are common. Sometimes the focal signature must be carefully looked for, because the clinical picture may be dominated by evidence of more global cerebral dysfunction due to multiple lesions, increased intracranial pressure, or involvement of the reticular activating system in the brainstem (135). Although hemispheric lesions frequently involve the basal ganglia (e.g., as in toxoplasmosis), classical signs of extrapyramidal disease such as hemiballismus (245,246), tremor (247), bradykinesia rigidity (248,249), and other involuntary movements (171,172,250) are uncommon. Brainstem and cerebellar lesions cause nystagmus, diplopia, gaze palsy, dysphagia, ataxia, and "crossed" syndromes in which some signs occur ipsilateral to the lesion while others are contralateral (50,65,141). Fever may occur with either tumor or infection and is therefore not helpful diagnostically.

It is usually impossible to determine clinically the nature of the specific pathogen or even whether a focal lesion is due to infection or tumor. Although it is often said that deterioration caused by tumor occurs more rapidly than that caused by infection, this dictum is completely unreliable in the immunodeficient patient.

Meningitis

Meningitis manifests in both acute and chronic forms. Acute manifestations include headache, photophobia, confusion, lethargy, and seizures. Papilledema may be present. In chronic meningitis, headache is often less prominent, and encephalopathic features (lethargy, impaired mentation) are correspondingly more common. Communicating hydrocephalus with increased intracranial pressure occurs frequently, and infarction may result from inflammatory arteritis. Chronic meningitis may lead to abscess formation, usually near a meningeal surface, with accompanying focal signs. Meningitis or ependymitis inconsistently results in diffuse enhancement of the meninges or ventricular lining (97,100) (Fig. 2).

Metabolic disturbances sometimes mimic the encephalopathy of chronic meningitis. When asterixis or multifocal myoclonus is present, it should strongly suggest a metabolic disorder. Common causes of metabolic encephalopathy in AIDS patients include chronic hypoxia, liver and kidney failure, and hyponatremia. Wernicke's encephalopathy has been reported in association with zidovudine therapy (79), and the pathological features of thiamine deficiency were incidentally noted at autopsy in another patient (65).

Spinal Cord

The most common cause of spinal cord dysfunction in HIV infection is the vacuolar myelopathy associated with ADC (204). Myelopathy can also result from compression due to epidural infection or tumor (5,251) (Fig. 11), viral myelitis (205,214,252,253), or, rarely, bacterial (254,255) or parasitic (256,257) infection of the cord itself. Some cases of severe peripheral neuropathy have been associated with sufficient retrograde degeneration to produce myelopathic signs and symptoms (212).

Clinical features of myelopathy include bilateral symptoms and signs with the legs more affected than the

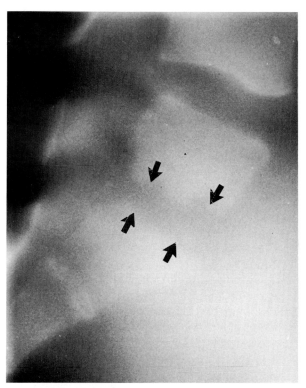
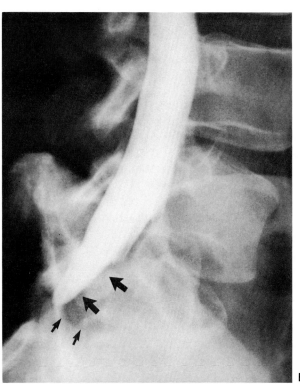

A

B

FIG. 11. A: Tomogram of L5-S1 interspace showing destruction of disc space. **B:** Myelogram shows indentation of dye column from a mass that was proved to be *M. tuberculosis* infection in a 31-year-old HIV-infected man, who had radicular pain and a positive PPD. (From ref. 251, with permission.)

arms. A transverse sensory level is often present, usually on the trunk, and sensory loss below this is usually greater for pin and light touch than for other modalities. Leg weakness is usually worse proximally, and if the disease process is sufficiently chronic, muscle tone is likely to be increased and spontaneous flexor spasms of the legs can be observed. Stretch reflexes are hyperactive below the level of the lesion, and the plantar reflexes are typically extensor. Patients with spinal cord disease complain early of urinary urgency and increased frequency and, as the myelopathy worsens, they develop complete loss of bladder and bowel function. Occasionally, patients note a change in sweat pattern, or they report radicular pain or a belt-like tightness around the chest at the involved level. When spinal cord compression occurs from epidural tumor or infection, there is usually localized pain or tenderness at the involved level. In patients with infection of the bone or epidural space, careful examination of the back may reveal an area of warmth or tenderness when the vertebral processes are percussed.

In cases of neoplastic meningitis, spinal nerve roots are commonly involved by tumor deposits, usually at multiple levels, and this results in radicular pain, segmental sensory loss, and areflexia. Some cases of CMV radiculitis simulate a conus lesion with radiating sacral pain followed by sacral numbness and then loss of bladder and bowel control with urinary retention (258).

Neuromuscular Syndromes

Distinguishing features of the various disorders affecting the peripheral nervous system are summarized in Table 3. Disorders of peripheral nerves cause both sen-

TABLE 3. *Localization of neurologic symptoms*

Symptom		Features	Cause
Weakness	Proximal	↑ Reflexes, Babinski	Myelopathy
		↓ Reflexes	Myopathy
	Isolated	↓ Reflexes Proximal or distal May be asymmetric	Mononeuritis multiplex
	Distal	↓ NCV[a] slowed ↓ Amplitude, NCV nl or slow	Neuropathy (inflammatory) (HIV related)
Pain	Bandlike	Usually thoracic	Myelopathy (compressive mass)
	Patchy	Radicular, can involve cranial nerves	Carcinomatous meningitis
	Cramps	Exertional ↑ CPK	Myopathy
	Distal feet > hands	Burning, numb, tingling	Neuropathy (HIV related)
Numbness	Distal (stocking/glove)	↓ All modalities ↓ Amplitude ↓ Velocity on NCV[a]	Neuropathy (HIV related)
	Spinal level	Usually thoracic ↓ Pin, touch	Myelopathy (cord compression)
Urination change	Urgency, frequency	Culture negative, constipation	Myelopathy, rarely hydrocephalous
	Incontinence, dribbling	Flaccid bladder	CMV sacral radiculitis or cauda equina mass
Pathologic reflexes	Bilateral Babinski		Myelopathy
	Unilateral Babinski		Brain (mass or PML)
	Bilateral Babinski with snout, grasp, glabellar		Brain (dementia, usually HIV)

[a] NCV, nerve conduction velocity.
[b] CMV, cytomegalovirus.

sory and motor symptoms, but strength and sensation are often affected unequally. In peripheral polyneuropathy, there is symmetric, distal loss of cutaneous sensation in a "glove-and-stocking" distribution. The sensory loss may affect only one modality (e.g., pin or light touch). When individual nerves are damaged ("mononeuritis"), there is weakness and sensory loss limited to the distribution of the affected nerve(s). Muscle disease causes limb weakness without sensory symptoms or signs. Stretch reflexes can be diminished or lost whenever the lower motor neuron or muscle is affected and are not helpful in specifying the site of the pathological process in the absence of other data.

Mononeuritis can result from localized vasculitis (47–49,228). A severe polyneuropathy of unknown cause has produced a clinical picture simulating progressive muscular atrophy with widespread weakness and atrophy (222). Some patients taking zidovudine have developed weakness without cramps from a mitochondrial myopathy, which probably results from competition by zidovudine with thymidine for the polymerase required in mitochondrial DNA replication (77). Symptoms of zidovudine myopathy resolve 1–8 weeks following drug withdrawal, although CPK levels may remain elevated longer. DDI causes a peripheral neuropathy in some but not all patients. In affected individuals, severity of the neuropathy is proportional to both the daily dose and cumulative dose. Most patients recover when the drug is stopped, although there may be temporary intensification of symptoms following drug withdrawal. DDI should be used cautiously in patients with preexisting neuropathy. Cramps on exertion may be nonspecific symptoms of anemia and hypoxia.

SEIZURES

Seizures are always symptoms of brain dysfunction and may be caused by focal cerebral lesions, meningitis or encephalitis, or metabolic derangements (especially hypoglycemia and hyponatremia). Sleep deprivation and alcohol use may lower seizure threshold in susceptible individuals. If a correctable cause is not found (e.g., metabolic abnormality), antiepileptic drug therapy should be started. Because most seizures in AIDS patients have a focal origin, drugs of choice are phenytoin or carbamazepine. In acute situations, therapeutic phenytoin levels can be achieved rapidly by loading with 1–1.5 g orally or, if necessary, intravenously. When given intravenously, phenytoin should not be administered at rates faster than 40–50 mg/min, and ECG and blood pressure should be monitored continuously during the infusion. Blood levels should be determined frequently if the patient is systemically ill or taking other medications. About 15–20% of patients taking carbamazepine develop a benign leukopenia that is not clinically significant, even in immunosuppressed patients.

SPECIFIC OPPORTUNISTIC INFECTIONS

Protozoan Infections

Toxoplasmosis

Toxoplasmosis is the most frequent CNS opportunistic infection among adult patients with AIDS (1,2,4,5, 96,137,244,259). Up to 30% of Americans have asymptomatic infection with *Toxoplasma gondii* as determined by serologic testing (260). Encephalitis develops in up to 30% of patients with AIDS who have toxoplasma antibodies (261), and this is usually not accompanied by a rise in serum antibody titer (99). The incidence of toxoplasma encephalitis or meningitis is higher in Haitians, Europeans, and intravenous drug users (IVDUs) than in other HIV-infected groups (104,137,259).

The clinical presentation of brain involvement may be that of a mass lesion (60%) (261), confusion, personality change or lethargy, nonspecific symptoms of increased intracranial pressure, or, less frequently, meningitis (262) or panhypopituitarism (263). Combinations of symptoms and signs are common. Fever is inconsistently present, and seizures occur in 30% (261).

Presumptive clinical diagnosis is made by finding multiple nodular lesions on CT or MRI of the brain combined with a positive serum serology (99). Using special cell cultures, toxoplasma can be grown from blood (264). CSF examination is rarely helpful (261). Lesions are typically found in the cortex, especially at the gray–white matter junction, or in the basal ganglia. Computed tomography consistently underestimates the number of lesions compared to MRI or postmortem examination (94,98,259,261). Contrast infusion typically results in enhancement, although this may be absent (a poor prognostic sign) in patients not capable of reactive vascular proliferation or mounting more than a minimal inflammatory response. Scans done immediately after contrast infusion show peripheral ring enhancement, but delayed scans may result in more homogeneous enhancement of the lesion. The amount of surrounding edema varies, and CT is more accurate than MRI in delineating the lesion's boundaries (94,98,105).

Neuropathological findings include necrotizing abscesses with vascular proliferation. Occasionally, thrombosed blood vessels and petechial hemorrhages are seen.

Once suspected, the diagnosis of CNS toxoplasmosis is confirmed empirically by observing the response to appropriate treatment. Clinical and radiographic improvement, as judged by resolution of neurological abnormalities and a measurable decrease in the size and number of lesions and in the associated edema, occurs within 2 or 3 weeks (103) (Fig. 12). If new lesions emerge on treatment, or if there is no change in existing ones, the diagnosis must be regarded as suspect, and brain biopsy becomes necessary (103). Special techniques for processing

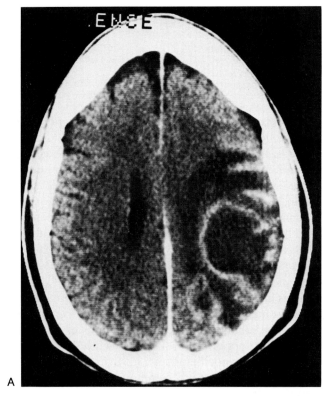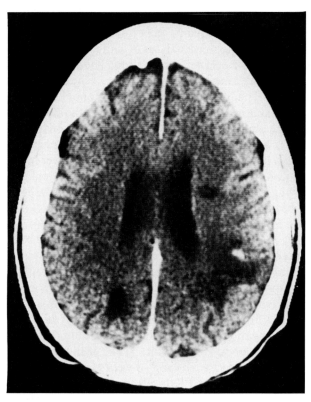

A   B

FIG. 12. A: Contrast-enhanced brain CT scan showing large left parietal ring-enhancing lesion with surrounding edema and gyral enhancement of the adjacent cortex. B: Same patient after 6 weeks of therapy for toxoplasmosis showing small area of calcification and an irregular low-density lesion in the same region as well as in the right occipital lobe and the left basal ganglia.

brain biopsy specimens are often required (261). Differentiating lymphoma from toxoplasmosis may be especially difficult when the organism is not visualized.

Standard treatment is pyrimethamine (50–100 mg/day following a loading dose of 100–200 mg) and sulfadiazine. Life-long therapy is recommended, although lower doses may be used for maintenance (99,104). In patients allergic to sulfa, clindamycin can be effectively substituted (103,261). Pyrimethamine alone, even at high doses, may be inadequate to prevent relapse (99). Folinic acid is given concomitantly with pyrimethamine to prevent hematologic toxicity (104).

Use of corticosteroids should be avoided unless required to prevent herniation. Therapeutic trials can be misleading if specific anti-infective agents are combined with corticosteroids, because apparent improvement may be due only to nonspecific beneficial effects of corticosteroids on edema and the blood–brain barrier.

Toxoplasmosis is uncommon in children with HIV infection, probably because its occurrence usually depends on reactivation of latent infection, and children may not yet have been exposed. Toxoplasma serological status should be determined in adults at the time HIV infection is diagnosed. If there is no evidence of toxo-

plasma infection, patients should be warned of the usual routes of transmission through accidental ingestion of cat feces or by consuming undercooked infected meat.

Other Parasitic Infections

Parasitic disease other than toxoplasmosis has only rarely involved the nervous system (3,244,265,266). Two cases of cysticercosis were discovered on autopsy in a series reported from Miami (3,244). Acanthamoeba meningoencephalitis has been reported (267,268), which may resemble toxoplasmosis on CT (268). Trypanosomiasis (Chagas' disease) presenting as a cerebral tumor was diagnosed at surgery and successfully treated with nifurtimox (266).

Fungal Infections

Which fungal infection a patient acquires reflects, in part, environmental exposure, thereby explaining why children have proportionally fewer fungal infections, although they are at increased risk for candida meningitis (95,269).

Cryptococcus

Cryptococcus neoformans is an encapsulated yeast found worldwide, especially in the soil of areas that support large pigeon populations. In patients with impaired T-cell immunity, *C. neoformans* causes a chronic meningitis that accounts for the majority of CNS fungal infections. Among AIDS patients, the prevalence of cryptococcal meningitis ranges from 4 to 25% (1,4,5,8,193, 270–272). Although the organism gains entry through the lungs, pulmonary infection is usually asymptomatic. Dissemination to other organs, including the brain, occurs via the bloodstream. Meningitis is the most common manifestation, occurring in 67–84% of patients with cryptococcosis (270,272), and it is frequently the presenting illness that leads to a diagnosis of AIDS. Although the CDC has reported that intravenous drug users have an incidence of cryptococcal meningitis almost three times higher than that of other HIV-infected groups, this was not confirmed in the series by Malouf et al. (6).

Cryptococcal meningitis usually begins insidiously, and signs or symptoms typical of meningeal irritation are minimal. Stiff neck and photophobia occur in a minority of patients (270–273). Usually, there is a history of malaise, lethargy, low-grade fever, altered mentation, or behavioral changes for several weeks or even months before the diagnosis is made. Rarely, nausea, vomiting, and seizures occur (272). Infarction due to infective arteritis is not seen, although transient ischemic attacks occurred in one patient (274). Occasionally, cryptococcal brain involvement is associated with the formation of cryptococcal abscesses or cryptococcal granulomas (torulomas), which can act as mass lesions to produce symptoms and signs that reflect their location. These probably arise by direct extension from infected meninges or the ependymal lining of ventricles (4,8,65,135,245) (Fig. 4).

Diagnosis of cryptococcal meningitis depends on a high index of clinical suspicion, demonstrating cryptococcal antigen in the CSF using latex agglutination and, ultimately, by culture. Routine CSF markers for meningitis are unreliable in AIDS patients (271). Pleocytosis is variable. In one series, lymphocytosis of more than 20 cells/mm^3 was a predictor of good outcome (271). The protein content is usually moderately elevated, but it can be normal in about one-third of cases (272). Similarly, the CSF glucose level is low in only 30% of patients (270). India ink preparations of CSF provide a rapid means of making a presumptive diagnosis, as yeast forms can be identified in centrifuged samples in 75% of patients (112,272). However, false positives due to artifacts misinterpreted as yeast are common, and in some AIDS patients, the organism may be difficult to recognize because of an atypical appearance resulting from incomplete capsule formation (139) (Fig. 8).

Rarely, CSF cultures have been positive despite absence of detectable antigen (270). Very high titers of cryptococcal antigen (>1:10,000) are associated with increased mortality (112). Hyponatremia and symptomatic systemic disease are also poor prognostic features (270).

Treatment of choice is intravenous amphotericin B unless precluded by renal failure. Initially, 1.5 g is given over 6 weeks (271). Liposomal delivery is experimental at present but may reduce toxicity and facilitate CNS entry (275). Flucytosine has been used as adjunctive therapy, but it contributes to bone marrow suppression and does not seem to improve outcome (270). Relapses occur in 50% of cases (276), and these are especially likely if end-of-treatment CSF antigen titers are greater than 1:8 (271). Accordingly, maintenance suppression with fluconazole has been recommended (273). Fluconazole has a high degree of CSF penetration following oral administration. Relapses have occurred in patients receiving amphotericin B, even when given intrathecally (4), or ketoconazole (270). Despite its inability to cross the blood–brain barrier, ketoconazole has reduced mortality from recurrent cryptococcal meningitis, possibly by preventing blood-borne dissemination of the organism from extracranial foci (270).

Improvement is slow in patients treated with amphotericin or fluconazole, and clear indications of beneficial effect may not be evident for up to 3 weeks. Declining antigen titers in serum and CSF usually indicate successful treatment, although this is not invariable.

Candidiasis

Overall, *Candida* species are the most common cause of fungal infection in humans. They are part of the normal body flora but become pathogenic in the presence of depressed cellular immunity. Nearly 60% of AIDS patients have oral candidiasis or candida esophagitis (277). Despite this ubiquity, candida is only rarely responsible for brain infection. Meningitis has been reported in children who seem particularly predisposed to this complication (95,269), and brain microabscesses have been found at autopsy in adults who have other cerebral infections, including toxoplasmosis (1,3–5,9,102,138).

Diagnosis of candida brain abscess can be made in life only from biopsy specimens, which allow the organisms to be demonstrated microscopically, using PAS, methanamine, or silver stains, and cultured.

Amphotericin is the preferred treatment, but its effectiveness is hard to evaluate. Fluconazole may prove useful, especially because it allows discontinuing the intravenous catheters required for amphotericin, which are often a source of continuing candida infection (277).

Coccidioidomycosis

Coccidioides immitis is a fungus found mainly in the deserts of the southwestern United States and Mexico.

Infection is usually asymptomatic, but the organism can cause both self-limited and chronic respiratory disease. Up to 95% of the population in Arizona and southern California have positive skin tests to *C. immitis* (278,279). Disseminated coccidioidomycosis is rare but manifests as chronic meningitis in 30–50% of cases (280,281). Jarvik et al. (105) have described the MRI findings in an HIV-infected patient with a brain abscess due to *C. immitis.* Intrathecal amphotericin has been the mainstay of treatment (165).

Histoplasmosis

Histoplasmosis is the most common endemic mycosis in the United States, occurring mainly in the Caribbean and in the Mississippi, Missouri, and Ohio River valleys. It usually causes a self-limited pulmonary infection, but disseminated cases occur, especially in persons whose immune systems are suppressed (278). The most fulminant examples of dissemination have been reported in AIDS patients. The brain has been involved only rarely, but both chronic meningitis and focal cerebritis have been described (8,280). More often, metabolic encephalopathy from pulmonary or liver failure is encountered (278). Disseminated infection has been controlled in some patients with amphotericin B (281).

Mucormycosis

Mucormycosis accounts for about 15% of fungal infections in immunocompromised patients (282,283). It generally presents in a rhinocerebral form, with brain infection occurring by direct extension from infected nasal mucosa, orbits, and sinuses. Common neurological findings include ophthalmoplegia, corneal and upper face hypoesthesia, blindness, and mental changes due to frontal lobe involvement. Invasion of blood vessels can lead to thrombosis and cerebral infarction (283,284). Chronic meningitis may occur once intracranial integrity is breached. Isolated brain abscess is rare, but a predelection for the basal ganglia has been alleged (284–286).

Once cerebral manifestations are evident, the course is usually one of rapid progression; successful therapy is rare (285,286). Hyperbaric oxygen may improve response to treatment (283), but this has not yet been tried in AIDS patients.

Aspergillosis

Unlike in transplant recipients, *Aspergillus fumigatus* is a rare cerebral pathogen in AIDS patients. As of mid-1990, only six cases had been reported (287). Brain infection occurs by hematogenous spread from pulmonary aspergillosis. CNS aspergillosis results in necrotizing, suppurative abscesses, which may be single or multiple. One case involved spinal cord compression by an epidural abscess that formed by direct extension from infected lungs (287). Because the organism invades blood vessel walls, abscesses are often accompanied by hemorrhage or hemorrhagic infarction. In addition to abscesses, chronic meningitis can occur.

Antemortem diagnosis of CNS aspergillosis is difficult without biopsy. It can be suspected in a patient with known or probable pulmonary aspergillosis who develops a brain abscess or meningitis. CSF studies, including culture and precipitin titers, are not helpful. By the time CNS disease is recognized, it is almost invariably fatal. The usefulness of itraconazole (288) is presently under evaluation.

Viral Infections

Cytomegalovirus (CMV) Infection

CMV was originally believed to be the causative agent for the subacute encephalitis that occurred in AIDS patients (4,5,289). It is now recognized that most of the pathological findings considered "typical" for CMV encephalitis are equally characteristic of HIV infection (155,175,290,291). Furthermore, CMV may potentiate the spread and destructive effects of HIV (293). Nonetheless, CMV has likely been the primary cause for subacute encephalopathy in some patients, especially those with prominent brainstem involvement (292–294). More often, CMV causes demyelination and vasculitis of the spinal cord and nerve roots (205,211,215,295), particularly the cauda equina (258,296–299). Individual peripheral nerves (300), cranial nerves, or their branches (e.g., the laryngeal nerve) (301) can also be symptomatically infected. CMV retinitis probably accounts for most cases of visual loss in patients with AIDS (302). Finally, CMV can also infect the adrenal glands and rarely cause adrenal insufficiency (281).

Evidence for CMV infection in these cases includes positive CSF cultures for CMV (303,304), characteristic findings on routine and electron microscopic examination of affected tissue (215,291,295,298,305), and positive results from various molecular probes and immunohistochemical techniques for CMV (205,291,292, 294,306). CMV has also been isolated from blood, urine, and CSF from individual patients with myelitis (253), chorioretinitis (302), and an illness resembling Guillain-Barré syndrome (211). Routine serum serology is not helpful; rises in viral titer with CMV infection are only rarely documented.

Treatment with ganciclovir helps in controlling viremia and stabilizing retinitis or colitis (302). One patient with biopsy proved CMV encephalitis also improved (292). Its use is limited by neutropenia, and it cannot be given concurrently with zidovudine. Relapses are common when the drug is stopped or the dose lowered (302). Alpha-interferon was not beneficial (307). Granulocyte-macrophage colony stimulating factor (GM-CSF) combined with ganciclovir has helped reduce bone marrow toxicity (308).

Herpes Simplex Virus

Like syphilis, genital ulcers due to herpes simplex virus (HSV) may predispose to easier acquisition of HIV (309). Furthermore, the incidence of HSV infection seems to be increasing in HIV-infected populations (124). Both HSV-1 and HSV-2 can cause encephalitis, meningitis, or myelitis, although HSV-1 is more often the cause of encephalitis, and HSV-2 of meningitis and myelitis (253).

The presentation and course of HSV encephalitis in HIV-infected individuals are much more variable than in immunocompetent hosts. Although many patients present with the familiar acute features of fever, headache, seizures, and abrupt deterioration in behavior and mental status accompanied by CSF pleocytosis and focal changes on EEG and CT or MRI (310), others have a more indolent course extending over weeks. Patients with this subacute variant of HSV encephalitis present with a slowly progressive neurological syndrome in which lethargy, behavioral changes, weakness, and seizures predominate. Fever may be absent, the spinal fluid unremarkable, and EEG changes nonspecific. In other patients, clinically asymptomatic, autopsy examination has demonstrated HSV in the brain (305,311).

These differences in the clinical spectrum of disease must reflect a modified pathogenesis caused by immunodeficiency. Severely immunocompromised patients are incapable of mounting a massive inflammatory response, and as a result, the disease can be much more protracted and the evidence of inflammation less marked. The encephalitis may also be more diffuse and less localized to frontal and temporal lobes in AIDS patients, and this possibly reflects a different route of entry into the brain. CSF analysis using experimental techniques to assay viral antigen, or PCR to amplify viral DNA from lymphocytes, may be helpful in diagnosis. When necessary, brain biopsy remains the definitive procedure for establishing a diagnosis. Cultures can determine the viral strain and exclude other infections or neoplasms that may produce a similar clinical picture (312). Rapid diagnosis is possible using *in situ* hybridization and electron microscopy (124,304).

Treatment of choice is acyclovir (304). Relapses occur, even in patients with reasonable immune function (313). Fear of developing acyclovir-resistant HSV strains from long-term maintenance therapy appears well founded: 7% of AIDS patients treated chronically for herpetic anogenital lesions demonstrated resistance using a rapid nucleic acid hybridization method (314). Because there are presently no guidelines for maintenance therapy of patients treated for encephalitis with acyclovir, it is probably advisable to treat for 10–20 days and then observe patients carefully for new neurological symptoms. If a relapse occurs, acyclovir should be resumed. In acyclovir-resistant cases, foscarnet has been effective for skin lesions (315,316), but it has not been evaluated in patients with encephalitis.

Progressive Multifocal Leukoencephalopathy (PML)

PML is a progressive demyelinating disease of the brain due to reactivation of latent papovavirus infection, usually of JC type (317). Latent virus has been demonstrated in bone marrow and spleen and presumably spreads through the circulation to brain, where it infects oligodendroglia. PML occurs in patients with T-cell dysfunction due to a variety of causes (107,318); it was first described in a patient with AIDS in 1982 (125). In one series of 79 AIDS patients, PML occurred in 3.8% over a 4-year period (107).

Signs and symptoms of PML infection develop gradually and reflect progressive white matter disease. Initial symptoms are usually mental changes, weakness, visual loss, or ataxia. Hemiparesis or weakness of an arm or leg was the initial presentation in 12 of 25 patients reviewed by Berger et al. (318). There are never signs of meningitis or raised intracranial pressure. Although a disease of white matter, seizures have been reported (318–320). As suggested by the name, white matter lesions are classically multifocal, but only one area of demyelination can be demonstrated in about 10% of cases (125).

The mean survival of AIDS patients with PML has averaged approximately 4 months (107,318). There have been rare cases of survival longer than 3 years, and stable disease or partial recovery has been demonstrated (320). Prognosis is worse when demyelination affects mainly the brainstem or cerebellum. In one case, infection with JC papovavirus seemed to induce an accelerated form of HIV encephalitis, possibly by recruiting HIV-infected macrophages (321).

MR or CT brain imaging characteristically shows nonenhancing lesions with irregular borders that are confined to white matter and not associated with edema or mass effect (107,108,318) (Fig. 13). On T2-weighted MRI, additional lesions may be detected as irregular areas of high signal intensity within white matter (108,318). The lesions of PML as visualized by MRI are more discrete than the diffuse subcortical white matter changes that occur with HIV encephalitis (ADC). Early in the illness, it is not unusual for patients to appear sicker than imaging abnormalities would seem to indicate. The EEG demonstrates moderate to severe focal or multifocal slow wave abnormalities, with nonspecific

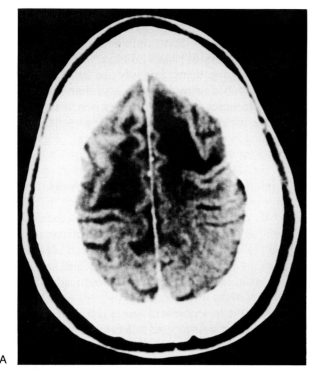 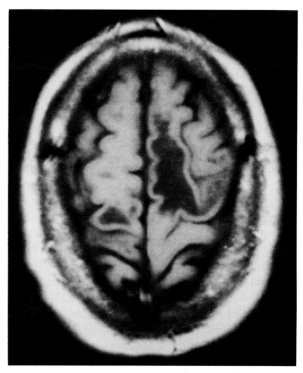

FIG. 13. A: Noncontrast CT scan of a 38-year-old HIV-infected man with mild dementia and progressive right hemiparesis, showing a hypodense lesion in the left frontal lobe. Enhanced scan did not show contrast in area. Presumed diagnosis was progressive multifocal leukoencephalopathy. **B:** T1-weighted brain MRI of same patient shows bilateral lesions without edema or mass effect.

diffuse changes later. Serological tests are not helpful in diagnosis, because 90% of adults have antibody titers to JC papovavirus (108). CSF examination reveals only mild protein elevation (<100 mg/dl) with no cellular response and a normal glucose level. Increased myelin basic protein can be demonstrated, and oligoclonal bands or increased IgG are found occasionally (107,125). If lymphocytic pleocytosis is present, it usually reflects HIV encephalitis or meningitis, or another separate process.

Neuropathological features include areas of demyelination of various ages and sizes that microscopically contain enlarged, bizarre multinucleated astrocytes, especially at the periphery, and hypertrophied oligodendroglia that contain characteristic intranuclear basophilic or eosinophilic inclusions. Sparing of axons is only relative, and in large lesions, there may be frank necrosis at the center with a phagocytic reaction (318,319). Immunofluorescent techniques usually demonstrate papovavirus antigen in the intranuclear inclusions (125). Electron microscopy reveals the typical virus particles within the intranuclear inclusions of oligodendrocytes (108,125).

So far, antiviral treatment using cytosine arabinoside (107), vidarabine (125), or acyclovir (318), and immunostimulation methods such as platelet transfusions (322) have been unsuccessful. Zidovudine has also been used, but results have not yet been reported. With all

therapies, interpretations of results is complicated by the rare occurrence of spontaneous remissions (322).

Herpes Zoster

The most common form of disease due to the varicella-zoster virus is shingles, which occurs in 5–10% of patients with HIV infection (1). Indeed, shingles often precedes development of severe immunodeficiency (2,323–327) and may be the symptom that calls attention to the underlying disorder. Both spinal and cranial nerve roots can be involved (5,6). Zoster encephalitis can develop following resolution of the rash (328), even in patients who completed a course of treatment with acyclovir. Myelitis can cause either segmental myoclonus or isolated leg weakness (171) when the infection is limited to cervical or lumbar dermatomes, or a more complete myelopathy with a level corresponding to the dermatome exhibiting shingles (171).

Although acyclovir may attenuate pain and limit spread from radicular involvement (329), resistance has emerged with chronic oral treatment (330). Furthermore, as already noted, encephalitis has developed following "appropriate" treatment (328). Patients with herpes zoster should be placed in strict isolation to avoid nosocomial transmission (281–331).

Mycobacterial Infection

Mycobacterial infection in AIDS patients is most often due to *M. avium-intracellulare* or *M. tuberculosis* but other atypical pathogens, such as *M. kansasii* and *M. leprae,* have been seen as well. Extrapulmonary involvement is common (332). *M. tuberculosis* is more frequent in Haitians (333) and parenteral drug users (334,335) than in other AIDS patients in the United States. All AIDS patients are at increased risk for atypical mycobacterial infection. Culture, which takes up to 4–6 weeks, has been required to determine which mycobacterium is present, but recently, genetic probes (113,336), anti-P32 antibody (117), and selective skin testing (337) have shown promise in making specific diagnosis more rapidly.

Mycobacterial infection typically causes meningitis or brain abscess (136,244,334) (Fig. 14). Intervertebral disc space infection and spinal epidural abscess have also been reported (251,255). Meningitis has been followed by tuberculoma formation (Fig. 14). Conversely, rupture of an abscess into the subarachnoid space or ventricle may lead to meningitis. Mycobacterial infection can also cause polymyositis (338), meningomyelitis (255), and peripheral neuropathy (339). Abscesses due to *M. avium-intracellulare* are more apt to occur in previously damaged brain (8) or in conjunction with other organisms such as toxoplasma (136,171,334).

Mycobacterial meningitis tends to be less fulminant and more subacute in AIDS patients than in non-HIV-infected groups and is more often associated with concurrent brain abscess. Thus patients often present with signs indicating both focal and diffuse neurological disease, and CT or MRI may demonstrate single or multiple mass lesions even in patients whose clinical course suggests a diffuse encephalopathy. Another cause for focal neurological abnormalities in patients with mycobacterial meningitis is cerebral infarction, a common complication that results from an associated infective arteritis of the major cerebral blood vessels (340). Inflammatory debris in the basilar cisterns and arachnoid granulations obstructs normal CSF circulation and leads to hydrocephalus (341).

CSF examination reveals increased protein content, variable lymphocytosis, and depressed sugar content. Acid-fast organisms can be found on stained smears of CSF in only 10% of cases, and CSF cultures are positive in less than 50% of cases. Special tests of CSF for the

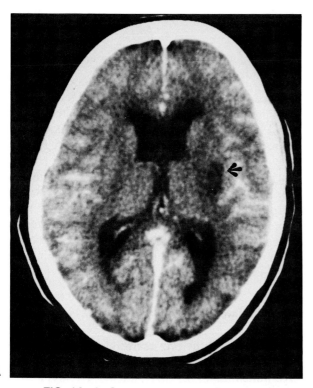
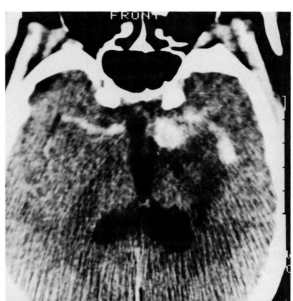

A   B

FIG. 14. A: Contrast-enhanced CT scan of the brain in a 30-year-old HIV-infected woman with headache, obtundation, and acute onset of right hemiplegia due to tuberculous meningitis. *Arrow* points to lacunar infarction of the left internal capsule. Meninges diffusely enhance with contrast. **B:** Contrast-enhanced scan of same patient after she developed decreased vision and impaired extraocular movements of the left eye despite 10 weeks of triple drug antituberculous therapy. The scan reveals a small densely enhancing round lesion adjacent to the middle cerebral artery. This eventually disappeared after several months of treatment with streptomycin in addition to isoniazid, ethambutol, and rifampin.

presence of anti-BCG cells (342), antibody to tuberculous antigens (116), or PCR (113) may increase the diagnostic yield but are not readily available. Organisms are recovered most often from tissue obtained by brain biopsy. In HIV-infected patients with tuberculosis of the central nervous system, tuberculin skin testing may or may not be positive, depending on the degree of immunosuppression (335,343,344).

Treatment of infection due to *M. tuberculosis* is usually successful, even in immunocompromised patients. The organism is typically sensitive to isoniazid, rifampin, and pyrazinamide, all of which cross the blood–brain barrier in effective concentrations (332, 345). Treatment failures occur most often when abscesses are present (334) or when patients are noncompliant with long-term therapy (332). Standard treatment regimens are of at least 9–12 months duration. Ventricular drainage or other CSF diversionary techniques may be necessary in patients with hydrocephalus. In non-AIDS patients, corticosteroids reduce morbidity from tuberculous meningitis, but they have not been systematically studied in AIDS patients.

In contrast, atypical mycobacterial infections in AIDS patients are notoriously resistant to most therapies. Combined drug regimens are almost always necessary, but results are almost invariably poor (279,337,346). Newer agents such as clofazimine, rifabutin, amikacin, and ciprofloxacin may prove more successful than have conventional anti-tuberculous drugs (281,335,346).

Spirochetal Infection

Syphilis

Syphilis and HIV infection are intimately related, and serologic tests for syphilis are positive in up to 30–50% of HIV-infected patients (71,120,347). A syphilitic chancre increases the risk of acquiring HIV, and syphilitic meningitis or syphilis-induced depression of cell-mediated immunity enhances the likelihood of HIV penetrating the brain (72). Other important issues related to coinfection with HIV and *Treponema pallidum* include the following:

1. HIV-immunocompromised patients may have falsely negative serological tests for syphilis, which hinders identification of infection (68,69,118,119, 348,349). The PCR test for *T. pallidum* (which is not yet generally available) should aid in more accurate detection.
2. Standard treatment to prevent progression may be ineffective (350,351), and relapses may occur in previously treated patients (71,72,119,352).
3. Neurological manifestations of syphilis in AIDS patients may occur early and may be unusual and include polyradiculopathy (351), transverse myelitis (353), or stroke (70,72,354,355,356).

Although there is general agreement that *Treponema pallidum* invades the CNS early in the course of syphilitic infection (347,357), it is not clear that the actual incidence of neurological manifestations is higher in HIV-infected patients (357). On the other hand, there is growing evidence that the course of syphilis in AIDS patients is more fulminant and atypical than in non-HIV-infected persons. CSF findings, especially early, do not always permit distinction between syphilitic and HIV brain infection (119). A positive CSF VDRL test, however, indicates neurosyphilis except when blood contaminates CSF, a well recognized cause of false-positive CSF serology (69,119,357).

Recommendations for treating primary syphilis and neurosyphilis in HIV-infected patients are still evolving (68,71,358), but penicillin continues to be the mainstay of therapy; resistance has not yet been documented (68,71). It is possible that high-dose penicillin regimens, such as 24 million units of penicillin iv daily for 10 days, are required for all AIDS patients with syphilis regardless of clinical stage or interval since infection (68,119), but this is unclear and not standard practice for disease outside the CNS. Maintenance treatment regimens (68,72) or use of a penicillin carrier combination that allows better passage across the blood–brain barrier (359) are additional areas for future study. Improved methods for detecting and monitoring active infection are also needed.

Borreliosis

There is one reported case of Lyme disease in an HIV-infected patient (360). This 39-year-old man had a typical annular rash, followed several weeks later by bilateral facial palsy and numbness. Specific antibody titers to *Borrelia burgdorferi* were present, and there was a good response to a standard treatment regimen. Potential clinical issues include false-negative serology in patients with coinfection; cross reactivity of *B. burgdorferi* with other spirochetes including *T. pallidum;* a possible need for more intensive antibiotic treatment; and confusion between neurological manifestations of Lyme disease with other, more common, causes of nervous system dysfunction in AIDS patients.

Bacterial Infections

Compared to the prevalence of infections caused by opportunistic organisms, bacterial infections are relatively uncommon in AIDS patients. Children, who have limited exposure to opportunistic organisms, are an exception in that they are more likely to develop bacterial infections, especially gram-negative meningitis (361). However, HIV may indirectly impair B-cell function in all patients, and drugs such as zidovudine or ganciclovir may lead to bone marrow suppression and neutropenia, all factors that may predispose to bacterial infection. Infections due to encapsulated bacteria occur with increased frequency, more acute presentations, and with greater tendency to relapse. Cerebral abscesses caused by *Listeria* (362), *Nocardia* (135,363), *Salmonella* (135), *Staphylococcus epidermidis* (138), *Streptococcus mitis* (364), and *Streptococcus pneumoniae* (361) have been recognized. Many of these were diagnosed only at autopsy. Spinal epidural abscess due to *S. aureus* or *S. epidermidis* fails to respond to antibiotic treatment alone and mandates surgery (251). Intramedullary spinal cord abscess due to *Pseudomonas cepacia* has been observed in one HIV-seropositive patient (254).

Listeria (365), *E. coli* (95,96,244,366), *S. pneumoniae,* and *H. influenzae* (281) have caused meningitis in HIV-infected patients (Fig. 2). Standard doses of penicillin or ampicillin have been successful in treating *Listeria* meningitis (365). Nath et al. (171) have described CNS Whipple's disease, presumably due to a bacilliform bacterium, in an AIDS patient. With the development of more sophisticated techniques to detect and culture fastidious organisms, recognition of unusual bacterial CNS infections may increase (367).

Intravenous drug users are at higher risk for bacterial infections than other HIV-infected groups, especially before severe immunosuppression develops. Risk factors include skin ulcers, endocarditis, and contaminated needles. Trauma often precedes cases of epidural spinal abscess (251). The incidence of infection following surgical procedures is higher in AIDS patients (2,7) than in non-HIV-infected individuals (Fig. 6B).

Diagnosis of meningitis requires lumbar puncture to obtain fluid for culture. CSF cultures can be positive even when Gram stains on centrifuged samples are negative. CT or MRI scans may suggest meningitis if they demonstrate meningeal enhancement (109). Suspicion of spinal epidural abscess necessitates either myelography followed by CT or spine MRI.

NEOPLASMS

Primary Brain Lymphoma

Primary brain lymphoma is a rare CNS tumor in the general population, but its increased frequency in patients with acquired immune suppression, including transplant recipients (368) and HIV-infected individuals (5,110,132,369–378), is now well established. In AIDS, the risk for developing primary brain lymphoma is nearly 100 times that in the general population (165,372,376). Lymphoma accounts now for 2–7% of the CNS complications in AIDS (1,4,5,190) and is secondary only to toxoplasmosis as a cause of mass lesion.

Reasons for the increased risk of lymphoma in this population are not fully understood, but most likely relate to defective internal surveillance mechanisms, oncogenic viruses, or dysfunction of immune regulation. De-

pression of T-cell numbers increases the likelihood that the immune system no longer effectively recognizes or destroys mutant, potentially neoplastic cells (369,379). The Epstein-Barr virus has been increasingly implicated in the development of CNS lymphoma (376,377,380). AIDS patients have impaired ability to suppress the growth of lymphocytes infected by Epstein-Barr virus (381,382). Other DNA viruses, including CMV, herpes simplex, and human papillomaviruses, may play a causative role in some patients, as may RNA viruses, including human T-cell leukemia virus-type I (369,376,377) and even possibly HIV itself. It is perhaps most reasonable to speculate that with sufficient derangement of the immune system, several viruses may play etiologic roles in the development of cancer.

Primary brain lymphoma presents mainly as a parenchymal mass lesion with signs reflecting its particular location and, often, increased intracranial pressure. Aphasia, hemiparesis, ataxia, and altered mentation are common early findings (376), and isolated oculomotor palsy has been described (383). Seizures occur in about one-third of patients, but they are more apt to occur as the illness evolves than at its presentation (376). Although meningeal involvement is common with metastatic spread from systemic lymphoma, it is infrequent with primary brain lymphoma (132).

The CSF is almost always abnormal but usually nonspecifically. The protein content is usually elevated, and some patients show mild pleocytosis (<50 cells/mm^3) and depressed glucose concentration (375). Because extensive meningeal infiltration does not usually occur with primary brain lymphoma, CSF cytology is almost always unhelpful.

Although the MRI or CT appearance of primary brain lymphoma is generally similar in AIDS and non-AIDS patients, some differences have been described (371). However, there are no pathognomonic features that reliably distinguish this mass lesion from that caused by toxoplasmosis. Lesions are usually deep with periventricular and cerebellar sites especially common (Fig. 4). Multifocal tumors are not rare. Primary brain lymphoma almost always shows enhancement after intravenous contrast administration, although the pattern is quite variable and may be nodular, patchy, or ringlike (371). Enhancement results from both local alterations in the blood–brain barrier and neoplastic angiogenesis. Surrounding edema and some element of mass effect are the rule, and, rarely, there may be diffuse gyral enhancement (371).

Primary brain lymphoma is exquisitely sensitive to corticosteroids, and their use may be associated with a rapid and sometimes dramatic reduction in lesion size (370). However, because diagnosis can only be made with certainty by biopsy, preoperative steroid administration may actually hinder attempts to locate the lesion (370). Biopsy is facilitated by using a CT-guided stereotactic approach (110). Attempts at complete resection have been disappointing and resulted in a high incidence of severe neurological sequelae (370).

Although radiation and corticosteroids almost always result in initial improvement and probably prolong survival, prognosis remains depressingly poor, and death usually occurs within a few months (4,5). Intensive chemotherapy is increasingly used after radiation (369, 370,384), but neurological and systemic toxicities are significant (369,373). Bermudez et al. (369) reported a 52% response rate and a median survival of 7 months using a MACOP-B regimen (methotrexate, adriamycin, cyclophosphamide, vincristine, prednisone, and bleomycin). Patients without previous or concurrent opportunistic infection survived longer (369). Gill et al. (385) had a similar response rate (54%) using M-BACOD (dexamethasone substituted for prednisone), but only a 33% response rate using high-dose cytosine arabinoside and methotrexate.

Metastatic Lymphoma and Other Tumors

Systemic non-Hodgkin's lymphomas also occur with increased frequency in AIDS patients, and the CNS is commonly involved, probably more often than in non-HIV-infected populations (386,387). The pattern of CNS involvement with metastatic lymphoma is usually leptomeningeal or epidural (376). Thus the presentation of intracranial metastatic lymphoma is usually that of subacute meningitis with headache, lethargy, and cranial nerve palsies (383). Tumor deposits on spinal nerve roots cause radicular pain and segmental symptoms or signs (5,370). Epidural metastases, most often to the midthoracic spine, are common and frequently lead to spinal cord compression (5). Back pain is almost invariable. Other common findings are sensory loss, sphincter dysfunction, and paraparesis.

Diagnosis of meningeal lymphoma is made by cytological examination of CSF. Intrathecal chemotherapy using methotrexate and cytosine arabinoside is the mainstay of treatment. With spinal cord compression, decompressive surgery and radiotherapy may also be required.

Kaposi's sarcoma and other tumors only rarely affect the nervous system, and always in the setting of metastatic spread from systemic involvement. The neurological complications of metastatic Kaposi's sarcoma have been described (1,98,102,388,389), and brain parenchyma, dura, spinal cord, and nerve roots have all been sites of involvement. Immunoblastic sarcoma (390) has also metastasized to brain, and we and others (391) have seen patients with nasopharyngeal tumors that involve the brain by direct extension (Fig. 15). Rhabdomyosarcoma (392), plasmacytoma (393), and immunoblastic sarcoma (5) have metastasized to the epidural space and produced spinal cord compression. Two HIV-

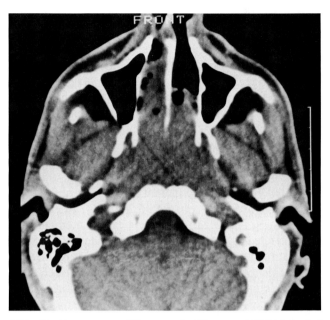

FIG. 15. Noncontrast CT scan of a 36-year-old HIV-infected man who presented with bilateral extraocular muscle palsies. Tumor mass fills the nasal passages and adjacent sinuses and, at higher levels, invaded the orbits (not shown). Biopsy revealed Burkitt's lymphoma.

seropositive patients developed rapidly progressive astrocytomas (394).

CEREBROVASCULAR DISEASE

Cerebral Infarction

Cerebral infarction and hemorrhage are not unusual in autopsy series of AIDS patients, with prevalence estimates ranging from 24% (66) to 34% (5,8,244,395). Nonetheless, cerebrovascular complications associated with AIDS have been diagnosed clinically in only 1.6% of adults (165) and 6% of children (66). Annual incidence rates of 0.75% (67) and 1.3% (66) have been estimated. Several reasons may account for the discrepancy between clinical and autopsy series. First, many cerebrovascular events probably occur late in the course of a patient's illness when new neurological symptoms or signs may be missed altogether, attributed to other, previously diagnosed neurological disease, or assumed to reflect preterminal hypoxia or hypotension. Second, cerebrovascular complications seem to be especially common in children with AIDS (66,95), an age group where they are not ordinarily suspected. Third, lesions may be "silent" because they are small or occur in areas of the brain that do not result in easily detectable clinical abnormalities (395). Finally, in our experience transient neurological disturbances occurring in patients with focal cerebral lesions are commonly attributed to seizures or postictal Todd's phenomena, often without adequate justification (67).

Cerebral infarction probably results from several mechanisms, although in half the cases, no presumptive cause can be identified (67). It is well established that mycobacteria, varicella zoster virus, and *T. pallidum* cause an infective arteritis that may lead to stroke (66,67,70,72,354,355) (Fig. 14), and that cryptococcal infection may be associated with transient ischemic attacks (274). In addition, occlusion of both small and medium to large vessels occurs from arteriopathies marked by endothelial prominence, fibrinoid deposits, intimal fibrodysplasia, and thickening of the vessel wall with variable inflammatory response (5,66,241–243,396–398). In some of these patients, the presence of intranuclear inclusions within endothelial or inflammatory cells, as well as more direct immunocytochemical evidence, have suggested an association with infective organisms, including CMV (19,215,294,399), the virus of PML (JC virus) (135), and, most convincingly, HIV (65). Vasculitis has been described in several patients with HIV infection, including one patient with simultaneous primary HIV and CMV infection (19), and another patient who developed a necrotizing vasculitis of the nervous system (399). Although it is tempting to speculate that some of the cerebrovascular complications seen in AIDS patients result from viral infection of vascular cells that either directly causes thrombotic occlusion (66,166,400) or indirectly mediates vascular injury through immune complex deposition (5,398,401,402), this mechanism remains hypothetical at the present time.

Cardiogenic emboli are another important cause of stroke in this group of patients. In addition to cardiomyopathy (66,403), both infective (2,6) and nonbacterial thrombotic (1,67) endocarditis may occur. Bacterial or fungal endocarditis is especially common in active intravenous drug users (2,6). Anticardiolipin antibodies or lupus anticoagulant (58,242) have been detected in up to half the AIDS patients surveyed, but the role of these "hypercoagulant" serum factors in producing cerebral infarction is unclear.

Cerebral Hemorrhage

Cerebral hemorrhage is easily diagnosed by CT scan (97) (Fig. 16), and additional cases are discovered at autopsy (8,9,56,244). Like cerebral infarction, there are several reasons for the increased frequency of hemorrhage in AIDS patients. Both adults and children with AIDS develop idiopathic thrombocytopenic purpura (ITP) on an autoimmune basis (56,57). ITP may appear early or late in the course of HIV infection and is often asymptomatic. However, Landonio et al. (56) rated the thrombocytopenia as severe in 5.3% of a group of HIV-seropositive drug users. Ratner et al. (54) found platelet

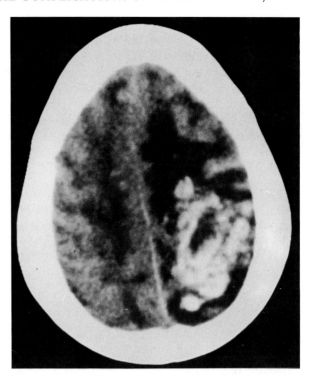

FIG. 16. Noncontrast scan of 28-year-old HIV-infected woman with thrombocytopenia who collapsed with sudden onset of right hemiplegia and the rapid development of coma. There is a large, multilobulated hyperdense area with surrounding edema and mass effect consistent with intraparenchymal hemorrhage.

counts less than 100,000/mm³ in 9% of intravenous drug users and in 3% of homosexual men who were HIV seropositive. Development of thrombocytopenia correlated with falling CD4 cell counts.

Hemophilia (57), aneurysmal dilatation (66), mycotic aneurysms (usually in intravenous drug users) (6), and CNS aspergillosis predispose to cerebral hemorrhage. Bleeding into metastatic Kaposi's sarcoma has been described (388,389).

CONCLUSION

Although HIV infection has devastating consequences for the central and peripheral nervous systems, some specific therapies and preventive measures are being developed. In addition, mass lesions, meningitis, and spinal cord disease caused by opportunistic infections or lymphoma are now well characterized, clinically diagnosable, and often treatable. It is important that all clinicians be aware of how HIV infection affects the nervous system and have an organized approach to diagnosis and treatment whenever possible. All patients can, at the least, be offered symptomatic relief and meaningful supportive care.

ACKNOWLEDGMENTS

I thank my husband, Dr. Timothy A. Pedley, for editing the manuscript and watching our children. I am grateful to Ken Bailey for excellent photography; to Shirley Susarchick and Amelia Gulston for expert typing; and to the patients and staff of Metropolitan Hospital, especially Dr. Ted Lenox, for teaching me about AIDS and the nervous system.

REFERENCES

1. Levy RM, Bredesen DE, Rosenblum ML. Neurological manifestations of the acquired immunodeficiency syndrome (AIDS). Experience at UCSF and review of the literature. *J Neurosurg* 1985;62:475–95.
2. McArthur JC. Neurologic manifestations of AIDS. *Medicine* 1987;66:408–37.
3. Berger JR, Moskowitz L, Fischl M, Kelley RE. Neurologic disease as the presenting manifestation of acquired immunodeficiency syndrome. *South Med J* 1987;80:683–6.
4. Koppel BS, Wormser GP, Tuchman AJ, Maayan S, Hewlett D Jr, Daras M. Central nervous system involvement in patients with acquired immunodeficiency syndrome (AIDS). *Acta Neurol Scand* 1985;71:337–53.
5. Snider WD, Simpson DM, Nielsen S, Gold JWM, Metroka CE, Posner JB. Neurological complications of acquired immunodeficiency syndrome. Analysis of 50 patients. *Ann Neurol* 1983;14:403–18.
6. Malouf R, Jacquette G, Dobkin J, Brust JCM. Neurologic disease in human immunodeficiency virus-infected drug abusers. *Arch Neurol* 1990;47:1002–7.
7. Lantos PL, McLaughlin JE, Scholtz CL, Berry CL, Tighe JR. Neuropathology of the brain in HIV infection. *Lancet* 1989;1:309–11.
8. Anders KH, Guerra WF, Tomiyasu U, Verity MA, Vinters HV. The neuropathology of AIDS. UCLA experience and review. *Am J Pathol* 1986;124:537–58.
9. Lemann W, Cho E-S, Nielsen S, Petito C. Neuropathologic findings in 104 cases of acquired immune deficiency syndrome (AIDS): an autopsy study. *J Neuropathol Exp Neurol* 1985;44:349A.
10. Levy RM, Bredesen DE, Rosenblum ML. Opportunistic central nervous system pathology in patients with AIDS. *Ann Neurol* 1988;23(suppl):S7–12.
11. Wechsler AF, Ho DD. Bilateral Bell's palsy at the time of HIV seroconversion. *Neurology* 1989;39:747–8.
12. Vendrell J, Heredia C, Pujol M, Vidal J, Blesa R, Grans F. Guillain-Barré syndrome associated with seroconversion for anti-HTLV-III. *Neurology* 1987;37:544.
13. Carne CA, Smith A, Elkington SG, et al. Acute encephalopathy coincident with seroconversion for anti-HTLV-III. *Lancet* 1985;1206–8.
14. Calabrese LH, Proffitt MR, Levin KH, Yen-Lieberman B, Starkey C. Acute infection with the human immunodeficiency virus (HIV) associated with acute brachial neuritis and exanthematous rash. *Ann Intern Med* 1987;107:849–51.
15. Elder G, Dalakas M, Pezeshkpour G, Sever J. Ataxic neuropathy due to ganglioneuronitis after probable acute human immunodeficiency virus infection. *Lancet* 1986;2:1275–6.
16. Dodson D. Transverse myelitis and spastic paraparesis in a patient with HIV infection. *N Engl J Med* 1990;322:1322.
17. Denning D, Anderson J, Rudge P, et al. Acute myelopathy associated with primary infection with human immunodeficiency virus. *Br Med J* 1987;294:143–4.
18. Piette AM, Tusseau F, Vignon D, Chapman A, Parrot G, Leibowitch J, Montagnier L. Acute neuropathy coincident with seroconversion for anti-LAV/HTLV-III. *Lancet* 1986;1:852.
19. Meyrhas M-C, Roullet E, Rouzioux C, Aymard A, Pelosse B, Eliascriwicz M, Frottier J. Cerebral venous thrombosis and dual primary infection with human immunodeficiency virus and cytomegalovirus. *J Neurol Neurosurg Psychiatry* 1989;52:1010–16.
20. del Rio C, Soffer O, Widell JL, Judd RL, Slade BA. Acute human immunodeficiency virus infection temporally associated with rhabdomyolysis, acute renal failure, and nephrosis. *Rev Infect Dis* 1990;12:282–5.
21. Koralnik IJ, Beaumanoir A, Hansle R, et al. A controlled study of early neurologic abnormalities in men with asymptomatic human immunodeficiency virus infection. *N Engl J Med* 1990;323:864–70.
22. Resnick L. Sleep disorders may be early sign of CNS infection with AIDS virus. 3rd International Conference on AIDS, Washington, DC, June 1987, abstract.
23. Rosenhall U, Hokansson C, Lowhagen G-B, Hanner P, Jonsson-Ehk B. Otoneurological abnormalities in asymptomatic HIV-seropositive patients. *Acta Neurol Scand* 1989;79:140–5.
24. Frank Y, Vishnubhakut SM, Pahwa S. Brainstem auditory evoked responses in infants and children with acquired immunodeficiency syndrome. *Ann Neurol* 1990;28:460A.
25. Goodin DS, Aminoff MJ, Chernoff DN, Hollander H. Long latency event-related potentials in patients infected with human immunodeficiency virus. *Ann Neurol* 1990;27:414–9.
26. Ollo C, Johnson R Jr, Grafman J. Signs of cognitive change in HIV disease: an event-related brain potential study. *Neurology* 1991;41:209–15.
27. Mayeux R, Dooneief G, Todak G, et al. A prospective study of magnetic resonance in parenteral drug users with human immunodeficiency virus. *Ann Neurol* 1990;28:221A.
28. Sonnerborg A, Saaf J, Alexius B, Strannegard O, Wahlund LO, Wetterberg L. Quantitative detection of brain aberrations in human immunodeficiency virus type I infected individuals by magnetic resonance imaging. *J Infect Dis* 1990;162:1245–51.
29. Singer E, Syndulko K, Ruane P, Fahy-Chandon B, Silbar C, Resnick L, Tourtellotte WW. Magnetic resonance imaging findings in human immunodeficiency virus-positive and high-risk seronegative subjects. *Ann Neurol* 1989;26:154A.
30. McArthur JC, Kumar AJ, Johnson R Jr, et al. Incidental white matter hyperintensities on magnetic resonance imaging in HIV-1 infection. *J AIDS* 1990;3:252–9.
31. Kieburtz KD, Ketonen L, Zettelmaier AE, Kido D, Kaine ED, Simon JH. Magnetic resonance imaging findings in HIV cognitive impairment. *Arch Neurol* 1990;47:643–5.
32. Grant I, Atkinson JH, Hesselink JR, et al. Evidence for early central nervous system infection in the acquired immunodeficiency syndrome (AIDS) and other human immunodeficiency virus (HIV) infections. *Ann Intern Med* 1987;107:828–36.
33. Rolfs A, Schumacher HC. Early findings in the cerebrospinal fluid of patients with HIV-1 infection of the central nervous system. *N Engl J Med* 1990;323:418–9.
34. Elovaara I, Iivanainen M, Valle S-L, Suni J, Terro T, Lahdevirt J. CSF protein and cellular properties in various stages of HIV infection related to neurological manifestations. *J Neurol Sci* 1987;78:331–42.
35. Goudsmit J, Paul DA, Lange JMA, et al. Expression of human immunodeficiency virus antigen (HIV-Ag) in serum and cerebrospinal fluid during acute and chronic infection. *Lancet* 1986;2:177–80.
36. McArthur JC, Cohen BA, Farzedegan H. Cerebrospinal fluid abnormalities in homosexual men with and without neuropsychiatric findings. *Ann Neurol* 1988;23:S34–7.
37. Shaunak S, Albright RE, Klotman ME, Henry SC, Bartlett JA, Hamilton JD. Amplification of HIV-1 provirus from cerebrospinal fluid and its correlation with neurologic disease. *J Infect Dis* 1990;161:1068–72.
38. Schielke E, Tatsch K, Pfister W, et al. Reduced cerebral blood flow in early stages of human immunodeficiency virus infection. *Arch Neurol* 1990;47:1342–5.
39. Wilkie FL, Eisdorfer C, Morgan R, Loewenstein DA, Szapolznik J. Cognition in early human immunodeficiency virus infection. *Arch Neurol* 1990;47:433–40.
40. Janssen RS, Saykin AJ, Kaplan JE, et al. Neurological complications of human immunodeficiency virus infection in patients with lymphadenopathy syndrome. *Ann Neurol* 1988;23:49–55.

41. Mayeux R, Stern Y, Marder K, et al. Cognitive manifestations precede other neurological signs with human immunodeficiency virus. *Ann Neurol* 1989;26:152.

42. Cornblath DR, McArthur JC, Kennedy PGE, Witte AS, Griffin JW. Inflammatory demyelinating peripheral neuropathies associated with human T-cell lymphotropic virus type III infection. *Ann Neurol* 1987;21:32–40.

43. Miller RG, Parry G, Lang W, Lippert R, Kiprov DD. AIDS-related inflammatory polyradiculo-neuropathy. Successful treatment with plasma exchange. *Neurology* 1986;36(suppl):206.

44. Miller RG, Kiprov DD, Parry G, Bredesen DG. Peripheral nervous system dysfunction in acquired immunodeficiency syndrome. In: Rosenblum LP, et al, eds. *AIDS and the nervous system.* New York: Raven Press; 1988:65–78.

45. Dalakas MC, Pezeshkpour GH. Neuromuscular disease associated with human immunodeficiency virus infection. *Ann Neurol* 1988;23:1538–48.

46. Kiprov D, Pfaeffl W, Parry G, Lippert R, Lang W, Miller R. Antibody-mediated peripheral neuropathies associated with ARC and AIDS: successful treatment with plasmapheresis. *J Clin Apheresis* 1988;4:3–7.

47. Said G, Lacroix-Ciando C, Fujimura H, Blas C, Faux N. The peripheral neuropathy of necrotizing arteritis: a clinicopathological study. *Ann Neurol* 1988;23:461–5.

48. Lipkin WI, Parry G, Kiprov D, Abrams D. Inflammatory neuropathy in homosexual men with lymphadenopathy. *Neurology* 1985;35:1479–83.

49. Gherardi R, Lebargy F, Gaulard P, et al. Necrotizing vasculitis and HIV replication in peripheral nerves. *N Engl J Med* 1989;321:685–6.

50. Belec L, Gherardi R, Georges AJ, et al. Peripheral facial paralysis and HIV infection: report of four African cases and review of the literature. *J Neurol* 1989;236:411–4.

51. Dalakas MC, Pezeshkpour GH, Grant M, et al. Polymyositis associated with AIDS retrovirus. *JAMA* 1986;256:2381–3.

52. Simpson DM, Bender AN, Farraye J, Mendelson S, Wolfe DE. AIDS wasting syndrome may represent a treatable myopathy. *Neurology* 1990;40:535–8.

53. Nath A, Kerman RH, Novak IS, Wolinsky JS. Immune studies in human immunodeficiency virus infection with myasthenia gravis: a case report. *Neurology* 1990;40:581–3.

54. Ratner L. Human immunodeficiency (virus-associated) autoimmune thrombocytopenic purpura: a review. *Am J Med* 1989;86:194–8.

55. Pena JM, Arnalich F, Barbado FJ, Diminguez A, Mostazi J, Valencia ME, Vazquez JJ. Successful zidovudine therapy for HIV-related severe thrombocytopenia. *Acta Haematol (Basel)* 1990;83:86–8.

56. Landonio G, Galli M, Nosari A, et al. HIV-related severe thrombocytopenia in intravenous drug users: prevalence, response to therapy in a medium-term follow-up, and pathogenetic evaluation. *AIDS* 1990;4:29–34.

57. Ragni MV, Bontempo FA, Myers DJ, Kiss JE, Oral A. Hemorrhagic sequelae of immune thrombocytopenic purpura in human immunodeficiency virus-infected hemophiliacs. *Blood* 1990;75:1267–72.

58. Gold JE, Haubenstock A, Zalusky R. Lupus anticoagulant and AIDS. *N Engl J Med* 1986;314:1252–3.

59. Levy JA. Human immunodeficiency viruses and the pathogenesis of AIDS. *JAMA* 1989;261:2997–3006.

60. Centers for Disease Control. Revision of the CDC surveillance case definition for acquired immunodeficiency syndrome. *MMWR* 1987;36(suppl):1S–15S.

61. Navia BA, Cho E-S, Petito CK, Price RW. The AIDS dementia complex II. Neuropathology. *Ann Neurol* 1986;19:525–35.

62. Navia BA, Jordan BD, Price RW. The AIDS dementia complex I. Clinical features. *Ann Neurol* 1986;19:517–24.

63. Price RW, Sidtis J, Rosenblum M. The AIDS dementia complex: some current questions. *Ann Neurol* 1988;23(suppl):S27–33.

64. McArthur JC, Becker PS, Parisi JE. Neuropathological changes in early HIV-I dementia. *Ann Neurol* 1989;26:681–4.

65. Rosemberg S, Lopes MBS, Tsanaclis AM. Neuropathology of acquired immunodeficiency syndrome (AIDS). Analysis of 22 Brazilian cases. *J Neurol Sci* 1986;76:187–98.

66. Park YD, Belman AL, Kim TS. Stroke in pediatiric acquired immunodeficiency syndrome. *Ann Neurol* 1990;28:303–11.

67. Engstrom JW, Lowenstein DH, Bredesen DE. Cerebral infarctions and transient neurologic deficits associated with acquired immunodeficiency syndrome. *Am J Med* 1989;86:528–32.

68. Tramont EC. Neurosyphilis and HIV infection. *N Engl J Med* 1987;317:1475.

69. Matlow AG, Rachlis AR. Syphilis serology in human immunodeficiency virus-infected patients with symptomatic neurosyphilis. Case report and review. *Rev Infect Dis* 1990;12:703–7.

70. Morgello S, Laufer H. Quaternary neurosyphilis. *N Engl J Med* 1988;319:1549–50.

71. Musher DM, Hamill RJ, Baughn RE. Effect of human immunodeficiency virus (HIV) infection on the course of syphilis and on the response to treatment. *Ann Intern Med* 1990;113:872–81.

72. Johns DR, Tierney M, Felsenstein D. Alteration in the natural history of neurosyphilis by concurrent infection with the human immunodeficiency virus. *N Engl J Med* 1987;316:1569–72.

73. Schaumburg HH, Arezz J, Berger A. Dideoxycytidine (DDC) in HIV infections: a report of 52 patients. *Neurology* 1990;40(suppl 1):248.

74. Lambert JS, Seidlin M, Reichman RC, et al. 2′3′-Dideoxyinosine (ddI) in patients with the acquired immunodeficiency syndrome or AIDS-related complex: a phase I trial. *N Engl J Med* 1990;322:1333–40.

75. Bach MC. Clinical responses to dideoxyinosine in patients with HIV infection resistant to zidovudine. *N Engl J Med* 1990;323:275.

76. Gertner E, Thurn JR, Williams DN, Simpson M, Balfour HH Jr, Rhame F, Henry K. Zidovudine-associated myopathy. *Am J Med* 1989;86:814–8.

77. Arnaudo E, Dalakas M, Shanske S, Moraes CT, DiMauro S, Schon EA. Depletion of muscle mitochondria DNA in AIDS patients with AZT-induced myopathy. *Lancet* 1991;1:508–11.

78. Dalakas MC, Illa I, Pezeshkpour GH, Laukaitis JP, Bohen B, Griffin JL. Mitochondrial myopathy caused by long-term zidovudine therapy. *N Engl J Med* 1990;332:1098–105.

79. Davtyan DG, Vinters HV. Wernicke's encephalopathy in AIDS patient treated with zidovudine. *Lancet* 1987;1:919–20.

80. Harris PJ, Caceras CA. Azidothymidine in the treatment of AIDS. *N Engl J Med* 1989;318:250.

81. Richman DD, Fischl MA, Grieco MH. The toxicity of azidothymidine (AZT) in the treatment of patients with AIDS and AIDS-related complex. *N Engl J Med* 1987;317:192–7.

82. Yarchoan R, Klecker RW, Weinhold KJ, et al. Administration of 3′-azido-3′-deoxythymidine, an inhibitor of HTLV-III LAV replication, to patients with AIDS or AIDS-related complex. *Lancet* 1986;1:575–80.

83. Gold JWM, Leyland-Jones B, Urmacher C, Armstrong D. Pulmonary and neurologic complications of treatment with FIAC (2′-fluoro-5-iodo-aracytosine) in patients with acquired immunodeficiency syndrome (AIDS). *AIDS Res* 1987;1:243–52.

84. Garcia PA, Messing RO, Simon RP. Acute compound Q neurotoxicity in previously asymptomatic HIV seropositive patients. *Neurology* 1990;40(suppl):235.

85. Joffe AM, Farley JD, Linden D, Goldsand GS. Trimethoprim-sulfamethoxazole-associated aseptic meningitis: case reports and review of the literature. *Am J Med* 1989;87:332–8.

86. Helmich CG, Green JK. Pentamidine-associated hypotension and route of administration. *Ann Intern Med* 1985;103:480.

87. Sands M, Kron MA, Brown RB. Pentamidine: a review. *Rev Infect Dis* 1985;7:625–34.

88. Wong MC, Suite NDA, Labar DR. Seizures in human immunodeficiency virus infection. *Arch Neurol* 1990;47:640–2.

89. Holtzman DM, Kaku DA, So YT. New-onset seizures associated with human immunodeficiency virus infection: causation and clinical features in 100 cases. *Am J Med* 1989;87:173–7.

90. Edelstein H, Knight RT. Severe parkinsonism in two AIDS patients taking prochlorperazine. *Lancet* 1987;2:341–2.

91. Hollander H, Golden J, Mendelson T, Cortland D. Extrapyramidal symptoms in AIDS patients given low dose metoclopramide or chlorpromazine. *Lancet* 1985;2:1186.

92. Britton CB, Marquardt MD, Koppel B, Garvey G, Miller JR. Neurologic complications of the gay immunosuppressed syn-

drome. Clinical and pathological features. *Ann Neurol* 1982;12:80A.

93. Roue R, Debord T, Denamur E, et al. Diagnosis of toxoplasma encephalitis in absence of neurologic signs by early computed tomographic scanning in patients with AIDS. *Lancet* 1984; 2:1472.

94. de la Paz R, Enzmann D. Neuroradiology of acquired immunodeficiency syndrome. In: Rosenblum ML, Levy RM, Bredesen D, eds. *AIDS and the nervous system.* New York: Raven Press; 1988:121–53.

95. Belman AL, Ultmann MH, Horoupian D, et al. Neurological complications in infants and children with acquired immunodeficiency syndrome. *Ann Neurol* 1985;18:560–6.

96. Post MJD, Kursunoglu SJ, Hensley GT, Chan JC, Moskowitz LB, Hoffman TA. Cranial CT of the acquired immune deficiency syndrome (AIDS): spectrum of disease and optimal contrast enhancement technique. *Am J Roent* 1985;145:929–40.

97. Elkin CM, Leon E, Grenell SL, Leeds NE. Intracranial lesions in the acquired immunodeficiency syndrome. Radiological (computed tomographic) features. *JAMA* 1985;253:393–6.

98. Post MJD, Sheldon JJ, Hensley GT, et al. Central nervous system disease in acquired immunodeficiency syndrome: prospective correlation using CT, MR imaging and pathologic studies. *Radiology* 1986;158:141–8.

99. Navia BA, Petito CK, Gold JWM, Cho E-S, Jordan BD, Price RW. Cerebral toxoplasmosis complicating the acquired immune deficiency syndrome: clinical and neuropathological findings in 27 patients. *Ann Neurol* 1986;19:224–38.

100. Whelan MA, Kricheff II, Handler M, Ho V, Crystal K, Gopinathan G, Laubenstein LL. Acquired immunodeficiency syndrome: cerebral computed tomographic manifestations. *Radiology* 1983;149:477–84.

101. Enzmann DR, Brant-Zawadzki M, Britt RM. CT of central nervous system infections in immunocompromised patients. *AJNR* 1980;1:239–43.

102. Kelly WM, Brant-Zawadzki, Britt RH. CT of central nervous system infections in immunocompromised patients. *Am J Radiol* 1980;135:263–7.

103. Cohn JA, McMeeking A, Cohen W, Jacobs J, Holzman RS. Evaluation of the policy of empiric treatment of suspected toxoplasma encephalitis in patients with the acquired immunodeficiency syndrome. *Am J Med* 1989;86:521–7.

104. Leport C, Raffi F, Matheron S, et al. Treatment of central nervous system toxoplasmosis with pyrimethamine/sulfadiazine combination in 35 patients with the acquired immunodeficiency syndrome. Efficacy of long-term continuous therapy. *Am J Med* 1988;84:94–9.

105. Jarvik JG, Hesselink JR, Kennedy C, et al. Acquired immunodeficiency syndrome. Magnetic resonance patterns of brain involvement with pathologic correlation. *Arch Neurol* 1988;45:731–6.

106. Levy RM, Rosenbloom S, Perrett LV. Neuroradiological findings in acquired immunodeficiency syndrome (AIDS): a review of 200 cases. *AJNR* 1986;7:833–9.

107. Krupp LB, Lipton RB, Swerdlow ML, Leeds NE, Llena J. Progressive multifocal leukoencephalopathy: clinical and radiographic features. *Ann Neurol* 1985;17:344–9.

108. Chaisson RE, Griffin DE. Progressive multifocal leukoencephalopathy in AIDS. *JAMA* 1990;264:79–82.

109. Chang KH, Han MH, Roh JK, Kim IO, Han MC, Kim C-W. Gd-DTPA-enhanced MR imaging of the brain in patients with meningitis: comparison with CT. *AJNR* 1990;11:69–76.

110. O'Neill BP, Kelly PJ, Earle JD, Scheithauer B, Banks PM. Computer-assisted stereotaxic biopsy for the diagnosis of primary central nervous system lymphoma. *Neurology* 1987;37:1160–4.

111. Denton IC, Stevens EA, Seidenfeld SM, Cramer CR, Esber JW, Weathers SB. The diagnosis of intracranial lesions in AIDS. *JAMA* 1985;253:3398.

112. Zuger A, Louie E, Holzman RS, Simberkoff MS, Rahal JJ. Cryptococcal disease in patients with acquired immunodeficiency syndrome: diagnostic features and outcome of treatment. *Ann Intern Med* 1986;104:234–40.

113. Eisenach KD, Cave MD, Bates JH, Crawford JT. Polymerase chain reaction amplification of a repetitive DNA sequence spe-

cific for *Mycobacterium tuberculosis. J Infect Dis* 1990;161: 977–81.

114. Portegies P, Epstein LG, Hung STA, de Gans J, Goudsmit J. Human immunodeficiency virus type I antigen in cerebrospinal fluid. *Arch Neurol* 1989;46:261–4.

115. Schmid P, Conrad A, Tourtellotte WW, Syndulko K, Singer E, Singer P. Polymerase chain reaction of cerebrospinal fluid in human immunodeficiency virus neurological disease. *Ann Neurol* 1990;28:252A.

116. Prabhakar S, Oommen A. ELISA using mycobacterial antigens as a diagnostic aid for tuberculous meningitis. *J Neurol Sci* 1987;78:203–11.

117. Farber C-M, Yernault J-C, Legros F, Debruyn J, Van Vooren J-P. Detection of anti-p32 mycobacterial IgG antibodies in patients with AIDS. *J Infect Dis* 1990;162:279–80.

118. Haas JS, Bolan G, Larsen SA, Clement MJ, Bacchetti P, Moss AR. Sensitivity of treponemal tests for detecting prior treated syphilis during human immunodeficiency virus infection. *J Infect Dis* 1990;162:862–6.

119. Davis LE. Neurosyphilis in the patient infected with human immunodeficiency virus. *Ann Neurol* 1990;27:211–2.

120. Berger JR, McCarthy M. Neurosyphilis in patients infected with human immunodeficiency virus. *Ann Neurol* 1990;27:213.

121. Chiodi F, Asjo B, Fenyo EM, Norkrans G, Hagberg L, Albert J. Isolation of human immunodeficiency virus from cerebrospinal fluid of antibody-positive virus carrier without neurological symptoms. *Lancet* 1986;2:1276–7.

122. Resnick L, DiMarzo-Veronese F, Schupbach J, et al. Intrablood–brain-barrier synthesis of HTLV-III-specific IgG in patients with neurologic symptoms associated with AIDS or AIDS-related complex. *N Engl J Med* 1985;313:1498–504.

123. Van Wielink G, McArthur JC, Moench T, Farzadegan H, McArthur JH, Johnson RT, Saah A. Intrathecal synthesis of anti-HIV IgG: correlation with increasing duration of HIV-I infection. *Neurology* 1990;40:816–9.

124. Whitley RJ. Viral encephalitis. *N Engl J Med* 1990;323:242–50.

125. Miller JR, Barrett RE, Britton CB, et al. Progressive multifocal leukoencephalopathy in a male homosexual with T-cell immune deficiency. *N Engl J Med* 1982;307:1436–8.

126. Levy JA, Shimabukuro J, Hollander H, Mills J, Kaminsky L. Isolation of AIDS-associated retroviruses from cerebrospinal fluid and brain of patients with neurological symptoms. *Lancet* 1985;2:586–8.

127. Ho DD, Rota MA, Schooley RT, et al. Isolation of HTLV-III from cerebrospinal fluid and neural tissues of patients with neurological syndromes related to acquired immunodeficiency syndrome. *N Engl J Med* 1985;313:1493–7.

128. Gabuzda DH, Levy SR, Chiappa KH. Electroencephalography in AIDS and AIDS-related complex. *Clin EEG* 1988;19:1–6.

129. Parisi A, Strosselli M, DiPerri G, et al. Electroencephalography in the early diagnosis of HIV-related subacute encephalitis: analysis of 185 patients. *Clin EEG* 1989;20:1–5.

130. Parisi A, DiPerri G, Strossell M, Nappi G, Minol L, Rondanelli EG. Usefulness of computerized electroencephalography in diagnosing, staging and monitoring AIDS-dementia complex. *AIDS* 1989;3:209–13.

131. Emerson R, Kairam R, Younger D, Labar D, Pedley TA. Median nerve somatosensory evoked potentials in patients with human immunodeficiency virus infection. *J Clin Neurophys* 1989;72:97.

132. Ioachim HL. Biopsy diagnosis in human immunodeficiency virus infection and acquired immunodeficiency syndrome. *Arch Pathol Lab Med* 1990;114:284–94.

133. Moskowitz LB, Hensley GT, Chan JC, Conley FK, Post MJD, Gonzalez-Arias SM. Brain biopsies in patients with acquired immune deficiency syndrome. *Arch Pathol Lab Med* 1984;108: 368–71.

134. Wormser GP. Multiple opportunistic infections and neoplasms in the acquired immunodeficiency syndrome. *JAMA* 1984;253: 3441–2.

135. Sharer LR, Kapila R. Neuropathologic observations in acquired immunodeficiency syndrome (AIDS). *Acta Neuropathol (Berl)* 1985;66:188–98.

136. Fischl MA, Pitchenik AE, Spira TJ. Tuberculous brain abscess

and toxoplasma encephalitis in a patient with the acquired immunodeficiency syndrome. *JAMA* 1985;253:3428–30.

137. Pitchenik A, Fischl M, Walls K. Evaluation of cerebral mass lesions in acquired immunodeficiency syndrome. *N Engl J Med* 1983;308:1099.

138. Pitlik SD, Rios A, Hersh EM, Bolivar R, Mansell PWA. Polymicrobial brain abscess in a homosexual man with Kaposi's sarcoma. *South Med J* 1984;77:271–2.

139. Bottone EJ, Toma M, Johansson BE, et al. Capsule-deficient *Cryptococcus neoformans* in AIDS patients. *Lancet* 1985;1:400.

140. Case records of the Massachusetts General Hospital, Case Number 33 1989. *N Engl J Med* 1989;321:454–63.

141. Bredesen DE, Lipkin WI, Massing R. Prolonged recurrent aseptic meningitis with prominent cranial nerve abnormalities: a new epidemic in gay men. *Neurology* 1981;31(suppl 2):85.

142. Hollander H, Stringari S. Human immunodeficiency virus-associated meningitis. *Am J Med* 1987;83:813–6.

143. Sharer RW, Offitt TK, Macris NJ, et al. Possible risk of steroid administration in patients at risk for AIDS. *Lancet* 1985;1:934–5.

144. Heyes MP, Rubinow D, Lane C, Markey SP. Cerebrospinal fluid quinolinic acid concentrations are increased in acquired immune deficiency syndrome. *Ann Neurol* 1989;26:275–7.

145. Heyes MP, Brew BJ, Martin A, et al. Quinolinic acid in cerebrospinal fluid and serum in HIV-1 infection: relationship to clinical and neurological status. *Ann Neurol* 1991;29:202–9.

146. Heyes MP, Mefford IN, Quearry BJ, Dedhia M, Lackner A. Increased ratio of quinolinic acid to kynurenic acid in cerebrospinal fluid of D retrovirus-infected rhesus macaques: relationship to clinical and viral status. *Ann Neurol* 1990;27:666–75.

147. Brew BJ, Bhalla RB, Paul M, Gallardo H, McArthur JC, Schwartz MK, Price RW. Cerebrospinal fluid neopterin in human immunodeficiency virus type I infection. *Ann Neurol* 1990;28:556–60.

148. Griffin DE, McArthur JC, Cornblath DR. Neopterin and interferon-gamma in serum and cerebrospinal fluid of patients with HIV associated neurologic disease. *Neurology* 1991;41:69–74.

149. Ho DD, Bredesen DE, Vinters HV, Daar ES. The acquired immunodeficiency syndrome (AIDS) dementia complex. *Ann Intern Med* 1989;111:400–10.

150. Grimaldi LME, Martino GV, Franciotta DM, Brustia R, Castagna A, Pristera R, Lazzarin A. Elevated alpha-tumor necrosis factor levels in spinal fluid from HIV-1-infected patients with central nervous system involvement. *Ann Neurol* 1991;29:21–5.

151. Brew BJ, Bhalla RB, Fleisher M, et al. Cerebrospinal fluid beta-2-microglobulin in patients infected with human immunodeficiency virus. *Neurology* 1989;39:830–4.

152. Harter DH. Neuropsychological status of asymptomatic individuals, seropositive to HIV-1. *Ann Neurol* 1989;26:589–91.

153. Sidtis JJ, Price RW. Early HIV-1 infection and the AIDS dementia complex. *Neurology* 1990;40:323–6.

154. Selnes OA, Miller E, McArthur J, et al. HIV-I infection: no evidence of cognitive decline during the asymptomatic stages. *Neurology* 1990;40:204–8.

155. Price RW, Brew B, Sidtis J, Rosenblum M, Scheck AC, Cleary P. The brain in AIDS: central nervous system HIV-I infection and AIDS dementia complex. *Science* 1988;239:586–92.

156. Currie J, Benson E, Ramsden B, Perdico M, Cooper D. Eye movement abnormalities as a predictor of the acquired immunodeficiency syndrome dementia complex. *Arch Neurol* 1988;45:949–53.

157. Deickon RF, Hubesch B, Jensen PC, et al. Alterations in brain phosphate metabolite concentrations in patients with human immunodeficiency virus infection. *Arch Neurol* 1991;48:203–9.

158. Brunetti A, Berg G, Yarchoan R, et al. PET-FDG studies in patients with AIDS related dementia: effect of treatment with azidothymidine. *J Nucl Med* 1988;29:163.

159. Rottenberg DA, Moella JR, Strother SC, et al. The metabolic pathology of the AIDS dementia complex. *Ann Neurol* 1987;22:700–6.

160. Yarchoan R, Berg G, Brouwers P, et al. Response of human-immunodeficiency-virus associated neurological disease to 3'-azido-3'-deoxythymidine. *Lancet* 1987;1:132–5.

161. Johnson KA, Worth J, Holman L, Navia B. SPECT in AIDS dementia complex. *Neurology* 1991;41(suppl):253.

162. Kramer EL, Sanger JJ. Brain imaging in acquired immunodeficiency syndrome dementia complex. *Semin Nucl Med* 1990;20:353–63.

163. Shaw GM, Harper ME, Hahn BH, et al. HTLV-III infection in brains of children and adults with AIDS encephalopathy. *Science* 1985;227:177–82.

164. Gabuzda DM, Ho DD, de la Monte SM, Hirsch MS, Rota TR, Sobel RA. Immunohistochemical identification of HTLV-III antigen in brain of patients with AIDS. *Ann Neurol* 1986;20:289–95.

165. Levy RM, Bredesen DE. Central nervous system dysfunction in acquired immunodeficiency syndrome. In: Rosenblem ML, et al, eds. *AIDS and the nervous system*. New York: Raven Press; 1988:29–63.

166. Epstein LG, Sharer LR, Joshi VV, Fojas MM, Koenigsberger MR, Oleske JM. Progressive encephalopathy in children: acquired immune deficiency syndrome. *Ann Neurol* 1985;17:488–96.

167. Scott GB, Hutto C, Makuch RW, et al. Survival in children with perinatally acquired human immunodeficiency virus type I infection. *N Engl J Med* 1989;321:1791–6.

168. Ultmann MH, Belman AL, Ruff HA, et al. Developmental abnormalities in infants and children with acquired immune deficiency syndrome (AIDS) and AIDS-related complex. *Dev Med Child Neurol* 1985;27:563–71.

169. Chamberlain MC, Press GA, Nichols S, Chase C. Pediatric acquired immunodeficiency syndrome: comparative magnetic resonance and computed tomographic brain imaging. *Ann Neurol* 1990;28:459.

170. Ketzler S, Weis S, Haung H, Budka H. Loss of neurons in the frontal cortex in AIDS brains. *Acta Neuropathol (Berl)* 1990;80:92–4.

171. Nath A, Jankovic J, Pettigrew LC. Movement disorders and AIDS. *Neurology* 1987;37:37–41.

172. Metzer WS. Movement disorders with AIDS encephalopathy: case report. *Neurology* 1987;37:1438.

173. Singer C, Sanchez-Ramos J, Rey G, Levin B, Weiner WJ. Acquired immune deficiency syndrome dementia complex presenting as an unusual unilateral hand tremor, clumsiness, and posturing. *Ann Neurol* 1990;28:301A.

174. De La Monte SM, Moore T, Hedley-Whyte ET. Vacuolar encephalopathy of AIDS. *N Engl J Med* 1986;315:1549–50.

175. Ho DD, Pomeratz RJ, Kaplan JC. Pathogenesis of infection with human immunodeficiency virus. *N Engl J Med* 1987;317:278–86.

176. Peudenier S, Hery C, Montagnier L, Tardieu M. Human microglial cells: characterization in cerebral tissue and in primary culture, and study of their susceptibility to HIV-I infection. *Ann Neurol* 1991;29:152–61.

177. Harouse JM, Wroblewska Z, Laughlin MA, Hickey WF, Schonwetter BS, Gonzalez-Scarano F. Human choroid plexus cells can be latently infected with human immunodeficiency virus. *Ann Neurol* 1989;25:406–11.

178. Wiley CA, Schrier RD, Nelson JA, Lampert PW, Oldstone MBA. Cellular localization of human immunodeficiency virus infection within the brains of acquired immunodeficiency patients. *Proc Natl Acad Sci USA* 1986;83:7089–93.

179. Giulian D, Vaca K, Noonan CA. Secretion of neurotoxins by mononuclear phagocytes infected with HIV-I. *Science* 1990;250:1593–6.

180. Dreyer EB, Kaiser PK, Offermann JT, Lipton SA. HIV-I coat protein neurotoxicity prevented by calcium channel antagonists. *Science* 1990;1248:364–7.

181. Sabatier JM, Vives E, Mabrouk K. Evidence for neurotoxic activity of *Tat* from human immunodeficiency virus type 1. *J Virol* 1991;65:961–7.

182. Altstiel LD, Sperber K, Mayer L. Human glial cells infected with human immunodeficiency virus type 1 produce interleukin-6. *Ann Neurol* 1990;28:242A.

183. Lee MR, Ho DD, Gurney ME. Functional interaction and partial

homology between human immunodeficiency virus and neuro-leukin. *Science* 1987;237:1047–51.

184. Buzy JM, Brenneman DE, Siegal FP, Ruff MR, Pert CB. Cerebrospinal fluid from cognitively impaired patients with acquired immunodeficiency syndrome shows gp120-like neuronal killing *in vitro. Am J Med* 1989;87:361–2.

185. Brenneman DE, Westbrook GL, Fitzgerald JP, et al. Neuronal cell killing by the envelope protein of HIV and its prevention by vasoactive intestinal peptide. *Nature* 1988;335:639–42.

186. Pert CB, Smith CC, Ruff MR, Hill JM. AIDS and its dementia as a neuropeptide disorder: role of VIP receptor blockade by human immunodeficiency virus envelope. *Ann Neurol* 1988;23(suppl): S71–3.

187. Cheng-Mayer C, Levy JA. Distinct biological and serological properties of human immunodeficiency viruses from the brain. *Ann Neurol* 1988;23(suppl):S58–61.

188. Chiodi F, Valentin A, Keys B, et al. Biological characterization of paired human immunodeficiency virus type 1 isolates from blood and cerebrospinal fluid. *Virology* 1989;173(1):178–87.

189. Syndulko K, Singer EJ, Faby-Chandon B, Singer P, Tuico E, Tourtellotte WW. Drug–alcohol abuse history but no depression is associated with neuropsychological deficits in human immunodeficiency virus neurological disease. *Ann Neurol* 1990;28:280A.

190. Levy RM, Janssen RS, Bush TJ, Rosenblum ML. Neuroepidemiology of acquired immunodeficiency syndrome. *J Acquired Immune Deficiency Syndrome* 1988;1:31–40.

191. Cheng-Mayer C, Seto D, Tateno M, Levy JA. Biologic features of HIV-1 that correlate with virulence in the host. *Science* 1988;240:80–2.

192. Anand R. Natural variants of human immunodeficiency virus from patients with neurological disorders do not kill T4$^+$ cells. *Ann Neurol* 1988;23(suppl):S66–70.

193. Greene WC. The molecular biology of human immunodeficiency virus type 1 infection. *N Engl J Med* 1991;324:308–17.

194. Bolognesi DP. Prospects for prevention of and early intervention against HIV. *JAMA* 1989;261:3007–13.

195. Smith RD. The pathobiology of HIV infection. *Arch Pathol Lab Med* 1990;114:235–9.

196. Schmitt FA, Bigley JW, McKinnis R, Logue PE, Evans RW, Drucker JL, and the AZT collaborative working group. Neuropsychological outcome of zidovudine (AZT) treatment of patients with AIDS and AIDS-related complex. *N Engl J Med* 1988;319:1573–8.

197. Pizzo PA, Eddy J, Falloon J, et al. Effect of continuous intravenous infusion of zidovudine (AZT) in children with symptomatic HIV infection. *N Engl J Med* 1988;319:889–96.

198. Yarchoan R, Mitsuya H, Myers CE, Broder S. Clinical pharmacology of 3'-azido-3'-dideoxythmidine (zidovudine) and related dideoxynucleosides. *N Engl J Med* 1989;321:726–38.

199. Sharer LR, Epstein LG. Intravenous infusion of zidovudine (AZT) in children with HIV infection. *N Engl J Med* 1989;320:806.

200. Singer E, Wilkins J, Syndulko K, et al. Altered cerebrospinal fluid levels of cortisol and biogenic amines in acquired immunodeficiency syndrome dementia complex versus asymptomatic seropositives; partial correction with zidovudine therapy. *Ann Neurol* 1990;28:280.

201. Lipton SA. Calcium channel antagonists and human immunodeficiency virus coat protein-mediated neuronal injury. *Ann Neurol* 1991;30:110–4.

202. Kaiser PK, Offermann JT, Lipton SA. Neuronal injury due to HIV-1 envelope protein is blocked by anti-gp120 antibodies but not by anti-CD4 antibodies. *Neurology* 1990;40:1757–61.

203. Kim S, Scheerer S, Geyer MA, Howell SB. Direct cerebrospinal fluid delivery of an antiretroviral agent using multivesicular liposomes. *J Infect Dis* 1990;162:750–2.

204. Petito CK, Navia BA, Cho E-S, Jordan BD, George DC, Price RW. Vacuolar myelopathy pathologically resembling subacute combined degeneration in patients with the acquired immunodeficiency syndrome. *N Engl J Med* 1985;312:874–9.

205. Grafe MR, Wiley CA. Spinal cord and peripheral nerve pathology in AIDS: the roles of cytomegalovirus and human immunodeficiency virus. *Ann Neurol* 1989;25:561–6.

206. Kieburtz KD, Giang DW, Schiffer RB, Vakil N. Abnormal vitamin B12 metabolism in human immunodeficiency virus infection association with neurological dysfunction. *Arch Neurol* 1991;48:312–4.

207. Rosenblum M, Scheck AC, Cronin K, Brew BJ, Khan A, Paul M, Price RW. Dissociation of AIDS-related vacuolar myelopathy and productive HIV-1 infection of the spinal cord. *Neurology* 1989;39:892–6.

208. Maier H, Budka H, Lassmann H, Pohl P. Vacuolar myelopathy with multinucleated giant cells in the acquired immune deficiency syndrome (AIDS). *Acta Neuropathol* 1989;78:497–503.

209. Budka H, Maier H, Pohl P. Human immunodeficiency virus in vacuolar myelopathy of the acquired immunodeficiency syndrome. *N Engl J Med* 1988;319:1667–8.

210. Dickson DW, Belman AL, Kim TS, Horoupian DS, Rubinstein A. Spinal cord pathology in pediatric acquired immunodeficiency syndrome. *Neurology* 1989;39:227–35.

211. Singh BM, Levine S, Yarrish RL, Hyland MJ, Jeanty D, Wormser GP. Spinal cord syndromes in the acquired immune deficiency syndrome. *Acta Neurol Scand* 1986;73:590–8.

212. Rance N, McArthur JC, Cornblath DR, Landstrom D, Griffin JW, Price DL. Gracile tract degeneration in patients with sensory neuropathy and AIDS. *Neurology* 1988;38:265–71.

213. Kimbrough RD. Vacuolar myelopathy in patients with the acquired immunodeficiency syndrome. *N Engl J Med* 1985; 313:827.

214. Goldstick L, Mandybur TI, Bode R. Spinal cord degeneration in AIDS. *Neurology* 1985;35:103–6.

215. Pattee GL, Kleinschmidt-DeMasters BK, Sandberg EJ, Berry CD, Neville HE. CMV arteritis with acute necrotic thoracic myelitis in an AIDS patient. *Neurology* 1990;40(suppl 1):235.

216. Berger JR, Raffanti S, Svenningsson A, McCarthy M, Snodgrass S, Resnick L. The role of HTLV-I in HIV-1 neurologic disease. *Neurology* 1991;41:197–202.

217. Aboulafia DM, Saxton EH, Koga H, Diagne A, Rosenblatt JD. A patient with progressive myelopathy and antibodies to human T-cell leukemia virus type I and human immunodeficiency virus type 1 in serum and cerebrospinal fluid. *Arch Neurol* 1990;47:477–9.

218. McArthur JC, Griffin JW, Cornblath DR, et al. Steroid-responsive myeloneuropathy in a man dually infected with HIV-1 and HTLV-I. *Neurology* 1990;40:938–44.

219. Koppel BS, Williams S, Daras M, DePietro D, Kaplan M, Coronesi M, Hall W. Myelopathy in patients with the acquired immunodeficiency syndrome coinfected with human T-lymphotropic virus type I. *Ann Neurol* 1990;28:252.

220. Brew BJ, Hardy W, Zuckerman E, et al. AIDS-related vacuolar myelopathy is not associated with coinfection by human T-lymphotropic virus type I. *Ann Neurol* 1989;26:679–81.

221. Hoffmann PM, Festoff BW, Giron LT Jr, et al. Isolation of LAV/HTLV-III from a patient with amyotrophic lateral sclerosis. *N Engl J Med* 1985;313:324–5.

222. Verma RK, Ziegler DK, Kepes JJ. HIV-related neuromuscular syndrome simulating motor neuron disease. *Neurology* 1990;40: 544–6.

223. Cornblath DR. Treatment of the neuromuscular complications of human immunodeficiency virus infection. *Ann Neurol* 1988;23(suppl):S88–91.

224. So YT, Holtzman DM, Abrams DI, Olney RK. Peripheral neuropathy associated with acquired immunodeficiency syndrome. *Arch Neurol* 1988;45:945–8.

225. Lin-Greenberger A, Taneja-Uppal N. Dysautonomia and infection with the human immunodeficiency virus. *Ann Intern Med* 1987;106:167.

226. Freeman R, Roberts MS, Friedman LS, Broadbridge C. Autonomic function and human immunodeficiency virus infection. *Neurology* 1990;40:575–80.

227. Leger JM, Bouche P, Bolgert F, et al. The spectrum of polyneuropathies in patients infected with HIV. *J Neurol Neurosurg Psychiatry* 1989;52:1369–74.

228. Lange DJ, Britton CB, Younger DS, Hays AP. The neuromuscular manifestations of human immunodeficiency virus infections. *Arch Neurol* 1988;45:1084–8.

229. Bailey RO, Baltch AL, Venkatesh R, Singh JK, Bishop MB. Sen-

sory motor neuropathy associated with AIDS. *Neurology* 1988;38:886–91.

230. Parry GJ. Peripheral neuropathies associated with human immunodeficiency virus infection. *Ann Neurol* 1988;23(suppl):S49–53.

231. Dalakas MC, Yarchoan R, Spitzer R, Elder G, Sever JL. Treatment of human immunodeficiency virus-related polyneuropathy with 3′-azido-2′,3′-dideoxythymidine. *Ann Neurol* 1988; 23(suppl):S92–4.

232. Yarchoan R, Thomas RV, Grafman J, et al. Long-term administration of 2′-azido-3′-dideoxythymidine to patients with AIDS-related neurologic disease. *Ann Neurol* 1985;23(suppl):S82–7.

233. Buskila D, Gladman D. Musculoskeletal manifestation of infection with human immunodeficiency virus. *Rev Infect Dis* 1990;12:223–35.

234. Gonzalez MF, Olney RK, So YT. Subacute structural myopathy associated with human immunodeficiency virus infection. *Arch Neurol* 1988;45:585–7.

235. Wiley CA, Nerenberg M, Cros D, Soto-Aguilar MC. HTLV-1 polymyositis in a patient also infected with human immunodeficiency virus. *N Engl J Med* 1989;320:992–5.

236. Berman A, Espinoza LR, Diaz JD, et al. Rheumatic manifestations of human immunodeficiency virus infection. *Am J Med* 1988;85:59–64.

237. Espinoza LR, Berman A, Aguilar JL. Myalgias in human immunodeficiency virus-infected patients. *Am J Med* 1989;86:510–1.

238. Chad DA, Smith TW, Blumenfeld A, Fairchild PG, DeGirolami U. Human immunodeficiency virus (HIV)-associated myopathy: immunocytochemical identification of an HIV antigen (gp41) in muscle macrophages. *Ann Neurol* 1990;28:579–82.

239. Price L, Gominak S, Raphael SA, Lischner HW, Griffin JW, Grover WD. Acute demyelinating polyneuropathy in childhood human immunodeficiency virus infection. *Ann Neurol* 1990; 28:459–60A.

240. Cornblath DR, Chaudhry V, Griffin JW. Treatment of chronic inflammatory demyelinating polyneuropathy with intravenous immunoglobulin. *Ann Neurol* 1991;30:104–6.

241. Schwartz ND, So YT, Hollander M, Allen S, Fje KH. Eosinophilic vasculitis leads to amaurosis fugax in patients with acquired immunodeficiency syndrome. *Arch Intern Med* 1986; 146:2059–60.

242. Taillan B, Roul C, Fuzibet J-G, et al. Circulating anticoagulant in patients seropositive for human immunodeficiency virus. *Am J Med* 1989;87:238.

243. Weber CA, Figueroa JP, Calabro JJ, Marcus EM, Gleckman RA. Co-occurrence of the Reiter syndrome and acquired immunodeficiency syndrome. *Ann Intern Med* 1987;107:112–3.

244. Moskowitz LB, Hensley GT, Chan JC, et al. The neuropathology of acquired immunodeficiency syndrome. *Arch Pathol Lab Med* 1984;108:867–72.

245. Namer IJ, Tan E, Akalin E, et al. Hemiballismus with cryptococcal meningitis. *Rev Neurol* 1990;146:153–4.

246. Sanchez-Ramos JR, Factor SA, Weiner WJ, Marguez J. Hemichorea-hemiballismus associated with acquired immune deficiency syndrome and cerebral toxoplasmosis. *Movement Disorders* 1989;4:266–73.

247. Koppel BS, Daras M. "Rubral" tremor due to midbrain toxoplasma abscess. *Movement Disorders* 1990;5:254–6.

248. Carrazana EJ, Rossitch E Jr, Samuels MA. Parkinsonian symptoms in a patient with AIDS and cerebral toxoplasmosis. *JNNP* 1989;52:1445–57.

249. Carrazana E, Rossitch E Jr, Martinez J. Unilateral "akathisia" in a patient with AIDS and a toxoplasmosis subthalamic abscess. *Neurology* 1989;39:449–50.

250. Gonzalez GR, Herskovitz S, Rosenblum M, Kanner R, Foley K, Portenoy R, Brown A. Clinicopathologic correlation of Dejerine-Roussy syndrome (DRS) caused by CNS toxoplasmosis in patients with AIDS. *Neurology* 1990;40(suppl):437.

251. Koppel BS, Tuchman AJ, Mangiardi JR, Daras M, Weitzner I. Epidural spinal infection in intravenous drug abusers. *Arch Neurol* 1988;45:1331–7.

252. Britton CB, Mesa-Tejade R, Fenoglio CM, et al. A new complication of AIDS: thoracic myelitis caused by herpes simplex virus. *Neurology* 1985;35:1071–4.

253. Tucker T, Dix RD, Katzen C, Davis RL, Schmidley JW. Cyto-

megalovirus and herpes simplex virus ascending myelitis in a patient with acquired immunodeficiency syndrome. *Ann Neurol* 1985;18:74–9.

254. Koppel BS, Daras M, Duffy KR. Intramedullary spinal cord abscess. *Neurosurgery* 1990;26:145–6.

255. Woolsey RM, Chambers TJ, Chung HD, McGarry JD. Mycobacterial meningomyelitis associated with human immunodeficiency virus infection. *Arch Neurol* 1988;46:691–3.

256. Overhage JM, Greist A, Brown DR. Conus medullaris syndrome resulting from *Toxoplasma gondii* infection in a patient with the acquired immunodeficiency syndrome. *Am J Med* 1990;89: 814–5.

257. Mehren M, Burns PJ, Mamani F, Levy CS, Laureno R. Toxoplasmic myelitis mimicking intramedullary spinal cord tumor. *Neurology* 1988;38:1648–50.

258. Miller RG, Storey JR, Greco CM. Ganciclovir in the treatment of progressive AIDS-related polyradiculopathy. *Neurology* 1990; 40:569–74.

259. Post MJD, Chan JC, Hensley GT, Hoffman TA, Moskowitz LB, Lippmann S. Toxoplasma encephalitis in Haitian adults with acquired immunodeficiency syndrome: a clinical–pathological–CT correlation. *Am J Roent* 1983;140:861–8.

260. McCabe R, Remington JS. Toxoplasmosis: the time has come. *N Engl J Med* 1988;318:313–5.

261. Israelski DM, Remington JS. Toxoplasmic encephalitis in patients with AIDS. *Infect Dis Clin NA* 1988;2:429–45.

262. Farkash AE, Maccabee PJ, Sher JH. CNS toxoplasmosis in acquired immunodeficiency syndrome: a clinical–pathological-radiological review of 12 cases. *JNNP* 1986;49:744–8.

263. Milligan SA, Katz MS, Craven PC, et al. Toxoplasmosis presenting as panhypopituitarism in a patient with acquired immunodeficiency syndrome. *Am J Med* 1984;77:760–4.

264. Tirard V, Niel G, Rosenheim M, et al. Diagnosis of toxoplasmosis in patients with AIDS by isolation of the parasite from the blood. *N Engl J Med* 1991;324:634.

265. Curry A, Turner AJ, Lucas S. Opportunistic protozoan infections in human immunodeficiency virus disease: review highlighting diagnostic and therapeutic aspects. *J Clin Pathol* 1991;44: 182–93.

266. Del Castillo M, Mendoza G, Oviedo J, Biarco RPP, Anselmo AE, Silva M. AIDS and Chagas' disease with CNS tumor-like lesion. *Am J Med* 1990;88:693–4.

267. Wiley CA, Safrin RE, Davis CE, Lampert PW, Braude AI, Martinez AJ, Visvesvara G. Acanthamoeba meningoencephalitis in a patient with AIDS. *J Infect Dis* 1987;155:130–3.

268. Anzil AP, Rao C, Wrzolek MA, Visvesvara GS, Sher JH, Kozlowski PB. Amebic meningoencephalitis in a patient with AIDS caused by a newly recognized opportunistic pathogen. *Arch Pathol Lab Med* 1991;115:21–5.

269. Ehni WF, Ellison RT III. Spontaneous *Candida albicans* meningitis in a patient with acquired immunodeficiency syndrome. *Am J Med* 1987;83:806–7.

270. Chuck SL, Sande MA. Infections with *Cryptococcus neoformans* in the acquired immunodeficiency syndrome. *N Engl J Med* 1989;321:794–9.

271. Dismukes WE, Cloud G, Gallis MA, et al. Treatment of cryptococcal meningitis with combination amphotericin B and flucytosine for four as compared with six weeks. *N Engl J Med* 1987;317:334–41.

272. Kovacs JA, Kovacs AA, Polis M, et al. Cryptococcosis in the acquired immunodeficiency syndrome. *Ann Intern Med* 1985;103:533–8.

273. Bozzette SA, Larsen RA, Chin J, et al. A placebo-controlled trial of maintenance therapy with fluconazole after treatment of cryptococcal meningitis in the acquired immunodeficiency syndrome. *N Engl J Med* 1991;324:580–4.

274. Nowack WJ, Bradsher RW. Cryptococcal meningoencephalitis presenting transient focal cerebral symptoms. *South Med J* 1989;82:395–6.

275. Lopez-Berestein G. Liposomes as carriers of antimicrobial agents. *Antimicrob Agents Chemother* 1987;31:675–78.

276. Devita VT Jr, Broder S, Franci AS, Kovacs JA, Chabner BA. Developmental therapeutics and the acquired immunodeficiency syndrome. *Ann Intern Med* 1987;106:568–81.

277. Crislip MA, Edwards JE. Candidiasis. *Infect Dis Clin North Am* 1989;3:103–33.

278. Minamoto G, Armstrong D. Fungal infections in AIDS: histoplasmosis and coccidioidomycosis. *Infect Dis Clin North Am* 1988;2:447–56.

279. Bronnimann DA, Adam RD, Galgiani JN, Habib MP, Petersen EA, Porter B, Bloom JW. Coccidioidomycosis in the acquired immunodeficiency syndrome. *Ann Intern Med* 1987;106:372–9.

280. Anaissie E, Fainstein V, Samo T, Bodey GP, Sarosi GA. Central nervous system histoplasmosis: an unappreciated complication of the acquired immunodeficiency syndrome. *Am J Med* 1988;84:215–7.

281. Glatt AE, Chirgwin K, Landesman SM. Treatment of infections associated with human immunodeficiency virus. *N Engl J Med* 1988;318:1439–47.

282. Cuadrado LM, Guerrero A, Asenjo JALG, Martin F, Palan E, Urra DG. Cerebral mucormycosis in two cases of acquired immunodeficiency syndrome. *Arch Neurol* 1988;45:109–11.

283. Galetta SL, Wulc AE, Goldberg HI, Nichols CW, Glaser JS. Rhinocerebral mucormycosis: management and survival after carotid occlusion. *Ann Neurol* 1990;28:103–7.

284. Stave GM, Heimberger T, Kerkering TM. Zygomycosis of the basal ganglia in intravenous drug users. *Am J Med* 1989;86:115–7.

285. Micozzi MS, Wetli CV. Intravenous amphetamine abuse, primary cerebral mucormycosis, and acquired immunodeficiency. *J Forensic Sci* 1985;30:504–10.

286. Case records of the Massachusetts General Hospital. (Case 52-1990). *N Engl J Med* 1990;323:1823–33.

287. Woods GL, Goldsmith JC. Aspergillus infection of the central nervous system in patients with acquired immunodeficiency syndrome. *Arch Neurol* 1990;47:181–4.

288. Denning DW, Tucker RM, Hanson LH, Stevens DA. Treatment of invasive aspergillosis with itraconazole. *Am J Med* 1989;86:791–800.

289. Post JMD, Hensley GT, Moskowitz LB, Fischl M. Cytomegalic inclusion virus encephalitis in patients with AIDS: CT, clinical, and pathologic correlation. *AJR* 1986;146:1229–34.

290. Walker DG, Itagaki S, Berry K, McGeer PL. Examination of brains of AIDS cases for human immunodeficiency virus and human cytomegalovirus nucleic acids. *J Neurol Neurosurg Psychiatry* 1989;52:583–90.

291. Hawley DA, Schaefer JF, Schulz DM, Muller J. Cytomegalovirus encephalitis in acquired immunodeficiency syndrome. *Am J Clin Pathol* 1983;80:874–7.

292. Masdeu JC, Small CB, Weiss L, Elkin CM, Llena J, Mesa-Tejada R. Multifocal cytomegalovirus encephalitis in AIDS. *Ann Neurol* 1988;23:97–9.

293. Vinters HV, Kwok MK, Ho HW, Anders KH, Tomiyasu U, Wolfsen WL, Robert F. Cytomegalovirus in the nervous system of patients with the acquired immune deficiency syndrome. *Brain* 1989;112:245–68.

294. Fuller GN, Guiloff RJ, Scaravilli F, Harcourt-Webster JN. Combined HIV-CMV encephalitis presenting with brainstem signs. *J Neurol Neurosurg Psychiatry* 1989;52:975–9.

295. Moskowitz LB, Gregorios JB, Hensley GT, Berger JR. Cytomegalovirus-induced demyelination associated with acquired immunodeficiency syndrome. *Arch Pathol Lab Med* 1984;108:873–7.

296. Eidelberg D, Sotrel A, Vogel H, Walker P, Kleefield J, Crumpacker CS III. Progressive polyradiculopathy in acquired immunodeficiency syndrome. *Neurology* 1986;36:912–6.

297. Behar R, Wiley C, McCutchan JA. Cytomegalovirus polyradiculoneuropathy in acquired immune deficiency syndrome. *Neurology* 1987;37:557–61.

298. Said G, Lacroix C, Chemouilli P, Agoulon-Goeau C, Rouller E, Penaud D. Cytomegalovirus neuropathy in acquired immunodeficiency syndrome: a clinical and pathological study. *Ann Neurol* 1991;29:139–46.

299. Mahieux F, Gray F, Fenelon G, Gherardi R, Adams D, Guillard A, Poirier J. Acute myeloradiculitis due to cytomegalovirus as the initial manifestation of AIDS. *J Neurol Neurosurg Psychiatry* 1989;52:270–4.

300. Fuller GN, Jacobs JM, Guiloff RJ. Association of painful peripheral neuropathy in AIDS with cytomegalovirus infection. *Lancet* 1989;2:937–41.

301. Small PM, McPhaul LW, Sooy CD, Wofsky CB, Jacobson MA. Cytomegalovirus infection of the laryngeal nerve presenting as hoarseness in patients with acquired immunodeficiency syndrome. *Am J Med* 1989;86:108–9.

302. Collaborative DHPG Treatment Study Group. Treatment of serious cytomegalovirus infections with 9-(1,3-dihydroxy-2-propoxymethyl)guanine in patients with AIDS and other immunodeficiencies. *N Engl J Med* 1986;314:801–15.

303. Edwards RM, Messing R, McKendall RR. Cytomegalovirus meningoencephalitis in a homosexual man with Kaposi's sarcoma: isolation of CMV from CSF cells. *Neurology* 1985;35:560–2.

304. Dix RD, Bredesen DE. Opportunistic viral infection in acquired immunodeficiency syndrome. In: Rosenblum ML, ed. *AIDS and the nervous system.* New York: Raven Press; 1988:221–61.

305. Morgello S, Cho L, Nielsen S, Petito C. The pathology of cytomegalovirus (CMV) encephalitis. *J Neuropathol Exp Neurol* 1985;44:350A.

306. Wiley CA, Schrier RD, Denaro FJ, et al. Localization within the CNS of cytomegalovirus proteins and genome during fulminant infection in an AIDS patient. *J Neuropathol Exp Neurol* 1985;44:350.

307. Chou SW, Dylewski JS, Gaynon MW, Egbert PR, Merigan TC. Alpha-interferon administration in cytomegalovirus retinitis. *Antimicrobial Agents Chemother* 1984;25:25–8.

308. Grossberg HS, Bonnem EM, Buhles WC Jr. GM-CSF with ganciclovir for the treatment of CMV retinitis in AIDS. *N Engl J Med* 1989;320:1560.

309. Holmberg SD, Stewart JA, Gerber AR, Byers RH, Lee FK, O'Malley PM, Nahmins AJ. Prior herpes simplex virus type 2 infection as a risk factor for HIV infection. *JAMA* 1988;259:1048–50.

310. Pascual-Leone A, Dhuna A, Langendorf F. P238. *Herpes simplex encephalitis: early magnetic resonance imaging findings in the face of normal electroencephalogram.* *Ann Neurol* 1990;28:280.

311. Laskin OL, Stahl-Bayliss CM, Morgello S. Concomitant herpes simplex virus type 1 and cytomegalovirus ventriculoencephalitis in acquired immunodeficiency syndrome. *Arch Neurol* 1987;44:843–7.

312. Carrazana EJ, Rossitch E Jr, Schachter S. Cerebral toxoplasmosis masquerading as herpes encephalitis in a patient with acquired immunodeficiency syndrome. *Am J Med* 1989;86:730–2.

313. Van Landingham KE, Marsteller HB, Ross GW, Hayden FG. Relapses of herpes simplex encephalitis after conventional acyclovir therapy. *JAMA* 1988;259:1051–3.

314. Englund JA, Zimmerman ME, Swierkosz EM, Goodman JL, Scholl DR, Balfour HH Jr. Herpes simplex virus resistant to acyclovir. *Ann Intern Med* 1990;112:416–22.

315. Safrin S, Assaykeen T, Follansbee S, Mills J. Foscarnet therapy for acyclovir-resistant mucocutaneous herpes simplex virus infection in 26 AIDS patients: preliminary data. *J Infect Dis* 1990;161:1078–84.

316. Safrin S, Crumpacker C, Chatis P, et al. A controlled trial comparing foscarnet with vidarabine for acyclovir-resistant mucocutaneous herpes simplex in the acquired immunodeficiency syndrome. *N Engl J Med* 1991;325:551–5.

317. Richardson EP Jr. Progressive multifocal leukoencephalopathy 30 years later (ed). *N Engl J Med* 1988;318:315–7.

318. Berger JR, Kaszovitz B, Post JD, Dickinson G. Progressive multifocal leukoencephalopathy associated with human immunodeficiency virus infection. *Ann Intern Med* 1987;107:78–87.

319. Bernick C, Gregorios JB. Progressive multifocal leukoencephalopathy in a patient with acquired immune deficiency syndrome. *Arch Neurol* 1984;41:780–2.

320. Berger JR, Mucke L. Prolonged survival and partial recovery in AIDS-associated progressive multifocal leukoencephalopathy. *Neurology* 1988;38:1060–5.

321. Vayeux R, Cumont M, Girard PM, et al. Severe encephalitis resulting from coinfections with HIV and JC virus. *Neurology* 1990;40:944–8.

322. Blum LW, Chambers RA, Schwartzman RJ, Streletz LJ. Progressive multifocal leukoencephalopathy in acquired immune deficiency syndrome. *Arch Neurol* 1985;42:137–9.

323. Verroust F, Lemay D, Laurian Y. High frequency of herpes zos-

ter in young hemophiliacs (letter). *N Engl J Med* 1987; 316:166–7.

324. Cone LA, Schiffman MA. Herpes zoster and the acquired immunodeficiency syndrome (letter). *Ann Intern Med* 1984;100:462.

325. Sandor E, Croxson TS, Millman A, Mildvan D. Herpes zoster ophthalmicus in patients at risk for AIDS. *N Engl J Med* 1984;310:1118–9.

326. Cole EL, Meisler DM, Calabrese LH, Holland GN, Mondino BJ, Conant MA. Herpes zoster ophthalmicus and acquired immune deficiency syndrome. *Arch Ophthalmol* 1984;102:1027–9.

327. Melbye M, Grossman RJ, Goedert JJ, Eyster ME, Biggar RJ. Risk of AIDS after herpes zoster. *Lancet* 1987;1:728–31.

328. Ryder JW, Croen K, Kleinschmidt-DeMasters BK, Ostrove JM, Straus SE, Cohn DL. Progressive encephalitis three months after resolution of cutaneous zoster in a patient with AIDS. *Ann Neurol* 1986;19:182–8.

329. Balfour HH, Bean B, Laskin OL, et al. Acyclovir halts progression of herpes zoster in immunocompromised patients. *N Engl J Med* 1983;308:1448–53.

330. Jacobson MD, Berger TG, Fikrig S, Becherer P, Moohr JW, Stanat SC, Biron KK. Acyclovir-resistant varicella zoster virus infection after chronic oral acyclovir therapy in patients with the acquired immunodeficiency syndrome (AIDS). *Ann Intern Med* 1990;112:187–91.

331. Jura E, Chadwick EG, Josephs SH, et al. Varicella-zoster virus infections in children infected with human immunodeficiency virus. *Pediatr Infect Dis* 1989;8:586–90.

332. Small PM, Schecter GF, Goodman PC, Sande MA, Chaisson RE, Hopewell PC. Treatment of tuberculosis in patients with advanced human immunodeficiency virus infection. *N Engl J Med* 1991;324:289–94.

333. Stead WW, Senner JW, Reddick WT, Lofgren JP. Racial differences in susceptibility to infection by *Mycobacterium tuberculosis. N Engl J Med* 1990;322:422–7.

334. Bishburg E, Sunderam G, Reichman LB, Kapila R. Central nervous system tuberculosis with the acquired immunodeficiency syndrome and its related complex. *Ann Intern Med* 1986; 105:210–3.

335. Selwyn PA, Hartel D, Lewis VA, et al. A prospective study of the risk of tuberculosis among intravenous drug users with human immunodeficiency virus infection. *N Engl J Med* 1989;320: 545–50.

336. Guthertz LS, Damsker B, Bottone EJ, Ford EG, Midura TF, Janda JM. *Mycobacterium avium* and *Mycobacterium intracellulare* infections in patients with and without AIDS. *J Infect Dis* 1989;160:1037–41.

337. Horowitz EA. Recent trends in mycobacterial diseases. *Hosp Formul* 1988;23:892–7.

338. Pouchot J, Vinceneux P, Barge J, LaParre F, Boussougant Y, Michon C. Tuberculous polymyositis in HIV infection. *Am J Med* 1990;89:250–1.

339. Lamfers EJP, Bastiaans AH, Mravunac M, Rampen FHJ. Leprosy in the acquired immunodeficiency syndrome. *Ann Intern Med* 1987;107:111–2.

340. Molavi A, LeFrock JL. Tuberculous meningitis. *Med Clin North Am* 1985;69:315–31.

341. Trautmann M, Kluge W, Otto H-S, Loddenkemper R. Computed tomography in CNS tuberculosis. *Eur Neurol* 1986; 25:91–7.

342. Lu C-Z, Qiao J, Shen T, Link H. Early diagnosis of tuberculous meningitis by detection of anti-BCG secreting cells in cerebrospinal fluid. *Lancet* 1990;1:10–3.

343. Robert C-F, Hirschel B, Rochat T, Deglon J-J. Tuberculin skin reactivity in HIV-seropositive intravenous drug addicts. *N Engl J Med* 1989;321:1268.

344. Pitchenik AE, Burr J, Cole CH. Tuberculin testing for persons with positive serologic studies for HTLV-III. *N Engl J Med* 1986;314:447.

345. Cohn DL, Catlin BJ, Peterson KL, Judson FN, Sbarbaro JA. A 62-dose, 6-month therapy for pulmonary and extrapulmonary tuberculosis: a twice-weekly, directly observed, and cost-effective regimen. *Ann Intern Med* 1990;112:407–15.

346. Agins BD, Berman DS, Spicehandler D, El-Sadr W, Simberkott MS, Rahal JJ. Effect of combined therapy with ansamycin, clofa-

zimine, ethambutol, and isoniazid for *Mycobacterium avium* infection in patients with AIDS. *J Infect Dis* 1989;159:784–7.

347. Wolters EC, Hische EAH, Tutuarima JA, et al. Central nervous system involvement in early and late syphilis: the problem of asymptomatic neurosyphilis. *J Neurol Sci* 1988;88:229–39.

348. Feraru ER, Aronow HA, Lipton RR. Neurosyphilis in AIDS patients: initial CSF VDRL may be negative. *Neurology* 1990;40:541–3.

349. McIntosh K. Congenital syphilis—breaking through the safety net (ed). *N Engl J Med* 1990;323:1339–41.

350. Berry CD, Hooton TM, Collier AC, Lukehart SA. Neurologic relapse after benzathine penicillin therapy for secondary syphilis in a patient with HIV infection. *N Engl J Med* 1987;316:1587–9.

351. Lanska MJ, Lanska DJ, Schmidley JW. Syphilitic polyradiculpathy in an HIV-positive man. *Neurology* 1988;38:1297–301.

352. Whiteside CM. Persistence of neurosyphilis despite multiple treatment regimens. *Am J Med* 1989;87:225–7.

353. Lowenstein DH, Mills C, Simon RP. Acute syphilitic transverse myelitis. Unusual presentation of meningovascular syphilis. *Genitourin Med* 1987;63:333–8.

354. Reid SE, Anzarut A. Neurosyphilis and stroke in a patient with antibodies to the human immunodeficiency virus. *Am J Med* 1989;87:119–21.

355. Kase CS, Levitz SM, Wolinsky JS, Sulis CA. Pontine pure motor hemparesis due to meningovascular syphilis in human immunodeficiency virus-positive patients. *Arch Neurol* 1988;45:832c.

356. Engstom JW. Neurosyphilis as a cause of cerebral infarction in AIDS. *Am J Med* 1990;88:700–1.

357. Lukehart SA, Hook EW III, Baker-Zander SA, Collier AC, Critchlow CW, Handsfield IIIH. Invasion of the central nervous system by *Treponema pallidum:* implications for diagnosis and treatment. *Ann Intern Med* 1988;109:855–62.

358. CDC: treatment of syphilis. *MMWR* 1989;38:3–13.

359. Weintraub M. Orphan status for drug-carrier combinations. *Pharmacol Ther* 1990;15:1109.

360. Garcia-Monco JC, Frey HM, Fernandez Villar B, Golightly MG, Benach JL. Lyme disease concurrent with human immunodeficiency virus infection. *Am J Med* 1989;87:325–8.

361. Scott GB, Buck BE, Leterman JG, Bloom FL, Parks WP. Acquired immunodeficiency in infants. *N Engl J Med* 1984; 310:76–81.

362. Harris JO, Marquez J, Swerdloff MA, Magana IA. Listeria brain abscess in the acquired immunodeficiency syndrome. *Arch Neurol* 1989;46:250.

363. Adair JC, Beck AC, Apfelbaum RI, Baringer JR. Nocardial cerebral abscess in the acquired immunodeficiency syndrome. *Arch Neurol* 1987;44:548–53.

364. Reichert CM, O'Leary TJ, Levens DL, Simrell CR, Macher AM. Autopsy pathology in the acquired immune deficiency syndrome. *Am J Pathol* 1983;112:357–82.

365. Kales CP, Holzman RS. Listeriosis in patients with HIV infection: clinical manifestations and response to therapy. *J Acquired Immune Deficiency Syndrome* 1990;3:139–43.

366. Welch K, Finkbeiner W, Alpers CE, Blumenfeld W, Davis RL, Smuckler EA, Beckstead JH. Autopsy findings in the acquired immune deficiency syndrome. *JAMA* 1984;252:1152–9.

367. Eisenstein BI. New opportunistic infections—more opportunities (ed). *N Engl J Med* 1990;323:1625–7.

368. Hotson JR, Pedley TA. The neurological complications of cardiac transplantation. *Brain* 1976;99:673–94.

369. Bermudez MA, Grant KM, Rodvien R, Mendes F. Non-Hodgkin's lymphoma in a population with or at risk for acquired immunodeficiency syndrome: indications for intensive chemotherapy. *Am J Med* 1989;86:71–6.

370. DeAngelis LM, Yahalom J, Heinemann M-H, Cirrincione C, Thaler HT, Krol G. Primary CNS lymphoma: combined treatment with chemotherapy and radiotherapy. *Neurology* 1990;40: 80–6.

371. Lee Y-Y, Bruner JM, Van Tassel P, Libshitz HI. Primary central nervous system lymphoma: CT and pathologic correlation. *Am J Rad* 1986;147:747–52.

372. Kaplan LD. AIDS-associated lymphoma. *Baillieres Cin Haematology* 1990;3:139–51.

373. Bates S, McKeever P, Masur H, Levens D, Macher A, Armstrong G, Magrath IT. Myelopathy following intrathecal chemotherapy

in a patient with extensive Burkitt's lymphoma and altered immune status. *Am J Med* 1985;78:697–702.

374. Rosenblum ML, Levy RM, Bredesen DE, So YT, Warc W, Ziegler JL. Primary central nervous system lymphoma in patients with AIDS. *Am Neurol* 1988;23:S13–6.

375. So YT, Beckstead JH, Davis RL. Primary central nervous system lymphoma in acquired immune deficiency syndrome. A clinical and pathologic study. *Ann Neurol* 1986;20:566–72.

376. So YT, Choucair A, Davis RL, Warc WM, Ziegler JL, Sheline GE, Beckstead JH. Neoplasms of the central nervous system in acquired immunodeficiency syndrome. In: Rosenblum ML, ed. *AIDS and the nervous system.* New York: Raven Press; 1988:chap 13.

377. Ziegler JL, Beckstead JH, Volberding PA, et al. Non-Hodgkin's lymphoma in 90 homosexual men. Relation to generalized lymphadenopathy and the acquired immunodeficiency syndrome. *N Engl J Med* 1984;311:565–70.

378. Snider WD, Simpson DM, Aronyk KE, Neilsen JL. Primary lymphoma of the nervous system associated with acquired immune deficiency syndrome. *N Engl J Med* 1983;308:45.

379. Groopman JE, Scadden DT. Interferon therapy for Kaposi sarcoma associated with the acquired immunodeficiency syndrome (AIDS). *Ann Intern Med* 1989;110:335–7.

380. Hochberg CJ, Miller G, Schooley RT, Hirsch MS, Ferriro P, Henle W. Central-nervous-system lymphoma related to Epstein-Barr virus. *N Engl J Med* 1983;309:745–8.

381. Birx DL, Redfield RR, Tosato G. Defective regulation of Epstein-Barr virus infection in patients with acquired immunodeficiency syndrome (AIDS) or AIDS-related diseases. *N Engl J Med* 1986;314:874–6.

382. Pirsch JD, Stratta RJ, Sollinger HW, Hafez GR, D'Allesandro AM, Kalayoglu M, Belzer FO. Treatment of severe Epstein-Barr virus-induced lymphoproliferative syndrome with ganciclovir: two cases after solid organ transplantation. *Am J Med* 1989;86:241–4.

383. Jack MK, Smith T, Collier AC. Oculomotor cranial nerve palsy associated with acquired immunodeficiency syndrome. *Ann Ophthalmol* 1984;16:460–2.

384. Montalvo FW, Casanova R, Clavell LA. Treatment outcome in children with malignancies associated with human immunodeficiency virus infection. *J Pediatr* 1990;116:735–8.

385. Gill PS, Levine AM, Krails M, et al. AIDS-related malignant lymphoma: results of prospective treatment trials. *J Clin Oncol* 1987;5:1322–8.

386. Ioachim HL, Cooper MC, Hellman GC. Lymphoma in men at high risk for acquired immune deficiency syndrome (AIDS). A study of 21 cases. *Cancer* 1985;56:2831–42.

387. Pitlik SD, Fainstein V, Bolivar R, et al. Spectrum of central nervous system complications in homosexual men with acquired immune deficiency syndrome. *J Infect Dis* 1983;148:771–772.

388. Gorin FA, Bale JF, Hall-Miller M, Schwartz RA. Kaposi's sarcoma metastatic to the CNS. *Arch Neurol* 1985;42:162–5.

389. Nielsen SL, Davis RL. Neuropathology of acquired immunodeficiency syndrome. In: Rosenblum ML, ed. *AIDS and the nervous system.* New York: Raven Press; 1988:155–81.

390. Van Ness PC. Pentobarbital and EEG burst suppression in treatment of status epilepticus refractory to benzodiazepines and phenytoin. *Epilepsy* 1990;31:61–7.

391. Oksenhendler E, Lida H, D'Agay M-F, Morinet F, Pulik M, Davi F, Clauvel J-P. Tumoral nasopharyngeal lymphoid hyperplasia in human immunodeficiency virus infected patients. *Arch Intern Med* 1989;149:2359–61.

392. Case Records. Case 9-1986. *N Engl J Med* 1986;314:629–40.

393. Israel AM, Koziner B, Straus DJ. Plasmacytoma and the acquired immunodeficiency syndrome. *Ann Intern Med* 1983; 99:635–6.

394. Gasnault J, Roux FX, Vedrenne C. Cerebral astrocytoma in association with HIV infection. *J Neurol Neurosurg Psychiatry* 1988;51:422–4.

395. Misusawa H, Hirano A, Llena JF, Shintaku M. Cerebrovascular lesions in acquired immune deficiency syndrome (AIDS). *Acta Neuropathol (Berl)* 1988;76:451–7.

396. Frank Y, Lim W, Kahn E, Farmer P, Gorey M, Pahwa S. Multiple ischemic infarcts in a child with AIDS, varicella zoster infection, and cerebral vasculitis. *Pediatr Neurol* 1989;5:64–7.

397. Cho ES, Sharer LR, Peress NS, Little B. Intimal proliferation of leptomeningeal arteries and brain infarcts in subjects with AIDS. *J Neuropathol Exp Neurol* 1987;46:385.

398. Joshi VV, Pawel B, Connor E, Sharer L, Oleske JM, Morrison S, Martin-Garcia J. Arteriopathy in children with acquired immune deficiency syndrome. *Pediatr Pathol* 1987;7:261–75.

399. Vinters HV, Guerra WF, Eppolito L, Keith PE III. Necrotizing vasculitis of the nervous system in a patient with AIDS-related complex. *Neuropathol Appl Neurobiol* 1988;14:417–24.

400. Scaravilli F, Daniel SE, Harcourt-Webster N, Guiloff RJ. Chronic basal meningitis and vasculitis in acquired immune deficiency syndrome: a possible role for human immunodeficiency virus. *Arch Pathol Lab Med* 1989;113:192–5.

401. Yankner BA, Skolnik PR, Shoukimas GM, Gabuzda DH, Sobel RA, Ho DD. Cerebral granulomatous angiitis associated with isolation of human T-lymphotropic virus type III from the central nervous system. *Ann Neurol* 1986;20:362–4.

402. Krapf FE, Herrmann M, Leitmann W, Schwartlander B, Kalden JR. Circulating immune complexes in HIV-infected persons. *Klin Wochenschr* 1990;68:299–305.

403. Cohen IS, Anderson DW, Virmani R, et al. Congestive cardiomyopathy in association with the acquired immunodeficiency syndrome. *N Engl J Med* 1986;314:623–30.

AIDS and Other Manifestations of HIV Infection,
Second Edition, Edited by Gary P. Wormser.
Raven Press, Ltd., New York © 1992.

CHAPTER 21

Biopsychosocial Aspects of the HIV Epidemic

Mary Ann Adler Cohen

The human immunodeficiency virus (HIV) epidemic has created a multidimensional crisis that is challenging the health care system (1,2). This chapter gives an overview of the biopsychosocial aspects of the HIV epidemic and presents a comprehensive approach to management.

THE STIGMA OF AIDS

AIDS is a paradigm of a medical illness that requires a biopsychosocial approach (3–9). The HIV epidemic has created a crisis affecting not only persons with the virus, but also their loved ones, caregivers, and communities (9). The crisis is one of fear, anxiety, uncertainty, and stigmatization. Persons with HIV infection are confronted with discrimination in addition to devastating illnesses that result in profound emaciation, weakness, depression, confusion, pain, disfigurement, and, ultimately, death (7). There is no other illness that so frequently elicits such fear.

Hunter has concluded that the "epidemic of fear" is growing faster than the HIV epidemic itself (10,11). She points out (12) that while during the 1980s we struggled to understand the illness, in the 1990s we need to struggle to overcome the stigma of HIV infection. Discrimination, which was described early in the epidemic (13,14), continues to the present and is illustrated in the vignettes that follow.

Case 1. The patient was a 44-year-old journalist who had Kaposi's sarcoma and AIDS. Prior to his hospital admission, his landlord attempted to evict him from the apartment where he had lived for 15 years. He sought and obtained legal help and testified from his bedside on his own behalf. The legal battle continued during the course of his hospitalization, providing yet another stress for an individual who was coping with fever, weight loss,

disfigurement, pain, and weakness. By the time he won the case, his condition had deteriorated to such an extent that he required transfer to a chronic care facility and could never return to his home.

Case 2. A 42-year-old physician was hospitalized for pneumonia. Only hours after bronchoscopy confirmed a diagnosis of *Pneumocystis carinii* pneumonia and AIDS, the physician received a telephone call from the director of his service asking him to resign or "the hospital would become a ghost town." The physician resigned, reluctant to pursue legal action for fear of loss of anonymity (9).

Some of our patients have been victims of discrimination by landlords, employers, dentists, insurance agencies, families, and physicians. Hunter (10) believes that among the reasons for discrimination are ignorance about how HIV is transmitted, stigma associated with HIV-related illness, and financial issues. She states that insurance companies, doctors, dentists, nursing homes, landlords, and employers discriminate, in part, for fear of contamination and, in part, for fear that future bills may not be paid, productivity may diminish, or that the costs of care will be too high (10).

Discrimination by physicians has also been described. Wormser and Joline (15) studied the attitudes of attendees at a medical grand rounds at a teaching hospital. They found that more physicians would prefer to eat cookies baked by a person with leukemia (27%) than by a person with HIV infection (7%). Thompson (16) described a member of a HIV support group who wanted to bake Christmas cookies for the group but feared no one would eat them. Kelly et al. (17) found that physicians would be less willing to work in the same office, renew a lease, continue a friendship, allow children to visit, attend a party with a person with AIDS, or go to a party where a person with AIDS had prepared food. Some of the attitudes of physicians toward persons with AIDS may be related to homophobia (18). Whatever their origin, such attitudes are clearly detrimental to the health care provider–patient relationship.

M. A. Adler Cohen: Metropolitan Hospital Center-New York Medical College, New York, New York 10029.

At times, discrimination may be so severe that individuals who develop AIDS may be undomiciled. Some individuals have lost their homes and reside in shelters for the homeless. Once a diagnosis of AIDS is confirmed, they may no longer be eligible for some shelters and have no place to go at all.

Children with HIV infection have been ostracized and prevented from attending school. Some long-term-care facilities, such as nursing homes, chronic care hospitals, and homes for the terminally ill, do not accept persons with AIDS. Funeral homes may refuse to bury persons with HIV infection. The attitudes of families, landlords, employers, chronic care facilities, health professionals, and funeral directors are compounded by discrimination as well as fears and anxieties about contagion. As a result, some persons with AIDS have problems obtaining health care, finding a place to live while they can still care for themselves, or even finding a place to die.

Cassens (19) delineates the special social consequences of AIDS for gay men. He states: "In a society that scarcely accepts sexuality, even heterosexuality, the guilt associated with homosexuality and AIDS is crippling. . . . Persons with anxiety about AIDS frequently respond that they would be embarrassed by the diagnosis. . . . Guilt further magnifies the sense of isolation and estrangement that many gay men have experienced throughout their lives." He points out that coping is made far more difficult because of forced disclosure of sexual orientation with secrecy about homosexuality an "impossible luxury."

Discrimination against people with AIDS has been described (14) as a new form of discrimination called AIDSism. AIDSism is built on a foundation of homophobia, addictophobia, and a fear of contagion and death. Discrimination, stigma, and therapeutic nihilism have contributed to both the epidemic of fear and to the epidemic of AIDS. Health care providers should take the lead in combatting discrimination (20).

THE BIOPSYCHOSOCIAL APPROACH TO AIDS

The biopsychosocial approach to illness maintains a view of each patient as an individual who is a member of a family, community, and culture who deserves coordinated compassionate care and treatment with dignity. Medical illness is seen as a stressor with biological, psychological, and sociocultural aspects. Coping with AIDS, as with any severe illness, can be adaptive or maladaptive. The biopsychosocial approach can help persons with AIDS and their caregivers to cope more effectively.

HIV can cause severe life-threatening organic illness with devastating psychological impact, that is considerably worsened by the virus' special affinity for brain and neural tissue (21–39).

Psychiatric sequelae complicate the HIV epidemic,

TABLE 1. *Biopsychosocial aspects of AIDS*

Bio-	Psycho-	Social
Infections	Organic brain syndromes	Alienation
Protozoal	Delirium	
Pneumocystis carinii pneumonia	Dementia	Recent losses
Toxoplasma gondi encephalitis	Organic mood syndrome	Recent separation
T. gondi disseminated infection	Organic delusional syndrome	
Cryptosporidium enteritis		Lack of social and family network
	Affective disorders	
Fungal	Major depression	Homelessness
Candida esophagitis	Dysthymic disorder	
Disseminated candidiasis		Unemployment
Cryptococcal meningitis	Substance abuse disorder	Financial problems
Cryptococcal pneumonia		
Cryptococcal brain involvement	Personality disorders	Eviction
Cryptococcal disseminated infection	Antisocial personality disorder	
	Borderline personality disorder	Homophobia
Viral	Adjustment disorder	Discrimination
CNS HIV infection	With depressed mood	
Chronic mucocutaneous herpes simplex	With anxious mood	Rejection by friends
Disseminated herpes zoster infection		
Cytomegalovirus of the brain	Uncomplicated bereavement	
Cytomegalovirus of the retina		
Bacterial		
Disseminated *Mycobacterium avium-intracellulare*		
Cancers		
Kaposi's sarcoma		
CNS lymphoma		

affecting both the uninfected and the infected. The psychiatric manifestations of the uninfected include anxiety, phobia, factitious disorder, delusions, and Münchausen's AIDS. Psychiatric disorders associated with HIV infection include organic mental disorders, substance abuse disorder, affective disorders, adjustment disorders, anxiety disorders, and personality disorders. AIDS is a multifaceted syndrome that has a profound impact on persons with AIDS, their loved ones, caregivers, and communities. One health care worker, working alone, cannot possibly cope with all the severe and

multiple illnesses and psychologic problems that are associated with HIV infection. Both staff and patient are often overwhelmed by the sheer magnitude of problems, as well as the psychologic reactions to them. An integrated comprehensive program is necessary to provide coordination of clinical and teaching activities as well as support for staff. A biopsychosocial approach enables persons with HIV infection, their loved ones, and caregivers to meet the challenges of the HIV epidemic with compassion, optimism, and dignity.

Consultation-liaison psychiatric services should be in-

TABLE 2. *Biopsychosocial assessment*

	Symptoms	Signs	Ancillary data
Bio-			
Gastrointestinal	Anorexia	Cachexia	
	Weight loss	Diarrhea	
	Dysphagia	Weight loss	
	Odynophagia		Esophageal candida on
	White patches in mouth	Hairy leukoplakia	esophagoscopy
Skin	Rash	Herpes simplex lesions	
	Purple spots	Kaposi's sarcoma lesions	
	Pallor		
General	Swollen glands	Lymphadenopathy	Anemia
	Arthralgias	Sweating	Leukopenia
	Myalgias	Fever	Lymphopenia
Neurologic	Weakness		EEG slowing
	Leg weakness	Paraparesis	CT scan abnormalities
	Loss of vision	Cotton wool retinal exudates	MRI abnormalities
	Unsteady gait	Ataxia	
		Urinary and fecal incontinence	
Psycho-			
Affectivity and	Anxiety	Apathy	Lack of response to usual
mood	Uncertainty	Blunting	treatment for
	Mood swings	Affective liability	depression, such as
	Withdrawal	Mutism	therapy and
	Crying	Depression	antidepressants
	Sadness	Slowed speech	
	Suicidal ideation	Psychomotor retardation	
	Suicide attempts	Psychomotor hyperactivity	
	Sense of isolation	Agitation	
	Euphoria	Hostility	
	Guilt		
	Anger		
	Anhedonia		
	Loss of libido		
Thought content	Suspiciousness	Paranoid delusions	
Cognition	Forgetfulness	Impaired memory	MRI and CT abnormalities
	Confusion	Disorientation	EEG slowing
	Difficulty concentrating	Impaired abstraction	Low scores on:
		Impaired intellectual functioning	Cognitive capacity
		Short attention span	Screening examination
		Perseveration	Neuropsychological
			testing
			Mini-mental state
Social			
Social and historical	Risk behavior		
	Absence of family history		
	of affective disorders		
	and/or alcoholism		
	Recent losses		
	Recent stresses		

tegrated into both the leadership and functioning of comprehensive programs to provide a biopsychosocial approach and support for staff.

A biopsychosocial approach to a person with HIV infection enables the caregiver to get to know each individual as a person in the context of family and community. This provides a means of establishing a relationship and improving adherence to both medical regimens and risk-reduction programs. Understanding the psychiatric aspects of AIDS may lead to early recognition of HIV infection when the presenting symptoms are primarily psychiatric. Early recognition can help to prolong life through therapeutic measures, such as zidovudine (AZT) or prophylactic measures, such as aerosolized pentamidine to prevent *Pneumocystis carinii* pneumonia. Additionally, recognition of psychiatric and social complications may enable caregivers to provide the necessary care and alleviate problems whenever possible. Ultimately, this comprehensive approach leads to improvement of care. It may also be lifesaving when suicidal ideation is elicited by a primary care physician or when one of the signs or symptoms of *Pneumocystis carinii* pneumonia is recognized by a nonphysician.

Table 1 provides a summary of some of the more common diagnoses and problems encountered in persons with HIV infection. This general listing is meant to heighten awareness of the numerous potential complications of HIV infection and to demonstrate the scope of the major issues.

Table 2 is designed to provide the clinician with an abbreviated listing of signs, symptoms, and ancillary data that will lead toward early identification of medical and psychologic problems in the context of a social and historical matrix.

UNDERSTANDING THE ILLNESS

A comprehensive approach to HIV infection would not be complete without the concept of determining the patient's understanding of the illness. The patient's understanding of illness is always important, but it becomes even more significant in severe and life-threatening illnesses or in those that involve uncertainty. Developing the ability to elicit the patient's understanding of the illness is of help to both the health care provider and the patient. The initial stages of illness are frightening to the patient. A person with a risk behavior may have severe anxiety about AIDS even though there is no evidence of signs or symptoms. Anxiety about AIDS can be paralyzing and can cause severe psychiatric symptoms. It may also impair an individual's capacity to function at work or at home.

If an individual with a risk behavior does develop a symptom consistent with HIV infection, anxiety may lead to an immediate assumption that HIV infection must be the diagnosis, even prior to seeking medical attention. Defenses of denial, suppression, or avoidance may delay diagnosis. From the onset of the very first symptom of HIV infection, an individual with a risk behavior develops thoughts, worries, and fantasies about AIDS and its impact. Many persons with symptoms begin to plan and prepare for death, even when this is premature.

Some individuals cope as well as possible and mobilize themselves, their families, and caregivers. They may cooperate readily and form trusting relationships with their physicians and other caregivers. No matter what the individual's coping capacities, severity of symptoms, or psychopathology, the capacity of the health care provider to elicit the patient's understanding of the illness remains an important factor in communication, development of a supportive relationship, and improving adherence. It is frustrating to the health care worker and patient alike if there are barriers to communication. When a person with AIDS is encouraged to share his or her own perceptions, understanding, or theories of the illness, communication proceeds at the appropriate level and pace.

Eliciting an individual's understanding of an illness is not a static event. It is a process that begins from the moment of first contact and continues periodically throughout the illness. An early understanding is important because it gives the opportunity to begin a process of exploration that will result in education of both the patient and the health care provider. Often, the patient may suspect the diagnosis of AIDS. The health care provider then learns the specific ideas that the patient has about AIDS and what they mean to him or her. The patient may then gradually learn from the health care provider whether the understanding coincides with what is actually known about his or her own illness.

Although the concept of eliciting the patient's understanding of the illness is hardly unique to AIDS, AIDS makes the concept even more significant for the following reasons. Societal taboos against openness about sexuality and death and the illegal nature of intravenous (IV) drug use create a climate of discrimination and fear. These are heightened by the contagious nature of HIV and by the specific modes of transmission. Additionally, some persons with HIV infection may not have an ongoing relationship with a health care provider. The onset of symptoms may result in the first entry of a young person with a risk behavior into the health care system. This is particularly significant in young IV drug users who have received health care only on an emergency basis. The concept of the understanding of the illness when applied in the context of a supportive relationship may enhance the development of health care provider–patient rapport.

Health care providers need to be able to field responses to the question: "What is your understanding of your illness?" Patients frequently respond with "I don't know" or "You're the doctor, you tell me!" A health care provider may then point out that he or she is interested in learning what the patient thinks or what ideas or theories that the patient has about the illness.

Since persons with HIV infection are often in their 20s and 30s, it may be difficult for young health care providers not to overidentify with their patients. House officers are overwhelmed not only with the ethical dilemmas posed by AIDS, but also by having to tell a young, previously healthy individual of the diagnosis. Here, the consultation-liaison psychiatrist may provide support and help a house officer progress from overidentification to understanding and empathic concern. Physicians and other health professionals at all levels benefit from enabling patients to share with them an ever-evolving understanding of the illness. It is clear that sitting down and spending time with the patient, becoming familiar with the patient as a person, and learning the patient's own ideas and perceptions of HIV infection will save time in the long run and improve overall care.

When writer and editor Anatole Broyard developed prostatic carcinoma, he wrote (40): "I want to be a good story for my doctor, to exchange some of my art for his. . . . To most physicians my illness is a routine incident in their rounds, while for me it's the crisis of my life. . . . Just as he orders blood tests and bone scans of my body, I'd like my doctor to scan me, to grope my spirit as well as my prostate. . . . In learning to talk to his patients the doctor may talk himself back into loving his work. He has little to lose and much to gain by letting the sick man into his heart. If he does, they can share, as few others can, the wonder, terror, and exaltation of being on the edge of being, between the natural and the supernatural."

The understanding of the illness and the relationship that can develop when the doctor is "being whom the patient needs" (41) can serve to mitigate the overwhelming impact of AIDS.

SUICIDE AND AIDS

The nature and severity of the illnesses that complicate HIV infection are devastating to individuals, some of whom felt alienated and expendable even prior to learning of the diagnosis. They may react to the thought of AIDS with the thought of suicide. The thought of suicide is as universal as its taboo. In persons with AIDS, thoughts of suicide may be universal.

Some persons with AIDS have risk behaviors such as drug use that have led to alienation from families or communities. They felt isolated, lonely, alienated, and expendable, even before the diagnosis of AIDS. Marzuk et al. (42) studied the rate of suicide in New York City during 1985. He found that the suicide rate for men with AIDS from 20 to 59 years old was 36 times that of men from 20 to 59 without a diagnosis of AIDS. Kizer et al.

(43) studied death certificates in California in 1986 and found that men with AIDS from 20 to 39 had a suicide rate 21 times that of men without a diagnosis of AIDS. Perry et al. (44) assessed suicidal ideation in individuals with risk behaviors before and after HIV testing. He found that 30% of those studied had suicidal ideation before testing and that even with extensive pretest and post-test counseling, suicidal ideation persisted in over 15% of both seropositive and seronegative individuals. Although this area warrants further study, it is clear that persons with HIV infection as well as those with risk behaviors are more vulnerable to suicide than the general population, so that AIDS itself is a risk factor for suicide. The suicidal person with AIDS is in the midst of a crisis of expendability. The concept of expendability (45,46) is conveyed to the suicidal individual in verbal and nonverbal ways and hopelessness develops. Once the diagnosis of AIDS is confirmed, alienation and expendability compound the sense of hopelessness. Risk factors for suicide in the general population (Table 3) include the following (47–49): hopelessness, impulsivity, substance abuse disorder, recent illness, recent hospitalization, depression, living alone, and inexpressible grief.

Persons with AIDS are frequently ill and hospitalized. They feel alienated and isolated because of the discrimination against them (50). Hopelessness is heightened by the high mortality rate associated with AIDS and the devastating downhill course. Further complicating the picture are the issues of pain, disfigurement, blindness, weakness, and depression associated with some of the infections and cancers comprising AIDS. The organic brain syndromes associated with AIDS are often accompanied by impulsivity, impaired judgment, and diminution of the individual's capacity to understand and cope with AIDS. Suicidal ideation may be further suggested either consciously or unconsciously by loved ones who are unable to deal with AIDS or its social consequences.

Case 3. The patient was a 32-year-old unemployed man who stated that he would kill himself if he were found to have AIDS. A diagnosis of AIDS was made when *Pneumocystis carinii* pneumonia was diagnosed. A diagnosis of organic mood disorder with depression was made. The patient was treated with psychotherapy and psychotropic medication and remained on suicide precautions until he responded to treatment.

Although suicidal ideation can be a frequent early reac-

TABLE 3. *Risk factors for suicide*

Hopelessness
Impulsivity
Substance abuse disorder
Depression
Recent illness
Recent hospitalization
Living alone
Inexpressible grief

tion to learning of HIV seropositivity, suicide may be contemplated at any point during the course of HIV infection. Persons with AIDS have contemplated taking pills, jumping from windows, electrocution, and wrist-slashing at various points in their illness. As the illnesses progress, and hospitalizations become more frequent, some individuals may think of suicide as a way to control their destiny.

The management of the suicidal person with HIV infection is a sensitive and complex issue. It is crucial to remember that all suicidal individuals have mixed feelings about suicide and can vacillate from being preoccupied with hopelessness and suicide to thoughts of and plans for the future. No one is suicidal all the time. Suicide may be an effort to gain control or to alleviate pain or alienation. Suicide is also a symptom of major depression, organic mood disorder, and a reaction to a growing realization of loss of health, strength, and cognitive capacities.

The caregiver needs to feel comfortable with taking a suicide history and discussing suicide in depth with the person with HIV infection. The steps include the following: (a) establishment of a trusting relationship, (b) discussion of suicide and death in relation to AIDS and the patient's philosophies and religious beliefs, and (c) realization of the value of continuity of care and reassurance that the person with HIV infection will not be abandoned.

Suicide history-taking includes the following questions:

1. Have you ever thought about killing yourself?
2. What is it specifically that made you think of suicide?
3. Have you made any plans?
4. What are they?
5. Have you ever tried to kill yourself?
6. Do you feel like killing yourself now?
7. What would you accomplish?
8. Do you plan to rejoin someone who has died?
9. Do you know anyone who committed suicide?

Far from harming the patient, being able to speak about suicidal thoughts and feelings is highly cathartic. Persons with HIV infection may feel isolated and alienated. Thoughts of suicide, while on the one hand providing some measure of consolation and control, may be frightening and painful on the other. Sharing suicidal feelings with an empathic listener is not only relieving but may result in a different perspective.

There is no treatment for suicide, only prevention and education. In order to prevent suicide in AIDS, caregivers need to be able to take a suicide history, recognize and treat depression and organic brain syndromes, and provide continuous observation when indicated. In order to resolve a suicidal crisis, it is important to reestablish bonds and provide the patient with a supportive network of family, loved ones, friends, and caregivers. Crisis intervention, network formation, ongoing support, and family therapy may prevent suicide.

A multidisciplinary team approach may be helpful in providing support, crisis intervention, and education for persons with HIV infection.

THE METROPOLITAN HOSPITAL CENTER MULTIDISCIPLINARY AIDS PROGRAM

There is a need for a comprehensive and coordinated approach to the crisis of AIDS (51). Individuals who are HIV seropositive and persons with AIDS are confronted with uncertainty, severe illnesses, profound psychologic reactions, discrimination, and death. Each individual deserves the best medical and psychologic care available, as well as services of other disciplines where indicated. Each person with HIV infection may require the care and services of a physician in primary care internal medicine as well as physicians with specialties in infectious disease, hematology-oncology, psychiatry, neurology, pulmonary medicine, dermatology, pediatrics, gastroenterology, immunology, gynecology, and dentistry. There is probably no medical specialty or subspecialty that is not necessary, at times, for persons with AIDS. They may need the companionship of a nurse aide during a hospitalization as well as the skills of a nursing staff member on medical floors and intensive care units. The nursing care requirements vary but can become overwhelming as complications such as dementia and paralyses ensue. Besides the depression, regression, and dependency needs that often accompany chronic illness, nursing staff is also faced with persons who have frequent diarrhea, may be incontinent, and have complicated and unusual treatment regimens that may be accompanied by severe side effects, such as even more diarrhea and vomiting.

Persons with AIDS may require the services and care of social workers, psychologists, discharge planners, drug addiction counselors, respiratory therapists, chaplains, lawyers, laboratory technicians, and community agencies. A multidisciplinary AIDS program can provide a coordinated, humane approach to care and a comprehensive and systematic educational program throughout the hospital. The Metropolitan Hospital Center AIDS Program has been described as a comprehensive program for persons with AIDS (1,7,52). The goals and objectives of the program are outlined in the Appendix.

The need for improvement in coordination of services for people with HIV infection has been recognized. There are some general concepts that we have used in our program that may be helpful in the formation of a multidisciplinary program. The needs of each specific hospital and community may differ. The levels of resources, community organization, support, and discrimination may vary considerably. And, finally, the composition of the hospital staff, kind of hospital, and resource availability may vary. Each program should be tailored to meet the needs of the patients, their families, the hospital, medical school, and community.

In general, the following steps may be of help in development of multidisciplinary AIDS programs:

1. Identification of individuals willing to provide organization and leadership.
2. Identification of volunteers from as many areas and specialties as is appropriate.
3. Preliminary meeting to decide on permanent membership of those individuals involved in the care of persons with AIDS.
4. Presentation of the program to the director of medicine, director of the hospital, and medical school dean in order to enlist support and/or involvement.
5. Organization of multidisciplinary AIDS program:
   a. Choice of leadership.
   b. Review of literature.
   c. Organization of seminars.
   d. Invitations to persons experienced in working with persons with AIDS or visits to other centers.
6. Scheduling of meetings on a weekly basis.
7. Assessment of programs of surveillance in order to determine the needs of the institution and to design programs to meet those needs.
8. Incorporation of consultation-liaison psychiatry into the program leadership and organization.
   a. Provide for psychological care of persons with AIDS.
   b. Provide ongoing program of support for staff members.
   c. Provide for accurate psychiatric diagnosis and treatment.
   d. Provide for coordination of care.

A multidisciplinary AIDS program can include the following members: infectious disease specialists, consultation-liaison psychiatrists, general internists, oncologists, pulmonologists, gastroenterologists, gynecologists, pediatricians, dentists, nurses, psychologists, social workers, drug addiction counselors, respiratory therapists, dieticians, chaplains, discharge planners, administrators, house officers, and community affairs representatives. The members may be permanent or rotating with an identified core of permanent members who meet on an ongoing basis and provide coordination of clinical, education, and research activities throughout the hospital.

The Metropolitan Hospital Center AIDS Program was developed in order to provide a coordinated and humane approach to the care of persons with AIDS. A team comprised of physicians with specialties in infectious disease, hematology-oncology, consultation-liaison psy-

chiatry, epidemiology, neurology, pediatrics, and employee's health, along with nurses, social workers, discharge planners, and a respiratory therapist, a dietician, a psychologist, a chaplain, and an administrator, has been meeting weekly since 1983. The program has coordinated care and provided help for more than 3000 men, women, and children with HIV infection.

It has provided medical and psychological care and support, crisis intervention, and suicide prevention. It implements educational programs for patients, hospital staff, other hospitals, medical schools, and community agencies. At Metropolitan Hospital Center, persons with AIDS are treated on general medical, surgical, and pediatric floors and intensive care units with a nonsegregated approach. They are seen in all ambulatory settings. Persons with AIDS are in two-, four-, and six-bed rooms with persons with other diagnoses. They are isolated only when they are unable to control secretions or if respiratory or strict isolation is indicated (53). Although it is clear that there are many approaches and models for the care of a person with AIDS, the sense of isolation and alienation engendered by AIDS and societal responses to AIDS make further isolation in the hospital setting even more unbearable. At least in the hospital, on the inpatient units and in the ambulatory setting, persons with AIDS need to find a safe haven where they are free from discrimination and stigmatization.

Hospital settings are not, however, intrinsically free from any of these, and work needs to be done to help both professional and nonprofessional staff to overcome societal taboos (54–58).

The Metropolitan Hospital Center AIDS Program addresses the frustrations and anxieties of staff and campaigns for widespread education, programs of risk reduction, decreased discrimination, and increased resources. This program is a model approach for providing humane care for persons with AIDS and helping them, their loved ones, and caregivers to cope with the crisis.

The health care professionals caring for persons with AIDS have numerous conflicts, fears, and concerns (59–61). The consultation-liaison psychiatrist addresses these conflicts and, through a multidisciplinary AIDS program, can provide support for caregivers. House officers, particularly residents in internal medicine, may be in need of such support. The stress of internship and residency training has been recognized (62–65). Psychiatric assistance should be available to house officers as part of residency training (66,67), in order to alleviate stress and treat depression as well as to prevent some of the tragic consequences, such as drug use (68,69) and suicide (70–72). Wachter (73) suggests that the AIDS epidemic has added yet another stress to medical residency training. He documents a major impact on workload, on education, and on the feelings of house officers. A multidisciplinary AIDS program in conjunction with consultation-liaison psychiatry can provide support for house officers.

PSYCHIATRIC MANIFESTATIONS

At times, health care professionals have difficulties managing psychiatric disorders associated with AIDS. Recognition of specific psychiatric disorders frequently associated with HIV infection is important to provide (a) greater understanding of the behavior of persons with HIV infection; (b) early recognition and diagnosis of HIV infection; (c) improved adherence to medical regimens; (d) appropriate risk reduction interventions; and (e) improved patient well-being.

Psychiatric Manifestations of Those Who Are Not Infected with HIV

Individuals with no risk behavior, no likelihood of infection, and no evidence of infection may, nevertheless, have psychiatric manifestations associated with HIV infection. These manifestations are summarized in Table 4. Some of the definitions of psychiatric disorders are based on those in the *Diagnostic and Statistical Manual of Mental Disorders,* Third Edition, Revised (DSM-III-R) (74), while other are adapted and applied to AIDS-related issues.

AIDS Anxiety

AIDS anxiety is characterized by unrealistic and excessive apprehension about having or developing AIDS and about the consequences of infection. This is all-consuming and is manifested by symptoms of anxiety, such as trembling, restlessness, fatigue, shortness of breath, sweating, dry mouth, chills, frequent urination, trouble swallowing, difficulty concentrating, insomnia, and irritability. It is of note that many of these symptoms can also occur with HIV infection.

The treatment for AIDS anxiety includes individual and group psychotherapy.

TABLE 4. *Psychiatric manifestations of those who are not infected with HIV*

AIDS anxiety
AIDS phobia
AIDS delusions
Schizophrenia with delusions of AIDS
Major depression with mood congruent psychotic features
Factitious disorder
Factitious AIDS
Münchausen's AIDS
Malingering AIDS

AIDS Phobia

AIDS phobia (75,76) is characterized by a persistent fear of AIDS that interferes with usual activities or relationships. The individual recognizes that the fear is excessive or unreasonable. AIDS phobia responds well to psychotherapy.

AIDS Delusions

Delusional ideas about HIV infection can be associated with schizophrenia or major affective disorder with mood-congruent psychotic features (77–81). Although most authors describe major depression with mood-congruent psychotic features that center around AIDS or HIV infection, other authors have described different psychopathological themes. Brotman and Forstein (82) described five individuals with depression and AIDS obsessions. Others have described delusions with somatization (83) and paranoid psychosis (84). Treatment is directed not toward the delusions but toward the underlying cause, such as schizophrenia or major depression.

Factitious Disorder with AIDS

This disorder is characterized by intentional production or feigning of physical symptoms because of a psychologic need to maintain the sick role. There is no evidence of external incentives, such as economic gain, drugs, or disability. Baer (85) has described an individual with factitious medical illness presenting as Münchausen's syndrome.

Case 4. This was a 28-year-old man who presented with symptoms of shortness of breath and headache and gave a complicated history of AIDS, *Pneumocystis carinii* pneumonia, and cryptococcal meningitis. This patient had no current evidence of illness and had forged his letters of introduction. Ultimately the patient admitted that he had asthma and refused further care (85).

Other cases of factitious AIDS have been reported (86–88).

Malingering with AIDS

This disorder is characterized by intentional production of physical or psychologic symptoms of AIDS in order to obtain money, drugs, housing, or disability. An individual who was malingering in order to obtain entitlements and housing was admitted to our hospital (1).

Case 5. The patient was a 29-year-old unemployed actor and former Disney World Donald Duck character who was admitted with weight loss, cough, night sweats, and fever. He gave a history of *Pneumocystis carinii* pneumonia and AIDS. He was found to have no evidence of HIV infection or opportunistic infection, and his history could not be verified. He was living in an AIDS Resource Center apartment and had fabricated his history in order to obtain a place to live in New York, where he wished to pursue an acting career.

Treatment for both factitious disorder and malingering is long-term psychotherapy. It is often difficult to engage patients in treatment because of their need to maintain their facades of illness.

Psychiatric Manifestations Associated with HIV Infection

Psychiatric disorders may be the first (89–93) and, at times, the only (91–93) manifestation of HIV infection. Early diagnosis of central nervous system (CNS) HIV-related abnormalities can lead to timely introduction of specific treatment with antiretroviral agents such as zidovudine (94). Early neuropsychiatric disorders have been described (89–93), in addition to later manifestations of general psychopathology (95–101), dementia (102–119), psychosis (120–122), depression (123–124), and mania (125–128). The psychiatric manifestations of HIV infection are summarized in Table 5.

Psychiatric disorders can be a reaction to the knowledge of the diagnosis of AIDS and its stigma. Alternatively, psychopathology can be related to intrinsic involvement of the brain with HIV or other opportunistic infections or cancers, such as toxoplasmosis, cryptococcosis, or lymphoma. In addition, treatment modalities for opportunistic infections and cancers may have CNS side effects, including psychiatric symptoms, and further complicate the picture.

Psychopathology may play an important role in various aspects of HIV infection. IV drug use is a risk behavior that is associated with HIV infection. The affective disorders can result in the initiation of substance abuse. Khantzian and others (129,130) have proposed that IV drug users are depressed individuals who seek drugs in order to medicate their depressions. He and others have proposed the "self-medication" and "drug-of-choice" theories to explain use of IV drugs. The association of depression with the use of IV drugs, as well as the high incidence of suicide in major depression and substance abuse disorders, places these individuals at an increased risk for suicide. Easy access to drugs and to weapons make suicide a relatively accessible alternative.

Substance abuse disorders can impair judgment and lead to risky behaviors. Use of IV drugs with contaminated needles is the principle source of transmission of HIV in this population. Because male IV drug users may also transmit the virus sexually to their female partners, and since women may be IV drug users themselves, substance abuse disorders also play a major role in transmis-

TABLE 5. *Psychiatric disorders associated with HIV infection*

Organic mental disorders
  Dementia
    HIV-dementia or AIDS-dementia complex
    Dementia associated with opportunistic infections and cancers
      Infections
      (a) Fungal: Cryptococcoma, cryptococcal meningitis, candida abscesses, candidiasis, aspergillosis, coccidioidomycosis
      (b) Protozoal: toxoplasmosis
      (c) Bacterial: *Mycobacterium avium-intracellulare*
      (d) Viral: cytomegalovirus, herpes encephalitis, papovavirus progressive multifocal leukoencephalopathy
      Cancers
      (a) Primary cerebral lymphoma
      (b) Disseminated Kaposi's sarcoma
  Delirium
Organic delusional disorder
Organic mood disorder
  Depressed
  Manic
  Mixed
Affective disorders
  Major depression
  Dysthymic disorder
Adjustment disorders
  Adjustment disorder with depressed mood
  Adjustment disorder with anxious mood
Substance abuse disorder
Borderline personality disorder
Antisocial personality disorder
Bereavement

sion of HIV to children. The majority of infants and children with AIDS are the offspring of IV drug users or of mothers whose sexual partners are IV drug users.

The antisocial personality disorder is associated with the buying and selling of illegal drugs. Hence this disorder may perpetuate the spread of AIDS. The acting-out behaviors associated with this disorder may contribute to difficulties with management, disruptive behavior, and problems with compliance. Patients with antisocial personality disorder require special approaches in order to work toward risk reduction.

The organic brain syndromes associated with intoxication and long-term drug use contribute to and complicate the cognitive dysfunction associated with HIV infection. Cognitive dysfunction is a major impediment to understanding, coping with, and adapting to AIDS and prevents individuals from learning risk-reduction measures or complying with care.

Psychologic Factors as a Cause of Immunosuppression

Separation, loss, stress, and depression may be psychological cofactors in the onset of illness in asymptomatic HIV-seropositive individuals. The effects of separation, loss, depression, and stress on the immune system have been explored by Spitz (131,132), Engel (133), Schmale (134), Hofer (135), Holmes and Rahe (136), Rahe et al. (137), and Weiner (138). Silberstein (139) has proposed that the association of stress and depression, with alterations of cell-mediated immunity may be a cofactor in the cause of AIDS. Blumenfield (140) proposed that psychosocial factors play a role in the onset of opportunistic infection in persons with HIV infection. Fawzy et al. demonstrated less psychological distress (141) and improved immune system functions (142) when individuals with recently diagnosed malignant melanoma had group therapy for 6 weeks. Derogatis et al. (143) correlated psychological coping mechanisms with survival time in metastatic breast cancer. Spiegel and co-workers have shown (144–146) that group therapy improved survival time in metastatic breast cancer. Psychiatric intervention could have a similar beneficial impact on persons with HIV infection. Psychotherapeutic interventions should be incorporated into treatment as soon as possible after the onset of HIV infection (1,147,148). Further research into this area is indicated.

ORGANIC BRAIN SYNDROME

Despite their frequent occurrence in general hospital populations, organic brain syndromes frequently go undiagnosed (149). Even delirium, which is associated with a high mortality rate, is often overlooked. Consultation requests for persons with delirium are most often called for isolated psychiatric symptoms, management problems, or assessment of capacity to give informed consent or refuse treatment. Even in populations of elderly patients with multiple illnesses and many reasons for metabolic, endocrinologic, hypoxic, or pharmacologically induced encephalopathies, organic brain syndromes go unrecognized, undiagnosed, or incorrectly treated. The organic brain syndromes associated with HIV infection are even more elusive. It is probably difficult for young physicians to associate aberrant behavior, mood swings, or treatment refusal with the dementias and deliria associated with HIV infection.

Organic brain syndromes occur frequently in persons with AIDS. They may or may not be associated with neurological findings. The presence of CNS involvement with *Toxoplasma gondi, Cryptococcus neoformans,* HIV, or cerebral lymphoma may, or may not, be indicative of the presence of cognitive dysfunction. Although cerebral atrophy is associated with AIDS dementia, the degree of atrophy may not correlate with the severity of the dementia.

Delirium

Delirium is the most frequently encountered organic brain syndrome. Lipowski (150,151) describes delirium as a disorder of cognition including global cognitive impairment with concurrent disorders of memory, thinking, orientation, perception, disturbances of the sleep–wake cycle, and a characteristic course marked by rapid onset, relatively brief duration, and fluctuations in the severity of the disturbance. There is impaired ability to process, retain, retrieve, and apply information about the environment, body, and self. The patient's level of awareness is reduced. Thinking, perceiving, and remembering are all impaired in delirium.

Etiology of Delirium in AIDS

Factors predisposing to delirium in AIDS include addiction to alcohol or drugs, brain damage, and chronic illness. Facilitating factors are psychological stress, sleep deprivation, and sensory deprivation during intensive care unit admission. Organic factors (see Table 6) are the most frequent causes of delirium, including (a) hypoxia secondary to *Pneumocystis carinii* pneumonia and acute respiratory distress; (b) infections such as HIV encephalopathy, bacterial or fungal meningitis, or septicemia; (c) space-occupying lesions of the brain such as toxoplasmosis and CNS lymphoma; and (d) drugs, including opiates, as well as antibiotics and chemotherapeutic agents.

TABLE 6. *Organic causes of delirium in AIDS*

Intoxication
  Drugs: antibiotics, anticonvulsants, sedative-hypnotics, opiates, phencyclidine, antineoplastic drugs, anticholinergic agents, cocaine
  Alcohol
Alcohol or drug withdrawal
  Alcohol
  Opiates
  Sedative-hypnotics
Metabolic encephalopathy
  Hypoxia
  Hepatic, renal, pulmonary, pancreatic insufficiency
  Hypoglycemia
  Disorders of fluid, electrolyte, and acid–base balance, water intoxication, dehydration, hypernatremia, hypokalemia, hypocalcemia, hypercalcemia, alkalosis, acidosis
  Endocrine disorders
Infections
  Systemic: bacteremia, septicemia, subacute bacterial endocarditis, pneumonia, *Pneumocystis carinii* pneumonia, cryptococcal pneumonia, herpes zoster, disseminated *Mycobacterium avium-intracellulare,* disseminated candidiasis
  Intracranial: cryptococcal meningitis, HIV encephalitis, tuberculous meningitis, toxoplasmosis
Epilepsy
Head trauma
Space-occupying lesions of brain: CNS lymphoma, toxoplasmosis, cytomegalovirus infection, abscesses, cryptococcoma
Blood: anemia

Several standardized tests have been developed, including the Short Portable Mental Status Questionnaire (152), the Mini-Mental State Examination (153), and the Cognitive Capacity Screening Examination (154). These are all screening tests for moderate to severe cognitive dysfunction and do not detect subtle signs or mild degrees of impairment. Mild dementia requires careful psychiatric examination and neuropsychologic assessment.

Romano and Engel (155), Pro and Wells (156), and Obrecht et al. (157) have stressed the usefulness of the electroencephalogram (EEG) in helping to support a diagnosis of delirium. Decrease in frequency of the EEG background activity is indicative of delirium, possibly as a result of a reduction of brain metabolism. EEG changes virtually always accompany delirium and make the electroencephalogram a useful diagnostic tool in persons with AIDS who manifest a change in mental status (158,159). EEG testing may also be helpful in evaluating and monitoring the course of AIDS dementia (160). A recent controlled study (161) of men with asymptomatic HIV infection showed that EEG and other electrophysiologic tests were the most sensitive indicators of subclinical neurologic impairment.

Treatment of delirium consists first of treating the underlying cause and maintaining hydration, electrolyte balance, and nutrition. In addition, it is important to provide an optimal environment for the patient: a quiet, well-lit room with a dim light at night, radio or television, a calendar, clock, photographs and familiar objects, and, if possible, visits from familiar people. Medical and nursing support should be directed toward orientation and companionship as well as adequate sleep and sedation. Haloperidol 0.5–10 mg may be recommended as a standing order for sleep until identification and treatment of the underlying cause have been accomplished.

Dementia

Dementia is an organic brain syndrome characterized by loss of intellectual abilities that is sufficiently severe as to interfere with the individual's social and/or occupational functioning (74). Dementia (162) may be regarded as a global disorder of cognition, in the sense that several cognitive functions are impaired concurrently. These include memory, judgment, and abstract thinking, which are decreased in function relative to the individual's premorbid level of performance. Apraxia, agnosia, anomia, and constructional difficulty are accompanied by dropping things and poor concentration. Denial, memory impairment, and impairment of abstraction make it difficult for some patients to comprehend a diagnosis such as AIDS. Personality changes include alteration of the characteristic personality or accentuation of personality traits. Loss of cortical inhibitions may lead to promiscuity, assaultive behavior, or lack of awareness of social

amenities. There may be use of obscenities by individuals who were not known to use them before. A patient may be unaware that he or she is not adequately clothed or that breasts or genitalia are exposed. These changes have a profound impact on family members, loved ones, and caregivers who might expect to see such changes in the elderly, but not in young adults.

Other features include depression, psychosis, and anxiety. Delusions of persecution or jealousy can occur. When a patient is confronted with a difficult series of tasks, such as during careful psychiatric examination or neuropsychologic testing, a catastrophic reaction (163) may result. This can be averted by an aware examiner who employs a supportive approach during evaluation of cognitive capacities. The signs and symptoms of dementia are summarized in Table 7. The most frequent cause of dementia in AIDS is HIV encephalopathy (Table 8). In general, differentiation of delirium from dementia may be based on criteria that include normal state of consciousness in dementia, rapidly fluctuating course in delirium, and EEG slowing in delirium. Although delirium may be superimposed on dementia in AIDS, it is important to understand how to distinguish the two entities (Table 9).

Firesetting: An Unexpected Manifestation of HIV-Dementia

Firesetting is a dangerous concomitant of HIV-dementia (164). Although relatively rare, we have seen three firesetters with HIV-dementia. The first patient accidentally ignited his pajamas while smoking. The patient was wearing his own pajamas and they were not flame-retardant. He died in the burn unit of another hospital to which he was transferred after sustaining third-

TABLE 7. *Symptoms and signs of HIV dementia*

Early	Signs
Early	
Word-finding difficulty	Cognitive impairment
Forgetfulness	Apathy
Poor concentration	Regression
Confusion	Psychosis
Slowed thinking	Psychomotor retardation
Difficulty performing complex learned tasks	Difficulty with abstract thinking
Loss of balance	Ataxia
Poor handwriting	Tremor
Leg weakness	Paresis
Dropping things	
Late	
Disorientation	Mutism
Severe confusion	Incontinence
	Seizures
	Perseveration
	Severe regression
	Carphologia (picking)

TABLE 8. *Causes of dementia in AIDS*

Brain involvement
  Cancers
    Primary cerebral lymphoma
    Kaposi's sarcoma
  Infections
    Viral
      HIV encephalopathy
      Herpes simplex encephalopathy
      Herpes zoster encephalopathy
      Cytomegalovirus encephalopathy
      Papovavirus progressive multifocal
        leukoencephalopathy
    Fungal
      Cryptococcal meningitis
      Cryptococcoma
      Candida abscesses
      Candidiasis
      Aspergillosis
      Coccidioidomycosis
    Protozoal
      Toxoplasma encephalitis
      Toxoplasma abscesses
    Bacterial
      Mycobacterium avium-intracellulare
  Systemic involvement
    Metabolic
      Hypoxic or anoxic encephalopathy
    Toxic substances
      Chronic abuse of drugs

degree burns over 70% of his body. The second patient survived after deliberately setting himself on fire at home. The third patient had HIV-dementia and antisocial personality disorder and is presented in the vignette that follows.

Case 6. The patient was a 49-year-old unemployed security guard with HIV-dementia who was transferred from the AIDS unit of a long-term-care facility because of firesetting and belligerent behavior. The patient had used IV heroin for 26 years and had been incarcerated many times. He had disseminated *Mycobacterium avium-intracellulare* infection, oral candidiasis, chronic hiccups, paraparesis, and fecal incontinence. He was cachectic, wheelchair-bound, and had impaired orientation, memory, and concentration. He responded well to supportive therapy, behavior modification, and close supervision. Chlorpromazine 150 mg twice daily and valproic acid 500 mg twice daily stabilized his behavior and eliminated hiccups. He showed no firesetting behavior during his stay at our hospital but was refused readmission to the long-term-care facility.

Dementia may be associated with specific personality or behavioral manifestations if there is invasion of certain brain areas by the infectious agents or tumors associated with AIDS. If the frontal lobes are involved, then the characteristics may include reduced drive, diminished self-concern, inability to delay gratification, impulsivity, lack of judgment, shallow blunted affect, persev-

eration, concrete thinking, and inability to change mental set (165).

It is important to provide the necessary support, psychotherapy, and family therapy for AIDS-associated dementia. Persons with dementia may benefit from ongoing therapy and may have a less precipitous course. Therapy is primarily supportive. Haloperidol can help to alleviate anxiety and agitation as well as psychotic symptomatology. Therapy should also include the family and should provide caregivers with enough information about dementia so that they will be able to understand the patient's behavior and help to orient and educate the patient as much as possible.

Treatment of dementia is similar to that of delirium. Although not all AIDS-related dementias are reversible at the present time, it is important to make an effort to identify and treat underlying causes.

Organic Mood Disorder

Organic mood disorder is a disorder in which there is a disturbance of mood with symptoms of a major depressive or manic episode. There is an underlying organic cause for the disturbance of mood, but no evidence of either delirium or dementia.

The following example illustrates organic mood disorder in a person with AIDS.

Case 7. The patient was a 30-year-old artist who was admitted to the psychiatric unit because of depression with suicidal ideation. History revealed that he had been hospitalized twice within the year prior to admission because of depression. There was no family history of affec-

TABLE 9. *Differentiation of delirium and dementia in AIDS*[a]

Indicators	Delirium	Dementia
EEG background slowing	+	−
Fluctuation of symptoms	+	−
Drowsiness	+	−
Illusions	+	−
Hallucinations	+	−
Confusion	+	−
Carphologia (picking)	+	−
Insomnia	+	+
Impaired attention	+	+
Impaired concentration	+	+
Slow speech	−	+
Slow motor responses	−	+
Delusions	−	+
Ataxia	−	+
Leg weakness	−	+

[a] Please note that the differentiation is *not* absolute and there is occasional overlap of symptoms and frequent appearance of delirium superimposed on preexisting dementia in AIDS. The features listed were chosen because they are more often different in the two categories than most other features.

tive disorder and no history of substance abuse in the patient or family. The patient was found to have recurrent major depression. He was treated with antidepressants and psychotherapy but did not respond. He was treated with electroshock therapy and continued to remain depressed and withdrawn with anorexia, weight loss, and suicidal ideation. He developed a fever and was found to have cryptococcal pneumonia and AIDS. Psychiatric evaluation revealed organic mood disorder with depression. He responded well to psychotherapy and antidepressants and was discharged and lost to follow-up for a period of 1 year. At the end of that year, he was hospitalized at another hospital, where he was described as acting aggressively and bizarrely. He was brought to our hospital where he was found to be alert and oriented, talkative, with pressure of speech, tangentiality, and euphoric mood. He was grandiose, with mood-congruent delusions. He was extremely agitated at times. He was treated with psychotherapy and trifluoperazine, to which he responded well. He was found to have cryptococcal meningitis and disseminated *Mycobacterium avium-intracellulare* infection. He deteriorated rapidly, became depressed, and died during this admission. His psychiatric diagnosis was organic mood disorder with recurrent manic and depressive episodes probably associated with CNS HIV infection and cryptococcal disease.

Initial treatment includes treating underlying opportunistic infections or cancers. The treatment of organic mood disorder includes individual psychotherapy and, at times, use of psychotropic medication. The tricyclic antidepressants, such as imipramine, may be used in doses as low as 10–25 mg or up to 75–200 mg at bedtime. Neuroleptics may be used in low doses, when necessary. Haloperidol 0.5–10 mg at bedtime or trifluoperazine 1–30 mg daily may be recommended.

Organic Delusional Disorder

In organic delusional disorder, delusions are the predominating symptom and are generally paranoid and grandiose. One patient believed that he was Jesus Christ. He had CNS toxoplasmosis. Treatment includes specific chemotherapy for the underlying opportunistic infections or cancers, psychotherapy, and neuroleptic medication.

Major Depression

Major depression is a disorder characterized by depressed mood, guilt, loss of interest in most activities (anhedonia), and hopelessness. There can be insomnia or hypersomnia and psychomotor retardation or agitation. There is diminution of self-esteem, feelings of worthlessness and hopelessness, and there may also be evidence of diminished ability to think or concentrate and suicidal ideation.

Treatment for major depression includes individual and family therapy and psychotropic medications.

Uncomplicated Bereavement

Although uncomplicated bereavement is defined in DSM-III-R in relationship to the loss of a loved one, in AIDS, as in other severe illnesses, the losses of health, functioning, body integrity, and anticipatory loss of life may result in the same reaction. Additionally, many persons with AIDS have also suffered the loss of their loved ones, or of friends who have died of AIDS.

A full depressive syndrome can be an expected reaction to such a loss, with feelings of depression and such

TABLE 10. *Differentiation of major depression and bereavement*

	Uncomplicated bereavement	Major depression
General	Exhaustion, lack of strength, restlessness, inability to sit still, aimless moving, decreased capacity for organized living, "going through the motions," insomnia	Insomnia, psychomotor retardation or agitation, diminished ability to function, decreased libido, headache, backache
Gastrointestinal	Empty feeling in abdomen, anorexia, tightness in throat, dysphagia, constipation	Somatic delusions ("my insides are rotting away"), anorexia, weight loss, constipation
Respiratory	Sighing respirations, dyspnea	
Emotional	Sorrow, sadness, guilt over survival, loss of warmth in other relations, hostility, preoccupation with image of deceased	Sadness, depressed, worthlessness, hopelessness, helplessness, decreased self-esteem, suicidal thoughts or acts
Course	Self-limiting	Requires intervention
Treatment	Working through of ambivalent feelings to achieve freedom from bondage to the deceased, readjustment to environment without the deceased, formation of new relationships, no medication	Therapy, antidepressants

associated symptoms as poor appetite, weight loss, and insomnia. However, morbid preoccupation with worthlessness, prolonged and marked functional impairment, and psychomotor retardation are uncommon and suggest that the bereavement is complicated by the development of a major depression (Table 10).

In uncomplicated bereavement, guilt, if present, is chiefly about things done or not done at the time of the death by the survivor; thoughts of death are usually limited to the individual's thinking that he or she would be better off dead or that he or she should have died with the person who died. The individual with uncomplicated bereavement generally regards the feeling or depressed mood as "normal," although he or she may seek professional help for relief of such associated symptoms as insomnia and anorexia.

The duration of "normal" bereavement varies considerably among different individuals and cultures.

PSYCHIATRIC TREATMENT APPROACHES TO PERSONS WITH HIV INFECTION

The anxiety, fear, problems in coping, psychologic reactions, and psychopathology associated with AIDS all indicate a need for intervention. There are many levels and kinds of intervention, and each needs to be tailored to the needs of the individual.

The gay community has taken the lead in developing programs and resources for persons with AIDS. Even before AIDS was described in the medical literature, a group of gay men in New York City began to meet to discuss the recent deaths of some of their close friends (166). These meetings resulted in the formation of the Gay Men's Health Crisis (GMHC). Similar organizations have formed throughout the United States. They offer services to any person with AIDS or individual with AIDS-related concerns. Services are not limited to gay or bisexual men. GMHC offers many services, including crisis intervention, counseling, AIDS therapy groups, care partners' groups, parents' support groups, social activities, buddy support systems, religious counseling, financial advocacy program, and psychiatric consultation. GMHC and other similar organizations have also provided leadership in education for risk reduction.

Consultation-liaison psychiatry can provide help for persons with HIV infection in the inpatient and outpatient settings of the general hospital (167,168). Psychiatrists and other mental health professionals can provide services in outpatient clinics and private offices. Persons with AIDS are responsive to therapy and are rewarding to work with. Models for treatment include all forms of therapy and should incorporate the services of programs such as GMHC.

Crisis intervention may be indicated when an individual and loved ones first learn of the diagnosis. Crisis intervention is also effective during initial stages and if suicidal ideation develops. It is also helpful for both patients and families at the time of death and afterward, during the period of mourning.

Supportive therapy and group therapy (169–171) are extremely effective for persons with HIV infection.

Individual therapy directed toward treatment of specific psychiatric problems or resolution of conflicts and bereavement is effective in helping individuals to cope and function at the highest possible level.

Family therapy and multiple family groups are extremely effective in resolution of serious family conflicts that often accompany HIV infection. Family therapy is one of the most effective interventions with other severe and potentially fatal illnesses (172–174), and this form of therapy can help to reconcile issues in families who have rejected a person with AIDS.

Finally, psychotropic medications may be effective as adjuncts to therapy when they are indicated for the psychiatric problems described (Table 11). Specific issues in prescribing psychotropic medications include the weight and medical condition of the patient. In particular, concern for the respiratory depressant potential must be recognized. In addition, persons with AIDS may be suicidal, and prescriptions for medications should take this into account. Persons with HIV infection are vulnerable to the extrapyramidal side effects of neuroleptic medications (175). Use of benzodiazepines is relatively contraindicated because of their depressive potential. Benzodiazepines also depress cortical function and can worsen dementia or produce a superimposed delirium.

It is best to give psychotropic medications on a routine rather than an as-needed basis. This is particularly important in the management of chronic pain associated with AIDS. It is upsetting to be in pain, but it is even more upsetting to be in pain and have to be faced on a

TABLE 11. *Indications for psychopharmacologic intervention with HIV*

Diagnosis	Examples of recommended medication and daily dose range
HIV-dementia with agitation	Haloperidol 0.5–10 mg
	Thioridazine 10–200 mg
	Trifluoperizine 1–30 mg
	Valproic acid 250–1000 mg
Organic delusional disorder	Haloperidol 0.5–10 mg
	Chlorpromazine 10–200 mg
Organic affective disorder	
With mania	Haloperidol 0.5–10 mg
	Trifluoperazine 1–30 mg
With depression	Imipramine 10–150 mg
	Desipramine 10–150 mg
	Nortriptyline 10–150 mg
Major depression	Imipramine 10–150 mg
	Desipramine 10–150 mg
	Nortriptyline 10–150 mg

regular basis with the humiliation of having to ask for pain medication. Once it is clear that a person with AIDS is experiencing pain, an effective regimen of pain medication should be provided on an around-the-clock basis.

Religious counseling should be available to persons with HIV infection throughout the course of the illness.

ETHICAL ISSUES IN AIDS

The biopsychosocial approach to persons with AIDS may be implemented through a multidisciplinary AIDS program. This enables persons with AIDS to be treated with love, respect, and dignity, and it provides caregivers and loved ones with the support they need throughout this process. Through educational programs, the painful and tragic societal responses of discrimination and rejection may change. However, during this transitional phase, persons with AIDS and HIV seropositivity are confronted with ethical dilemmas that may be catastrophic or overwhelming. Their caregivers are confronted with similar dilemmas. Only those ethical issues with practical relevance for a multidisciplinary AIDS program will be raised, although there are many other ethical dimensions (176).

Confidentiality

Our patients have taught us, all too poignantly, how important confidentiality is. An individual who is struggling with as devastating an illness as AIDS deserves not only humane care but also confidentiality. This is especially important in a society in which individuals may be discriminated against simply because they have AIDS. It is crucial that a patient's rights to privacy and confidentiality remain protected in the hospital setting, as well as in the community. The nature of the illness, however, poses several difficulties. Special containers for needles and special red plastic bags are employed in order to help hospital personnel take appropriate precautions. These markers may allow other people to guess the diagnosis. Use of universal precautions can combat this problem. The vital importance of confidentiality must be stressed to all employees at initial orientation and during ongoing educational programs.

Sexual partners of persons with HIV infection are at risk for AIDS. Although a person with HIV infection should be encouraged to inform a partner or potential partners and should be taught methods of risk reduction, health care providers should obtain consent from patients before informing partners or tracing contacts. This becomes further complicated when infected persons are illegal aliens or fugitives. In general, most people with HIV infection are eager to inform their partners and to take whatever precautions are necessary to prevent the spread of the illness. Unfortunately, not all infected persons have the courage, wisdom, or cognitive capacities to enable them to cooperate in this way. Issues of confidentiality can be exquisitely painful and may not always have simple answers.

Employees or Students with AIDS or Other Manifestations of HIV Infection

Employers need to develop policies in order to prevent discrimination against employees with HIV infection. When the employers are hospitals and medical schools, AIDS policies need to emphasize confidentiality. The rights of employees to confidentiality must be protected. Employees or students with HIV infection should be treated in the same way as all other employees. Persons with HIV infection should be allowed to attend school or work until severe illness, disability, incapacitation, or death intervenes. The burdens and losses associated with HIV infection are painful enough. There is no reason to add more losses. Employees with AIDS within our hospital system have worked for as long as they were able to and left work only because they chose to do so. This policy was reinforced by the support of both medical staff and administration. The preservation of a job enables a person with AIDS to continue to support himself or herself financially, to maintain dignity and self-respect, and to have a sense of purpose. If the patient is also supporting a family, they too will be protected.

Ethics of HIV Testing

The HIV test is a test for antibodies to the AIDS virus. Although most individuals develop antibodies and become HIV seropositive within 6 weeks to 6 months after exposure, it can take up to several years to develop antibodies in a small fraction of cases. This latency period can present a public health hazard by falsely reassuring an individual who is infected that he or she is not. On the other hand, there are also rare false positives that may lead to unnecessary anxiety in an individual who is, in fact, uninfected.

HIV testing should be voluntary and anonymous, and it should not be used to screen prospective employees, insurance applicants, marriage license applicants (177), or students. HIV testing should be done with both pre-test and post-test counseling and written informed consent (178). Confidentiality of HIV test results should be carefully maintained and these results should not be disclosed without a specific written release of information.

Early detection of HIV seropositivity can lead to early prophylactic medical intervention, prolong life, and prevent transmission of HIV (179). Voluntary anonymous testing of individuals with risk behaviors should be encouraged.

**Ethical Issues Involved with Foregoing
Life-Sustaining Treatment**

The person with HIV infection needs to be able to maintain dignity and humanity from the day of diagnosis until the day of death. Caregivers should discuss issues of heroic measures and cardiopulmonary resuscitation with persons with AIDS and their loved ones. Since *Pneumocystis carinii* pneumonia is a treatable opportunistic infection, physicians need to explore very carefully the difference between intubation as part of a treatment plan versus intubation as part of a heroic attempt to keep a dying person alive. It may be helpful to be specific with those persons who have a clear idea of how they want to be cared for once they can no longer care for themselves. They may want to write a living will and designate a health care proxy agent to make medical decisions when they can no longer do so.

Ask a person who has been intubated or suctioned repeatedly through an endotracheal tube if he or she would willingly endure the process again. The answer might be "yes" if there was hope for recovery, but if there were none, then it might be "what on earth for."

Persons with AIDS vary in how they approach the process of dying. Some individuals want to be resuscitated and wish for every heroic measure possible (180–182). Others want no heroics. Plans need to be discussed so that patients can express feelings and explore the process with loved ones and caregivers. Plans then can be tailored to fit the individual's wishes and circumstances.

The ethical issues in AIDS demonstrate the importance of humanism and compassion in the care of those infected with HIV.

OVERCOMING THE STIGMA OF AIDS

In order to prevent the spread of HIV infection we need to overcome both the stigma of AIDS and the epidemic of fear. The only methods we have are education and compassion.

Barriers to Education

Epidemic of Denial

De Buono et al. (183) and MacDonald et al. (184) reported the results of surveys of the sexual behavior of college students in the United States and Canada, respectively. These surveys revealed that although condom use had increased, it had not even reached 50% by 1989. They also indicated (184) that women still tended to use contraceptive pills to prevent pregnancy and did not use condoms regularly despite awareness of HIV transmission. In three groups of college women who attended a student health service in 1975, 1986, and 1989, respectively, no significant differences were found in the num-

bers of total sexual partners or frequency of anal intercourse (183). One report (185) indicated that college students lie for sex and would lie about having a negative HIV-antibody test. These results indicate that denial and dishonesty are major factors in sexual behavior.

Epidemic of Ignorance

The Kinsey Institute New Report on Sex (186) revealed that 55% of nearly 2000 Americans failed a test on sexual knowledge. This 18-item test included important questions related to HIV transmission. Fifty percent of those tested did not know that petroleum jelly (or other oil-based lubricants) should not be used as a lubricant for condoms. Only 5% knew that nonoxynol-9 is a spermicide that has been shown to kill HIV *in vitro*. Fifty percent believed they could get AIDS from anal intercourse even if their partner were *not* infected with HIV.

Epidemic of Therapeutic Nihilism About Drug Addiction

A large proportion of HIV transmission occurs through sharing of contaminated needles by intravenous drug users (IVDUs). This is the primary mode of parenteral transmission in the United States and indirectly accounts for the majority of the spread of HIV from mother to fetus and among heterosexuals. Despite awareness of the growing epidemic among IVDUs, there are inadequate programs to treat drug users and a dearth of prevention programs targeted at this population. Part of this is based on the belief that substance users will not change their behavior. However, our own experience as well as that of others (187,188) has shown that comprehensive programs of treatment and education are effective in changing behavior in this population.

Attitudes of Health Care Workers Toward HIV Infection

Physicians and other health care professionals are not immune to the epidemics of AIDS, fear, and discrimination. In 1982, when the AIDS epidemic began at Metropolitan Hospital Center, fear and anxiety led to neglect in the care of persons with AIDS. One of the earliest manifestations was reluctance of health care professionals and ancillary staff to enter the room of a person with AIDS. When I responded to my first consultation on a person with AIDS, I discovered "the sticky floor syndrome." My shoes stuck to the floor of the room and make loud noises as I walked toward the bedside of the patient. The floor was sticky from an accumulation of spilled food, beverages, water, and body fluids. These layers accumulated because of fear on the part of the hospital maintenance staff. Nurses requested transfers and called in sick. As a result we developed the Metropolitan Hospital Center AIDS Program to address both the clinical and educational needs of staff. Nurses on the floor with the largest number of persons with AIDS were in need of support. A stress group for nurses and a comprehensive multidisciplinary program were established. However, AIDS education poses exceptional challenges for teachers and students (189). Because the disease entails both highly technical and highly emotionally charged information, AIDS education requires a biopsychosocial approach.

Biopsychosocial Approach to Education About AIDS

There is a need for a comprehensive and integrated educational approach for persons with HIV infection, their loved ones, and also hospital staffs and communities. Education should be geared not only toward giving factual information about AIDS and about risk reduction, but also toward anxiety reduction. Educators need to be comfortable with discussing sexual issues as well as with imparting specific facts about infection control. Educators also need to come to terms with and understand their feelings about AIDS, fears of contagion, and feelings about sexuality and intravenous drug use.

An organized educational program needs to examine carefully the attitudes of the teachers. These are best discussed in small group settings that give permission to be open with feelings and enable teachers to share feelings without blame, shame, or embarrassment. There is no room in the teaching of patients, families, staff, or communities for judgmental attitudes. Judgmental attitudes are as detrimental in the educational process as they are in the care of persons with AIDS. It is helpful to attempt to resolve these issues prior to embarking on an educational process. Education for physicians should begin during the first year of medical school and continue through graduation and residency (189–194).

Educational programs need to address the anxieties and fears of the learners. A well-organized program of training will be forgotten if the anxiety level is too high. Directors of residency training programs are often aware that house officers may remember little from their day of orientation because of the high level of anxiety on the first day of internship. The same concept applies to AIDS education, and it is helpful to address the anxieties and estimate their levels. Educational programs need to encompass the biopsychosocial aspects of AIDS as well as stress the importance of risk reduction. With intravenous drug users, it is necessary to involve the families or loved ones in the educational program.

Education for the community needs to begin with community agencies, centers, and community organizations. This education will help reduce anxiety as well as risk. But the most important program, that of primary prevention, needs to begin in elementary school, where

systematic programs of sex and health education, as well as education about the dangers of substance abuse, should begin in kindergarten and continue through high school and college. The programs can be tailored to the level of understanding of each group.

Educational programs about AIDS need to be tailored specifically toward the level of understanding of the learners. In AIDS, as in any illness, it is important to determine the understanding of the illness, whether it is for educational programs or direct patient care.

Medical students are in a unique position in the health care system (189). They are young enough to be ideal role models for high school and college students and mature enough to be responsible educators. A student-run AIDS education program (189) has been described. The concept of student-led volunteer educational programs can be used in high schools, colleges, and communities. Training should emphasize both anxiety reduction and risk reduction. The method includes a small-group approach that is nonjudgmental and nonauthoritarian and tailored to the level of understanding of the learners.

"The HIV epidemic has affected the experience of training in internal medicine dramatically, forcing us to confront the implicit purpose of clinical education" (195). The American Board of Internal Medicine (196) requires compassion and empathy as well as clinical skills. But physicians can be compassionate and caring only if they themselves feel supported and cared about. Cooke and Sande (195) believe that the HIV epidemic could catalyse much needed reforms in house officer training and lead to improvement in working conditions. They recommend adequate programs of universal precautions and infection control as well as widely available disability benefits and life insurance. Trainees need education about universal precautions and infection control and ready availability of equipment needed to follow guidelines. We have developed policies to address employees' concerns about needlesticks and other exposures to HIV. Medical students, house officers, physicians, nurses, and all hospital personnel need to have a support system in place in order to address concerns about accidental exposure. We developed an Employee Assistance Program (EAP) to provide services for employees. Our EAP has been providing support and counseling on a confidential basis. In addition to support from EAP and our AIDS program, employees need resources to protect themselves from infection. Boxes for disposal of needles and sharp instruments need to be emptied regularly so that accidental needlesticks do not occur when a needle is being placed in an overfilled container. Health care facilities, medical schools and hospitals need to take responsibility for assuring that there are adequate and readily accessible resources (197) in order to protect employees from exposure.

It should be noted that infection control guidelines are continually evolving in an effort to find the safest possible practice. A recent study (198) revealed that switching needles during blood culture phlebotomy did not have a significant impact on preventing contamination of blood culture bottles. Since there was no difference in the rate of contamination with or without switching needles, it is not necessary to do so. This may diminish chances for needlestick exposure during this procedure. New devices and methods of protection are being developed and could prove to be effective barriers to exposure. Postexposure zidovudine use is now being evaluated (199,200), although some recent reports have indicated that it may not be protective against infection (201,202).

Employees need to be educated and reeducated as new information becomes available. Postexposure zidovudine is recommended almost immediately (1 hr or less) after exposure. All employees on all shifts must be aware of the availability of zidovudine, its risks and benefits, and where to obtain it. In order for employees to have easy accessibility, policies, procedures, and resources to implement them must be in place on a round-the-clock basis.

AIDS has been described as an occupational disease (203), although the risk of infection after exposure is extremely low (204–210). A supportive institutional environment provides education and resources and can prevent the tragedy of an adversarial relationship developing between an employee and a health care facility (211).

The care of persons with HIV infection can be rewarding for caregivers. When orientation, education, resources, and ongoing support are available, institutions, caregivers, and patients benefit. When a physician can get to know a patient with AIDS as a person, the development of an ongoing caring relationship can diminish the barriers of discrimination and help combat the epidemics of fear and AIDS.

CONCLUSION

> We shall assume that everyone is much more simply human than otherwise . . . man—however undistinguished biologically—as long as he is entitled to the term human personality, will be very much more like every other instance of human personality than he is like anything else in the world. As I have tried to hint before, it is to some extent on this basis that I have become occupied with the science, not of individual differences, but of human identities or parallels, one might say. In other words, I try to study the degrees and patterns of things which I assume to be ubiquitously human. (212)

Harry Stack Sullivan's statement about persons with psychopathology and their psychiatrists is relevant to persons with AIDS and their caregivers.

AIDS takes a toll on patients, their loved ones, caregivers, and communities. AIDS and other manifestations of HIV infection are exquisitely painful and may

have tragic consequences. We need to work closely together to provide networks of support for patients and caregivers alike in order to cope with the crisis of AIDS. The biopsychosocial approach helps to combat the epidemics of AIDS and AIDSism. A multidisciplinary AIDS program addresses the frustrations and anxieties of staff and implements programs of education and risk reduction. A biopsychosocial approach enables persons with HIV infection, their loved ones, and caregivers to meet the challenges of AIDS with optimism and dignity.

APPENDIX: GOALS AND OBJECTIVES OF A MULTIDISCIPLINARY AIDS PROGRAM

Goals

1. To improve the care of persons with HIV infection by means of a biopsychosocial approach that maintains a view of each individual as a member of a family and community, who deserves a coordinated approach to care and treatment with dignity.
2. To improve communication and diminish alienation and expendability by means of a multidisciplinary team approach.
3. To provide ongoing programs of education for persons with HIV infection and their families, for hospital staff, and for the community.
4. To provide programs of risk reduction for individuals, schools, and community organizations.
5. To prevent transmission of HIV and to prevent discrimination against persons with HIV infection.

Enabling Objectives

1. Identification of volunteers from all areas of the hospital.
2. Formation of a multidisciplinary team.
3. Development of a comprehensive program.
   a. Clinical care of patients.
   b. Staff education.
   c. Faculty development.
   d. Liaison with outside agencies.
4. Development of methods to provide comprehensive care.
   a. Regular rounds on patients with HIV infection.
   b. Special AIDS rounds on a weekly basis to meet with all staff involved.
   c. Identification of psychological and social problems frequently encountered in HIV-infected persons.
5. Development of educational programs for persons with HIV infection.
   a. Regular seminars.
   b. Special meeting with all members of the team.

6. Educational programs of risk reduction for drug users.
   a. Special programs for IV drug users.
   b. Methadone maintenance program members.
   c. Patients in drug detoxification units.
7. Community programs of education and risk education.
   a. For schools.
   b. For community organizations.
8. Integration of inpatient and outpatient care.
   a. Home care.
   b. Home visits.
   c. Coordination of community services.

Terminal Objectives

1. Heightened awareness of psychologic problems encountered in persons with HIV infection and their families.
2. Heightened awareness in staff of psychological reactions to persons with HIV infection.
3. Improvement in health care provider–patient communication.
4. Opening avenues of communication among health professionals dealing with persons with HIV infection.
5. Humane approach to persons with HIV infection by both professional and nonprofessional hospital staff.
6. Identification and treatment of psychologic problems through individual, couple, family, group, and psychopharmacologic therapy.
7. Abstinence from needle sharing or use of IV drugs.
8. Abstinence from exchange of body fluids.
9. Diminution of discrimination against persons with HIV infection.
10. Improvement and increased availability of services for persons with HIV infection.
11. Integration of a comprehensive program of care for persons with HIV infection enabling individuals to remain as functional and healthy as possible within the family setting.
12. Primary prevention of HIV infection through elementary school education.

ACKNOWLEDGMENTS

This chapter is dedicated to the men, women, and children with AIDS and other manifestations of HIV infection at Metropolitan Hospital Center. I give special thanks to Dr. Asher D. Aladjem, without whom there would be no Metropolitan AIDS Program. My thanks to Drs. Frederick P. Duncanson, Natalie Klein, and Theodore Lenox for their outstanding contributions to the care of persons with AIDS. I thank Steven C. Cohen for his editorial assistance and Karen Crider for her technical assistance.

REFERENCES

1. Cohen MA. A biopsychosocial approach to the human immunodeficiency virus epidemic. *Gen Hosp Psychiatry* 1990;12:98–123.
2. Winerip M. For a teacher fighting AIDS, love and loss. *The New York Times,* August 24, 1990:B1.
3. Lipowski ZJ. The holistic approach to medicine. In: Lipowski ZJ, ed. *Psychosomatic medicine and liaison psychiatry.* New York: Plenum Press; 1985.
4. Engel GL. The need for a new medical model: a challenge for biomedicine. *Science* 1977;196:129–36.
5. Kimball CP. *The biopsychosocial approach to the patient.* Baltimore: Williams & Wilkins; 1981.
6. Engel GL. The biopsychosocial model and medical education: who are the teachers? *N Engl J Med* 1982;306:802–5.
7. Cohen MA, Weisman HW. A biopsychosocial approach to AIDS. *Psychosomatics* 1986;27:245–9.
8. Cohen MA. Psychiatric aspects of AIDS: a biopsychosocial approach. In: Wormser GP, Stahl RE, Bottone EJ, eds. *AIDS and other manifestations of HIV infection.* Park Ridge, NJ: Noyes Publications; 1987.
9. Cohen MA, Weisman HW, Vazquez C. The acquired immunodeficiency syndrome: a psychiatric crisis. *NY Med Q* 1988;8:53–8.
10. Hunter ND. *Epidemic of fear: a survey of AIDS discrimination in the 1980s and policy recommendations for the 1990s.* American Civil Liberties Union AIDS Project. New York: ACLU; 1990.
11. Reference 10, p 1.
12. Reference 10, p 5.
13. Blendon RJ, Donelan K. Discrimination against people with AIDS: the public's perspective. *N Engl J Med* 1988;319:1022–6.
14. Cohen MA. AIDSism, a new form of discrimination. *AMA News* January 20, 1989:43.
15. Wormser GP, Joline C. Would you eat cookies prepared by an AIDS patient? Survey reveals harmful attitudes among professionals. *Postgrad Med* 1989;86:174–84.
16. Thompson LM. Dealing with AIDS and fear: would you accept cookies from an AIDS patient? *South Med J* 1987;80:228–32.
17. Kelly JA, St. Lawrence JS, Smith S Jr, et al. Stigmatization of AIDS patients by physicians. *Am J Public Health* 1987;77:789–91.
18. Nichols SE. The social climate when AIDS developed. In: Nichols SE, Ostrow DG, eds. *Psychiatric implications of acquired immune deficiency syndrome.* Washington, DC: American Psychiatric Press; 1984:85–92.
19. Cassens B. Social consequences of acquired immunodeficiency syndrome. *Ann Intern Med* 1985;103:768–71.
20. Nichols SE. Psychosocial reactions of persons with the acquired immunodeficiency syndrome. *Ann Intern Med* 1985;103:765–7.
21. Ho DD, Rota TR, Schooley RT, et al. Isolation of HTLV-III from cerebrospinal fluid and neural tissues of patients with neurological syndromes related to the acquired immunodeficiency syndrome. *N Engl J Med* 1985;313:1493–7.
22. Resnik L, di Marzo-Veronese F, Schupbach J, et al. Intra-blood-brain barrier synthesis of HTLV-III-specific IgG in patients with neurological symptoms associated with AIDS or AIDS-related complex. *N Engl J Med* 1985;313:1498–504.
23. Black PH. HTLV-III, AIDS and the brain. *N Engl J Med* 1985;313:1538–40.
24. Gabuzda DH, Hirsch MS. The neurological manifestations of infection with human immunodeficiency virus. *Ann Intern Med* 1987;107:383–91.
25. Montagnier L. Lymphadenopathy-associated virus: from molecular biology to pathogenicity. *Ann Intern Med* 1985;103:689–93.
26. Barre-Sinoussi F, Chermmann JC, Rey R, et al. Isolation of a T-lymphotropic retrovirus from a patient at risk for an acquired immune deficiency syndrome (AIDS). *Science* 1983;220:868–71.
27. Gallo RC, Salahuddin SZ, Popovic M, et al. Frequent detection and isolation of cytopathic retroviruses (HTLV-III) from patients with AIDS and at risk for AIDS. *Science* 1984;224:500–3.

28. Montagnier L, Chermann JC, Barre-Sinoussi F, et al. A new human T-lymphotropic retrovirus: characterization and possible role in lymphadenopathy and acquired immune deficiency syndromes. In: Gallo RC, Essex M, Gross L, eds. *Human T-cell leukemia/lymphoma virus.* Cold Spring Harbor Laboratory Press, New York; 1984:363–70.

29. Ho DD, Pomerantz RJ, Kaplan JC. Pathogenesis of infection with human immunodeficiency virus. *N Engl J Med* 1987; 317:278–86.

30. Popovic M, Sarngadharan MC, Read E, et al. Detection, isolation, and continuous production of cytopathic retroviruses (HTLV-III) from patients with AIDS and pre-AIDS. *Science* 1984;224:497–500.

31. Levy JA, Hoffman AD, Kramer SM, et al. Isolation of lymphocytopathic retroviruses from San Francisco patients with AIDS. *Science* 1984;225:840–2.

32. Curran JW, Morgan WM, Hardy AM, et al. The epidemiology of AIDS: current status and future prospects. *Science* 1985;229: 1352–7.

33. Sivak SL, Wormser GP. How common is HTLV-III infection in the United States? *N Engl J Med* 1984;313:1352.

34. Coolfont report: a PHS plan for prevention and control of AIDS and the AIDS virus. *Public Health Record* 1986;101:341–8.

35. Centers for Disease Control. *Pneumocystis* pneumonia—Los Angeles. *MMWR* 1981;30:250–2.

36. Centers for Disease Control. Kaposi's sarcoma and *Pneumocystis* pneumonia among homosexual men—New York City and California. *MMWR* 1981;30:305–8.

37. Gottlieb MS, Scharoff R, Schanker HM, et al. *Pneumocystis carinii* pneumonia and mucosal candidiasis in previously healthy homosexual men: evidence of a new acquired cellular immunodeficiency. *N Engl J Med* 1981;305:1425–31.

38. Blattner WA, Biggar RJ, Weiss SH, et al. Epidemiology of human T-lymphotropic virus type III and the risk of the acquired immunodeficiency syndrome. *Ann Intern Med* 1985;103:665–70.

39. Selik RM, Haverkos HW, Curran JW. Acquired immune deficiency syndrome (AIDS) trends in the United States, 1978–82. *Am J Med* 1984;76:493–500.

40. Broyard A. Doctor—talk to me. *The New York Times Magazine,* August 26, 1990:32–6.

41. Zinn W. Transference phenomena in medical practice: being whom the patient needs. *Ann Intern Med* 1990;113:293–8.

42. Marzuk PM, Tierney H, Tardiff K, et al. Increased risk of suicide in persons with AIDS. *JAMA* 1988;259:1333–7.

43. Kizer KW, Green M, Perkins CI, Doebbert G, Hughes MJ. AIDS and suicide in California. *JAMA* 1988;250:1881.

44. Perry S, Jacobsberg L, Fishman B. Suicidal ideation and HIV testing. *JAMA* 1990;263:679–82.

45. Cohen MA, Merlino JP. The suicidal patient on the surgical ward: a multidisciplinary case conference. *Gen Hosp Psychiatry* 1983;5:65–71.

46. Sabbath J. The suicidal adolescent: the expendable child. *J Am Acad Child Psychiatry* 1969;8:272–89.

47. Beck AT, Steer RA, Kovacs M, et al. Hopelessness and eventual suicide. *Am J Psychiatry* 1985;142:559–63.

48. Miles CP. Conditions predisposing to suicide: a review. *J Nerv Ment Dis* 1977;164:231–46.

49. Barraclough B, Bunch J, Nelson B, et al. A hundred cases of suicide: clinical aspects. *Br J Psychiatry* 1974;125:355–73.

50. Leibenluft E, Goldberg RL. The suicidal terminally ill patient with depression. *Psychosomatics* 1988;29:379–86.

51. Landesman SH, Ginzburg HM, Weiss SH. The AIDS epidemic. *N Engl J Med* 1985;312:521–5.

52. Deuchar N. AIDS in New York City with particular reference to the psychosocial aspects. *Br J Psychiatry* 1984;145:612–9.

53. Conte JE, Hadley WK, Sande M. Infection control guidelines for patients with the acquired immunodeficiency syndrome (AIDS). *N Engl J Med* 1983;309:741–4.

54. Cox C. Peer review: face to face with AIDS phobia. *Nurs Times* 1985;81:22.

55. Rubinow DR. The psychological impact of AIDS. *Top Clin Nurs* 1984;6:26–30.

56. Simmons-Alling S. AIDS: psychosocial needs of the health care worker. *Top Clin Nurs* 1984;6:31–7.

57. Lusby G. AIDS: the impact on the health worker. *Front Radiat Ther Oncol* 1985;19:164–7.

58. Polan JH, Hellerstein D, Amchin J. Impact of AIDS-related cases on an in-patient therapeutic milieu. *Hosp Community Psychiatry* 1985;36:173–6.

59. Wellisch DK. UCLA psychological study of AIDS. *Front Radiat Ther Oncol* 1985;19:155–8.

60. Rosse RB. Reactions of psychiatric staff to an AIDS patient. *Am J Psychiatry* 1985;142:523.

61. Batten CP, Tabor R. Nursing the patient with AIDS. *Can Nurs* 1983;79:19–22.

62. Small GW. House officer stress syndrome. *Psychosomatics* 1981;22:860–9.

63. Ford CV. Emotional distress in internship and residency: a questionnaire study. *Psychiatric Med* 1983;1:143–50.

64. Valko RJ, Clayton PJ. Depression in internship. *Dis Nerv Syst* 1975;36:26–9.

65. McCue J. Distress of internship: causes and prevention. *N Engl J Med* 1985;312:449–52.

66. Borenstein DB, Cook K. Impairment prevention in the training years. *JAMA* 1982;247:2700–3.

67. Borenstein DB. Should physician training centers offer formal psychiatric assistance to house officers: a report on the major findings of a prototype program. *Am J Psychiatry* 1985;142: 1053–7.

68. Modlin HC, Montes A. Narcotics addiction in physicians. *Am J Psychiatry* 1964;121:358–63.

69. Putnam PL, Ellinwood EH Jr. Narcotic addiction among physicians: a ten-year follow-up. *Am J Psychiatry* 1966;122:745–8.

70. Epstein LC, Thomas CB, Shaffer JW, et al. Clinical prediction of physician suicide based on medical student data. *J Nerv Ment Dis* 1973;156:19–29.

71. Craig AG, Pitts FN. Suicide by physicians. *Dis Nerv Syst* 1969;29:763–72.

72. Steppacher RC, Mausner JS. Suicide in male and female physicians. *JAMA* 1974;228:323–8.

73. Wachter RM. The impact of the acquired immunodeficiency syndrome on medical residency training. *N Engl J Med* 1986;314:177–80.

74. American Psychiatric Association: *Diagnostic and statistical manual of mental disorders,* 3rd ed., revised (DSM-III-R). Washington, DC: American Psychiatric Association; 1987.

75. Miller D, Green J, Farmer R, et al. A "pseudo-AIDS" syndrome following from fear of AIDS. *Br J Psychiatry* 1985;146:550–1.

76. Freed E. AIDophobia. *Med J Aust* 1983;2:479.

77. Mahorney SL, Cavenar JO. A new and timely delusion: the complaint of having AIDS. *Am J Psychiatry* 1988;145:1130–2.

78. Colenda CC, Kryanowski L, Klinger R. Major depression in late life with AIDS delusions—a case report and review. *Gen Hosp Psychiatry* 1990;12:207–9.

79. Miller JD, Green J, Falmer R, Carroll G. A "pseudo-AIDS" syndrome following fear of AIDS. *Br J Psychiatry* 1985;146:550–51.

80. Shetty GC. Depressive illness with delusions of AIDS. *Am J Psychiatry* 1988;145:765.

81. Jenicke M, Pato C. Disabling fear of AIDS responsive to imipramine. *Psychosomatics* 1986;27:143–4.

82. Brotman AW, Forstein M. AIDS obsessions in depressed heterosexuals. *Psychosomatics* 1988;29:428–31.

83. O'Brien G, Hassanyeh F. AIDS-panic: AIDS-induced psychogenic states. *Br J Psychiatry* 1985;147:91.

84. Todd J. AIDS as a current psychopathological theme. A report on five heterosexual patients. *Br J Psychiatry* 1989;154:253–5.

85. Baer JW. Case report: Munchausen's AIDS. *Gen Hosp Psychiatry* 1987;9:75–6.

86. Miller F, Weiden P, Sacks M, et al. Two cases of factitious acquired immune deficiency syndrome (letter). *Am J Psychiatry* 1986;143:1483.

87. Robinson EN, Latham RH. A factitious case of acquired immunodeficiency syndrome. *Sex Transm Dis* 1987;14:54–57.

88. Nickoloff SE, Neppe VM, Ries RK. Factitious AIDS. *Psychosomatics* 1989;30:342–5.

89. Thomas CS, Szabadi E. Paranoid psychosis as the first presentation of a fulminating lethal case of AIDS. *Br J Psychiatry* 1987;151:693–5.

90. Halevie-Goldman BD, Potkin SG, Poyourow P. AIDS-related complex presenting as psychosis. *Am J Psychiatry* 1987;144:7.
91. Beckett A, Summergrad P, Manschreck T, et al. Symptomatic HIV infection of the CNS in a patient without clinical evidence of immune deficiency. *Am J Psychiatry* 1987;144:1342-4.
92. Jones HR, Ho DD, Forgacs P, et al. Acute fulminating fatal leukoencephalopathy as the only manifestation of human immunodeficiency virus infection. *Ann Neurol* 1988;23:519-22.
93. Navia BA, Price RW. The acquired immunodeficiency syndrome dementia as the presenting or sole manifestation of human immunodeficiency virus infection. *Arch Neurol* 1987;44:65-9.
94. Parisi A, DiPerri G, Strosselli M, Cairoli S, Minoli L. Instrumental evidence of zidovudine effectiveness in the treatment of HIV-associated subacute encephalitis. *AIDS* 1988;2:482-3.
95. Shaw GM, Harper ME, Hahn BH, et al. HTLV-III infection in brains of children and adults with AIDS encephalopathy. *Science* 1985;227:177-82.
96. Nurnberg HG, Prudic J, Fiori M, et al. Psychopathology complicating acquired immune deficiency syndrome (AIDS). *Am J Psychiatry* 1984;141:95-6.
97. Perry SW, Tross S. Psychiatric problems of AIDS in patients at the New York Hospital: preliminary report. *Public Health Rep* 1984;99:200-5.
98. Dilley JW, Ochitill HN, Perl M, et al. Findings in psychiatric consultations with patients with acquired immune deficiency syndrome. *Am J Psychiatry* 1985;142:82-96.
99. Polan HJ, Hellerstein D, Amchin J. Impact of AIDS-related cases on an inpatient therapeutic milieu. *Hosp Community Psychiatry* 1985;36:173-6.
100. Price WA, Forejt J. Neuropsychiatric aspects of AIDS: a case report. *Gen Hosp Psychiatry* 1986;8:7-10.
101. Ostrow D, Grant I, Atkinson H. Assessment and management of the AIDS patient with neuropsychiatric disturbances. *J Clin Psychiatry* 1988;49:14-22.
102. Cummings JL, Benson F. Subcortical dementia. Review of an emerging concept. *Arch Neurol* 1984;41:874-9.
103. Kermani E, Drob S, Alpert M. Organic brain syndrome in three cases of acquired immune deficiency syndrome. *Compr Psychiatry* 1984;25:294-7.
104. Hoffman RS. Neuropsychiatric complications of AIDS. *Psychosomatics* 1984;25:393-400.
105. Nurnberg HG, Prudic J, Fiori M, Freedman EP. Psychopathology complicating acquired immune deficiency syndrome (AIDS). *Am J Psychiatry* 1984;141:95-6.
106. Kleihues P, Lang W, Burger PC, et al. Progressive diffuse leukoencephalopathy in patients with acquired immune deficiency syndrome (AIDS). *Acta Neuropathol (Berl)* 1985;68:333-9.
107. Levy RM, Bredesen DE, Rosenblum ML. Neurological manifestations of the acquired immunodeficiency syndrome (AIDS): experience at UCSF and review of the literature. *J Neurosurg* 1985;62:475-95.
108. Navia BA, Jordan BD, Price RW. The AIDS dementia complex. *Ann Neurol* 1986;19:517-24.
109. Beresford TP, Blow FC, Hall RCW. AIDS encephalitis mimicking alcohol dementia and depression. *Biol Psychiatry* 1986;21:394-7.
110. Navia BA, Jordan BD, Price RW. The AIDS dementia complex: I. Clinical features. *Ann Neurol* 1986;109:517-24.
111. Navia BA, Cho BS, Petito CK, Price RW. The AIDS dementia complex: II. Neuropathology. *Ann Neurol* 1986;19:525-35.
112. Price RW, Brew BJ. The AIDS dementia complex. *J Infect Dis* 1988;158:1079-83.
113. Levy RM, Bredesen DE. Central nervous system dysfunction in acquired immunodeficiency syndrome. *J AIDS* 1988;1:41-64.
114. Price RW, Brew B, Sidtis J, Rosenblum M, Scheck AC, Cleary P. The brain in AIDS: central nervous system HIV-I infection and the AIDS dementia complex. *Science* 1988;239:586-92.
115. Tross S, Price RW, Navia BA, et al. Neuropsychological characterization of the AIDS dementia complex: a preliminary report. *AIDS* 1988;2:81-8.
116. Milner GL. Organic reaction in AIDS. *Br J Psychiatry* 1989;154:255-7.
117. Ho DD, Bredesen DE, Vinters HV, Daar ES. The acquired immunodeficiency syndrome (AIDS) dementia-complex. *Ann Intern Med* 1989;111:400-10.
118. Perry SW. Organic mental disorders caused by HIV: update on early diagnosis and treatment. *Am J Psychiatry* 1990;147:696-710.
119. Westreich L. AIDS dementia complex for the primary physician. *Resident Staff Physician* 1990;36:47-53.
120. Holmes VF. Treatment of monosymptomatic hypochondriacal psychosis with pimozide in an AIDS patient. *Am J Psychiatry* 1989;146:554-5.
121. Halstead S, Riccio M, Harlow P, Oretti R, Thompson C. Psychosis associated with HIV infection. *Br J Psychiatry* 1988;153:618-23.
122. Buhrich N, Cooper DA, Freed E. HIV infection associated with symptoms indistinguishable from functional psychosis. *Br J Psychiatry* 1988;152:649-53.
123. Rundell JR, Wise MG, Ursano RJ. Three cases of AIDS-related psychiatric disorders. *Am J Psychiatry* 1986;143:777-8.
124. Price WA, Forejt J. Neuropsychiatric aspects of AIDS: a case report. *Gen Hosp Psychiatry* 1986;8:7-10.
125. Kermani EJ, Borod JC, Brown PH, Tunnell G. New psychopathologic findings in AIDS. *J Clin Psychiatry* 1985;46:240-1.
126. Gabel RH, Barnard N, Norko M, O'Connell RA. AIDS presenting as mania. *Compr Psychiatry* 1986;27:251-4.
127. Johannesen DJ, Wilson LG. Mania with cryptococcal meningitis in two AIDS patients. *J Clin Psychiatry* 1988;49:200-1.
128. Maxwell S, Scheftner WA, Kessler HA, Busch K. Manic syndrome associated with zidovudine treatment. *JAMA* 1988;259:3406-7.
129. Khantzian EJ. The self-medication hypothesis of addictive disorders: focus on heroin and cocaine dependence. *Am J Psychiatry* 1985;142:1259-64.
130. Wurmser L. The question of specific psychopathology in compulsive drug use. *Ann NY Acad Sci* 1982;398:33-43.
131. Spitz RA. Hospitalism, an inquiry into the genesis of psychiatric conditions in early childhood. *Psychoanal Study Child* 1945;I:53-74.
132. Spitz RA. Anaclitic depression. *Psychoanal Study Child* 1946;II:313-17.
133. Engel GL. A life-setting conducive to illness: the giving-up complex. *Ann Intern Med* 1968;69:293-300.
134. Schmale AH. Relation of separation and depression to disease I. A report on hospitalized medical population. *Psychosom Med* 1958;20:259-77.
135. Hofer M. *The roots of human behavior. An introduction to the psychobiology of early development.* San Francisco: Freeman; 1981.
136. Holmes TH, Rahe RH. The social readjustment rating scale. *J Psychosom Res* 1967;11:213-8.
137. Rahe RH, Meyer M, Smith M, et al. Social stress and illness onset. *J Psychosom Res* 1964;8:35-44.
138. Weiner H. *Psychobiology and human disease.* New York: Elsevier/North-Holland; 1977.
139. Silberstein C. Psychobiological considerations in the development of acquired immunodeficiency syndrome. *Einstein J Biol Med* 1985;3:136-43.
140. Blumenfield M. Letter to the editor. *Gen Hosp Psychiatry* 1986;8:217.
141. Fawzy FI, Cousins N, Fawzy NW, Kemeny ME, Elashoff R, Morton D. A structured psychiatric intervention for cancer patients. I. Changes over time in methods of coping and affective disturbance. *Arch Gen Psychiatry* 1990;47:720-5.
142. Fawzy FI, Kemeny M, Fawzy NW, et al. A structured psychiatric intervention for cancer patients. II. Changes over time in immunological measures. *Arch Gen Psychiatry* 1990;47:729-35.
143. Derogatis LR, Abeloff MD, Melisataros N. Psychological coping mechanisms and survival time in metastatic breast cancer. *JAMA* 1979;242:1504-8.
144. Spiegel D, Bloom J, Yalom ID. Group support for patients with metastatic breast cancer. *Arch Gen Psychiatry* 1981;38:527-33.
145. Spiegel D, Bloom JR, Kraemer HC, Gottheil E. Effect of psychosocial treatment on survival of patients with metastatic breast cancer. *Lancet* 1989;2:888-91.

146. Speigel D. Can psychotherapy prolong cancer survival? *Psychosomatics* 1990;31:361–6.

147. Fernandez F, Holmes VF, Levy JK, Ruiz P. Consultation-liaison psychiatry and HIV-related disorders. *Hosp Community Psychiatry* 1989;40:146–53.

148. Wolcott DL, Fawzy FI, Pasnau RO. Acquired immune deficiency syndrome (AIDS) and consultation-liaison psychiatry. *Gen Hosp Psychiatry* 1985;7:280–92.

149. McEvoy JP. Organic brain syndromes. *Ann Intern Med* 1981;95:212–20.

150. Lipowski ZJ. Delirium (acute confusional states). In: Fredericks JAM, ed. *Handbook of clinical neurology,* vol 2. (46) Neurobehavioral disorders. New York: Elsevier; 1985.

151. Lipowski ZJ. *Delirium: acute brain failure in man.* Springfield, IL: Charles C Thomas; 1980.

152. Pfeiffer E. A short portable mental status questionnaire for the assessment of organic brain deficits in elderly patients. *J Am Geriatr Soc* 1975;23:433–41.

153. Folstein MF, Folstein SE, McHugh PR. Mini-mental state—a practical method for grading the cognitive state of patients for the clinician. *J Psychiatry Res* 1975;12:189–98.

154. Jacobs JN, Bernhard MR, Delgado A, Strain JJ. Screening for organic mental syndromes in the medically ill. *Ann Intern Med* 1977;86:40–6.

155. Romano J, Engel GL. Delirium I. Electroencephalographic data. *Arch Neurol Psychiatry* 1944;51:227–55.

156. Pro JD, Wells CE. The use of the electroencephalogram in the diagnosis of delirium. *Dis Nerv Syst* 1977;38:807–8.

157. Obrecht R, Okhominia FOA, Scott DF. Value of EEG in acute confusional states. *J Neurol Neurosurg Psychiatry* 1970;42:75–7.

158. Snider WD, Simpson DM, Nielsen S, et al. Neurological complications of acquired immune deficiency syndrome: analysis of 50 patients. *Ann Intern Med* 1983;14:403–18.

159. Holland JC, Tross S. The psychosocial and neuropsychiatric sequelae of the acquired immunodeficiency syndrome and related disorders. *Ann Intern Med* 1985;103:760–4.

160. Parisi A, DiPerri G, Stroselli M, Nappi G, Minoli L, Rondanelli EG. Usefulness of computerized electroencephalography in diagnosing, staging, and monitoring AIDS-dementia complex. *AIDS* 1989;3:209–23.

161. Koralnik IJ, Beaumanoir A, Hausler R, et al. A controlled study of early neurologic abnormalities in men with asymptomatic human immunodeficiency virus infection. *N Engl J Med* 1990;323:864–70.

162. Lipowski ZJ. The concept and psychopathology of dementia. In: Lipowski ZJ, ed. *Psychosomatic medicine and liaison psychiatry.* New York: Plenum; 1985:307–13.

163. Goldstein K. Functional disturbances in brain damage. In: Arieti S, Reiser MF, eds. *American handbook of psychiatry,* 2nd ed, vol 4. New York: Basic Books; 1975:182–207.

164. Cohen MA, Aladjem AD, Brenin D, Ghazi M. Firesetting by patients with the acquired immunodeficiency syndrome (AIDS). *Ann Intern Med* 1990;112:386–7.

165. Loewenstein RJ, Sharfstein SS. Neuropsychiatric aspects of acquired immune deficiency syndrome. *Int J Psychiatry Med* 1984;13:255–60.

166. Tavares R, Lopez DJ. *Response of the gay community to acquired immune deficiency syndrome.* Washington, DC: American Psychiatric Press; 1984:106–10.

167. Barbuto J. Psychiatric care of seriously ill patients with acquired immune syndrome. In: Nichols SE, Ostrow DG, eds. *Psychiatric implications of acquired immune deficiency syndrome.* Washington, DC: American Psychiatric Press; 1984:72–76.

168. Perry S, Jacobsen P. Neuropsychiatric manifestations of AIDS-spectrum disorders. *Hosp Community Psychiatry* 1986;37:135–42.

169. Newmark DA. Review of a support group for patients with AIDS. *Top Clin Nurs* 1984;6:38–44.

170. Nichols SE. Social and support groups for patients with acquired immune deficiency syndrome. In: Nichols SE, Ostrow DG, eds. *Psychiatric implications of acquired immune deficiency syndrome.* Washington, DC: American Psychiatric Press; 1984: 78–82.

171. Aladjem A. AIDS: mind and body. *Issues Law Med* 1988;4:359–65.

172. Minuchin S, Rosman B, Baker L. *Psychosomatic families: anorexia nervosa in context.* Cambridge, MA: Harvard University Press; 1981.

173. Minuchin S, Baker L, Rosman B, et al. A conceptual model of psychosomatic illness in children: family organization and family therapy. *Arch Gen Psychiatry* 1985;32:559–63.

174. Minuchin S. *Families and family therapy.* Cambridge, MA: Harvard University Press; 1981.

175. Swenson RJ, Erman M, Labelle J, et al. Extra-pyramidal reactions—neuropsychiatric mimics in patients with AIDS. *Gen Hosp Psychiatry* 1989;11:248–53.

176. Steinbrook R, Lo B, Tirpack J, et al. Ethical dilemmas in caring for patients with the acquired immunodeficiency syndrome. *Ann Intern Med* 1985;103:787–90.

177. Turnock BJ, Kelly CJ. Mandatory premarital testing for human immunodeficiency virus—the Illinois experience. *JAMA* 1989;261:3415–8.

178. Lo B, Steinbrook RL, Cooke M, et al. Voluntary screening for human immunodeficiency virus (HIV) infection—weighing the benefits and harms. *Ann Intern Med* 1989;110:727–33.

179. Drotman DP. Earlier diagnosis of human immunodeficiency virus (HIV) infection and more counseling. *Ann Intern Med* 1989;110:680–1.

180. Steinbrook R, Lo B, Moulton J, et al. Preferences of homosexual men with AIDS for life-sustaining treatment. *N Engl J Med* 1986;314:457–60.

181. Brown JH, Henteleff P, Barakaf S, et al. Is it normal for terminally ill patients to desire death? *Am J Psychiatry* 1986;143: 208–11.

182. Miles SH, Singer PA, Siegler M. Conflicts between patients' wishes to forgo treatment and the policies of health care facilities. *N Engl J Med* 1989;321:48–50.

183. De Buono BA, Zinner SH, Daamen M, McCormack WM. Sexual behavior of college women in 1975, 1986 and 1989. *N Engl J Med* 1990;322:821–5.

184. MacDonald NE, Wells GA, Fisher WA, et al. High-risk STD/HIV behavior among college students. *JAMA* 1990;263:3155–9.

185. Cochran SD, Mays VM. Sex, lies and HIV. *N Engl J Med* 1990;22:774–5.

186. Reinisch JM, Beasley R. *The Kinsey Institute new report on sex. What you must know to be sexually literate.* New York: St Martin's Press; 1990.

187. Freidland G, Selwyn P. Intravenous drug use and HIV infection. *AIDS Clin Care* 1990;2:29–32.

188. Samuels J. Can IVDUs comply with conventional HIV care? *AIDS Clin Care* 1990;2:34.

189. Cohen MA, Cohen SC. AIDS education and a volunteer training program for medical students. *Psychosomatics* 1991;32:187–90.

190. Bowles LT. The AIDS epidemic (editorial). *J Med Educ* 1987;62:541.

191. Bowen OR. The war against AIDS. *J Med Educ* 1987;62:543–8.

192. Kelly JA, St Lawrence JS, Smith S, et al. Medical students' attitudes toward AIDS and homosexual patients. *J Med Educ* 1987;62:549–56.

193. Goldman JD. An elective seminar to teach first-year students the social and medical aspects of AIDS. *J Med Educ* 1987;62:557–61.

194. Whalen JP. Participation of medical students in the care of patients with AIDS. *J Med Educ* 1987;62:53–4.

195. Cooke M, Sande MA. The HIV epidemic and training in internal medicine. *N Engl J Med* 1989;321:1334–7.

196. Subcommittee on evaluation of humanistic qualities in the internist, American Board of Internal Medicine. Evaluation of humanistic qualities in the internist. *Ann Intern Med* 1983; 99:720–4.

197. Friedland G. AIDS and compassion. *JAMA* 1988;259:2898–9.

198. Krumholz HM, Cummings S, York M. Blood culture phlebotomy: switching needles does not prevent contamination. *Ann Intern Med* 1990;113:290–2.

199. Public Health Service statement on management of occupational exposure to human immunodeficiency virus, including considerations regarding zidovudine postexposure use. *MMWR* 1990; 39(RR1):13–4.

200. Henderson DK, Geberding JL. Prophylactic zidovudine after occupational exposure to the human immunodeficiency virus: an interim analysis. *J Infect Dis* 1989;160:321–7.

201. Lange JMA, Boucher CAB, Hollak CEM, et al. Failure of zidovudine prophylaxis after accidental exposure to HIV. *N Engl J Med* 1990;322:1375–7.

202. Looke DFM, Grove DI. Failed prophylactic zidovudine after needlestick injury. *Lancet* 1990;335:1280.

203. Brennan TA. The acquired immunodeficiency syndrome (AIDS) as an occupational disease. *Ann Intern Med* 1987;107:581–3.

204. Henderson DK. HIV-1 in the health care setting. In: Mandell GL, Douglas RG Jr, Bennett JE, eds. *Principles and practice of infectious disease,* 3rd ed. New York: Churchill Livingstone; 1990:2221–36.

205. Marcus R, CDC Cooperative Needlestick Surveillance Group. Surveillance of health care workers exposed to blood from patients infected with the human immunodeficiency virus. *N Engl J Med* 1988;319:1118–23.

206. Henderson DK, Saah AJ, Zak BJ, et al. Risk of nosocomial infection with human T-cell lymphotropic virus type III/lymphadenopathy-associated virus in a large cohort of intensively exposed health care workers. *Ann Intern Med* 1986;104:644–7.

207. Update: acquired immunodeficiency syndrome and human immunodeficiency virus infection among health-care workers. *MMWR* 1988;37:229–34,239.

208. Guidelines for prevention of transmission of human immunodeficiency virus and hepatitis B virus to health-care and public-safety workers. *MMWR* 1989;38(suppl S-6):1–37.

209. Recommendations for prevention of HIV transmission in health-care settings. *MMWR* 1987;36(suppl 2S):1S–18S.

210. Update: universal precautions for prevention of transmission of human immunodeficiency virus, hepatitis B virus, and other blood borne pathogens in health-care settings. *MMWR* 1988;37:377–82,387–8.

211. Aoun H. When a house officer gets AIDS. *N Engl J Med* 1989;321:693–6.

212. Sullivan HS. *The interpersonal theory of psychiatry.* New York: Norton; 1953:32–3.

AIDS and Other Manifestations of HIV Infection,
Second Edition, Edited by Gary P. Wormser.
Raven Press, Ltd., New York © 1992.

CHAPTER 22

The AIDS Dementia Complex

Richard W. Price and John J. Sidtis

Infection by human immunodeficiency virus type 1 (HIV-1) is complicated by a variety of neurological disorders. Among the most common and, from the standpoint of both morbidity and pathobiology of HIV-1 infection, one of the most important and most intriguing of these is the AIDS dementia complex (ADC), which presents as a "subcortical dementia" with a characteristic constellation of cognitive, motor, and, at times, behavioral dysfunction (1,2). While its pathogenesis remains puzzling in a number of critical aspects, ADC likely relates in a fundamental way to the effects of HIV-1 itself, rather than to a secondary opportunistic infection by another organism (3,4).

TERMINOLOGY

ADC was clinically recognized early in the AIDS epidemic and subsequently has been designated by a variety of terms, including *subacute encephalitis, subacute encephalopathy, HIV-dementia,* and *HIV encephalopathy* (5–8). This uncertainty in terminology is indicative of a number of unresolved issues. Thus specific diagnostic criteria have not yet been formalized nor have the limits of the condition been defined with respect to severity and the inclusion of particular symptoms and signs. Most importantly, its etiology and pathogenesis, including whether it truly represents a single disease process, remain uncertain.

The term *AIDS dementia complex* was introduced to describe a clinical syndrome, that is, a cohesive constellation of symptoms and signs, rather than a clearly established, uniform etiopathogenetic disease entity (1,9). It remains both appropriate and useful to adhere to this original intent. It is particularly important to segregate the concept of ADC, on the one hand, from that of HIV-1 brain infection, on the other; the latter refers to a pathobiological process rather than a clinical condition. As discussed below, HIV-1 clearly infects the CNS and likely accounts for at least one of the pathological subtypes of ADC, and thus ADC and HIV-1 brain infection overlap, but they are not synonymous and the two terms should not be used interchangeably.

The distinct character of the ADC cognitive change, which includes prominent mental slowing and inattention, along with concomitant affliction of motor performance, underlies ADC's classification among the *subcortical dementias,* which also include the cognitive impairment found in Parkinson's disease, Huntington's disease, hydrocephalus, and progressive supranuclear palsy (10); this is in contradistinction to the cortical dementias, such as Alzheimer's disease, in which memory impairment predominates, or Creutzfeldt-Jakob disease, which variously presents with aphasia, apraxia, or other focal features (11). While the anatomical justification of this designation remains to be fully demonstrated, it is a clinically useful distinction and emphasizes the inappropriateness of applying to ADC the definitions and measurement tools that were originally targeted to Alzheimer's disease. It also draws attention to similarities of the ADC cognitive deficits with those of the other subcortical dementias and suggests that some of the same anatomical pathways may be affected.

With respect to nomenclature, each of the three components of the term ADC was chosen for a particular reason. Thus *AIDS* was included because the morbidity of the condition may be comparable to that of other AIDS-defining complications of HIV-1 infection. *Dementia* was included because acquired and persistent cognitive decline is the most common and generally the most disabling manifestation; additionally, this cognitive difficulty is characteristically unaccompanied by alterations in the level of alertness. The third component, *complex,* was added because the syndrome also impor-

R. W. Price and J. J. Sidtis: Department of Neurology, University of Minnesota Health Science Center, Minneapolis, Minnesota 55455-0323.

tantly includes impaired motor performance and, at times, behavioral change and therefore is not simply an isolated dementia (6). Myelopathy, *but not peripheral neuropathy,* and organic psychosis, *but not "reactive" anxiety or depression,* were included within this umbrella term because they may coexist with, or be difficult to separate from, the "core" cognitive and motor abnormalities.

For both clinical and investigative studies, we have found it very useful to apply a staging scheme based on functional severity in the cognitive and motor spheres, once the diagnosis of ADC is established (Table 1) (2,12). This staging relies on relatively simple functional evaluation and has proved a pivotal step in an iterative strategy to characterize the significance of various symptoms and

signs and to interpret the results of formal neuropsychological evaluations. Moreover, this scheme provides a common vocabulary for practical clinical use and for comparing patients assessed by different physicians. It also provides a simple framework for correlations with various laboratory studies, including both virological and pathological results.

Recently, the World Health Organization (WHO) introduced a new terminology that is in some ways more cumbersome but also has certain useful features omitted from previous classifications (13). This WHO classification can also be roughly "translated" into the ADC staging scheme. WHO introduced the term *HIV-1 associated cognitive/motor complex* to encompass the full constellation of ADC and added subcategories to refer to patients with predominantly cognitive (*HIV-1 associated dementia*) or myelopathic (*HIV-1 associated myelopathy*) presentations of sufficient severity to interfere with work or activities of daily living (hence severe enough to qualify as stage 2 or greater in ADC staging). The term *HIV-1 associated minor cognitive/motor disorder* was introduced to designate patients with mild symptoms and signs and only minimal functional impairment of work or activities of daily living (stage 1 ADC). In addition to the advantage of attempting to separate the patients with predominant myelopathy from those with cognitive changes, this terminology restricts the term *dementia* to patients with a level of cognitive impairment consistent with that used in other formal definitions of dementias. It should also simplify reporting the condition as an AIDS-defining disorder (14), which can now be logically restricted to patients with sufficient functional severity to be termed *HIV-1 associated dementia* or *HIV-1 associated myelopathy.* The requirement for this level of severity (equivalent to stage 2 or greater in the ADC terminology) is probably also biologically and prognostically consistent with other AIDS-defining conditions. It also does not make the implicit assumption that the disorder is a single disease entity differing only in severity.

TABLE 1. *Staging scheme for the AIDS dementia complex (ADC)*

ADC stage	Characteristics
Stage 0 (Normal)	Normal mental and motor function.
Stage 0.5 (Equivocal/ subclinical)	Either minimal or equivocal *symptoms* of cognitive or motor dysfunction characteristic of ADC, or mild signs (snout response, slowed extremity movements) but *without impairment of work or capacity to perform activities of daily living* (ADL). Gait and strength are normal.
Stage 1 (Mild)	Unequivocal evidence (symptoms, signs, neuropsychological test performance) of functional intellectual or motor impairment characteristic of ADC, but able to perform *all but the more demanding aspects of work or ADL.* Can walk without assistance.
Stage 2 (Moderate)	Cannot work or maintain the more demanding aspects of daily life but able to perform *basic activities of self-care.* Ambulatory but may require a single prop.
Stage 3 (Severe)	*Major intellectual incapacity* (cannot follow news or personal events, cannot sustain complex conversation, considerable slowing of all output) *or motor disability* (cannot walk unassisted, requiring walker or personal support, usually with slowing and clumsiness of arms as well).
Stage 4 (End stage)	*Nearly vegetative.* Intellectual and social comprehension and responses are at a rudimentary level. Nearly or absolutely mute. Paraparetic or paraplegic with double incontinence.

CLINICAL PRESENTATION

Although both the severity and the relative prominence of certain symptoms and signs may vary, the general character of ADC adheres to a consistent pattern and affects cognition, motor performance, and, at times, behavior (1). Most often, patients' earliest symptoms consist of difficulties with concentration and memory. They complain of losing track of their train of thought or conversation and that they need to keep lists to maintain their daily schedules. For example, they may get up and go into another room and then be unable to recall the reason. Symptoms that are normally experienced intermittently in association with fatigue or minor illness now become constant and intrude on activities of everyday life. Many patients complain of "slowness" in thinking and note that more complex tasks at work or in the home are increasingly difficult, must now be broken down into simpler components, and take longer to complete. Reading may become more difficult because of the attentional deficit; sentences, paragraphs, or pages must be gone over several times before registering. For this reason, recreational reading may be abandoned because of the extra work required.

Very early in the course, patients may perform within the normal range on common bedside mental status testing such as the "mini-mental status" examination (15) but are slower and less facile despite the overall accuracy. With advancing disease, they have increasing difficulty with tasks requiring concentration and attention, such as word and digit reversals and serial subtraction. Eventually, a larger array of bedside and more formal mental status tests are abnormal, and psychomotor slowing becomes more prominent.

Motor abnormalities, including particularly slowing of rapid successive and alternating movements of the extremities and eyes, are frequent and early findings on examination. Perhaps, the simplest bedside abnormality is slowness in efforts to oppose the thumb and forefinger rapidly and repeatedly. Abnormal reflexes are also common, including generalized hyperreflexia (in the absence of concomitant neuropathy) and "release" signs, such as snout or glabellar responses. With progression there may be symptomatic difficulty with balance or coordination. In still more advanced disease, ataxia and, subsequently, leg weakness limit ambulation. Patients with early or predominating spastic–ataxic gait usually will be shown to have vacuolar myelopathy pathologically (16). In those with a severe progressive course, the terminal stage of the ADC is nearly vegetative (stage 4); patients lie in bed with a vacant stare, paraparesis, and incontinence. Unless intercurrent illness develops, their level of arousal is usually preserved.

Psychological depression appears to be surprisingly infrequent in these patients. While they may frequently appear disinterested and lack initiative, dysphoria and other aspects of true depression are not present. In an interesting subgroup of ADC patients, a more agitated organic psychosis with manic features may be the presenting or predominant aspect of the illness accompanying the cognitive and motor dysfunction.

While this chapter confines itself to adult disease, children with AIDS suffer a parallel condition with the same general features but in the context of the developing brain (17,18). Its progressive form is characterized by loss of previously acquired developmental milestones with continued decline leading to frank cognitive and motor abnormalities, the latter ranging from spastic paraparesis to quadriplegia, pseudobulbar palsy, and rigidity. Acquired microcephaly is almost universal.

NEUROPSYCHOLOGICAL TESTING

Formal neuropsychological testing may be useful in assessing ADC, particularly in the context of clinical research studies of epidemiology and treatment, but, at times, for practical patient diagnosis and management as well (19,20). Appropriately chosen neuropsychological assessments target the same cardinal dysfunction sought by the AIDS-directed clinical examination but provide a formal, quantitative methodology for following patients serially. Indeed, it is most useful to consider this methodology as a *quantitative neurological examination.* In the case of ADC, such tests focus on alterations in motor speed, concentration, mental manipulation, and, to a lesser degree, memory. Their major purpose is to provide practical and accurate serial assessment of HIV-1-infected patients.

The need for an "ADC test battery" has been raised by some but has given rise to some confusion among clinicians regarding the use of such testing in patient management. It is important to understand that the results of neuropsychological assessments are not used as the sole or even major criteria for diagnosis and thus do not substitute for the clinical neurological evaluation. The results of these assessments are not disease-specific and should always be interpreted in the full clinical context. There are clearly some dysfunctional HIV-1-infected patients whose test performance falls within the population norms, just as there are HIV-1-infected patients who perform poorly on testing for reasons other than ADC. However, with proper interpretation, such studies may provide ancillary data useful to diagnosis, usually in substantiating that the magnitude and profile of the functional deficit is consistent with ADC and clinical staging.

NEUROIMAGING

In evaluated patients with suspected ADC, laboratory studies are generally most useful in the process of differential diagnosis, and, more particularly, in ruling out confounding conditions. This is true of neuroimaging procedures, CSF examination, and most other clinical laboratory studies. In the case of anatomic neuroimaging modalities, one is therefore usually assessing the presence or absence of other disorders, which might mimic ADC. However, there are also certain radiographic findings that are frequently present and can even be considered "consistent with" a diagnosis of ADC. Most notable on both MRI and CT scanning is cerebral atrophy, which is present in virtually all ADC patients, particularly those with stage 2 or greater severity (1,21–23). While increase in the size of cortical sulci and ventricles is not diagnostically specific and, by itself, should not be used to make a clinical diagnosis, absence of atrophy in a patient suspected to suffer ADC should raise questions regarding the diagnosis.

MRI scanning similarly detects atrophy and, in addition, may also reveal increased signal in the white matter or basal ganglia of some AIDS patients (1,24). Such signal changes can be patchy or "fluffy" in appearance, or in the white matter may have a more homogeneous "ground-glass" appearance. While it is reasonable to speculate that increase in brain water concentration relates to direct HIV-1 brain infection, correlation of MRI findings and histopathological findings has not been established. In children with AIDS, mineralization of the basal ganglia is often prominent (25).

Metabolic imaging of ADC has also been reported using both positron emission tomography (PET) and single photon emission computed tomography (SPECT) scanning but their diagnostic utility remains to be clearly delineated (26–28). In the case of PET, improvement in the alterations in cerebral metabolism have been used to corroborate therapeutic effect (29).

CEREBROSPINAL FLUID (CSF)

The overall clinical value of CSF analysis in ADC patients parallels that of neuroimaging. Abnormalities are frequent but lack specificity, and the major practical utility of lumbar puncture is in ruling out other diagnoses, particularly cryptococcal meningitis. Of biological interest, analysis of CSF has provided interesting information regarding the interaction of HIV-1 and the CNS. Indeed, in the absence of serial sampling of brain, and particularly in the absence of anatomic sampling of brain early in disease, the CSF has provided a unique window into events in the CNS (30–34).

The CSF of ADC patients may show a variable elevation in CSF protein and mild mononuclear pleocytosis. However, because studies of asymptomatic HIV-1 seropositives also exhibit similar abnormalities, these findings are of limited diagnostic value. Studies of asymptomatic seropositives have also shown more specific reactions to HIV-1, with intrathecal production of antibodies against viral antigens. Additionally, HIV-1 can be isolated from CSF in 10–30% of asymptomatic subjects. These observations indicate that the virus reaches the CNS relatively early in the course of systemic infection and elicits local responses, yet brain function appears to remain normal. From a pathogenetic perspective, it is important to understand how the virus within the brain is controlled during this stage of infection and why such infection is apparently innocent with respect to alteration in brain function. In a more practical vein, these "background" abnormalities must be taken into account when interpreting CSF results of HIV-1-infected patients. Mild pleocytosis or elevated protein does not necessarily imply another infection. Likewise, isolation of

HIV-1 from CSF does not indicate ADC or HIV-1 encephalitis.

In some severely affected ADC patients, HIV-1 p24 antigen may be detected by immunoassay in the CSF (35). This is usually of limited practical utility since the diagnosis is most often clinically quite evident in such patients. Of perhaps greater potential value, certain "markers" of immune-cell activation have been noted to increase in the CSF of ADC patients, with concentrations correlating, to some extent, with clinical severity. These surrogate markers include β_2-microglobulin (β_2M; a noncovalently bound portion of the class 1 major histocompatibility complex) and neopterin (a product of pteridine metabolism that appears to be released by activated macrophages) (36,37). Quinolinic acid is similarly elevated (38); this product of tryptophan metabolism can be induced by γ-interferon and perhaps other cytokines and can act at the N-methyl-D-aspartate (NMDA) receptor as an endogenous excitotoxin. It has been speculated that quinolinic acid may contribute to CNS injury of ADC patients. More recently, α-tumor necrosis factor in CSF during late HIV-1 infection has been reported (39), but this has not yet been correlated with ADC stage, and, indeed, this elevation has not been confirmed in other studies (40). Of pathogenetic interest, elevation of these surrogate markers in CSF indicate that, although AIDS patients are immunosuppressed, certain immune-cell responses are upregulated as disease progresses. This occurs in both the blood and CSF compartments, reflecting systemic and CNS disease, respectively. Since these markers may be increased by the action of cytokines, these observations raise the question of whether cytokine-related reactions can actually be involved in the production of CNS injury (see below).

Assessment of these surrogate markers may also turn out to be clinically useful, although further study is needed to clearly delineate such utility. Studies thus far indicate that elevated levels of β_2M, neopterin, and quinolinic acid in the CSF are *not diagnostically specific;* these markers are also elevated in the CSF of patients with opportunistic CNS infections and CNS lymphoma (36–38). However, in the absence of these conditions, increased concentrations of these markers may be helpful in assessing mild or equivocal ADC. They may also prove useful in following the effects of therapy since, for example, zidovudine (AZT) treatment lowers the elevated CSF concentration of these markers in ADC patients (37,38).

DIFFERENTIAL DIAGNOSIS

The problems of differential diagnosis of ADC often vary somewhat according to whether either mild or more severe forms are suspected. When confronting early ADC (WHO minor cognitive/motor disorder), practical diagnosis often focuses on the issue of whether the condition is present or whether the patient is simply suffering from the effects of fatigue, anxiety, depression, or even hypochondriasis. Indeed, the border between fatigue and ADC may be difficult to define and they both may result from similar processes. It is often very useful to obtain independent testimony regarding the patient's functional ability in establishing the presence of ADC in such patients. Formal neuropsychological testing may also be useful in this setting, particularly if the history is unreliable and some objective measure of performance is needed; such assessment also provides a valuable baseline for subsequent evaluations. We have generally been conservative in the diagnosis of early ADC and if symptoms are of equivocal importance and functional impairment is uncertain, we have used the ADC stage 0.5 designation. This is also used when "soft" neurological signs are present but functional ability remains intact.

In more advanced ADC, differential diagnosis most commonly centers on distinction from the other neurological complications noted in HIV-1-infected patients (41) or, less commonly, from dementing or myelopathic neurological disease, which can occur in the normal population. Preserved consciousness and the absence of focal neurological deficits are important clinical features of ADC, although these may be unhelpful in the patient with coexisting CNS disease of other types. Primary CNS lymphoma, when deep and bilateral, may produce a similar picture, although sleepiness may be more notable than in ADC. CMV or diffuse microscopic toxoplasmosis may cause subacute "diffuse" cerebral dysfunction, although again, consciousness is often blunted in these conditions. MRI scans showing white matter abnormalities may raise the question of progressive multifocal leukoencephalopathy (PML), but the clinical picture of this opportunistic viral infection is quite different from that of ADC. PML is characterized by major focal neurological deficits (e.g., hemiparesis, hemianopia). Alzheimer's-type dementia most often includes predominantly amnestic features rather than the characteristic "subcortical" dementia of ADC. Likewise, vacuolar myelopathy encompassed in the ADC syndrome differs from more focal transverse myelopathies of epidural tumor or varicella-zoster virus infections, which include a segmental sensory level. Both neuroimaging procedures and cerebrospinal fluid (CSF) examination are frequently essential aspects of evaluation, particularly in pursuing macroscopic focal lesions of the brain or spinal cord.

EPIDEMIOLOGY AND NATURAL HISTORY

The epidemiology of ADC, including its prevalence at various stages of systemic HIV-1 infection, is not yet clearly defined (4). Current understanding derives largely from clinical case series (1,42) rather than from more rigorously controlled prospective epidemiological investigations. Several recent studies of the latter type have, however, more clearly characterized some of the neurological and neuropsychological aspects of asymptomatic HIV-1-seropositive subjects (12,43,44). Additionally, the epidemiology of ADC may be undergoing modification related to the widespread early use of antiviral therapy (45).

Available information, nonetheless, probably allows some approximations of the prevalence of ADC at different phases of untreated systemic HIV-1 infection. Both the prevalence and severity of ADC increase as systemic disease progresses and helper (CD4+) lymphocyte counts fall. Thus our own impression is that ADC is a frequent and significant clinical problem in the late stages of systemic HIV-1 infection, and prior to death the majority of AIDS patients exhibit neurological symptoms and signs, with perhaps one-half of these showing functionally important (stages 2–4) disability. Somewhat earlier in the evolution of systemic illness, when patients first present with AIDS-defining opportunistic infections (e.g., *Pneumocystis carinii* pneumonia), mild (stage 1) ADC is detectable in perhaps 10–30% of patients while more severe neurological impairment (stages 2–4) is present in perhaps another 5–15%. In the transitional phase of HIV-1 infection, when immunosuppression begins to manifest with constitutional symptoms and the AIDS-related complex, subclinical abnormalities (stage 0.5) may be present in one-third or more, although probably less than 10% exhibit features of stage 1 or higher. In contrast, during the clinical "latent" period, when patients are constitutionally well, functionally significant abnormalities are rare, although some asymptomatic seropositives (<15%) may exhibit mild signs (stage 0.5).

The course of ADC is also highly variable. Steadily progressive and severe disease (stages 2–4) develops principally in individuals with advanced immunosuppression, while the course in those with latent or transitional phase systemic disease is more likely to be indolently progressive or even static (stages 0.5–1). Exceptional patients may progress to stage 2–4 ADC without experiencing major systemic complications of HIV-1, although characteristically, laboratory evidence of severe immunosuppression is present and most have suffered with constitutional, although not AIDS-defining, symptoms and signs before or concomitant with neurological deterioration (46). At the other extreme, some patients remain neurologically intact and continue to function at a high level despite recurrent, severe episodes of opportunistic infections. Thus the link between severe progressive ADC and systemic immunosuppression is not absolute and other factor(s) must be involved in determining the development of ADC.

PATHOGENESIS OF ADC: RELATION TO HIV-1 INFECTION OF THE CNS AND IMMUNE RESPONSES

Neither the viral pathogenesis of ADC nor the full spectrum of interactions of HIV-1 with the CNS are yet clearly defined. As emphasized earlier, ADC is not synonymous with HIV-1 brain infection. Analysis of CSF from asymptomatic seropositives indicates early exposure of the CNS to HIV-1 with a seeming absence of concomitant neurological sequelae, at least at this stage of infection. However, later in the course of infection, ADC emerges and appears to relate to HIV-1 infection, although with a heterogeneous pathological and virological substrate.

Neuropathology of ADC

The neuropathology of ADC includes at least three overlapping "subsets" of major abnormalities: (a) central gliosis and white matter pallor, (b) multinucleated-cell encephalitis, and (c) vacuolar myelopathy (4,9,47–52). These abnormalities can generally be correlated with the clinical manifestations and severity of ADC and also with respect to the demonstrable presence of productive virus infection (Table 2). Central gliosis and white matter pallor are almost universal findings in ADC patients and, in isolation, are the major abnormalities in clinically milder patients (stages 0.5–2). Rarely, they will be the only abnormalities in patients with even more severe clinical symptoms and signs (stage 3 or 4). Studies using immunohistochemistry to demonstrate viral antigens or in situ hybridization to detect viral nucleic acid have generally been negative in brains in which this is the sole pathology (52).

Multinucleated-cell encephalitis is characterized by the presence of perivascular and, at times, parenchymal cell reactions, which include macrophages and microglial cells, along with multinucleated cells derived from fusion of these two cell types. Multinucleated-cell encephalitis is generally found in patients with more severe

and progressive ADC (stages 2–4). This pathology can legitimately be termed HIV-1 encephalitis, since the multinucleated-cell formation appears to reflect direct viral cytopathology (4). Indeed, the multinucleated cells are likely the in vivo counterpart of cell fusion and syncytia formation noted in vitro in certain HIV-1-infected cell culture systems and result from the interactions of the HIV-1 glycoprotein gp120 with the CD4 receptor and the fusion glycoprotein gp41.

Vacuolar myelopathy, while defined pathologically, can also often be distinguished clinically on the basis of patients' predominant myelopathic symptoms and signs (16). Such patients usually present with spastic–ataxic gait difficulty but with proportionally little sensory disturbance and no definable sensory "level." Histologically, it closely resembles the subacute combined spinal cord degeneration that accompanies vitamin B_{12} deficiency. Our own studies have failed to show a relation of the vacuolar changes to productive HIV-1 infection of the spinal cord, at least to the type of infection causing multinucleated-cell formation (53).

Virology

As noted previously, anatomic studies of brain have shown that productive HIV-1 infection is confined largely, if not exclusively, to macrophages, microglia (or cells of macrophage lineage with microglial morphology), and derivative multinucleated cells (4,54–63). Controversy exists as to whether vascular endothelial cells are infected, and likely neurons, oligodendrocytes, and astrocytes are not productively infected in vivo; earlier reports suggesting that these major "functional elements" of the brain were infected probably relate to imprecise cell identification (58,64). This contrasts with certain tissue culture studies, which show that in addition to lymphocytes, macrophages, and microglia (65), various primary neuroectodermal cells and cell lines can be infected (66,67). However, most of these in vitro infections have been characterized by low viral yields and absence of CD4-dependent virus–cell interaction. Whether such observations bear on the pathogenesis of infection in vivo awaits further study.

An additional important question relates to the possible role of viral variants, the neuropathic strains, of HIV-1 in the genesis of brain infection and ADC. While initially the search for viral strains with a predilection to cause neurological disease focused on isolates that infected cells of neuroectodermal origin (66), most attention now is directed toward the study of viral strains that replicate well in macrophages or microglia (68–74). It is speculated that the poor fidelity of the viral reverse transcriptase leads to constant generation of viral variants within individual patients and consequently to eventual selection and emergence of macrophage-trophic strains

TABLE 2. *Some general correlations of clinical neuropathological and virological findings*

Clinical	Pathology	Virology
Mild ADC (stages 0.5–2)	Gliosis/pallor	Negative for productive infection
Severe ADC (stages 2–4)	Multinucleated-cell encephalitis	Productive infection
Myelopathic ADC (stages 1–4) (predominant paraparesis)	Vacuolar myelopathy	Negative for productive infection

that might be particularly prone to cause infection within the CNS in some patients. This might be a second major determinate, in addition to immunosuppression, of the variation in ADC prevalence. A number of studies of viral isolates, including isolates cloned directly from brain (74), provide support for this speculation, although whether such isolates are more importantly the result or the cause of brain infection remains to be established.

Immunology

As noted previously, the immune system is an additional important variable in the development of ADC, which increases in both prevalence and severity with more advanced immunosuppression and lower CD4+ lymphocyte counts. This suggests that loss of immunity to HIV-1 itself may have an important *permissive* effect on the development of ADC. In this sense, severe ADC and multinucleated-cell HIV-1 encephalitis may be an opportunistic infection after all, although one in which systemic infection by the same organism first creates the opportunity by virtue of its effects on the immune system.

A second, less clearly established role for the immune system might relate to immunopathological processes, likely chiefly mediated through the actions of cytokines, in causing neurological injury. The elevated concentrations of markers of immune activation in CSF discussed earlier provide suggestive evidence in this regard. Thus increases in β_2M, neopterin, and quinolinic acid likely reflect upregulation of certain pathways in immune cells. Elsewhere, we have presented a model of virus-immune interactions, which outlines a scheme whereby progressive loss of effective immune defenses might result in increased virus production, which in turn signals further immune activation (3). This activation might then result in production of neurotoxic molecules. In this model, loss of effective anti-HIV-1 immune responses removes the negative feedback inhibiting both viral production and activation of the remaining immune cells.

Target: the Central Nervous System

While the virus and the immune system appear to be the principal agonists in causing ADC, the nature and mechanisms of brain injury remain unresolved. While no other organism or process has been implicated in producing ADC, clearly it is not simply a manifestation of HIV-1 brain infection in the same way that poliovirus infection of the spinal cord and brain causes paralytic poliomyelitis. The relationship of HIV-1 infection to brain injury and clinical symptoms involves processes other than virus-induced killing of infected neurons, oligodendrocytes, or astrocytes.

Pathological studies have not yet precisely defined the principal targets of ADC-related brain injury. Thus it is uncertain whether white matter or grey matter is the major functional target. Likewise, if grey matter is the target, the susceptible neuronal population has not been delineated. The distribution of gliosis, white matter pallor, and, when present, multinucleated cells is not homogeneous but seems to favor deeper brain structures, including the basal ganglia and deeper white matter (47,52,75). This is in keeping with the "subcortical dementia" noted clinically. However, the explanation for this regional distribution remains uncertain.

If functional brain cells are not injured by direct infection and virus-mediated cell lysis, what then leads to neurological symptoms and signs? Speculation centered on the role of toxins released by either infected or reactive cells has been supported by several recent observations in the laboratory. This includes a study showing that the HIV-1 external glycoprotein gp120 is toxic to neurons in cell culture through a calcium channel-mediated mechanism (76). Another study has demonstrated that a small molecule produced by infected macrophage-like cell lines, but not by infected lymphocytes and hence likely not a viral gene product, also is toxic to neurons, in this case via interaction with the N-methyl-D-aspartate (NMDA) receptor (77). Additionally, a further study has shown that HIV-1-infected macrophages release toxin(s) into the cell culture medium, which alter both neuronal and glial elements of aggregate brain cultures (78). Cytokines released by reactive cells might have similar effects and explain CNS toxicity in the absence of demonstrable productive infection. Such mechanisms might hold importance not only for ADC but also for other neurological disorders in which immune or inflammatory mechanisms appear to be pathogenetically important.

TREATMENT

Whatever the details of pathogenetic mechanisms, it appears that the *prime mover* in ADC pathogenesis is HIV-1 infection, located either directly within the CNS or outside the brain. Hence the major line of therapy has involved antiretroviral drugs. Before outlining the results of treatment efforts thus far, it is useful to articulate briefly the objectives of ADC therapy (20).

Objectives of Treatment

The immediate clinical objectives of treatment include (a) alleviating symptomatic ADC and (b) preventing ADC in susceptible subjects. An additional suggested rationale relates to the prospect of "eradication" of HIV-1 infection from the CNS. This concept derives from analogy with the treatment of childhood leukemia in which targeted CNS prophylaxis was developed to prevent CNS relapse of "systemically cured" patients. The mechanism of such relapse in the case of leukemia involves the sequestration of malignant cells within the CNS, where they are protected from chemotherapy by the blood–brain barrier. However, the extent to which this analogy can be applied to HIV-1 infection is uncertain. As discussed earlier, there is evidence that the CNS is frequently exposed to HIV-1 early in the course of systemic infection, but whether the virus then establishes latency in the CNS is not known. Moreover, even if the virus is latent in the brain, its capacity to cause parallel latent infection throughout the body might far overshadow the effect of such a CNS reservoir. Additionally, major progressive ADC with underlying multinucleated-cell encephalitis usually develops in the setting of poorly controlled systemic infection accompanied by active viremia and evolution of genetic variants; thus this stage is characterized by continued, high-level reexposure of the CNS to an expanding quantity and array of HIV-1's. Earlier latent infection is probably eclipsed by these late developments and there is no evidence that late CNS infection derives from latent virus that reached the brain early in infection. Finally, since there are presently no means to eradicate latent HIV-1 from infected cells either within or outside the brain, or even the prospect of developing such means, this issue currently lacks practical significance.

Treatment Modalities and Efficacy

There is now accumulating evidence that ADC can be treated and perhaps prevented, at least to some extent, by antiretroviral drug therapy. The first report of effective therapy for ADC involved anecdotal cases encountered in phase 1 trials of AZT (79). Subsequently, Schmitt and colleagues reported the results of neuropsychological testing in the original Burroughs Wellcome-sponsored controlled trial of AZT in patients with AIDS or AIDS-related complex (ARC)(80). Although the patients in this trial were not selected for dementia, both the AIDS and ARC groups scored in the low-average range at baseline, and on several measures of attention, psychomotor performance, and recall, those treated with AZT demonstrated significantly greater improvement from baseline at 8 and 16 weeks than did those given placebo. In a pediatric trial employing constant infusion AZT, Pizzo and colleagues also showed dramatic improvement in neuropsychological performance in a group of pediatric patients with and without overt neurodevelopmental abnormalities (81,82). More recently, a placebo-controlled trial in adults with ADC, in which two high doses of AZT (1000 and 2000 mg/day) were studied, showed improvement in neuropsychological test performance in the two AZT-treated groups compared to placebo (83). Of relevance to the issue of pre-

vention, a study of the epidemiology of ADC in The Netherlands suggested that AZT, in fact, reduced the incidence of new cases when it was first introduced into widespread clinical practice (45).

Unresolved issues with AZT include the question of optimal dose in both prophylactic and therapeutic situations. In the absence of precise dosage guidelines, conventional dosage (500–600 mg/day) is recommended. In patients who deteriorate neurologically on this dose, the clinician may either attempt to increase the dose to 1000 mg or more of AZT per day or switch to another antiretroviral such as dideoxyinosine (DDI). The efficacy of DDI in ADC is now under investigation. Again anecdotal reports suggest some therapeutic efficacy in adults, and the early pediatric experience appears to substantiate such an effect (84). However, at this point, further studies are still needed to establish the place of DDI and other newer antiretrovirals in this condition.

The possible role of toxins in the genesis ADC has also given rise to proposals attempting to block the effects of these putative intermediaries in ADC. For example, the calcium channel blocker, nimodipine, which appeared to block the neuronal toxicity of HIV-1 gp120 in cell culture (76), is now being considered for clinical trial.

Finally, symptomatic management is also important in ADC patients. In the subset of patients who present with mania, lithium or neuroleptics may be helpful. However, ADC patients may be unusually susceptible to the side effects of neuroleptics and other psychotropic drugs, and thus treatment should be cautious and begin with low doses.

ACKNOWLEDGMENTS

Our research program studying the AIDS dementia complex is supported by U.S. Public Health Service grant NS-25701.

REFERENCES

1. Navia BA, Jordan BD, Price RW. The AIDS dementia complex: I. Clinical features. *Ann Neurol* 1986;19:517–24.
2. Price RW, Brew BJ. The AIDS dementia complex. *J Infect Dis* 1988;158:1079–83.
3. Price RW, Brew BJ, Rosenblum M. The AIDS dementia complex and HIV-1 infection: a pathogenetic model of virus-immune interaction. In: BH Waksman, ed. *Immunologic mechanisms in neurologic and psychiatric disease.* New York: Raven Press; 1989: 269–90.
4. Price RW, Brew BJ, Sidtis J, Rosenblum M, Scheck AC, Cleary P. The brain in AIDS: central nervous system HIV-1 infection and AIDS dementia complex. *Science* 1988;239:586–92.
5. Horowitz SL, Benson DF, Gottleib MS, Davos I, Bentson JR. Neurological complications of gay-related immunodeficiency disorder. *Ann Neurol* 1982;12:80 (abst).
6. Gopinathan G, Laubenstein LJ, Mondale B, Krigel RG. Central nervous system manifestations of the acquired immunodeficiency (AID) syndrome in homosexual men. *Neurology* 1983;33(suppl 2):105 (abst).

7. Snider WD, Simpson DM, Neilsen S, Gold JW, Metroka CE, Posner JB. Neurological complications of acquired immune deficiency syndrome: analysis of 50 patients. *Ann Neurol* 1983; 14:403–18.

8. Britton CB, Miller JR. Neurologic complications in acquired immunodeficiency syndrome (AIDS). *Neurol Clin* 1984;2:315–39.

9. Navia BA, Cho E-W, Petito CK, Price RW. The AIDS dementia complex: II. Neuropathology. *Ann Neurol* 1986;19:525–35.

10. Cummings JL, Benson DF. Subcortical dementia—review of an emerging concept. *Arch Neurol* 1984;41:874–9.

11. Benson DF. The spectrum of dementia: a comparison of the clinical features AIDS/dementia and dementia of the Alzheimer type. *Alzheimer Dis Assoc Disorders* 1987;1(4):217–20.

12. Price RW, Sidtis JJ. Early HIV infection and the AIDS dementia complex. *Neurology* 1990;40:323–6.

13. World Health Organization consultation on the neuropsychiatric aspects of HIV-1 infection. Geneva, 11–13 January 1990. *AIDS* 1990;4(9):935–6.

14. Centers for Disease Control. Revision of the CDC surveillance case definition for acquired immunodeficiency syndrome. *MMWR* 1987;36:1S–14S.

15. Folstein M, Folstein S, McHugh PR. "Mini-mental status." A practical method for grading the cognitive state of patients for the clinician. *J Psychiatr Res* 1975;12:189–98.

16. Petito CK, Navia BA, Cho E-S, Jordan BD, George DC, Price RW. Vacuolar myelopathy pathologically resembling subacute combined degeneration in patients with acquired immunodeficiency syndrome (AIDS). *N Engl J Med* 1985;312:874–9.

17. Belman AL, Ultmann MH, Horoupian D, et al. Neurological complications in infants and children with acquired immune deficiency syndrome. *Ann Neurol* 1985;18:560–6.

18. Epstein LG, Sharer LR, Joshi VV, Fojas MM, Koenigsberger MR, Oleske JM. Progressive encephalopathy in children with acquired immune deficiency syndrome. *Ann Neurol* 1985;17:488–96.

19. Tross S, Price RW, Navia BA, Thaler HT, Gold J, Hirsch DA, Sidtis JJ. Neuropsychological characterization of the AIDS dementia complex: a preliminary report. *AIDS* 1988;2:81–8.

20. Price RW, Sidtis JJ. Evaluation of the AIDS dementia complex in clinical trials. *J AIDS* 1990;3(suppl 2):S51–60.

21. Post MJ, Tate LG, Quencer RM, Hensley GT, Berger JR, Sheremata WA, Maul G. CT, MR, and pathology in HIV encephalitis and meningitis. *AJR* 1988;151:373–80.

22. Jakobsen J, Gyldensted C, Brun B, Bruhn P, Helweg-Larsen S, Arlien-Soborg P. Cerebral ventricular enlargement relates to neuropsychological measures in unselected AIDS patients. *Acta Neurol Scand* 1989;79:59–62.

23. Moeller AA, Backmund HC. Ventricle brain ratio in the clinical course of HIV infection. *Acta Neurol Scand* 1990;81:512–5.

24. Jarvik JG, Hesselink JR, Kennedy C, et al. Acquired immunodeficiency syndrome. Magnetic resonance patterns of brain involvement with pathologic correlation. *Arch Neurol* 1988;45(7):731–6.

25. Belman AL, Lantos G, Horoupian D, et al. Calcification of the basal ganglia in infants and children. *Neurology* 1986;36:1192–9.

26. Rottenberg DA, Moeller JR, Strother SC, et al. The metabolic pathology of the AIDS dementia complex. *Ann Neurol* 1987;22(6):700–6.

27. Kramer EL, Sanger JJ. Brain imaging in acquired immunodeficiency syndrome dementia complex. *Semin Nucl Med* 1990; 20(4):353–63.

28. Pohl P, Vogl G, Fill H, Rossler H, Zangerle R, Gerstenbrand F. Single photon emission computed tomography in AIDS dementia complex. *J Nucl Med* 1988;29(8):1382–6.

29. Brunetti A, Berg G, DiChiro G, et al. Reversal of brain metabolic abnormalities following treatment of AIDS dementia complex with 3′-azido-2′,3′-dideoxythymidine (AZT, zidovudine): a PET-FDG study. *J Nucl Med* 1989;30(5):581–90.

30. Marshall DW, Brey RL, Cahill WT, Houk RW, Zajac RA, Boswell RN. Spectrum of cerebrospinal fluid findings in various stages of human immunodeficiency virus infection. *Arch Neurol* 1988; 45:954–8.

31. McArthur JC, Cohen BA, Farzadegan H, et al. Cerebrospinal fluid abnormalities in homosexual men with and without neuropsychiatric findings. *Ann Neurol* 1988;23(suppl):S34–7.

32. Resnick L, Berger JR, Shapshak P, Tourtellotte WW. Early penetration of the blood–brain-barrier by HIV. *Neurology* 1988;38: 9–14.

33. Elovaara I, Iivanainen M, Sirkka-Liisa V, et al. CSF protein and cellular profiles in various stages of HIV infection related to neurological manifestations. *J Neurol Sci* 1987;78:331–42.

34. Ho DD, Rota TR, Schooley RT, et al. Isolation of HTLV-III from cerebrospinal fluid and neural tissues of patients with neurologic syndromes related to the acquired immunodeficiency syndrome. *N Engl J Med* 1984;313(24):1493–7.

35. Paul MO, Brew BJ, Khan A, Gallardo M, Price RW. Detection of HIV-1 in cerebrospinal fluid (CSF): correlation with presence and severity of the AIDS dementia complex. 5th International Conference on AIDS, Montreal, Canada, June 1989 (abst 238).

36. Brew BH, Bhalla RB, Fleisher M, et al. Cerebrospinal fluid β_2 microglobulin in patients infected with human immunodeficiency virus. *Neurology* 1989;39:830–4.

37. Brew BJ, Bhalla RB, Paul M, Gallardo H, McArthur JC, Schwartz MK, Price RW. Cerebrospinal fluid neopterin in human immunodeficiency virus type 1 infection. *Ann Neurol* 1990;28:556–60.

38. Heyes MP, Brew BJ, Martin A. Quinolinic acid in cerebrospinal fluid and serum in HIV-1 infection: relationship to clinical and neurological status. *Ann Neurol* 1991;29:202–9.

39. Grimaldi LME, Martino GV, Franciotta DM, Brustia R, Castagna A, Pristera R, Lazzarin A. Elevated α-tumor necrosis factor levels in spinal fluid from HIV-1-infected patients with central nervous system involvement. *Ann Neurol* 1991;29:21–5.

40. Gallo P, Piccinno MG, Krzalic L, Tavolato B. Tumor necrosis factor α (TNF α) and neurological diseases. Failure in detecting TNF α in the cerebrospinal fluid from patients with multiple sclerosis, AIDS dementia complex, and brain tumours. *J Neuroimmunol* 1989;23(1):41–4.

41. Price RW, Brew BJ. Management of the neurological complications of HIV infection and AIDS. In: Sande M, Volberding P, eds. *The medical management of AIDS,* 2nd ed. Philadelphia: Saunders; 1990:161–81.

42. Clifford DB, Jacoby RG, Miller JP, Seyfried WR, Glicksman M. Neuropsychometric performance of asymptomatic HIV-infected subjects. *AIDS* 1990;4(8):767–74.

43. Selnes OA, Miller E, McArthur J, and the Multicenter AIDS Cohort Study. HIV-1 infection: no evidence of cognitive decline during the asymptomatic stages. *Neurology* 1990;40:204–8.

44. Miller EB, Selnes OA, McArthur JC, et al. Neuropsychological performance in HIV-1-infected homosexual men: the multi-center AIDS Cohort Study (MACS). *Neurology* 1990;40:197–203.

45. Portegies P, de Gans J, Lange JM, et al. Declining incidence of AIDS dementia complex after introduction of zidovudine treatment. *Br Med J* 1989;299:819–21.

46. Navia BA, Price RW. The acquired immunodeficiency syndrome dementia complex as the presenting or sole manifestation of human immunodeficiency virus infection. *Arch Neurol* 1987;44: 65–9.

47. Rosenblum MK. Infection of the central nervous system by the human immunodeficiency virus type 1. Morphology and relation to syndromes of progressive encephalopathy and myelopathy in patients with AIDS. *Pathol Annu* 1990;25(pt 1):117–69.

48. Petito CK, Cho E-S, Lemann W, Navia BA, Price RW. Neuropathology of acquired immunodeficiency syndrome (AIDS): an autopsy review. *J Neuropathol Exp Neurol* 1986;45:635–46.

49. Budka H, Costanzi G, Cristina S, Lechi A, Parravicini C, Trabattoni R, Vago L. Brain pathology induced by infection with the human immunodeficiency virus (HIV). A histological, immunocytochemical and electron microscopical study of 100 autopsy cases. *Acta Neuropathol (Berl)* 1987;75:185–98.

50. Budka H. Human immunodeficiency virus (HIV)-induced disease of the central nervous system: pathology and implications for pathogenesis. *Acta Neuropathol (Berl)* 1989;77:225–36.

51. Budka H. Neuropathology of HIV encephalitis. *Brain Pathol* 1991;1:163–75.

52. Cronin KC, Rosenblum M, Brew BJ, Price RW. HIV-1 brain infection: distribution of infection and clinical correlates. 5th International Conference on AIDS, Montreal, Canada, June 1989 (abst 599).

53. Rosenblum M, Scheck AC, Cronin K, Brew BJ, Khan A, Paul M, Price RW. Dissociation of AIDS-related vacuolar myelopathy and

productive HIV-1 infection of the spinal cord. *Neurology* 1989;39:892–6.

54. De La Monte SM, Ho DD, Schooley RT, Hirsch MS, Richardson EP. Subacute encephalomyelitis of AIDS and its relation to HTLV-III infection. *Neurology* 1987;37:562–9.

55. Epstein LG, Sharer LR, Cho ES, et al. HTLV-III/LAV like retrovirus particles in the brains of patients with AIDS encephalopathy. *AIDS Res* 1984;1:447–54.

56. Gabuzda DH, Ho DD, De La Monte SM, et al. Immunohistochemical identification of HTLV-III antigen in brains of patients with AIDS. *Ann Neurol* 1986;20:289–95.

57. Michaels J, Price RW, Rosenblum MK. Microglia in the human immunodeficiency virus encephalitis of acquired immune deficiency syndrome: proliferation, infection and fusion. *Acta Neuropathol* 1988;76:373–9.

58. Pumarola-Sune T, Navia BA, Cordon-Cardo C, et al. HIV antigen in the brains of patients with the AIDS dementia complex. *Ann Neurol* 1987;21:490–6.

59. Stoler MH, Eskin TA, Benn S, et al. Human T cell lymphotropic virus type III infection of the central nervous system—a preliminary *in situ* analysis. *JAMA* 1986;256:2360–4.

60. Vazeux R, Brousse N, Jarry A, et al. AIDS subacute encephalitis: identification of HIV-infected cells. *Am J Pathol* 1987;126: 403–10.

61. Wiley CA, Schrier RD, Nelson JA, et al. Cellular localization of human immunodeficiency virus infection within the brains of acquired immune deficiency syndrome patients. *Proc Natl Acad Sci USA* 1986;83:7089–93.

62. Koenig S, Gendelman HE, Orenstein JM, et al. Detection of AIDS virus in macrophages in brain tissue from AIDS patients with encephalopathy. *Science* 1986;233:1089–93.

63. Peudenier S, Hery C, Montagnier L, Tardieu M. Human microglial cells: characterization in cerebral tissue and in primary culture, and study of their susceptibility to HIV-1 infection. *Ann Neurol* 1991;29:152–61.

64. Gyorkey F, Melnick JL, Gyorkey P. Human immunodeficiency virus in brain biopsies of patients with AIDS and progressive encephalopathy. *J Infect Dis* 1987;155:870–6.

65. Watkins B, Dorn HH, Kelly WB, et al. Specific tropism of HIV-1 for microglial cells in primary human brain cultures. *Science* 1990;249:549–53.

66. Cheng-Mayer C, Rutka JT, Rosenblum ML, et al. Human immunodeficiency virus can productively infect cultured human glial cells. *Proc Natl Acad Sci USA* 1987;84:3526–30.

67. Shapshak P, Sun NC, Resnick L, et al. HIV-1 propagates in human neuroblastoma cells. *J AIDS* 1991;4(3):228–37.

68. Gartner S, Markovits P, Markovitz DM, Betts RF, Popovic M. Virus isolation from and identification of HTLV-III/LAV producing cells in brain tissue from a patient with AIDS. *JAMA* 1986;256:2365–71.

69. Cheng-Mayer C, Weiss C, Seto D, Levy JA. Isolates of human immunodeficiency virus type 1 from the brain may constitute a special group of the AIDS virus. *Proc Natl Acad Sci USA* 1989;86:8575–9.

70. Koyanagi Y, Miles S, Mitsuyasu RT, Merrill JE, Vinters HV, Chen ISY. Dual infection of the central nervous system by AIDS viruses with distinct cellular tropisms. *Science* 1987;236:819–22.

71. O'Brien WA, Koyanagi Y, Namazie A, et al. HIV-1 tropism for mononuclear phagocytes can be determined by regions of gp120 outside the CD4-binding domain. *Nature* 1990;348:69–73.

72. Pang S, Koyanagi Y, Miles S, Wiley C, Vinters HV, Chen ISY. High levels of unintegrated HIV-1 DNA in brain tissue of AIDS dementia patients. *Nature* 1990;348:85–9.

73. Shioda T, Levy JA, Cheng-Mayer C. Macrophage and T cell-line tropisms of HIV-1 are determined by specific regions of the envelope gp120 gene. *Nature* 1991;349:167–9.

74. Li Y, Kappes JC, Conway JA, Price RW, Shaw GM, Hahn BH. Molecular characterization of human immunodeficiency virus type-1 cloned directly from uncultured human brain: identification of replication competent and defective viral genomes. *J Virol* 1991;65:3973–85.

75. Kure K, Weidenheim KM, Lyman WD, Dickson DW. Morphology and distribution of HIV-1 gp41-positive microglia in subacute AIDS encephalitis. Pattern of involvement resembling a multisystem degeneration. *Acta Neuropathol* 1990;80:393–400.

76. Dreyer EV, Kaiser PK, Offermann JT, Lipton SA. HIV-1 coat protein neurotoxicity prevented by calcium channel antagonists. *Science* 1990;248:364–7.

77. Giulian D, Vaca K, Noonan CA. Secretion of neurotoxins by mononuclear phagocytes infected with HIV. *Science* 1990;250: 1593–6.

78. Pulliam L, Herndier BG, Tang HM, McGrath MS. Human immunodeficiency virus-infected macrophages produce soluble factors that cause histological and neurochemical alterations in cultured human brains. *J Clin Invest* 1991;87:503–12.

79. Yarchoan R, Berg G, Brouwers P, et al. Response of human immunodeficiency virus associated neurological disease to 3'-azido-3'-deoxythymidine. *Lancet* 1987;1:132–5.

80. Schmitt FA, Bigley JW, McKinnis R, Logue PE, Evans RW, Drucker JL, AZT Collaborative Working Group. Neuropsychological outcome of zidovudine (AZT) treatment of patients with AIDS and AIDS-related complex. *N Engl J Med* 1988;319: 1573–8.

81. Pizzo PA, Eddy J, Falloon J, et al. Effect of continuous intravenous infusion of zidovudine (AZT) in children with symptomatic HIV infection. *N Engl J Med* 1988;319:889–96.

82. Brouwers P, Moss H, Wolters P, Eddy J, Balis F, Poplack DG. Effect of continuous-infusion zidovudine therapy on neuropsychologic functioning in children with symptomatic human immunodeficiency virus infection. *J Pediatr* 1990;116:908–85.

83. Sidtis JJ, Gatsonis C, Price RW, et al. Zidovudine treatment of the AIDS dementia complex: results of a placebo-controlled trial. [Submitted].

84. Yarchoan R, Mitsuya H, Thomas RV, et al. *In vivo* activity against HIV and favorable toxicity profile of 2',3'dideoxyinosine. *Science* 1989;245:412–5.

*AIDS and Other Manifestations of HIV Infection,
Second Edition,* Edited by Gary P. Wormser.
Raven Press, Ltd., New York © 1992.

CHAPTER 23

Toxoplasmosis in AIDS

Peter Mariuz and Benjamin J. Luft

Toxoplasma gondii, an obligate intracellular protozoan, is probably the most common cause of infection of the central nervous system in humans. Depending on the mode of acquisition (e.g., congenital, acute acquired) and the immunological status of the host, it may cause significant morbidity and mortality in both humans and animals. In 1937, *Toxoplasma* was established as a cause of neonatal encephalitis in humans, and in 1942, it was shown that the infection was congenitally acquired (1–3). With the development of sensitive and specific serological tests, the ubiquitous nature of the infection and the wide spectrum of clinical manifestations due to infection could fully be appreciated. In adults, *Toxoplasma* has been reported sporadically and infrequently to be a cause of encephalitis in the nonimmunocompromised host (4). However, among patients receiving immunosuppressive drugs for malignancies, organ transplantation, or collagen vascular diseases, *Toxoplasma* has been recognized as a cause of encephalitis in an increasing number of patients. In patients with the acquired immunodeficiency syndrome (AIDS), *Toxoplasma* is the most common opportunistic infection involving the brain (5). In order to treat, diagnose, and prevent *Toxoplasma* infection effectively, it is important to understand the organism's life cycle as well as the pathogenesis of the diseases it causes.

ETIOLOGY

Toxoplasma is a coccidian of the Eimeria suborder. Although there is strain variation in respect to rate of multiplication, propensity toward tissue cyst formation, and virulence in animals, all strains appear to be antigenically similar. The organism exists in three forms: (a) the tachyzoite (trophozoite), (b) the tissue cyst (which con-

tains bradyzoites), and (c) the oocyst (which contains sporozoites). The cat family of mammals is the only definitive host for *Toxoplasma.* The organism can undergo its complete life cycle including both an enteroepithelial cycle and an extraintestinal cycle only in the cat (6,7). After the cat ingests food contaminated with either tissue cysts or oocysts, *Toxoplasma gondii* is released and invades the epithelial cells of the small intestine. In the intestine the organism undergoes sequential stages of asexual and sexual development and multiplication, resulting in the formation of oocysts that are discharged into the feces. The prepatent period to oocyst production varies between 3 and 24 days, depending on the form of the organism originally ingested by the cat. Millions of oocysts are excreted in the feces for approximately 2–3 weeks. Only after the oocyst sporulates does it become infectious. Sporogony occurs after the oocysts have been discharged into the environment and requires 2–21 days.

In humans, and other incidental hosts, the organism has only an extraintestinal phase of development. In these hosts, the organism is ingested by eating raw or undercooked meat containing the tissue cysts or foods contaminated with the oocysts. The cyst wall is then disrupted by peptic or tryptic digestion, liberating the organism that invades the intestinal mucosa, replicates as tachyzoites, and disseminates throughout the body. The tachyzoite is an obligate intracellular parasite that can infect every type of mammalian cell, and therefore all tissues and organs are susceptible to infection. The organism multiplies by endodyogeny, a process in which two daughter cells develop within a mother cell. The tachyzoites proliferate intracellularly within the parasitopherous vacuole until 8–16 organisms accumulate, which then lyse the cell. Tachyzoites may form pseudocysts, which accumulate in host cells for a prolonged period of time without forming a true tissue cyst. Eventually, true tissue cysts are formed; these contain bradyzoites, which slowly divide by endodyogeny. The cyst's

P. Mariuz and B. J. Luft: Health Sciences Center, SUNY at Stony Brook, Stony Brook, New York 11794-8153.

outer membrane is composed of host and parasitic material. Tissue cysts appear to be immunologically inert and in the chronically infected host they rarely induce an inflammatory response. Although a particular tissue tropism for *Toxoplasma* has never been demonstrated, cysts are found most commonly in brain and muscle tissue. It is believed that the cyst may persist for the life of the host. The mechanisms involved in the transformation of actively dividing tachyzoites to slowly dividing bradyzoites have not yet been delineated.

Besides ingestion of foods contaminated with tissue cysts or oocysts, toxoplasmosis may be acquired as a result of organ transplantation (e.g., cardiac transplantation) (8,9), blood transfusion (10,11), or laboratory accidents (12,13).

EPIDEMIOLOGY

Toxoplasma gondii is an ubiquitous pathogen found throughout the world. The prevalence of infection varies among different populations and is dependent on environmental (e.g., altitude, climatic conditions), cultural (e.g., preference for raw or undercooked meat), and socioeconomic (sanitation) conditions. For instance, in areas of western Europe such as France, Germany, Italy, and Spain, the seroprevalence of *Toxoplasma* infection in adults varies between 50 and 80%, whereas in the United States, the seroprevalence of infection is between 15 and 30% (14). In more tropical areas such as Central America and Equatorial Africa, the seroprevalence is high and may approach 80%.

The development of encephalitis occurs predominantly in two patient populations, the neonate as a result of congenital infection and the immunocompromised host. Rare sporadic cases of toxoplasmic encephalitis in nonimmunocompromised adults have also been reported (4).

The most common underlying neoplastic disorders associated with toxoplasmic encephalitis are those involving the reticuloendothelial system, in particular, Hodgkin's disease (5). Encephalitis has also been reported in cardiac, kidney, bone marrow, and liver transplant recipients (5). The most frequent predisposing condition for the development of significant *Toxoplasma* infection is the acquired immunodeficiency syndrome (15). Toxoplasmic encephalitis occurs in approximately 30% of AIDS patients seropositive for *T. gondii* (16). Therefore clinically apparent *T. gondii* infection varies among different groups of HIV-infected patients in accordance with the *Toxoplasma* seroprevalence and has been reported to occur in 5–40% of patients (17). Thus it is understandable that toxoplasmic encephalitis has been observed with very high frequency in Haitians (17,18), Africans (19,20), and certain Europeans (14) with AIDS. In the United States, toxoplasmic encephalitis is three

times more frequent in black, nonintravenous drug using, heterosexual males (usually of African or Haitian origin) than in white homosexual males. It has also been suggested that toxoplasmic encephalitis occurs more frequently among intravenous drug users (21).

Host Defense

The lymphocyte–monocyte–macrophage axis is the dominant host defense mechanism against *Toxoplasma* (22); antibody is not critical in the immune surveillance of chronic infection (23). The organism has developed certain strategies to evade the host's immune response, including the ability: to invade all mammalian cells; to avoid triggering the oxidative burst; to prevent phagosome–lysosome fusion and acidification with phagocytes; and to induce downregulation of the immune response. Lymphokines, such as γ-interferon, activate macrophages and other cells to kill *Toxoplasma* (24) and exogenous γ-interferon confers resistance against *Toxoplasma* in a murine model (25). Interleukin-2 has also been found to have a protective effect against *T. gondii* infection in mice (26). Administration of anti-γ-interferon to animals acutely infected with *T. gondii* inhibits the host's ability to resist infection and may lead to recrudescence of disease in the chronically infected animal (27–32).

Agents that impair cell-dependent immunity, such as corticosteroids, cytotoxic drugs, or anti-lymphocyte agents, depress the host's ability to control acute infection and allow reactivation of latent infection. In addition, certain malignancies of the reticuloendothelial or hematological systems, which are associated with defects in cell-mediated immunity, are strongly associated with a risk of severe disease from *T. gondii* (5). Patients with AIDS who have profound CD4 T-lymphocyte depletion and numerous qualitative abnormalities in lymphocyte function, are at particularly high risk for the development of toxoplasmic encephalitis. In experimental encephalitis, Vollmer et al. showed that depletion of humoral immunity using anti-Ia antibody did not alter survival in *Toxoplasma*-infected mice and reactivation of chronic infection occurred despite high titers of circulating anti-*Toxoplasma* antibody (23). Sharma et al. (33) reported that inhibition of specific IgG and IgM responses did not hinder the development of resistance to *T. gondii* in experimentally infected mice.

Pathogenesis

Our knowledge of the pathogenesis of *Toxoplasma* infection in the immunocompromised host is largely dependent on studies of experimental infection. In animals exposed to *Toxoplasma*, tachyzoites disseminate throughout the body, multiply, and eventually transform into tissue cysts. It has been speculated that *Toxoplasma* tachyzoites are less efficiently cleared from the brain of mice than from extraneural sites, even with the development of cell-mediated and humoral immune responses. With the development of cell-mediated and humoral immunity, tachyzoites are destroyed and the tissue cyst becomes the only demonstrable form of the organism. There is also evidence to suggest that, in chronically infected animals, active recurrent infection is responsible for the life-long persistence of antibodies and cell-mediated immunity to *Toxoplasma*. Lainson (34) and Van der Waaj (35) studied the development of tissue cysts in the brains of mice infected with *Toxoplasma* and found that daughter cysts develop in close proximity to larger cysts and that no inflammatory reaction accompanied this process. Therefore chronic infection in animal models is not a static state in which tissue cysts persist inertly for the life of the host. Rather, it appears that a dynamic process is occurring with the intercurrent rupturing of cysts releasing organisms and the formation of new cysts. This process may cause persistent antigenic stimulation, which may account for the high titers of antibody seen for the life of the host.

The effect of immunosuppression on the pathogenesis of toxoplasmic encephalitis has been studied by numerous investigators. Frankel et al. (28,29) first provided convincing experimental evidence that pharmacological suppression of cell-mediated immunity resulted in the recrudescence of toxoplasmosis in chronically infected animals. The pathological features of this process were similar to those seen in natural infection in immunocompromised humans. Histologically, the encephalitis was a focal necrotizing process consistent with the rupturing of tissue cysts in close proximity to one another. This caused the release of tachyzoites, which resulted in infection of surrounding neurons and astrocytes accompanied by an inflammatory infiltrate. The center of the inflammatory foci consisted of necrotic tissue, while toward the periphery there were large numbers of tachyzoites.

In humans, the combination of immunological abnormalities and chemotherapy associated with reticuloendothelial malignancies seems to enhance greatly the risk for development of necrotizing encephalitis. The most convincing evidence that recrudescence of latent infection is an important pathogenetic mechanism comes from recent studies in AIDS patients and bone marrow transplant recipients. Virtually all AIDS patients and bone marrow transplant recipients who develop toxoplasmic encephalitis are seropositive for *T. gondii* prior to the development of clinical disease. In contrast, in cardiac transplant recipients there is strong epidemiological evidence that acute acquisition of infection is the principal pathogenetic mechanism involved in development of toxoplasmosis (8,36). The donor heart appears to be the principal source of infection. Seronegative car-

diac transplant recipients receiving a heart from a seropositive donor may develop severe life-threatening infection. Clinically significant disease does not develop in those patients who are seropositive prior to transplantation. In addition, toxoplasmic encephalitis has been reported in four renal transplant recipients who were seronegative prior to transplantation (37). In these cases, as in the series described by Siegal et al. (10) of transfusion associated toxoplasmosis, the infection was widespread with multiorgan involvement.

Pathologic Changes of Toxoplasmic Encephalitis

Infection with *Toxoplasma* causes vascular proliferation and endothelial hyperplasia associated with a perivascular inflammatory infiltrate, which may progress to frank vasculitis and necrosis (32,38). There may be a profound response of microglial cells in various stages of activation, which form nodules. These nodules may occur in the absence of other evidence of acute inflammation; however, in areas remote from these nodules, there may be large zones of necrosis. Conley et al. (39) have shown that tachyzoites or *Toxoplasma* antigens are frequently associated with microglial nodules and are not found in the surrounding parenchyma. It should be noted that microglial nodules per se are not specific for toxoplasmosis and can be found in numerous other pathological processes including cytomegalovirus encephalitis, HIV encephalitis, and cerebral lymphoma (40). Although it is most common to find focal areas of encephalitis separated by normal brain tissue, diffuse necrotizing encephalitis has been reported (41,42).

The pathological features of toxoplasmic encephalitis are most often consistent with recrudescence of a latent infection. Histopathologically, three distinct zones have been identified (43). The central zone is an amorphous, avascular, necrotic area containing few identifiable organisms. When vessels are seen, they are necrotic and occluded by thrombi. The intermediate zone contains engorged blood vessels, areas of spotty necrosis, and numerous free extracellular and intracellular tachyzoites, but rarely cysts. There is prominent perivascular cuffing by inflammatory cells, with edema and vascular proliferation. In the outer zone, necrosis is rare and the vascular lesions are minimal. Here cysts are the predominant form of the organism. In studies using immunohistopathological methods for organism identification, tachyzoites and *Toxoplasma* antigens have been recognized more easily than with standard histological stains (44).

The severity of histopathological changes is variable and directly dependent on the degree of underlying immunodeficiency. Changes can vary from a well localized indolent granulomatous process (45–47) to a diffuse necrotizing encephalitis (47,48). In patients who are severely immunocompromised, the ability to contain the infection by developing an organized, encapsulated abscess is low. Lesions can be unifocal or multifocal and can vary in size from microscopic to encompassing an entire hemisphere. Both white and gray matter, as well as every part of the central nervous system, may be involved. There is a propensity toward localization in the basal ganglia, corticomedullary junction, thalamus, and white matter. The pituitary gland and the hypothalamus may also be involved. In contrast to congenital toxoplasmosis, the meninges are usually not involved except as part of a localized reaction to the underlying cortical process.

CLINICAL MANIFESTATIONS

Toxoplasma has a predilection to cause severe necrotizing encephalitis in patients with AIDS and is the most frequent cause of intracerebral mass lesions (49) and encephalitis (2). It has been estimated that by the end of 1991, 20,000–40,000 cases of toxoplasmic encephalitis will have been diagnosed in the United States alone. Toxoplasmosis is the AIDS-defining illness in approximately 5% of patients and almost always results from reactivation of a chronic, latent infection (1).

The clinical manifestations are protean with signs and symptoms of focal or generalized neurological dysfunction, or more commonly a mixture of both. Clinical manifestations are a function of the number and size of the lesions coupled with the host's response. Focal abnormalities include hemiparesis, hemiplegia, focal seizures, ataxia, diplopia, visual field deficits, cranial nerve palsies, cerebellar tremor, extrapyramidal movements, hemisensory loss, and aphasia; these findings correlate with the anatomical area of focal encephalitis. Generalized abnormalities include psychosis, lethargy, confusion, anxiety, and global cognitive impairment similar to AIDS dementia, with decreased recent memory, impaired attention span, and slowed verbal and motor responses (44,49–56). The clinical presentation can evolve insidiously over several weeks to an acute confusional state, with or without focal neurological abnormalities. Although the majority of patients develop signs of focal neurological disease as the infection progresses, some patients have been described who present with a rapidly progressive and fatal, global cerebral dysfunction in the absence of focal deficits and who do not have focal lesions on neuroradiographic studies (41). Macroscopically the brain was normal in three of four cases, with numerous microglial nodules mainly involving the grey matter noted on microscopic examination, most with central *Toxoplasma* cysts or free tachyzoites. An autopsy study of 55 cases of cerebral toxoplasmosis revealed diffuse toxoplasmic encephalitis without abscesses in seven patients (42). CT scans are frequently negative in patients with diffuse encephalitis. This appears to be a form of toxoplasmic encephalitis unique to AIDS patients.

Other symptoms associated with cerebral toxoplasmosis include headache, which can be focal or generalized and may be unremitting. Fever is variably present, noted in only 1 of 15 patients in one series (57) but in 15 of 27 patients in another series (52). *Toxoplasma* infection is predominantly intra-axial so that significant meningeal involvement is rare, making signs of meningeal irritation unusual and examination of cerebrospinal fluid (CSF) unrewarding, except to exclude other diseases. Rare complications of toxoplasmic encephalitis include secondary hydrocephalus (58), the syndrome of inappropriate antidiuretic hormone secretion (52,59), and panhypopituitarism (59). Toxoplasmic myelitis has been described in two patients, one who had cervical involvement with numbness and weakness of the left arm (60) and the other who manifested a corpus medullaris syndrome (61).

Toxoplasmosis Outside the Central Nervous System

In AIDS patients, toxoplasmosis primarily affects the CNS while other organ involvement is uncommon. Cases of pulmonary toxoplasmosis (62–67) account for less than 1% of pulmonary complications in HIV-infected patients (68). The clinical manifestations of *T. gondii* lung infection are generally similar to those seen with *P. carinii* pneumonia (PCP). Patients may have fever, dyspnea, a nonproductive cough, and occasionally hemoptysis (67). However, the onset of disease tends to be more rapid, and patients may present in respiratory failure with a clinical picture mimicking septic shock with hypotension, metabolic acidosis, and disseminated intravascular coagulation (67,69). The chest roentgenogram typically reveals bilateral interstitial infiltrates, but single nodules or nodular infiltrates, and hilar adenopathy have also been described (65,67,69). Concurrent encephalitis may or may not be present and multiorgan involvement, including heart, bone marrow, liver, testis, and stomach, can occur. Pathologically, *T. gondii* in tissue is most often associated with necrosis and mixed inflammation. Both intracellular and free tachyzoites, bradyzoites, and cysts may be found (69–71). The diagnosis is made using Giemsa or eosin-methylene blue fast stains of bronchoalveolar lavage fluid or a lung biopsy specimen. Improved detection of the organism has been reported using the peroxidase antiperoxidase method (69). *T. gondii* pneumonia is thought to result from reactivation of latent infection, but it is uncertain as to whether the presence of the organism in the lung arises from cysts already there, or is a consequence of parasitemia originating from a distant site. Primary *Toxoplasma* myocarditis manifested by cardiac tamponade or biventricular failure has been reported (72,73), but cardiac infection is usually asymptomatic, occurring in the setting of disseminated disease, in which CNS abnormalities predominate clinically (74). Definitive diagnosis is inconvenient and difficult as it requires an endomyocardial biopsy, which may miss the diagnosis due to the small amount of tissue obtained and the patchy nature of the myocarditis. Retinochoroiditis, with or without concomitant encephalitis, can also occur (75–77). Orchitis has occasionally been reported (78,79).

DIAGNOSIS

Serology

Serologic diagnosis of toxoplasmosis is dependent to a large extent on the particular patient population in which the diagnosis is being entertained. In the nonimmunocompromised host, acute acquired toxoplasmosis is usually established by the demonstration of seroconversion from a negative to a positive antibody titer, or by a fourfold rise in antibody titer. Titers by either the Sabin Feldman dye test or the indirect fluorescent antibody assay (IFA) usually exceed 1:1024 within the first 2 weeks after infection. Although the presence of a high antibody titer is suggestive of acute infection, such titers may persist for years after acute infection. Therefore, in patients with stable high antibody titers, detection of an IgM antibody directed against *T. gondii* may suggest acute infection, although even these antibodies may remain elevated for as long as 1 year (80,81). Recent data suggest that an elevated anti-*Toxoplasma* IgA antibody (82) may be even a more specific indicator of acute acquired infection. The latter test may be particularly useful in the pregnant patient for whom it is essential to ascertain whether *Toxoplasma* was acquired during gestation. In the few cases in which serological data were available for the nonimmunocompromised host with toxoplasmic encephalitis, evidence of a brisk antibody response was present. Generally, the IgG antibody titer was greater than 1:1000. In one nonimmunocompromised patient who eventually died of toxoplasmic encephalitis, no serum anti-*Toxoplasma* antibody was demonstrated; however, *Toxoplasma* antibody was detected in cerebrospinal fluid. In this patient, *Toxoplasma* organisms were also observed in CSF (4).

In immunocompromised patient populations, the serologic diagnosis of toxoplasmic encephalitis depends on the specific pathogenesis of infection. For instance, in heart (8) and probably renal transplant recipients (37), toxoplasmic encephalitis most often occurs as a result of acute acquisition of the organism, through receipt of an organ from a donor who had previously been infected with *T. gondii*. Seronegative heart transplant recipients who seroconvert as a result of receiving a heart from a seropositive donor have developed severe symptomatic disease. In contrast, heart transplant recipients who were seropositive prior to transplantation often develop an

increase in titers of IgG and IgM antibodies to *T. gondii* in the post-transplantation period but remain asymptomatic. In the latter instance, a rise in antibody titer is not diagnostic for significant disease due to *T. gondii*. Knowledge of the serologic status of the organ donor and recipient is thus important both in determining which organ recipients are at greatest risk and in interpretating posttransplant serologic findings. Significant rises in antibody titers have been demonstrated in a variety of immunocompromised patients in the absence of clinical evidence of active toxoplasmosis (50,83,84). In patients with underlying immunocompromising conditions and nonspecific signs such as persistent fever and malaise, confirmation of active *Toxoplasma* infection should be sought by detection of parasitemia (85) or by histopathological demonstration of the organism.

Many patients with cerebral toxoplasmosis do not demonstrate either high or rising serum anti-*Toxoplasma* antibody titers and instead have stable low level titers. This serologic response is consistent with recrudescence of latent infection in a patient who is severely immunocompromised, most notably in bone marrow transplant recipients (86) and in AIDS patients. Almost uniformly, low but detectable levels of anti-*Toxoplasma* antibody were present for long periods prior to the development of encephalitis. A decline in antibody titer may occur in some of these patients as the encephalitis progresses. Anti-*Toxoplasma* IgM antibody is also rarely present in these patients. In the non-AIDS immunocompromised host in whom the frequency of toxoplasmic encephalitis is low, the usefulness of serology is also limited and diagnosis will most often require immunohistopathologic examination of a sample of brain tissue.

The most important feature of toxoplasmic serology in AIDS patients is its predictive value. At least 97% of AIDS patients with toxoplasmic encephalitis have *Toxoplasma* antibody titers of between 1:8 and 1:1024. This antibody level is not discernibly different from that found in AIDS patients without evidence of encephalitis. However, the predictive value of a positive serology in a patient with characteristic abnormalities on neuroradiographic studies may be as high as 80% in the United States (87). Therefore it has become standard clinical care to initiate a therapeutic trial of anti-*Toxoplasma* chemotherapy in HIV-infected patients who have a compatible neuroradiographic and/or clinical picture and a positive serology. In HIV-infected patient populations in whom other central nervous system processes are more prevalent than toxoplasmosis, the predictive value of a positive *Toxoplasma* serology is diminished (88). Furthermore, in populations in which the overall seroprevalence for *T. gondii* is very high, the predictive value of a positive serology to distinguish toxoplasmic encephalitis from other similar appearing infectious and noninfectious etiologies is reduced. As a rule of thumb, a clinical and/or neuroradiographic response should be evident within the first 2 weeks of therapy. The outcome of empiric therapy is therefore in and of itself an excellent diagnostic modality.

CSF serology may be a useful adjunctive test in selected patients (89), particularly if intrathecal production of anti-*Toxoplasma* antibody can be demonstrated. The following formula can be used: [CSF dye test titer (reciprocal)/total CSF globulin] × [total serum globulin/ serum dye test titer (reciprocal)]. Intrathecal production of anti-*Toxoplasma* antibody is indicated by a value greater than 1, except in patients with high levels of anti-*Toxoplasma* antibody in their serum (i.e., ≥1:1024). This is probably because there is not a sufficiently disproportionate increase in CSF levels in these patients.

Neuroradiographic Studies

Computerized axial tomography (CAT) (66,90–92) and magnetic resonance imaging (MRI) (90,93–95) have been extremely useful in delineating CNS lesions due to toxoplasmic encephalitis. Characteristically, on CAT scan the lesions of toxoplasmic encephalitis are rounded, single or multiple, and isodense or hypodense. Most often the lesions are ring enhancing. In approximately 75% of cases, the lesions are multiple and are most often localized in the corticomedullary junction and basal ganglia, although any part of the central nervous system may be involved. The lesions are frequently associated with edema and mass effect; cerebral hemorrhage has been noted in rare instances (91,92). Some investigators believe that a double-dose delayed contrast study may be a more sensitive method for delineating the true extent of disease. In several cases the immediate CAT scan was reported as negative whereas the delayed study demonstrated enhancing lesions. The increasing use of MRI has revealed limitations of CAT scanning in delineating the true extent of disease (32,93–96). MRI has detected lesions in patients with active toxoplasmic encephalitis in whom CAT scans were normal. MRI should be considered in patients with neurological symptoms and positive *Toxoplasma* serology if the CAT scan is negative. The neuroimaging features of the lesions on either the CAT scan or MRI, are not pathognomonic for toxoplasmic encephalitis and can be seen in a variety of infectious and noninfectious processes including intracerebral lymphoma, Kaposi's sarcoma, cryptococcoma, and tuberculoma. It has been suggested that the presence of multiple ring-enhancing lesions are more suggestive of *Toxoplasma* compared to single, partial, or non-contrast-enhancing lesions, which favor lymphoma. However, in a recent review, 40% of CNS lymphomas were observed to be multicentric and almost 50% had ring enhancement (97).

MRI or CAT scans are useful to assess the response to empiric anti-*Toxoplasma* therapy. Improvement on sequential neuroimaging strongly suggests the diagnosis of toxoplasmic encephalitis. Although complete resolution of abnormalities on CAT scan may take up to 6 months, patients responding to therapy usually have radiographic evidence of improvement within 2–3 weeks of initiation of treatment. Peripheral CNS lesions tend to resolve more quickly than deeper lesions. Often the radiographic response to therapy lags behind the clinical response. It is important to note that other processes of an infectious or malignant nature can occur concomitantly with toxoplasmic encephalitis; therefore partially resolving lesions, or new lesions developing while older ones are resolving, warrant consideration of a brain biopsy.

Identification of the Organism

Definitive diagnosis of toxoplasmic encephalitis requires demonstration of the tachyzoite in a clinical specimen. With the exception of AIDS patients and heart transplant recipients (for reasons indicated above), the diagnosis of toxoplasmic encephalitis in immunocompromised hosts in whom the infection is rare, is usually made by a brain biopsy. Intraoperative sonography and needle biopsy with a stereotactic device have proved useful in identifying the site of infection and decreasing operative morbidity. However, the amount of tissue obtained by needle biopsy is small, limiting the extent of immunohistological examination that can be performed. Since the histological changes associated with *Toxoplasma* may at times closely resemble those of viral encephalitis, and tachyzoites may be difficult to discern from nuclear debris, diagnosis of toxoplasmic encephalitis often requires specialized immunohistochemical techniques in order to detect the organism or its antigens. In addition, the reactive round cell infiltrate in toxoplasmic encephalitis may be difficult to differentiate from lymphoma (22,96). Therefore it is recommended that if a needle biopsy sample does not definitively indicate *T. gondii* infection or an alternative diagnosis, further tissue should be obtained for more extensive immunohistological studies utilizing pathogen- and cell-specific antibodies. Pseudocysts and tachyzoites are more readily identified at the periphery of a lesion or within normal brain tissue, compared to the central necrotic area.

Occasionally patients with toxoplasmic encephalitis have a concomitant pneumonitis and the pathogen can be detected in bronchoalveolar lavage fluid (66). Also, in the rare patient in whom there is meningeal involvement, the organism can be isolated from cerebrospinal fluid (98). Recently, the organism has been isolated from blood cultures of patients with, and without, evidence of an ongoing encephalitis (99,100). In the past, isolation of *T. gondii* from clinical specimens required inoculation into a laboratory animal, most commonly a mouse (99).

However, this technique is labor intensive and requires up to 6 weeks to demonstrate the organism. Tissue culture systems commonly used for viral isolation are also useful for isolation of *T. gondii* from clinical specimens. Another diagnostic methodology being explored is the selective amplification by polymerase chain reaction of DNA fragments specific to *T. gondii* (100). This latter technique may provide a sensitive, specific, and rapid assay for the direct identification of *T. gondii* in clinical specimens. Preliminary reports indicate that PCR may be helpful in the detection of *Toxoplasma* in amniotic fluid and in confirming congenital infection. The utility of this extremely sensitive technique in identifying the pathogen in cerebrospinal fluid in toxoplasmic encephalitis remains to be determined (101).

TREATMENT

The mainstay of therapy for toxoplasmic encephalitis is the combination of pyrimethamine and sulfadiazine. These two drugs sequentially block folic acid metabolism and thereby act synergistically against *T. gondii*. Among the sulfonamides, sulfadiazine, sulfamethazine, and sulfamerazine are equally efficacious (22).

Recent studies of pyrimethamine levels in patients with AIDS and toxoplasmic encephalitis have shown that serum drug levels were erratic (102,103). Recently, we examined the pharmacokinetics of pyrimethamine in five patients with toxoplasmic encephalitis treated with 75 mg of pyrimethamine per day. The half-life of pyrimethamine varied between 26 and 90 hr and the serum levels varied between 500 and 2000 ng/ml (*unpublished data*). The factors that influence serum pyrimethamine levels and half-life are unknown. Furthermore, no studies have correlated serum levels of anti-*Toxoplasma* chemotherapeutic agents with either clinical response or drug toxicity. Sulfadiazine is rapidly absorbed from the gastrointestinal tract and serum levels peak within 3–6 hr after ingestion. Both pyrimethamine and sulfadiazine cross the blood–spinal fluid barrier. Currently, pyrimethamine is administered orally as a 100–200-mg loading dose with a subsequent daily dose of 50–75 mg for the first 3–6 weeks of therapy. Sulfadiazine is given by mouth at a dose of 4–6 g/day in four divided doses. The combination of these drugs is highly active against the tachyzoite form of the organism but has no effect on the cyst form. Therefore patients who remain severely immunocompromised are at risk of relapse upon discontinuation of therapy. As a rule of thumb, therapy for toxoplasmic encephalitis is continued until it is clinically apparent that an adequate cell-mediated immune response has been reestablished. Since HIV-infected patients have an inexorable decline of cell-mediated immunity, life-long prophylaxis is necessary. The maintenance phase of therapy usually requires much lower doses of pyrimethamine and sulfadiazine. A variety of regimens have been administered for maintenance therapy, which have included pyrimethamine, 25–50 mg, plus sulfadiazine, 2–4 g, given daily to two to three times weekly (104,105). More studies are needed to optimize dosing schedules for both acute and long-term therapy. Folinic acid at a dose of 5–15 mg daily is added to this regimen to prevent hematologic toxicity from antifolate therapy.

Side effects of pyrimethamine–sulfadiazine therapy are common. Over 40% of patients treated with the drug combination will develop a significant level of toxicity, often necessitating discontinuation of this therapy (49). During the acute phase of treatment, skin rash is the most prominent adverse reaction and is expected to occur in up to 20% of patients. Drug-induced hematologic toxicity usually occurs later and may be exacerbated by the concomitant use of antiretroviral chemotherapy with zidovudine (AZT) (106). Currently, patients receiving long-term suppressive therapy for toxoplasmic encephalitis may be given AZT up to a dose of 500 mg/day, if monitored carefully for evidence of hematologic toxicity (cytopenias). Crystalluria, hematuria, radiolucent stones, and renal failure are well known adverse effects of sulfonamides. Treatment includes hydration, alkalinization of urine, and decreasing the dose of sulfadiazine (107).

The high frequency of toxicity associated with pyrimethamine–sulfadiazine has fueled a search for alternative chemotherapeutic agents. Clindamycin has long been recognized as an effective drug for the treatment of murine toxoplasmosis (108). Several reports describe patients with AIDS and toxoplasmic encephalitis who were effectively treated with pyrimethamine (25–75 mg/day) and oral (109–111) or intravenous clindamycin (1200–4800 mg/day)(112). Recently, a prospective study by the California University-Wide Task Force on AIDS reported that clindamycin (1200 mg iv Q6h) plus pyrimethamine (75 mg orally per day) was equally effective as standard therapy for treatment of toxoplasmic encephalitis (113). Furthermore, there was a trend toward less toxicity with the clindamycin–pyrimethamine regimen.

Other chemotherapeutic agents have recently been shown to have efficacy in murine models of *Toxoplasma* infection (114–118). These agents have included investigational macrolides, such as roxithromycin, azithromycin, and clarithromycin, as well as doxycycline. In a pilot study of 13 AIDS patients, the combination of pyrimethamine and clarithromycin appeared effective, although adverse reactions, primarily increased transaminase levels and hearing loss, were noted (119). The exact role of these drugs in the treatment of toxoplasmosis remains to be determined. Other investigational agents that may prove to be effective for the treatment of toxoplasmic encephalitis are the highly lipid-soluble dihydrofolate reductase inhibitors, for example, trimetrexate or pitrexin

(118,119). These drugs have a higher affinity for *T. gondii*'s dihydrofolate reductase than does pyrimethamine. However, it has been reported that toxoplasmic encephalitis recrudesces during the course of treatment with trimetrexate when used as a single agent (120). Preliminary studies of the investigational agent BW566C80 (Burroughs Wellcome Company) have shown promising results in murine toxoplasmosis; this agent also possesses activity against the tissue cyst stage (121). It remains to be determined whether these agents either individually or in drug combinations, will be useful modalities for the treatment of toxoplasmic encephalitis, especially for the subpopulation of patients who are unable to tolerate, or respond poorly to, pyrimethamine plus sulfadiazine.

REFERENCES

1. Wolf A, Cowen D. Granulomatous encephalomyelitis due to encephalitozoan (encephalitozoic encephalomyelitis). A new protozoan disease of man. *Bull Neurol Inst NY* 1937;6:306–9.
2. Sabin A, Olitski P. *Toxoplasma* and obligate intracellular parasitism. *Science* 1937;85:336–8.
3. Paige BH, Cowen D, Wolff A. Toxoplasmic encephalitis. V. Further observations of infantile toxoplasmoses: intra-uterine inception of the disease: visceral manifestation. *Am J Dis Child* 1942;63:474–8.
4. Luft BJ, Remington JS. Toxoplasmosis of the central nervous system. In: Remington JS, Swartz MN, eds. *Current topics in infectious disease*, vol 6. New York: McGraw-Hill; 1985.
5. Luft BJ, Brooks RG, Conley FK, et al. Toxoplasmic encephalitis in patients with AIDS. *JAMA* 1984;252:913–7.
6. Frenkel JK. Toxoplasmosis: parasite life cycle, pathology and immunology. In: Hammond DM, ed. *The coccidia*. Baltimore: University Park Press; 1973:343–7.
7. Dubey JP, Miller NL, Frenkel JK. The *Toxoplasma gondii* oocyst from cat feces. *J Exp Med* 1970;133:636–40.
8. Luft BJ. Primary and reactivated *Toxoplasma* infection in patients with cardiac transplants: clinical spectrum and problems in diagnosis in a defined population. *Ann Intern Med* 1983;99:27–31.
9. Rose AC, Vys CJ, Novitsky D, Cooper DKC, Barnard CN. Toxoplasmosis of donor and recipient hearts after heterotopic cardiac transplantation. *Arch Pathol Lab Med* 1983;107:368–73.
10. Siegal SE, Lunde MN, Gelderman AH, et al. Transmission of toxoplasmosis by leukocyte transfusion. *Blood* 1971;37:388–94.
11. Beauvais B, Garin JF, Lariviere M, Languillat G, Galal H. Toxoplasmose et transfusion. *Ann Parasitol (Paris)* 1976;51:625–35.
12. Kayhoe DE, Jacobs L, Beye HK, McCullough NB. Acquired toxoplasmosis; observations on two parasitologically proved cases treated with pyrimethamine and triple sulfonamides. *N Engl J Med* 1957;257:1247–54.
13. Frenkel JK, Weber RW, Lunde MN. Acute toxoplasmosis. Effective treatment with pyrimethamine, sulfadiazine, leucovorin calcium and yeast. *JAMA* 1960;173:1471–6.
14. McCabe R, Remington JS. Toxoplasmosis: the time has come. *N Engl J Med* 1988;318:313–5.
15. Luft BJ, Remington JS. Toxoplasmic encephalitis. *J Infect Dis* 1988;157:1–6.
16. Grant IH, Gold JWM, Rosenblum M, et al. *Toxoplasma gondii* serology in HIV-infected patients: the development of central nervous system toxoplasmosis in AIDS. *AIDS* 1990;4:519–23.
17. Viera J, Frank E, Spira TJ, Landesman SH. Acquired immune deficiency in Haitians: opportunistic infections in previously healthy Haitian immigrants. *N Engl J Med* 1983;308:125–9.
18. Moskowitz IB, Corey P, Chan J, et al. Unusual causes of death in Haitians residing in Miami. High prevalence of opportunistic infections. *JAMA* 1983;250:1187–91.
19. Clumeck N, Sonnet J, Taelman H, et al. Acquired immunodeficiency syndrome in African patients. *N Engl J Med* 1984;310:492–7.
20. Carme B, M'Pele P, Mbitsi A, et al. Opportunistic parasitic diseases and mycoses in AIDS. Their frequencies in Brazzaville (Congo). *Bull Soc Pathol Exot. Filiales* 1988;81:311–6.
21. Ambros RA, Leo EY, Sharer LR, et al. The acquired immunodeficiency syndrome in intravenous drug abusers and patients with a sexual risk: clinical and postmortem comparisons. *Hum Pathol* 1987;18:1109–14.
22. Luft BJ. *Toxoplasma gondii*. In: Walzer PD, Gertz RM, eds. *Parasitic infections in the compromised host*. New York: Marcel Dekker; 1989:179–279.
23. Vollmer TL, Waldor MK, Steiman L. Detection of T-4+ lymphocytes with monoclonal antibody reactivates toxoplasmosis in the central nervous system: a model of superinfection in AIDS. *J Immunol* 1987;138:3737–41.
24. Pfefferkorn ER, Guyre PM. Inhibition of growth of *Toxoplasma gondii* in cultured fibroblasts by human recombinant gamma interferon. *Infect Immun* 1984;44:211–6.
25. McCabe RE, Luft BJ, Remington JS. Effect of murine interferon gamma on toxoplasmosis. *J Infect Dis* 1984;150:961–3.
26. Sharma SD, Hofflin JM, Remington JS. *In vivo* recombinant interleukin 2 administration enhances survival against a lethal challenge with *Toxoplasma gondii*. *J Immunol* 1985;135(6):4160–3.
27. Suzuki Y, Orellona MA, Schreiber RD, Remington JS. Interferon γ: the major mediator of resistance against *Toxoplasma gondii*. *Science* 1988;240:516–8.
28. Frenkel JK. Effects of cortisone total body irradiation and mitogen mustered on chronic, latent toxoplasmosis. *Am J Pathol* 1957;33:618–9.
29. Frenkel JK, Nelson BM, Arias-Stelle J. Immunosuppression and toxoplasmic encephalitis: clinical and experimental aspects. *Hum Pathol* 1975;6:97–111.
30. Stahl W, Modification of subclinical toxoplasmosis in mice by cortisone, t-mercaptopurine and splenectomy. *Am J Trop Med Hyg* 1966;15:869–72.
31. Strannegard O, Lycke E. Effect of antithymocyte serum on experimental toxoplasmosis in mice. *Infect Immun* 1972;5:769–74.
32. Stahl W. Effect of heterologous antithymocyte serum on *Toxoplasma gondii* infection in mice. I. Potentiation of primary nonlethal infection. *Jpn J Parasitol* 1978;27:231–4.
33. Sharma S, Budzich T, Profitt M, et al. Regulation of natural killer activity by anti-I region monoclonal antibodies. *Cell Immunol* 1984;85:125–9.
34. Lainson R. Observations on the development and nature of pseudocysts and cysts of *Toxoplasma gondii*. *Trans R Soc Trop Med Hyg* 1958;12:221–5.
35. Van der Waaj D. Formation, growth and multiplication of *Toxoplasma gondii* cysts in mouse brains. *Trop Geogr Med* 1959;11:345–9.
36. Nagington J, Martin AL. Toxoplasmosis and heart transplantation. *Lancet* 1983;2:679–82.
37. Reynolds ES, Walls KW, Pfieffer RI. Generalized toxoplasmosis following renal transplantation. *Arch Intern Med* 1966;118:401–5.
38. Casado-Naranjo I, Lopez-Trigo J, Ferrandiz A, Cervello A, Navarro V. Hemorrhagic abscess in a patient with the acquired immunodeficiency syndrome. *Neuroradiology* 1989;31:289–92.
39. Conley FK, et al. *Toxoplasma gondii* infection of the central nervous system. *Hum Pathol* 1981;12:690–8.
40. Matthiessen L, Cabrousse F, Marche C, et al. Morphology and etiology of microglial nodules in 27 AIDS autopsy cases. *Clin Neuropathol* 1988;7:187–92.
41. Gray F, Gherardi R, Wingate E, et al. Diffuse "encephalitic" cerebral toxoplasmosis in AIDS. *J Neurol* 1989;236:273–7.
42. Khuong MA, Matherson S, Marche C, et al. Diffuse toxoplasmic encephalitis without abscess in AIDS patients. Interscience Conference on Antimicrobial Agents and Chemotherapy #1157, Atlanta, Georgia, 1990.
43. Post MJD, Chan JC, Hensley GT, et al. Toxoplasma encephalitis in Haitian adults with acquired immunodeficiency syndrome: a clinical–pathologic–CT correlation. *AJR* 1983;140:861–8.

44. Wanke C, Tuazon CV, Kovacs A, et al. *Toxoplasma* encephalitis in patients with acquired immune deficiency syndrome: diagnosis and response to therapy. *Am J Trop Med Hyg* 1987;36:509–16.

45. Koeze TH, Klinger GH. Acquired toxoplasmosis. *Arch Neurol* 1964;11:191–3.

46. Ghatak NR, Sawyer DR. A morphologic study of opportunistic cerebral toxoplasmosis. *Acta Neuropathol* 1978;42:217–21.

47. Tavolato B, et al. *Toxoplasma* encephalitis in the adult. *Acta Neurol (Napoli)* 1978;33:321–6.

48. Townsend J, Wolinsky JS, Baringer JR, Johnson PC. Acquired toxoplasmosis. *Arch Neurol* 1975;32:335–43.

49. Luft BJ, Remington JS. Toxoplasmic encephalitis. *J Infect Dis* 1988;157(1):1–6.

50. Luft BJ, Hafner R. Toxoplasmic encephalitis. Editorial comment. *AIDS* 1990;4:593–5.

51. Levy RM, Bredesen DE, Rosenblum MC. Neurological manifestations of the acquired immunodeficiency syndrome (AIDS). Experience at UCSF and review of the literature. *J Neurosurg* 1985;62:475–95.

52. Navia BA, Petito CK, Gold JWM, Cho ES, Jordan BD, Price RW. Cerebral toxoplasmosis complicating the acquired immunodeficiency syndrome: clinical and neuropathological findings in 27 patients. *Ann Neurol* 1989;19:224–38.

53. Wong MD, Gold JWM, Brown AE, et al. Central nervous system toxoplasmosis in homosexual men and parenteral drug abusers. *Ann Intern Med* 1984;100:36–42.

54. Levy RM, Janssen RS, Bush TJ, Rosenblum MD. Neuroepidemiology of acquired immunodeficiency syndrome. In: Rosenblum ML, ed. *AIDS and the nervous system.* New York: Raven Press; 1988:13–27.

55. Snider WD, Simpson DM, Nielsen SN. Neurological complications of acquired immune deficiency syndrome: analysis of 50 patients. *Ann Neurol* 1983;14:403–18.

56. Luft BJ, Brooks RG, Conley FK. Toxoplasmic encephalitis in patients with the acquired immune deficiency syndrome. *JAMA* 1984;252:913–7.

57. McArthur JC. Neurologic manifestations of AIDS. *Medicine (Baltimore)* 1987;66:407–37.

58. Nolla-Sallas J, Ricart C, D'Ohlaberringue L, et al. Hydrocephalus: an unusual CT presentation of cerebral toxoplasmosis in a patient with acquired immunodeficiency syndrome. *Eur Neurol* 1987;27:130–2.

59. Milligan SA, Katz MS, Craven PC. Toxoplasmosis presenting as panhypopituitarism in a patient with the acquired immune deficiency syndrome. *Am J Med* 1984;77:760–4.

60. Mehren M, Burn DO, Maurami CS. Toxoplasmic myelitis mimicking intramedullary spinal cord tumor. *Neurology* 1988;38:1648–50.

61. Overhage JM, Griest A, Brown D. Conus medullaris syndrome resulting from *Toxoplasma gondii* infection in a patient with the acquired immunodeficiency syndrome. *Am J Med* 1990;89:814–5.

62. Tourni JM, Isreal-Biet D, Venet A, Andrieu JM. Unusual pulmonary infection in a puzzling presentation of AIDS (letter). *Lancet* 1985;1:189–93.

63. Touboul JL, Salmon D, Lancastre F, et al. Pneumopatic a *Toxoplasma gondii* chez un patient affient de sindrome d'immunodepression acquins: mise en evidence der parasite par lavage bronchiolo-alveolar. *Rev Rheumol Clin* 1986;42:150–2.

64. Mendelson MH, Finkel LJ, Meyers BR, et al. Pulmonary toxoplasmosis in AIDS. *Scand J Infect Dis* 1987;19:703–6.

65. Tawney S, Masci J, Berger HW, et al. Pulmonary toxoplasmosis: an unusual nodular radiographic pattern in a patient with AIDS. *Mt Sinai J Med* 1986;53:683–5.

66. Derouin F, Sarfati C, Beauvais B, et al. Laboratory diagnosis of pulmonary toxoplasmosis in patients with acquired immunodeficiency syndrome. *J Clin Microbiol* 1989;27:1661–3.

67. Oskenhendler E, Cadranel J, Sarfati C, et al. *Toxoplasma gondii* pneumonia in patients with the acquired immunodeficiency syndrome. *Am J Med* 1989;88(5M):18–21.

68. Murray JF, Folton CP, Garay SM, et al. Pulmonary complications of the acquired immunodeficiency syndrome. *N Engl J Med* 1984;310:1682–8.

69. Catterall JR, Hofflin JM, Remington JS. Pulmonary toxoplasmosis. *Am Rev Respir Dis* 1986;133:704–5.

70. Tschirhart D, Klatt E. Disseminated toxoplasmosis in the acquired immunodeficiency syndrome. *Arch Pathol Lab Med* 1988;112:1237–41.

71. Marche C, Mayorga R, Trophilme D, et al. Pathological study of extraneurological toxoplasmosis in AIDS. 4th International Conference on AIDS, Stockholm, Sweden, June 1988.

72. Adair OV, Randive N, Krasnow N. Isolated *Toxoplasma* myocarditis in acquired immunodeficiency syndrome. *Am Heart J* 1989;118(4):856–7.

73. Moskowitz L, Hemsley GT, Chan JC, et al. Immediate causes of death in acquired immunodeficiency syndrome. *Arch Pathol Lab Med* 1985;109:735–8.

74. Roldan EO, Moskowitz L, Hemsley GT. Pathology of the heart in acquired immunodeficiency syndrome. *Arch Pathol Lab Med* 1987;111:943–6.

75. Weiss A, Margoan C, Ledford D, et al. Toxoplasmic retinochoroiditis. An initial manifestation of the acquired immune deficiency syndrome. *Am J Ophthalmol* 1984;101(2):248–9.

76. Parke DW, Font RC. Diffuse toxoplasmic retinochoroiditis in a patient with AIDS. *Arch Ophthalmol* 1968;104:571–5.

77. Friedman AH. Retinal lesions in the acquired immunodeficiency syndrome. *Trans Am Ophthalmol Soc* 1984;82:447–91.

78. Nistal M, Santana A, Paniaqua R, et al. Testicular toxoplasmosis in two men with the acquired immunodeficiency syndrome (AIDS). *Arch Pathol Lab Med* 1986;110:744–6.

79. Crider SR, Horstman WG, Massey GS. *Toxoplasma* orchitis: report of a case and a review of the literature. *Am J Med* 1988;95:421–4.

80. Welch PC, Masur H, Jones TC, et al. Serologic diagnosis of acute lymphadenopathic toxoplasmosis. *J Infect Dis* 1980;142:256–60.

81. Peacock JE, Folds J, Orringer E, et al. *Toxoplasma gondii* and the compromised host: antibody response in the absence of clinical manifestations of disease. *Arch Intern Med* 1983;143:1235–7.

82. Stepick-Biek P, Thulliez P, Araujo FG, Remington JS. IgA antibodies for diagnosis of acute congenital and acquired toxoplasmosis. *J Infect Dis* 1990;162(1):270–3.

83. Vogel CL, Lunde MN. *Toxoplasma* serology in patients with malignant diseases of the reticuloendothelial system. *Cancer* 1969;25:637–43.

84. Lunde MN, Gelderman AH, Hayes SL, Vogel CL. Serological diagnosis of active toxoplasmosis complicating malignant disease. *Cancer* 1970;25:637–43.

85. Shepp DH, Hackman RC, Conley FK, et al. *Toxoplasma gondii* reactivation identified by a detection of parasitemia in tissue culture. *Ann Intern Med* 1985;103:218–21.

86. Lowenberg B, Van Gijn J, Prins E, Polderman AM. Fatal cerebral toxoplasmosis in a bone marrow transplant recipient with leukemia. *Transplantation* 1983;35:30–4.

87. Cohn JA, McMeeking A, Cohen W, et al. Evaluation of the policy of empiric treatment for suspected *Toxoplasma* encephalitis in patients with the acquired immunodeficiency syndrome. *Am J Med* 1989;86:521–7.

88. Bishburg E, Eng RH, Slim J, et al. Brain lesions in patients with acquired immunodeficiency syndrome. *Arch Intern Med* 1989;149:941–3.

89. Potsman I, Resnick I, Luft BJ, Remington JS. Intrathecal production of antibodies against *Toxoplasma gondii* in patients with toxoplasmic encephalitis and the acquired immunodeficiency syndrome (AIDS). *Ann Intern Med* 1988;108:49–51.

90. Levy RM, Rosenbloom S, Perrett LV. Neuroradiological findings in the acquired immunodeficiency syndrome (AIDS). A review of 200 cases. *AJNR* 1986;7:833–9.

91. Chaudhari AB, Singh A, Jindal S, et al. Haemorrhage in cerebral toxoplasmosis. *Sam J* 1989;76:272–4.

92. Casado Naranjo I, Lopoz Trigo J, Forrandiz A, et al. Hemorrhagic abscess in a patient with the acquired immunodeficiency syndrome. *Neuroradiology* 1989;31:289–92.

93. Whelan MA, Kricheff II, Handler M, et al. A.I.D.S.: cerebral computed tomographic manifestations. *Radiology* 1983;149:477–84.

94. Jarvik JG, Hessolink JR, Kennedy C, et al. Acquired immunode-

ficiency syndrome. Magnetic resonance patterns of brain involvement with pathologic correlation. *Arch Neurol* 1988;45:731–6.

95. Ostertun B, Dewes W, Suss H, Steudel A, Brassel H, Harder T. MR tomography of non-tumor diseases of the brain and cervical cord. *ROFO* 1988;148:408–14.

96. Gill PS, Graham KA, Boswell W, Meyer P, Krailo M, Levine AM. A comparison of imaging, clinical, and pathologic aspects of space-occupying lesions within the brain in patients with acquired immune deficiency syndrome. *Am J Physiol Imaging* 1986;1:134–41.

97. Remick SC, Diamond BS, Migliozzi JA. Primary central nervous system lymphoma in patients with and without AIDS. *Medicine (Baltimore)* 1989;69(6):345.

98. DeMent SH, Cox MD, Gupta PK. Diagnosis of central nervous system *Toxoplasma gondii* from the cerebrospinal fluid in a patient with acquired immunodeficiency syndrome. *Diagn Cytopathol* 1987;3:148–51.

99. Derouin F, Mazeron MC, Garin YJF. Comparative study of tissue culture and mouse inoculation methods for demonstration of *Toxoplasma gondii*. *J Clin Microbiol* 1987;25:1597–600.

100. Burg JL, Grover CM, Pouletty P, Boothroyd JC. Direct and sensitive detection of a pathogenic protozoan, *Toxoplasma gondii*, by polymerase chain reaction. *J Clin Microbiol* 1989;27:1787–92.

101. Holliman RE, Johnson JD, Savra D. Diagnosis of cerebral toxoplasmosis in association with AIDS using the polymerase chain reaction. *Scand J Infect Dis* 1990;22:240–4.

102. Leport C, Meulemans A, Gameron G, Matheron S, Katlama C, Robine D. Levels of pyrimethamine in serum of AIDS patients treated for toxoplasmic encephalitis. Proceedings for the IV European Congress of Clinical Microbiology, Nice, May 1989.

103. Weiss LM, Harris C, Berger M, Tanowitz HB, Wittner M. Pyrimethamine concentrations in serum and cerebrospinal fluid during treatment of acute *Toxoplasma* encephalitis in patients with AIDS. *J Infect Dis* 1988;157:580–3.

104. Leport C, Raffi F, Matheron S, et al. Treatment of central nervous system toxoplasmosis with pyrimethamine/sulfadiazine combination in 35 patients with the acquired immunodeficiency syndrome: efficacy of long-term continuous therapy. *Am J Med* 1988;84:94–108.

105. Pedrol E, Gonzalez-Clemente JM, Gatell J, et al. Central nervous system toxoplasmosis in AIDS patients: efficacy of an intermittent maintenance therapy. *AIDS* 1990;4:511–7.

106. Leport C, Chakroun M, Matheron S, Rozenbaum W, Dournon E, Rognier B. Zidovudine efficacy and tolerance in 32 patients with cerebral toxoplasmosis in the acquired immunodeficiency syndrome (letter). *Presse Med* 1988;17:1813–4.

107. Oster S, Hutchinson F, McCabe R. Resolution of acute renal failure in toxoplasmic encephalitis despite continuance of sulfadiazine. *Rev Infect Dis* 1990;12(4):618–20.

108. Hofflin JM, Remington JS. Clindamycin in a murine model of toxoplasmic encephalitis. *Antimicrob Agents Chemother* 1986;31:492–6.

109. Leport C, Bastuji-Garin S, Perronne C, et al. An open study of the pyrimethamine–clindamycin combination in AIDS patients with brain toxoplasmosis. *J Infect Dis* 1989;160:557–8.

110. Danneman BR, Israelski DM, Remington JS. Treatment of toxoplasmic encephalitis with intravenous clindamycin. *Arch Intern Med* 1988;148:2477–82.

111. Rolston KV, Hoy J. Role of clindamycin in the treatment of central nervous system toxoplasmosis. *Am J Med* 1987;83:551–4.

112. Rolston KV. Clindamycin in cerebral toxoplasmosis (letter). *Am J Med* 1988;85:285.

113. Danneman BR, Israelski DM, McCutchan JA, et al. Treatment of toxoplasmic encephalitis in AIDS: Primary Report of the California Collaborative Treatment Group Randomized Trial of Pyrimethamine plus Sulfanamides versus Pyrimethamine plus Clindamycin. 28th Interscience Conference on Antimicrobial Agents and Chemotherapy, Los Angeles, 1988.

114. Chan J, Luft BJ. RU28965: an effective drug in the treatment of murine toxoplasmosis. *Antimicrob Agents Chemother* 1986;30:323–7.

115. Araujo FG, Remington JS. Azithromycin: a macrolide with potent activity against *Toxoplasma gondii*. *Antimicrob Agents Chemother* 1988;32:755–7.

116. Luft BJ. Potent *in vivo* activity of aprinocid, a purine analog, against murine toxoplasmosis. *J Infect Dis* 1986;154:692–5.

117. Kovacs JA, Allegia CJ, Chabner BA, et al. Potent effect of trimetrexate, a lipid soluble antifolate on *Toxoplasma gondii*. *J Infect Dis* 1987;155:1027–32.

118. Araujo FG, Guptill DR, Remington JS. *In vivo* activity of pitrexin against *Toxoplasma gondii*. *J Infect Dis* 1987;156:828–30.

119. Leport C, Fdez-Maartin J, Morlat P, et al. Combination of pyrimethamine–clarithromycin for acute therapy of toxoplasmic encephalitis (TE): a pilot study. *Intersci Conf Antimicrob Agents Chemother* 1990;279:1158.

120. Polis MA, Masur H, Tuazon C, et al. Salvage trial of trimetrexate–leucovorin for treatment of cerebral toxoplasmosis in AIDS patients. *Clin Res* 1989;37:437A.

121. Araujo FG, Gutteridge WE, Remington JS. Remarkable activity of 566C80 against *Toxoplasma gondii*. *Clin Res* 1990;38(3):779A.

AIDS and Other Manifestations of HIV Infection,
Second Edition, Edited by Gary P. Wormser.
Raven Press, Ltd., New York © 1992.

CHAPTER 24

Cryptococcus neoformans Infections in the Era of AIDS

Joseph R. Masci, Michael Poon, Gary P. Wormser, and Edward J. Bottone

Cryptococcus neoformans was first described as a human pathogen in 1894 (1). Over the ensuing nine decades, great strides were made in understanding the organism and its complex interrelationships with the human host. Epidemiologic features, diagnostic modalities, and treatment approaches were carefully determined through years of meticulous study. Many excellent reviews have been published summarizing these efforts (2–17).

What, then, is the purpose of providing another review of the same subject, 11 years into the acquired immunodeficiency syndrome (AIDS) epidemic? To paraphrase an earlier remark made by Campbell and Mackenzie (18), probably no yeast has produced as many surprises as has *C. neoformans*. Stated less abstractly, the pathobiology of this organism has been so immensely influenced by the advent of human immunodeficiency virus (HIV) infection as to necessitate a broad reexamination of current knowledge of this mycotic infection.

The most obvious impact of HIV infection has been to increase the number of cases of cryptococcosis so immensely as to dwarf the number of background cases occurring unrelated to AIDS. Such a dramatic change in frequency and in epidemiology has not been reported for the other systemic mycoses. Prior to AIDS, the annual incidence of cryptococcal infection in the United States

and areas in western Europe was estimated to be 1 to 2 new cases per 1 million inhabitants (19). One-half of these patients had no known underlying immunosuppressive disease. In contrast, among AIDS patients the reported frequency of cryptococcosis has ranged from 1.9% to 9% with an average value of approximately 6–7% (2,20). Using these figures plus census data for the number of U.S. residents (approximately 249 million) and the Public Health Service tabulation of the number of AIDS cases diagnosed during 1990 (approximately 43,000), it follows that the ratio of cases of cryptococcosis in AIDS to those in non-AIDS patients is now at least 5 to 1. In some areas actual figures appear to be much higher. At the City Hospital Center at Elmhurst in Queens, New York, 36 cases of cryptococcosis were diagnosed during an 8-year period (1980–1988). All but three patients belonged to established risk groups for AIDS. At this study center (and in many others in New York City and elsewhere), *C. neoformans* is now the most common cause of culture-positive meningitis in adults. According to Public Health Service projections, by the end of 1993 an estimated 390,000–480,000 Americans will have developed AIDS (21,22). Approximately 25,000–31,000 of these patients can be expected to develop clinically apparent cryptococcal infection, if current trends continue.

Because of AIDS, cryptococcal meningitis is no longer a rare disease. Therefore, it is imperative to have a current perspective on this pathogen and the diseases it causes, and to give special emphasis to cryptococcosis in the context of HIV infection. This dramatic change in underlying disease has significantly altered prior tenets about cryptococcal infections. For example, previous recommendations on treatment found in standard medical textbooks, which were based on careful investigations done in an earlier era (8,9), are invalid today. This topic

J. R. Masci: Division of Infectious Diseases, Department of Medicine, City Hospital Center at Elmhurst, Elmhurst, New York 11373.

M. Poon and E. J. Bottone: Clinical Microbiology Laboratories, The Mount Sinai Hospital; New York, New York 10029-6574.

G. P. Wormser: Division of Infectious Diseases, Department of Medicine, Westchester County Medical Center, Valhalla, New York 10595.

M. Poon: present address is Division of Cardiology, Department of Medicine, The Mount Sinai Hospital, New York, New York 10029-6574.

TABLE 1. *Comparison of selected characteristics of* Cryptococcus neoformans *varieties* neoformans *and* gattii

Characteristic	*Cryptococcus neoformans*	
	Var. neoformans	Var. gattii
Capsular serotype	A and D	B and C
Blastospore (yeast cell) shape	Spherical	Ovoid
Basidiospore shape	Ovoid	Bacillary
Growth at 37°C	Good	Slow–poor
Geographic distribution	Global	Tropical, subtropical climates
Reservoir in nature	Pigeon droppings, soil	Flowering *Eucalyptus camaldulensis* trees

and others pertinent to the impact of HIV infection will be discussed in detail in this chapter.

TAXONOMY

The genus *Cryptococcus* comprises at least 17 species of which *C. neoformans,* because of its pathogenic potential for humans, has served as the focal point for scientific study. Taxonomic studies by Kwon-Chung (23,24) have identified two morphologically and physiologically distinct perfect (sexual) states of *C. neoformans* for which the genus *Filobasidella* was created to include the varieties *F. neoformans* var. *neoformans* and *F. neoformans* var. *bacillispora*. *F. neoformans* is obtained when compatible strains of *C. neoformans* capsular serotypes A and D are mated whereas *F. bacillispora* is the perfect state of viable matings of *C. neoformans* serotypes B and C. Because of the discovery of two morphologically and physiologically distinct perfect states of *C. neoformans,* two varieties were delineated, namely *C. neoformans* var. *neoformans* (serotypes A and D) and *C. neoformans* var. *gattii* (serotypes B and C) (25). Table 1 summarizes selected characteristics of the two varieties of *C. neoformans.*

SEROGROUP DISTRIBUTION OF *Cryptococcus neoformans* IN PATIENTS WITH AIDS

One of the most intriguing and perplexing enigmas of cryptococcosis in patients with AIDS is the almost exclusive occurrence of the A/D serogroup of *C. neoformans* even in areas of the world [California, Australia, central Africa (Zaire)] where the B/C serogroup predominates (26–28) and the natural habitat for this variety, flowering *Eucalyptus camaldulensis* trees, are also found (29).

Indeed, Rinaldi et al. (30) and Shimizu et al. (31), on the basis of a biochemical identification method (32) of a total of 48 *C. neoformans* isolates from patients with AIDS residing in B/C endemic areas of California (San Francisco and Los Angeles) and Texas (San Antonio), showed that *C. neoformans* var. *neoformans* (serogroup A/D) was the only variety isolated. Similarly, in our study (33) of 55 *C. neoformans* isolates from patients with AIDS (51 from New York State and one isolate

TABLE 2. *Emerging trend in varietal distribution of 191* Cryptococcus neoformans *isolates in patients with AIDS*

Investigator (ref.)	Geographic locale	*Cryptococcus neoformans* endemic prevalence		AIDS patients (no. strains)
		High	Low	
Rinaldi et al., 1986 (30)	San Francisco	A/D	B/C[a]	A/D (28)
Shimizu et al., 1986 (31)	Los Angeles	B/C (50%)	A/D (50%)	A/D (20)
Swinne et al., 1986 (28)	Zaire (central Africa)	B/C (1981)[b]	A/D	A/D (34)
Bottone et al., 1987 (33)	New York (61)	A/D	B/C (rare)	A/D (65)
	New Orleans (1)			
	Washington, D.C. (1)			
	San Francisco (1)			
	Australia (1)			
D. Marriott[c]	Australia	B/C	A/D	A/D (10)
Kapend'a et al., 1987 (34)	Rwanda (central Africa)	B/C	A/D	A/D (30)
				B/C (1)
Kwon-Chung and Varma, 1989 (34a)	Zaire	B/C		
	Canada (travel to Mexico)?			
	Los Angeles	B/C (50%)	A/D (50%)	B/C (3)

[a] Bennett et al., 1977.
[b] Since 1981 A/D serogroup predominating.
[c] Personal communication. Isolates biochemically identified as *C. neoformans* var. *gatti* or var. *neoformans.*

each from New Orleans, San Francisco, Washington, D.C., and Sydney, Australia), all were biochemically identified as *C. neoformans* var. *neoformans* (Table 2). Furthermore, Swinne et al. (28) reported that 34 isolates of *C. neoformans* from patients with AIDS in central Africa (Zaire) recovered since 1981 have been *C. neoformans* var. *neoformans* (serogroup A/D). Additionally, Kapend'a and colleagues (34), in the course of describing the first case of *C. neoformans* var. *gattii* (serotype B) in an AIDS patient from Zaire, noted that 30 previous strains isolated from Rwandese patients in central Africa with AIDS were *C. neoformans* var. *neoformans* (serogroup A/D). Even in Australia, an endemic focus for *C. neoformans* var. *gattii* (serogroup B/C) (27), *C. neoformans* var. *neoformans* was the exclusive isolate recovered from ten patients with AIDS (D. Marriott, personal communication).

Taken in total, 187 of 191 reported cases of cryptococcosis in patients with AIDS in which the isolate was biochemically identified or specifically serotyped have been attributed to *C. neoformans* var. *neoformans* (serogroup A/D). This includes ten additional isolates of ours from patients residing in New York that were of the A/D variety, and three isolates of the B/C serogroup reported by Kwon-Chung and Varma (34a). Factors accounting for the overwhelming predominance of the *neoformans* variety in patients with AIDS include the widespread environmental distribution of *C. neoformans* var. *neoformans,* including even the gastrointestinal tract of cockroaches (35). Hence, in contrast to the variety *gattii,* which is found in focal geographic areas in association with eucalyptus trees (29), more frequent exposure to environmental sources of *C. neoformans* var. *neoformans* (even in endemic areas for *C. neoformans* var. *gattii*) may increase the risk of overt infection in immunologically incompetent hosts. Less frequent exposure to the *gattii* variety, however, does not fully explain the preponderance of *C. neoformans* var. *neoformans* (serogroup A/D) among clinical isolates in endemic areas for the *gattii* variety. While there may be undefined epidemiologic correlates underscoring this ecologic shift, which in Zaire began in 1969 and has been noted worldwide since, it is equally plausible that the unique form of immunosuppression associated with HIV infection accounts for a selective propensity to infection with *C. neoformans* var. *neoformans.*

CAPSULE AND PATHOGENESIS

The extracellular polysaccharide capsule of *C. neoformans* has been shown to play a significant role in numerous host–fungus interactions, in diagnostic and prognostic assessment of the patient, and in serotyping of *C. neoformans* strains.

The *C. neoformans* capsular polysaccharide is a polyvalent anionic gel composed of a mannose backbone with xylose, galactose, and uronic acid that encircles the cryptococcal cell wall. The cell itself is round or oval, measuring from 4–6 μm in diameter, whereas the surrounding capsule usually ranges in diameter from 1 μm to 15 μm (36). In rare instances cells may achieve 20 μm in diameter and highly encapsulated strains are encountered in which the total cell plus capsule diameter may measure up to 55 μm (37,38) (Fig. 1). Nonencapsulated strains of *C. neoformans* occur in natural habitats such as soil and pigeon droppings (39,40) but on occasion may be isolated from clinical specimens (41).

The role of cryptococcal encapsulation as a virulence factor has been the subject of numerous studies and a comprehensive review (42). Biologic functions ascribed to the presence and size of the capsule include: (1) the prevention of Fc-mediated attachment of *C. neoformans* to macrophages in the presence of cell-wall-bound opsonizing antibodies by blocking contact between opsonic ligands bound to sites beneath the capsule and their receptors on phagocytes (43); and (2) the passive inhibition of phagocytosis as a function of capsule size. In the absence of anticapsular antibody, capsule-deficient cells are readily phagocytized, while large encapsulated cells are more slowly ingested by macrophages (44) and neutrophils (45,46). The importance of cryptococcal polysaccharide in antiphagocytic activity was initially studied by Bulmer and Sans (45,47), who noted that the presence of a capsule was critical to virulence. This observation was further strengthened by Kozel (48), who showed that the addition of purified cryptococcal polysaccharide to washed formalinized suspensions of nonencapsulated yeast cells restored antiphagocytic activity. The added polysaccharide bound to specific surface receptors on the nonencapsulated cells.

Ikeda et al. (49) subsequently showed that specific immunoglobulin G (IgG) anticapsular antibody is opsoniz-

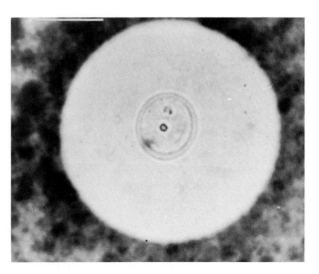

FIG. 1. India ink preparation of gelatinous material from pulmonary nodule from non-AIDS patient showing markedly encapsulated *C. neoformans*. Scale bar = 17 μm.

ing for heavily encapsulated cryptococci via activation of the classical complement pathway with C3b deposition on the capsular surface. More recently, however, Kozel et al. (50) demonstrated that binding of C3 fragments is necessary but not sufficient for phagocytosis by neutrophils of encapsulated *C. neoformans* strains. In the nonimmune host with infection due to poorly encapsulated cells, the alternative complement pathway appears to play the major role in opsonization.

Encapsulation serves as a major diagnostic clue for the presence of this fungus. Cryptococcosis in different patient populations ranging from normal individuals to those profoundly immunodeficient, as exemplified by patients with AIDS, is often diagnosed by demonstrating an encapsulated yeast cell in India ink preparations, with little regard paid to the size of the capsule, just to its presence.

The host factors that contribute to the degree of in vivo *C. neoformans* capsule synthesis following inhalation of sparsely or nonencapsulated *C. neoformans* particles from environmental sources are poorly understood. Similarly, little attention has been paid to the degree of encapsulation of *C. neoformans* causing human infections as a function of the host's immune status. In our laboratory we have consistently observed that *C. neoformans* from cerebrospinal fluid of AIDS patients are poorly encapsulated as contrasted to *C. neoformans* from other patient populations (Fig. 2) (51,52). Poorly encapsulated *C. neoformans* was seen in cryptococcal infections in AIDS patients from all risk groups for HIV

infection. Of the 33 patients studied to date, 20 were intravenous drug abusers, 12 male homosexuals, and 1 a blood transfusion recipient.

The association of poorly encapsulated cryptococci in patients with AIDS has also been noted by Gal and colleagues (53). These investigators, working in southern California (Los Angeles) measured the capsule plus cell size of cryptococci in the cerebrospinal fluid (CSF) of eight consecutive untreated patients and noted that the yeast cell including the capsule measured only 5.1 μm (2.0–8.0 μm, SD = 2.2 μm). Poorly encapsulated cryptococci were also noted in bronchoalveolar lavage and bone marrow specimens from some of these patients.

The observations of the latter investigators (53) are significant for several reasons. First, the presence of poorly encapsulated cryptococci infecting patients with AIDS, when specifically looked for, seems widespread. Second, since the California isolates were even less well encapsulated than those in New York, geographic origin of the cryptococcal organism may also influence this biologic characteristic. It is important to note, however, that poorly encapsulated cryptococci are not, per se, restricted to patients with AIDS (54–57).

Our human and animal (mouse) (58,59) experimentation data suggest that a fundamental relationship exists between host immune status and degree of *C. neoformans* encapsulation in vivo. Prior to inhalation, cryptococci exist in nature in a poorly or unencapsulated state with cell diameters ranging from 0.65 μm to 5 μm in diameter (46,60,61). After inhalation, capsule synthesis

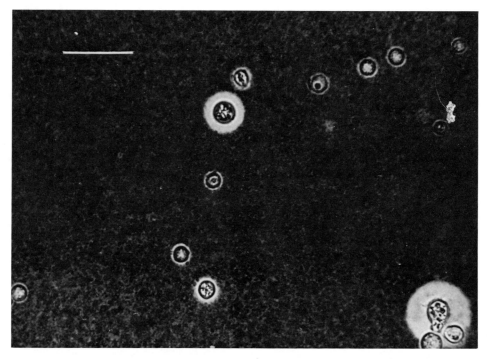

FIG. 2. India ink preparation of cerebrospinal fluid from a patient with AIDS showing numerous poorly encapsulated cryptococci. Scale bar = 17 μm.

begins promptly within the first 10 hours (39). In the early host–fungus interactions, the degree of cryptococcal encapsulation may be critical, as an inverse relationship exists between capsule size and inhibition of phagocytosis (62). Although the putative host factors that bear on in vivo capsule synthesis are unknown, it would appear that ordinary host selective pressures favor the survival of cryptococcal cells expressing maximal encapsulation. Therefore, in patients with AIDS, the profound immunodeficiency state would exert little selective pressure on inhaled poorly encapsulated cryptococci. Paradoxically, the survival of these poorly encapsulated strains may directly contribute to the florid presentation of cryptococcosis in many patients with AIDS, as these organisms, because of their small size, may more readily enter the blood stream and disseminate widely (63).

EPIDEMIOLOGY OF CRYPTOCOCCOSIS IN AIDS PATIENTS

To date, little attention has been devoted to the epidemiology and risk factors associated with cryptococcosis in HIV-infected patients. Poon et al. (64) undertook a retrospective analysis of patients with AIDS in New York City who presented with primary extrapulmonary cryptococcosis and assessed social, racial, sexual, and other demographic variables as risk factors for cryptococcosis.

This study, updated to 1986, comprised 485 patients with cryptococcosis as their first AIDS-defining diagnosis (primary cryptococcosis) among a total of 8,690 patients with AIDS reported to the NYC AIDS Surveillance Unit between 1980 and 1986. (The 163 cases in which cryptococcosis occurred as a secondary or tertiary diagnosis were excluded from this analysis.)

The study showed a steady increase in prevalence of primary cryptococcosis from 3.9% (5/128) of total AIDS cases in 1981 to a peak of 7.0% (220/3,147) at the close of 1986. The prevalence of primary cryptococcosis cases differed significantly ($p < 0.05$) from other AIDS cases in the distribution of ethnic groups involved (favoring blacks and Hispanics), sexual preference (more heterosexuals), and a history of intravenous drug abuse (more likely) (Table 3). No significant differences were noted in patient sex, age, or disease seasonality. The crude odds ratio for primary cryptococcosis as the presenting infection in heterosexual as compared with homosexual/bisexual patients with AIDS was 3.18 ($p < 0.05$) and for intravenous drug users (IVDU), irrespective of sexual preference, as compared with non IVDU's with AIDS was 2.79 ($p < 0.05$).

Horsburgh and Selik reviewed 3,022 cases of extrapulmonary cryptococcosis among AIDS patients reported to Centers for Disease Control between 1981 and 1987 (65). Blacks had an increased frequency of cryptococcal infection, which persisted despite controlling for intravenous drug use. Conversely, intravenous drug users had an increased frequency of cryptococcal infection despite controlling for race. Men, however, were not at higher risk than women. Cryptococcosis was seen more frequently in the East South Central United States. The explanation for these epidemiological features of cryptococcal infection among AIDS patients is unknown.

CLINICAL PATTERNS

Clinical features of cryptococcal infection in AIDS patients differ in important ways from those seen in non-AIDS patients. Reported mortality and relapse rates are higher in AIDS and such typical signs of infection as CSF leukocytosis and depression of CSF glucose levels are often lacking in AIDS-related cases (Table 4).

CENTRAL NERVOUS SYSTEM DISEASE

As in non-AIDS patients with cryptococcal infection, the central nervous system (CNS) is the most common

TABLE 3. *Statistically significant risk factors for primary cryptococcosis among patients with AIDS in New York City (1980–1986) by univariate analysis[a]*

	No. cryptococcal cases/ no. AIDS cases	Prevalence (%)	Statistical evaluation (p by Chi square)
Ethnic group			
Haitian	29/226	12.8	
Black	210/2,521	8.3	
Hispanic	140/2,079	6.7	<0.001
White	105/3,811	2.8	
Unknown	1/53	1.9	
Sexual preference			
Heterosexual	294/2,983	9.9	
Homosexual	177/5,333	3.3	<0.05
Intravenous drug history			
Intravenous drug abuse	292/3,118	9.4	
No intravenous drug abuse	185/5,172	3.6	<0.05

[a] Insignificant risk factors for cryptococcosis: seasonality, age, sex.

TABLE 4. *Comparison of features of cryptococcal meningitis in AIDS and non-AIDS patients*

	AIDS		Non-AIDS[a]	
	% With finding	No. patients (ref)	% With finding	No. patients (ref)
Laboratory result				
CSF				
Leukocyte count <5/mm³	65	17 (66)	15	20 (8)
Protein >45 mg/dl	69	16 (66)	95	20 (8)
Glucose <50 mg/dl	65	26 (67)	83	18 (8)
India ink prep positive	82	17 (66)	64	89 (96)
Culture positive	95	43 (66, 67)	70	23 (8)
Blood				
Culture positive	35	26 (66)	21	76 (96)
Extraneural involvement (coexistent)	17	44 (66, 67)	25	23 (8)
Mortality from active disease (treated)	33	21 (67)	21	19 (8)
Relapse rate				
With suppressive therapy	0	7 (67)	NA	NA
Without suppressive therapy	44	18 (66, 67)	14	107 (96)

[a] NA, nonapplicable.

site of recognized involvement in patients with AIDS. Thirty-four of 36 (94%) AIDS patients with cryptococcal infection in our series presented with meningitis (J. Masci, unpublished data). In two recent reports, which included a total of 53 AIDS patients with cryptococcal infection (66,67), 40 (75%) had CNS involvement.

In those series, as well as in our patients, fever and headache were the most common presenting complaints in patients with CNS infection, each occurring in approximately 90% of cases. Meningismus, photophobia, and mental status changes were each seen in approximately 25% of cases. Nausea, vomiting, and seizures were less common and focal neurological defects were rare. Neither cranial nerve involvement, which has been reported with high frequency (66%) in non-AIDS patients with cryptococcal infection (8), nor hydrocephalus, which has been described as a late posttreatment phenomenon in non-AIDS patients (17), was noted in these series.

EXTRANEURAL DISEASE

Concomitant involvement of sites outside the CNS is relatively common in patients with AIDS. The extent of extraneural infection in these patients may not be fully appreciated at presentation since the various manifestations of extraneural cryptococcosis may mimic other, more common, opportunistic infections or malignancies. Only 2 of our 36 patients presented solely with extraneural disease. Additional patients in our series, all of whom died during the first 48 hours of therapy from cryptococcal meningitis and cryptococcemia, had, at autopsy, widespread extraneural infection. In reported clinical series (66,67), 22 of 53 patients with AIDS had

extraneural cryptococcal infections, including nine with concomitant CNS infection.

Autopsy examinations have been helpful in elucidating the spectrum of extraneural cryptococcal infection. In four published reports that describe a total of 102 postmortem examinations in AIDS patients (68–71) with a variety of opportunistic infections, 11 patients were found to have cryptococcal infection at one or more extraneural sites including the lungs, lymph nodes, adrenal glands, spleen, kidneys, and myocardium. Clinical reports of AIDS patients suggest that the respiratory tract is the extraneural site in which cryptococcal infection is most commonly diagnosed premortem (67).

In one retrospective series (72), 441 of 1,067 AIDS patients had serious pulmonary abnormalities. Eight (2%) of these patients had cryptococcal infection, in each instance coexisting with *Pneumocystis carinii* pneumonia. Interstitial infiltrates and hilar lymphadenopathy either alone or in combination are the radiographic patterns most often seen in association with pulmonary cryptococcosis in AIDS (73). More unusual manifestations include mediastinal lymph node involvement mimicking lymphoma (74), empyema (75–77), and the adult respiratory distress syndrome complicating cryptococcemia (77a). Two of our 36 AIDS patients with cryptococcosis presented with isolated pulmonary cryptococcal infection, one with mediastinal lymph node involvement and the other with a solitary lung nodule. Both patients presented with unexplained fever without respiratory complaints. Cryptococcal antigen was detected in the serum but not the CSF in both cases. The diagnosis was confirmed in each case by percutaneous biopsy of the lesion.

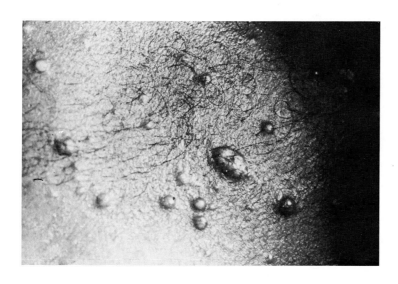

FIG. 3. Hypopigmented raised molluscum contagiosum-like papules caused by *Cryptococcus neoformans* in a patient with AIDS. From ref. 137, with permission.

Pulmonary cryptococcosis in non-AIDS patients has been associated with a wide variety of radiographic findings. As the incidence of AIDS continues to rise, these clinical syndromes may also be encountered in AIDS patients with cryptococcosis. Kerkering et al. (78) described 41 non-AIDS patients with pulmonary cryptococcal infection. Twenty-nine patients, 28 of whom were considered immunocompromised, had concomitant extrapulmonary infection. Of the 12 patients without extrapulmonary involvement, 6 (50%) were immunocompromised. Several different radiographic patterns were seen including multiple small, rounded opacities, platelike atelectasis, interstitial infiltrates, abscess cavities, large mass lesions, and pleural effusions.

Several types of skin lesions have been associated with cryptococcal infection in AIDS patients (Figs. 3–5) (79–82). Rico and Penneys (82) described hypopigmented umbilicated papules resembling molluscum contagiosum on the face of a Haitian man with AIDS. The patient died of disseminated cryptococcal infection involving the lungs, kidneys, liver, and gastrointestinal tract; organisms were identified in the papillary dermis of the

involved skin at autopsy. Concus et al. (81) also described a Haitian patient with AIDS and cutaneous cryptococcosis mimicking molluscum contagiosum. This patient also had pulmonary involvement. Early diagnosis through biopsy resulted in specific therapy and resolution of infection at both sites.

Borton and Wintroub (79) reported herpetiform lesions due to cryptococcal infection in an AIDS patient. Cutanous cryptococcosis has also been associated with a wide variety of other types of skin lesions in non-AIDS patients including papules, nodules, nonhealing ulcers, ecchymoses, acneform lesions, gummatous lesions, cellulitis, and subcutaneous abscesses (80; N. S. Penneys, personal communication), all of which can be anticipated in AIDS patients as well. Coexistence of cryptococcal infection and Kaposi's sarcoma within the same skin lesion has been described (83). Rarely, cryptococcus has been isolated from oral lesions (84) and anal ulcerations (85).

Cryptococcal infection at a variety of other sites has been reported in AIDS patients. Cardiac involvement, including myocarditis (86) with organisms contained

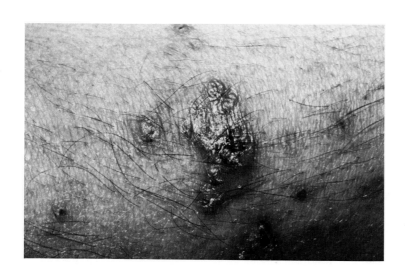

FIG. 4. Lichenoid lesions on leg in patient with disseminated cryptococcosis. Note resemblance to cutaneous Kaposi's sarcoma. Photograph courtesy of Dr. Neal S. Penneys.

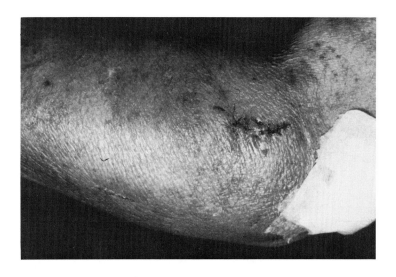

FIG. 5. Cellulitis of forearm of patient with disseminated cryptococcosis. Photograph courtesy of Dr. Neal S. Penneys.

within myocytes, and pericarditis (87) diagnosed by culture and cryptococcal antigen determination of pericardial fluid have been described.

Evidence exists that the genitourinary tract may act as a reservoir of cryptococcal infection. Prostatic infection (20,88,89) and positive cultures of seminal fluid have been documented following standard therapy (90). Persistent infection in the prostate may account for systemic relapses in some AIDS patients (88).

Uncommon sites of involvement that have been described include the eyes (91,92), placenta (93), joints (80), mesenteric lymph nodes (94), and thyroid (95).

DIAGNOSIS

Central Nervous System Disease

Clinical and Laboratory Findings

Once suspected, the diagnosis of cryptococcal CNS infection is seldom difficult to confirm. It should be considered in patients at risk for AIDS presenting with headache, meningismus, photophobia, mental status changes, and seizures or focal neurological deficits, as well as in those with fever of obscure origin or cerebral mass lesions identified by computerized tomography (CT).

Examination of the CSF is necessary to confirm the diagnosis. Characteristic CSF findings in AIDS are qualitatively similar to those in non-AIDS-related cryptococcal meningitis and include a mild-to-moderate lymphocytic pleocytosis, an elevated protein level, and a depressed glucose level. However, all of these abnormalities tend to be less severe in AIDS patients than in non-AIDS patients (Table 4), reflecting, most likely, the extreme impairment of host defenses seen in AIDS. Several of our patients, including two who presented with overwhelming meningitis and cryptococcemia and died

within 48 hours, had no cellular response and normal glucose and protein levels in CSF. In these individuals the diagnosis of cryptococcal infection was initially made only because organisms were visualized in the CSF.

India ink examination of the CSF is an important diagnostic technique, but lacks sensitivity. Recent series indicate that 60–80% of AIDS patients with cryptococcal meningitis have positive examinations (66,67) and, as in non-AIDS patients (96), this finding was associated with a poor prognosis (67). A positive India ink examination should be confirmed by culture and serological methods,

TABLE 5. *AIDS-related infections and malignancies that may be mimicked by cryptococcal infection*

Organ system	Disease
Central nervous system	Toxoplasmosis
	Lymphoma
	Progressive multifocal leukoencephalopathy
	Tuberculous meningitis
	HIV encephalopathy
	HIV meningitis
Respiratory system	*Pneumocystis carinii* pneumonia
	Cytomegalovirus pneumonia
	Tuberculosis
	Lymphoma
	Kaposi's sarcoma
	Toxoplasmosis
	Histoplasmosis
	Strongyloidiasis
	Lymphocytic interstitial pneumonitis
Cardiovascular system	Tuberculous pericarditis
	HIV cardiomyopathy
Skin	Molluscum contagiosum
	Herpes simplex
	Kaposi's sarcoma
	Bacterial cellulitis
	Mycobacterial infection
	Lymphoma

since lymphocytes or erythrocytes in the CSF, or non-cryptococcal yeast cells contaminating the India ink, may cause false-positive results. Cryptococci may be visible in gram-stained preparations as gram-negative or lavender-colored structures containing gram-positive granules (97).

Detection of cryptococcal antigen is a more sensitive and specific means of diagnosis (98). Although patients who test positive for rheumatoid factor may have positive tests for cryptococcal antigen when tested for by latex agglutination, the sensitivity and specificity of the test are both greater than 90% if controls are performed. Antigen was detected in serum and/or CSF in all of our cases of culture-proven cryptococcal infection diagnosed between 1980 and 1988. In two other recent series, antigen was detected in CSF in 100% (66) and 92% (67) and in serum in 75% (66) and 94% (67) of AIDS patients with cryptococcal meningitis. The median CSF antigen titer was reported to be 200 by Zuger et al. (67) in 22 patients. Diamond et al. (96) reported a mean CSF titer of 27.5 in a series of 81 non-AIDS patients. High titers of antigen in CSF have been associated with a poor prognosis in AIDS (66) and non-AIDS patients (99). Initial antigen titers of three of our patients who died within 48 hours of diagnosis ranged from 22,480 to 128,000 in CSF and 2,560 to 32,000,000 in serum, reflecting the overwhelming numbers of cryptococci in these patients. In contrast, initial serum and CSF titers averaged 1,076 and 939, respectively, in patients who had a partial response to therapy and 576 and 100, respectively, in patients who had a complete response to therapy.

Serum cryptococcal antigen determination may be an important screening tool for early infection. Four of 88 (4.5%) asymptomatic HIV-positive patients with CD4 lymphocyte counts less than 250/mm³ had detectable antigen (titer 16–2,560) at our institution. Three of these patients had active meningitis with positive India ink preparations and cultures of CSF. The other patient had a cryptococcal lung nodule.

Cerebrospinal fluid cultures are a reliable means of diagnosis, and are almost always positive in AIDS patients with cryptococcal meningitis. Organisms were isolated from the CSF in 95% of AIDS patients with other diagnostic criteria for cryptococcal meningitis in recent series (66,67). Cryptococcemia was detected in 50% of our AIDS-related cases and in 35% of cases reported by Kovacs et al. (66) (Table 4), in comparison with a frequency of 21% among non-AIDS patients with cryptococcal meningitis described by Diamond et al. (96).

Roentgenographic Findings

Cryptococcal infection of the CNS is not associated with specific abnormalities on CT and rarely produces mass lesions, even when infection is present within the brain substance. In one series by Post et al. (99a), only two of ten AIDS patients with CNS cryptococcal infection had positive CT scans, in both cases due to the presence of a second process (toxoplasmosis, lymphoma). Among the eight patients with negative scans were two in whom perivascular infiltration of the brain with cryptococci was seen at autopsy. Whelan et al. (100) described nine AIDS patients with cryptococcal meningitis. None had structural lesions on CT scan. Mild sulcal prominence and mild ventricular dilatation were seen, however. Two of these patients were found to have yeast cells in the brain parenchyma at autopsy. Other authors (101,102) have described enlargement of the cerebral ventricles and sulci spaces. Zuger et al. (67) described three patients with structural abnormalities seen on CT scan. Two had multiple ring-enhancing lesions that were proved by biopsy to be cryptococcomas, and one had a single hyperdense lesion in the temporal lobe that resolved with antifungal therapy.

Non-Central Nervous System Disease

Clinical patterns in extraneural cryptococcal infection in AIDS are less specific than in CNS disease. Cryptococcal pneumonia, for example, may mimic or even coexist with *P. carinii* infection, a far more common infection in AIDS patients. Cryptococcal skin lesions are nonspecific and may resemble a variety of other processes. Cryptococcal infection may be seen in the setting of multiple, simultaneous opportunistic infections. For example, in our experience, 4 of 20 consecutive patients with cryptococcal meningitis had concomitant *P. carinii* pneumonia. One of these patients also had cerebral toxoplasmosis, and three other patients had other concomitant serious opportunistic infections, including disseminated forms of histoplasmosis, tuberculosis, and herpes zoster infections.

Cryptococcal antigen determination is of somewhat less value in the diagnosis of extraneural infection than in the diagnosis of cryptococcal meningitis. Serum antigen determination was negative in four of nine patients with extraneural disease in one recent series (66), including one patient with cryptococcemia.

Serum antigen determinations, however, may provide the only clue to the presence of occult cryptococcal infection. The detection of antigen, as well as positive cultures from any site in patients at risk for AIDS, warrants a thorough search for CNS infection and the prompt institution of antifungal therapy.

Histopathological Findings

Cryptococcal tissue infections in AIDS and non-AIDS patients are marked histologically by a striking absence of inflammatory response. Yeast cells are seen individu-

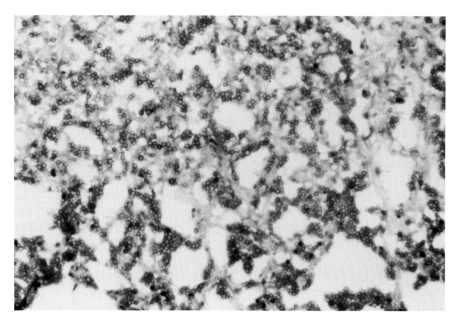

FIG. 6. Mucicarmine-stained histologic section of spleen of a patient with AIDS with disseminated cryptococcosis showing massive numbers of cryptococci supplanting and destroying normal tissue architecture.

ally or in masses with either no cellular infiltrate (Fig. 6), a thin layer of surrounding lymphocytes or, rarely, focal infiltrates of polymorphonuclear leukocytes. In chronic lesions, fibrotic or granulomatous changes may be seen (103). The organisms stain poorly with hematoxylin and eosin but are generally well seen with periodic acid-Schiff or Gomori methenamine silver (GMS). *Cryptococcus,* including smaller and poorly encapsulated forms, can be distinguished from other yeasts or from

artifacts with the mucicarmine stain, which colors the capsule red but does not stain other similar fungi (36,53). For capsule-deficient cryptococci, however, the Fontana-Masson silver stain is superior to the mucicarmine stain (104). Budding with a narrow-neck connection between the parent and single daughter cells may be seen. Confusion with *P. carinii* in lung specimens is possible, since both organisms stain with GMS and may, in fact, coexist in the same tissue (Fig. 7). However, the distinc-

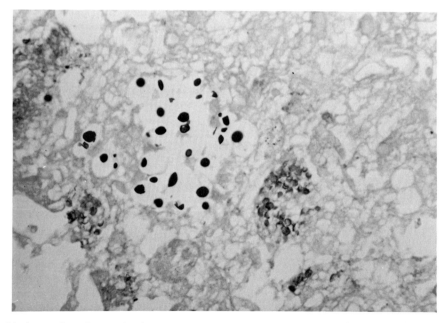

FIG. 7. Methenamine silver stain of lung biopsy of patient with AIDS showing oval budding yeast cells of *Cryptococcus neoformans* (*center*) and smaller masses of whole and collapsed cysts of *Pneumocystis carinii.* ×800. Photograph courtesy of Dr. Antonio Subietas.

tion can usually be made by an experienced pathologist. *Pneumocystis carinii* does not produce budding forms. Grossly, cryptococcal lesions may appear gelatinous due to the capsular polysaccharide.

In the central nervous system, foci of organisms may be found in the subarachnoid space, the cerebellum, or the gray matter near the pons and basal ganglia.

Differential Diagnosis

As noted, cryptococcal infection may share clinical features with a number of other disease processes seen in AIDS patients (Table 5). CNS infection may occasionally be associated with intracerebral mass lesions and thus mimic the radiographic features of toxoplasmosis, lymphoma, or tuberculosis. CSF characteristics in cryptococcal infections may be misleading. The cellular response (predominantly lymphocytic) is similar to that seen with tuberculous, syphilitic, or lymphomatous meningitis, and the depressed CSF glucose with elevated protein levels may suggest toxoplasmosis or tuberculosis. In addition, lymphocytic pleocytosis with an elevated CSF protein level may also be seen in HIV encephalitis.

Respiratory infection with cryptococcus may produce a variety of roentgenographic patterns, including diffuse infiltrates mimicking *P. carinii* pneumonia (76,105).

Cryptococcal pericarditis may mimic that due to tuberculosis or histoplasmosis, and skin lesions of cryptococcal infection may resemble molluscum contagiosum, Kaposi's sarcoma, cutaneous lymphoma, mycobacterial disease, or bacterial cellulitis (79–81; N. S. Penneys, personal communication).

TREATMENT

Antifungal Susceptibility

Because *C. neoformans* recovered from patients with AIDS differs in colonial morphology and in capsule size from most non-AIDS isolates, it is reasonable to ask if there might also be a difference in antifungal susceptibility. Poon and colleagues (106) tested 26 recent isolates of *C. neoformans* var. *neoformans* (serogroup A/D) from 26 patients with AIDS for susceptibility to amphotericin B, flucytosine, ketoconazole, and miconazole by the broth dilution method of Shadomy et al. (107). For comparative purposes three non-AIDS *C. neoformans* isolates were also tested.

Ninety percent (MIC_{90}) of all isolates were inhibited after a 48-hour incubation by concentrations of amphotericin B (1 $\mu g/ml$) (range, 0.25–2 $\mu g/ml$), flucytosine (32 $\mu g/ml$) (range, 1–>64 $\mu g/ml$), ketoconazole (0.5 $\mu g/ml$) (range, 0.06–1 $\mu g/ml$), and miconazole (0.25 $\mu g/ml$) (range, 0.06–0.5 $\mu g/ml$) within achievable serum levels. However, the minimum fungicidal concentration of

these antifungal agents necessary to kill 90% of the isolates exceeded usual drug levels in CSF. No differences in antifungal susceptibility to the four agents tested could be discerned between the *C. neoformans* from patients with AIDS and those from non-AIDS patients. Furthermore, these results were unaffected by degree of encapsulation of the studied strains.

In these susceptibility tests, 28 of the 29 *C. neoformans* were of the *neoformans* variety (serogroup A/D) and one was *C. neoformans* var. *gattii* serotype B (37); all isolates were recovered from patients residing in the New York City area. Shadomy et al. (108), using data from previous studies, noted that 90% of 48 (28 A/D, 20 B/C) clinical isolates of *C. neoformans* from patients without AIDS from diverse geographic locales were inhibited by 0.05–0.39 $\mu g/ml$ of amphotericin B as determined by agar dilution. For flucytosine, these investigators tested 53 isolates (32 A/D, 21 B/C), and noted that the B/C serogroup appeared more resistant to this antifungal agent after 48 hours and 72 hours of incubation. With continued incubation (72 hours) the MIC_{90} for the A/D serogroup was 25 $\mu g/ml$ as contrasted to an MIC_{90} of 50 $\mu g/ml$ for the B/C serogroup. Fromtling et al. (109), however, found no difference in flucytosine susceptibility between serotypes A/D and B/C. Differences in methodology (broth versus agar dilution), assessment of endpoints (turbidity versus colony size), and length of incubation (48 hours versus 72 hours) may account for the differences in susceptibilities observed in the various studies. It is important to note, however, that little correlation exists between in vitro antifungal susceptibility testing and clinical efficacy.

Therapy

Within the past several years, efforts to determine the optimal therapeutic approach for cryptococcal infection in AIDS patients have intensified. Because of the considerable toxicity of previously established therapeutic regimens and the high rate of relapse of cryptococcal meningitis in AIDS patients, new drugs, particularly the triazole compounds fluconazole and itraconazole, have received much attention.

Based on the work of Utz et al. (110) and Bennett et al. (111), amphotericin B, either alone or in combination with 5-flucytosine has become the established mode of therapy for cryptococcal meningitis in non-AIDS patients and has substantially reduced mortality. Diamond and Bennett (96) reported a 71% response rate in patients treated with amphotericin B in a series prior to the AIDS epidemic, and Bennett et al. (111) reported a 68% response rate in non-AIDS patients treated with a regimen consisting of amphotericin B (0.3 mg/kg/day) and 5-flucytosine (150 mg/kg/day in four divided doses) given for 6 weeks. Therapy with this regimen, or with amphotericin B alone given at higher doses and for longer periods of time, was judged to be satisfactory if cultures reverted to negative and if antigen determinations became negative or fell significantly. Recently, in a prospective, randomized study, Dismukes et al. (112) found a higher relapse rate (27% versus 16%) in patients treated with a 4-week regimen of amphotericin B (0.3 mg/kg/day) and 5-flucytosine when compared with those treated for 6 weeks. Only 2 of 91 patients studied, however, were AIDS patients.

Amphotericin B may be administered directly into the CSF, and this approach has been recommended for patients who do not respond to systemic therapy (113) or who develop intolerable side effects. Polsky et al. (114) in a small retrospective review, found that five of six patients treated with both intraventricular and systemic amphotericin B and 5-flucytosine survived compared with only one of seven patients receiving systemic therapy alone. This study was uncontrolled, however, and included only one AIDS patient. In addition, the mortality rate seen with patients receiving systemic therapy alone was substantially higher than has been reported in most other series (Table 4).

Therapy of cryptococcal infections in AIDS patients has been frustrated by incomplete responses and high rates of fatal relapses following conventional therapy. Zuger et al. (67) reported a 12.5% mortality rate from active disease during therapy with either the combination of amphotericin B and 5-flucytosine, or amphotericin B alone. Kovacs et al. (66) reported that 9 of 24 patients (38%) died of cryptococcal infection during or within 4 weeks of the completion of therapy with amphotericin B and that an additional 5 patients (20%) had either persistently positive cultures on therapy or developed positive cultures within 4 weeks of completion and subsequently died. Overall relapse rates in these series were 50% and 60%, respectively, among patients who received no chronic suppressive antifungal therapy, and 88% of relapses were fatal. In contrast, a relapse rate of only 14% was seen in a study of 107 non-AIDS patients, and 87% of these patients were cured on retreatment (113).

Of the 15 patients treated with amphotericin B alone in our series, 6 (40%) died of cryptococcosis during the first 4 weeks of therapy, including 3 who died during the first 48 hours from overwhelming cryptococcemia. Of the 60% who survived beyond 4 weeks of therapy, 33% had an incomplete response with persistent high titers of antigen in CSF despite having received more than 3 g of amphotericin B intravenously. One additional patient suffered relapses at 15 and 30 months after an initial response and responded to retreatment both times.

5-Flucytosine, which when used in dual regimens in non-AIDS patients may permit lower doses of amphotericin B (111), causes bone marrow depression (115) and may have limited utility in AIDS patients, because of the low initial blood counts in these individuals. In addition, emergence of resistance to this agent during therapy, even when it is used in combination with amphotericin B, has been described (112).

Two imidazole compounds, miconazole and ketoconazole, show in vitro activity against isolates of *C. neoformans,* but data concerning the therapy of human infections with these drugs are extremely limited. Weinstein and Jacoby (116) described a non-AIDS patient with cryptococcal meningitis who was cured with intravenous miconazole after failing to respond to a 40-day course of amphotericin B and 5-flucytosine. Graybill and Levine (117) described a patient who responded to intraventricular miconazole after failing to respond to a 5-week course of amphotericin B and 5-flucytosine. It has been pointed out (118) that neither of these patients received miconazole alone, and that these favorable results have not yet been duplicated in controlled trials. Ketoconazole, an oral agent, has been shown to be effective in the therapy of five of seven non-AIDS patients with pulmonary cryptococcal infection and in four non-AIDS cases with meningitis due to *Coccidioides immitis* (119). Adequate CSF levels have been demonstrated in some patients (120) but not in others (121) receiving oral therapy. Clinical data on initial treatment of cryptococcal meningitis with ketoconazole are limited, however, and progression of infection during therapy has been described (122).

Both fluconazole and itraconazole, two recently developed triazole compounds, possess in vitro activity against *C. neoformans* (123,124) and have shown efficacy in the mouse model of meningocerebral cryptococcosis (125,126).

Fluconazole, but not itraconazole, attains high CSF concentrations in rabbits (127) and humans (128) and also achieves excellent serum concentrations with oral dosing. For these reasons fluconazole has received the most attention as a potential therapeutic agent. Stern et al. (129) using oral doses of 100–400 mg/day reported sterilization of CSF in two of two patients who received fluconazole as primary therapy for cryptococcal meningitis and two of three patients who received fluconazole after failing therapy with amphotericin B. It is of concern, however, that two additional patients with extraneural cryptococcosis in this series developed meningitis while receiving fluconazole.

In a randomized, prospective study comparing oral fluconazole (400 mg daily for 10 weeks) with the combination of amphotericin B (0.7 mg/kg daily for 1 week, then three times weekly for 9 weeks) and flucytosine (150 mg/kg daily in four divided doses for 9 weeks), 8 of 14 (57%) patients receiving fluconazole were considered treatment failures (defined as neurologic deterioration necessitating withdrawal from the study drug or positive CSF cultures after 10 weeks of therapy), while all six patients receiving amphotericin B and flucytosine responded ($p = 0.04$) (130). In addition, the time to sterilization of CSF cultures was significantly longer in patients receiving fluconazole. Two patients receiving fluconazole but none receiving amphotericin B and flucytosine died of cryptococcal meningitis. Although the U.S. Food and Drug Administration licensed fluconazole for the treatment of cryptococcal infections in early 1990, the role of this new agent in primary disease has not yet been defined (131).

Viviani et al. (132) described suppression of clinical symptoms of cryptococcal meningitis in three AIDS patients treated with itraconazole after initial therapy with amphotericin B. In addition, in a recent study of 20 patients with cryptococcal meningitis, 13 had a complete response to itraconazole (200 mg twice daily) (133). Itraconazole has not yet been licensed in the United States.

The frequent finding of persistent high antigen titers after prolonged treatment courses in AIDS patients, and the high rate of fatal relapses, have led to strategies of long-term suppression of cryptococcal infection after initial therapy.

Results using amphotericin B for chronic suppression have been equivocal. In the series by Zuger et al. (134), 2 of 13 patients had fatal relapses while receiving suppressive amphotericin B in doses ranging from 40 mg/week to 100 mg/week over follow-up periods of 7–77 weeks. However, none of six patients who discontinued suppressive therapy relapsed during 8–98 weeks of follow-up. The likelihood of relapse could not be predicted by the duration of initial treatment in these patients.

Oral fluconazole has emerged as an effective suppressive agent. When it has been used in maintenance therapy of cryptococcal meningitis after initial therapy with amphotericin B, clinical relapse rates of 7–10% over periods of follow-up of 9–64 months have been reported (129,135). In a controlled trial, relapses were seen in only 1 of 34 (3%) patients receiving suppressive therapy with oral fluconazole (100–200 mg daily) followed for a mean of 164 days (range, 14–529) after initial therapy with amphotericin B alone or in combination with flucytosine. In contrast, 10 of 27 patients (37%) receiving placebo relapsed ($p < 0.001$) during a mean period of observation of 117 days (136). Although generally well tolerated, long-term therapy with oral fluconazole may be associated with liver function abnormalities or thrombocytopenia, necessitating interruption of therapy.

CONCLUDING PERSPECTIVE

Few microorganisms described at the turn of the century have enjoyed the renaissance that *C. neoformans* has. The unbridled interest shown in this yeast-like fungus is closely linked to the interest in AIDS. Cryptococcosis and disseminated mycobacterial infections are encroaching on *P. carinii* as the primary life-threatening opportunistic infections in these afflicted individuals. Although the first decade of the AIDS epidemic is behind

us, numerous challenges still face the medical and general communities. Paramount among these is maintenance of the life of AIDS patients while medical science unravels newer, more effective preventive and therapeutic modalities. As *C. neoformans* approaches its centennial, it has, unfortunately, found a new forum to trumpet its presence that challenges medical resourcefulness.

Cryptococcus neoformans was first described in 1894. During the ensuing nine decades the clinical, epidemiologic, mycologic, diagnostic, and therapeutic correlates underscoring this mycotic infection were elucidated. With the advent of AIDS, however, infections with this yeast-like fungus have been so altered as to deem cryptococcosis in patients with AIDS a new fungal disease.

For example, the incidence of cryptococcosis as the primary etiology of meningitis has so dramatically risen that it is now the leading cause of culture-positive meningitis in adults in many urban areas. In New York City, the major risk factors for AIDS-related cryptococcosis are intravenous drug use and non-white ethnic background. Globally, the serogroup distribution of *C. neoformans* causing infections in patients with AIDS is almost exclusively the A/D serogroup (*C. neoformans* var. *neoformans*) even in geographic locales where the B/C serogroup (*C. neoformans* var. *gattii*) is endemic. Even the morphologic presentation of this yeast-like fungus is distinct, as poorly encapsulated strains predominate in clinical specimens derived from patients with AIDS. Unlike infection in patients prior to the AIDS epidemic, cryptococcosis now is an often fulminant illness with multiorgan involvement. Antigenemia is profound and relapse is common following conventional therapy.

REFERENCES

1. Sanfelice F. Sull'azione patogena de blastomiceti como contributo alla etiologica dei tumori maligni. Nota preliminare II. *Policlinico* 1895;2:204–11.
2. Anonymous. Cryptococcosis and AIDS. *Lancet* 1988;1:1434–6.
3. Benham R. The genus *Cryptococcus*. *Bacteriol Rev* 1956;20:189–201.
4. Binford CH. Torulosis of the central nervous system; a review of recent literature and report of a case. *Am J Clin Pathol* 1941;11:242–51.
5. Evans EE, Harrell ER Jr. Cryptococcosis (torulosis); a review of recent cases. *Univ Mich Med Bull* 1982;18:43–63.
6. Fromtling RA, Shadomy JH. Immunity in cryptococcosis: an overview. *Mycopathologica* 1982;77:183–190.
7. Kozel TR, Pfrommer GST, Guerlain A, Highison BA, Highison GJ. Role of the capsule in phagocytosis of *Cryptococcus neoformans*. *Rev Infect Dis* 1988;10:436–9.
8. Lewis JI, Rabinowich SH. The wide spectrum of cryptococcal infections. *Am J Med* 1972;43:315–22.
9. Littman ML, Zimmerman LE. *Cryptococcosis: torulosis or European blastomycosis,* New York: Grune & Stratton, 1956.
10. Littman ML, Walter JE. Cryptococcosis: current status. *Am J Med* 1968;45:922–32.
11. McCullough NB, Louria DB, Hilbish TF, Thomas LB, Emmons C. Cryptococcus: clinical staff conference at the National Institutes of Health. *Ann Intern Med* 1958;49:642–61.
12. Miller GPG. The immunology of cryptococcal disease *Semin Respir Infect* 1986;1:45–52.

13. Mosberg WH Jr, Arnold JG Jr. Torulosis of the central nervous system: review of literature and report of five cases. *Ann Intern Med* 1950;32:1153–83.

14. Murphy JW. Influence of cryptococcal antigens on cell-mediated immunity. *Rev Infect Dis* 1988;10:432–5.

15. Nichols DR, Martin WF. Cryptococcosis: clinical features and differential diagnosis. *Ann Intern Med* 1955;43:767–80.

16. Sheppe W. Torula infection in man. *Am J Med Sci* 1942;167: 91–108.

17. Stoddard JL, Cutler EG. Torula infection in man. *Rockefeller Inst Med Res Monogr* 1916;62:1–98.

18. Campbell CK, Mackenzie DWR. *Cryptococcus neoformans*— pathogen and saprophyte. *Soc Appl Bacteriol Symp Ser* 1980;9: 249–58.

19. Scholer HG. Diagnosis of cryptococcosis and monitoring of chemotherapy. *Mykosen* 1985;28:5–16.

20. CDC. Update: acquired immunodeficiency syndrome—United States. *MMWR* 1986;35:17–21.

21. Heyward WL, Curran JW. The epidemiology of AIDS in the U.S. *Sci Am* 1988;259:72–81.

22. CDC. HIV prevalence estimates and AIDS projections for the United States: report based on a workshop. *MMWR* 1990;39: 1–31.

23. Kwon-Chung KJ. A new genus, *Filobasidiella*, the perfect state of *Cryptococcus neoformans*. *Mycologia* 1975;67:1197–2000.

24. Kwon-Chung KJ. A new species of *Filobasidiella*, the sexual state of *Cryptococcus neoformans* B and C serotypes. *Mycologia* 1976;68:942–6.

25. Kwon-Chung KJ, Bennett JE, Theodore TS. *Cryptococcus bacillisporus* sp. nov.: serotype B-C of *Cryptococcus neoformans*. *Am J Epidemiol* 1977;105:582–6.

26. Bennett JE, Kwon-Chung KJ, Howard DH. Epidemiologic differences among serotypes of *Cryptococcus neoformans*. *Am J Epidemiol* 1977;105:582–6.

27. Ellis DH. *Cryptococcus neoformans* var. *gattii* in Australia. *J Clin Microbiol* 1987;25:430–1.

28. Swinne D, Nkurikiyinfura JB, Muyembe T. Clinical isolates of *Cryptococcus neoformans* from Zaire. *Eur J Clin Microbiol* 1986;5:50–1.

29. Ellis DH, Pfeiffer TJ. Natural habitat of *Cryptococcus neoformans* var. *gattii*. *J Clin Microbiol* 1990;28:1642–4.

30. Rinaldi MG, Drutz DJ, Howell A, Sande MA, Hadley WK. Serotypes of *Cryptococcus neoformans* in patients with AIDS [Letter]. *J Infect Dis* 1986;153:642.

31. Shimizu RY, Howard DH, Clancy MN. The variety of *Cryptococcus neoformans* in patients with AIDS [Letter]. *J Infect Dis* 1986;154:1042.

32. Salkin IF, Hurd NJ. New medium for differentiation of *Cryptococcus neoformans* serotype pairs. *J Clin Microbiol* 1982;15: 169–71.

33. Bottone EJ, Salkin IF, Hurd NJ, Wormser GP. Serogroup distribution of *Cryptococcus neoformans* in patients with AIDS [Letter]. *J Infect Dis* 1987;156:242.

34. Kapend'a K, Komichelo K, Swinne D, Vandepitte J. Meningitis due to *Cryptococcus neoformans* biovar *gattii* in a Zairean AIDS patient. *Eur J Clin Microbiol* 1987;6:320–1.

34a. Kwon-Chung KJ, Varma A. *Cryptococcus neoformans*—ecology and epidemiology. In: *3rd symposium on topics in mycology; mycosis in AIDS patients.* Paris: Pasteur Institute, November 1989;55–56 (abst).

35. Swinne D, Mulumba M, Alilou M. Pathogénicité comparée de souches de *Cryptococcus neoformans* var. *neoformans* Belges et Africaines d'origine saprophytique. *Bull Soc Fran Mycol Med* 1985;14:231–4.

36. Diamond RD. *Cryptococcus neoformans.* In: Mandell GI, Douglas RG Jr, eds. *Principles and practice of infectious disease.* New York: John Wiley & Sons, 1985;1460–8.

37. Bottone EJ, Kirschner PA, Salkin IF. Isolation of highly encapsulated *Cryptococcus neoformans* serotype B from a patient in New York City. *J Clin Microbiol* 1986;23:186–8.

38. Cruickshank JG, Cavil R, Jelbert M. *Cryptococcus neoformans* of unusual morphology. *Appl Microbiol* 1973;25:309–12.

39. Farhi F, Bulmer GS, Tacker JR. *Cryptococcus neoformans* IV. The not-so-encapsulated yeast. *Infect Immun* 1970;1:526–31.

40. Ruiz A, Fromtling RA, Bulmer GS. Distribution of *Cryptococcus neoformans* in a natural state. *Infect Immun* 1981;31:560–3.

41. Levinson DJ, Slicox DC, Rippon JW, Thomsen S. Septic arthritis due to nonencapsulated *Cryptococcus neoformans* with coexisting sarcoidosis. *Arthritis Rheum* 1974;17:1037–47.

42. Bhattacharjee AK, Bennett JE, Glaudemans CPS. Capsular polysaccharides of *Cryptococcus neoformans*. *Rev Infect Dis* 1984;6: 619–24.

43. McGaw TG, Kozel TR. Opsonization of *Cryptococcus neoformans* by human immunoglobulin G: masking of immunoglobulin G by cryptococcal polysaccharide. *Infect Immun* 1979;25: 262–7.

44. Mitchell TG, Friedman L. In vitro phagocytosis and intracellular fate of variously encapsulated strains of *Cryptococcus neoformans*. *Infect Immun* 1972;5:491–8.

45. Bulmer GS, Sans MD. *Cryptococcus neoformans* II. Phagocytosis by human leukocytes. *J Bacteriol* 1967;94:1480–3.

46. Diamond R, Root RK, Bennett JE. Factors influencing killing of *Cryptococcus neoformans* by human leukocytes in vitro. *J Infect Dis* 1972;125:367–76.

47. Bulmer GS, Sans MD. *Cryptococcus neoformans.* III. Inhibition of phagocytosis. *J Bacteriol* 1968;95:5–8.

48. Kozel TR. Non-encapsulated variant of *Cryptococcus neoformans.* II. Surface receptors for cryptococcal polysaccharide and their role in inhibition of phagocytosis by polysaccharide. *Infect Immun* 1977;16:99–106.

49. Ikeda R, Shinoda T, Kagaya K, Fukazawa Y. Role of serum factors in the phagocytosis of weakly or heavily encapsulated *Cryptococcus neoformans* strains by guinea pig peripheral blood leukocytes. *Microbiol Immunol* 1984;28:51–61.

50. Kozel TR, Pfrommer GST, Guerlain AS, Highison BA, Highison GJ. Strain variations in phagocytosis of *Cryptococcus neoformans:* dissociation of susceptibility to phagocytosis from activation and binding of opsonic fragments of C3. *Infect Immun* 1988;56:2794–800.

51. Bottone EJ, Toma M, Johansson BE, Wormser GP. Capsule-deficient *Cryptococcus neoformans* in AIDS patients [Letter]. *Lancet* 1985;1:400.

52. Bottone EJ, Toma M, Johansson BE, Wormser GP. Poorly encapsulated *Cryptococcus neoformans* from patients with AIDS. I. Preliminary observations. *AIDS Res* 1986;2:211–8.

53. Gal AA, Evans S, Meyer PR. The clinical laboratory evaluation of cryptococcal infections in the acquired immunodeficiency syndrome. *Diagn Microbiol Infect Dis* 1987;7:249–54.

54. Mackenzie DWR, Hay RJ. Capsule-deficient *Cryptococcus neoformans* in AIDS patients [Letter]. *Lancet* 1985;1:642.

55. Fromtling RA, Bulmer GS. Capsule-deficient *Cryptococcus neoformans* in AIDS patients [Letter]. *Lancet* 1985;1:988.

56. Benbow EW, Stoddart RW. Capsule-deficient *Cryptococcus neoformans* in AIDS patients [Letter]. *Lancet* 1985;1:988.

57. Benn J, Monro PS, Duncan G. Capsule-deficient *Cryptococcus neoformans* in AIDS patients [Letter]. *Lancet* 1985;1:989.

58. Bottone EJ, Wormser GP. Capsule-deficient cryptococci in AIDS [Letter]. *Lancet* 1985;2:553.

59. Bottone EJ, Wormser GP. Poorly encapsulated *Cryptococcus neoformans* from patients with AIDS. II: Correlation of capsule size observed directly in cerebrospinal fluid with that after animal passage. *AIDS Res* 1986;2:219–25.

60. Neilson JB, Fromtling RA, Bulmer GS. *Cryptococcus neoformans:* size range of infectious particles from aerosolized soil. *Infect Immun* 1977;17:634–8.

61. Powell KE, Dahl BA, Weeks RJ, Tosh FE. Airborne *Cryptococcus neoformans:* particles from pigeon excreta compatible with alveolar deposition. *J Infect Dis* 1972;125:412–5.

62. Kozel TR, Gotschlich EC. The capsule of *Cryptococcus neoformans* passively inhibits phagocytosis of the yeast by macrophages. 1982;129:1675–80.

63. Dykstra MA, Friedman L, Murphy JW. Capsule size of *Cryptococcus neoformans:* control and relationship to virulence. *Infect Immun* 1977;16:129–35.

64. Poon M, Cronin DC II, Smith DA, Stoneburner R, Bottone EJ. Interscience Conference of Antimicrobial Agents and Chemotherapy, New York, 1987.

65. Horsburgh CR, Selik RM. Interscience Conference on Antimicrobial Agents and Chemotherapy, Los Angeles, 1988.

66. Kovacs JA, Kovacs AA, Polis M, et al. Cryptococcosis in the acquired immunodeficiency syndrome. *Ann Intern Med* 1985; 103:533–8.

67. Zuger A, Louie E, Holzman RS, Simberkoff MS, Rahal JJ. Cryptococcal disease in patients with the acquired immunodeficiency syndrome. *Ann Intern Med* 1986;104:234–40.

68. Glasgow BJ, Steinsapir KD, Anders K, Layfield LJ. Adrenal pathology in the acquired immunodeficiency syndrome. *Am J Clin Pathol* 1985;84:497–594.

69. Pass HI, Macher AM, Shelhammer JH, et al. Thoracic manifestations of the acquired immunodeficiency syndrome. *J Thorac Cardiovasc Surg* 1984;88:654–8.

70. Reichert CM, O'Leary TJ, Levens DL, Simrell CR, Macher AM. Autopsy pathology in the acquired immunodeficiency syndrome. *Am J Pathol* 1982;112:357–82.

71. Welch K, Finkbeiner W, Aplers CE, et al. Autopsy findings in the acquired immunodeficiency syndrome. *JAMA* 1984;252:1152–9.

72. Murray JF, Felton CP, Garay SM, et al. Pulmonary complications of the acquired immunodeficiency syndrome. *N Engl J Med* 1984;310:1682–8.

73. Miller WT Jr, Edelman JR, Miller WT. Cryptococcal pulmonary infection in patients with AIDS: radiographic appearance. *Radiology* 1990;175:725–8.

74. Torres RA. Cryptococcal mediastinitis mimicking lymphoma in the acquired immune deficiency syndrome. *Am J Med* 1987;83:1004–5.

75. Newman TG, Soni A, Acaron S, Huang CT. Pleural cryptococcosis in the acquired immune deficiency syndrome. *Chest* 1987;91:459–61.

76. Wasser L, Talavera W. Pulmonary cryptococcosis in AIDS. *Chest* 1987;92:692–5.

77. Katz AS, Niesenbaum L, Mass B. Pleural effusion as the initial manifestation of disseminated cryptococcosis in acquired immune deficiency syndrome. Diagnosis by pleural biopsy. *Chest* 1989;96:440–1.

77a. Murray RJ, Becker PK, Furth P, Criner GJ. Recovery form cryptococcemia and the adult respiratory distress syndrome in the acquired immunodeficiency syndrome. *Chest* 1988;93:1304–6.

78. Kerkering TM, Duma RJ, Shadomy S. The evolution of pulmonary cryptococcosis: clinical implications from a study of 41 patients with and without compromising host factors. *Ann Intern Med* 1981;94:611–6.

79. Borton LK, Wintroub BU. Disseminated cryptococcosis presenting as herpetiform lesions in a homosexual man with the acquired immunodeficiency syndrome. *J Am Acad Dermatol* 1984; 10:387–90.

80. Chu AD, Hay RG, MacDonald DM. Cutaneous cryptococcosis. *Br J Dermatol* 1980;121:901–2.

81. Concus AP, Helfand RA, Imber MJ, Lerner EA, Sharpe RJ. Cutaneous cryptococcus mimicking molluscum contagiosum in a patient with AIDS. *J Infect Dis* 1988;158:897–8.

82. Rico MJ, Penneys NS. Cutaneous cryptococcosis resembling molluscum contagiosum in a patient with AIDS. *Arch Dermatol* 1985;121:901–2.

83. Sofman MS, Heilman ER. Simultaneous occurrence of Kaposi's sarcoma and cryptococcus within a cutaneous lesion in a patient with acquired immunodeficiency syndrome. *Arch Dermatol* 1990;16:683–4.

84. Glick M, Cohen SG, Cheney RT, Crooks GW, Greenberg MS. Oral manifestations of disseminated *Cryptococcus neoformans* in a patient with acquired immunodeficiency syndrome. *Arch Dermatol* 1990;16:683–4.

85. Van Calck M, Motte S, Rickaert F, Serruys E, Alder M, Wybran J. Cryptococcal anal ulceration in a patient with AIDS. *Am J Gastroenterol* 1988;83:1306–8.

86. Cammarosano C, Lewis W. Cardiac lesions in acquired immune deficiency syndrome (AIDS). *J Am Coll Cardiol* 1985;5:703–6.

87. Schuster M, Valentine F, Holzman R. Cryptococcal pericarditis in an intravenous drug abuser [Letter]. *J Infect Dis* 1985;152:842.

88. Larsen RA, Bozzette S, McCutchan JA, et al. Persistent *Cryptococcus neoformans* infection of the prostate after successful treatment of meningitis. *Ann Intern Med* 1989;111:125–8.

89. Lief M, Sarfarazi J. Prostatic cryptococcosis in acquired immune deficiency syndrome. *Urology* 1986;28:318–9.

90. Staib F, Seibold M, L'age M, et al. *Cryptococcus neoformans* in the seminal fluid of an AIDS patient. A contribution to the clinical course of cryptococcosis. *Mycoses* 1989;32:171–80.

91. Lipson BK, Freeman WR, Beniz J, et al. Optic neuropathy associated with cryptococcal arachnoiditis in AIDS patients. *Am J Opthalmol* 1989;107:523–7.

92. Carney MD, Combs JL, Waschler W. Cryptococcal choroiditis. *Retina* 1990;10:27–32.

93. Kida M, Abramowsky CR, Santoscoy C. Cryptococcosis of the placenta in a woman with acquired immunodeficiency syndrome. *Hum Pathol* 1989;20:920–1.

94. Scalfano FP Jr, Prichard JG, Lamki N, Athey PA, Graves RC. Abdominal cryptococcoma in AIDS: a case report. *J Comput Tomogr* 1988;12:237–9.

95. Machac J, Nejatheim M, Goldsmith SJ. Gallium-67 citrate uptake in cryptococcal thyroiditis in a homosexual male. *J Nucl Med Allied Sci* 1985;29:283–5.

96. Diamond RD, Bennett JE. Prognostic factors in cryptococcal meningitis: a study of 111 cases. *Ann Intern Med* 1974;80: 176–81.

97. Bottone EJ. *Cryptococcus neoformans:* pitfalls in diagnosis through evaluation of gram-stained smears of purulent exudates. *J Clin Microbiol* 1980;12:790–1.

98. Chuck SL, Sande MA. Infection with *Cryptococcus neoformans* in the acquired immunodeficiency syndrome. *N Engl J Med* 1989;321:794–9.

99. Goodman JS, Kaufman L, Loening LM. Diagnosis of cryptococcal meningitis: value of immunologic detection of cryptococcal antigen. *N Engl J Med* 1971;285:434–6.

99a. Post MJD, Kursunoglu SJ, Hensley GT, Chan JC, Moskowitz LB, Hoffman TA. Cranial CT in acquired immunodeficiency syndrome: spectrum of diseases and optimal contrast enhancement technique. *AJR* 1985;145:929–49.

100. Whelan AM, Kricheff II, Handler M, et al. Acquired immunodeficiency syndrome: cerebral computed tomographic manifestations. *Radiology* 1983;149:477–84.

101. Kelly WM, Brant-Zawadski M. Acquired immunodeficiency syndrome: neuroradiologic findings. *Radiology* 1983;149: 484–91.

102. Levy RM, Bredesen DE, Rosenblum ML. Neurological manifestations of the acquired immunodeficiency syndrome (AIDS): experience at UCSF and review of the literature. *J Neurosurg* 1985;62:475–95.

103. Wilson JW, Plunkett OA. Cryptococcosis. In: *The fungus diseases of man.* Berkeley: University of California Press, 1965;111–29.

104. Ro JY, Lee SS, Ayala AG. Advantage of Fontana-Masson stain in capsule-deficient cryptococcal infection. *Arch Pathol Lab Med* 1987;111:53–7.

105. Loerinc AM, Bottone EJ, Finkel LJ, Teirstein AS. Primary cryptococcal pneumonia mimicking *Pneumocystis carinii* pneumonia in a patient with AIDS. *Mt Sinai J Med (NY)* 1988;56:181–6.

106. Poon M, Cronin DC II, Wormser GP, Bottone EJ. In vitro susceptibility of *Cryptococcus neoformans* isolates from patients with acquired immunodeficiency syndrome. *Arch Pathol Lab Med* 1988;112:161–2.

107. Shadomy S, Espinel-Ingroff A, Cartwright RF. Laboratory studies with antifungal agents: susceptibility tests and bioassays. In: Lennette EH, Balows A, Hausler WJ Jr, Shadomy HJ, eds. Manual of clinical microbiology, 4th ed. Washington, DC: American Society for Microbiology, 1985;991–9.

108. Shadomy HJ, Wood-Helie S, Shadomy S, Dismukes WE, Chan RY. Biochemical serogrouping of clinical isolates of *Cryptococcus neoformans*. *Diagn Microbiol Infect Dis* 1987;6:131–8.

109. Fromtling RA, Abruzzo LR, Bulmer GS. *Cryptococcus neoformans:* comparison of in vitro antifungal susceptibilities of serotype AD and BC. *Mycopathologica* 1986;94:27–30.

110. Utz JP, Garriques IL, Sande MA, et al. Therapy of cryptococcosis with a combination of flucytosine and amphotericin B. *J Infect Dis* 1975;13:368–73.

111. Bennett JE, Dismukes WE, Duma RJ, et al. A comparison of amphotericin B alone and combined with flucytosine in the treat-

ment of cryptococcal meningitis. *N Engl J Med* 1979;301:
126–31.

112. Dismukes WE, Cloud G, Gallis HA, et al. Treatment of cryptococcal meningitis with combination amphotericin B and flucytosine for four as compared with six weeks. *N Engl J Med*
1987;317:334–41.

113. Diamond RD, Bennett JE. A subcutaneous reservoir for intrathecal therapy of fungal meningitis. *N Engl J Med* 1973;288:186–8.

114. Polsky B, Depman MR, Gold JWM, Galicich JH, Armstrong D.
Intraventricular therapy of cryptococcal meningitis via a subcutaneous reservoir. *Am J Med* 1986;81:24–8.

115. Kauffman CA, Frame PT. Bone marrow toxicity associated with
5-flucytosine therapy. *Antimicrob Agents Chemother* 1977;11:
244–7.

116. Weinstein L, Jacoby I. Successful treatment of cerebral cryptococcoma and meningitis with miconazole. *Ann Intern Med*
1980;93:569–71.

117. Graybill JR, Levine HB. Successful treatment of cryptococcal
meningitis with intraventricular miconazole. *Arch Intern Med*
1978;138:814–6.

118. Bennett JE, Remington JS. Miconazole in cryptococcosis and
systemic candidiasis: a word of caution. *Ann Intern Med*
1981;94:708–9.

119. Kerkering TA, Kaplowitz LG, Cloud G, Bowles C, Shadomy S.
Treatment of systemic mycoses with ketoconazole: emphasis on
toxicity and clinical response in 52 patients: National Institute of
Allergy and Infectious Diseases Collaborative Antifungal Study.
Ann Intern Med 1983;98:13–20.

120. Craven PC, Graybill Jr, Jorgensen JH, Dismukes WE, Levine BE.
High-dose ketoconazole for treatment of fungal infections of the
central nervous system. *Ann Intern Med* 1983;10:160–7.

121. Mes TP, Hadley WK, Wofsy CB. 3rd International Conference
on AIDS, Washington, DC, June, 1987.

122. Perfect JR, Durack DT, Hamilton JH, Gallis HA. Failure of ketoconazole in cryptococcal meningitis. *JAMA* 1982;247:3349–51.

123. Perfect JR, Savani DV, Durack DT. Comparison of itraconazole
and fluconazole in treatment of cryptococcal meningitis and candida pyelonephritis in rabbits. *Antimicrob Agents Chemother*
1986;29:579–83.

124. Dupont B, Drouhet E. Cryptococcal meningitis and fluconazole
[Letter]. *Ann Intern Med* 1987;106:778.

125. Palou de Fernandez E, Patino MM, Graybill JR, Tarbit MH.
Treatment of cryptococcal meningitis in mice with fluconazole. *J
Antimicrob Chemother* 1986;18:261–70.

126. Van Cutsem J, Van Gerven F, Janssen PAJ. Activity of orally,
topically, and parenterally administered itraconazole in the treatment of superficial and deep mycoses: animal models. *Rev Infect
Dis* 1987;9:S15–S32.

127. Perfect JR, Durack DT. Penetration of imidazoles and triazoles
into cerebrospinal fluid of rabbits. *J Antimicrob Chemother*
1985;16:81–6.

128. Arndt CAS, Walsh TJ, McCully CI, Balis FM, Pizzo PA, Poplack
DG. Fluconazole penetration into cerebrospinal fluid: implica-
tions for treating fungal infections of the central nervous system.
J Infect Dis 1988;157:178–80.

129. Stern JJ, Hartman BJ, Sharkey P, et al. Oral fluconazole therapy
for patients with acquired immunodeficiency syndrome and
cryptococcosis: experience with 22 patients. *Am J Med*
1988;85:477–80.

130. Larsen RA, Leal MAE, Chan LS. Fluconazole compared with
amphotericin B plus flucytosine for cryptococcal meningitis in
AIDS. A randomized trial. *Ann Intern Med* 1990;113:183–7.

131. Galgiani JN. Fluconazole, a new antifungal agent. *Ann Intern
Med* 1990;113:177–9.

132. Viviani MA, Tortorano AM, Giani PC, et al. Itraconazole for
cryptococcal infection in the acquired immunodeficiency syndrome [Letter]. *Ann Intern Med* 1987;106:166.

133. Denning DW, Tucker RM, Hanson LH, Hamilton JR, Stevens
DA. Itraconazole therapy for cryptococcal meningitis and cryptococcosis. *Arch Intern Med* 1989;149:2301–8.

134. Zuger A, Schuster M, Simberkoff MS, Rahal JJ, Holzman RS.
Maintenance amphotericin B for cryptococcal meningitis in the
acquired immunodeficiency syndrome (AIDS). *Ann Intern Med*
1988;109:592–3.

135. Sugar AM, Saunders C. Oral fluconazole as suppressive therapy
of disseminated cryptococcosis in patients with acquired immunodeficiency syndrome. *Am J Med* 1988;85:481–9.

136. Bozette SA, Larsen RA, Chiu J, et al. A placebo-controlled trial of
maintenance therapy with fluconazole after treatment of cryptococcal meningitis in the acquired immunodeficiency syndrome.
N Engl J Med 1991;324:580–4.

137. Penneys NS. *Skin manifestations of AIDS.* London: Martin Dun-
itz Ltd, 1990.

*AIDS and Other Manifestations of HIV Infection,
Second Edition,* Edited by Gary P. Wormser.
Raven Press, Ltd., New York © 1992.

CHAPTER 25

Progressive Multifocal Leukoencephalopathy and HIV-1 Infection

Lauren B. Krupp, Anita L. Belman, and Paul S. Shneidman

Progressive multifocal leukoencephalopathy (PML) is a rare but devastating demyelinating disease of the brain associated with papovavirus infection. The target of this opportunistic viral infection is the oligodendrocyte, the myelin-producing cell of the central nervous system (CNS). Infection results in cellular dysfunction, cytopathic changes, and ultimately cell death. The clinical syndrome that results is one of progressive neurologic deterioration, usually fatal within 6 months.

PML was first described in 1958 (1). Initially it was recognized in patients with lymphoproliferative disorders. Subsequently it has been reported in patients with sarcoidosis, tuberculosis, neoplasms, other immunosuppressive conditions including chronic steroid therapy (2–4), and more recently in patients with HIV-1 infection and AIDS (5–13). Since the onset of the AIDS epidemic increasing numbers of patients with HIV-1 disease and coincidental PML have been identified; a 3–7% incidence in AIDS is estimated from clinical and pathological series (14–23). New manifestations of the illness have been recognized (24), the spectrum of radiographic findings has widened (25–27), and a greater understanding of its pathogenesis is emerging (28).

In this chapter we describe the neurological, neuroimaging, and neuropathological features of PML and review the clinical findings in 50 patients with coexisting PML and HIV-1 infection. Recent data pertaining to the molecular and biologic properties of JC virus (JCV), the etiologic agent of PML, and new approaches to therapy for this disease are also discussed.

L. B. Krupp and A. L. Belman: Department of Neurology, State University of New York at Stony Brook, Stony Brook, New York 11794.

P. S. Shneidman: Department of Neuropathology, University of Pennsylvania School of Medicine, Philadelphia, Pennsylvania 10904.

PML AND PAPOVAVIRUS

The viral etiology of PML was suggested in 1965 when ultrastructural studies of brain tissue from patients with PML revealed crystalline arrays of particles within oligodendrocytes that were identical in size and morphology to papovavirus (29). Initial attempts to recover virus by conventional techniques were unsuccessful. It was not until 1971 that viruses of the papovavirus group were isolated from brain extracts of patients with PML. The virus was named JC, after the initials of the first patient from whom it was recovered (30). (In retrospect this terminology was a poor choice, as it has frequently caused confusion with the unrelated Jakob-Creutzfeld disease). Shortly thereafter another papovavirus, simian virus 40 (SV40), was isolated from the brains of two other patients (31). However, while JCV has subsequently been isolated from numerous patients with PML, SV40 has been identified only in the two patients described above (4,32).

Compelling evidence from various investigations has established that PML is caused by JCV infection of the CNS. These data include identification of viral particles within oligodendrocytes by electron microscopic studies of brains of patients with PML (4), localization of viral antigen by immunohistochemical techniques (33), demonstration of nucleotide sequences by in situ hybridization (33,34), amplification of JCV DNA sequences by the polymerase chain reaction (PCR) (35,36), and recovery of virus from the brain of numerous affected patients (32,37).

BIOLOGICAL AND MOLECULAR PROPERTIES OF JC VIRUS

At least two issues involving the biology of JCV are crucial to understanding the clinical syndrome caused by this virus. First, how does the virus establish dormancy or latency only to escape this state after immunosuppression? Second, what is the basis for the tropism for oligodendroglia?

The human population is the natural reservoir for JCV (4). Infection by JCV is ubiquitous, and greater than 75% of the U.S. population has been exposed to the virus by middle adulthood (4). However, PML is the only recognized clinical syndrome associated with the virus. The tissue in which viral replication occurs is not well defined. The kidney is one possible site of latency, since the virus has been recovered occasionally from the urine of immunocompetent people and pregnant women (4). JCV infects and replicates in vitro at low efficiency in human uroepithelial cells as well as a few other human cell types (38). However, it grows efficiently in vitro only in human fetal glial cells (38). Therefore, it remains unclear exactly where the virus lies dormant.

Recent work has provided a possible explanation for how JCV may gain access to the brain. Houff and colleagues (28) studied two patients with PML and found JCV antigens and nucleic acid in mononuclear cells and B lymphocytes in the bone marrow. They also found JCV nucleic acid and antigen in the kidney and spleen of one patient. The authors hypothesized that B cells and other mononuclear cells can under certain conditions harbor JCV and, after reactivation of the virus, could carry JCV to the brain.

Molecular biological experiments have attempted to explain why JCV is so specific for glial cells (the class of cell to which oligodendroglia belong) (39–45). A number of studies have compared JCV with SV40, a papovavirus that is less restricted in its host range. The structure of JCV is closely related to SV40, and the viruses share a 69% homology on a DNA sequence level (42,43). Both contain small circular double-stranded DNA genomes of about 5,000 base pairs that code for six proteins. The large T antigen (or T protein) is an essential replication factor, and is expressed early in infection, prior to DNA replication. The other viral products are capsid and structural proteins and are expressed late, after the onset of DNA replication. The early and late transcription units are transcribed from divergently oriented promoters at either end of an intergenic regulatory region. This region contains DNA sequences that augment transcription (enhancers), as well as sequences that act in concert with the T protein, as an origin of DNA replication. The sequences of SV40 and JCV differ most in their respective enhancer regions.

Despite many shared structural characteristics between the two viruses, certain molecular biologic properties may explain why JCV can productively infect only primary human fetal glial cells, whereas SV40 infects many human and simian primary and tissue culture cells. Transgenic mice containing the early promoter and the T-antigen gene of JCV express T antigen only in oligodendroglia, astrocytes, or embryonic neural crest. Transgenic mice containing the analogous portions of the SV40 genome show a more widespread tissue and cell-type expression of the SV40 T antigen (40). Gene transfer experiments have demonstrated that JCV early and late promoters are active only in glial cell lines. In contrast, the analogous promoter sequences of SV40 are active in many differentiated cell lines (38,41,45).

Investigators have also examined the respective T proteins of the two viruses (46). In terms of DNA replication, the JCV T protein binds less well to either the SV40 or JCV replication origin as compared with the binding of SV40 T protein (43). Furthermore, even after binding, JCV T antigen probably interacts less efficiently than SV40 T antigen with the other cellular replication elements (43).

Another possible explanation for the selectivity of JCV may lie in its enhancer region. Most of the DNA sequences in the 98-base pair enhancer region of JCV act to increase transcription in glial cells, but some may act to decrease transcription in nonglial cells (45). Biochemical studies show that multiple site-specific DNA binding factors interact with this region (47), and it is probably through a combination of positively and negatively acting transcription factors targeted to this area that the virus is able to display its cell-type-restricted transcriptional activity.

NEUROLOGIC PRESENTATION AND COURSE

Neurologic dysfunction begins insidiously. The most frequent early signs and symptoms include mental status changes (personality change, disturbance of memory and language), weakness, and sensory loss. Aphasia, dysarthria, and headache may also occur as initial manifestations. Approximately 10% of patients present with coordination difficulties, poor balance, or other manifestations of cerebellar or brainstem involvement. In a review of 230 pathologically confirmed cases of PML in patients with a variety of immunosuppressive disorders, initial findings consisted of mental dysfunction (36%), visual field deficits (35%), and mono- or hemiparesis (33%). Seizures were uncommon as a presenting manifestation (6%) (48). Although neurologic dysfunction begins insidiously, it is usually relentlessly progressive and fatal. Over 80% of patients are dead by 8 months (48). However, it is noteworthy that there have been rare reports of patients, often with transient or mild immunodeficiencies, that have survived for 10 years (49) or longer (4).

NEUROIMAGING FINDINGS

Neuroimaging plays a central role in the evaluation of patients with HIV-1 infection who develop signs and symptoms of neurologic dysfunction (50–63). However, it must be kept in mind that although neuroimaging may suggest PML, histologic confirmation is required for definitive diagnosis, as well as to exclude other treatable conditions.

Computerized Tomography

The characteristic findings of PML on computerized tomography (CT) examination of the head are discrete regions of decreased attenuation confined to the white matter. These lesions demonstrate no mass effect, do not enhance after injection of contrast material, and their location bears no relationship to the vascular distribution or to the ventricular system (54–57) (Fig. 1). Early in the disease, the CT may be normal or show only a small hypodense area. As the disease progresses, the areas enlarge, often extending to the subcortical gray–white junction, and assume a scalloped appearance. Similar lesions may appear in the cerebellum (58,59). There are exceptions to this pattern, and both contrast enhancement (26) and mild mass effect may occur.

Early in the course of PML the clinical signs may indicate more extensive disease than is visualized on CT scan, or so-called CT-clinical dissociation (57). The CT lesions progressively enlarge over time but may lag behind the clinical evolution.

Magnetic Resonance Imaging

Magnetic resonance imaging (MRI) has become the neuroimaging procedure of choice in the evaluation of a patient with suspected PML. Due to its increased sensitivity, MRI can detect focal lesions in the white matter that are either missed on CT or are underestimated in size by CT (25,52,53,60). In addition, MRI may show lesions prior to the development of clinical signs and symptoms.

On T2-weighted images, the typical MRI features of PML include focal or multifocal asymmetric areas of increased signal, located predominantly in the white matter, that may or may not be confluent. They usually assume a scalloped appearance and spare the gray matter. Typically there is little to no mass effect (Fig. 2). The most common site of involvement is the parietal–occipital region. In a recent MRI study of patients with PML and HIV-1 infection, the parietal lobe was most commonly affected, followed by the occipital, frontal, and temporal lobes (25). Lesions may also be seen in the basal ganglia, cerebellum, brainstem, and corpus callosum.

Angiography

Angiography is less useful than CT or MRI in the diagnostic evaluation of PML. Abnormal patterns described

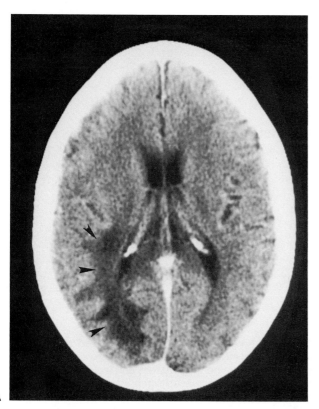

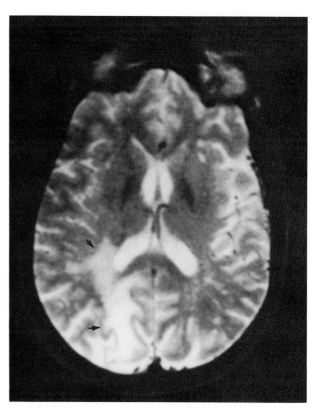

A

B

FIG. 1. A: Axial CT after administration of contrast material demonstrates a nonenhancing lucency involving the parietal–occipital white matter with undulated margins (*arrowheads*). **B:** Axial MRI long TR/TE (2,040/80) through the same area shows hyperintensity in the white matter lesion. PML was confirmed at postmortem examination.

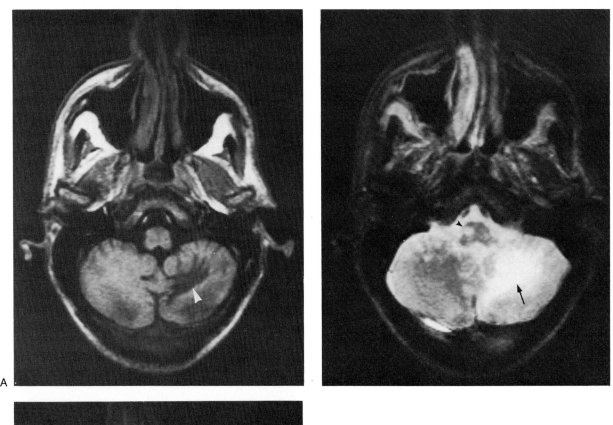

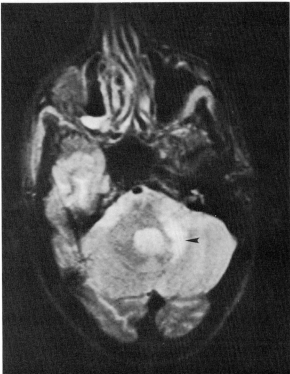

FIG. 2. A: The short TR/TE (600/200) image of a 27-year-old homosexual man, who presented with coordination and gait difficulty, shows an area of decreased signal intensity involving the left cerebellar white matter. The lesion has a typical scalloped appearance, spares the gray matter, and lacks mass effect. **B:** Long TR/TE images (1,966/100) of the same patient shows increased signal intensity in the lesion. An additional smaller hyperintense lesion is seen on the right side of the medulla. This is not seen on the short TR/TE (600/20) image (Fig. 2A). Note the lack of mass effect. **C:** At a higher level an area of increased signal on the long TR/TE (1,966/100) image is present in the middle cerebellar peduncle. PML was confirmed at postmortem examination.

include avascular zones (54); dilation of medullary veins, small arteries, or arterioles; or faint vascular blush (57). Rarely, a mild mass effect with stretching and separation of arterial branches occurs (61). More commonly, however, the angiogram is normal.

NEUROPHYSIOLOGICAL FINDINGS

Clinical neurophysiological studies are often abnormal in patients with PML but the findings are usually nonspecific (62). At times, the electroencephalograph (EEG) may be positive before CT findings appear, but normal EEGs in the setting of abnormalities on MRI may also be observed (6). Abnormal findings include focal polymorphic slowing in the theta or delta frequencies, or diffuse slowing such as disruption of the background activity (62). Focal polymorphic slowing probably reflects destructive lesions in the hemispheric white matter due to PML. However, background slowing is nonspecific and may occur in AIDS–dementia complex, many metabolic derangements, and systemic diseases.

When PML involves the posterior fossa, the EEG is usually normal. However, brainstem auditory evoked potentials may detect posterior fossa involvement in PML (58), even when the CT shows only limited findings. Despite this application of evoked potentials, MRI is more useful in the evaluation of posterior fossa pathology.

CEREBROSPINAL FLUID FINDINGS

Cerebrospinal fluid (CSF) analyses are usually normal or reveal only mild elevation in protein content. Hypoglycorrhachia or CSF pleocytosis suggests a process other than PML, or an additional process, and warrants further evaluation.

PATHOLOGY

Gross inspection of the brain from PML patients reveals foci of demyelination ranging from pinhead-sized lesions to extensive areas of leukomalacia. The variation in size and the frequent finding of small foci adjacent to larger ones suggest that, as the disease advances, small lesions coalesce to form larger demyelinated areas. The cerebral hemispheres are generally more affected than the cerebellum or brainstem, but in some cases this distribution is reversed. The histopathologic features are distinctive and characteristic. The most striking finding is the presence of oligodendrocytes containing nuclei two to three times their normal size. With hematoxylin and eosin staining, these cells have a dense and often glassy appearance. The swollen infected oligodendrocytes surround demyelinated zones and contain abundant viral particles (2,3,37).

Morphological studies (63) suggest that following adsorption and penetration, the virus enters the cell nucleus and initiates viral assembly. As production of viral progeny proceeds, the cell's cytoplasm becomes increasingly vacuolated. The ribosomes disappear and mitochondria swell; eventually the nuclear membrane disintegrates, the cell undergoes cytolysis, and virions are released to infect nearby cells.

One of the earliest findings of PML in affected brains is glial cells staining positive for T antigen, the JC regulatory protein whose synthesis occurs early in viral transcription. Since it is a regulatory and not a structural protein, it is not found in the final virion (64–66). Glial cells staining for T antigen can be found in clusters in normal tissue and along the leading edge of an advancing lesion (64). They are somewhat less frequent in more advanced areas of infection. In these more advanced areas the large infected oligodendrocytes stain positively for the viral capsid antigen. The disassociation in the appearance of early and late viral proteins suggests a relatively indolent pace to the infection (64).

In early stages of infection, there is a normal amount of myelin basic protein (MBP) and myelin-associated glycoprotein (MAG). In more advanced areas where large swollen oligodendrocytes containing virus occur, MAG begins to disappear. Since MAG is synthesized in the oligodendrocyte perikaryon, its loss reflects viral spread into oligodendroglia cytoplasm and processes (67). The relative distribution of MAP and MBP helps distinguish PML from other demyelinating conditions such as multiple sclerosis and acute measles encephalitis (68).

As oligodendroglia continue to degenerate and their myelin sheaths break down, macrophages and giant astrocytes accumulate while oligodendrocytes are lost. Gradually, with disease progression, scattered demyelinated areas enlarge and become confluent. In chronic "burnt-out" lesions, demyelination is complete and oligodendrocytes and viral particles are rarely found. The chronic lesions contain many macrophages and reactive astrocytes. These older lesions often contain another characteristic histopathologic feature of PML—abnormal giant astrocytes with multilobulated, hyperchromatic, and pleomorphic nuclei, which assume a bizarre and often malignant appearance. The appearance of the abnormal astrocytes, coupled with the fact that JCV is known to produce tumors in other species, has led to speculation about JCV's oncogenic potential in man. However, an association between JCV and human glioma has never been demonstrated.

Pathological studies in patients with PML and HIV-1 infection have been compared with patients who have PML associated with other immunodeficiency states, and have provided insight into the respective roles of JCV and HIV-1 in CNS disease (70a,64,69,70). In an autopsy series of ten PML cases with AIDS and ten PML cases with other immunodeficiency states, the demyelination secondary to HIV-1 infection was easily distinguishable from the PML lesions by histopathological criteria (69). However, some minor differences in the areas affected by JCV were noted between AIDS and non-AIDS cases. Autopsy material from AIDS cases showed more numerous and larger areas of demyelination and necrosis. There was also more perivascular mononuclear infiltration of the white matter in brains from AIDS patients. However, in some of the AIDS autopsy specimens, other infections, such as HIV-1-related encephalitis or toxoplasmosis, were also present and may have accounted for the more prominent perivascular infiltration.

Certain features were common to the AIDS and non-AIDS patient groups. The extensive changes of the oligodendrocytes were seen in all brains. Both patient groups on autopsy had some extension of the PML lesions into the gray matter, and JCV capsid antigen and JCV DNA were readily identified in the gray matter. Bizarre astrocytes were noted in both AIDS and non-AIDS PML lesions.

In summary, PML in HIV-1-infected patients shares many pathological characteristics with PML associated with other immunodeficiency states. However, in AIDS patients there is greater white matter destruction from PML than in non-AIDS patients. Although white matter abnormalities other than PML are also present in the brains of AIDS patients (70a,70), they can be distinguished from PML by histopathologic criteria.

CLINICAL FINDINGS IN PML ASSOCIATED WITH HIV-1 INFECTION

In general, the clinical findings of PML in patients with HIV-1 infection are similar to features of PML described in the setting of other immunodeficiency states. However, patients with HIV-1 infection and PML present unique challenges because of the range of possible coexisting CNS infections. Therefore, we reviewed the clinical and neuroimaging findings of 50 patients with PML and HIV-1 infection reported between 1983 and 1990 (5–13,23,24,28,31,44,57–59,64,70–77). There were 46 men and four women, with an average age of 36.8 years (range, 22–58 years). The most frequent risk factors for HIV infection were male homosexuality (64%), intravenous drug use (IVDU) (20%), or both (4%). In the remaining patients, risk factors included heterosexual contact (4%), blood transfusion (2%), or were not stated (6%).

PML was the initial opportunistic infection in 44% of the patients. Conditions that preceded the development of PML in the other patients included *Pneumocystis carinii* pneumonia (22%), oral candidiasis (8%), Kaposi's sarcoma (8%), herpes zoster (6%), varied skin disorders (6%), tuberculosis (6%), cryptococcal infection (4%), cy-

tomegalovirus infection (4%), intestinal infections (4%), multiple unspecified infections (2%), and toxoplasmosis (2%).

The presenting neurologic manifestations are summarized in Table 1. The most common findings were monoparesis or hemiparesis (42%), visual disturbance such as visual field deficits or visual loss (22%), and cognitive impairment (including impaired concentration, confusion, or progressive dementia) (18%).

The average survival after the diagnosis of PML was 4.7 months (range, 1–30 months). Some patients had a rapidly progressive course and died within 1 month of diagnosis. Although uncommon, several patients had prolonged survival and even partial remission (7,71; J. R. Berger, personal communication). One of these patients had an initially deteriorating course but improved following treatment with zidovudine and survived at least 11 months (71). Two patients died 3 years after PML was diagnosed (J. R. Berger, personal communication). A fourth patient is still alive at the time of this writing, 5 years since diagnosis of PML, and has experienced partial remission from PML without specific therapy (J. R. Berger, personal communication). Clinical improvement was associated with a decrease in both the size and number of lesions visualized on neuroimaging studies (7,71).

CT was performed in 47 of the 50 patients reviewed. Twenty-one (44.7%) had a single lesion and 17 (36.2%) had multiple lesions. The majority of CT lesions had the typical radiographic appearance of PML described above. Atypical findings included mild mass effect in two cases, and contrast enhancement in two cases. In nine patients (19.1%), the initial CT scans revealed no lesion. However, a follow-up CT in three patients showed one or more PML lesions, and an MRI was positive in each of the four patients in whom it was performed.

MRI was carried out in 16 of the 50 patients. White matter lesions compatible with PML were identified in all. Twelve patients (75%) had multiple areas of in-

TABLE 1. *Progressive multifocal leukoencephalopathy (PML) in HIV infection: clinical characteristics in 50 patients*

Initial neurologic presentation	No. (%)
Mono- or hemiparesis	21 (42)
Visual deficits	11 (22)
Cognitive deficits	9 (18)
Clumsiness/poor coordination	7 (14)
Dysarthria	8 (16)
Headache	7 (14)
Aphasia	6 (12)
Ataxia	5 (10)
Seizures	4 (8)
Involuntary movements	3 (6)
Stupor	2 (4)

creased signal intensity, while four (25%) had a single focus. Additional findings included a diffuse pattern of white matter involvement (one patient); gray matter involvement (three patients); gadolinium enhancement (one patient); and mild mass effect (one patient).

Similar MRI findings in ten HIV-1 infected patients with pathologically confirmed PML were reported by Mark et al. (25). Unifocal areas of increased signal intensity were found in the white matter in six patients and multifocal lesions in four. Five patients had increased signal intensity in the gray matter in addition to the white matter abnormalities, and one patient had increased signal intensity in the thalamus, globus pallidus, and surrounding subcortical white matter. Another MRI demonstrated significant mass effect, which may have been secondary to hemorrhage into the lesion (25).

EEGs performed in 21 of the 50 patients with PML and HIV-1 infection showed diffuse generalized slowing in ten (50%) and focal slowing in seven (33%). Four patients had normal EEGs.

CSF findings were reported in 38 patients and were abnormal in 15. Abnormalities included mild protein elevation (seven), increased IgG or IgG index (five), oligoclonal bands (two), and mild lymphocytic pleocytosis (three). One patient who had concurrent cryptococcal meningitis had a positive India ink test. In 23 patients the CSF was normal.

Not surprisingly, our review indicates that the clinical features of PML in patients with HIV-1 infection are similar to the manifestations of PML described in association with other causes of immunodeficiency. Most patients will have focal neurologic signs and an abnormal MRI. It is important to note that PML may be the first manifestation of HIV-1 infection.

DIFFERENTIAL DIAGNOSIS

The differential diagnosis of PML in a patient with HIV-1 infection who develops progressive cognitive or motor dysfunction and a focal lesion(s) on neuroimaging studies includes other infectious etiologies (e.g., toxoplasmosis, abscess, mycobacterial or fungal infection), neoplasm (primary or metastatic CNS lymphoma, more rarely, Kaposi's sarcoma), stroke, and AIDS–dementia complex (17,50). In non-AIDS patients who have PML in association with neoplasms, the differential diagnosis additionally includes metastatic disease, or complications of cancer treatment such as methotrexate leukoencephalopathy or CNS radiation necrosis.

Often the clinical examination or history may help in distinguishing PML from the entities mentioned above. PML often presents with focal neurological signs that are usually absent in AIDS–dementia complex. Strokes can be differentiated from PML by their abrupt onset and temporal evolution. However, clinical examination alone may not be sufficient to distinguish PML from other etiologies of multifocal neurologic dysfunction that occur in the setting of HIV infection, such as toxoplasmosis or CNS lymphoma.

Neuroimaging is often helpful in the differential diagnosis. Characteristic CT features of toxoplasmosis include multiple ring lesions that enhance after injection of contrast material, as well as typical lesion location at the cerebral gray–white junction and/or the basal ganglia. There may or may not be mass effect. T2-weighted MRI studies usually show multiple focal areas of abnormal increased signal intensity along the cerebral gray–white junction and/or in basal ganglia (60). The presence of gadolinium enhancement and the location in the gray matter help to distinguish these lesions from PML. Occasionally toxoplasmosis may show a diffuse or punctate MRI pattern, which is not typically described in PML (25,52,60).

CT characteristics of lymphoma are variable and include hyperdense or isodense mass lesions, which may or may not enhance after injection of contrast material; diffusely infiltrating contrast-enhancing lesions; and periventricular contrast-enhancing lesions. Multiple lesions are common. On T2-weighted MRI studies, primary CNS lymphoma usually appears as an area of increased signal intensity often associated with mass effect and surrounding edema in the white matter. The presence of mass effect and enhancement following administration of gadolinium helps to differentiate lymphoma from PML.

Distinguishing PML from other leukoencephalopathies in the HIV-1-infected patient may be more difficult. The most common MRI finding in HIV-1-infected patients is an abnormality of the cerebral white matter. This can be due to a variety of processes including cytomegalovirus (CMV) encephalitis, AIDS–dementia complex, and nonviral infections (52). Identifying the pattern of white matter involvement may help in differential diagnosis (52). For example, the usual pathologic correlate of a "diffuse" pattern of increased signal in the cerebral white matter is primary HIV-1 infection of the brain. In one study correlating the MRI patterns of white matter abnormalities in HIV-1-infected patients with pathological findings at postmortem, 21 of 32 (72%) patients with the diffuse MRI pattern had pathologic findings consistent with AIDS–dementia complex, 4 had CMV encephalitis, and 1 each had toxoplasmosis and cryptococcal meningitis. None of the 32 patients with this diffuse pattern had PML (52).

Abnormalities in the white matter that appear diffuse, patchy, or punctate on T2-weighted MRI are more likely to be due to HIV-1 CNS disease, toxoplasmosis, or CMV encephalitis than to PML. However, focal areas of white matter involvement are consistent with PML. Careful interpretation of the MRI may guide in the differential diagnosis of PML, although definitive diagnosis always requires pathologic confirmation.

DIAGNOSIS

Stereotactic CT or MRI guided biopsies generally provide rapid diagnosis (78). If insufficient tissue is obtained, a repeat stereotactic biopsy or an open biopsy should be considered. In cases of cerebellar involvement, open biopsy is the method of choice. Although stereotactic biopsy may be complicated by small hemorrhages or focal seizures, serious complications rarely occur (78). Diagnostic findings on biopsy are focal demyelination, bizarre-appearing enlarged astrocytes, and swollen oligodendrocytes with inclusions. Further confirmation involves demonstration of virus by electron microscopic examination, immunohistochemistry, in situ hybridization, or PCR. In some laboratories PCR and in situ hybridization have supplemented electron microscopy in providing a rapid diagnosis (36).

TREATMENT

Having established the diagnosis of PML, one is faced with the problem of treatment. Currently, there is no proven therapy for PML. Most published therapeutic attempts have been empiric, uncontrolled, with variable results and no definite benefit (4). Favorable responses for biopsy-proven cases of PML treated with cytarabine (cytosine arabinoside) have occasionally been reported. However, there are numerous cases in which cytarabine has had no benefit (57). Currently, a protocol under Dr. J. Berger, at the University of Miami, investigating the efficacy of α-interferon for treatment of PML in HIV-infected patients is in progress (J. R. Berger, personal communication). The protocol involves high-dose α-interferon and zidovudine (AZT). Patients are treated with AZT 100 mg every four hours, and recombinant α-2a-interferon 18 million units, administered subcutaneously daily. The α-2a interferon is initiated as 1 million units and increased every other day by 2 million units until the total dosage is achieved. Treatment is then continued indefinitely.

To date, 12 patients have been treated with the α-interferon protocol (J. R. Berger, personal communication). Preliminary findings suggest that in patients with very aggressive PML there is no benefit. However, in patients with more gradual deterioration, some improvement in their course has been observed. Several patients have survived in excess of 6 months (J. R. Berger, personal communication). If these preliminary findings can be confirmed in a larger series, there may be a therapeutic option for this otherwise usually progressive and fatal disease.

REFERENCES

1. Astrom KE, Mancall EL, Richardson EP Jr. Progressive multifocal leukoencephalopathy. *Brain* 1958;81:93–111.
2. Richardson EP. Progressive multifocal leukoencephalopathy. *N Engl J Med* 1961;265:815–23.
3. Richardson EP. Progressive multifocal leunoencephalopathy. In: Vinken PJ, Bruyn GW, eds. *Handbook of clinical neurology,* vol 9. Amsterdam: Elsevier Publishers, 1970;489–99.
4. Walker DL. Progressive multifocal leukoencephalopathy. In: Koetsier JC, eds. *Handbook of clinical neurology,* vol 47. New York: Elsevier Publishers, 1985;503–29.
5. Bedri J, Weinstein W, DeGregorio P, et al. Progressive multifocal leukoencephalopathy in acquired immunodeficiency syndrome. *N Engl J Med* 1983;309:492–3.
6. Berger JR, Kasozovitz B, Post JD, Dickinson G. Progressive multifocal leukoencephalopathy associated with human immunodeficiency virus infection. A review of the literature with a report of sixteen cases. *Ann Intern Med* 1987;107:78–87.
7. Berger JR, Mucke L. Prolonged survival and partial recovery in AIDS-associated progressive multifocal leukoencephalopathy. *Neurology* 1988;38:1060–4.
8. Bernick C, Gregorios JB. Progressive multifocal leukoencephalopathy in a patient with acquired immune deficiency syndrome. *Arch Neurol* 1984;41:780–2.
9. Blum LW, Chambers RA, Schwartzman RS. Progressive multifocal leukoencephalopathy in acquired immunodeficiency syndrome. *Arch Neurol* 1985;42:137–9.
10. Chaisson RE, Griffin DE. Progressive multifocal leukoencephalopathy in AIDS. *JAMA* 1990;264:79–82.
11. England JD, Hsu CY, Garen PD, Goust JM, Biggs PJ. Progressive multifocal leukoencephalopathy occurring with the acquired immune deficiency syndrome. *South Med J* 1984;77:1041–3.
12. Ho JL, Plldre PA, McEnry D, et al. Acquired immunodeficiency with progressive multifocal leukoencephalopathy and monoclonal B-cell proliferation. *Ann Intern Med* 1984;100:693–6.
13. Speelman JD, ter Schegget J, Bots G. Progressive multifocal leukoencephalopathy in a case of acquired immunodeficiency syndrome. *Clin Neurol Neurosurg* 1985;87:27–33.
14. Amberson JB, DiCarlo EF, Metroka CE, Koizumi JH, Mouradian JA. Diagnostic pathology in the acquired immunodeficiency syndrome. *Arch Pathol Lab Med* 1985;109:345–51.
15. Helweg-Larsen S, Jakobsen J, Boesen F, Arlien-Soborg P. Neurological complications and concomitants of AIDS. *Acta Neurol Scand* 1986;74:467–74.
16. Lang W, Miklossy J, Deruax JP, et al. Neuropathology of the acquired immune deficiency syndrome (AIDS): a report of 135 consecutive autopsy cases from Switzerland. *Neuropathologica* 1989;379–90.
17. Levy AM, Bredsen DE, Rosenblum ML. Neurological manifestations of the acquired immunodeficiency syndrome (AIDS): experience at UCSF and review of the literature. *J Neurosurg* 1985;62:475–95.
18. Moskowitz LB, Hensley GT, Chan JC, Gregorios J, Conley FK. The neuropathology of acquired immunodeficiency syndrome. *Arch Pathol Lab Med* 1984;108:867–72.
19. Niedt GW, Schinelle RA. Acquired immunodeficiency syndrome: clinicopathologic study of 56 autopsies. *Arch Pathol Lab Med* 1985;109:727–34.
20. Petito CK, Cho ES, Lemann W, Navia BA, Price RW. Neuropathology of acquired immunodeficiency syndrome (AIDS): an autopsy review. *J Neuropathol Exp Neurol* 1986;45:635–46.
21. Reichert CM, O'Leary TJ, Levens DL, Simrell CR, Macher AM. Autopsy pathology in the acquired immune deficiency syndrome. *Am J Pathol* 1983;112:357–82.
22. Rodesch G, Parizel PM, Farber CM, et al. Nervous system manifestations and neuroradiologic findings in acquired immunodeficiency syndrome (AIDS). *Neuroradiology* 1989;31:33–9.
23. Snider WD, Simpson DM, Nielson S, Gold JWM, Metroka CE, Posner JB. Neurological complications of acquired immune deficiency syndrome: analysis of 50 patients. *Ann Neurol* 1983;14:403–18.
24. Ledoux S, Libman I, Robert F, Just N. Progressive multifocal leukoencephalopathy with gray matter involvement. *Can J Neurol Sci* 1989;16:200–2.
25. Mark AS, Atlas SW. Progressive multifocal leukoencephalopathy in patients with AIDS: appearance on MR images. *Radiology* 1989;173:517–20.

26. Saxton CR, Farkis RA, Helderman K. Progressive multifocal leukoencephalopathy in a renal transplant recipient—increased sensitivity of CT scanning by double dose contrast with delayed films. *Am J Med* 1984;77:333–7.

27. Shafran B, Roke ME, Barr RM, Cairncross JG. Contrast enhancing lesions in progressive multifocal leukoencephalopathy: a clinicopathological correlation. *Can J Neurol Sci* 1987;14:600–2.

28. Houff SA, Major EO, Katz DA, et al. Involvement of JC virus-infected mononuclear cells from the bone marrow and spleen in the pathogenesis of progressive multifocal leukoencephalopathy. *N Engl J Med* 1988;5:301–5.

29. Zurhein GM, Chou SM. Particles resembling papovaviruses in human cerebral demyelinating disease. *Science* 1965;148:1477–9.

30. Padgett BL, Walker DL, Zurhein GM, Eckroade RJ, Dessel BH. Cultivation of papova-like virus from human brain with progressive multifocal leukoencephalopathy. *Lancet* 1971;1:1257–60.

31. Weiner LP, Herndon RM, Narayan O, et al. Isolation of virus related to SV40 from patients with progressive multifocal leukoencephalopathy. *N Engl J Med* 1972;286:385–90.

32. Padgett BL, Walker DL, Zurhein RJ, Houdach AE, Chou SM. JC papovavirus in progressive multifocal leukoencephalopathy. *J Infect Dis* 1976;133:686–90.

33. Aksamit AJ, Sever JL, Major EO. Progressive multifocal leukoencephalopathy: JC virus detection by in situ hybridization compared with immunohistochemistry. *Neurology* 1986;36:499–504.

34. Aksamit AJ, Mourrain P, Sever JL, Major EO. Progressive multifocal leukoencephalopathy: investigation of three cases using in situ hybridization with JC virus biotinylated DNA probe. *Ann Neurol* 1985;18:490–6.

35. Arthur RR, Dagostin S, Shah KV. Detection of BK virus and JC virus in urine and brain tissue by the polymerase chain reaction. *J Clin Microbiol* 1989;27:1174–9.

36. Telenti A, Aksamit AJ, Proper J, Smith TF. Detection of JC virus DNA by polymerase chain reaction in patients with progressive multifocal leukoencephalopathy. *J Infect Dis* 1990;162:858–61.

37. Johnson RT. Evidence for polyoma viruses in human diseases. In: Sever JL, Madden DL, eds. *Polyoma viruses and human diseases.* New York: Alan R. Liss, 1983.

38. Kenny S, Natarajan, Strike D, Khoury G, Salzman NP. JC virus enhancer-promoter active in human brain cells. *Science* 1984;226:1337–9.

39. Ahmed S, Chowdhury M, Khalili K. Regulation of a human neurotropic virus promoter, JCV: identification of a novel activator domain located upstream from the 98 bp enhancer promoter region. *Nucleic Acids Res* 1990;18:7417–23.

40. Beggs AH, Miner JH, Scangos GA. Cell type-specific expression of JC virus T antigen in primary and established cell lines from transgenic mice. *J Gen Virol* 1990;71:151–64.

41. Feigenbaum L, Khalili K, Major E, Khoury G. Regulation of the host range of human papovavirus JCV. *Proc Natl Acad Sci USA* 1987;84:3695–8.

42. Frisque RJ, Bream GL, Canella MT. Human polyomavirus JC virus genome. *J Virol* 1984;51:458–69.

43. Lynch KJ, Frisque RJ. Factors contributing to the restricted DNA replicating activity of JC virus. *Virology* 1991;180:306–17.

44. Tada H, Lashgari MS, Khalili K. Promoter function: evidence that a pentanucleotide "silencer" repeat sequence AGGGAAGGGA down-regulates transcription of the JC virus late promoter. *Virology* 1991;180:327–38.

45. Tada H, Lashgari M, Rappaport J, Khalili K. Cell type-specific expression of JC virus early promoter is determined by positive and negative regulation. *J Virol* 1989;63:463–6.

46. Lashgari MS, Tada H, Amini S, Khalili K. Regulation of JCV-L promoter function: transactivation of JCV-L promoter by JCV and SV40 early proteins. *Virology* 1989;170:292–5.

47. Kalili K, Rappaport J, Khoury G. Nuclear factors in human brain cells bind specifically to the JCV regulatory region. *EMBO J* 1988;7:1205–10.

48. Brooks BR, Walker DL. Progressive multifocal leukoencephalopathy. *Neurol Clin North Am* 1984;2:299–313.

49. Kepes JJ, Chou SM, Price LW. Progressive multifocal leukoencephalopathy with 10 year survival in a patient with nontropical sprue. *Neurology* 1975;25:1006–12.

50. Britton CB, Miller JR. Neurologic complications in acquired immunodeficiency syndrome (AIDS). *Neurol Clin North Am* 1984;2:315–39.

51. Elkin CM, Leon E, Grenell SL, et al. Intracranial lesions in the acquired immunodeficiency syndrome: radiological (computed tomographic) features. *JAMA* 1985;253:393–6.

52. Olsen WL, Longo FM, Mille CM, Norma D. White matter disease in AIDS: findings at MR imaging. *Radiology* 1988;169:445–8.

53. Post MJD, Sheldon JJ, Hensley GT, et al. Central nervous system disease in acquired immunodeficiency syndrome: prospective correlation using CT, MR imaging, and pathologic studies. *Radiology* 1986;158:141–8.

54. Carroll BA, Lane B, Norman D, et al. Diagnosis of progressive multifocal leukoencephalopathy by computed tomography. *Radiology* 1977;122:137–41.

55. Conomy JP, Weinstein MA, Agamanolis D, et al. Computed tomography in progressive multifocal leukoencephalopathy. *AJR* 1976;127:663–5.

56. Durham DS, Freyer JA, O'Neil BJ, et al. Progressive multifocal leukoencephalopathy: CT and pathological features. *Med J Aust* 1980;2:502–4.

57. Krupp LB, Lipton RB, Swerdlow MD, Leeds NE, Llena J. Progressive multifocal leukoencephalopathy: clinical and radiographic features. *Ann Neurol* 1985;17:344–9.

58. Lipton RB, Krupp L, Horoupian D, Hershkovitz S, Arezzo JC, Kurtzberg D. Progressive multifocal leukoencephalopathy of the posterior fossa in an AIDS patient: clinical, radiographic and evoked potential findings. *Eur Neurol* 1988;28:258–61.

59. Miller JR, Barret RB, Britton CB, et al. Progressive multifocal leukoencephalopathy in a male homosexual with T-cell immune deficiency. *N Engl J Med* 1982;307:1436–7.

60. Sze G, Zimmerman RD. The magnetic resonance imaging of infections and inflammatory diseases. *Radiol Clin North Am* 1988;26:839–58.

61. Heinz EB, Dreyer BP, Haenggell CA, et al. Computed tomography in white matter disease. *Radiology* 1979;130:371–8.

62. Farrell DF. The EEG in progressive multifocal leukoencephalopathy. *Electroencephalogr Clin Neurophysiol* 1972;26:357–60.

63. Mazlo M, Tariska I. Morphological demonstration of the first phase of polyomavirus replication in oligodendroglia cells of human brain in progressive multifocal leukoencephalopathy (PML). *Acta Neuropathol (Berl)* 1980;49:133–43.

64. Stoner GL, Soffer D, Ryschkewitsch CF, Walker DL, Webster HD. A double-label method detects both early (T-antigen) and late (capsid) proteins of JC virus in progressive multifocal leukoencephalopathy brain tissue from AIDS and non-AIDS patients. *J Neuroimmunol* 1988;19:223–36.

65. Stoner GL, Ryschkewitsch CF, Walker DL, Soffer D, Webster HD. A monoclonal antibody to SV40 large T-antigen labels a nuclear antigen in JC virus-transformed cells in progressive multifocal leukoencephalopathy (PML) brain infected with CJ virus. *J Neuroimmunol* 1988;17:331–45.

66. Stoner GL, Ryschkewitsch CF, Walker DL, Webster HD. JC papovavirus large tumor (T)-antigen expression in brain tissue of acquired immune deficiency syndrome (AIDS) and non-AIDS patients with progressive multifocal leukoencephalopathy. *Proc Natl Acad Sci USA* 1986;83:2271–5.

67. Itoyama Y, Webster H deF, Sternberger NH, et al. Distribution of papovavirus, myelin-associated glycoprotein, and myelin basic protein in progressive multifocal leukoencephalopathy lesions. *Ann Neurol* 1982;11:396–407.

68. Gendelman HE, Pezeshkpour GH, Pressman NJ, et al. A quantitation of myelin-associated glycoprotein and myelin basic protein loss in different demyelinating diseases. *Ann Neurol* 1986;11:396–407.

69. Aksamit AJ, Gendelman HE, Orenstein JM, Pezeshkpour GH. AIDS-associated progressive multifocal leukoencephalopathy (PML): Comparison to non-AIDS PML with in situ hybridization and immunohistochemistry. *Neurology* 1990;40:1073–8.

70. Vazeux R, Cumont M, Girar PM, et al. Severe encephalitis resulting from coinfections with HIV and JC virus. *Neurology* 1990;40:944–8.

70a. Wiley CA, Grafe M, Kennedy C, Nelson JA. Human immunodeficiency virus (HIV) and JC virus in acquired immune deficiency syndrome (AIDS) patients with progressive multifocal leukoencephalopathy. *Acta Neuropathol (Berl)* 1986;71:150–3.

71. Conway B, Halliday WC, Brunham RC. Human immunodeficiency virus-associated progressive multifocal leukoencephalopathy: apparent response to 3'-azido-3'-deoxythymidine. *Rev Infect Dis* 1990;12:479–82.

72. Jakobsen J, Diemer NH, Gaub J, Brun B, Helweg-Larsen S. Progressive multifocal leukoencephalopathy in a patient without other clinical manifestations of AIDS. *Acta Neurol Scand.* 1987;75:209–13.

73. Lechenberg R, Sher JH. *AIDS in the nervous system.* New York: Churchill Livingston, 1988;85–90.

74. Macher AB, Parisi JE, Aksamit AJ, et al. AIDS case for diagnosis. *Military Med* 1986;151:25–32.

75. Snow RB, Lavyne MH. Intracranial space-occupying lesions in acquired immune deficiency syndrome patients. *Neurosurgery* 1985;16:148–53.

76. Suhrland MJ, Koslow M, Perchick A, et al. Cytologic findings in progressive multifocal leukoencephalopathy. *Acta Cytol* 1987;31:505–11.

77. Voutsinas L. Case of the season. *Semin Roentgenol* 1986;4:243–4.

78. Apuzzo ML, Sabshin JK. Computed tomographic guidance stereotaxis in the management of intracranial lesions. *Neurosurgery* 1983;12:277–84.

79. Rhodes RH, Ward JM, Duard WL, Ross A. Progressive multifocal leukoencephalopathy and retroviral encephalitis in acquired immunodeficiency syndrome. *Arch Pathol Lab Med* 1988;112:1207–13.

AIDS and Other Manifestations of HIV Infection,
Second Edition, Edited by Gary P. Wormser.
Raven Press, Ltd., New York © 1992.

CHAPTER 26

Gastrointestinal Manifestations of AIDS

Brad M. Dworkin

Patients with the acquired immunodeficiency syndrome (AIDS) frequently have gastrointestinal complaints including diarrhea and weight loss (1–9). In one series up to 85% of AIDS patients had GI complaints, and diarrhea, present in over half of cases, is a frequent reason for seeking medical attention (1–3,9). The scope of gastrointestinal pathology in AIDS is wide and for the purposes of this chapter will be divided into three broad categories: (1) infectious agents, (2) neoplasms, and (3) other derangements related to human immunodeficiency virus (HIV) infection. This chapter will provide a broad clinical overview of the gastrointestinal conditions associated with HIV infection.

GI INFECTIOUS AGENTS

Enteric pathogens are frequently found in HIV-infected patients with or without diarrhea or other symptoms (1,2,10–12) (Table 1). Bacterial, viral, fungal, or protozoal organisms have been found in the gastrointestinal tract of 10–39% of AIDS cases without diarrhea and in up to 85% of cases with diarrhea (10–13). The symptom of diarrhea per se has seen estimated to be only 70% sensitive and 62% specific for the presence of pathogens (12). Diagnosis of these disorders is complicated by the need for specialized techniques to detect certain agents (11,14). Furthermore, even when detected, treatment may be inadequate, usually due to lack of efficacious therapy (10,11). This has led some authors to suggest, based on an analysis of cost effectiveness, that the use of symptomatic therapy with minimal diagnostic evaluations is the approach of choice (15). However, this approach could delay a specific effective treatment and increase the risk of additional morbidity, including

worsening nutritional status (10,16,17). Clinicians need to be aware of the spectrum of infectious complications in HIV infection, including how they are most readily diagnosed and treated.

FUNGAL INFECTIONS

Candida

Oroesophageal candidiasis is one of the earliest and most common opportunistic infections associated with the advanced immunodeficiency state of HIV infection (18–22). *Candida albicans* is the most common species of candida recovered, which is not surprising since it can be found in the oropharynx of approximately 50% of the normal population (23,24). Oral candidiasis has been reported to occur in about 75% of persons with AIDS (23). In HIV-infected patients without AIDS, the presence of oral candidiasis carries a poor prognosis. In some studies as many as 59% of persons with oral candidiasis developed other more serious opportunistic infections or Kaposi's sarcoma within 3 months (21,25).

The exact relationship between oral candidiasis and esophageal involvement in the HIV-infected patient is less clear, since esophageal involvement may be present in the absence of the characteristic symptoms of dysphagia or odynophagia (26). Porro et al. (27) recently noted that 40% of patients with endoscopically documented candida esophagitis had no esophageal symptoms. Thrush is not always present in HIV-infected patients with candida esophagitis but has been observed in 71–88% (27) of cases. The combination of oral thrush plus esophageal symptoms is highly specific (approaches 100%) for the diagnosis of candida esophagitis, whereas oral thrush alone is only about 80% specific (27,28).

Several methods are available to document the presence of candida esophagitis. These include barium x-ray studies, endoscopy, and blind cytologic brushing or

B. M. Dworkin: Section of Nutrition, Sarah C. Upham Division of Gastroenterology, New York Medical College, Valhalla, New York 10595.

TABLE 1. *Common GI infectious agents in HIV disease*

Fungal
    Candidiasis
    Histoplasmosis
Viral
    Cytomegalovirus
    Herpes simplex
    Epstein-Barr virus (rare)
    Adenovirus
Bacterial
    Mycobacterium avium-intracellulare
    Mycobacterium tuberculosis
    Other bacteria with atypical clinical features
        Salmonella
        Shigella
        Helicobacter pylori
        Campylobacter
        Clostridium difficile
Protozoan
    Cryptosporidium
    Microsporidium
    Isospora belli
    Nonopportunisitic parasites
        Giardia lamblia
        Entamoeba histolytica
        Strongyloides stercoralis (a helminth)

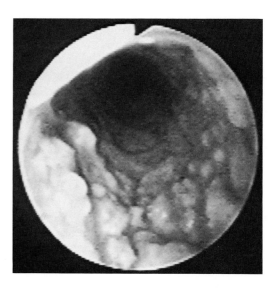

FIG. 1. Endoscopic view of candida esophagitis with white "cheesy" plaques of candida lining the esophagus.

esophageal lavage (24–31). Air-contrast barium studies should be performed when looking for esophagitis, as these have significantly higher sensitivity than single-contrast exams (31). However, even with these techniques, the radiographic findings are often nonspecific (21,24,30,31). Likewise, blind brushings and esophageal lavage may result in false-positive results, presumably due to oral contamination (28). Endoscopy with both brush cytology and biopsy should be performed when a definitive diagnosis is required (20,21,24,29). The typical endoscopic appearance is that of multiple white or grey plaques, which may be present as discrete lesions or as dense confluent exudates (32) (Figure 1). The plaques are usually adherent, and the intervening mucosa may be either normal in appearance or be erythematous and friable. Even this characteristic appearance, however, is not entirely specific (24,32). Therefore, the exudate should be brushed and a microscopic examination of a potassium hydroxide preparation done to confirm the presence of candida-like organisms. Biopsy specimens should also be examined using silver or periodic acid-Schiff stains to confirm the presence of fungal elements (24,32). Culture alone is not adequate to establish the diagnosis due to the high likelihood of oral contamination with candida (32,33).

Initial therapy of oroesophageal candidiasis is usually successful in HIV-infected patients although relapses often occur if antifungal therapy is discontinued (18,24,34–36). Nystatin oral suspension or clotrimazole troches if given 4 or 5 times daily are usually adequate treatment for oral thrush (24). For esophageal disease, oral therapy with either ketoconazole or fluconazole is recommended. Therapeutic failure with ketoconazole has been reported and could either be due to resistant strains of candida or malabsorption of drug secondary to the hypochlorhydria that is commonly seen in AIDS patients (34,35). Fluconazole may still be effective in such cases, particularly if hypochlorhydria is the reason for ketoconazole failure, since gastric acidity is not required for fluconazole absorption. In refractory cases, therapy with amphotericin is indicated (24,29).

Other fungal infections seen in HIV-infected patients infrequently involve the GI tract. Patients with disseminated histoplasmosis may have diarrhea in up to 14% of cases, but this is usually attributable to coinfection with other organisms (37). Even in patients with proven gastrointestinal histoplasmosis, diarrhea may be absent (37).

VIRAL INFECTIONS

Acute and chronic viral infections are common causes of morbidity in HIV-infected patients (2,5,6,9–11,38,39). However, many of the viral agents well known to cause diarrhea in non-HIV-infected persons, including rotaviruses, enteric adenoviruses, Norwalk agent, coronavirus, coxsackieviruses, and others are infrequently found in North American patients with HIV infection (9–11,40,41). Even when these viruses are identified, their importance as a cause of diarrhea is ill defined (41). Cunningham et al. (40) isolated enteroviruses from 54% of a group of Australian men with symptomatic HIV disease who had diarrhea. However, 50% of patients without diarrhea also harbored these viruses (40). Therefore, the pathogenicity of these agents in AIDS remains questionable. On the other hand certain viral agents, such as cytomegalovirus and herpes simplex, can clearly cause several types of gastrointestinal disease in AIDS patients (2,5,9–13).

Cytomegalovirus

Cytomegalovirus (CMV) rarely causes gastrointestinal disease in healthy persons, but severe disease involving almost any organ of the GI tract has been reported in immunocompromised hosts, including patients with AIDS (2,4,9,42–49). Autopsy series have documented that disseminated CMV is one of the most common opportunistic infections in AIDS (50–52). Jacobson et al. (43) reported a 2.2% incidence of symptomatic CMV GI disease over a 1-year period among 760 AIDS patients. In another series, 13% of gastrointestinal biopsies in AIDS cases showed CMV (44). The colon appears to be the most common site of involvement in patients with HIV infection, but any level of the GI tract may be affected (42–52).

Symptomatic GI involvement due to CMV is generally characterized by ulceration, sometimes with secondary bacterial or fungal infections (50). Therefore, symptoms of CMV are nonspecific, reflecting an acute inflammatory process in the involved organ.

There are several methods available to diagnose CMV infection (53). These include serologic testing for antibody, viral culture, radiologic diagnosis (54,55), and various histologic methods, including routine staining with hematoxylin and eosin (H&E), immunohistochemical assays, and in situ hybridization for CMV DNA (53,56,57). Serologic testing to establish a diagnosis of active CMV infection is of almost no value in HIV-infected patients (56). This is due to the very high baseline prevalence of seropositivity and the abnormal humoral immune response in this patient population (56). Likewise, because of the high incidence of CMV culture positivity in asymptomatic HIV-infected patients, a positive culture by itself does not establish clinically relevant disease (58). In addition, in direct comparison to histology, culture also appears to be less sensitive (42,45,56). Therefore, the diagnosis of CMV disease of the GI tract is preferentially made by histologic examination of a tissue sample (56,57). On H&E stain typical large cells with intranuclear or paranuclear inclusions are found (57). However, the sensitivity of H & E diagnosis is variable and observer dependent. Other methods, including immunohistochemical techniques and (more recently) CMV DNA probes can lead to further increases in sensitivity and specificity (57).

Because CMV infections of the GI tract may involve multiple sites the clinical presentation is variable. In the esophagus, the principal symptom is odynophagia, with or without dysphagia (43). Barium contrast radiology may show ulceration in the mid- or distal esophagus, a

finding indistinguishable from herpes simplex esophagitis (54). However, the presence of large flat or ovoid ulcers that can be several centimeters in length is strongly suggestive of CMV esophagitis (54,55). The endoscopic findings reveal esophageal ulceration, frequently with a solitary large shallow ulcer (32,45). As reviewed above, the diagnosis of CMV must not be based on gross appearance alone.

Colonic involvement with CMV in AIDS is usually characterized by diarrhea. Patients may also complain of abdominal pain and rectal bleeding (42,43,44,48,59). In severe cases bowel perforation leading to an acute abdomen or massive hemorrhage requiring emergency colectomy can occur (42,59). Barium enema exams may reveal nonspecific colitis sometimes with deep ulcerations, but can occasionally be normal (60). Abdominal computed tomography (CT) scans may reveal bowel wall thickening, which can be focal or diffuse (60). Endoscopic findings in CMV colitis are varied, ranging from normal-appearing mucosa to varying degrees of inflammation, with or without ulcerations (43,56,61,62). The ulcerations can be solitary or multiple and occasionally have an appearance consistent with pseudomembranous colitis (61–63a) (Figure 2). The yield of rectal biopsy in establishing the diagnosis may approximate 80% (56). Because the disease is often patchy, multiple biopsy samples are recommended.

CMV may also involve pancreas, liver, gallbladder, and the biliary tree. (63a, b) Patients with biliary tract involvement may present with abdominal pain and raised levels of alkaline phosphatase. Ultrasonography of the biliary tree is frequently normal and endoscopic retrograde cholangiopancreatography (ERCP) is the diagnostic modality of choice. A picture resembling idiopathic primary sclerosing cholangitis, papillary stenosis,

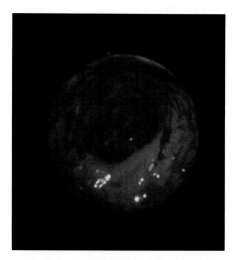

FIG. 2. Colonoscopic appearance of colitis due to cytomegalovirus (CMV). Note diffusely erythematous mucosa with some friability and hemorrhage and white lacy exudate suggestive of pseudomembranes. Biopsy was positive for CMV.

or biliary strictures may be present (63a–d). There may be concomitant cryptosporidial infection of the upper intestine or biliary tree.

At the present time, ganciclovir is the primary treatment for CMV infections of the GI tract in AIDS patients (42,43,45,63a,64–67). Clinical response rates of up to 75% have been reported, usually associated with a positive virologic response as well (45,64–67). The principal toxicity is hematologic, particularly leukopenia (64–67), especially if zidovudine (AZT) is also given, which is usually not recommended (65).

Foscarnet (trisodium phosphonoformate) has also been reported to be of clinical benefit in GI CMV infections in AIDS and has the advantage of avoiding significant bone marrow toxicity (42,43,45,63a,64). A sentinel problem in the treatment of CMV infections in AIDS is that relapses occur in up to 50% of cases (42,63a,64,66). Maintenance therapy with ganciclovir (or foscarnet) may be needed, but has been associated with neutropenia (42,43). In addition, emergence of CMV strains resistant to ganciclovir may be as high as 38% of patients on therapy for greater than 3 months who continue to excrete virus, or 7.6% of treated patients overall (68). Finally, patients with CMV esophagitis have a particularly poor long-term prognosis, with a 1-year mortality rate of over 90%, usually due to comorbid factors (45).

Herpes Simplex Virus

Herpes simplex virus (HSV) has long been recognized as an important cause of gastrointestinal disease in non-immunosuppressed individuals including homosexual men, and is also a well-established cause of significant morbidity in HIV-infected patients (5,10,11,18,21, 36,69–74). As is true in non-AIDS cases, HSV infections can present with several different GI clinical syndromes depending on the area of involvement. Sites of infection include the rectosigmoid colon, oropharynx, esophagus, and perianal skin (18).

HSV type 1 may be associated with ulcerated lesions of the esophagus (21,53,73,74). These are usually, but not always, associated with odynophagia and herpetic lesions in the oropharynx (21,53,74). However, some patients may have only oropharyngeal candidiasis. Double-contrast barium esophograms will show esophageal ulceration in more than 50% of cases (75). Definitive diagnosis requires endoscopy with cytologic examination of brushings or histologic examination of a tissue sample.

A second pattern of HSV infection in AIDS patients is proctitis (10,11,18). HSV is usually not a significant cause of diarrhea, but is the most common infectious cause of proctitis (11). HSV type 2 is most commonly responsible for proctitis (70). Patients may have anorectal pain as well as mucoid or bloody stools, often with

tenesmus. Perianal vesicles or ulcerations may also be present (70,76). The endoscopic findings show a nonspecific proctitis (71,76). Cytologic brushings and biopsy are required to establish the diagnosis.

The third clinical syndrome with HSV and GI disease in AIDS patients is perianal ulceration (73,77–79). The lesions begin as vesicles, which rupture, ulcerate, and frequently coalesce (77). Large, painful, clean-based ulcers may result (73,78). The virus is readily cultured from the ulcer sites. The lesions rarely subside spontaneously, but do respond virologically and clinically to acyclovir (36,73,80). Topical therapy may be useful, but in some cases oral or intravenous acyclovir is indicated (80). Because recurrence is common, chronic therapy is often required. In addition, acyclovir-resistant mucocutaneous HSV infection has been reported (81). Clinical response to foscarnet is as high as 81% in these cases (82).

Epstein-Barr Virus

Epstein-Barr virus (EBV) has rarely been implicated in causing significant GI illness in HIV-infected patients (73). Ulcerative esophagitis has been reported in association with EBV, which was confirmed by DNA in situ hybridization (83). Oral hairy leukoplakia may also be related to EBV infection (84,85). If EBV induced esophagitis is suspected, therapy with acyclovir may be tried, although there is little evidence for clinical efficacy in this infection. (85).

BACTERIA

Bacterial agents are major causes of GI morbidity in HIV-infected patients (1,2,5,9–15,18–20,36,38,39, 73,86–88). As is true for other pathogens, GI bacterial infections in AIDS patients are characterized by atypical or chronic disease with organisms that usually cause self-limited or no illness in normal individuals.

Salmonella infections in HIV-infected patients differ in several important aspects from non-AIDS individuals (88–91). First, these infections are much more common in the setting of HIV (approximately 20-fold) (91); second, the incidence of salmonella bacteremia is higher; and third, the bacteremia may be persistent or recurrent despite treatment with appropriate antimicrobial therapy (88–91). Life-long (maintenance) antibiotic therapy may be required. In a small uncontrolled study norfloxacin has shown promise in eradicating persistent salmonella infection in AIDS patients (92).

Campylobacter infection has also been described in HIV-infected patients (93–95). This infection may result in diarrhea or frank colitis and (rarely) may be associated with bacteremia. Coinfection with other bowel pathogens is common (11,94). Antibody responses in these patients are poor and infection may persist despite antibiotic therapy in up to 33% of cases (94). Such chronic infections have been associated with the emergence of antibiotic-resistant strains (93–95).

Shigella infections in AIDS patients may also have atypical clinical features (86). Whereas shigella bacteremia is rare in normal hosts, it may occur with increased frequency in AIDS patients (96). In addition, the course of the disease may be protracted, even though an antibody response may be present and appropriate antibiotic therapy given (96,97).

Mycobacterium avium-intracellulare (MAI) frequently involves the GI tract in AIDS patients (1,2,10–12,14,18,73,86–88,98–101). Diarrhea and weight loss are common and GI malabsorption, as documented by abnormal D-xylose tests, occurs in 50% or more of patients (1,14,99,100). Systemic infection, usually associated with fever, bacteremia, abnormal liver function tests, lymphadenopathy, and bone marrow involvement is common (99). The small bowel is the most common site of GI involvement, but any level of the GI tract including the esophagus may be affected (99). Stool cultures are positive for MAI in up to 86% of infected cases, although the organism may take weeks to grow (99). More rapid diagnosis is made by endoscopic biopsy with appropriate staining for acid-fast bacilli. A unique pathologic picture may accompany MAI of the GI tract. Granuloma formation is poor in these patients, and therefore specific staining for acid-fast bacilli must be done with (or without) the presence of granulomas (1,98,99). In addition, occasionally a picture mimicking Whipple's disease, including periodic acid-Schiff (PAS)-positive macrophages, has been seen (100). Electron microscopy, stains for acid-fast organisms, and appropriate culture should distinguish the two diseases (100,102).

Treatment for MAI remains problematic (98,103). In limited studies, multidrug regimens with amikacin, ethambutol, rifampin, and ciprofloxacin, with or without clofazimine, have been shown to reduce bacteremia and improve clinical symptoms (104,105).

Although much attention has been focused on MAI infection of the GI tract in AIDS, it is important to remember that *Mycobacterium tuberculosis* can also cause extensive GI disease in HIV-infected patients (106–109). This is particularly important in those HIV-infected patients with the highest rates of prior (or recent) exposure to *M. tuberculosis* (109). Extrapulmonary and disseminated tuberculosis are common in these patients (109,110). Because of cutaneous anergy, the purified protein derivative (PPD) skin test is of limited diagnostic value (109). Definitive diagnosis is made by culture of the organism. Tuberculosis in HIV-infected patients responds well to standard therapy, including isoniazid and rifampin (109). However, treatment may need to be prolonged (109).

Helicobacter pylori is a common pathogen in normal hosts that is associated with acute and chronic gastritis and peptic ulcer disease (111–113). The organism generally does not invade the gastric mucosa (111). HIV-infected patients are no more likely to be infected with this organism than are age-matched controls (114). Likewise, in most AIDS cases, this organism is not invasive, and is associated with gastritis, as seen in non-AIDS patients (114). However, *H. pylori* was reported to have invaded the lamina propria of one AIDS patient, producing severe GI symptoms and a radiographic appearance suggestive of gastric lymphoma (115). Response to therapy with antibiotics and bismuth subsalicylate seems adequate (115).

Clostridium difficile is not particularly common in AIDS, but may be an important pathogen in some patients because it is the principal cause of antibiotic-associated pseudomembranous colitis (10–13,116–118). This endoscopic picture is not, however, pathognomonic for *C. difficile* infection and can occur with other diseases including CMV colitis (61–63). Of particular note in HIV-infected patients is that the disease has been reported in an individual who received no drugs other than acyclovir and zidovudine (119). Therefore, use of conventional antibiotics is not always an antecedent factor, and stool studies for *C. difficile* toxin should be done for HIV-infected patients with diarrhea or proctitis (11,119).

PROTOZOA

The protozoan parasites include a variety of pathogens that collectively are the most frequent causes of infectious diarrhea in HIV-infected patients (1,10–14,87,120). Male homosexuals have an increased risk of exposure to certain enteric protozoan pathogens. Protozoan infections may have an atypical course in HIV-infected patients as a result of the underlying immune deficiency (10–14,69–71,86,120–122).

Cryptosporidium has only recently been recognized as a human pathogen (123). In immunocompetent persons it usually presents as an acute self-limited gastroenteritis, with resolution of diarrhea in 1–2 weeks (123–126). Contact with farm animals or contaminated water is not a prerequisite for infection, and fecal–oral spread is likely (123–128). In nonimmunosuppressed persons there may be an asymptomatic carrier state, thus resulting in a potential human reservoir for the disease (129). In AIDS patients chronic diarrhea and wasting are hallmarks of cryptosporidium infection (123,130–132). Cryptosporidia are among the most common pathogens identified in AIDS patients with diarrhea, found in up to 19% of cases (10–15,87,120,123,130,131). It is estimated that 3–4% of patients with AIDS in the United States have cryptosporidia compared with rates as high as 50% in Haiti or Africa (123).

Cryptosporidium is not an invasive organism, but does attach to the plasma membrane of epithelial cells

(133). Light microscopic changes often show evidence of small intestinal injury including partial villous atrophy (120). These changes can be accompanied by significant malabsorption of both lactose and D-xylose (120,123). Cryptosporidium has been identified throughout the luminal GI tract (120,123,131). Patients usually present with diarrhea, with or without abdominal cramps. The diarrhea can be massive, leading to dehydration. Fever, leukocytosis, or GI bleeding are uncommon (123). Because malabsorption is common, symptoms may be exaggerated by eating. Although transient improvement may occur, the course is generally chronic and the infection persistent (130,131).

Extraluminal gastrointestinal disease can also occur with cryptosporidium, most notably in the biliary tree (63b, c,134,135). Cholestasis, cholangitis, and acalculous cholecystitis may occur. ERCP may yield findings clinically indistinguishable from primary sclerosing cholangitis (63b, c,123,134,135).

A variety of methods are available to diagnose cryptosporidium (120,122–133). GI radiologic studies are usually normal or show only nonspecific changes (123,131). Although these organisms can be detected on light microscopy of small intestinal or rectal biopsy specimens, multiple specially processed and stained stool examinations can usually establish the diagnosis without the need for invasive procedures (1,120,123,130,131).

At present, the greatest challenge lies in the treatment of cryptosporidium infection (15). Nonspecific therapy with antidiarrheal agents, such as diphenoxylate, can reduce stool volumes (15,131). Antibiotic therapy with erythromycin or spiramycin has also produced transient reduction in diarrhea, but results are not uniformly successful (123,131,136). Octreotide acetate, a parenterally administered somatastatin analog, can reduce diarrhea by its antisecretory effects, but it is expensive, requires multiple parenteral doses, does not clear the organism, and is not uniformly successful in reducing diarrhea (131,137). Clearance of the organism from the stool associated with a clinical response has been reported in one patient treated with hyperimmune bovine colostrum (138). Improving the underlying immunodeficiency may also be an effective therapeutic approach, as illustrated by several reports of response to AZT (131,139,140).

Isospora belli infection is a well recognized but uncommon cause of diarrhea among HIV-infected patients in the United States and Great Britain, probably accounting for only 1% of cases, and absent altogether from many series (1,10–14,120,123,141). However, it may be present in 15% of Haitian AIDS patients with diarrhea (142). In the United States, the source of infection is unclear, but sexual transmission via homosexual contact may be possible (142,143). Clinically, the disease is indistinguishable from cryptosporidiosis except that Charcot-Leyden crystals may be evident in the stool (123). Diag-

nosis is made by examination of a concentrated stool specimen. As for most intestinal parasite infections, yield is likely to be increased by examining multiple stool samples (144). Therapy with oral trimethoprim-sulfamethoxazole usually results in a prompt clinical response (142). Relapse is common, but also usually responds to retreatment (142). In those unable to tolerate that therapy, metronidazole may be partially effective (145).

Microsporidia can produce disease in small mammals and humans. Serologic studies have suggested a high incidence of exposure to microsporidia among homosexual men (146). Data are limited on the true prevalence of this infection in HIV-infected patients, undoubtedly because of the extreme difficulty in making the diagnosis (14,120). Kotler et al. (120) estimated a minimum 7.5% incidence in AIDS patients with diarrhea in New York City. Electron microscopy of a tissue sample from the small intestine may be the most reliable means of establishing the diagnosis, although the organism can be detected with difficulty by light microscopy (14,120,133, 147–149). The microscopic findings are consistent with the specific organism, *Enterocytozoon bieneusi* (14,120, 149). Studies suggest that this organism may be responsible for some cases previously classified as "AIDS enteropathy," in that chronic diarrhea and wasting are common (14,120,148,149). Infection with microsporidia may result in small bowel inflammatory changes including prominent intraepithelial lymphocyte infiltration (14). Malabsorption is also common (120,148). At the present time no specific therapy is of proven benefit in the treatment of microsporidia infection.

Several nonopportunistic protozoal parasites are commonly seen in AIDS patients, often in combination with other organisms (1,2,5,10–15,18,87,88,141). *Giardia lamblia* is frequently encountered in homosexual men and is considered a cause of diarrhea in approximately 5–15% of HIV-infected patients (10–13,15,69,70). Approximately 13% of infected persons may be asymptomatic (11,159). Giardiasis is commonly associated with structural and functional changes in the small bowel, resulting in malabsorption of fat, D-xylose, lactose, and vitamins that is reversible upon eradication of the organism (150–153). The disease is usually associated with crampy upper abdominal pain and loose stools consistent with malabsorption. Blood and mucous in the stool are rare, as is high fever (150). Eosinophilia is generally not present (150). Immunodeficiency has long been recognized as a predisposing factor to persistent giardia infection including hypogammaglobulinemic disorders and intestinal IgA deficiency (121,150–153). T-cell function may also be important in clearing the organism, which may explain its pathogenicity in AIDS (153). The diagnosis is established either by visualizing the organism in stool, or, if negative, in duodenal fluid, usually obtained at the time of small bowel biopsy. Either duodenal aspirate or biopsy may yield positive results when stool studies are negative (10–12,144,150). Therapy with metronidazole is usually effective in eradicating the organism in AIDS patients, although stools should be reexamined following therapy, as treatment failures do occur (10–12,86,141).

Entamoeba histolytica is another nonopportunistic pathogen sometimes associated with diarrhea in HIV-infected patients (10–15,87). Similar to giardiasis, there is a high prevalence of amebiasis among male homosexuals, many of whom are asymptomatic carriers of the organism (69–71,86,87). However, infection with *E. histolytica* differs from that due to giardia in many important respects. *E. histolytica* primarily affects the colon. Ameba can produce a wide spectrum of disease, from self-limited diarrhea to invasive colitis characterized by bloody diarrhea that can progress to toxic megacolon (154,155). The clinical picture can sometimes mimic idiopathic inflammatory bowel disease (156). Endoscopically, a nonspecific colitis or discrete ulcers, often with a red rim and white exudate on the base, may be present (76). Amebiasis may also produce several syndromes not associated temporally with colitis or diarrhea per se. These include a cecal mass or ameboma and an hepatic abscess, usually in the right lobe (154,155). These are not particularly common in AIDS (87). Diagnosis of amebiasis is based on stool examinations, which will confirm the presence of the organism in most cases (154). Serology is of value in invasive amebiasis only and will often be negative in homosexual men harboring the organism without frank colitis (86). Histologic examination of tissue from the margin of an amebic ulcer can also establish the diagnosis (76). Treatment of amebiasis is the same as for non-HIV-infected patients and is generally effective (10,12,13,15,86,87,157). If diarrhea persists after treatment, a thorough search for other causes should be considered (141).

Strongyloides stercoralis infection is endemic in subtropical and tropical areas of the world and is also prevalent (although uncommon) in sexually active homosexual men (158). Persons infected with this helminth in the setting of immunodeficiency may develop the hyperinfection syndrome, which is associated with gram-negative bacterial sepsis and meningitis. This syndrome has been reported infrequently in HIV-infected patients (158,159). Similarly, strongyloides is also a rarely identified cause of diarrhea in HIV-infected patients, being found in less than 1% of cases (1,3,4,10–14,120,141). The apparent underrepresentation of this organism as a cause of morbidity and mortality in AIDS is unexplained (158).

NEOPLASMS

Immunodeficiency has clearly been recognized as a risk factor for the development of human malignancy (160). However, few other diseases of humans have been associated with as high an incidence of neoplasm as has AIDS (161). For the GI tract this includes several different tumor types including Kaposi's sarcoma (KS), non-Hodgkin's lymphoma, and carcinomas (5,73,88,161–166) (Table 2). The GI tract may be involved as part of disseminated disease, or may be the primary organ of presentation. The diagnosis and treatment of GI tumors are common reasons for GI endoscopy and abdominal surgery in AIDS patients (61,88,167–173).

Kaposi's Sarcoma

Kaposi's sarcoma is the most frequent neoplasm encountered in AIDS patients (161,165). The incidence of KS varies with the different epidemiologic groups at risk for AIDS but is highest among male homosexuals (165,174–177).

The GI tract is recognized to be involved in 30–50% of AIDS patients with KS during life (162,178,179), and in an even larger proportion (up to 70%) at postmortem (51,52). GI tract involvement is most common when extensive skin disease is present (162,179). However, GI disease can occur in the absence of KS in other locations and without concomitant involvement of the oropharynx (180–182).

Despite the high frequency of GI involvement in KS, clinical disease is uncommon (88,162,165,178,183). Most lesions are clinically silent. However, a wide array of GI symptoms have been reported with KS, including upper or lower GI bleeding, abdominal pain, diarrhea, intussusception, obstruction, and perforation (162,167–173,180,181).

The diagnosis of GI KS generally requires endoscopy. Barium radiography may miss early lesions and later findings may be indistinguishable from GI lymphoma or other solid tumors (162,184) (Fig. 3). Abdominal CT scanning may demonstrate focal bowel wall thickening from KS (185). Additionally, abdominal lymphadenopathy can be identified, and fine needle aspiration biopsy employed to establish the diagnosis (185). The endoscopic appearance of KS is varied (82,162–183). Most commonly, purple or red nodules are evident, sometimes associated with ulceration or hemorrhage. Polypoid masses can occur, sometimes with central umbilication or volcano-like lesions, similar in appearance to gastric lymphoma. In the colon, flat hemorrhagic lesions

TABLE 2. *Neoplasms involving the GI tract in HIV-infected patients*

Kaposi's sarcoma
Non-Hodgkin's lymphoma
Hodgkin's disease
Squamous cell carcinoma of the anus
Associated with human papillomavirus (HPV)

indistinguishable from colitis, or mass lesions that can even be mistaken for hemorrhoids, have been described (162,179–183,186). Because of these varied appearances, reliance on visual diagnosis can be misleading and tissue samples should be obtained whenever possible. However, biopsies are frequently negative, probably due to the submucosal nature of the disease (38,162) (Figure 3).

The decision to treat intestinal KS is usually based on whether or not symptoms are present, since significant morbidity or mortality is rare from intestinal KS per se. Obviously, emergent surgical therapy must be given as required (167–172). KS is often radiosensitive and may also be amenable to various chemotherapeutic regimens (162,165,187). Finally, high-dose recombinant α-interferon has activity in KS in certain AIDS patients, with rare reports of complete remission of visceral KS (162,188).

Patients with HIV infection are also predisposed to develop non-Hodgkin's lymphoma (161,162,166,189, 190), which is typically associated with extranodal disease and specifically with GI tract involvement in up to 31% of cases (189,190). These lymphomas may occur at all levels of the GI tract from oral to perianal areas (162,191–195). The liver is commonly involved as well (189,190). The tumors are generally of B-cell origin, and most are classified as high-grade lymphomas (189). KS may coexist with lymphoma in up to 20% of cases (189,196), and various opportunistic infections may develop concomitantly (189,196–198).

Because involvement may occur throughout the GI tract, signs and symptoms will depend on the location of the tumor. Dysphagia, GI bleeding, bowel obstruction, abdominal pain, diarrhea, and cachexia can all occur.

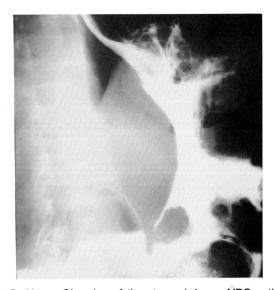

FIG. 3. Upper GI series of the stomach in an AIDS patient showing multiple large mucosal and submucosal masses. These proved positive on biopsy for Kaposi's sarcoma.

Because of overlapping symptoms with other AIDS syndromes, delay in diagnosis is common (193). Radiographic studies are often abnormal but nonspecific; endoscopy with biopsy is the most useful method to establish the diagnosis (162,184,185). Laparotomy may be required for cases not endoscopically accessible (193).

GI lymphoma in AIDS has generally been treated with combination chemotherapy, and complete response rates as high as 52% have been reported, depending on the histologic grade of the lymphoma (189). Recurrence is more likely in patients with HIV infection compared with other patients, and the overall prognosis is poor (189,199). Most patients die with recurrent lymphoma, with a median survival for all histologic grades of under 1 year (189,193,195).

Hodgkin's disease also occurs in HIV-infected patients, although not at unexpectedly high frequency (189,200). This tumor seems to differ from Hodgkin's disease in non-HIV-infected patients in its aggressive clinical course and rapidly fatal outcome (189). No clear data have emerged concerning specific GI involvement with Hodgkin's disease in HIV infection, but extranodal disease and hepatic involvement are common (189).

A variety of other tumors of the GI tract have occasionally been reported in HIV-infected patients including pancreatic and colon cancer (161,201). However, neoplastic involvement of the pancreas is most commonly due to KS or lymphoma as part of disseminated disease, and is usually subclinical (201).

Homosexual men in particular may be at higher risk for the development of squamous cell carcinoma of the anus in association with human papillomavirus infection (HPV) (202). The immunosuppression associated with HIV infection may promote the oncogenicity of HPV and lead to a higher incidence of neoplasia (203–204). Palefsky et al. (163) recently reported a 54% incidence of HPV infection in stage IV HIV-infected homosexual men, along with a 15% incidence of neoplasia. Abnormal cytology was associated with lower CD4+ cell counts (163). Although not as yet a proven association, HIV-positive homosexual men are likely to be at risk for the development of anal cancer (88,162,163).

OTHER DERANGEMENTS RELATED TO HIV INFECTION

AIDS Enteropathy

As discussed above, diarrhea and GI malabsorption are common in patients with AIDS (1,8,14,15,73,88). Although between 50% and 85% of patients with this constellation of symptoms have identifiable bowel pathogens or tumors, there remains a subset of patients in whom no such diseases are present (1,7,8,10–15, 120,205–207). This group of patients has been considered to have AIDS enteropathy (7). Nonspecific histologic changes are common in small bowel tissue samples from these patients and malabsorption of a variety of nutrients including fat, D-xylose, lactose, and vitamins and minerals can occur (1,7,8,120,206–209).

It has been postulated that HIV infection itself, either directly, or by secondary effects on immune function, plays a role in the enteropathy syndrome (7,8,14,206,207). Certain patients with HIV infection develop idiopathic esophageal or colonic ulcerations (210–212). HIV RNA has been found in lymphocytes and mononuclear cells from the base of ulcers in two patients and taken as evidence that HIV may have an etiologic role in the development of these ulcers (212). It is also possible that these cells are innocent bystanders with no direct pathogenic significance. Electron microscopy of these ulcerative lesions was not reported (210–212). HIV RNA has also been detected in the lamina propria of rectal and sigmoid tissue samples (213). However, Fox et al. (213) found that epithelial cells were not involved, with most HIV activity within macrophages. In contrast, Nelson et al. (214) and Levy et al. (215) found HIV-infected cells in gut argentaffin-staining cells, strongly suggesting that enterochromaffin cells are targets of HIV infection. Abnormalities of these cells could theoretically result in diarrhea and malabsorption (214,215).

Another potential mechanism for the AIDS enteropathy syndrome is altered gut immunology (216). Several studies have documented abnormalities of T-cell subpopulations in the GI tract of AIDS patients (216–218). In addition, abnormal activation of epithelial lymphocytes and deficiency of T-mast cells (tryptase-positive mast cells, the predominant type in normal GI mucosa) in gut epithelium of AIDS patients have been described (219,220). Also, a significant decrease in intestinal IgA-containing plasma cells has been reported, although not correlated with specific GI symptoms (221). The exact mechanisms by which these various local immunologic derangements might lead to the enteropathy syndrome are not clear (14,216). Among others, bacterial overgrowth, autoimmunity, and an innocent bystander graft-versus-host-like reaction have been postulated as possible pathogenic mechanisms (7,14,216,218). The latter phenomenon has been reported in other T-cell deficiency states (222,223). Certainly, gastrointestinal disease has long been recognized in association with other immune deficiency states (224–226). The exact pathophysiologic relationships in HIV infection, which will undoubtedly be complex and multifactorial, are still awaiting full elucidation.

Several other factors may also contribute to AIDS enteropathy. One is malnutrition per se. Hypoalbuminemia is common in AIDS patients and has been postulated as a cause of diarrhea (1,227). Protein energy malnutrition per se, often associated with vitamin and mineral deficiencies, can cause GI malabsorption, which could contribute to an AIDS enteropathy (209,228,229). This has important therapeutic implications in the nutritional care of AIDS patients (229).

Finally, it is entirely likely that, as diagnostic tests improve, other heretofore unrecognized pathogens are likely to emerge and cause some cases of AIDS enteropathy to be reclassified (88). Certainly electron microscopy has added greatly to our ability to detect microsporidia (14,120). Similarly, adenovirus has recently been identified in AIDS patients and postulated as a cause for diarrhea (230). It is possible as time progresses that the number of true idiopathic enteropathy cases will diminish.

NUTRITIONAL CONSIDERATIONS IN AIDS

Severe and progressive wasting has long been recognized as a serious complication of HIV infection. The causes are complex and undoubtedly multifactorial, being related to anorexia, GI malabsorption, and altered metabolism due to either opportunistic infection, tumor, or HIV infection per se (1,16,17,209,231,232). Poor nutritional status may directly impact on survival in AIDS (16,209,233). The nutritional support of these patients should be an integral part of overall therapy and should progress in a stepwise fashion according to the clinical needs of the patient (209,232). Every attempt should be made to maintain normal nutrition and address nutritional needs before the onset of severe cachexia.

The first step in this approach is an evaluation of baseline nutritional status and dietary intake (232). Factors capable of affecting the spontaneous intake of a balanced diet should be actively sought. These include obvious medical conditions such as pharyngitis, but should also extend to other domains. Examples include poverty, alcoholism, poor dentition, and depression. Dietary counseling can aid the patient with proper food selection. Oral nutritional supplements may be useful if diet alone is inadequate, but may not be helpful in the individual with anorexia.

Megestrol acetate has been shown to improve intake in some individuals and could be tried in those capable of oral intake but whose consumption is inadequate (234). Enteral feedings should be reserved for individuals showing evidence of progressive malnutrition as demonstrated by weight loss coupled with an inability to consume adequate nutrients spontaneously. Tube feeding may improve nutritional status in AIDS patients, but is often technically difficult to maintain due to diarrhea and other factors (209,235). There are only limited data on the use of total parenteral nutrition (TPN) in HIV-infected patients (209). Nutritional repletion by TPN is possible in some, but not all AIDS patients (209, 236,237). Those with severe infectious complications do not readily replete lean body mass (236). Although clinical improvement may occur, survival advantage has not been shown with parenteral nutrition in AIDS and the frequency of complications, particularly catheter sepsis, can be high (209,236–238). Therefore, although most agree that nutritional support is an important component in the management of AIDS patients, and that poor nutritional status is a comorbid factor, the exact methods and criteria for patient selection for nutritional therapy remain poorly defined (209).

REFERENCES

1. Dworkin BM, Wormser GP, Rosenthal WS, et al. Gastrointestinal manifestations of the acquired immunodeficiency syndrome: a review of 22 cases. *Am J Gastroenterol* 1985;80:774–8.
2. Gelb A, Miller S. AIDS and gastroenterology. *Am J Gastroenterol* 1986;81:619–22.
3. Pape JW, Liautaud B, Thomas F, et al. Characteristics of the acquired immunodeficiency syndrome (AIDS) in Haiti. *N Engl J Med* 1983;309:945–50.
4. Malebranche R, Guerin JM, Laroche AC, et al. Acquired immunodeficiency syndrome with severe gastrointestinal manifestations in Haiti. *Lancet* 1983;2:873–7.
5. Selwyn P. AIDS: what is now known. III. Clinical aspects. *Hosp Pract* 1986;21:119–53.
6. Gottlieb M. Nonneoplastic AIDS syndromes. *Semin Oncol* 1984;11:40–6.
7. Kotler D, Gaetz HP, Lange M, Klein M, Holt P. Enteropathy associated with the acquired immunodeficiency syndrome. *Ann Intern Med* 1984;101:421–8.
8. Gillin JS, Shike M, Alcock N, et al. Malabsorption and mucosal abnormalities of the small intestine in the acquired immunodeficiency syndrome. *Ann Intern Med* 1985;102:619–22.
9. Tunoff EN, Smith PD. Perspectives on gastrointestinal infections in AIDS. *Gastroenterol Clin North Am* 1988;17:451–63.
10. Smith P, Lane C, Gill VJ, et al. Intestinal infections in patients with the acquired immunodeficiency syndrome (AIDS). *Ann Intern Med* 1988;108:328–33.
11. Laughon BE, Druckman DA, Vernon A, et al. Prevalence of enteric pathogens in homosexual men with and without acquired immunodeficiency syndrome. *Gastroenterology* 1988;94:984–93.
12. Rene E, Marche C, Regnier B, et al. Intestinal infections in patients with acquired immunodeficiency syndrome. A prospective study in 132 patients. *Dig Dis Sci* 1989;34:773–80.
13. Rolston KV, Rodriguez S, Hernandez M, Bodey G. Diarrhea in patients infected with the human immunodeficiency virus. *Am J Med* 1989;86:137–8.
14. Greenson JK, Belitosis PC, Yardley JH, Barlett JG. AIDS enteropathy: occult enteric infections and duodenal mucosal alterations in chronic diarrhea. *Ann Intern Med* 1991;114:366–72.
15. Johanson JF, Sonnenberg A. Efficient management of diarrhea in the acquired immunodeficiency syndrome (AIDS). *Ann Intern Med* 1990;112:942–8.
16. Chlebowski RT, Grosvenor MB, Bernhard NH, Morales LS, Bulcavage MB. Nutritional status, gastrointestinal dysfunction and survival in patients with AIDS. *Am J Gastroenterol* 1989;84:1288–93.
17. Dworkin BM, Wormser GP, Axelrod F, Pierre N, Schwarz E, Seaton T. Dietary intake in patients with acquired immunodeficiency syndrome (AIDS), patients with AIDS-related complex, and serologically positive human immunodeficiency virus patients: correlations with nutritional status. *J Parenter Ent Nutrit* 1990;14:605–9.
18. Smith PD. Gastrointestinal infections in patients with acquired immunodeficiency syndrome. *Viewpoints Dig Dis* 1986;18:1–4.
19. Wormser GP, Krupp LB, Hanrahan JP, Gavis G, Spira TJ, Cunningham-Rundles S. Acquired immunodeficiency syndrome in male prisoners. *Ann Intern Med* 1983;98:297–303.
20. Quinn TC. Gastrointestinal manifestations of AIDS. *Prac Gastroenterol* 1985;9:23–4.
21. Kaufman JP. Odynophagia dysphagia in AIDS. *Gastroenterol Clin North Am* 1988;17:599–614.
22. Maayan S, Wormser GP, Hewlett D, et al. Acquired immunodeficiency syndrome (AIDS) in an economically disadvantaged population. *Arch Intern Med* 1985;145:1607–12.
23. Greenspan D, Greenspan J. Oral clinical features of HIV infection. *Gastroenterol Clin North Am* 1988;17:535–43.
24. Haulk AA, Sugar AM. Candida esophagitis. *Adv Intern Med* 1991;36:307–18.
25. Klein RS, Harris CA, Small CB, et al. Oral candidiasis in high-risk patients as the initial manifestation of the acquired immunodeficiency syndrome. *N Engl J Med* 1984;311:354–8.
26. Tavitian A, Ranfaran JF, Rosenthal LE. Oral candidiasis as a marker for esophageal candidiasis in the acquired immunodeficiency syndrome. *Ann Intern Med* 1986;104:54–5.
27. Porro GB, Parente F, Cernuschi M. The diagnosis of esophageal candidiasis in patients with acquired immune deficiency syndrome: is endoscopy always necessary? *Am J Gastroenterol* 1989;84:143–6.
28. Bonacini M, Laine L, Gal A, Lee MH, Martin SE, Strigle S. Prospective evaluation of blind brushing of the esophagus for candida esophagitis in patients with human immunodeficiency virus infection. *Am Coll Gastroenterol* 1990;85:385–9.
29. Walsh TJ, Hamilton SR, Belitsos N. Esophageal candidiasis. Managing an increasingly prevalent infection. *Postgrad Med* 1988;84:193–204.
30. Wall SD, Ominsky S, Altman DF, et al. Multifocal abnormalities of the gastrointestinal tract in AIDS. *AJR* 1986;146:1–5.
31. Levine MS, Macones AJ, Laufen I. Candida esophagitis: accuracy of radiologic diagnosis. *Radiology* 1985;154:581–7.
32. Blackstone MO. *Endoscopic interpretation.* New York: Raven Press, 1984;19–33.
33. Kodsi BE, Wickremesinghe PC, Kozinn PJ, et al. Candida esophagitis: a prospective study of 27 cases. *Gastroenterology* 1976;71:715–9.
34. Tavilian A, Rauffman JP, Rosenthal LE, et al. Ketoconazole resistant candida esophagitis in patients with acquired immunodeficiency syndrome. *Gastroenterology* 1986;90:443–5.
35. Lake-Bakaar G, Tom W, Lake-Bakaar D, et al. Gastropathy and ketoconazole malabsorption in the acquired immunodeficiency syndrome (AIDS). *Ann Intern Med* 1988;109:471–3.
36. Armstrong D, Gold JWM, Dryjanski J, et al. Treatment of infections in patients with the acquired immunodeficiency syndrome. *Ann Intern Med* 1985;103:738–43.
37. Johnson PC, Khardori N, Najjar AF, Butt F, Mansell PWA, Sarosi GA. Progressive disseminated histoplasmosis in patients with acquired immunodeficiency syndrome. *Am J Med* 1988;85:152–8.
38. Gottlieb MS, Groopman JE, Weinstein WM, et al. The acquired immunodeficiency syndrome. *Ann Intern Med* 1983;99:208–20.
39. Fauci AS, Macher AM, Longo DL, et al. Acquired immunodeficiency syndrome: epidemiologic, clinical, immunologic and therapeutic considerations. *Ann Intern Med* 1984;100:92–106.
40. Cunningham AL, Grohman GS, Harkness J, et al. Gastrointestinal viral infections in homosexual men who were symptomatic and seropositive for human immunodeficiency virus. *J Infect Dis* 1988;158:386–91.
41. Kaljot KT, Ling JP, Gold JWM, et al. Prevalence of acute enteric viral pathogens in acquired immunodeficiency syndrome patients with diarrhea. *Gastroenterology* 1989;97:1031–2.
42. Jacobson MA, Mills J. Serious cytomegalovirus disease in the acquired immunodeficiency syndrome (AIDS). Clinical findings, diagnosis and treatment. *Ann Intern Med* 1988;108:585–94.
43. Jacobson MA, O'Donnell JJ, Porteous D, et al. Retinal and gastrointestinal disease due to cytomegalovirus in patients with the acquired immune deficiency syndrome: prevalence, natural history, and response to ganciclovir therapy. *Q J Med* 1988;67:473–86.
44. Francis ND, Boylston AW, Roberts AHG, Parkin JM, Pinching AJ. Cytomegalovirus infection in gastrointestinal tracts of patients infected with HIV-1 or AIDS. *J Clin Pathol* 1989;42:1055–64.
45. Wilcox CM, Diehl DL, Cello JP, et al. CMV esophagitis in patients with AIDS. *Ann Intern Med* 1990;113:589–93.
46. Jacobson MA, Cello JP, Sande MA. Cholestasis and dissemi-

nated cytomegalovirus disease in patients with the acquired immunodeficiency syndrome. *Am J Med* 1988;84:218–24.

47. Wilcox MC, Forsmark CE, Grendell JH, Darragh TM, Cello JP. Cytomegalovirus-associated acute pancreatic disease in patients with acquired immunodeficiency syndrome. Report of two patients. *Gastroenterology* 1990;99:263–7.

48. Weber JN, Thom S, Barrison I, Unwin R, et al. Cytomegalovirus colitis and oesophageal ulceration in the context of AIDS: clinical manifestations and preliminary report of treatment with foscarnet. *Gut* 1987;28:482–7.

49. Yarrish RL. Cytomegalovirus infections. In: Wormser GP, Stahl RE, Bottone EJ (eds). *AIDS and other manifestations of HIV infection.* Park Ridge, NJ: Noyes Publications, 1987;478–517.

50. Reichert CM, O'Leary TJ, Levens DL, Simrell CR, Macher AM. Autopsy pathology in the acquired immune deficiency syndrome. *Am J Pathol* 1983;112:357–82.

51. Welch K, Finkbeiner W, Alpers C, et al. Autopsy findings in the acquired immune deficiency syndrome. *JAMA* 1984;252:1152–9.

52. Guarda LA, Luna MA, Smith JL, Mansell PWA, Gyorkey F, Roca AN. Acquired immune deficiency syndrome: postmortem findings. *Am J Clin Pathol* 1984;81:549–57.

53. Cockerill FR. Diagnosing cytomegalovirus infection. *Mayo Clin Proc* 1985;60:636–8.

54. Levine MS. Interest rising in radiologic diagnosis of esophagitis. *Contemp Gastroenterol* 1990;3:47–56.

55. Balthazow EJ, Megiban AJ, Hirbiek DH, et al. Cytomegalovirus esophagitis in AIDS; radiographic features in 16 patients. *AJR* 1987;149:919.

56. Culpepper-Morgan JA, Kotler DP, Scholes JV, Tierney AR. Evaluation of diagnostic criteria for mucosal cytomegalic inclusion disease in the acquired immune deficiency syndrome. *Am J Gastroenterol* 1987;82:1264–70.

57. Wu GD, Shintaku PI, Chien K, Geller SA. A comparison of routine light microscopy, immunohistochemistry, and in situ hybridization for the detection of cytomegalovirus in gastrointestinal biopsies. 1989;84:1517–20.

58. Quinnan RU, Masur H, Rook AH, et al. Herpes virus infections in the acquired immunodeficiency syndrome. *JAMA* 1984;252:72–7.

59. Wexner SD, Smithy WB, Trillo C, Hopkins BS, Dailey TH. Emergency colectomy for cytomegalovirus ileocolitis in patients with the acquired immune deficiency syndrome. *Dis Colon Rectum* 1988;31:755–61.

60. Teixidor HS, Honig CL, Norsoph E, Albert S, Mouradian JA, Whalen JP. Cytomegalovirus infections of the alimentary canal: radiologic findings with pathologic correlation. *Radiology* 1987;163:317–23.

61. Lumb BJ, Hunt RH. Miscellaneous disorders of the colon. In: Sivak MV (ed). *Gastroenterologic endoscopy.* Philadelphia: WB Saunders Co., 1987;946–59.

62. Blackstone MO. *Endoscopic interpretations.* New York: Raven Press, 1984;495–509.

63. Gertler SL, Pressman J, Price P, et al. Gastrointestinal cytomegalovirus infection in a homosexual man with severe acquired immunodeficiency syndrome. *Gastroenterology* 1983;85:102–6.

63a. Connolly GM. Cytomegalovirus disease of the gastrointestinal tract in AIDS. *Baillieres Clin Gastroenterology* 1990;4:405–23.

63b. Cello JP. Acquired immunodeficiency syndrome cholangiopathy: spectrum of disease. *Am J Med* 1989;86:539–46.

63c. Schneiderman DJ, Celo JP, Laing FC. Papillary stenosis and sclerosing cholangitis in the acquired immunodeficiency syndrome. *Ann Intern Med* 1987;106:546–9.

63d. Viteri AI, Green JF. Bile duct abnormalities in the acquired immunodeficiency syndrome. *Gastroenterology* 1987;92:2014–8.

64. Myers JD. Management of cytomegalovirus infection. *Am J Med* 1988;85:102–6.

65. Hochster H, Dieterich D, Bozzette S, et al. Toxicity of combined ganciclovir and zidovudine for cytomegalovirus disease associated with AIDS. An AIDS Clinical Trials Group Study. *Ann Intern Med* 1990;113:111–7.

66. Dieterich DT, Chachoua A, Lafleur F, Worrell C. Ganciclovir treatment of gastrointestinal infections caused by cytomegalovi-

rus in patients with AIDS. *Rev Infect Dis* 1988;10[Suppl 3]:S532–7.

67. Chachoua A, Dieterich D, Kransinski K, et al. 9-(1,3-Dihydroxy-2-propoxymethyl) guanine (ganciclovir) in the treatment of cytomegalovirus gastrointestinal disease with the acquired immunodeficiency syndrome. *Ann Intern Med* 1987;107:133–7.

68. Drew LW, Miner RC, Busch DF, et al. Prevalence of resistance in patients receiving ganciclovir for serious cytomegalovirus infection. *J Infect Dis* 1991;163:716–9.

69. Weller IVD. The gay bowel. *Gut* 1985;26:869–75.

70. Baker RW, Peppercorn MA. Gastrointestinal ailments of homosexual men. *Medicine* 1982;61:390–405.

71. Quinn TC, Corey L, Chaffee RG, Schuffler MD, Brancato FP, Holmes KK. The etiology of anorectal infections in homosexual men. *Am J Med* 1981;71:395–406.

72. Rene E, Verdon R. Upper Gastrointestinal Infections in AIDS. *Baillieres Clin Gastroenterol* 1990;4:339–59.

73. Kotler DP. Intestinal and Hepatic Manifestations of AIDS. *Adv Intern Med* 1989;34:43–72.

74. Owensby LC, Stammer JL. Esophagitis associated with herpes simplex infection in an immunocompetent host. *Gastroenterology* 1978;74:1305–6.

75. Levine MS, Locuner LA, Saul SH, et al. Herpes esophagitis; sensitivity of double contrast esophagography. *AJR* 1988;154:57.

76. Waye JD. The differential diagnosis of inflammatory and infectious colitis. In: Sivak MV (ed). *Gastroenterologic Endoscopy.* Philadelphia: WB Saunders Co., 1987;881–99.

77. Rein MF. Clinical Approach to Urethritis, mucocutaneous lesions and Inguinal Lymphadenopathy in Homosexual Men. *Med Clin North Am* 1986;70:587–609.

78. Siegal FP, Lopez C, Hammer GS, et al. Severe acquired immunodeficiency in male homosexuals manifested by chronic perianal ulcerative herpes simplex lesions. *N Engl J Med* 1981;305:1439–44.

79. Maier JA, Bergman A, Ross MG. Acquired immunodeficiency syndrome manifested by chronic primary genital herpes. *Am J Obstet Gynecol* 1986;155:756–8.

80. Saral R. Management of mucocutaneous herpes simplex virus infections in immunocompromised patients. *Am J Med* 1988;85[Suppl 2A]:57–60.

81. Erlich K, Mills J, Chatis P, et al. Acyclovir resistant herpes simplex virus infections in patients with the acquired immunodeficiency syndrome. *N Engl J Med* 1989;320:293–6.

82. Safrin S, Assaykeen T, Follansbee S, Mills J. Foscarnet therapy for acyclovir-resistant mucocutaneous herpes simplex virus infection in 26 AIDS patients: preliminary data. *J Infect Dis* 1990;161:1078–84.

83. Kitchen VS, Helbert M, Francis ND, et al. Epstein-Barr virus associated oesophageal ulcers in AIDS. *Gut* 1990;31:1223–5.

84. Greenspan JS, Greenspan D, Lennette ET, et al. Replication of Epstein-Barr virus within the epithelial cells of oral "hairy" leukoplakia, an AIDS-associated lesion. *N Engl J Med* 1985;313:1564–71.

85. Anderson J, Ernberg I. Management of Epstein-Barr virus infections. *Am J Med* 1988;85[suppl 2A]:107–15.

86. Quinn TC. Clinical approach to intestinal infections in homosexual men. *Med Clin North Am* 1986;70:611–34.

87. Smith PD, Janoff EN. Infectious diarrhea in human immunodeficiency virus infection. *Gastroenterol Clin North Am* 1988;17:587–98.

88. Friedman SL, Owen RL. Gastrointestinal manifestations of AIDS and other sexually transmissible diseases. In: Sleisenger MH and Fordtran JS (eds), *Gastrointestinal disease* 4th ed. Philadelphia: WB Saunders Co., 1989;1242–80.

89. Bottone EJ, Wormser GP, Duncanson FP. Nontyphoidal salmonella bacteremia as an early infection in acquired immunodeficiency syndrome. *Diagn Microbiol Infect Dis* 1984;2:247–50.

90. Profeta S, Forrester C, Eng RHK, et al. Salmonella infections in patients with acquired immunodeficiency syndrome. *Arch Intern Med* 1985;145:670–2.

91. Ceium CL, Chaisson RE, Rutherford GW, Barnhart JL. Incidence of salmonellosis in patients with AIDS. *J Infect Dis* 1987;156:998–1001.

92. Heseltine PNR, Causey DM, Appleman MD, Corrados ML, Lee-

dom JM. Norfloxacin in the eradication of enteric infections in AIDS patients. *Eur J Cancer Clin Oncol* 1988;24[Suppl 1]:525–8.

93. Dworkin B, Wormser GP, Abdoo RA, Cabello F, Aguero ME, Sivak SL. Persistence of multiply antibiotic-resistant *Campylobacter jejuni* in a patient with the acquired immune deficiency syndrome. *Am J Med* 1986;80:965–70.

94. Bernard E, Roger PM, Charles D, Bonaldi V, Fournier JP, Dellamonica P. Diarrhea and *Campylobacter* infections in patients infected with the human immunodeficiency virus. *J Infect Dis* 1989;159:143–4.

95. Perlman DM, Ampel NM, Schifman RB, et al. Persistent *Campylobacter jejuni* infections in patients infected with human immunodeficiency virus (HIV). *Ann Intern Med* 1988;108:540–6.

96. Baskin DH, Lax JD, Barenberg D. Shigella bacteremia in patients with the acquired immune deficiency syndrome. *Am J Gastroenterol* 1987;82:338–41.

97. Blaser MJ, Hale TL, Formal SB. Recurrent shigellosis complicating human immunodeficiency virus infection: failure of pre-existing antibodies to confer protection. *Am J Med* 1989; 86:105–7.

98. Green JB, Sidhu GS, Lewin S, et al. *Mycobacterium avium-intracellulare:* a cause of disseminated life-threatening infection in homosexuals and drug abusers. *Ann Intern Med* 1982;97:539–46.

99. Gray JR, Rabeneck L. Atypical mycobacterial infection of the gastrointestinal tract in AIDS patients. *Am J Gastroenterol* 1989;84:1521–4.

100. Gillin SJ, Urmacher C, West R, Shike M. Disseminated *Mycobacterium avium-intracellulare* infection in acquired immunodeficiency syndrome mimicking Whipple's disease. *Gastroenterology* 1983;85:1187–91.

101. Rosengart TK, Coppa GF. Abdominal mycobacterial infections in immunocompromised patients. *Am J Surg* 1990;159:125–31.

102. Maliha GM, Hepps KS, Maria DM, et al. Whipple's disease can mimic chronic AIDS enteropathy. *Am J Gastroenterol* 1991;86:79–81.

103. Klein NC, Duncanson FP, Damsker B. *Mycobacterium avium-intracellulare* infections in AIDS. In: Wormser GP, Stahl RE, Bottone EJ (eds). *AIDS and other manifestations of HIV infection.* Park Ridge, NJ: Noyes Publications, 1987;539–47.

104. Chiu J, Nussbaum J, Bozzette S, et al. Treatment of disseminated *Mycobacterium avium* complex infections in AIDS with amikacin, ethambutol, rifampin, and ciprofloxacin. *Ann Intern Med* 1990;113:358–61.

105. Benson CA, Kessler HA, Pottage JC, Trenholme GM. Successful treatment of acquired immunodeficiency syndrome-related *Mycobacterium avium* complex disease with a multiple drug regimen including amikacin. *Arch Intern Med* 1991;151:582–5.

106. Israel HC. The respiratory system, In: Berk JE (ed). *Bockus Gastroenterology,* 4th ed. Philadelphia: WB Saunders Co., 1985;4584–97.

107. Paustian FF, Marshall JB. Intestinal tuberculosis. In: Berk JE (ed). *Bockus Gastroenterology,* 4th ed. Philadelphia: WB Saunders Co., 1985;2018–36.

108. Tabrisky J, Lindstrom RR, Peters R. Tuberculosis enteritis: a review of a protean disease. *Am J Gastroenterol* 1975;63:49–57.

109. Duncansan FP, Klein NC. Tuberculosis in AIDS. In: Wormser GP, Stahl RE, Bottone EJ (eds). *AIDS and other manifestations of HIV infection.* Park Ridge, NJ: Noyes Publications, 1987;530–8.

110. Sunderam G, McDonald RJ, Maniatis T, Oleske J, Kapila R, Reichman LB. Tuberculosis as a manifestation of the acquired immunodeficiency syndrome (AIDS). *JAMA* 1986;256:362–6.

111. Chodos JE, Dworkin BM, Smith F, Van Horn K, Weiss L, Rosenthal WS. *Campylobacter pylori* and gastroduodenal disease. A prospective endoscopic study and comparison of diagnostic tests. *Am J Gastroenterol* 1988;83:1226–30.

112. Perez-Perez GI, Dworkin BM, Chodos JE, et al. *Campylobacter pylori* antibodies in humans. *Ann Intern Med* 1988;109:11–7.

113. Dworkin BM, Chodos JE, Fernandez ME, et al. Use of plasmid profiles in the investigation of a patient with *Helicobacter pylori* infection and peptic ulcer disease. *Am J Gastroenterol* 1991;86:354–6.

114. Battan R, Raviglione MC, Palagiano A, et al. *Helicobacter pylori* infection in patients with acquired immune deficiency syndrome. *Am J Gastroenterol* 1990;85:1576–9.

115. Meiselman MS, Miller-Catchpole R, Christ M, Randall E. *Campylobacter pylori* gastritis in the acquired immunodeficiency syndrome. *Gastroenterology* 1988;95:209–12.

116. Bartlett JG, Chang TW, Gurwith M, Gorbach SL, Onderdonk AB. Antibiotic-associated pseudomembranous colitis due to toxin-producing clostridia. *N Engl J Med* 1978;298:531–4.

117. Tedesco FJ. Pseudomembranous colitis pathogenesis and therapy. *Med Clin North Am* 1982;66:655–64.

118. Tedesco FJ. Antibiotic associated pseudomembranous colitis with negative proctosigmoidoscopy examination. *Gastroenterology* 1979;77:295–7.

119. Colarian J. *Clostridium difficile* colitis following antiviral therapy in the acquired immunodeficiency syndrome. *Am J Med* 1988;84:1081.

120. Kotler DP, Francisco A, Clayton F, Scholes JV, Orenstein JM. Small intestinal injury and parasitic diseases in AIDS. *Ann Intern Med* 1990;113:444–9.

121. Boyd WP, Brachman BA. Gastrointestinal infections in the compromised host. *Med Clin North Am* 1982;66:743–53.

122. Pearce RB. Intestinal protozoal infections and AIDS. *Lancet* 1983;2:51.

123. Soave R, Johnson WD. Cryotosporidium and *Isospora belli* infections. *J Infect Dis* 1988;157:225–9.

124. Cryptosporidiosis. *Lancet* 1984;1:492–3.

125. Jokipii L, Pohjola S, Jokipii AMM. Cryptosporidium: a frequent finding in patients with gastrointestinal symptoms. *Lancet* 1983;2:358–60.

126. Hunt DA, Shannon R, Palmer SR, Jephcott AE. Cryptosporidiosis in an urban community. *Br Med J* 1984;289:814–5.

127. Current WL, Reese NC, Ernst JV, Bailey WS, Heyman MB, Weinstein WM. Human cryptosporidiosis in immunocompetent and immunodeficient persons. *N Engl J Med* 1983;308:1252–7.

128. Soave R, Danner RL, Honig CL, et al. Cryptosporidiosis in homosexual men. *Ann Intern Med* 1984;100:504–11.

129. Roberts WG, Green PHR, Ma J, Carr M, Ginsberg AM. Prevalence of cryptosporidiosis in patients undergoing endoscopy: evidence of an asymptomatic carrier state. *Am J Med* 1989;87:537–9.

130. Soave R. Cryptosporidiosis in AIDS. In: Wormser GP, Stahl RE, Bottone EJ (eds). *AIDS and Other Manifestations of HIV Infection.* Park Ridge, NJ: Noyes Publications, 1987;713–35.

131. Connolly GM, Dryden MS, Shanson DC, Gazzard BG. Cryptosporidial diarrhoea in AIDS and its treatment. *Gut* 1988;29:593–7.

132. Andreani T, Charpentier YL, Brouet JC, et al. Acquired immunodeficiency with intestinal cryptosporidiosis; possible transmission by Haitian whole blood. *Lancet* 1983;1:1187–91.

133. Dobbins WO, Weinstein WM. Electron microscopy of the intestine and rectum in acquired immunodeficiency syndrome. *Gastroenterology* 1985;88:738–49.

134. Margulis SJ, Honig CL, Soave R, et al. Biliary tract obstruction in the acquired immunodeficiency syndrome. *Ann Intern Med* 1986;105:207–10.

135. Cappell MS. Hepatobiliary manifestations of the acquired immune deficiency syndrome. *Am J Gastroenterol* 1991;86:1–15.

136. Mittenberg DF, Miller NW, Vander Ende J. Spiramycin is not effective in treating cryptosporidium diarrhea in infants. *J Infect Dis* 1989;159:131–2.

137. Cook DJ, Keltan JG, Stanisz AM, et al. Somatostatin treatment for cryptosporidial diarrhea in AIDS. *Ann Intern Med* 1988;108:708–9.

138. Ungar BLP, Ward DJ, Fayer R, Quinn CA. Cessation of cryptosporidium-associated diarrhea in an acquired immunodeficiency syndrome patient after treatment with hyperimmune bovine colostrum. *Gastroenterology* 1990;98:486–9.

139. Greenberg RE, Mir R, Bank S, Siegal FP. Resolution of intestinal cryptosporidiosis after treatment of AIDS with AZT. *Gastroenterology* 1989;97:1327–0.

140. Sogni P. Treatment of intestinal cryptosporidiosis in AIDS. *Gastroenterology* 1990;99:602–9.

141. Connolly GM, Shanson D, Hawkins DA, Webster JN, Gazzard BG. Non-cryptosporidial diarrhoea in human immunodeficiency virus (HIV) infected patients. *Gut* 1989;30:195–200.

142. DeHovitz JA, Pape JW, Boncy M, Johnson WD. Clinical mani-

festations and therapy of *Isospora belli* infection in patients with the acquired immunodeficiency syndrome. *N Engl J Med* 1986;315:87–90.

143. Ma P, Kaufman D. *Isospora belli* diarrheal infection in homosexual men. *AIDS Res* 1984;1:327–38.

144. Thomson RB, Haas RA. Intestinal parasites: the necessity of examining multiple stool specimens. *Mayo Clin Proc* 1984;59:641–2.

145. Romeu J, Clotet B, Tural C, Carles J, Roz M. Therapeutic challenge for *Isospora belli* enteritis in an AIDS patient who developed Lyell syndrome after co-trimoxazole therapy. *Am J Gastroenterol* 1989;84:207–9.

146. Berquist A, Morfeldt-Monsan L, Pehpson PO, et al. Antibody against *Encephalitozoon cuniculi* in Swedish homosexual men. *Scand J Infect Dis* 1984;16:389–91.

147. Rupstone AC, Canning EU, Vankete RJ, et al. Use of light microscopy to diagnose small-intestinal microsporidiosis in patients with AIDS. *J Infect Dis* 1988;157:827–31.

148. Modigliani R, Bories C, Charpentier YL, et al. Diarrhoea and malabsorption in acquired immune deficiency syndrome: a study of four cases with special emphasis on opportunistic protozoan infections. *Gut* 1985;26:179–87.

149. Orenstein JM, Chiang J, Steinberg W, et al. Intestinal microsporidiosis as a cause of diarrhea in human immunodeficiency virus-infected patients: a report of 20 cases. *Hum Pathol* 1990;21:475–81.

150. Wolfe MS. Giardiasis. *N Engl J Med* 1978;298:319–21.

151. Ament ME, Rubin CE. Relation of giardiasis to abnormal intestinal structure and function in gastrointestinal immunodeficiency syndromes. *Gastroenterology* 1972;62:216–26.

152. Hartong WA, Gourley WK, Arvanitakis C. Giardiasis: clinical spectrum and functional-structural abnormalities of the small intestinal mucosa. *Gastroenterology* 1979;77:61–9.

153. Battles against giardia in gut mucosa. *Lancet* 1982;2:2527–8.

154. Krogstad DJ, Spencer HC, Healy GR. Amebiasis. *N Engl J Med* 1978;298:262–5.

155. Adams EB, MacLeod IN. Invasive amebiasis. *Medicine* 1977;56:315–34.

156. Blumerman H, Kaser L, Rowen J, et al. Role of endoscopy in suspected amebiasis. *Am J Gastroenterol* 1983;78:15–8.

157. Rosenblatt JE, Edson RS. Metronidazole. *Mayo Clin Proc* 1983;58:154–7.

158. Maayan S, Wormser GP, Widerhorn J, Sy ER, Kim EH, Ernst JA. *Strongyloides stercoralis* hyperinfection in a patient with the acquired immune deficiency syndrome. *Am J Med* 1987;83:945–7.

159. Armignacco O, Capecchi A, DeMori P, Spallanzani OL, Grillo LR. *Strongyloides stercoralis* hyperinfection and the acquired immunodeficiency syndrome. *Am J Med* 1989;86:258.

160. Filipovich AH, Spector B, Kersey J. Immunodeficiency in humans as a risk factor in the development of malignancy. *Prev Med* 1980;9:252–9.

161. Kaplan MH, Susin M, Pahwa SG, et al. Neoplastic complications of HTLV-III Infection. *Am J Med* 1987;82:389–96.

162. Fordman SL. Gastrointestinal and hepatobiliary neoplasms in AIDS. *Gastroenterol Clin North Am* 1988;17:465–86.

163. Palefsky MD, Gonzales J, Greenblatt RM, Ahn DK, Hollander H. Anal intraepithelial neoplasia and anal papillomavirus infection among homosexual males with group IV HIV disease. *JAMA* 1990;263:2911–6.

164. Volberding PA. Kaposi's sarcoma and the acquired immunodeficiency syndrome. *Med Clin North Am* 70:665–75.

165. Hymes KB, Kaposi's sarcoma. In: Wormser GP, Stahl RE, Bottone EJ (eds). *AIDS and other manifestations of HIV infection*. Park Ridge, NJ: Noyes Publications, 1987.

166. Ahmed T. Tumors associated with AIDS. In: Wormser GP, Stahl RE, Bottone EJ (ed). *AIDS and other manifestations of HIV infection*. Park Ridge, NJ: Noyes Publications, 1987;736–46.

167. LaRaja RD, Rothenberg RE, Odom JW, Mueller SC. The incidence of intra-abdominal surgery in acquired immunodeficiency syndrome: a statistical review of 904 patients. *Surgery* 1989;105:175–9.

168. Barone JE, Gingold BS, Nealon TF, Arvanitis ML. Abdominal pain in patients with acquired immune deficiency syndrome. *Ann Surg* 1986;204:619–23.

169. Wexner SD, Smithy WB, Milson JW, Dailey TH. The surgical management of anorectal diseases in AIDS and pre-AIDS patients. *Dis Colon Rectum* 1986;29:719–23.

170. Wilson SE, Robinson G, Williams RA, et al. Acquired immune deficiency syndrome (AIDS). Indications for abdominal surgery, pathology and outcome. *Ann Surg* 1989;210:428–34.

171. Macho JR. Gastrointestinal surgery in the AIDS patient. *Gastroenterol Clin North Am* 1988;17:563–71.

172. Cello JP, Wilcox CM. Evaluation and treatment of GI tract hemorrhage in patients with AIDS. *Gastroenterol Clin North Am* 1988;17:639–48.

173. Ranfuman JF, Straus EW. Endoscopic procedures in the AIDS patient: risks, precautions, indications and obligations. *Gastroenterol Clin North Am* 1988;17:495–586.

174. Des Jarlais DC, Marmor M, Thomas P, Chamberland M, Zolla-Pazner S, Sencer DJ. Kaposi's sarcoma among four different AIDS risk groups. *N Engl J Med* 1984;310:1119–20.

175. Friedman-Kien AE, Laubenstein LJ, Rubinstein P, et al. Disseminated Kaposi's sarcoma in homosexual men. *Ann Intern Med* 1982;96:693–700.

176. Jaffe HW, Choi K, Thomas PA, et al. National case-control study of Kaposi's sarcoma and *Pneumocystis carinii* pneumonia in homosexual men. Part 1, Epidemiologic results. *Ann Intern Med* 1983;99:145–51.

177. Rogers MF, Morens DM, Stewart JA, et al. National case-control study of Kaposi's sarcoma and *Pneumocystis carinii* pneumonia in homosexual men: Part 2, Laboratory results. *Ann Intern Med* 1983;99:152–8.

178. Safai B, Johnson KG, Myskowski PL, et al. The natural history of Kaposi's sarcoma in the acquired immunodeficiency syndrome. *Ann Intern Med* 1985;103:744–50.

179. Saltz RK, Kurtz RC, Lightdale CJ. Kaposi's sarcoma; gastrointestinal involvement and correlation with skin findings and immunologic function. *Dig Dis Sci* 1984;29:817–23.

180. Biggs BA, Crowe SM, Lucas CR, et al. AIDS related Kaposi's sarcoma presenting as ulcerative colitis and complicated by toxic megacolon. *Gut* 1987;28:1302–6.

181. Khan AA, Ravalli S, Vincent RA, et al. Primary Kaposi's sarcoma simulating hemorrhoids in a patient with acquired immune deficiency syndrome. *Am J Gastroenterol* 1989;84:1592–3.

182. Lustbader I, Sherman A. Primary gastrointestinal Kaposi's sarcoma in a patient with acquired immune deficiency syndrome. *Am J Gastroenterol* 1987;82:894–5.

183. Friedman SL, Wright TC, Altman DF. Gastrointestinal Kaposi's sarcoma in patients with acquired immunodeficiency syndrome. Endoscopic and autopsy findings. *Gastroenterology* 1985;89:102–8.

184. Wall SD. Gastrointestinal imaging in AIDS—luminal gastrointestinal tract. *Gastroenterol Clin North Am* 1988;17:523–33.

185. Jeffrey RB. Gastrointestinal imaging in AIDS—abdominal computed tomography and ultrasound. *Gastroenterol Clin North Am* 1988;17:507–21.

186. Blackstone MO. *Endoscopic interpretation*. New York: Raven Press, 1984;155–7.

187. Volberding P, Conant MA, Sticker RB, et al. Chemotherapy in advanced Kaposi's sarcoma. *Am J Med* 1983;74:652–6.

188. Krown SE, Real FX, Cunningham-Rundles S, et al. Preliminary observations on the effect of recombinant leukocyte alpha interferon in homosexual men with Kaposi's sarcoma. *N Engl J Med* 1983;308:1071–6.

189. Knowles DM, Chamulak GA, Subar M, et al. Lymphoid neoplasia associated with the acquired immunodeficiency syndrome (AIDS). *Ann Intern Med* 1988;108:744–53.

190. Ziegler JL, Bedstead JA, Volberding PA, et al. Non-Hodgkin's lymphoma in 90 homosexual men. Relationship to generalized lymphadenopathy and the acquired immunodeficiency syndrome. *N Engl J Med* 1984;311:565–70.

191. Ioachim HL, Weinstein MA, Robbins RD, et al. Primary anorectal lymphoma. A new manifestation of the acquired immune deficiency syndrome (AIDS). *Cancer* 1987;60:1449–53.

192. Morrison JG, Scharfenberg JC, Timmcke AE. Perianal lym-

phoma as a manifestation of the acquired immune deficiency syndrome. *Dis Colon Rectum* 1989;32:521–3.

193. Steinberg JJ, Bridges N, Feiner HD, et al. Small intestinal lymphoma in three patients with acquired immune deficiency syndrome. *Am J Gastroenterol* 1985;80:21–6.

194. Bernal A, del Junco GW. Endoscopic and pathologic features of esophageal lymphoma: a report of four cases in patients with acquired immune deficiency syndrome. *Gastrointest Endosc* 1986;32:96–9.

195. Burkes L, Meyer PR, Gill PS, et al. Rectal lymphoma in homosexual men. *Arch Intern Med* 1986;146:913–5.

196. Ciobanu N, Andreeff M, Safai B, et al. Lymphoblastic neoplasia in a homosexual patient with Kaposi's sarcoma. *Ann Intern Med* 1983;98:151–5.

197. Burkes RL, Gal AA, Stewart ML, et al. Simultaneous occurrence of *Pneumocystis carinii* pneumonia, cytomegalovirus infection, Kaposi's sarcoma and B-immunoblastic sarcoma in a homosexual man. *JAMA* 1985;253:3425–8.

198. Wormser G. Multiple opportunistic infections and neoplasms in the acquired immunodeficiency syndrome. *JAMA* 1985;253:3441–2.

199. Dworkin B, Lightdale CJ, Weingrad DN, et al. Primary gastric lymphoma. A review of 50 cases. *Dig Dis Sci* 1982;27:986–92.

200. Mitsuyasu RT, Colman F. Simultaneous occurrence of Hodgkin's disease and Kaposi's sarcoma in a patient with the acquired immune deficiency syndrome. *Am J Med* 1986;80:954–8.

201. Schwartz MS, Brandt LJ. The spectrum of pancreatic disorders in patients with the acquired immune deficiency syndrome. *Am J Gastroenterol* 1989;84:459–62.

202. Wexner SD, Milsam JW, Dailey TH. The demographics of anal cancers are changing; identification of a high-risk population. *Dis Colon Rectum* 1987;30:942–6.

203. Sonnabend J, Witkin ST, Purtilo DT. Acquired immunodeficiency syndrome, opportunistic infections, and malignancies in male homosexuals. A hypothesis of etiologic factors in pathogenesis. *JAMA* 1983;249:2370–4.

204. Frazer IH, Medley G, Crapper RM, et al. Association between anorectal dysplasia, human papillomavirus and human immunodeficiency virus infection in homosexual men. *Lancet* 1986;2:657–60.

205. Diarrhea and malabsorption associated with the acquired immunodeficiency syndrome (AIDS). *Nutr Rev* 1985;43:235–7.

206. Ullrich R, Zeitz M, Heise W, et al. Small intestinal structure and function in patients infected with human immunodeficiency virus (HIV): evidence for HIV-induced enteropathy. *Ann Intern Med* 1989;111:15–21.

207. Miller ARO, Griffin GE, Batman P, et al. Jejunal mucosal architecture and fat absorption in male homosexuals infected with human immunodeficiency virus. *Q J Med* 1988;69:1009–19.

208. Harriman GR, Smith PD, Horne MK, et al. Vitamin B12 malabsorption in patients with acquired immunodeficiency syndrome. *Arch Intern Med* 1989;149:2039–41.

209. Raiten DJ. Nutrition and HIV infection. Life Sciences Research Office. *Fed Am Soc Exp Biol* 1990;17–54.

210. Bach MC, Howell DA, Valenti AJ, et al. Aphthous ulceration of the gastrointestinal tract in patients with the acquired immunodeficiency syndrome (AIDS). *Ann Intern Med* 1990;112:465–6.

211. Pedro-Botet J, Miralles R, Sauleda J, et al. Idiopathic ulcer of the esophagus in the AIDS syndrome: a potential life-threatening complication. *Gastrointest Endosc* 1989;35:470–1.

212. Kotler DP, Wilson CS, Haroutiounian G, et al. Detection of human immunodeficiency virus-1 by ^{35}S-RNA in situ hybridization in solitary esophageal ulcers in two patients with the acquired immune deficiency syndrome. *Am J Gastroenterol* 1989;84:313–7.

213. Fox CH, Kotler D, Tierney A, et al. Detection of HIV-1 in the lamina propria of patients with AIDS and gastrointestinal disease. *J Infect Dis* 1989;159:467–71.

214. Nelson JA, Reynolds-Kohler C, Margaretten W, et al. Human immunodeficiency virus detected in bowel epithelium from patients with gastrointestinal symptoms. *Lancet* 1988;1:259–62.

215. Levy JA, Margaretten W, Nelson J. Detection of HIV in enterochromaffin cells in the rectal mucosa of an AIDS patient. *Am J Gastroenterol* 1989;84:787–9.

216. Rodgers VD, Kagnoff MF. Abnormalities of the intestinal immune system in AIDS. *Gastroenterol Clin North Am* 1988;17:487–94.

217. Rodgers VD, Fassett R, Kagnoff MF. Abnormalities in intestinal mucosal T cells in homosexual populations including those with the lymphadenopathy syndrome and acquired immunodeficiency syndrome. *Gastroenterology* 1986;90:552–8.

218. Budhraja M, Levendoglu H, Kocka F, et al. Duodenal mucosal T cell subpopulation and bacterial cultures in acquired immune deficiency syndrome. *Am J Gastroenterol* 1987;82:427–31.

219. Weber JR, Dobbins WO. The intestinal and rectal epithelial lymphocyte in AIDS. An electron-microscopic study. *Am J Surg Pathol* 1986;10:627–39.

220. Irani AA, Craig SS, DeBlois G, et al. Deficiency of the tryptase-positive, chymase-negative mast cell type in gastrointestinal mucosa of patients with defective T lymphocyte function. *J Immunol* 1987;138:4381–6.

221. Kotler DP, Scholes JV, Tiernay AR. Intestinal plasma cell alterations in acquired immunodeficiency syndrome. *Dig Dis Sci* 1987;32:129–38.

222. Snover DC, Filipovich AH, Ramsay NKC, et al. Graft-versus-host-disease-like histopathological findings in pre-bone-marrow transplantation biopsies of patients with severe T cell deficiency. *Transplantation* 1985;39:95–7.

223. Elson CO, Reilly RW, Rosenberg IH. Small intestinal injury in the graft versus host reaction: an innocent bystander phenomenon. *Gastroenterology* 1977;72:886–9.

224. Hermans PE, Diaz-Buxo JA, Stobo JD. Idiopathic late-onset immunoglobulin deficiency. Clinical Observations in 50 patients. *Am J Med* 1976;61:221–37.

225. Ament ME, Ochs HD, Davis SD. Structure and function of the gastrointestinal tract in primary immunodeficiency syndromes. A study of 39 patients. *Medicine* 1973;52:227–48.

226. Ross IN, Asquith P. Primary immune deficiency. In: Asquith P (ed). *Immunology of the GI tract*. New York: Churchill Livingston, 1979;152–62.

227. Brinson RR. Hypoalbuminemia, diarrhea, and the acquired immunodeficiency syndrome. *Ann Intern Med* 1985;102:413.

228. Tornn B, Viteri FE. Protein-energy malnutrition. In: Shils ME, Young VR (eds). *Modern nutrition in health and disease*. Philadelphia: Lee & Febiger, 1988;746–73.

229. Benkov KD, Stawski C, Storlin SM, et al. Atypical presentation of childhood acquired immune deficiency syndrome mimicking Crohn's disease: nutritional considerations and management. *Am J Gastroenterol* 1985;80:260–5.

230. Janoff EN, Orenstein JM, Manischewitz JF, et al. Adenovirus colitis in the acquired immunodeficiency syndrome. *Gastroenterology* 1991;100:976–9.

231. Greene JB. Clinical approach to weight loss in the patient with HIV infection. *Gastroenterol Clin North Am* 1988;17:573–86.

232. Hickey MS, Weaver KE. Nutritional management of patients with ARC or AIDS. *Gastroenterol Clin North Am* 1988;17:545–61.

233. Kotler DP, Tierney AR, Wang J, et al. Magnitude of body cell mass depletion and the timing of death from wasting in AIDS. *Am J Clin Nutr* 1989;50:444–7.

234. Von Roenn JH, Murphy RL, Weber KM, et al. Megestrol acetate for treatment of cachexia associated with human immunodeficiency virus (HIV) infection. *Ann Intern Med* 1988;109:840–1.

235. Kotler DP, Tierney AR, Ferrano R, et al. Enteral alimentation and repletion of body cell mass in malnourished patients with acquired immunodeficiency syndrome. *Am J Clin Nutr* 1991;53:149–54.

236. Kotler DP, Tierney AR, Culpepper-Morgan JA, et al. Effect of home total parenteral nutrition on body composition in patients with acquired immunodeficiency syndrome. *J Parenter Ent Nutr* 1990;14:454–8.

237. Singer P, Rothkopf MM, Kvetan V, et al. Risks and benefits of home parenteral nutrition in the acquired immunodeficiency syndrome. *JPEN* 1991;15:75–9.

238. Raviglione MC, Battan R, Pablos-Mendez A, et al. Infections associated with Hickman catheters in patients with acquired immunodeficiency syndrome. *Am J Med* 1989;86:780–6.

AIDS and Other Manifestations of HIV Infection,
Second Edition, Edited by Gary P. Wormser.
Raven Press, Ltd., New York © 1992.

CHAPTER 27

Cryptosporidiosis, Isosporiasis, and Microsporidiosis in AIDS

Abdollah Bijan Naficy and Rosemary Soave

CRYPTOSPORIDIOSIS IN AIDS

In 1981–1982, 47 patients with the acquired immunodeficiency syndrome (AIDS) and cryptosporidiosis were reported to the Centers for Disease Control (CDC) (1). Cryptosporidiosis with diarrhea persisting for more than 1 month was subsequently incorporated into the surveillance definition of AIDS, as proposed by CDC. Prior to 1981, only seven human cases of cryptosporidiosis had been reported, mostly in immunocompromised patients (2–8). Improved methods for diagnosis introduced since the AIDS epidemic have led to reports of cryptosporidiosis in animal handlers (9), travelers (10,11), and immunocompetent hosts (12), and to an appreciation of the organism's distribution worldwide (13–16).

Cryptosporidium, a coccidian protozoan, was first described and named by Tyzzer in 1907 when he identified it in the gastric glands of asymptomatic laboratory mice (17). The name *Cryptosporidium,* Greek for *hidden spore,* denotes an organism with spores (sporozoites) concealed within an oocyst. Initially thought to be a benign commensal of animals, it was first recognized as a cause of diarrhea in poultry in 1955 (18). Subsequently, *Cryptosporidium* was found to cause disease in several other animal species and is currently responsible for major agricultural losses each year (14–16,19).

The Organism

The life cycle of *Cryptosporidium* (Fig. 1) differs from that of other coccidia in that it occurs entirely within a

single host (monoxenous). Infection is initiated by the ingestion or perhaps inhalation (20,21) of oocysts. The oocyst is 2–5 μm in diameter and when fully mature (sporulated) contains four naked (no sporocyst) sporozoites (Fig. 2). With appropriate environmental conditions, dissolution of the oocyst wall results in the release (excystation) of the thin, flat, elliptical sporozoites (Fig. 3). The sporozoites move by gliding and flexing and implant within the host epithelial cell, where they develop into trophozoites, in a unique intracellular but extracytoplasmic position (Fig. 4). Sporozoites have an apical complex at their anterior end. This complex contains electron-dense organelles that may have a secretory function during penetration of the host cell. Asexual multiplication (merogony) ensues with the formation of type I and type II meronts (schizonts). Type I meronts release six to eight merozoites that can reinvade uninfected host cells and repeat merogony or alternatively, develop into type II meronts. Type II meronts release four merozoites that differentiate into micro (male) and macro (female) gametocytes and initiate sexual multiplication (gametogony). Aflagellar but motile microgametes fertilize macrogametes that develop into diploid oocysts that can either reinfect the same host or exit in search of a new host. Thin-walled oocysts are reported to reinfect, whereas the more numerous hardy thick-walled oocysts are expelled into the environment (22). It is this great potential for reinfection within a single host that provides the mechanism for the sustained infection manifested by the immunocompromised host.

The genus *Cryptosporidium* has been classified in the phylum Apicomplexa, class Sporozoasida, subclass Coccidiasina, order Eucoccidiorida, suborder Eimeriorina (23). Other related protozoa within the suborder Eimeriorina include *Isospora, Toxoplasma, Sarcocystis,* and *Eimeria* species. Several species of *Cryptosporidium* were named according to the host in which they were

---

A. B. Naficy: Division of Infectious Diseases, Elmhurst Hospital, Elmhurst, New York 11373.

R. Soave: Division of Infectious Diseases, The New York Hospital-Cornell Medical Center, New York, New York 10021.

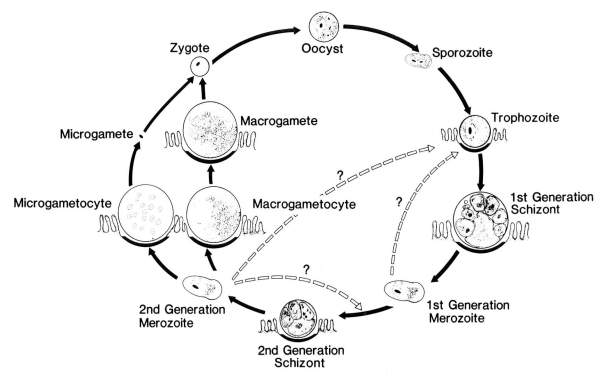

FIG. 1. Proposed life cycle of *Cryptosporidium.* From Navin and Juranek (58).

identified. Cross-transmission studies have demonstrated an absence of host specificity (24). Based upon oocyst size, two different species have been reported to infect cattle (25). The smaller *C. parvum* is considered the cause of infection in humans.

Epidemiology

Transmission of *Cryptosporidium* to humans can be from animals (9,26,27), from fecal contamination of water (28–30), or from person-to-person (fecal–oral)

spread, as reported in day care center attendees (14,31–34), household contacts of index cases (11,12,19,32,35), hospitalized patients, and health care personnel (36–39). Transmission by fomites and house flies has been speculated (40).

Contamination of environmental waters has been found in several states (41,42) as well as in treated and untreated sewage (43). *Cryptosporidium* oocysts are resistant to chlorination and numerous disinfectants including 5% formaldehyde, iodophor, 2–5% sodium hypochlorite, cresylic acid, and benzalkonium chloride. Prolonged treatment (18 hours) with bleach, heating at 65°C or freezing below 0°C for 30 minutes, or 10% for-

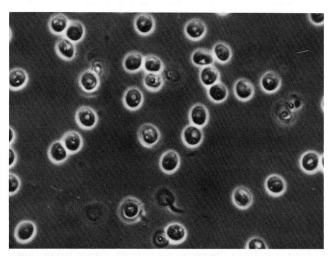

FIG. 2. Human stool-derived *Cryptosporidium* oocysts. Phase contrast, ×630.

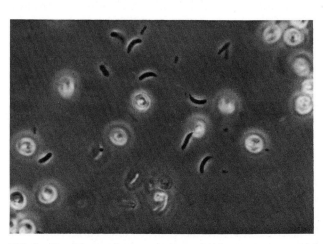

FIG. 3. *Cryptosporidium* sporozoites. Phase contrast, ×630.

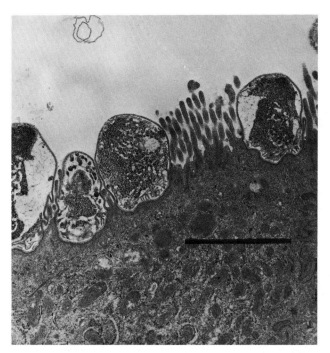

FIG. 4. Endogenous stages of *Cryptosporidium* in the brush border of the small intestine of an AIDS patient. Scale bar = 5 μm; ×10,000.

malin combined with either bleach or 5% ammonia appear to eliminate infectivity (14,19).

The true prevalence of human cryptosporidiosis is not known. Estimates vary according to the population studied, and can differ within the same population as a function of the diagnostic techniques that are used. In industrialized countries, infection is estimated to occur in approximately 2.5% of individuals with diarrhea and less than 1% of asymptomatic individuals. In developing countries, these estimates increase to approximately 8% and 3.5%, respectively (34,40). Prevalence rates fall with increasing age. In patients with AIDS, prevalence rates from 3% to 16% have been reported within the United States, and up to 41% in other nations such as Haiti (40,44,45).

Clinical Manifestations

The incubation period for human cryptosporidiosis appears to be between 2 and 14 days. The spectrum of clinical illness is quite variable, ranging from asymptomatic carriage to fulminant cholera-like enteritis. The predominant symptoms of infection include watery diarrhea, cramping abdominal pain, weight loss, anorexia, flatulence, and malaise. A variety of other complaints, such as nausea, vomiting, myalgias, and fever may also be present. Intermittent exacerbations often occur, sometimes following the ingestion of food. Physical examination may reveal signs of dehydration. Blood and leuko-

cytes are usually absent in feces. The severity and duration of illness are determined by the status of the host's immunologic defenses (9,12–16,46,47). Typically, for the immunocompetent host, symptoms have an explosive onset and last for approximately 2 weeks (12). Fecal clearance of the parasite frequently lags behind clinical resolution of illness by 1–2 weeks (48). Certain hosts, e.g., malnourished children, may have a protracted illness requiring hospitalization.

In patients with AIDS or other types of immunocompromise (e.g., congenital), the onset of illness is insidious and there is an inexorable progression as immune function deteriorates (3,4,47,49). Symptoms may include frequent (up to 25), voluminous (up to 25 liters) daily bowel movements, severe abdominal pain, and significant weight loss (>25% of the total body weight). Hospitalization is often required for dehydration, electrolyte imbalance, and cachexia.

AIDS patients with biliary cryptosporidiosis present with right upper quadrant and epigastric abdominal pain, nausea, and vomiting. Jaundice and hepatomegaly are usually absent (49–52). Respiratory cryptosporidiosis has been described in AIDS patients with pulmonary symptoms. The parasite has been detected in sputum or attached to bronchial epithelium; however, it may be that access to the bronchial tree occurred secondary to contamination from the gastrointestinal tract (53–56).

Pathology and Pathogenesis

Cryptosporidia have been detected in the pharynx, esophagus, stomach, duodenum, small intestine, appendix, colon, rectum (3–8,13–16,47,49,50,57–59), gallbladder, pancreas, and bile and pancreatic ducts (49–52,60,61), in colonic submucosal blood vessels (62), and within the respiratory tract (53–56) of immunocompromised patients (Fig. 5).

Intestinal histological changes include blunting or loss of villi, fusion of some villi, lengthening of the crypts, and infiltration of the lamina propria with lymphocytes, polymorphonuclear leukocytes, and plasma cells. These nonspecific changes are variable and do not correlate with the severity of infection. Electron microscopy reveals that during merogony and gametogony the parasite is separated from the cytoplasm of the enterocyte by a parasitophorous vacuole membrane and a sheet of microfilaments (63,64) (Fig. 4).

In patients with biliary cryptosporidiosis, organisms are found in bile and adherent to gallbladder epithelium. Usually there is edema, lymphocytic infiltration, and destruction of the underlying mucosa (49–52). At times, concomitant infection with cytomegalovirus is present (51,52). Although *Cryptosporidium* has been detected in specimens from the respiratory tract, concomitant gastrointestinal involvement and the presence of other pul-

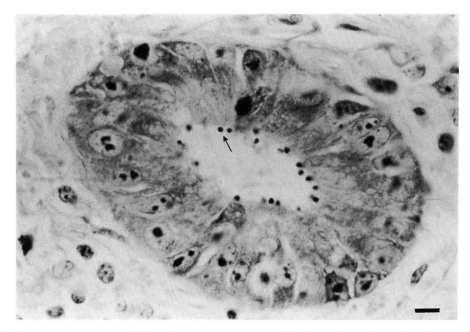

FIG. 5. Numerous cryptosporidial bodies (*arrow*) on crypt epithelium of small intestine. Scale bar = 20 μm; Giemsa stain.

monary pathogens makes it difficult to distinguish true infection from colonization or contamination (53–56). Neither biliary nor pulmonary cryptosporidiosis has been described in immunocompetent individuals.

The pathogenetic mechanism whereby *Cryptosporidium* causes disease is unknown. The voluminous secretory diarrhea suggests an enterotoxin-mediated mechanism; however, malabsorption associated with physical destruction of the brush border may also play a role.

Diagnosis

Microscopic examination of intestinal tissue biopsy specimens is no longer necessary for a diagnosis of intestinal cryptosporidiosis (Fig. 5). Since 1981, there have been numerous reports of different staining techniques for detecting the oocysts of *Cryptosporidium* in fecal smears (1,48,65–71). Most popular have been several modifications of the acid-fast technique that differentiate red staining cryptosporidial oocysts from the morphologically similar but non-acid-fast yeasts that stain green. Despite some variability in stain uptake, experienced observers have little difficulty in detecting the oocysts. Recently, a sensitive and specific direct fluorescent antibody stain that uses a murine monoclonal antibody (IgG) against the oocyst wall became available commercially (72,73). Studies comparing the sensitivity and specificity of the various staining techniques on stool samples with histologic findings on intestinal biopsy material have not been performed. The number of negative stool specimens required to exclude cryptosporidial infection

reliably is also unknown. As oocyst excretion can be intermittent, and because the limits of detection have not been characterized, at least two specimens should be stained (48). Concentration techniques such as zinc sulfate or Sheather's sucrose flotation optimize oocyst detection in specimens in which they are scarce (e.g., asymptomatic contacts and environmental samples). These techniques, which pose a risk of exposure by aerosolization, are usually not necessary for diagnosis during acute, severe illness.

Utilizing immunofluorescent and enzyme-linked immunosorbent assays (IFA and ELISA), serum antibodies to cryptosporidia have been detected in immunocompetent and immunocompromised hosts (74). With the IgG and IgM ELISA, 95% of patients presenting with cryptosporidiosis (including patients with AIDS) were found to have detectable antibody (75). Although the ELISA is not helpful in the immediate diagnosis of acute illness, it should be useful in epidemiologic studies.

Nonspecific findings associated with cryptosporidial enteritis include steatorrhea, D-xylose, and vitamin B_{12} malabsorption, reversible lactose intolerance, and radiographic features consistent with disordered motility and malabsorption (e.g., barium flocculation, mucosal thickening, and small bowel dilatation).

With biliary cryptosporidiosis, serum levels of alkaline phosphatase and γ-glutamyl transpeptidase are elevated, while serum bilirubin and transaminase levels remain normal. Radiographic findings include a dilated gallbladder with thickened walls and dilated bile ducts with luminal irregularities resembling sclerosing cholangitis.

Treatment

Currently there is no known efficacious therapy for human cryptosporidiosis. Supportive management via fluid and electrolyte replacement is essential. Termination of iatrogenic immunosuppression such as with corticosteroids leads to resolution of infection. Because of the accelerated wasting that is associated with chronic infection in AIDS patients, parenteral hyperalimentation can provide significant palliation. In cases of lactose intolerance, dietary control measures often lead to symptomatic improvement. Antidiarrheal agents such as kaolin plus pectin, bismuth subsalicylate, loperamide, diphenoxylate, or opiates have varying degrees of efficacy from patient to patient and for the same individual over time. Whether motility-altering agents are safe for *Cryptosporidium*-infected individuals has not been determined. Several patients have responded to parenteral administration of the long-acting somatostatin analog octreotide acetate. Some of these patients were coinfected with the Microsporidium, *Enterocytozoon bieneusi*. In patients with biliary cryptosporidiosis, transient improvement of symptoms and laboratory abnormalities has been observed following cholecystectomy or endoscopic papillotomy.

A variety of antimicrobial and immunomodulating agents have been administered to *Cryptosporidium*-infected AIDS patients with widely variable results (76).

Despite some improvement with the ornithine decarboxylase inhibitor α-difluoromethylornithine (DFMO), severe bone marrow and gastrointestinal toxicity has limited further studies (77). There have been numerous anecdotal reports of success with paromomycin, and controlled studies using this drug are currently being planned (77a).

Anecdotal reports of success with oral spiramycin (78) have not been confirmed in a placebo-controlled trial. Pharmacokinetic data suggest that the poor bioavailability of oral spiramycin may have contributed to the lack of efficacy. This prompted a single-blind placebo-controlled study of intravenous spiramycin that was sponsored by the National Institutes of Health AIDS Clinical Trials Group Program. The study has recently been completed and is undergoing analysis. Also recently terminated was a study of the benzeneacetonitrile derivative diclazuril. This drug, which is useful for the prevention of poultry coccidiosis, was not shown to be effective in a placebo-controlled trial involving 60 patients, but this may have been due to poor bioavailability rather than drug inactivity (79). A trial of a more absorbable diclazuril congener, letrazuril, is about to be opened.

Reports suggesting that breastfeeding protects against the acquisition of *Cryptosporidium* (34,46) have provided the rationale for using hyperimmune bovine colostrum. Use of this agent has resulted in symptomatic im-provement for some patients (80); however, total clinical and parasitologic cure has been reported in only a single AIDS patient with cryptosporidiosis (81). A controlled trial of oral bovine dialyzable leukocyte extract (transfer factor) for cryptosporidiosis in AIDS patients demonstrated a statistically significant improvement in symptoms and change in body weight. Oocyst eradication from fecal smears approached but did not reach statistical significance (82). Transfer factor is the cell-free supernatant obtained from a single-cell suspension of lymph nodes from immunized cows. The active components of transfer factor and bovine colostrum have not been characterized.

The lack of a small animal model of symptomatic disease and the absence of an in vitro method for propagation of the organism have impeded testing of novel therapeutic agents and elucidation of the mechanisms of disease pathogenesis. Limited growth of *Cryptosporidium* in differentiated HT-29 (human colon adenocarcinoma) cells has been achieved (83); however, further refinement of this system is necessary to enable the testing of potential therapeutic agents. Recently described models of chronic symptomatic cryptosporidiosis in adult athymic, and in T-cell-depleted mice, should also prove useful (84).

ISOSPORIASIS IN AIDS

Isospora belli, also a coccidian protozoan, is widely distributed in the animal kingdom; however, its prevalence in humans is unknown.

Isosporiasis has been reported in less than 0.2% of AIDS patients in the United States, and in 15% of AIDS patients in Haiti (85). One might expect higher prevalence rates if the organism was carefully searched for in all patients. Infection is endemic in certain parts of South America, Southeast Asia, and Africa (86,87). Institutional outbreaks (87) and travelers' diarrhea (88) have been reported in the United States.

The life cycle of *I. belli* is similar to that of *Cryptosporidium* in that only one host is required for its completion. Unsporulated oocysts undergo maturation in the soil and contain two sporulated sporocysts when fully infective. Infection occurs through ingestion of sporulated oocysts and the release of four sporozoites from each sporocyst. Asexual (schizogony) and sexual (gametogony) phases occur in the cytoplasm of the intestinal epithelial cells, and unsporulated oocysts are shed in the feces. The oocysts are ovoid, with tapered ends, and they measure 20–33 μm long and 10–19 μm wide (Fig. 6).

Clinical manifestations of isosporiasis include diarrhea (watery without blood or polymorphonuclear leukocytes), steatorrhea, cramping abdominal pain, and weight loss. Eosinophilia has been reported. An acute self-limited enteritis may progress to a severe protracted

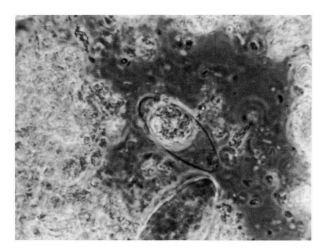

FIG. 6. *Isospora belli* oocyst (×630) in fecal sample from an AIDS patient.

illness in AIDS patients (89,90), as well as in infants and children without AIDS (91). Extraintestinal involvement of lymph nodes has been reported in cats (92) and in one patient with AIDS (89).

Like cryptosporidiosis, the pathogenesis of isosporiasis is unknown. Histological findings include atrophy of the small intestinal mucosa with villous blunting, hypertrophic crypts, and infiltration of the lamina propria with inflammatory cells, especially eosinophils (86,93,94). With electron microscopy, organisms may be found intracellularly within cytoplasmic vacuoles (95).

Diagnosis is made via detection of *Isospora* oocysts in stool specimens. Acid-fast techniques used to identify cryptosporidial oocysts will also identify the larger morphologically dissimilar oocysts of *Isospora*. *Isospora* oocyst shedding is intermittent and may not coincide with clinical symptoms.

Fortunately, unlike cryptosporidiosis, there are therapeutic options for isosporiasis. Complete clinical and parasitological cure has been obtained with a 7-day course of oral trimethoprim–sulfamethoxazole (TMP–SMX) (160 mg TMP–800 mg SMX administered four times daily) (85,96). Relapse is common in AIDS patients, and despite adequate responses to retreatment with TMP–SMX, chronic suppressive therapy with TMP–SMX at a lower dose or with weekly pyrimethamine–sulfadoxine (Fansidar) is usually required (96). Therapeutic responses have been reported with the use of pyrimethamine (97), and the experimental macrolide roxithromycin (98). Mixed results have been observed with other agents including metronidazole, quinacrine, and nitrofurantoin (86,90,93,99).

MICROSPORIDIOSIS IN AIDS

Microsporidia are ubiquitous, obligate intracellular protozoan parasites that lack mitochondria. There are hundreds of genera of microsporidia but only four have been implicated in human disease: *Nosema*, *Pleistophora*, *Encephalitozoon*, and *Enterocytozoon*. It has not been possible to classify several species into the known genera; hence the genus *Microsporidium* was designated to encompass these species. Infection with microsporidia is widespread within the animal kingdom.

The first conclusive evidence for human infection with microsporidia was reported in 1959, and involved a Japanese boy with no known immunodeficiency who presented with fever and a seizure disorder (100). Very few human cases have been reported in patients with no known immunodeficiency. In these cases infection was limited to the cornea (101–103) except in one case in which the presentation was again that of a seizure disorder (104).

The first case of microsporidiosis in an immunocompromised host was reported in 1979 and involved disseminated infection in an infant with thymic aplasia (105). Subsequently, almost all infections in immunocompromised hosts have involved patients with AIDS. Despite reports of corneal infection (106,107), hepatitis (108), and peritonitis (109) in patients with AIDS, it appears that the most common site of infection is the jejunum (110,111). *Enterocytozoon bieneusi* is the new genus and species that was created in 1985 to encompass those isolates detected in patients with AIDS. Certain morphologic and developmental features distinguish *E. bieneusi* from other microsporidia and thus form the basis for creating a new genus (112,113). *Enterocytozoon bieneusi* has only been identified in humans with AIDS. Although *E. bieneusi* has been implicated as the cause of severe diarrhea and weight loss in patients with AIDS, the pathogenicity of this organism awaits further confirmation. The prevalence of intestinal infection in patients with AIDS is unknown; however, estimates from uncontrolled case series have ranged from 0% to 30% (111).

The spores of *E. bieneusi* measure approximately 1.5 by 0.5 μm. Following ingestion, undefined intestinal stimuli cause the coiled polar tube to evert, penetrate the enterocyte, and inject the sporoplasm through the tube into the host intestinal cell. Merogony and sporogony ensue, with the formation of sporoblasts that mature into new spores. Development of *E. bieneusi* occurs in direct contact with the host cell cytoplasm, unlike *Encephalitozoon cuniculi*, which develops within a parasitophorous vacuole (114). New spores may be excreted in the feces with possible subsequent fecal–oral transmission.

Enterocytozoon bieneusi can be identified in small intestinal biopsy specimens with light microscopic examination of routine hematoxylin and eosin-stained paraffin-embedded sections by skilled individuals. Identification of organisms may be enhanced with methylene blue–azure II followed by basic fuschin or with toluidine blue stain of semithin sections (110). Giemsa-stained touch preparations of biopsy material has been described as an alternative method for diagnosis (115). Electron microscopy is often needed for definitive diagnosis with demonstration of the characteristic coiled polar tube, and for differentiation of microsporidian species. Spores of *E. bieneusi* have been recovered from feces and may prove to obviate the need for intestinal biopsy (116). Serologic assays are currently available only for *E. cuniculi*, and their sensitivity and specificity are unknown.

The clinical manifestations of infection with *E. bieneusi* are indistinguishable from cryptosporidiosis. As with cryptosporidiosis, there is no known efficacious therapy for microsporidiosis. There have been anecdotal reports of symptomatic improvement with pyrimethamine (115), metronidazole (115), and TMP–SMX (117). There have been recent reports of success with albendazole therapy (118). The development of specific serologic assays and the evaluation of potentially useful therapeutic agents are contingent upon successful propagation of *E. bieneusi* in vitro.

REFERENCES

1. CDC. Cryptosporidiosis: assessment of chemotherapy of males with acquired immune deficiency syndrome (AIDS). *MMWR* 1982;31:589–92.
2. Nime FA, Burek JD, Page DL, et al. Acute enterocolitis in a human being infected with the protozoan *Cryptosporidium. Gastroenterology* 1976;70:592–8.
3. Meisel JL, Perea DR, Meligro C, et al. Overwhelming watery diarrhea associated with a *Cryptosporidium* in an immunosuppressed patient. *Gastroenterology* 1976;70:1156–60.
4. Lasser KH, Lewin KJ, Ryning FW. Cryptosporidial enteritis in a patient with congenital hypogammaglobulinemia. *Hum Pathol* 1979;10:234–40.
5. Stemmermann CN, Hayashi T, Glober GA, et al. Cryptosporidiosis. Report of fatal case complicated by disseminated toxoplasmosis. *Am J Med* 1980;69:637–42.
6. Tzipori S, Angus KW, Gray EW, et al. Vomiting and diarrhea associated with cryptosporidial infection. *N Engl J Med* 1980;303:818.
7. Weinstein L, Edelstein SM, Madara JL, et al. Intestinal cryptosporidiosis complicated by disseminated cytomegalovirus infection. *Gastroenterology* 1981;81:584–91.
8. Weisburger WR, Hutcheon DF, Yardley JH, et al. Cryptosporidiosis in an immunosuppressed renal transplant recipient with IgA deficiency. *Am J Clin Pathol* 1979;72:473–8.
9. Current WL, Reese NC, Ernst JV, et al. Human cryptosporidiosis in immunocompetent and immunodeficient persons: studies of an outbreak and experimental transmission. *N Engl J Med* 1983;308:1252–7.
10. Jokipii L, Pohjola S, Valle SL, et al. Cryptosporidiosis associated with traveling and giardiasis. *Gastroenterology* 1985;4:838–42.
11. Soave R, Ma P. Cryptosporidiosis: traveler's diarrhea in two families. *Arch Intern Med* 1985;145:70–2.
12. Wolfson JS, Richter JM, Waldron MA, et al. Cryptosporidiosis in immunocompetent patients. *N Engl J Med* 1985;312:1278–82.
13. Tzipori S. Cryptosporidiosis in perspective. *Adv Parasitol* 1988;27:63–129.
14. Fayer R, Ungar BLP. *Cryptosporidium* spp. and cryptosporidiosis. *Microbiol Rev* 1986;50:458–83.
15. Soave R, Armstrong D. *Cryptosporidium* and cryptosporidiosis. *Rev Infect Dis* 1986;8:1012–23.
16. Janoff EN, Barth Reller L. *Cryptosporidium* species, a protean protozoan. *J Clin Microbiol* 1987;25:967–75.
17. Tyzzer EE. A sporozoan found in the peptic glands of the common mouse. *Proc Soc Exp Biol Med* 1907–1908;5:12–3.
18. Slavin D. *Cryptosporidium meleagridis* (sp. nov.) *J Comp Pathol Ther* 1955;65:262–6.
19. Tzipori S. Cryptosporidiosis in animals and humans. *Microbiol Rev* 1983;47:84–96.
20. Blagburn BL, Current WL. Accidental infection of a researcher with human *Cryptosporidium* [Letter]. *J Infect Dis* 1983;148: 772–3.
21. Hojlyng N, Holten-Andersen W, Jepsen S. Cryptosporidiosis: a case of airborne transmission. *Lancet* 1987;2:271–2.
22. Current WL, Haynes TB. Complete development of *Cryptosporidium* in cell culture. *Science* 1984;224:603–5.
23. Levine ND. Taxonomy and review of the coccidian genus *Cryptosporidium* (Protozoa, Apicomplexa). *J Protozool* 1984;31:94–8.
24. Tzipori S, Angus KW, Campbell I, et al. *Cryptosporidium:* evidence for a single-species genus. *Infect Immun* 1980;30:884–6.
25. Upton SJ, Current WL. The species of *Cryptosporidium* (Apicomplexa: Cryptosporididae) infecting mammals. *J Parasitol* 1985;71:625–9.
26. Hart CA, Baxby D, Blundell N. Gastroenteritis due to *Cryptosporidium:* a prospective survey in a children's hospital. *J Infect* 1984;9:264–70.
27. Koch KL, Shankey TV, Weinstein GS, et al. Cryptosporidiosis in a patient with hemophilia, common variable hypogammaglobulinemia, and the acquired immunodeficiency syndrome. *Ann Intern Med* 1983;99:337–40.
28. Ma P, Kaufman DL, Helmick CG, et al. Cryptosporidiosis in tourists returning from the Caribbean. *N Engl J Med* 1985;312:647–8.
29. D'Antonio RG, Winn RE, Taylor JP, et al. A waterborne outbreak of cryptosporidiosis in normal hosts. *Ann Intern Med* 1985;103:886–8.
30. Gallaher MM, Herndon JL, Nims LJ, et al. Cryptosporidiosis and surface water. *Am J Public Health* 1989;79:39–42.
31. CDC. Cryptosporidiosis among children attending day-care centers—Georgia, Pennsylvania, Michigan, California, New Mexico. *MMWR* 1984;33:599–601.
32. Heijbel H, Slaine K, Seigel B, et al. Outbreak of diarrhea in a day care center with spread to household members: the role of *Cryptosporidium. Pediatr Infect Dis J* 1987;6:532–5.
33. Stehr-Green JK, McCaig L, Remsen HM, et al. Shedding of oocysts in immunocompetent individuals infected with *Cryptosporidium. Am J Trop Med Hyg* 1987;36:338–42.
34. Navin TR. Cryptosporidiosis in humans: review of recent epidemiologic studies. *Eur J Epidemiol* 1985;1:77–83.
35. Collier AC, Miller RA, Meyers JD. Cryptosporidiosis after marrow transplantation: person-to-person transmission and treatment with spiramycin. *Ann Intern Med* 1984;101:205–6.
36. Dryjanski J, Gold JW, Ritchie MT, et al. Cryptosporidiosis. Case report in a health team worker. *Am J Med* 1986;80:751–2.
37. Koch KL, Phillips DJ, Aber RC, et al. Cryptosporidiosis in hospital personnel. Evidence for person-to-person transmission. *Ann Intern Med* 1985;102:593–6.
38. Baxby D, Hart CA, Taylor C. Human cryptosporidiosis: a possible cause of hospital cross-infection. *Br Med J* 1983;287:1760–1.
39. Martino P, Gentile G, Caprioli A, et al. Hospital acquired cryptosporidiosis in a bone marrow transplantation unit. *J Infect Dis* 1988;158:647–9.
40. Crawford FG, Vermund SH. Human cryptosporidiosis. *CRC Crit Rev Microbiol* 1988;16:113–59.
41. Madore MS, Rose JB, Gerba CP, et al. Occurence of *Cryptosporidium* oocysts in sewage effluents and select surface waters. *J Parasitol* 1987;73:702–5.
42. Ongerth JE, Stibbs HH. Identification of *Cryptosporidium* oocysts in river water. *Appl Environ Microbiol* 1987;53:672–6.
43. Rose JB, Cifrino A, Madore MS, et al. Detection of *Cryptosporidium* from wastewater and freshwater environments. *Water Sci Tech* 1986;18:233–9.
44. Smith PD, HC Lane, VJ Gill, et al. Intestinal infections in patients with the acquired immunodeficiency syndrome (AIDS). *Ann Intern Med* 1988;108:328–33.
45. Laughon BE, Druckman DA, Vernon A, et al. Prevalence of en-

teric pathogens in homosexual men with and without acquired immunodeficiency syndrome. *Gastroenterology* 1988;94:984–93.

46. Mata L, Bolanos H, Pizarro D, et al. Cryptosporidiosis in children from some highland Costa Rican rural and urban areas. *Am J Trop Med Hyg* 1984;33:24–9.

47. Soave R, Danner RL, Honig CL, et al. Cryptosporidiosis in homosexual men. *Ann Intern Med* 1984;110:504–11.

48. Jokipii L, Jokipii AMM. Timing of symptoms and oocyst excretion in human cryptosporidiosis. *N Engl J Med* 1986;315:1643–7.

49. Pitlik SD, Fainstein V, Garza D, et al. Human cryptosporidiosis: spectrum of disease. Report of six cases and review of the literature. *Arch Intern Med* 1983;143:2269–76.

50. Guarda LA, Stein SA, Cleary KA, et al. Human cryptosporidiosis in the acquired immune deficiency syndrome. *Arch Pathol Lab Med* 1983;107:562–6.

51. Blumberg RS, Kelsey P, Perrone T, et al. Cytomegalovirus- and cryptosporidium-associated with acalculous gangrenous cholecystis. *Am J Med* 1984;76:1118–23.

52. Margulis SJ, Honig CL, Soave R, et al. Biliary tract obstruction in the acquired immunodeficiency syndrome. *Ann Intern Med* 1986;105:207–10.

53. Kocoshis SA, Cibull ML, Davis TE, et al. Intestinal and pulmonary cryptosporidiosis in an infant with severe combined immune deficiency. *J Pediatr Gastroenterol Nutr* 1984;3:149–57.

54. Forgacs P, Tarshis A, Ma P, et al. Intestinal and bronchial cryptosporidiosis in an immunodeficient homosexual man. *Ann Intern Med* 1983;99:793–4.

55. Miller RA, Wasserheit JN, Kirihara J, et al. Detection of *Cryptosporidium* oocysts in sputum during screening for mycobacterium. *J Clin Microbiol* 1984;20:1992–3.

56. Ma P, Villanueva TG, Kaufman D, et al. Respiratory cryptosporidiosis in the acquired immune deficiency syndrome. *JAMA* 1984;252:1298–301.

57. Lefkowitch JH, Krumholz S, Feng-Chen K-C, et al. Cryptosporidiosis of the human small intestine: a light and electron microscopic study. *Hum Pathol* 1984;15:746–52.

58. Navin TR, Juranek DD. Cryptosporidiosis: clinical, epidemiologic, and parasitologic review. *Rev Infect Dis* 1984;6:313–27.

59. Sloper KS, Dourmashkin RR, Bird RB, et al. Chronic malabsorption due to cryptosporidiosis in a child with immunoglobulin deficiency. *Gut* 1982;23:80–2.

60. Schneiderman DJ, Cello JP, Laing FC. Papillary stenosis and sclerosing cholangitis in the acquired immunodeficiency syndrome. *Ann Intern Med* 1987;106:546–9.

61. Davis JJ, Heyman MB, Ferrell L, et al. Sclerosing cholangitis associated with chronic cryptosporidiosis in a child with a congenital immunodeficiency disorder. *Am J Gastroenterol* 1987;82:1196–202.

62. Gentile G, Baldassarri L, Caprioli A, et al. Colonic vascular invasion as a possible route of extraintestinal cryptosporidiosis. *Am J Med* 1987;82:574–5.

63. Vetterling JM, Takeuchi A, Madden PA. Ultrastructure of *Cryptosporidium wrairi* from the guinea pig. *J Protozool* 1971;18:248–60.

64. Pohlenz J, Benrick WJ, Moon HW, et al. Bovine cryptosporidiosis: a transmission and scanning electron microscopic study of some stages in the life cycle and of the host-parasite relationship. *Vet Pathol* 1978;15:417–27.

65. Henricksen SA, Pohlenz JFL. Staining of cryptosporidia by a modified Ziehl-Neelsen technique. *Acta Vet Scand* 1981;22:594–6.

66. Ma P, Soave R. Three-step stool examination for cryptosporidiosis in 10 homosexual men with protracted watery diarrhea. *J Infect Dis* 1983;147:824–8.

67. Garcia LS, Bruckner DA, Brewer TC, et al. Techniques for the recovery and identification of *Cryptosporidium* oocysts from stool specimens. *J Clin Microbiol* 1983;18:185–90.

68. Baxby D, Blundell N. Sensitive, rapid, simple methods for detecting *Cryptosporidium* in feces. *Lancet* 1983;2:1149.

69. Horen WP. Detection of *Cryptosporidium* in human fecal specimens. *J Parasitol* 1983;69:622–4.

70. Bronsdon MA. Rapid dimethyl sulfoxide-modified acid-fast stain of *Cryptosporidium* oocysts in stool specimens. *J Clin Microbiol* 1984;19:952–3.

71. McNabb SJ, Hensel DM, Welch DF, et al. Comparison of sedimentation and flotation techniques for identification of *Cryptosporidium* sp. oocysts in a large outbreak of human diarrhea. *J Clin Microbiol* 1985;22:587–9.

72. Sterling CR, Arrowood MJ. Detection of *Cryptosporidium* sp. infections using a direct immunofluorescent assay. *Pediatr Infect Dis* 1986;5:5139–2.

73. Garcia LS, Brewer TC, Bruckner DA. Fluorescence detection of *Cryptosporidium* oocysts in human fecal specimens by using monoclonal antibodies. *J Clin Microbiol* 1987;25:119–21.

74. Campbell PM, Current WL. Demonstration of serum antibodies to *Cryptosporidium* sp. in normal and immunodeficient humans with confirmed infections. *J Clin Microbiol* 1983;18:165–9.

75. Ungar BL, Soave R, Fayer R, et al. Enzyme immunoassay detection of immunoglobulin M and G antibodies to *Cryptosporidium* in immunocompetent and immunocompromised patients. *J Infect Dis* 1986;153:570–8.

76. Soave R. Treatment strategies for cryptosporidiosis. *Ann NY Acad Sci* 1990;616:442–51.

77. Soave R, Sjoerdsma A, Cawein MJ. Treatment of cryptosporidiosis in AIDS patients with DFMO. International Conference on AIDS, Atlanta, Georgia, 1985.

77a. Gathe J, Piot D, Hawkins K, et al. Treatment of gastrointestinal cryptosporidiosis with paromomycin. 6th International Conference on AIDS, San Francisco, June, 1990;2121(abst).

78. Portnoy D, Whiteside ME, Buckley E III, et al. Treatment of intestinal cryptosporidiosis with spiramycin. *Ann Intern Med* 1984;101:202–4.

79. Soave R, Dieterich D, Kotler D, et al. Oral diclazuril for cryptosporidiosis. 6th International Conference on AIDS, San Francisco, June, 1990;520(abst).

80. Tzipori S, Roberton D, Chapman C. Remission of diarrhea due to cryptosporidiosis in an immunodeficient child treated with hyperimmune bovine colostrum. *Br Med J* 1986;293:1276–7.

81. Ungar BLP, Ward DJ, Fayer R, et al. Cessation of *Cryptosporidium*-associated diarrhea in an acquired immunodeficiency syndrome patient after treatment with hyperimmune bovine colostrum. *Gastroenterology* 1990;98:486–9.

82. McMeeking A, Borkowsky W, Klesius PH, et al. A controlled trial of bovine dialyzable leukocyte extract for cryptosporidiosis in patients with AIDS. *J Infect Dis* 1990;161:108–12.

83. Soave R, Harrison EM. Factors influencing the development of *Cryptosporidium* in vitro. *Clin Res* 1988;36:471(abst).

84. Ungar BLP, Burris JA, Quinn CA, et al. New mouse models for chronic *Cryptosporidium* infection in immunodeficient host. *Infect Immun* 1990;58:961–9.

85. DeHovitz JA, Pape JW, Boncy M, et al. Clinical manifestations and therapy of *Isospora belli* infection in patients with acquired immunodeficiency syndrome. *N Engl J Med* 1986;315:87–90.

86. Brandborg LL, Goldberg SB, Briedenbach WC. Human coccidiosis—a possible cause of malabsorption. The life cycle in small-bowel mucosal biopsies as a diagnostic feature. *N Engl J Med* 1970;283:1306–13.

87. Faust EC, Giraldo LE, Caicedo G, et al. Human isosporosis in the Western hemisphere. *Am J Med* 1983;10:343–9.

88. Shaffer N, Moore L. Chronic travelers diarrhea in a normal host due to *Isospora belli*. *J Infect Dis* 1989;159:596–7.

89. Restrepo C, Macher AM, Radany EH. Disseminated extraintestinal isosporiasis in a patient with acquired immunodeficiency syndrome. *Am J Clin Pathol* 1987;87:536–42.

90. Forthal DN, Guest SS. *Isospora belli* enteritis in three homosexual men. *Am J Trop Med Hyg* 1984;33:1060–4.

91. Faria JA, Brust MB. Human isosporiasis caused by *Isospora belli*, Wenyon 1923. Salvador-Bahia. *Rev Inst Med Trop Sao Paulo* 1983;251:47–9.

92. Dubey JP, Frenkel JK. Extra-intestinal stages of *Isospora felis I. rivolta* (Protozoa: Eimeridiae) in cats. *J Protozool* 1972;19:89–92.

93. Trier JS, Moxey PC, Schimmel EM, et al. Chronic intestinal coccidiosis in man: intestinal morphology and response to treatment. *Gastroenterology* 1974;66:923–35.

94. Webster BH. Human isosporiasis: a report of three cases with necropsy findings in one case. *Am J Trop Med* 1957;6:86–9.

95. Liebman WM, Thaler MM, DeLorimier A, et al. Intractable diarrhea of infancy due to intestinal coccidiosis. *Gastroenterology* 1980;78:579–84.

96. Pape JW, Verdier R, Johnson WD. Treatment and prophylaxis of *Isospora belli* infection in patients with the acquired immunodeficiency syndrome. *N Engl J Med* 1989;320:1044–7.

97. Weiss LM, Perlman DC, Sherman J, et al. *Isospora belli* infection. Treatment with pyrimethamine. *Ann Intern Med* 1988;109:474–5.

98. Musey KL, Chidiac C, Beaucaire G, et al. Effectiveness of roxithromycin for treating *Isospora belli* infection. *J Infect Dis* 1988;158:646.

99. Ma P, Kaufman D, Montana J. *Isospora belli* diarrheal infection in homosexual men. *AIDS Res* 1984;1:327–38.

100. Matsubayashi H, Koike T, Mikata T, et al. A case of *Encephalitozoon* like body infection in man. *Arch Pathol* 1959;67:181–7.

101. Ashton N, Wirasinha PA. Encephalitozoonosis (nosematosis) of the cornea. *Br J Ophthalmol* 1973;57:669–74.

102. Pinnolis M, Egbert PR, Font RL, et al. Nosematosis of the cornea. *Arch Ophthalmol* 1981;99:1044–7.

103. Davis RM, Font RL, Keisler MS, et al. Corneal microsporidiosis: a case report including ultrastructural observations. *Ophthalmology* 1990;97:953–7.

104. Bergquist NR, Stintzing G, Smedman L, et al. Diagnosis of encephalitozoonosis in man by serological tests. *Br Med J* 1984;288:902.

105. Margileth AM, Strano AJ, Chandra R, et al. Disseminated nosematosis in an immunologically compromised infant. *Arch Pathol* 1973;95:145–50.

106. Friedberg DN, Stenson SM, Orenstein JM, et al. Microsporidial keratoconjunctivitis in acquired immunodeficiency syndrome. *Arch Ophthalmol* 1990;108:504–8.

107. Lowder CY, Meisler DM, McMahon JT, et al. Microsporidia infection of the cornea in an HIV-positive man. *Am J Ophthalmol* 1990;109:242–4.

108. Terada S, Reddy R, Jeffers LJ, et al. Microsporidian hepatitis in the acquired immunodeficiency syndrome. *Ann Intern Med* 1987;107:61–2.

109. Zender HO, Arrigoni E, Eckert J, et al. A case of *Encephalitozoon cuniculi* peritonitis in a patient with AIDS. *Am J Clin Pathol* 1989;92:352–6.

110. Orenstein JM, Chiang J, Steinberg W, et al. Intestinal microsporidiosis as a cause of diarrhea in human immunodeficiency virus-infected patients. *Hum Pathol* 1990;21:475–81.

111. Bryan RT, Cali A, Owen RL, et al. Microsporidia: opportunistic pathogens in patients with AIDS. In: Sun T, ed. *Progress in clinical parasitology,* 2. Philadelphia: Field and Wood, 1990;1–26.

112. Modigliani R, Bories C, Le Charpentier Y, et al. Diarrhea and malabsorption in acquired immunodeficiency syndrome: a study of four cases with special emphasis on opportunistic protozoan infestations. *Gut* 1985;26:179–87.

113. Desportes I, Le Charpentier Y, Galian A, et al. Occurrence of a new microsporidian: *Enterocytozoon bieneusi* n g, n sp, in the enterocytes of a human patient with AIDS. *J Protozool* 1985;32:250–4.

114. Canning EU, Hollister WS. *Enterocytozoon bieneusi* (Microspora): prevalence and pathogenicity in AIDS patients. *Trans R Soc Trop Med Hyg* 1990;84:181–6.

115. Rijpstra AC, Canning EU, Van Ketel RJ, et al. Use of light microscopy to diagnose small-intestinal microsporidiosis in patients with AIDS. *J Infect Dis* 1988;157:827–31.

116. Van Gool T, Hollister WS, Schattenkerk JE, et al. Diagnosis of *Enterocytozoon bieneusi* microsporidiosis in AIDS patients by recovery of spores from faeces. *Lancet* 1990;336:697–8.

117. Current WL, Owen RL. Cryptosporidiosis and microsporidiosis. In: Farthing MJG, Keusch GT, eds. *Enteric infection: mechanisms, manifestations, and management.* London: Chapman and Hall Medical, 1989;223–49.

118. Blanshard C, Peacock C, Ellis D, et al. Treatment of intestinal microsporidiosis with albendazole. 7th International Conference on AIDS, Florence, Italy, June, 1991;W.B.2265 (abst).

AIDS and Other Manifestations of HIV Infection,
Second Edition, Edited by Gary P. Wormser.
Raven Press, Ltd., New York © 1992.

CHAPTER 28

Neoplastic Complications of HIV Infection

Alexandra M. Levine, Parkash S. Gill, and Syed Zaki Salahuddin

PATHOGENESIS AND TREATMENT OF AIDS-RELATED KAPOSI'S SARCOMA

Prior to the AIDS epidemic, Kaposi's sarcoma (KS) was a rare tumor. It was seen in certain geographic regions in well-defined population groups, such as classic KS in older men from the Eastern European and Mediterranean regions, and in adult men and children from Central Africa (1). Since the beginning of the acquired immunodeficiency syndrome (AIDS) epidemic, KS has been reported in 20–50% of AIDS patients (2). Homosexual and bisexual men with AIDS develop KS more frequently than other HIV-infected populations (3). It is unclear as to the factors that predispose homosexual men to the development of KS, or why there has been a steady decline in the incidence of KS since the beginning of the epidemic.

This decline may be related to changes in life style that have occurred in the male homosexual population, such as a decrease in high-risk sexual behaviors, number of sexual partners, use of recreational drugs, and occurrence of other sexually transmitted diseases. It is possible that a general diminution in chronic stimuli to the immune system may reduce the incidence of KS, due to a reduction of growth initiation factors liberated from activated T lymphocytes and monocytes. Furthermore, the use of zidovudine (AZT) may play a significant role in reducing these growth factors through inhibition of human immunodeficiency virus (HIV), which may act directly and indirectly as a mitogen to those cells that produce the KS growth initiation factors. These possibilities, however, remain speculative at present and need to be addressed through appropriate scientific inquiry.

It is also possible that the reported decline in incidence

of KS may be artifactual, due to more frequent clinical diagnoses of KS, without biopsy confirmation, and to underreporting of KS, when it is diagnosed after an earlier AIDS-defining opportunistic infection. It is clear that formal studies are warranted to confirm the decline in incidence, and to ascertain the cofactors involved in development of KS.

The pathologic characteristics of epidemic, AIDS-associated KS are similar to KS when it occurs in other epidemiologic settings. The clinical course is different, however, being often progressive with frequent visceral involvement. Although KS causes mortality only in patients with extensive visceral involvement, it contributes significantly to morbidity. Treatment modalities should be guided by tumor burden, immunologic status of the patient, and toxicity of the therapy. Early KS, particularly with a relatively intact immune status, can be treated with antiretroviral agents combined with immune modulators (e.g., AZT + α-interferon). Rapidly progressive disease or advanced KS requires systemic chemotherapy alone or in combination with antiretroviral agents. However, bone marrow suppression is a dose-limiting toxicity of such therapy, which may be circumvented with the combined use of hematopoietic growth factors [such as granulocyte–macrophage colony-stimulating factor (GM-CSF) or granulocyte colony-stimulating factor (G-CSF)]. Kaposi's sarcoma often relapses following discontinuation of therapy, emphasizing the need for discovery of a safe and effective form of maintenance therapy.

Pathogenesis

KS is a multifocal, polyclonal hyperplastic neoplasm that is perhaps influenced by hormones, cytokines, and other humoral factors in immune-compromised individuals. It does not behave as an ordinary soft tissue tumor, which is characterized by local growth and eventual me-

A. M. Levine, P. S. Gill, and S. Z. Salahuddin: Division of Hematology, Department of Internal Medicine, University of Southern California School of Medicine, Los Angeles, California 90033.

tastasis. Skin is the most commonly involved site, but KS lesions can occur in any organ, although rarely in brain or bone marrow. KS is a tumor of mixed cellularity, consisting of spindle-like cells, small vascular spaces, numerous dilated abnormal lymphocytics, blood vessels, and extravasated red cells present in slit-like vascular structures. A variety of mononuclear cells may also be present in these lesions such as T cells, plasma cells, and phagocytic macrophages. Often there is associated edema. Histologically, KS lesions are remarkably similar, regardless of anatomic location (skin, lymph nodes, respiratory tract, and/or intestine).

Major breakthroughs in the pathogenesis of KS have occurred in the past 3 years through the work of Salahuddin et al. (4) and Nakamura et al. (5) in the Laboratory of Tumor Cell Biology at the National Cancer Institute. Salahuddin and associates have successfully established cultures of primary human KS tumor from AIDS patients. This was accomplished through the use of conditioned media, utilizing the supernatants of T-cell lines that had been transformed by various known human retroviruses. The supernatants were found to contain what appears to be a novel growth factor, which is currently undergoing characterization. This conditioned media was found to enhance the growth of KS-derived spindle cells. These investigators also showed that glucocorticoids enhance the proliferation of KS-derived spindle cells, parallel to the clinical reports of either development of KS or enhancement of the growth of existing KS in a variety of clinical states (renal transplant recipients, collagen vascular diseases, and AIDS) following steroid use (6). Work pertaining to the role of previously known angiogenic factors has also been very informative. Thus KS-derived spindle cells synthesize angiogenic factors that include basic fibroblast growth factor (bFGF) and interleukin-1 (IL-1), both of which can in turn enhance the growth of the KS-derived spindle cells from which they were synthesized. In addition, tumor necrosis factor (TNF) also acts as a growth factor for KS. These findings suggest that tumor cells make autocrine and paracrine growth factors.

On the basis of evidence collected to date, it is reasonable to assume that there are preexisting cells in lymph node, skin, and other sites that can respond to humoral factors such as cytokines and hormones. Furthermore, as discussed, KS may be a neoplasm induced by such soluble mediators. Thus, in AIDS-associated KS, it would be reasonable to assume that, among many factors, HIV-1 may be directly or indirectly associated with the induction and/or maintenance of these lesions. In the setting of underlying HIV infection, activated T cells would release various soluble factors, which could induce the activation and proliferation of KS progenitor cells. Endothelial cells of lymphatic as well as vascular origin, connective tissue cells, and infiltrating leukocytes could also be stimulated. In addition, this cascade of events would also stimulate the replication of HIV-1 in situ, releasing not only virus particles but also HIV-1 tat protein.

An important study regarding the pathogenesis of KS was reported by Vogel et al. (7), who introduced the tat gene under the control of HIV long terminal repeat (LTR) into the germ line of mice, and studied the expression of tat gene in various tissues. Tat expression was detectable only in skin. Furthermore, male mice carrying the tat gene developed hyperplasia of the dermis and epidermis, and 15% of these male offspring also developed vascular cutaneous lesions resembling KS after 12–18 months. Direct analysis of tumor tissue showed tat gene expression, while cell lines derived from the tumor had no detectable tat gene messenger RNA. These findings suggest that the accessory cells expressing the tat gene may also produce various growth factors that induce the vascular KS-like tumor. Furthermore, development of vascular tumors in male mice may be relevant to the preponderance of KS in men, and provides a model to study the pathogenetic effects of various hormones.

Recent reports of the effect of HIV-1 tat protein on cultured spindle cells may indeed be the critical link between the virus and the subsequent development and promotion of KS lesions in AIDS-associated KS (8). The stimulated spindle cells are of central significance in these lesions. Although these cells do not actively replicate, they produce a number of important cytokines such as IL-1, IL-6, GM-CSF, and other factors that promote chemotaxis, chemoinvasion, and vascular permeability (9). The spindle cells both release and respond to these factors as measured by their in vitro replication and by other functional assays. The spindle cells also provide stimulation to other cells in the KS lesion, contributing to the maintenance and growth of these lesions. Thus cultured spindle cells obtained from human KS biopsy tissue, when transplanted into nude mice, induce a KS-like lesion of murine origin (4).

The various forms of presentation of KS, such as nodular, plaque, or mixed morphology, could result from differences in the quality and/or quantity of various mediating cytokines within the specific lesion. The exact nature and origin of the spindle cells in vivo, and the cultured cells in vitro, still remain unresolved. Older studies have suggested a variety of origins, including vascular, endothelial, lymphatic, and/or vascular smooth muscle. Current data would favor vascular smooth muscle as the cell of origin of the critical KS spindle cell (10).

Infectious agents, particularly cytomegalovirus (CMV), have been considered in the pathogenesis of KS. At this point, it appears unlikely that CMV has a direct role in the development of KS. However, it is possible that lytic herpes viruses may contribute to the disease indirectly, through the activation of leukocytes and induction of soluble factors. Furthermore, the search for another, yet unidentified infectious agent is in progress in various laboratories.

Pathology

The cutaneous lesions of Kaposi's sarcoma are classified into patch, plaque, and/or nodular lesions (11). Early on, KS of the skin begins as a small, flat purple lesion (patch lesion). The lesion may broaden and become elevated to form a plaque. A plaque may enlarge progressively to become a nodule. Histopathologic studies show that earlier lesions are located in the reticular (upper) dermis, with subdermal involvement in some cases.

In very early stages of KS, the lesions may resemble granulation tissue, with patchy distribution in the reticular dermis. Vessel proliferation is composed of irregular jagged vessels dissecting the collagen bundles of the dermis. The nuclei of the endothelial cells are flat, elongated, and darkly stained. They are frequently surrounded by plasma cells and scattered lymphocytes and neutrophils. As the vascular structures proliferate, plaque lesions develop. Nodular lesions are quite different histologically from the patch and plaque lesions, and consist predominantly of spindle cells, giving a sarcomatous appearance. These spindle cells are arranged in interwoven fascicles. The spindle cells themselves are generally not strikingly atypical, although they are often pleomorphic, and may be seen in mitosis. Areas of necrosis may be observed. Nodular lesions also express extensive perivascular infiltration of lymphocytes, plasma cells, and macrophages. Red cell extravasation into the slit-like spaces among the spindle cells is characteristic of KS lesions, and may help to distinguish them from other lesions.

Various investigators have attempted to define the etiology and cell of origin using immunocytochemistry (11) and in situ hybridization techniques (12). As discussed above, KS was previously considered to originate from small vascular structures, possibly from endothelial cells. Endothelial cells express various antigens including FVIIIR antigen. Immunohistochemical studies of both frozen and fixed tissues have failed to show a uniform staining for FVIIIR antigen in KS cells, suggesting one of two possibilities: (1) that the cell of origin is not endothelial; or (2) that the tumor cell, although of endothelial cell origin, is at a different stage of differentiation and does not express FVIIIR antigen. Several other markers, including various antigens (HLA-DR immune region-associated antigen, macrophage–endothelial antigens), enzymes (5'-nucleotidase, adenosine triphosphatase, alkaline phosphatase), and binding of the lectin *Ulex europaeus* I, have been used to help define the cell of origin (13). KS spindle cells express markers that are shared with lymphatic endothelium including 5'-nucleotidase and *U. europaeus* I lectin. Rutgers et al. (14) described three monoclonal antibodies (E92, OKM5, HCL-1) that react with normal vascular, but not lymphatic, endothelium and react with the vascular lining of KS. Two of these antibodies (E92, OKM5) also react with the spindle cell component of the tumor, supporting the idea that KS originates from vascular endothelium. Scully et al. (15) have described two other monoclonal antibodies (B721 and E431) that recognize endothelial cell surface antigens. These antibodies stain both large and small normal blood vessel endothelial cells and also stain KS tissue. The intensity of staining is variable, more intense in the lining cells of abnormal vascular structures than in the spindle cell component. These antibodies also stain a subset of activated CD4 lymphocytes. The lymphatic structures appeared negative, again suggesting a vascular origin for KS. Other investigators (16) have suggested that KS originates from primitive pluripotent mesenchymal cells that may differentiate into more specialized cell types, including endothelial, smooth muscle, fibroblast, and myofibroblasts. These authors suggest that KS originates from small vascular structures, possibly endothelial cells, although, as discussed above, definitive evidence for the cell of origin remains to be established, and has clearly not yet been elucidated by means of these various immunocytochemical techniques.

Clinical Manifestations

The epidemic form of KS is seen predominantly in young homosexual men. The lesions may affect any site of the body, although the skin is the most common site for initial presentation. The lesions are multifocal. Sites of presentation in the absence of skin involvement include lymph nodes, gastrointestinal tract, oral mucosa, conjunctiva, and lungs (17,18).

Cutaneous lesions often first appear as small, fleshy, flat lesions that progress to reddish or purple nodules. They are generally painless, nonpruritic, and often linear, following the pattern of cutaneous lymphatic drainage (Fig. 1). The lesions may be associated with local edema, suggesting lymphatic obstruction; they may coalesce to form large infiltrating lesions, and may even ulcerate and cause local pain. The soles of the feet are often affected, where the lesions appear less purple or red. Surprisingly, the palms are rarely involved.

Sites other than skin are frequently involved and correlate with advanced or progressive cutaneous disease. The oral cavity is involved in nearly one-third of cases, often located on the palate and less frequently the gingiva and the tongue (Fig. 2). Although common, the true fre-

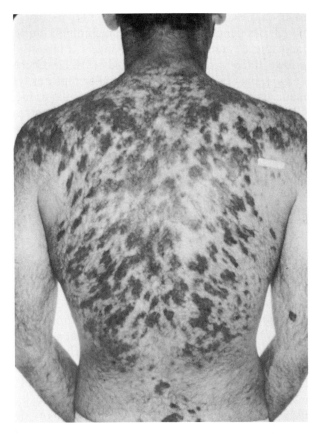

FIG. 1. Raised, reddish-purple cutaneous lesions of Kaposi's sarcoma on the skin. Note the symmetric pattern of distribution.

quency of lymph node involvement is not known because of the lack of routine node biopsy in all KS cases. Visceral involvement, particularly in the gastrointestinal tract, occurs in nearly 50% of cases and may involve the esophagus, stomach, duodenum, colon, and rectum. Advanced gastrointestinal involvement may cause abdominal pain, early satiety, and even bleeding. Asymptomatic

gastrointestinal involvement does not affect survival, and routine evaluation is not needed in the absence of symptoms. However, symptomatic gastrointestinal involvement should be evaluated with endoscopy, since barium contrast studies often produce false-negative findings.

Pulmonary involvement has also been reported with increasing frequency in the past several years, and has occurred in 20–50% of KS cases (19). Pulmonary involvement can often be diagnosed with bronchoscopy without biopsy, due to the classic appearance of these lesions, and the likelihood of complications from the risk of bleeding. Open lung biopsy is rarely necessary to make the diagnosis. Patients with significant involvement often complain of exertional dyspnea, dry cough, and (rarely) chest pain. Radiographic findings may be abnormal and include diffuse interstitial infiltrates, mediastinal adenopathy, pulmonary nodules, and/or pleural effusions, in order of decreasing frequency. Patients with advanced pulmonary involvement have a poor prognosis, with a median survival of only 3 months.

Cardiac involvement has rarely been reported, but may lead to cardiac tamponade and death (20). Nearly all organs have been shown to be involved with KS, including the brain (rarely).

Staging System

Several methods to define the extent and bulk of KS have been proposed, in order to provide guidelines for treatment, prognosis, and uniform response criteria. Several pitfalls exist, due to: (1) the multifocal manifestations of disease; (2) the difficulty in objectively determining tumor response due to residual hyperpigmentation even after successful therapy; and, most importantly, (3) the infectious complications of immune deficiency and their impact on tumor response. Most recently, Krown

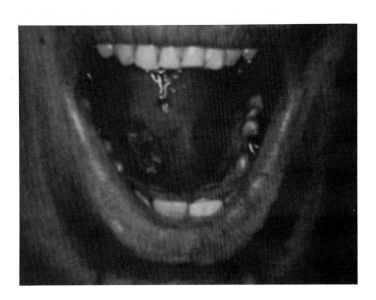

FIG. 2. Kaposi's sarcoma lesion within the mucous membranes of the mouth.

and associates (21) have devised a modified staging system that attempts to incorporate these complex parameters, particularly tumor bulk, with or without local complications; presence of visceral disease; and status of the immune system, particularly the CD4 lymphocyte count; history of opportunistic infection; and the presence or absence of constitutional "B" symptoms.

Prognostic Features

The survival of patients with AIDS/KS is predominantly related to the underlying immunologic status and multiplicity of infectious complications that may have occurred. KS is often the source of serious morbidity, due to cosmetic problems, local edema, pain, and even ulceration. Although visceral KS is often asymptomatic, gastrointestinal and pulmonary involvement can lead to bleeding, organ dysfunction, and death.

Several investigators have defined various prognostic parameters that predict for response and survival. Lane and DeWit (22,23) have shown that patients with CD4 counts above $400/mm^3$ are more likely to respond to α-interferon, while response rates decline rapidly with CD4 counts below $200/mm^3$. Chachoua and colleagues (24), in a large database of 212 AIDS/KS cases, have shown that significant prognostic variables include the presence of systemic constitutional symptoms ("B" symptoms), ($p = 0.001$), prior or coexistent opportunistic infections ($p = 0.02$), and CD4 lymphocyte counts less than $300/mm^3$ ($p = 0.02$). They have suggested that based upon these features, AIDS/KS cases may be subdivided into the following groups:
1. No prior or coexistent opportunistic infections, no systemic symptoms, CD4 $\geq 300/mm^3$: expected median survival of 31 months;
2. No prior or coexistent opportunistic infections, no systemic symptoms, CD4 $< 300/mm^3$: median survival of 20 months;
3. No prior or coexistent opportunistic infections, presence of systemic symptoms, median survival of 15 months;
4. Prior or coexistent opportunistic infections: median survival of 7 months.

Treatment

The management of KS should be designed based on consideration of several aspects. First, one must define any complications related to HIV, such as acute opportunistic infections, AIDS dementia complex, status of bone marrow function, and concurrent use of various myelosuppressive agents. Secondly, one must define the extent of KS, such as the number of cutaneous lesions; local complications such as edema, ulceration, or super-

infections; visceral sites of involvement; and the severity of such involvement. For example, symptomatic pulmonary KS requires immediate attention, with use of systemic cytotoxic therapy. Thirdly, the immunologic status of the patient should be established at baseline, including the number of peripheral blood CD4 lymphocytes, in order to predict response to certain treatment modalities (such as α-interferon) and the risk of opportunistic infections.

Radiation Therapy

The role of radiotherapy in localized cutaneous disease for cosmetic purposes and for local pain control is well established (25,26). However, radiation therapy rarely produces complete resolution of large lesions. Furthermore, radiation therapy of KS lesions in the oral cavity may result in severe mucositis and should therefore be discouraged.

Interferon

Recombinant α-interferon has been studied extensively in the treatment of AIDS/KS, due to its immunoregulatory, antitumor, and antiviral activity. Specifically, α-interferon inhibits HIV replication in vitro, through interference with viral assembly at the cell membrane. Furthermore, in vitro, α-interferon acts synergistically with AZT in HIV inhibition. α-Interferon has been used at a dose of 1 mU to 52 mU per day with response rates ranging between 25% and 50%. Tumor regression begins 4–8 weeks after initiation of therapy and major response is achieved in 12–24 weeks. Upon analyzing CD4 lymphocyte counts as a parameter to predict response to interferon, it is clear that patients with CD4 counts above $400/mm^3$ are most likely to achieve tumor response (23,24). More recently, combinations of AZT and α-interferon have been evaluated in AIDS-KS. Kovacs and associates (27) studied AZT at 50, 100, or 250 mg every 4 hours, with α-interferon at various escalating dosages. Thirty-seven patients were entered into the trial. The maximum tolerated dose of interferon when combined with AZT at 100 mg every 4 hours ranged between 10 mU and 15 mU when given every day. Half of the patients who received a stable dose of the two drugs achieved major response (partial or complete). In a phase I study, Krown and associates (28) similarly showed that the maximum tolerated dose of interferon when given with AZT at 100 mg every 4 hours is 18 mU/day, and at an AZT dose of 200 mg every 4 hours it was 4.5 mU/day. Larger phase II studies are in progress to determine the response rates in AIDS-KS when both drugs are given in combination.

Chemotherapy

Systemic cytotoxic chemotherapy should be reserved for patients with extensive or rapidly progressive KS, particularly patients with symptomatic visceral involvement. Single-agent chemotherapy has been associated with modest responses. Thus, vinblastine used alone has produced responses in less than one-third of cases (29). Other agents studied alone include etoposide (30), doxorubicin, and alternating vinblastine and vincristine (31). As shown by Gill et al. (32,33), a combination of doxorubicin (20 mg/m^2), bleomycin (10 mg/m^2), and vincristine (2 mg) given every 2 weeks is well tolerated, with responses in over 80%, while adriamycin alone at the same dose and schedule produced major responses in just under 50% of the cases. Combinations of bleomycin and vincristine at the above dosages and schedule can be administered, even when patients have compromised bone marrow function (33). Patients with symptomatic pulmonary KS have a predicted survival of approximately 3 months without therapy, but may respond to combination chemotherapy with improved survival (19). In a retrospective analysis, combinations of AZT with bleomycin and vincristine have been well tolerated with high response rates (34); predominant toxicity consists of anemia and neutropenia. Prospective studies of chemotherapy and AZT, with or without hematopoietic growth factors such as GM-CSF, are currently in progress.

A major problem relates to the fact that KS almost always relapses shortly after discontinuation of chemotherapy. Thus, safe and effective maintenance therapy short of cytotoxic chemotherapy will be needed to maintain tumor response. α-Interferon alone has limited activity in this regard, and studies using combinations of AZT and interferon following chemotherapy are currently in progress.

Several angiostatic compounds have been discovered recently, and are undergoing in vitro and preclinical evaluation at present. These compounds may soon be available for clinical evaluation.

Conclusions

Kaposi's sarcoma occurs in a significant number of HIV-infected individuals. The cell of origin and the etiology of the malignancy are still poorly understood. However, significant advances have occurred during the last few years regarding the pathogenesis of KS and the role of HIV in its development. In addition, the demonstration of various known autocrine and paracrine growth factors produced by the KS cell, as well as the existence of one or more novel growth factors for KS, has further expanded our understanding of the initiation and progression of this neoplasm. These findings allow for the possibility of novel treatment regimens, which would be designed to block the effects of these various growth factors.

AIDS-ASSOCIATED LYMPHOMA

Although lymphoma primary to the central nervous system was considered one of the initial criteria for the diagnosis of AIDS, it was not until 1985 that sufficient epidemiologic data were available to indicate a statistical increase in systemic lymphoma as well (35). Based upon these data, the Centers for Disease Control changed the case definition of AIDS in October 1985, to include cases of intermediate or high-grade B-cell lymphoma in AIDS risk group members (36). At the present time, such cases in the setting of HIV seropositivity would indicate the development of full-blown AIDS. This delayed recognition of systemic lymphoma as a criterion for AIDS is consistent with the hypothesis that lymphoma is a relatively late manifestation of infection by HIV, a concept that has recently been supported by data from the National Cancer Institute (37). Thus, as demonstrated by Pluda et al. (37), eight of 55 patients with symptomatic HIV infection developed high-grade, B-cell lymphoma after a median of 23.8 months from the institution of antiretroviral therapy, given as part of various therapeutic trials at the National Cancer Institute. Using Kaplan and Meier analyses, the estimated probability of developing lymphoma by 30 months was 28.6%, and by 36 months was 46.4% (CI = 19.6–75.5%). Although patient numbers are very small, and the precise incidence of lymphoma over time is yet to be truly defined, it is still apparent that ever increasing numbers of HIV-infected patients with lymphoma are to be expected. This follows directly from the enhanced patient survival being witnessed, due to effective antiretroviral therapy and prophylaxis, early recognition, and therapy for the various complicating opportunistic infections (38).

Pathologic Characteristics

Approximately 70–90% of patients with AIDS lymphoma are diagnosed with "high-grade" pathologic types of disease, including immunoblastic lymphoma, and/or small noncleaved lymphoma ("undifferentiated"), which may be of the Burkitt or non-Burkitt types (39–44). This very unique pathologic spectrum of disease may be appreciated by review of prior experience at the University of Southern California (USC) and the Working Formulation for Clinical Usage (45,46). In these very large series of well over 1,000 cases diagnosed prior to the 1980s, immunoblastic or small noncleaved lymphomas comprised approximately 10% of all cases.

Although the vast majority of AIDS lymphomas are immunoblastic or small noncleaved lymphomas, approximately 10–30% are at an "intermediate grade," usually the large noncleaved type. The precise meaning of this distinction is somewhat problematic, especially considering the subtle nature of pathologic distinction, and the well-appreciated difficulties in reproducibility of pathologic diagnosis. Furthermore, although some investigators have found certain clinicopathologic correlates of disease in the intermediate versus high-grade types (41), these correlates have not been confirmed in other series (47), and at the present time it is probably justified to consider patients with either intermediate or high-grade disease similarly, with regard to prognosis and therapy.

A small number of patients with underlying HIV infection have also been diagnosed with low-grade lymphomas, including chronic lymphocytic leukemia, multiple myeloma, and small cleaved lymphoma. There are no epidemiologic data to suggest that these cases represent anything other than chance occurrence. Furthermore, these patients appear to behave identically to patients without HIV infection, in regard to prognosis and therapeutic outcome (40,41,47). Likewise, several HIV-infected patients with various types of T-cell lymphoma have also been reported; once again, there is no statistical evidence to indicate that these cases represent anything other than chance occurrence, especially considering the fact that the most commonly reported of these lymphomas, lymphoblastic lymphoma, is expected to occur in young males (48).

Immunobiologic Features

AIDS lymphomas are expected to be of B-lymphoid origin, as reported initially by Levine et al. (39) in 1984, and confirmed by all subsequent studies (41,42). In the series from USC of 93 cases, 31% marked as the monoclonal κ immunophenotype; 13% were monoclonal λ; 8% were both κ and λ positive; 14% were other B-cell marker positive; 5% were nonmarking; and the remainder (29%) were not studied (47). In the series from New York University (NYU), 25/26 patients tested were positive for B-cell antigens, and one had T-cell antigen expression. Seventy-seven percent of small noncleaved lymphomas were common ALL antigen (CALLA) positive, while 13% of the large noncleaved cases expressed the CALLA marker (49).

Interestingly, immunoglobulin gene rearrangement studies, performed by Southern blot technology, have indicated that, while the majority of cases demonstrate one clonal heavy chain gene rearrangement, consistent with immunogenotypic monoclonality, many cases have multiple clonal B-cell expansions (49), similar to what has previously been described in transplantation-associated lymphoma. These data have implications related to the etiology and pathogenesis of lymphoma in the setting of underlying immunodeficiency.

Epidemiology

Unlike Kaposi's sarcoma, in which the predominant group affected appears to be homosexual or bisexual men, AIDS-associated lymphoma may be seen equally in any group at risk for HIV infection (50,51). Thus, homosexual males, hemophiliacs, intravenous drug users, and transfusion recipients have all been at risk for development of lymphoma. Interestingly, the clinical and pathologic characteristics of disease appear identical in all population groups. Furthermore, as noted above, the incidence of AIDS-related lymphoma is expected to rise in all of these groups over time, as the epidemic proceeds.

Clinical Characteristics

Approximately 70–80% of patients with AIDS lymphoma present with systemic "B" symptoms (52), including unexplained fever, drenching night sweats, and/or weight loss, in excess of 10% of normal body weight (39–44). This type of presentation may be quite problematic, as the clinician searches for the presence of what is assumed to be an occult opportunistic infection, or even considers underlying HIV infection, per se. It is important to recognize that such systemic symptoms may be an indication of underlying lymphomatous disease as well. Conversely, in the patient with known lymphoma, the presence of such symptoms cannot be assumed to be lymphoma-related, until a careful evaluation for infection, such as *Mycobacterium avium-intracellulare* infection or others, has been performed.

Patients with AIDS-associated lymphoma classically present with widespread lymphomatous disease, involving multiple extranodal sites (39–44). Thus, in the series from USC (47), 84% of individuals presented with lymphoma in extranodal sites. In Ziegler's report from several institutions, 95% had evidence of lymphomatous disease in extranodal sites (44), while investigators at NYU reported such a finding in 87% (41), and Kaplan et al. (42) from San Francisco General Hospital noted extranodal presentations in 97% of cases.

The unique nature of such widespread lymphomatous disease at presentation may be appreciated from older experiences published by Jones et al. in 1973 (53). In this series of 405 lymphoma patients, all diagnosed prior to the AIDS epidemic, 39% were found to have extranodal lymphoma at the time of initial diagnosis. One of the distinguishing features of AIDS-related lymphoma, then, is the widespread nature of lymphomatous involvement, even at initial presentation. It is not unusual, for example, to see a patient with extensive involvement of the entire gastrointestinal tract, from mouth to anus.

Not only do affected individuals present with extranodal disease, but they are also distinguished by the very unusual sites of lymphomatous involvement that have been reported (39–44). Lymphoma in the myocardium, bile ducts, ear lobes, orbit, popliteal fossa, gingiva, appendix, and rectum have been seen. In addition to these sites, other areas of involvement are observed with some regularity. Thus, in the series from USC, central nervous system involvement has been noted in approximately 32%; gastrointestinal tract in 26%; bone marrow in 25%; liver in 12%; and kidney and lung in 9% each. Other series have had consistent findings. One of the challenges in treating such individuals is the frequent occurrence of extensive organ involvement and even of organ failure, and the necessity of utilizing chemotherapeutic agents that in themselves may cause organ dysfunction, especially related to the bone marrow and liver.

Prognostic Factors for Survival

Several investigators have reported pretherapy characteristics that were found to be associated with shorter survival in patients with HIV-related lymphoma. The results of these various series have been remarkably consistent. As noted by Ziegler et al. (44) in a retrospective, multiinstitutional trial, the presence of an AIDS diagnosis prior to diagnosis of lymphoma predicted shorter survival, a finding also noted by Lowenthal et al. (43), Levine (54), and Kaplan et al. (42). In a large retrospective study from the University of California San Francisco, Kaplan et al. (42) performed multivariate analysis and found that a low CD4 count (less than $100/mm^3$), history of prior AIDS, Karnofsky performance status (KPS) of 70% or less, and presence of extranodal disease each predicted for decreased survival. In a retrospective study of 60 cases of systemic lymphoma in known HIV-seropositive individuals, all of whom were treated with curative intent, Levine (54) defined three poor prognostic indicators on multivariate analysis, including a KPS less than 70%; an AIDS diagnosis prior to development of lymphoma; and the presence of bone marrow involvement. Lower CD4 counts, on a continuous scale, were also a significant predictor of shorter survival.

It is apparent from this information that both HIV-related factors (CD4 count; history of prior AIDS; KPS less than 70%) and lymphoma-related factors (bone marrow involvement; presence of extranodal disease) are important in determining prognosis in the HIV-infected patient with systemic lymphoma.

Therapeutic Considerations

In recent years, the importance of dose intensity has been recognized in attempts to define optimal therapy of the patient with non-HIV-related lymphoma (55). Thus successive chemotherapeutic regimens reported in the 1980s have been increasingly intensive, with use of multiple additional agents, given at higher than usual doses, and at shorter time intervals. While the full impact of these regimens, when compared with those used earlier, has still to be learned, this initial information led various investigators to consider the use of such dose-intensive therapy in the patient with AIDS-related lymphoma whose disease was likely to be bulky and extensive, and of "high grade" or aggressive pathologic type.

With these considerations in mind, Gill et al. (56), from USC, embarked upon an intensive regimen of multiagent chemotherapy, reported in 1987. High-dose cytosine arabinoside, methotrexate, and cyclophosphamide were used, along with other traditional agents, in an attempt to provide early central nervous system therapy, as well as to give attention to systemic sites of disease. Despite the known efficacy of these agents in other settings, the regimen was essentially ineffective in patients with HIV-related disease, associated with a complete remission (CR) rate of only 33%, and evidence of CNS progression in 66%. Furthermore, the regimen was simply too toxic in these individuals, with complicating opportunistic infections developing in 78%, leading to demise in all. Due to these results the trial was terminated early.

Other investigators have also noted poor treatment results after use of very intensive regimens. Thus, the NYU group reported a 20% CR rate after use of the intensive ProMACE-MOPP regimen, which also required extensive delays and dose reductions, due to the underlying HIV-related immunodeficiency. Furthermore, Kaplan et al. (42) treated 38 patients with COMET-A, consisting of high-dose cytosine arabinoside, cyclophosphamide, methotrexate, and other agents, similar to those reported by Gill et al. (56). Median survival for patients treated with this regimen was significantly shorter than that for patients who had received other, less intensive regimens. Additionally, on multivariate analysis of those factors associated with decreased survival, patients receiving high-dose cyclophosphamide (greater than 1 g/m^2) on any regimen had a significantly shorter survival than patients who had received less than 1 g/m^2 (42), again confirming the observation that HIV-infected patients with lymphoma simply cannot tolerate the dose-intensive therapy that has been commonly employed in other settings.

There has been one published report of the efficacious use of intensive therapy in HIV-infected patients with lymphoma. The MACOP-B regimen was employed by Bermudez et al. (58) in 12 patients, 8 of whom (67%) attained complete remission. It is noteworthy that 6/8 had a KPS of 100%, and only one had a KPS less than 80%. Furthermore, only one had a history of AIDS prior to the diagnosis of lymphoma. It is certainly possible, then, that selected individuals, with none of the predictors of poor prognosis, may be able to tolerate such dose-intensive therapy with good response. However, in the majority of individuals with more severe HIV-related disease (history of prior AIDS; low CD4 cells; low KPS), such dose-intensive therapy is likely to be quite toxic, and ineffective, as discussed above.

With these considerations in mind, Levine et al. (59) embarked upon a study of low-dose chemotherapy, with early CNS prophylaxis. Using a low-dose modification of the M-BACOD regimen (Table 1) (60), a total of 42 patients were accrued as part of the AIDS Clinical Trials Groups (ACTG) of the NIAID. With 35 evaluable patients, a complete remission rate of 46% was achieved, with only 4/16 complete remission patients experiencing relapse, after a median follow-up period of over 14 months. The median survival of complete responders has not yet been reached, but will be in excess of 14 months. Although nadir granulocyte counts less than 500/mm^3 were seen in approximately 20%, only one patient experienced bacterial sepsis, and a total of approximately 20% developed opportunistic infections, consisting of *Pneumocystis carinii* pneumonia (PCP) in all. Prior series of chemotherapy-treated patients with AIDS-related lymphoma or Kaposi's sarcoma have reported the development of PCP in between 40% and 78% of treated subjects. Thus, although the results with low-dose M-BACOD are still not optimal, the regimen appears tolerable and associated with the likelihood of long-term, lymphoma-free survival, even in patients presenting with a history of prior AIDS, low CD4 count, low KPS, and/or bone marrow involvement.

It is important to note that even though long-term lymphoma-free survival was achieved in this study, patients were still at risk for development of additional HIV-related illness, including opportunistic infections and/or HIV wasting syndrome, after completion of all chemotherapy. It is thus apparent that long-term, "event-free" survival will require not only effective chemotherapy, but effective antiretroviral therapy as well. To this end, several on-going therapeutic trials are now studying the use of concomitant chemotherapy and antiviral therapy, with or without the use of hematopoietic growth factor support. The results of these studies are awaited with interest.

Primary Central Nervous System Lymphoma

Primary CNS lymphoma usually presents with one or two mass lesions in the brain; any parenchymal area may be involved (61,62). Symptoms include seizures, focal neurologic dysfunction, headache, and/or cranial nerve palsies. Interestingly, affected patients may present with altered mental status, even of a very subtle nature, as the only clinical manifestation of disease.

Radiographic evaluation usually reveals one or two relatively large (2–4 cm) homogeneous or heterogeneous lesions within the parenchyma. Ring enhancement may be seen on double-dose contrast studies, and, in general, the lesions are enhancing (61,62). Although CT scans of the brain may be similar in patients with cerebral toxoplasmosis, these individuals often have multiple, smaller lesions than those seen in primary CNS lymphoma (61). It is not unusual for such patients to receive empiric therapy for cerebral toxoplasmosis, with repeat of the CT scan within 1–2 weeks. With definite improvement documented, the patient may be safely assumed to have cerebral toxoplasmosis. However, with similar or worsening disease parameters after this period of empiric therapy, a brain biopsy is indicated, to confirm the diagnosis of primary CNS lymphoma, or some other pathologic process.

The prognosis of the HIV-infected patient with primary CNS lymphoma is quite poor. In fact, in the retro-

TABLE 1. *Treatment protocols for lymphoma^a in HIV-infected patients*

	Current regimen	M-BACOD regimen (ref. 60)
Bleomycin	4 mg/m^2, day 1 IV	4 mg/m^2, day 1, IV
Doxorubicin	25 mg/m^2, day 1 IV	45 mg/m^2, day 1, IV
Cyclophosphamide	300 mg/m^2, day 1 IV	600 mg/m^2, day 1, IV
Vincristine	1.4 mg/m^2, day 1 IV (not to exceed 2 mg)	1.0 mg/m^2, day 1, IV
Dexamethasone	3 mg/m^2 days 1–5, po	6 mg/m^2, days 1–5, po
Methotrexate (MTX)	500 mg/m^2 day 15, IV with folinic acid rescue, 25 mg po Q6H × 4, beginning 6 hours after completion of MTX	3,000 mg/m^2, day 14, IV with folinic acid rescue, 10 mg/m^2 IV or po Q6H for 72 hours, beginning 24 hours after completion of MTX.
Cytosine arabinoside	50 mg, intrathecal, days 1, 8, 21, 28	0
Helmet field radiotherapy	2,400 cGy with marrow involvement; 4,000 cGy with known CNS involvement	0
Zidovudine (AZT)	200 mg every 4 hours for 1 year; starting after chemo	0
Total treatment	4–6 cycles, at 28-day intervals	10 cycles, at 21-day intervals

^{a} Excluding primary central nervous system lymphoma.

spective series published by Levine (54), the survival of these individuals, even when treated, was significantly shorter than that for patients with systemic HIV-related lymphoma. Interestingly, patients with primary CNS disease had significantly more severe underlying HIV-related disease, as reflected by the fact that 73% had a prior diagnosis of AIDS, and the median CD4 count at diagnosis of lymphoma was only 34/mm^3.

Although radiation therapy may be associated with complete remission in approximately 50% of these patients, survival beyond 6 months is unusual, due to intercurrent opportunistic infections and the presence of multiple on-going neuropathologic processes (63). Clearly, effective antiretroviral therapy must be a part of future therapeutic trials, used early in the treatment schema. Additionally, the use of cytotoxic chemotherapy in addition to radiation must be explored.

MISCELLANEOUS CANCERS

Hodgkin's Disease

Although there are no epidemiologic data to demonstrate a statistical increase in Hodgkin's disease since the onset of AIDS, it is apparent that the course of disease in an HIV-infected patient is altered. This is fully consistent with the previously understood relationship between host immunity and the specific clinicopathologic characteristics of Hodgkin's disease in a given patient.

In the patient with underlying HIV infection, Hodgkin's disease is likely to be widespread, often involving extranodal sites, such as bone marrow, liver, and/or lung (64,65). Although unusual sites of disease have been described, such as the rectum, clearly this is the exception, in contrast to the experience with AIDS-associated lymphoma. Aside from widespread disease, affected patients are often symptomatic ("B" symptoms), with fever, night sweats, and/or unexplained weight loss. Mixed cellularity and lymphocyte depletion subtypes are seen most frequently.

Therapy of such patients may be problematic, due to underlying bone marrow dysfunction secondary to HIV, or in some cases, due to involvement by Hodgkin's disease itself. Multiagent chemotherapy may further compromise hematologic parameters, with the risk of neutropenia and resulting bacterial and/or opportunistic infections (which may occur even in the patient without underlying HIV infection). Despite all of the potential difficulties of multiagent chemotherapy in this setting, the likelihood of symptomatic, disseminated disease is so high that the majority of these patients do require such therapeutic intervention. The median survival of HIV-infected patients with Hodgkin's disease has been in the range of 2 years (64,65), in comparison with the strong likelihood of cure in the majority of such patients who

are not infected by HIV. Clearly, alternative strategies are required, such as the concomitant use of chemotherapy with hematopoietic growth factors. Such trials are currently under way.

MISCELLANEOUS SOLID CANCERS

Miscellaneous cancers have been reported in patients with HIV infection, and although there is no statistical evidence to suggest an epidemic of these tumors, it is wise to follow such cases and gather statistics over time, to ascertain their true incidence and significance.

Experience in patients with organ transplantation provides a model for the development of such cancers (66). Presumably because of iatrogenically induced immunosuppression, organ transplantation recipients are at increased risk for a variety of cancers, including Kaposi's sarcoma, lymphoma, squamous cell carcinomas of the mouth and skin, and carcinomas of the vulva and perineum, kidney and hepatobiliary tract, as well as various sarcomas. Interestingly, the degree of immunosuppression may be predictive of the specific type of malignancy that develops, with the more immunosuppressive regimens more likely to be associated with lymphomas, occurring relatively early in the posttransplantation period. In general, the average interval between renal transplantation and the development of Kaposi's sarcoma is approximately 20 months, while that of lymphoma is 33 months, miscellaneous other tumors is approximately 67 months, and cancers of the vulva and perineum occur approximately 107 months after transplantation (66).

Patients with underlying HIV infection have now been described with squamous cell carcinomas of the skin and oral and anogenital regions; basal cell carcinomas of the skin; melanomas; germinal testicular tumors; gastric adenocarcinomas; and others (67). Since the transplantation model would predict ever increasing numbers of these cancers in the years ahead, it is important to document such cases, with information obtained regarding specific immune status, clinical and pathologic correlates, presence of coinfections such as papilloma virus infection, and therapeutic outcome.

REFERENCES

1. Reynolds WA, Winkelmann RK, Soule EH. Kaposi's sarcoma. *Medicine* 1965;44:419–43.
2. Fauci AS, Masur H, Gelman EP, et al. The acquired immunodeficiency syndrome. An update. *Ann Intern Med* 1985;102:800–13.
3. Krigel RL, Friedman-Kien AE. In: DeVita VT, Hellman S, Rosenberg SA, eds. *Cancer: principles and practice of oncology,* 2nd ed. Philadelphia: JB Lippincott, 1985.
4. Salahuddin SZ, Nakamura S, Biberfeld P, et al. Angiogenic properties of Kaposi's sarcoma-derived cells after long-term culture in vitro. *Science* 1988;242:430–3.
5. Nakamura S, Salahuddin SZ, Biberfeld P, et al. Kaposi's sarcoma cells: long-term culture with growth factor from retrovirus-infected CD4+ T cells. *Science* 1988;242:426–30.

6. Gill PS, Loureiro C, Bernstein-Singer M, Rarick MU, Sattler F, Levine AM. Clinical effects of glucocorticoids on Kaposi's sarcoma related to the acquired immunodeficiency syndrome (AIDS). *Ann Intern Med* 1989;110:937–40.

7. Vogel J, Hinrichs SH, Reynolds RK, Luciw PA, Jay G. The HIV tat gene induces dermal lesions resembling Kaposi's sarcoma in transgenic mice. *Nature* 1988;335:606–11.

8. Ensoli B, Barillari G, Salahuddin SZ, Gallo RC, Wong-Staal F. Tat protein of HIV-1 stimulates growth of cells derived from Kaposi's sarcoma lesions of AIDS patients. *Nature* 1990;344:84–6.

9. Sakurada S, Nakamura S, Markham PD, Gallo RC, Salahuddin SZ. unpublished data, 1991.

10. Weich HA, Salahuddin SZ, Nakamura S, Gallo RC, Folkman J. unpublished data, 1991.

11. Facchetti F, Lucini L, Gavazzoni R, Callea F. Immunomorphologic analysis of the role of blood vessel endothelium in the morphogenesis of cutaneous Kaposi's sarcoma: a study of 57 cases. *Histopathology* 1988;12:581–93.

12. Grody WW, Lewin KJ, Naeim F. Detection of cytomegalovirus DNA in classic and epidemic Kaposi's sarcoma by in situ hybridization. *Hum Pathol* 1988;19:524–8.

13. Beckstead JH, Wood GS, Fletcher V. Evidence for the origin of Kaposi's sarcoma from lymphatic endothelium. *Am J Pathol* 1985;119:294–300.

14. Rutgers JL, Wieczorek R, Bonetti F, Kaplan KS, Posnett DN, Friedman-Kien AE, Knowles DM II. The expression of endothelial cell surface antigens by AIDS-associated Kaposi's sarcoma. Evidence for a vascular endothelial cell origin. *Am J Pathol* 1986;122:493–9.

15. Scully PA, Steinman HK, Kennedy C, Trueblood K, Frisman DM, Voland JR. AIDS-related Kaposi's sarcoma displays differential expression of endothelial surface antigens. *Am J Pathol* 1988;130:244–51.

16. Niemi M, Mustakallio KK. The fine structure of the spindle cell in Kaposi's sarcoma. *Acta Pathol Microbiol Immunol Scand* 1965;63:567–75.

17. Hymes KB, Cheng T, Greene JB, et al. Kaposi's sarcoma in homosexual men: a report of eight cases. *Lancet* 1981;2:598–600.

18. Friedman-Kien AE, Laubenstein LJ, Rubinstein P, et al. Disseminated Kaposi's sarcoma in homosexual men. *Ann Intern Med* 1982;96:693–700.

19. Gill PS, Akil B, Colletti P, et al. Pulmonary Kaposi's sarcoma: clinical findings and results of therapy. *Am J Med* 1989;87:57–61.

20. Steigman CK, Anderson DW, Macher AM, Sennesh JD, Virmani R. Fatal cardiac tamponade in acquired immunodeficiency syndrome with epicardial Kaposi's sarcoma. *Am Heart J* 1988;116:1105–7.

21. Krown WE, Metroka C, Wernz JC. Kaposi's sarcoma in the acquired immunodeficiency syndrome: a proposal for uniform evaluation, response, and staging criteria. *J Clin Oncol* 1989;7:1201–7.

22. DeWit R, Boucher CB, Veenhof KN, Schattenkerk J, Bakker P, Danner S. Clinical and virological effects of high dose recombinant interferon-alpha in disseminated AIDS related Kaposi's sarcoma. *Lancet* 1988;2:1214–7.

23. Lane HC, Feinberg J, Davey V, et al. Anti-retroviral effects of interferon-alpha in AIDS-associated Kaposi's sarcoma. *Lancet* 1988;2:1218–22.

24. Chachoua A, Krigel R, Lafleur F, et al. Prognostic factors and staging classification of patients with epidemic Kaposi's sarcoma. *J Clin Oncol* 1989;7:745–8.

25. Hill DR. The role of radiotherapy for epidemic Kaposi's sarcoma. *Semin Oncol* 1987;14[Suppl 3]:19–22.

26. Chak LY, Gill PS, Levine AM, Meyer PR, Anselmo JA, Petrovich Z. Radiation therapy for acquired immunodeficiency syndrome related Kaposi's sarcoma. *J Clin Oncol* 1988;6:863–7.

27. Kovacs JA, Deyton L, Davey R, et al. Combined zidovudine and interferon-alpha therapy in patients with Kaposi's sarcoma and the acquired immunodeficiency syndrome (AIDS). *Ann Intern Med* 1989;111:280–7.

28. Krown SE, Gold JWM, Niedzwiecki D, et al. Interferon-alpha with zidovudine: safety, tolerance, and clinical and virologic effects in patients with Kaposi's sarcoma associated with the acquired immunodeficiency syndrome (AIDS). *Ann Intern Med* 1990;112:812–21.

29. Volberding PA, Abrams DI, Conant M, et al. Vinblastine therapy for Kaposi's sarcoma in the acquired immunodeficiency syndrome. *Ann Intern Med* 1985;103:335–8.

30. Laubenstein LJ, Krigel RL, Odajnk CM, et al. Treatment of epidemic Kaposi's sarcoma with etoposide or a combination of doxorubicin, bleomycin, and vinblastine. *J Clin Oncol* 1984;2:1115–20.

31. Kaplan L, Abrams D, Volberding P. Treatment of Kaposi's sarcoma in acquired immunodeficiency syndrome with an alternating vincristine-vinblastine regimen. *Cancer Treat Rep* 1986;70:1121–2.

32. Gill PS, Rarick MU, Espina B, et al. Advanced acquired immunodeficiency syndrome related Kaposi's sarcoma. Results of pilot studies using combination chemotherapy. *Cancer* 1990;65:1074–8.

33. Gill PS, Rarick M, Bernstein-Singer M, et al. Treatment of advanced Kaposi's sarcoma using a combination of bleomycin and vincristine. *Am J Clin Oncol* 1990;13:315–9.

34. Rarick MU, Gill PS, Montgomery T, Bernstein-Singer M, Jones B, Levine AM. Treatment of epidemic Kaposi's sarcoma with combination of chemotherapy (vincristine and bleomycin) and zidovudine. *Ann Oncol* 1990;1:147–9.

35. Ross RK, Dworsky RL, Paganini-Hill A, et al. Non-Hodgkin's lymphomas in never married men in Los Angeles. *Br J Cancer* 1985;52:785–97.

36. CDC: Revision of the case definition of acquired immunodeficiency syndrome for national reporting—United States. *MMWR* 1985;34:373–5.

37. Pluda JM, Yarchoan R, Jaffe ES, et al. Development of lymphoma in a cohort of patients with severe human immunodeficiency virus (HIV) infection on long term antiretroviral therapy. *Ann Intern Med* 1990;113:276–82.

38. Fischl MA, Richman DD, Greico MH, et al. The efficacy of azidothymidine (AZT) in the treatment of patients with AIDS and AIDS related complex. *N Engl J Med* 1987;317:185–91.

39. Levine AM, Meyer PR, Begandy MK, et al. Development of B-cell lymphoma in homosexual men: clinical and immunologic findings. *Ann Intern Med* 1984;100:7–13.

40. Levine AM, Gill PS, Meyer PR, et al. Retrovirus and malignant lymphoma in homosexual men. *JAMA* 1985;254:1921–5.

41. Knowles DM, Chamulak GA, Subar M, et al. Lymphoid neoplasia associated with the acquired immunodeficiency syndrome (AIDS): the New York University experience. *Ann Intern Med* 1988;108:744–53.

42. Kaplan LD, Abrams DI, Feigal E, et al. AIDS-associated non-Hodgkin's lymphoma in San Francisco. *JAMA* 1989;261:719–24.

43. Lowenthal DA, Straus DJ, Campbell SW, et al. AIDS-related lymphoid neoplasia: the Memorial Hospital Experience. *Cancer* 1988;61:2325–37.

44. Ziegler JL, Beckstead JA, Volberding PA, et al. Non-Hodgkin's lymphoma in 90 homosexual men: relationship to generalized lymphadenopathy and acquired immunodeficiency syndrome (AIDS). *N Engl J Med* 1984;311:565–70.

45. Lukes RJ, Parker JW, Taylor CR, et al. Immunologic approach to non-Hodgkin's lymphomas and related leukemias. Analysis of the results of multiparameter studies of 425 cases. *Semin Hematol* 1978;15:322–51.

46. Non-Hodgkin's Lymphoma Pathologic Classification Project. National Cancer Institute sponsored study of classifications of non-Hodgkin's lymphomas: summary and description of a working formulation for clinical usage. *Cancer* 1982;49:2112–35.

47. Levine AM. Reactive and neoplastic lymphoproliferative disorders and other miscellaneous cancers associated with HIV infection. In: DeVita VT Jr, Hellman S, Rosenberg SA, eds. *AIDS: etiology, diagnosis, treatment and prevention.* Philadelphia: JP Lippincott, 1988;263–75.

48. Rosen PG, Feinstein KI, Pattengale PF, et al. Convoluted lymphocytic lymphomas in adults: a clinicopathologic entity. *Ann Intern Med* 1978;89:319–24.

49. Raphael BG, Knowles DM. Acquired immunodeficiency syndrome-associated non-Hodgkin's lymphoma. *Semin Oncol* 1990;17:361–6.

50. Ragni M, Kingsley L, Duzyk A, Obrams I. HIV associated malig-

nancy in hemophiliacs: preliminary report from the Hemophilia Malignancy Study (HMS). *Blood* 1988;74:38a.

51. Monfardini S, Vaccher E, Tirelli U. AIDS associated non-Hodgkin's lymphoma in Italy: intravenous drug users versus homosexual men. *Ann Oncol* 1990;1:208–11.

52. Carbone PP, Kaplan HS, Musshoff K, et al. Report of the committee on Hodgkin's disease staging classification. *Cancer Res* 1971;31:1860–1.

53. Jones SE, Fulks Z, Bullm M, et al. Non-Hodgkin's lymphomas. IV. Clinicopathologic correlation of 405 cases. *Cancer* 1973;31:806–23.

54. Levine AM. HIV-related lymphoma: prognostic factors predictive of survival. *Blood* 1988;72:247a.

55. Frei E III, Canellos GP. Dose: a critical factor in cancer chemotherapy. *Am J Med* 1980;69:585–94.

56. Gill PS, Levine AM, Krailo M, et al. AIDS-related malignant lymphoma: results of prospective treatment trials. *J Clin Oncol* 1987;5:1322–8.

57. Dugan M, Subar M, Odajnyk C, et al. Intensive multiagent chemotherapy for AIDS related diffuse large cell lymphoma. *Blood* 1986;68:124a.

58. Bermudez MA, Grant KM, Rodvien R, Mendes F. Non-Hodgkin's lymphoma in a population with or at risk for acquired immunodeficiency syndrome: indications for intensive chemotherapy. *Am J Med* 1989;86:71–6.

59. Levine AM, Wernz JC, Kaplan L, et al. Low dose chemotherapy with central nervous system prophylaxis and zidovudine maintenance in AIDS-related lymphoma: a multi-institutional trial. *Blood* 1989;74:897a.

60. Skarin AT, Canellos GP, Rosenthal DS, et al. Improved prognosis of diffuse histiocytic and undifferentiated lymphoma by use of high dose methotrexate alternating with standard agents (M-BACOD). *J Clin Oncol* 1983;1:91–8.

61. Gill PS, Graham RA, Boswell W, et al. A comparison of imaging, clinical and pathologic aspects of space occupying lesions within the brain in patients with acquired immunodeficiency syndrome. *Am J Physiol Imaging* 1986;1:134–41.

62. So YT, Beckstead JH, Davis RL. Primary central nervous system lymphoma in acquired immune deficiency syndrome: a clinical and pathological study. *Ann Neurol* 1986;20:566–72.

63. Formenti SC, Gill PS, Lean E, et al. Primary central nervous system lymphoma in AIDS: results of radiation therapy. *Cancer* 1989;63:1101–7.

64. Schoppel SL, Hoppe RT, Dorfman RF, et al. Hodgkin's disease in homosexual men with generalized lymphadenopathy. *Ann Intern Med* 1985;102:68–70.

65. Italian Cooperative Group for AIDS-related tumors. Malignant lymphomas in patients with or at risk for AIDS in Italy. *J Natl Cancer Inst* 1988;80:855–60.

66. Penn, I. Cancers complicating organ transplantation [Editorial]. *N Engl J Med* 1990;323:1767–9.

67. Levine AM, Gill PS, Kaplan L, Cohen P. Cancer in the acquired immunodeficiency syndrome. *Curr Opin Oncol* 1989;1:55–72.

AIDS and Other Manifestations of HIV Infection,
Second Edition, Edited by Gary P. Wormser.
Raven Press, Ltd., New York © 1992.

CHAPTER **29**

Hematologic Findings in HIV Infection

Dania Caron, Daniel Jacobson, and Christina Walsh

Peripheral blood and bone marrow abnormalities often accompany human immunodeficiency virus (HIV) infection, and are frequently multifactorial in origin. Opportunistic infections, tumor infiltration, antiretroviral, antimicrobial, or antitumor therapy, and possibly direct insult or suppressive effects by the HIV virus itself, may all affect hematologic parameters. The syndrome of HIV-related idiopathic thrombocytopenia purpura (ITP) will be discussed separately below.

ANEMIA AND LEUKOPENIA

All combinations of cytopenias may occur in HIV-infected patients. Anemia is seen in about 70% of AIDS patients and 10–20% of asymptomatic HIV-seropositive individuals (1–4). The degree of anemia tends to worsen throughout the course of the HIV infection, as the immune deterioration progresses. The anemia is usually normochromic and normocytic, although both anisocytosis and poikilocytosis occur. Rouleaux formation may be seen, probably resulting from the polyclonal hypergammaglobulinemia that is often present. Iron stores and ferritin are frequently increased (consistent with an anemia of chronic disease), although in a third of cases iron stores are reduced (5). Although hemolytic anemia is unusual in HIV-infected individuals, there is an increased incidence of positive direct antiglobulin tests (3). These antibodies may react with specific red cell antigens or may be antiphospholipid antibodies.

Leukopenia is present in up to 85% of patients with symptomatic HIV infection and 20% of healthy HIV-seropositive individuals (2). Lymphopenia is the most common type of leukopenia (1,2), occurring in 65–80% of AIDS patients. Typically, the number of CD4-positive cells is reduced and the CD4:CD8 ratio (normally >1) is reversed. Neutropenia occurs in 20–50% of AIDS patients (2,6) and in some asymptomatic seropositive individuals. Antineutrophil antibodies have been found in some neutropenic patients (6), suggesting an autoimmune mechanism. Neutrophil function may be impaired, as shown in vitro by decreased chemotaxis (7). Monocytopenia is seen in 30% of AIDS patients (2). Circulating monocytes may be vacuolated or morphologically abnormal (1,2).

BONE MARROW FINDINGS

No bone marrow changes are pathognomonic for HIV infection. The marrow is often difficult to aspirate (a "dry tap"). Reticulin may be focally or diffusely increased (1,5). The bone marrow is usually normocellular or hypercellular, although hypocellularity has been reported in 5% of patients (3). Plasmacytosis and benign-appearing lymphoid aggregates are commonly present (3,5). Eosinophils and monocytes in the marrow are often increased. Erythroid dysplasia with megaloblastic change is often seen. Rarely, ringed sideroblasts are noted (3), and granulocytic dysplasia may be found. Poorly formed granulomas may result from *Mycobacterium avium-intracellulare* infection, or other infectious agents associated with granulomatous inflammation. Marrow aspiration or biopsy occasionally reveals fungal infections (e.g., *Cryptococcus neoformans* or *Histoplasma capsulatum*). Lymphoid neoplasms often infiltrate the marrow.

D. Caron: Department of Clinical Affairs, Immunex Corporation, Seattle Washington 98101.

C. Walsh: Department of Medicine, Kaplan Cancer Center, Division of Oncology, New York University Medical Center, New York, New York 10016

D. Jacobson: Division of Oncology, New York University Medical Center, New York, New York 10016; and Research Service, New York VA Medical Center, New York, New York 10010.

DRUG EFFECTS

Zidovudine (AZT) frequently causes anemia and myelosuppression (8–10). In one study, 24% of 145 AZT-treated AIDS or AIDS-related complex (ARC) patients (dosage of AZT, 1,500 mg/day) developed significant anemia after 6 weeks of therapy, compared with 4% of controls, and 21% of the AZT-treated patients required multiple red blood cell transfusions, compared with 4% of controls (8). Sixteen percent of the AZT-treated patients developed neutropenia, compared with 2% of controls. AZT treatment was associated with an increase in mean corpuscular volume (MCV) and megaloblastic changes. The MCV increased to over 110 μm^3 in 60 (41%) of 145 AZT recipients, and to between 100 μm^3 and 110 μm^3 in an additional 40 (28%). The anemia was dose-dependent, and it generally improved when AZT was stopped or the dosage was lowered. Patients who entered the study with low CD4 counts, low serum B_{12} levels, or preexisting cytopenias were more likely to have hematologic side effects. Supplemental B_{12} does not alleviate the suppressive effects of AZT on the bone marrow (4). Lower doses of AZT (600–1,200 mg/day) are less likely to cause bone marrow depression (10).

The development of anemia was examined in a group of patients with Kaposi's sarcoma receiving AZT (9). A fall in the reticulocyte count was the earliest peripheral blood indicator of toxicity. The MCV increased in patients who did not develop anemia, but remained stable, or increased only slightly, in those who became anemic. Bone marrow aspiration and biopsies done on the patients who developed transfusion requiring anemia showed selective hypoplasia or aplasia of the erythroid series. These anemic patients were found to have elevated serum levels of erythropoietin (EPO).

Other myelosuppressive drugs frequently used in AIDS patients include ganciclovir, pentamidine, trimethoprim–sulfamethoxazole, pyrimethamine–sulfadiazine, and various chemotherapeutic agents (4).

POSSIBLE MECHANISMS OF MARROW SUPPRESSION

The mechanism by which HIV infection directly causes bone marrow suppression and abnormal hematopoiesis is unknown. Donahue et al. (11) reported that anti-HIV antibodies suppressed the in vitro proliferation of bone marrow progenitors from AIDS/ARC patients, but had no effect on marrow cultures from HIV-seronegative persons. Leiderman et al. (12) identified an 84-kd glycoprotein in the conditioned medium of nucleated bone marrow cells from AIDS/ARC patients that inhibited the colony growth of granulocyte–macrophage progenitor cells (CFU–GMs) from normal individuals in

vitro. HIV immune sera did not react with this purified glycoprotein, suggesting that it was a host protein produced in response to HIV infection, rather than a product of the viral genome. CFU–GMs from HIV-seropositive patients had reduced proliferative capacity in this study. Stella et al. (13) also found reduced in vitro proliferative potential of marrow precursor cells from patients with AIDS/ARC. Depletion of T cells from the bone marrow cultures enhanced colony production. The readdition of autologus T cells suppressed progenitor colony growth.

Folks et al. (14) purified CD34-positive progenitor cells from normal bone marrow and successfully infected them in vitro with HIV-1 (14). These cells were devoid of mature myeloid or T-cell markers. Viral production was detected after 40–60 days by transmission electron microscopy and reverse transcriptase activity. Phenotypically, the infected cells had differentiated into CD4-positive monocytes. More recently, von Laer analyzed bone marrow cell populations from 14 AIDS/ARC patients (15). Polymerase chain reaction (PCR) was used as a highly sensitive method to detect HIV-1 proviral DNA. CD34-positive progenitors were HIV positive in only one patient, while CD4-positive helper cells were positive in all patients. Using in situ hybridization, Sun et al. (16) also detected HIV-associated nucleic acid in the bone marrow of AIDS/ARC patients (16). Scadden and coworkers (17) recently reported the in vitro infection of primary human bone marrow stromal fibroblasts with HIV-1 and HIV-2 (17). These cells were capable of passing HIV to cells of lymphoid or myeloid lineage. How these various factors interact and influence the marrow suppression that accompanies HIV infection remains to be determined. Susceptibility of megakaryocytes to HIV infection is discussed later.

THERAPY

The use of hematopoietic growth factors represents a promising therapeutic approach to the myelosuppression seen in HIV infection. Administration of recombinant GM colony-stimulating factor (GMCSF) to leukopenic AIDS patients resulted in dose-dependent increases in circulating neutrophils, eosinophils, and monocytes (18). Despite in vitro studies indicating that GMCSF can enhance virus production in monocytes/macrophages, GMCSF treatment had no effect on the ability to culture HIV from peripheral mononuclear cells (19). In a clinical trial of recombinant (r)GMCSF in neutropenic AIDS/ARC patients taking AZT, total white blood cell and polymorphonuclear leukocyte counts increased significantly, indicating that GMCSF restored granulopoiesis in AIDS patients taking AZT (20). No evidence of HIV stimulation as measured by serum HIV p24 antigen or virus cultured from peripheral blood mononuclear cells was detected in the patients receiving rGMCSF. Miles et al. (21) reported that in patients with advanced HIV disease treated with GCSF, increases in hemoglobin, reticulocytes, and burst-forming units–erythion (BFU–E) were seen, in addition to an increase in neutrophils, suggesting that GCSF produced a multilineage effect in these patients.

Erythropoietin has been shown to decrease transfusion requirements and to increase hemoglobin concentration in AZT-treated AIDS patients compared with placebo-treated controls (22). This advantage of EPO therapy was noted only in those patients with baseline serum EPO levels of less than 500 mU/ml.

HIV-ASSOCIATED IDIOPATHIC THROMBOCYTOPENIA PURPURA

A syndrome of thrombocytopenia in homosexual men was first reported in 1982. Morris et al. (23) described 11 cases of ITP seen in homosexual men in New York City in 1980 and 1981. Salient clinical features in this group included elevated levels of platelet-associated IgG, decreased helper/suppressor T-cell ratios, and elevated levels of circulating immune complexes. The link with HIV infection was firmly established later when serologic testing became available (24). Several subsequent series have been published, the largest of which came from the San Francisco General Hospital (25). The ITP syndrome has also been reported in intravenous drug users and in hemophiliacs in association with HIV infection (26,27). A recent report of 1,004 HIV-infected patients from a Washington DC clinic found that 18% of persons with diagnosed AIDS and 9% of HIV-seropositive persons without AIDS had a platelet count < 150,000/mm^3 (28). Patients with all known risk factors were included; the likelihood of thrombocytopenia was unrelated to the presumed mode of infection. A longitudinal study of hemophiliacs found that 11% of HIV-infected patients had abnormal platelet counts on at least two occasions (29). Though the laboratory finding of a low platelet count is a common occurrence in HIV-infected patients, only a minority of these patients will require treatment for thrombocytopenia, which is generally reserved for patients with bleeding manifestations or platelet counts < 20,000/mm^3. However, the relatively high rate of at least mild thrombocytopenia encourages the hope that research into its mechanism may give insight about basic issues in the pathogenesis of HIV infection.

Mechanisms

One of the earliest findings in the study of thrombocytopenia in homosexual men was the observation that these patients had very high levels of IgG and complement on their platelets. Levels of IgG, C3, and C4 on their platelets were three to four times higher than the levels found on the platelets of female patients with classic autoimmune thrombocytopenic purpura (ATP) (30). This finding, coupled with the demonstration of high levels of immune complexes in the serum of these patients, raised the question of whether the bound IgG might be in the form of immune complexes, rather than autoantibody directed at a specific platelet antigen. Initial work done at New York University supported this concept. Serum fractionation experiments showed that the platelet-binding activity in the serum of these patients was not in the IgG fraction, as it is in the sera of classic ATP patients. In addition, though antiplatelet IgG could be eluted from the platelets of classic ITP patients, no antiplatelet IgG could be eluted from the platelets of HIV-infected homosexual men with ITP. Thus, in this latter group of patients, evidence suggested a role for immune complexes rather than antiplatelet antibody in the etiology of thrombocytopenia (30). When the serum of intravenous drug users with thrombocytopenia was studied with the same techniques, the results were somewhat different. These patients appeared to have antiplatelet antibody in the IgG serum fraction as well as high levels of immune complexes (4). Hemophiliacs with thrombocytopenia had findings similar to those found in classic ATP patients, with serum antiplatelet activity found predominantly in the IgG serum fraction (31). Thus, there may be more than one mechanism contributing to thrombocytopenia in HIV infection. The evidence for immune complex binding to platelets as an etiologic factor is strongest in the HIV-infected homosexual group.

Stricker et al. (32) reported the detection of a specific antiplatelet autoantibody in the serum of HIV-infected homosexual men with ITP. Using a sensitive immunoblotting technique, they found an antibody in the serum of these patients that appeared to bind to a specific 25,000-dalton platelet antigen. However, since this antibody was also found in the serum of 15 of 16 nonthrombocytopenic HIV-infected patients with lymphadenopathy or AIDS, its role in the etiology of thrombocytopenia is not clear (32).

In additional studies (33), anti-HIV-1 antibody has been demonstrated in serum immune complexes and in platelet eluates from thrombocytopenic patients in the homosexual and narcotic addict groups. Antibodies directed against the anti-HIV-1 antibody have also been found (34). Despite the presence of anti-HIV-1 antibodies in platelet eluates, no known HIV antigens have been detected on the surface of platelets, and no HIV-1 proviral DNA has been demonstrated in platelets, using the PCR technique. It thus appears that antibody–antibody complexes, which may be part of an immune regulatory network, may be binding to platelets and possibly contributing to shortened platelet survival.

Accelerated platelet destruction may not be the only factor leading to thrombocytopenia in HIV-infected persons. A recent investigation (35) addressed the issue of platelet production in a group of thrombocytopenic patients receiving AZT. As will be discussed further below, AZT treatment elevates the platelet count in a high percentage of patients with HIV-associated thrombocytopenia. Ballem et al. (35) studied platelet turnover in two subgroups of thrombocytopenic patients. The first was receiving no therapy, and the second was receiving AZT at a dose of 1,200 mg daily. In the patients receiving no therapy, platelet turnover was decreased compared with normal controls. The patients taking AZT, most of whom had increased platelet counts on therapy, had normal or increased platelet turnover. In addition, two patients were studied before and after the initiation of AZT therapy. Platelet count increases were accompanied by marked increases in platelet turnover without an increase in platelet survival (35). The results suggest that marrow production of platelets is depressed in certain HIV-infected patients; production may be improved by AZT treatment.

The means by which HIV infection suppresses platelet production at the marrow level is not known. Karpatkin and coworkers (36) have demonstrated the presence of the CD4 receptor on megakaryocytes. In their study, about 25% of marrow cells staining as megakaryocytes also had the CD4 receptor by a fluorescence-activated cell sorting (FACS) analysis. This molecule could presumably provide a binding site for direct entry of HIV into megakaryocytes.

Zucker-Franklin et al. (37) detected HIV-1 viral RNA in megakaryocytes of HIV-infected persons by in situ hybridization. After coculture of normal human bone marrow and platelets with HIV-infected H9 cells in vitro, viral particles could be detected by electron microscopy in megakaryocytes (38); however, integrated proviral DNA has not yet been demonstrated in megakaryocytes.

Therapy

The first therapy used for patients with HIV-associated ITP was prednisone at doses of 20–60 mg daily. An increase in platelet count to greater than 50,000/mm³ was regularly seen but few patients could be successfully tapered off steroids without a marked decline in platelet count (24,25). Although long-standing concern has been raised about potential detrimental immunosuppressive effects of steroids, there is little evidence that such therapy hastens the time course for progression of clinical AIDS. With the advent of additional therapeutic choices, including AZT, prednisone has been used less often, but it remains a potential option in patients with severe thrombocytopenia or bleeding.

Splenectomy is generally considered for patients with platelet counts < 20,000/mm³ who have been refractory to another treatment modality. Long-term follow-up data are limited. Two early series reported maintenance of normal platelet counts in 10 of 10 and 10 of 14 splenectomized patients at 10 months of follow-up (24,39). Oksenhendler et al. (40) recently reported the outcome at a mean follow-up of 40 months. They found that 37 of 45 splenectomized patients had a persistent increase in platelet count, but the exact numerical value was not provided (40). Again, no data have linked splenectomy to an accelerated rate of progression to AIDS.

Intravenous gamma globulin has been used successfully to elevate the platelet count acutely but has drawbacks for long-term use. Rarick et al. (41) studied a schedule of 1 g/kg on days 1, 2, and 15, followed by maintenance doses at 3-week intervals. In a group of eight patients whose mean baseline platelet count was 18,000/mm³, a mean count of 71,000/mm³ was achieved on day 2 with a later peak mean value of 170,000/mm³. However, all counts dropped dramatically before the first planned maintenance dose. Bussel et al. (42) treated 23 patients and found that 20 of 23 had a platelet count >50,000/mm³ within 1 week. They found that γ-globulin maintenance doses were required every 2 weeks. Maintenance is not effective in all patients and, even when effective, is costly. Intravenous γ-globulin is frequently used in acutely bleeding patients or in patients who require a surgical procedure.

The use of anti-Rh immunoglobulin has been reported recently for HIV-infected patients with thrombocytopenia. In Oksenhendler's experience (43) doses of 12–15 μg/kg intravenously on 2 consecutive days resulted in 9 of 14 patients having a rise in platelet count to >50,000/mm³ by days 3–12. The concomitant fall in hemoglobin ranged from 0.4 to 2.2 g/dl (43). Cattaneo and coworkers (44) reported a response rate of 65% to treatment with 13 μg/kg for 3 days with an IV preparation. They also found that a maintenance dose of 6 μg/kg per week IM was effective in some patients.

Limited data are available on the use of other immunomodulators. Because α-interferon therapy has resulted in improved platelet counts in non-HIV-related immune thrombocytopenia, Luzzati et al. (45) studied a dose of 3 mU/m² three times weekly for at least 12 weeks. In a group of nine patients with HIV infection they found an increase in mean platelet count at 4, 8, and 12 weeks. Interferon preparations deserve further study in view of their possible additional antiretroviral activity. Bussel et al. (46) have reported the use of an anti-Fc receptor monoclonal antibody in HIV-infected patients with cytopenias. Increases in leukocyte and platelet counts were observed in two of three patients.

The advent of AZT has significantly changed the treatment picture for HIV-associated thrombocytopenia. In 1988 Hymes et al. (47) observed platelet count rises after institution of AZT therapy in a small number of HIV-infected patients. The Swiss Group for Clinical Studies in AIDS evaluated the effect of AZT on HIV-associated thrombocytopenia. Ten patients with platelet counts from 10,000 to 100,000/mm^3 were studied. The dose of AZT was 2 g daily for 2 weeks followed by 1 g daily for an additional 6 weeks. Using a cross-over design, patients received both drug and placebo, each for 8 weeks. Average platelet counts rose by at least 20,000/mm^3 within 1 month of starting AZT (48). Several subsequent studies have confirmed that more than 50% of thrombocytopenic patients have a response to AZT (40,49,50). Unresolved issues in this regard are defining the most appropriate dose of AZT and determining the expected duration of platelet count improvement. An AZT dose of 500–600 mg daily is less toxic than doses of 1 g or more and is now the recommended dose for most HIV-infected persons (51). AZT in this dose range has also been shown to be effective in elevating platelet counts (40,52). Duration of response is uncertain, but reports to date have shown improvement lasting a year or more (49,50).

Optimal therapy for the HIV-infected patient with a platelet count of <20,000/mm^3 or with bleeding symptoms is not known. Controlled trials have not been performed. Studies with AZT usually report platelet count improvement within 3–4 weeks of initiating therapy (48). Intravenous γ-globulin, and possibly prednisone, may improve the count more rapidly. If these modalities are selected, AZT can be utilized for maintenance. A trial of AZT can be considered as the initial option in asymptomatic patients.

THROMBOTIC THROMBOCYTOPENIC PURPURA

Thrombotic thrombocytopenic purpura (TTP) has also been reported in HIV-infected individuals (53–55). There are only small numbers of reported cases, but several publications have documented responses to standard therapy with combinations of steroids, plasmapheresis, and antiplatelet agents. Despite much speculation, the mechanism of TTP in HIV infection is not known. Among six early cases reported, four were tested for platelet agglutinating factors but none was detected. No abnormalities were found in von Willebrand factor multimer distribution in two patients tested in the acute phase or in the one patient tested during convalescence (53,54). Whether the incidence of TTP is increased in HIV infection remains to be proved, but this diagnosis must be considered in seropositive or at-risk patients presenting with combinations of fever, mental status changes, anemia, and thrombocytopenia. Further study is necessary to evaluate the possible role of immune complexes in causing platelet or endothelial injury in these patients.

LUPUS ANTICOAGULANT

The lupus anticoagulant is commonly found in patients with HIV infection (56–59). In 1986 Cohen et al. (56) reported laboratory evidence of a circulating anticoagulant in 10 of 50 AIDS patients tested. The diagnosis of lupus-type anticoagulant was supported by prolonged dilute thromboplastin inhibition assays and increased Russell viper venom clotting times. Most patients had active opportunistic infections at the time the anticoagulant was found, and an abnormal PTT was often detected as part of a coagulation screen prior to invasive procedures. These authors reported no evidence that the presence of lupus anticoagulant alone was associated with bleeding complications. However, they evaluated bleeding times, levels of coagulation factors, and platelet counts, and patients with hypoprothrombinemia, thrombocytopenia, or platelet dysfunction were treated prophylactically prior to invasive procedures. Isolation of immunoglobulin fractions from the sera of seven patients showed that either monoclonal IgG or polyclonal IgM could have inhibitory activity. These authors and others have reported that lupus anticoagulant activity may disappear with the resolution of acute infection (56,59). Reports of thrombotic complications in HIV-infected patients with anticoagulants are rare (57), and it may be that recurrent thromboses are less likely in this group.

REFERENCES

1. Spivak JL, Bender BS, Quinn TC. Hematologic abnormalities in the acquired immunodeficiency syndrome. *Am J Med* 1984;77: 224–8.
2. Treacy M, Lai L, Costello C, Clark A. Peripheral blood and bone marrow abnormalities in patients with HIV related disease. *Br J Haematol* 1987;65:289–94.
3. Zon LI, Arkin C, Groopman JE. Haematologic manifestations of the human immune deficiency virus. *Br J Haematol* 1987;66: 251–6.
4. Scadden DT, Zon LI, Groopman JE. Pathophysiology and management of HIV-associated hematologic disorders. *Blood* 1989;74:1455–63.
5. Castella A, Croxson TS, Mildvan D, et al. The bone marrow in AIDS: A histologic, hematologic and microbiologic study. *Am J Clin Pathol* 1985;84:425–31.
6. Murphy MF, Metcalfe P, Waters AH, et al. Incidence and mechanism of neutropenia and thrombocytopenia in patients with human immunodeficiency virus infection. *Br J Haematol* 1987;66: 337–40.
7. Ellis M, Gupta S, Vandeven C, et al. Decreased polymorphonuclear chemotaxis secondary to serum inhibition and abnormal bacterial killing in preacquired immunodeficiency syndrome (pre-AIDS) and AIDS. *Blood* 1985;66:110a.
8. Richman DD, Fischl MA, Grieco MH, et al. The toxicity of azidothymidine (AZT) in the treatment of patients with AIDS and AIDS-related complex. A double-blind, placebo-controlled trial. *N Engl J Med* 1987;317:192–7.
9. Walker RE, Parker RI, Kovacs JA, et al. Anemia and erythropoiesis in patients with the acquired immunodeficiency syndrome (AIDS) and Kaposi's sarcoma treated with zidovudine. *Ann Intern Med* 1988;108:372–6.
10. Fischl M, Parker CB, Pettinelli C, et al. A randomized controlled trial of a reduced daily dose of zidovudine in patients with the

acquired immunodeficiency syndrome. *N Engl J Med* 1990;323:1009–14.

11. Donahue RE, Johnson MM, Zon LI, et al. Suppression of in vitro haematopoiesis following human immunodeficiency virus infection. *Nature* 1987;326:200–3.

12. Leiderman IZ, Greenberg ML, Adelsberg BR, Siegal FP. A glycoprotein inhibitor of in vitro granulopoiesis associated with AIDS. *Blood* 1987;70:1267–72.

13. Stella CC, Ganser A, Hoelzer D. Defective in vitro growth of the hemopoietic progenitor cells in the acquired immunodeficiency syndrome. *J Clin Invest* 1987;80:286–93.

14. Folks TM, Kessler SW, Orenstein JM, et al. Infection and replication of HIV-1 in purified progenitor cells of normal human bone marrow. *Science* 1988;242:919–22.

15. von Laer D, Hufert FT, Fenner TE, et al. CD34+ hematopoietic progenitor cells are not a major reservoir of human immunodeficiency virus. *Blood* 1990;76:1281–6.

16. Sun NC, Shapshak P, Lachant NA, et al. Bone marrow examination in patients with AIDS and AIDS related complex (ARC). Morphologic and in situ hybridization studies. *Am J Clin Pathol* 1989;92:589–94.

17. Scadden DT, Zeira M, Woon A, et al. Human immunodeficiency virus infection of human bone marrow stromal fibroblasts. *Blood* 1990;76:317–22.

18. Groopman JE, Mitsuyasu RT, DeLeo MJ, et al. Effect of recombinant human granulocyte-macrophage colony-stimulating factor on myelopoiesis in the acquired immunodeficiency syndrome. *N Engl J Med* 1987;317:593–8.

19. Koyanagi Y, O'Brien WA, Zhao JQ, et al. Cytokines alter production of HIV-1 from primary mononuclear phagocytes. *Science* 1988;241:1673–5.

20. Levine JD, Allan JD, Tessitore JH, et al. Granulocyte-macrophage colony stimulating factor ameliorates the neutropenia induced by azidothymidine in AIDS/ARC patients. *Proc Annu Meet Am Soc Clin Oncol* 1989;8:A3.

21. Miles SA, Mitsuyasu RT, Lee K, et al. Recombinant human granulocyte colony-stimulating factor increases circulating burst forming unit-erythion and red blood cell production in patients with severe human immunodeficiency virus infection. *Blood* 1990;75:2137–42.

22. Rudnick SA. Human recombinant erythropoietin (R-HUEPO): A double-blind, placebo-controlled study in acquired immunodeficiency syndrome (AIDS) patients with anemia induced by disease and AZT. *Proc Annu Meet Am Soc Clin Oncol* 1989;8:A7.

23. Morris L, Distenfeld A, Amorosi E, et al. Autoimmune thrombocytopenic purpura in homosexual men. *Ann Intern Med* 1982;96:714–7.

24. Walsh C, Krigel R, Lennette E, et al. Thrombocytopenia in homosexual patients. *Ann Intern Med* 1985;103:542–5.

25. Abrams D, Kiprov D, Goedert J, et al. Antibodies to HTLV III and development of AIDS in homosexual men presenting with immune thrombocytopenia. *Ann Intern Med* 1986;104:47–50.

26. Savona S, Nardi M, Lennette E, et al. Thrombocytopenic purpura in narcotic addicts. *Ann Intern Med* 1985;102:737–41.

27. Ratnoff O, Menitove J, Aster R, et al. Coincident classic hemophilia and "idiopathic" thrombocytopenic purpura in patients under treatment with concentrations of AHF. *N Engl J Med* 1983;308:439–42.

28. Sloand EM, Merritt SE, Hollingsworth C, Pierce P. The epidemiology of thrombocytopenia in individuals infected with the acquired immune deficiency virus (HIV). *Blood* 1989;74:924a.

29. Conlan MG, Hoots WK. Thrombocytopenia in HIV-infected hemophiliacs: Prevalence and natural history. *Proc Am Soc Hematol* 1989;74:88a.

30. Walsh C, Nardi M, Karpatkin S. On the mechanism of thrombocytopenic purpura in sexually active homosexual men. *N Engl J Med* 1984;311:635–9.

31. Karpatkin S, Nardi M. On the mechanism of thrombocytopenia in hemophiliacs multiply transfused with AHF concentrates. *J Lab Clin Med* 1988;111:441–8.

32. Stricker R, Abrams D, Corash L, et al. Target platelet antigen in homosexual men with immune thrombocytopenia. *N Engl J Med* 1985;313:1375–80.

33. Karpatkin S, Nardi M, Lennette E, et al. Anti-HIV-1 antibody complexes on platelets of seropositive thrombocytopenic homosexuals and narcotic addicts. *Proc Natl Acad Sci USA* 1988;85:9763–7.

34. Karpatkin S, Nardi M. Cross-reactive anti-idiotype antibody vs anti-HIVgp120 in HIV-1-thrombocytopenia: Correlation with thrombocytopenia. *Proc Am Soc Hematol* 1990;74:128a.

35. Ballem P, Belzberg A, Devine D, et al. Pathophysiology of HIV ITP and the mechanism of the response to AZT. *Proc Am Soc Hematol* 1988;72:261a(abst).

36. Basch R, Kouri Y, Karpatkin S. Human megakaryocytes have a CD4 receptor on their surface. *Proc Am Soc Hematol* 1989;74:206a.

37. Zucker-Franklin D, Cao Y. Megakaryocytes of HIV infected individuals express viral RNA. *Proc Natl Acad Sci USA* 1989;86:5595.

38. Zucker-Franklin D, Seremetis S, Zheng ZY. Internalization of human immunodeficiency virus type 1 and other retroviruses by megakaryocytes and platelets. *Blood* 1990;75:1920–3.

39. Oksenhendler E, Bierling P, Farcet J, et al. Response to therapy in 37 patients with HIV related thrombocytopenic purpura. *Br J Hematol* 1987;66:491–5.

40. Oksenhendler E, Bierling P, Archamebeaud MP, Delfraissy JF, Chevret S, Clauvel JP. HIV-related immune thrombocytopenia: Follow up and treatment of 157 patients. 6th International Conference on AIDS, San Francisco, June, 1990.

41. Rarick M, Loureiro C, Harb M, et al. IGIV in treatment of HIV related thrombocytopenia. *Proc Am Soc Hematol* 1988;72:359a(abst).

42. Bussel J, Hiami J, Cunningham-Rundles C. IVGG treatment of HIV related ITP. *Proc Am Soc Hematol* 1986;68:122a.

43. Oksenhendler E, Bierling P, Brossard Y, et al. AntiRh Ig therapy for HIV related ITP. *Blood* 1988;71:1499–502.

44. Santagostino E, Cattaneo M, Capitanio A, Gringeri A, Tradati F, Mannucci PM. Anti-D immunoglobulin for treatment of immune thrombocytopenic purpura (ITP): Comparison between HIV-related ITP and idiopathic ITP. 6th International Conference on AIDS, San Francisco, June, 1990.

45. Luzzati R, Di Perri G, Malena M, Mazzi R, Concia E, Bassett D. Alpha-interferon in treatment of severe HIV-related thrombocytopenia (TP). 6th International Conference on AIDS, San Francisco, June, 1990.

46. Bussel J, Khayat D, Cunningham-Rundles S, Kimberly R, Nachman R, Unkeless J. Alleviation of cytopenias in 3 HIV infected patients with infusion of a monoclonal anti-FCRIII antibody. *Proc Am Soc Hematol* 1989;74:89a.

47. Hymes K, Greene J, Karpatkin S. The effect of azidothymidine on HIV related thrombocytopenia. *N Engl J Med* 1988;318:516–7.

48. Swiss Group for Clinical Studies in AIDS. Zidovudine for the treatment of thrombocytopenia associated with HIV. *Ann Intern Med* 1988;109:718–21.

49. Carton JA, Carcaba V, Vicente P, Maradona JA, Llorente R. Efficacy of zidovudine in the treatment of HIV infection associated thrombocytopenia. 6th International Conference on AIDS, San Francisco, June, 1990.

50. Paola C, Lazzarin A, Landonio G, Gringeri A, Nosari AM, Moroni M. Medium-long term efficacy of zidovudine in HIV-related thrombocytopenia. 6th International Conference on AIDS, San Francisco, June, 1990.

51. Volberding PA, Lagakos SW, Koch MA, et al. Zidovudine in asymptomatic human immunodeficiency virus infection: a controlled trial in persons with fewer than 500 CD4-positive cells per cubic millimeter. *N Engl J Med* 1990;322:941–9.

52. Montaner J, Le T, Gelman K, et al. The effect of zidovudine on platelet count in HIV associated thrombocytopenia. 5th International Conference on AIDS, Montreal, Canada, June, 1989.

53. Leaf AN, Laubenstein LJ, Raphael B, Hochster H, Baez L, Karpatkin S. Thrombotic thrombocytopenic purpura associated with human immunodeficiency virus type 1 (HIV-1) infection. *Ann Intern Med* 1988;109:194–7.

54. Nair JMG, Bellevue R, Bertoni M, Dosik H. Thrombotic thrombocytopenic purpura in patients with the acquired immunodeficiency syndrome (AIDS)-related complex: a report of two cases. *Ann Intern Med* 1988;109:209–12.

55. DeNobriga J, Chu-Fong A, Elizalde A. Thrombotic thrombocyto-penic purpura (TTP) in a human immune deficiency virus (HIV)-positive patient: successful treatment with high dose gamma globulin (HDGG). *Proc Annu Meet Am Soc Clin Oncol* 1989;8:A21.

56. Cohen AJ, Philips TM, Kessler CM. Circulating coagulation inhibi-tors in the acquired immunodeficiency syndrome. *Ann Intern Med* 1986;104:175–80.

57. Bloom EJ, Abrams DI, Rodgers G. Lupus anticoagulant in the acquired immunodeficiency syndrome. *JAMA* 1986;256:491–3.

58. Kaye BR. Rheumatologic manifestations of infection with human immunodeficiency virus (HIV). *Ann Intern Med* 1989;111:158–67.

59. Gold JE, Haubenstock A, Zalusky R. Lupus anticoagulant and AIDS [Letter]. *N Engl J Med* 1986;314:1252–3.

AIDS and Other Manifestations of HIV Infection,
Second Edition, Edited by Gary P. Wormser.
Raven Press, Ltd., New York © 1992.

CHAPTER 30

Cutaneous and Histologic Signs of HIV Infection Other than Kaposi's Sarcoma

Clay J. Cockerell

Because the skin is so commonly affected in patients with human immunodeficiency virus (HIV) infection, it is of utmost importance that clinicians be able to recognize those skin conditions that may indicate the presence of underlying HIV infection or of superimposed infectious and neoplastic diseases. Appropriate antimicrobial or immunomodulatory therapy may be administered based on such findings.

This chapter will review many of the clinical and histopathologic manifestations of HIV infection that may occur in the skin, recognizing that new cutaneous manifestations of this disease are continually being described.

Skin manifestations of HIV infection other than Kaposi's sarcoma can be divided broadly into two groups: infectious diseases that affect the skin (Table 1) and noninfectious cutaneous disorders (Table 2). These will be discussed in sequence.

VIRAL INFECTIONS

Acute Exanthem of HIV Infection

Certainly the earliest cutaneous manifestation of HIV infection is the HIV exanthem (1). This eruption occurs soon after infection with HIV and is characterized by tiny pinkish macules and papules involving the trunk and extremities accompanied by fever and pharyngitis (1–3) (Fig. 1A). The eruption is somewhat less florid than other morbilliform viral eruptions such as measles. In many cases, the exanthem may go totally unnoticed.

Histologically, there is usually a superficial perivascular infiltrate consisting mostly of lymphocytes and histiocytes with slight spongiosis of the overlying epidermis and occasional individually necrotic keratinocytes (Fig. 1B) (4,5).

Cytomegalovirus Infection

Cytomegalovirus (CMV) is a common pathogen in HIV infection. The most common manifestations of CMV infection are systemic rather than cutaneous, but the skin may be involved. Petechiae and purpura related to thrombocytopenia, which may be induced by CMV, are common cutaneous signs of this systemic viral infection. Vesicular, bullous, and generalized morbilliform skin eruptions may also be associated with CMV infection (6). Other unusual signs of systemic CMV infection may occur. Hyperpigmented, indurated cutaneous plaques have been reported as heralding disseminated CMV infection (7), and there is one case report of a generalized bullous toxic epidermal necrolysis-like eruption that occurred in association with CMV hepatitis in a patient with AIDS (8). In contrast to adult infection, neonates with CMV may have bluish-red cutaneous papules and nodules, which consist of foci of extramedullary hematopoietic tissue (9). Such findings characteristically occur in association with congenital CMV infection in non-AIDS patients, but may also be encountered in neonatal HIV infection (9). An unusual cutaneous manifestation of CMV infection is persistent perianal ulceration resembling the perianal ulcerations of anogenital herpes simplex virus infection (Fig. 2A) (10,11). Unlike herpetic ulcerations, ulcers due to CMV do not respond to topical treatments such as sitz baths and compresses. Typically, patients with perianal CMV ulceration also have coexistent intractable CMV proctitis and/or CMV colitis (11).

C. J. Cockerell: Departments of Pathology (Division of Dermatopathology) and Dermatology, University of Texas Southwestern Medical Center at Dallas, Dallas, Texas 75235-9072.

TABLE 1. *Cutaneous and mucosal infections in HIV infection*

Abscesses
Bacillary epithelioid angiomatosis
Botryomycosis
Candida infection (thrush)
Condylomata acuminata
Cryptococcosis
Cytomegalovirus infection
Demodecosis
Dermatophyte infection
Ecthyma
Exanthem of HIV infection
Folliculitis
Furuncles
Hairy leukoplakia
Herpes simplex infection
Histoplasmosis
Impetigo
Molluscum contagiosum
Mycobacterial infection
Plantar warts
Pneumocystosis
Pyomyositis
Scabies
Staphylococcal scalded skin syndrome
Syphilis
Varicella-zoster infection
Verruca plana
Verruca vulgaris

The CMV ulcers most likely represent contiguous spread to the skin from the gastrointestinal tract. Patients with CMV ulcerations are usually thought to have persistent herpes simplex infection and light microscopic and electron microscopic examination of biopsy specimens and/or virus isolation are required to confirm the diagnosis. The finding of CMV-induced perianal ulcers often confers a grave prognosis. Although treatment with ganciclovir may be effective for some patients with this infectious complication (12,13), most of our patients have died within 2 months following the diagnosis.

Persistent ulceration of the perianal area not responsive to anti-herpes simplex or other empiric therapy should be biopsied. Microscopically, in CMV disease there is ulceration of the epithelium. In the dermis or lamina propria, depending on the site, there is a dense inflammatory response with numerous lymphocytes, histiocytes, neutrophils, eosinophils, and plasma cells. There is also abundant granulation tissue. On careful inspection, characteristic CMV-infected cells can be found (Fig. 2B). These are usually found in the deep portion of the biopsy rather than in the epithelium. These cells are usually one and one-half to two times the size of fibroblasts and/or endothelial cells. Inclusions may be found in either the cytoplasm, the nucleus, or both. Intranuclear inclusions are characteristically elongated geometric structures that appear purplish in hematoxylin and eosin-stained sections. Intracytoplasmic inclusions are small, purplish dots found in clusters within the cytoplasm. There may be many or relatively few cells that display the characteristic inclusions. The usual cell type is the fibroblast or the endothelial cell. Only rarely is a keratinocyte infected.

It should also be noted that occasionally ulcerations may be caused by more than one infectious agent. For example, it is not uncommon to find cells containing inclusions of CMV in conjunction with the characteristic multinucleated giant cells of herpes simplex infection. One case has been reported in which skin lesions were found to contain acid-fast bacilli as well as cells infected with CMV and herpes simplex virus (14). Thus, it is important to identify all infectious agents in a patient with HIV infection since specific therapies may differ significantly.

Herpes Zoster and Herpes Simplex

Herpes zoster infection is thought to result from reactivation of a latent infection of a dorsal root ganglion in

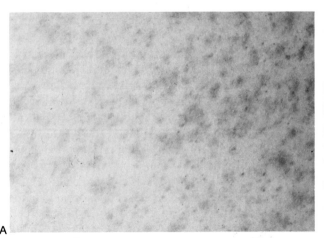 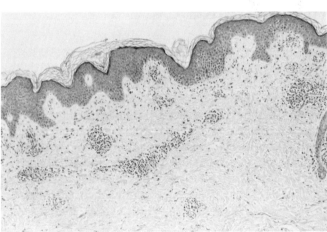

A   B

FIG. 1. A: A widely distributed eruption of pinkish macules and papules is characteristic of the acute exanthem of HIV infection. **B:** Histologic findings, acute exanthem of HIV infection. Note the superficial perivascular infiltrate of lymphoid cells with slight spongiosis. H&E, original magnification ×40.

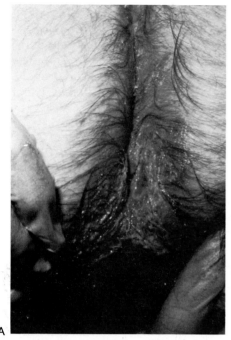
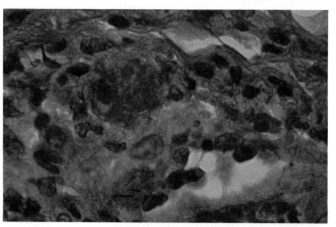

A

B

FIG. 2. A: Perianal ulcerations caused by cytomegalovirus infection. These ulcerations are nonspecific clinically and could be caused by a number of different organisms. When associated with persistent diarrhea in a patient with AIDS, a biopsy should be obtained to rule out cytomegalovirus infection. **B:** Fibroblasts infected with cytomegalovirus. Note the large rhomboidally shaped intranuclear inclusion and small granular cytoplasmic inclusions. The cells are several times normal size.

patients with previous varicella infection. It is usually manifested by painful clusters of vesicles in a localized neurodermatomal distribution. The vesicles often lie on a patch of erythema. In HIV-infected patients, the initially localized zoster infection may become generalized with widely disseminated vesicles appearing at sites distant from the originally involved dermatome (15). In some cases of disseminated zoster, lung and central nervous system involvement occurs for which the patient may require hospitalization. The severe zoster infections seen in patients with AIDS or AIDS-related complex (ARC) more often leave residual scars than do such conditions in non-HIV-infected patients, and the incidence of postherpetic neuralgia may be somewhat higher (16). Herpes zoster infections are also known to occur in individuals with defects in cell-mediated immunity other than those induced by HIV infection, such as in Hodgkin's disease, chronic lymphocytic leukemia, and iatrogenically induced immunosuppression for organ transplantation. Even otherwise "healthy" zoster patients exhibit a diminished in vitro cell-mediated response to the varicella-zoster viral antigen during acute disease (17). The occurrence of herpes zoster infection in a patient from a high-risk group should immediately alert the health care provider to consider the possibility of underlying HIV infection (17–19). Treatment of zoster consists of high-dose acyclovir (given either orally at a dose of 800 mg five times daily or 10 mg/kg IV every 8 hours for 7–10 days).

Patients with HIV infection and advanced immunodeficiency are not uncommonly affected by severe recurrent herpes simplex virus infection (HSV). These infections are often more extensive, persistent, and less responsive to antiviral therapy with acyclovir than HSV infections occurring in healthy hosts (Fig. 3) (20). Histopathological examination of tissue samples from sites of HSV or zoster infection typically show eosinophilic, rhomboidally shaped intracytoplasmic cellular inclusions, as well as margination of the nucleoplasm against the nuclear membrane. Multinucleated epithelial giant cells are also characteristic (Fig. 4). If an intact vesicle is present, these cells are acantholytic and found within the vesicle. The degree of inflammatory cell infiltrate varies in accordance with both the stage of the herpetic infection and the degree of immunodeficiency of the patient. A fully developed ulceration due to HSV infection is associated with a dense inflammatory cell infiltrate consisting of lymphocytes, histiocytes, eosinophils, neutrophils, and plasma cells. In severely immunocompromised patients, extensive, confluent epithelial necrosis may be seen with innumerable virally infected cells. Paradoxically, the inflammatory infiltrate may be sparse in such cases.

Although uncommon, disseminated HSV infection may occur in patients with AIDS, in which the entire skin surface may be studded with individual lesions and clusters of erythematous papules and vesicles. Such infections may be associated with visceral involvement

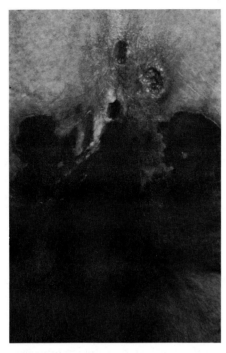

FIG. 3. Perianal ulcerations caused by herpes simplex virus infection. Deep, nonhealing ulcerations caused by this agent are characteristically seen in patients with AIDS. These may appear identical to ulcerations caused by cytomegalovirus infection.

and may necessitate hospitalization for intravenous acyclovir therapy.

Anogenital HSV infections are commonly encountered in HIV-infected patients. These infections can be prolonged and painful, sometimes leading to extensive necrotizing ulcers, which may become superinfected with bacteria (21). Patients with this degree of involvement require stool softeners and careful attention to maintenance of cleanliness in the infected area. These persistent herpetic infections often require treatment

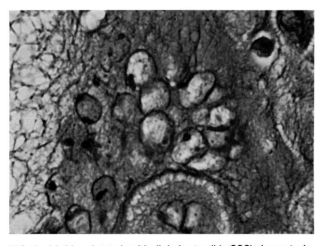

FIG. 4. Multinucleated epithelial giant cell (×800) characteristic of herpes virus infection.

with intravenous acyclovir in high doses, although a course of oral acyclovir (200 mg five times daily for 10 days) is usually tried first. Prophylaxis with oral acyclovir is beneficial for many patients to lessen the number and frequency of recurrent attacks.

Molluscum Contagiosum

Molluscum contagiosum is a poxvirus infection of the skin characterized by waxy yellowish papular lesions often with central umbilication. This infection is usually spread by close contact. In children infected by this virus, papules are commonly seen on any cutaneous surface. When seen in sexually active young adults, the pubic and inner thigh areas are most frequently involved. In patients with HIV infection, however, cutaneous infections with molluscum contagiosum may become widely disseminated. Lesions are often more numerous and can be several times larger than those seen in non-HIV infected children (22). Occasionally, the individual lesions may be confused with basal cell carcinomas and ordinary nevi (22). To make a definitive diagnosis, a biopsy may be required. Histopathologically, characteristic purplish oval-shaped molluscum bodies are seen within dilated infundibula of hair follicles. These follicles may coalesce to form the characteristic umbilicated papule. In general, molluscum papules are easily eradicated by simple curettage or cryosurgery using a topical application of liquid nitrogen. Lesions found in HIV-infected AIDS patients, however, are often refractory to treatment, tending to recur and to spread to other skin sites.

Human Papillomavirus Infections

Human papillomavirus (HPV) infections, such as verrucae vulgares, are often seen in patients with HIV infection. They tend to occur in the same distribution as in non-HIV infected healthy adults, but are present in greater number, and seem to be resistant to standard therapies. Insufficient data are currently available regarding the specific subtype of HPV that causes disease in these patients. However, skin lesions may be of several different clinical varieties: extensive flat and filiform warts, often found in the bearded area of the face (23); exuberant cauliflower-like plaques of confluent condylomata acuminata in the anogenital region (Fig. 5) (24); or multiple, large hyperkeratotic verrucae vulgares, commonly seen on or around the fingers (23). Multiple plantar warts have also been observed. If a biopsy is performed, the characteristic histologic pattern of verrucae vulgares or condylomata acuminata is found. Classically, digitated epidermal hyperplasia with dilated blood vessels and parakeratosis with hemorrhage at the tips of papillae are seen in common warts. There may also be

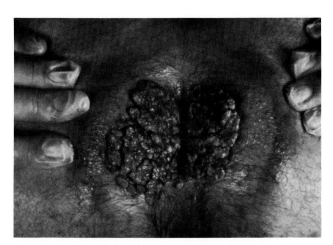

FIG. 5. Condyloma acuminata. Infections from this common human papillomavirus may be very severe and result in anal obstruction.

koilocytosis and hypergranulosis in the epidermis. A gently papillated, slightly acanthotic epidermis with dilated blood vessels in the lamina propria is a characteristic finding in condylomata acuminata. Occasionally numerous atypical mitotic figures may be seen within the field of such a lesion, which raises the possibility of a form of squamous cell carcinoma in situ, called Bowenoid papulosis. Bowenoid papulosis in the setting of HIV-induced immunodeficiency should be managed with vigorous therapeutic measures, such as complete surgical removal, in order to prevent the possible development of more aggressive cutaneous neoplasms.

Hairy Leukoplakia

An oral mucosal lesion known as hairy leukoplakia has been frequently described in patients with HIV infection. Whitish, corrugated verrucous plaques are characteristically seen on the lateral margins of the tongue

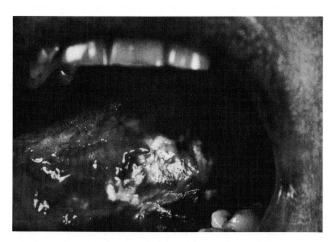

FIG. 6. Hairy leukoplakia. A whitish verrucous plaque that does not rub away is characteristic of this condition.

and buccal mucosa (Fig. 6) (25). Clinically, these lesions may resemble and may be misdiagnosed as candidiasis. Unlike thrush, when plaques of hairy leukoplakia are scraped with a tongue depressor or other blunt instrument, the whitish surface cannot be rubbed away. Histochemical and electron microscopic evidence have demonstrated the presence of Epstein-Barr virus in these lesions (26). Histologic examination of tissue is required for confirmation of the diagnosis. Microscopically, digitated epidermal hyperplasia with marked vacuolation of the mucosal epithelial cells is seen. Tortuous dilated blood vessels are present within digitations. Such lesions may be confused with a mucosal verrucae. Often pseudohyphae of *Candida albicans* are superimposed on lesions of hairy leukoplakia.

BACTERIAL AND PARASITIC INFECTIONS

Folliculitis, Abscesses, Furuncles, and Impetigo

Because the B-cell arm of the immune system is also defective in patients with HIV infection (27), infections caused by common bacterial organisms, as well as those caused by more virulent bacteria, may be responsible for several types of skin lesions in these patients. Acneiform papules and pustules may be widely distributed over the trunk, extremities, and face. Cultures of such lesions commonly yield *Staphylococcus aureus* or *Streptococcus pyogenes* (28). In some cases, unusual organisms such as *Rhodococcus* sp. have been found (29). Like many of the other infectious diseases encountered in patients with HIV infection, such bacterial infections are often refractory to usual therapeutic measures. Typical histologic findings include the presence of infundibula of follicles filled with neutrophils, occasional lymphocytes, and histiocytes, with or without rupture. Often there is a dense acute inflammatory cell response in the dermis surrounding the hair follicle.

Folliculitis may progress to form localized abscesses, furuncles, and even carbuncles (28). Occasionally, cellulitis may supervene. Whereas an immunocompetent patient is often treated with oral antibiotics as an outpatient, the patient with AIDS may require hospitalization for intravenous antimicrobial therapy, since the risk of systemic spread of infection is much greater.

When cultures are performed, the clinical laboratory should be alerted to the fact that the patient is immunocompromised so that a search for unusual opportunistic pathogens will be undertaken. Clinically, for example, one may not be able to distinguish a pyogenic infection caused by *Staphylococcus aureus* from one caused by *Mycobacteria* sp. Delays in accurate diagnosis are detrimental for the patient.

A common skin infection of childhood that is seen quite frequently among HIV-infected patients is impetigo, which is caused by *Staphylococcus aureus* or *Streptococcus pyogenes.* While impetigo in otherwise healthy children is seen most commonly on the face, in HIV-infected patients this infection is often found in the axillary and inguinal regions. Impetigo usually begins as painful red macules, which may develop into flaccid bullae that rupture, releasing serous or purulent fluid. A characteristic honey-colored surface crust forms and satellite and disseminated lesions may develop. When biopsy material is obtained from such a lesion and examined histopathologically, a subcorneal vesicle containing scattered acantholytic keratinocytes with neutrophils, plasma cells, and occasional bacteria is seen. When the lesions are fully crusted, a purulent scale-crust is present on the surface of an eroded epidermis. Usually, the infection responds readily to systemic and sometimes topical antibiotics. However, in HIV infection, the therapeutic response may be delayed.

In addition to these bacterial infections, a number of other conditions have been reported sporadically in patients with HIV infection. Botryomycosis, a rare condition caused by a deeply seated staphylococcal infection of skin and characterized by nondescript papules, may on occasion be encountered (30,31). Histologically, one sees a dense, mixed inflammatory infiltrate in the dermis with basophilic "grains" representative of the bacteria. Staphylococcal scalded skin syndrome (32), as well as pyomyositis (33,34), ecthyma and even toxic shock syndrome have all been reported in patients with HIV infection.

Bacillary Epithelioid Angiomatosis

A recently described bacterial infection known as bacillary epithelioid angiomatosis (BEA) may occur in HIV-infected patients (35,36). The skin is characteristically (but not exclusively) involved, and the most common cutaneous manifestations are small, reddish to purple papules with a clinical appearance similar to cherry angiomata or pyogenic granulomata. Individual lesions may be few in number or numerous and can involve mucosal surfaces as well as visceral organs (Fig. 7A). The eruption may be quite extensive, with skin lesions numbering in the thousands. Some lesions may be deeply seated, involving subcutaneous tissue, underlying muscle, and even bone (37); peliosis hepatis may develop in association with this infection (37a). It has been postulated that this disease is caused by a bacterium with similarities to both *Bartonella bacilliformis* and the cat scratch disease bacillus. Further characterization has shown the bacterium to be a previously uncharacterized rickettsia-like organism, closely related to *Rochalimaea quintana* (37b).

On biopsy, several different histologic patterns may be present, but the most common one is a diffuse vascular proliferation of round blood vessels with plump epithelioid cells in the interstitium (Fig. 7B and C) (37). Numerous neutrophils are characteristically seen infiltrating lesions, and scattered aggregates of purplish granular material are noted. With Warthin-Starry staining, such purplish material is shown to consist of colonies of bacteria (Fig. 7D). Although this condition may be very serious, sometimes even fatal, it responds well to treatment with erythromycin at a dosage of 500 mg four times a day orally for 2 weeks (37). Consequently, it is important to distinguish this infection from Kaposi's sarcoma.

Syphilis

Syphilis may assume a number of unusual features in patients with HIV infection. Although lesions of classic secondary syphilis may occur, in some cases very bizarre clinical manifestations are encountered. Some of the unusual skin manifestations that have been reported include sclerodermoid skin changes (38), pityriasis rubra pilaris-like eruption, lues maligna (39), rupial syphilis, and coexistent primary, secondary, and tertiary syphilis with palatal gummata (40). Adding further diagnostic confusion is the fact that serologic findings may be unreliable in some of these patients (41). In such cases, the diagnosis is made by performing special stains for spirochetes in tissue.

When tissue sections of patients with HIV infection and syphilis are examined histologically, a number of different findings have been observed. The classic superficial and deep perivascular infiltrate of mononuclear cells containing numerous plasma cells with psoriasiform hyperplasia of the epidermis is probably the most common histopathologic picture (38). However, other histologic patterns such as severe necrotizing vasculitis, very sparse inflammatory infiltrates containing almost no plasma cells with little epidermal change, or diffuse granulomatous inflammation have all been seen. Spirochetes may vary in number from few to numerous, regardless of the histologic pattern.

It is important to treat HIV-infected patients with syphilis aggressively, as neurosyphilis and other signs of late syphilis have occurred in some cases despite previous treatment with the standard antibiotic regimens recommended for immunocompetent patients (42,43).

Parasitic Infections

Several parasitic infections and infestations have been described in patients with HIV infection. Disseminated cutaneous toxoplasmosis has been seen in one individual (44). Clinical lesions were nondescript papules that were somewhat reddish and slightly indurated. The patient was shown to have concurrent central nervous system

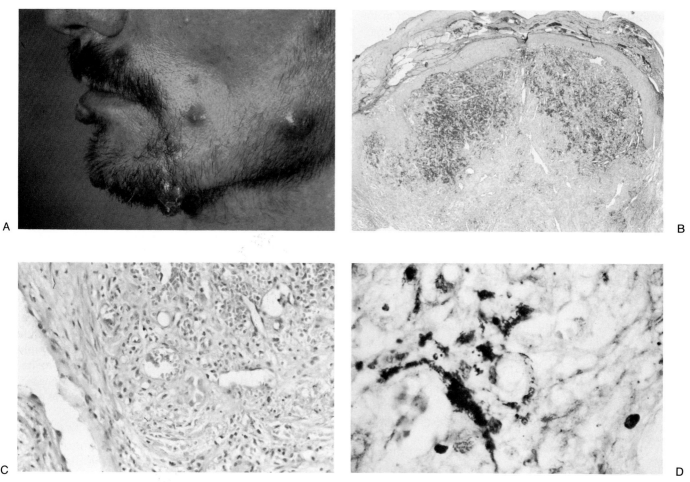

FIG. 7. Bacillary angiomatosis. **A:** There are reddish nodules on the skin surface some of which have a somewhat acuminant shape. Note the presence of crusting. **B:** Histology. There is a lobular proliferation of blood vessels with a collarette of epithelium and crusting on the surface. These features are reminiscent of a pyogenic granuloma. H&E, original magnification ×40. **C:** High magnification. Note the rounded blood vessels with the plump cuboidal "epithelioid" endothelial cells. There is also an admixture of inflammatory cells with occasional neutrophils. H&E, original magnification ×400. **D:** Warthin-Starry staining of lesions demonstrates clumps of bacteria present interstitially. These bacteria are closely related to rickettsiae. Warthin-Starry, original magnification ×400.

toxoplasmosis. The cutaneous eruption responded to treatment with pyrimethamine and sulfadiazine.

Cutaneous *Pneumocystis carinii* infection has been reported in several patients with AIDS. Most lesions have appeared clinically as dome-shaped nodules, primarily in areas such as the external ear and nasopharynx (45–47). Extrapulmonary *P. carinii* infection should be watched for in patients receiving aerosolized pentamidine for prophylaxis of *P. carinii* pneumonia, since this therapy does not protect against disseminated infection (48,49). We have encountered two such cases in HIV-infected patients, both of whom had eruptions of nondescript translucent umbilicated papules, which, when biopsied, showed the characteristic foamy exudate typical of *P. carinii* infection (50). The skin lesions responded to systemic treatment with trimethoprim-sulfamethoxazole or intravenous pentamidine.

Norwegian scabies occurs relatively frequently in patients with HIV infection; however, in these patients the skin eruption is quite different from that usually seen in patients with Norwegian scabies (51,52). A widespread reddish "papulosquamous" eruption may be encountered that may be confused with atopic dermatitis or seborrheic dermatitis. Patients usually complain of severe pruritus. Skin scrapings reveal innumerable mites and histologic sections show the characteristic perivascular and interstitial infiltrate of lymphocytes, histiocytes, and eosinophils with abundant organisms in the cornified layer. Treatment consists of topical lindane or pyrethrin preparations to eradicate the infestation. In spite of adequate scabicidal measures, however, the accompanying pruritus may persist for months. Treatment of the post-scabetic pruritus syndrome consists of application of topical steroid creams and ointments and administration of antihistamines. Papular urticaria may also develop following a bout of scabies, which may be long-standing.

Demodex folliculorum may multiply to large numbers in patients with HIV infection, leading to a skin eruption with a clinical appearance similar to that of sarcoptic mange in dogs. Several cases of florid pyoderma have also been associated with proliferation of demodectic mites (53). Therapeutic benefit may be obtained using topical metronidazole.

Mycobacterial Infections

AIDS patients with systemic mycobacterial infections may develop cutaneous lesions. Clinically, the mycobacterial skin lesions may have a number of different appearances that may lead to inaccurate clinical diagnoses. One manifestation is that of small papules and pustules that resemble folliculitis (54). Cultures and specially stained biopsy specimens consistently demonstrate mycobacteria. In six patients with AIDS and cutaneous mycobacterial disease seen at our institution, three were found to have *Mycobacterium tuberculosis,* and one each had *M. avium, M. kansasii,* and *M. chelonei.* In the patients with *M. tuberculosis,* pustular lesions of the skin were secondary to reactivated pulmonary foci. Other cutaneous manifestations of tuberculosis in HIV-infected individuals include ulcers, abscesses, indurated plaques, and lupus vulgaris.

When a mycobacterial cutaneous lesion is examined histopathologically, several different findings may be seen. In some instances there is a tuberculoid granulomatous dermatitis with numerous histiocytes, many of them multinucleated, surrounded by lymphocytes in the uppermost portion of the dermis, and extending into the mid- to lower reticular dermis with irregular psoriasiform hyperplasia and scale-crust. Alternatively, there may be a suppurative folliculitis in which neutrophils, histiocytes, and eosinophils are present in the infundibula of hair follicles that rupture causing a granulomatous response in the dermis surrounding the follicles.

In general, special stains for acid-fast bacilli are strongly positive in patients with HIV infection; however, it is important to alert the pathologist that a given patient is immunocompromised so that special stains will be performed when unusual histologic reaction patterns are observed.

It should be reemphasized that individual lesions may appear virtually identical to those of simple folliculitis. Since this diagnosis can be confirmed with certainty only by culture or examination of tissue stained for acid-fast bacilli, such studies should be performed for any HIV-infected patient with suggestive lesions.

FUNGAL INFECTIONS

Superficial Fungal Infections

White patches of the buccal mucosa or tongue in a patient at high risk for HIV infection are likely to be due to oral candidiasis (also called moniliasis and thrush). Thrush is a sign of advanced immunodeficiency and indicates a high probability of progressing to AIDS (55). Thrush is characterized by whitish, curd-like exudates on the dorsal or lateral tongue, oropharynx, or buccal mucosa that can be easily scraped away with a cotton swab or tongue depressor. A reddish friable surface that may be associated with a burning sensation is often found beneath the candidal exudate. Sometimes, only a beefy red, eroded surface of the tongue is seen. Microscopic examination of exudate scraped from the tongue surface treated with 10% potassium hydroxide solution shows numerous pseudohyphae and budding yeasts. If a biopsy specimen is obtained, a dense infiltrate of lymphocytes, histiocytes, and neutrophils is seen in the lamina propria with psoriasiform hyperplasia of the overlying epithelium. Spongiosis containing neutrophils with numerous yeast and pseudohyphae are seen in the uppermost portion of the epithelium. Organisms can be easily demonstrated with periodic acid-Schiff (PAS) or Gomori methenamine silver stains. Esophageal candidiasis occurs in some patients with thrush. This complication may be associated with dysphagia, which can lead to anorexia and consequently, malnutrition. Cutaneous, perianal, and especially vaginal candidal infections occasionally occur as well.

Treatment may need to be prolonged indefinitely since thrush typically recurs when therapy is discontinued. Oral administration of clotrimazole or nystatin may help to suppress candidal overgrowth. Ultimately, ketoconazole or fluconazole may be required.

In addition to *Candida albicans,* other fungi may cause severe cutaneous and/or systemic infections that fail to respond to available topical and systemic antifungal therapy (56). Widespread dermatophytosis, especially caused by *Trichophyton rubrum,* involving palms, soles, nails, and intertriginous areas has been observed in patients with HIV infection. The histopathology of such infections is identical to that seen in patients who are nonimmunocompromised. A variably dense lymphohistiocytic infiltrate is seen in the dermis with psoriasiform epidermal hyperplasia and slight spongiosis, sometimes containing neutrophils; parakeratosis containing neutrophils overlies the epidermis. With careful inspection, hyphae are often found between the parakeratotic and overlying basketweave orthokeratotic stratum corneum. Neither systemic griseofulvin nor topical antifungal medications have been found to be completely effective in eradicating such infections.

Systemic Fungal Infections

The systemic fungal infections most commonly found among patients with AIDS are due to *Cryptococcus neoformans* and *Histoplasma capsulatum.*

Cryptococcosis most often causes meningitis although the skin may be involved. This fungus may cause single or multiple red to purple, 5 mm to 1 cm, papules, nodules, or indurated plaques of the integument that resemble the cutaneous lesions of bacterial cellulitis. Superficial erosion and crusting of skin lesions may be found. Another, more common manifestation of cutaneous cryptococcosis, is an eruption consisting of widespread, skin-colored, dome-shaped, and sometimes slightly umbilicated papules that bear a striking resemblance to the papules of molluscum contagiosum (57). Occasionally, an HIV-infected patient has both molluscum contagiosum and cutaneous cryptococcosis simultaneously, and individual lesions of each may be clinically indistinguishable. It is often necessary to biopsy and culture suspicious molluscum contagiosum papules to exclude the more serious diagnosis of cryptococcosis. Cutaneous involvement with cryptococcosis is distinctive histopathologically. In the papillary and reticular dermis are numerous clear staining areas that contain within them small hyperchromatic bodies representing the viable component of the fungus. The clear staining material is the mucogelatinous capsule characteristic of *Cryptococcus neoformans*. There may be only a minimal inflammatory cell infiltrate in response to the fungus. The capsular material is demonstrated best with the mucicarmine stain, which colors the capsule a brilliant magenta. Patients with cryptococcosis are usually ill but may be entirely asymptomatic. On occasion, symptoms are quite minimal and elicited only by a careful history and neurologic examination, revealing subtle changes in personality, memory loss, thought disorders, or a poorly defined psychiatric illness. In such cases, cerebrospinal fluid examination including India ink examination, a test for cryptococcal antigen, and fungal culture are indicated. Treatment of cryptococcosis is difficult and requires systemic antifungal therapy with amphotericin B or fluconazole.

The incidence of cutaneous histoplasmosis is even rarer than that of cryptococcosis in patients with AIDS. Examination of the skin may reveal scattered acneiform papules, a widespread eruption of reddish macules and papules, or one to a few indurated, pinkish-red crusted plaques (58,59). A specific diagnosis can only be made with certainty by fungal culture and/or histopathologic evaluation of biopsy specimens. Such histopathologic examination may reveal only subtle manifestations. There may be an infiltrate of lymphocytes and histiocytes in the uppermost portion of the papillary dermis. Some of the histiocytes may have slightly vacuolated cytoplasm, and on careful inspection, small intracytoplasmic inclusions representative of the fungus can be seen. It is important to note that the fungus is often quite difficult to visualize in hematoxylin and eosin-stained sections, and special stains for fungi, as well as for acid-fast bacilli, should be performed routinely. As with cryptococcosis, the inflammatory cell infiltrate may be relatively sparse. This may be attributable to properties of the invading organism itself or to the compromised state of the pa-

tient. It is important to alert the pathologist that the patient has or is suspected of having HIV infection since the diagnosis of histoplasmosis can be overlooked even with microscopic examination. As in the case with cryptococcosis, patients with cutaneous histoplasmosis may not be acutely ill or have any evidence of systemic or pulmonary involvement. HIV-infected patients with cutaneous histoplasmosis are often not aware of prior pulmonary disease.

Any cutaneous infectious disease in patients with HIV infection may have an unusual appearance. Therefore, health care providers should maintain a high index of suspicion and perform biopsies and viral, bacterial, mycobacterial, and/or fungal cultures of any atypical skin lesion so as not to miss a potentially serious or even fatal infectious complication.

NONINFECTIOUS CUTANEOUS SIGNS

In addition to infectious diseases, a number of noninfectious cutaneous signs and symptoms have been described in HIV infected patients (Table 2). Included among these are nonspecific severe pruritus and hives. The presence of one of these conditions should also alert the health care practitioner to consider the possibility of underlying HIV infection.

Seborrheic Dermatitis-Like Eruption

One of the most commonly observed skin conditions associated with HIV infection is an eruption that resembles seborrheic dermatitis; this occurs in 32–83% of patients infected with HIV (60–62). The reason for its development is unknown. It has been postulated that physical or emotional stress may play a role. A more likely explanation is that an overgrowth of certain cutaneous fungi,

TABLE 2. *Noninfectious nonneoplastic cutaneous disorders in HIV infection*

Alopecia
Calciphylaxis
Eosinophilic pustular folliculitis
Erythema elevatum diutinum
Granuloma annulare
Hives
Ichthyosis
Leukocytoclastic vasculitis
Morbilliform drug eruption
Papular urticaria
Pityriasis rubra pilaris
Porphyria cutanea tarda
Prurigo nodularis
Pruritus
Psoriasis
Reiter's syndrome
Seborrheic dermatitis-like eruption
Transient acantholytic dermatosis
Xerosis

such as *Candida* (63) or *Pityrosporum* (64–66) secondary to the immunocompromise, either causes or contributes to the cause of this eruption. HIV-infected patients may develop this condition in association with preexisting seborrheic dermatitis simply because it is exacerbated, or it may develop de novo with the onset of HIV disease or its sequelae. The greater the degree of immunodepression, i.e., T-helper cell numbers less than 150 cells/mm³, the greater the tendency for development of this condition and the greater its severity.

Although the seborrheic dermatitis-like condition of HIV infection has features similar to common seborrheic dermatitis, there are, in many cases, distinct differences. The eruption is characteristically more florid and may be characterized by intense erythema and thick scaly plaques distributed not only in the usual "seborrheic dermatitis" areas but also in other locations such as the upper anterior chest, back, groin, and extremities (67,68) (Fig. 8A). The scalp may be involved in dramatic fashion by thick scaly erythematous plaques with accompanying oozing and weeping. In some patients, widespread eruptions may occur leading to diffuse erythroderma. Some cases may be associated with psoriasis but, in most, the characteristic seborrheic dermatitis-like nature of the eruption is maintained.

Histopathologically, this eruption differs from that of ordinary seborrheic dermatitis in several respects. Usually there is a superficial perivascular lymphohistiocytic infiltrate with occasional plasma cells in the dermis (Fig. 8B and 8C). There is slight psoriasiform hyperplasia of the epidermis with parakeratosis that usually extends across the entire specimen rather than only the edges of the follicular ostea as seen in non-HIV-related seborrheic dermatitis. There also may be scattered neutrophils present in the parakeratotic cornified layer. Of interest is that occasional individually necrotic keratinocytes are often present within the epidermis (Fig. 8D).

Although the condition usually resembles seborrheic dermatitis in immunocompetent patients, when it is especially florid, it may resemble psoriasis. Distinction can

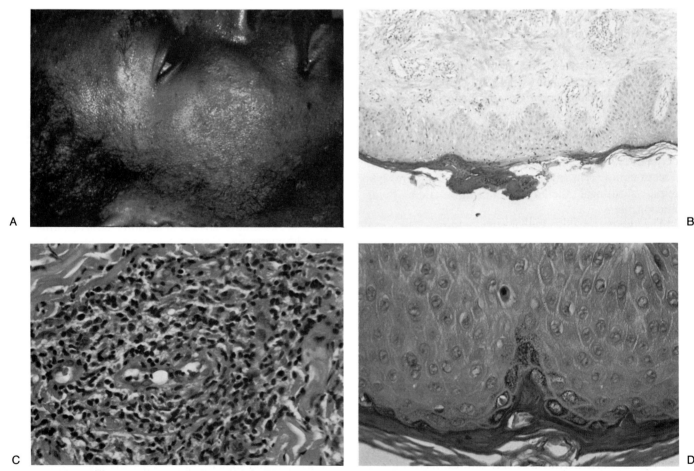

A

B

C

D

FIG. 8. Seborrheic dermatitis-like eruption. **A:** An extensive eruption of scaly pinkish plaques is characteristic. **B:** The epidermis is hyperplastic and there is scale and crust present over most of the specimen. **C:** An inflammatory cell infiltrate consisting of lymphocytes and plasma cells is highly characteristic of this condition. **D:** Occasionally, necrotic keratinocytes, as pictured here, are seen scattered at random throughout the epidermis. Original magnification ×500.

be made from psoriasis as seborrheic dermatitis does not usually involve extensor surfaces of the elbows and knees. Furthermore, there is characteristically a superficial scale or crust rather than the thick and "micaceous" scale of typical psoriasis. Nevertheless, patients with HIV infection may also develop psoriasis often of a severe and diffuse nature (69,70). In individuals with a prior history of psoriasis, this condition may be exacerbated and may become widespread (70). Reiter's syndrome may also occur in HIV-infected patients and may be the presenting sign of HIV infection (71,72). It is important not to treat this with methotrexate, since by doing so, profound immunosuppression and accelerated death may result (71).

Treatment of seborrheic dermatitis in HIV-infected patients is usually similar to that in immunocompetent patients. Applications of topical corticosteroid creams and ointments as well as topical antifungal preparations have been shown to be effective in some cases. However, in others, the condition is refractory to virtually any therapy. If response to treatment is seen, following its discontinuation, there may be prompt exacerbation. Scalp disease often requires keratolytic agents and selenium or tar shampoos with accompanying corticosteroid gels or solutions. In selected cases, ultraviolet phototherapy or treatment with grenz rays may be beneficial.

Although the seborrheic dermatitis-like condition may be a severe problem for HIV-infected patients, these individuals may also develop more classical seborrheic dermatitis that poses few clinical problems and responds well to therapy. Seborrheic dermatitis may be the presenting sign of HIV infection and clinicians should maintain a high index of suspicion for HIV disease in at-risk patients with severe or refractory lesions.

Eosinophilic Pustular Folliculitis

HIV-infected patients may develop eosinophilic pustular folliculitis, a widespread acneiform papular and pustular eruption that characteristically involves the face, trunk, neck, and extremities (73,74). Although the clinical appearance of this eruption is similar to that of bacterial folliculitis, the pruritus is usually much more severe. Because of the extensive pruritus, it is not uncommon for patients to present primarily with prurigo nodularis and lichen simplex chronicus as a consequence of rubbing and scratching.

The histopathologic findings are characteristic, showing innumerable eosinophils within the infundibula of hair follicles. On occasion, rupture of such follicles is seen resulting in perifolliculitis consisting of eosinophils, neutrophils, and sometimes multinucleated histiocytes. Fortunately, effective treatment for this severely pruritic condition has been found. Ultraviolet B (UVB) phototherapy analogous to that used for psoriasis is quite effec-

tive in alleviating the condition (75); however, such treatment should be undertaken with some caution as UVB may cause activation of latent HIV with an increase in HIV production (76), in addition to a reduction in cell number and function of Langerhans cells and CD4+ lymphocytes (77).

Morbilliform Drug Eruption

A widespread drug-related eruption consisting of pruritic, pinkish-red macules and papules, many often urticarial, frequently develops following the administration of certain drugs to patients with HIV infection. One agent that is especially likely to result in this complication is trimethoprim–sulfamethoxazole. Up to 70% of AIDS patients may develop a morbilliform drug eruption following administration of this medication (78). Although this drug eruption is similar to the drug eruption frequently seen in patients with infectious mononucleosis who have received ampicillin, no definite correlation with viral infection has been established. Usually the clinical diagnosis of drug eruption is quite easily made and for that reason, only rarely are such eruptions ever biopsied. However, a superficial perivascular and slightly interstitial mixed-cell infiltrate consisting of lymphocytes, histiocytes, and eosinophils with occasional plasma cells is the typical histologic pattern. In some cases, there may be slight spongiosis of the epidermis, and sometimes, the infiltrate in the dermis obscures the dermoepidermal junction. The eruption may persist for several weeks, even months, after the offending drug has been discontinued. Other agents that may be associated with morbilliform eruptions in these patients include clindamycin, cephalexin, rifabutin, and diphenylhydantoin, among others (79).

Papular Urticaria

A peculiar and unusual nonspecific cutaneous sign of HIV infection is "papular urticaria," characterized by the onset of itchy red to pink, urticarial, dome-shaped papules with widespread distribution, primarily involving the trunk and extremities (80). Individual lesions may resemble insect bites. Patients complain of severe pruritus, and like certain other conditions seen in these individuals, the symptoms, as well as the eruption, are not readily responsive to conventional treatment modalities. The eruption may persist for months, although the lesions may subside and recur intermittently. These cycles may continue relentlessly. Histopathologically, a superficial and sometimes deep perivascular and interstitial mixed-cell infiltrate containing lymphocytes, histiocytes, eosinophils, and occasional plasma cells is demonstrable. There may be slight spongiosis in the epidermis. There is often evidence of excoriation because of the intense pruritus. Although the histologic changes are nonspecific, they may be suggestive of responses to insect bites.

Other Unusual Manifestations

A number of other noninfectious conditions have been found in association with HIV infection (Table 2). Whether all of these are truly associated, or represent coincidental findings, has yet to be fully determined. Some of these conditions include transient acantholytic dermatosis (Grover's disease) (81), alopecia (82,83), calciphylaxis (84), cutaneous T-cell lymphoma (P.E. Leboit, personal communication, 1990), acquired ichthyosis (85), xerosis (86), asteatotic dermatitis (86), granuloma annulare (87), porphyria cutanea tarda (88), leukocytoclastic vasculitis (89), erythema elevatum diutinum (90), and pityriasis rubra pilaris (91).

CONCLUSIONS

In conclusion, many cutaneous conditions may be encountered in patients with HIV infection. It is essential that health care providers who deal with these patients be cognizant of both the clinical as well as the histopathological patterns of these entities. Even though the prognosis of HIV infection continues to be grave, it remains important to recognize and treat both the infectious and noninfectious conditions as promptly and as well as possible. By so doing, the severe morbidity and mortality these patients already face may be lessened, and the quality of life enhanced.

REFERENCES

1. Rustin MHA, Ridley CM, Smith MD, et al. The acute exanthem associated with seroconversion to human T-cell lymphotropic virus-III in a homosexual man. *J Infect* 1986;12:161–3.
2. Wantzin GRC, Lindhardt BO, Weismann K, et al. Acute HTLV-III infection associated with exanthema, diagnosed by seroconversion. *Br J Dermatol* 1986;115:602–6.
3. Calabrese L, Roffitt MR, Levin KH, et al. Acute infection with the human immunodeficiency virus (HIV) associated with acute brachial neuritis and exanthematous rash. *Ann Intern Med* 1987;107:849–51.
4. McMillan A, Bishop PE, Dennis A, Peutherer JF. Immunohistology of the skin rash associated with acute HIV infection. *AIDS* 1989;3:309–12.
5. Bremmer-Anderson E, Torssander J. The exanthema of acute (primary) HIV infection: identification of a characteristic histopathologic picture. *Acta Dermatovenereol (Stockh)* 1990;70:85–7.
6. Lin CS, Penha PD, Krishnan MN, et al. Cytomegalic inclusion disease of the skin. *Arch Dermatol* 1981;117:282–4.
7. Feldman PS, Walker AN, Baker R. Cutaneous lesions heralding disseminated cytomegalovirus infection. *J Am Acad Dermatol* 1982;7:545–8.
8. Muller-Stamou A, Senn HJ, Emody G. Epidermolysis in a case of severe cytomegalovirus infection. *Br Med J* 1974;3:609–10.
9. Medearis DN Jr. Cytomegalic inclusion disease: an analysis of the clinical features based on the literature and six additional cases. *Pediatrics* 1957;19:167–480.
10. Mintz L, Drew WL, Miner RC, et al. Cytomegalovirus infections in homosexual men. *Ann Intern Med* 1983;99:326–9.
11. Knapp AB, Horst DA, Eliopoulos G, et al. Widespread cytomegalovirus gastroenterocolitis in a patient with the acquired immunodeficiency syndrome. *Gastroenterology* 1983;85:1399–402.
12. Masur H, Lane HC, Palestine A, et al. Effect of 9-(1,3-dihydroxy-2-propoxymethyl) guanine on serious cytomegalovirus disease in eight immunosuppressed homosexual men. *Ann Intern Med* 1986;104:41–4.
13. Koretz SH, Buhler WC, Brewin A, et al. Treatment of serious cytomegalovirus infection with 9-(1,3-dihydroxy-2-propoxymethyl) guanine in patients with AIDS and other immunodeficiencies. *N Engl J Med* 1986;314:801–5.
14. Kwan TH, Kaufman HW. Acid-fast bacilli with cytomegalovirus and herpes virus inclusions in the skin of an AIDS patient. *Am J Clin Pathol* 1986;85:236–8.
15. Cohen PR, Beltrani VP, Grossman ME. Disseminated herpes zoster in patients with human immunodeficiency virus infection. *Am J Med* 1988;84:1076–80.
16. Sandor I, Croxson TS, Millman A, et al. Herpes zoster ophthalmicus in patients at risk for AIDS. *N Engl J Med* 1984;310:1118–9.
17. Friedman-Kien AE, LaFleur FL, Gendler EC, et al. Herpes zoster: a possible early clinical sign for development of acquired immunodeficiency syndrome in high risk individuals. *J Am Acad Dermatol* 1986;14:1023–8.
18. Melbye M, Grossman RJ, Goedert J, et al. Risk of AIDS after herpes zoster. *Lancet* 1987;1:728–31.
19. Colebunders R, Mann JM, Francis H, et al. Herpes zoster in African patients. A clinical predictor of human immunodeficiency virus infection. *J Infect Dis* 1988;157:314–8.
20. Quinnan GV, Masur H, Rook AH, et al. Herpes-virus infections in the acquired immune deficiency syndrome. *JAMA* 1984;252:72–7.
21. Siegal FP, Lopez C, Hammer GS, et al. Severe acquired immunodeficiency in male homosexuals, manifested by chronic perianal ulcerative herpes simplex lesions. *N Engl J Med* 1981;305:1439–44.
22. Fivenson DP, Weltman RE, Gibson SH. Giant molluscum contagiosum presenting as basal cell carcinoma in an acquired immunodeficiency syndrome patient. *J Am Acad Dermatol* 1988;19:912–4.
23. Cockerell CJ. Cutaneous manifestations of HIV infection other than Kaposi's sarcoma: clinical and histologic aspects. *J Am Acad Dermatol* 1990;22:1260–9.
24. Rudlinger R, Grob R, Buchmann P, et al. Anogenital warts of the condyloma acuminatum type in HIV-positive patients. *Dermatologica* 1988;176:277–81.
25. Hollander H, Greenspan D, Stringari S, et al. Hairy leukoplakia and the acquired immunodeficiency syndrome. *Ann Intern Med* 1986;104:892–7.
26. Greenspan JS, Greenspan D, Lennette ET, et al. Replication of Epstein-Barr virus within the epithelial cells of oral "hairy" leukoplakia, an AIDS associated lesion. *N Engl J Med* 1985;313:1564–71.
27. Lane HC, Masur H, Edgar LC, et al. Abnormalities of B-cell activation and immunoregulation in patients with the acquired immunodeficiency syndrome. *N Engl J Med* 1983;309:453–8.
28. Duvic M. Staphylococcal infections and the pruritus of AIDS-related complex. *Arch Dermatol* 1987;123:1599–1602.
29. Kaplan MH, Sadick N, McNutt NS, et al. Dermatologic findings and manifestations of acquired immunodeficiency syndrome (AIDS). *J Am Acad Dermatol* 1987;16:485–506.
30. Patterson JW, Kitces EN, Neafie RC. Cutaneous botryomycosis in a patient with acquired immunodeficiency syndrome. *J Am Acad Dermatol* 1987;16:238–42.
31. Toth IR, Kazal HL. Botryomycosis in acquired immunodeficiency syndrome. *Arch Pathol Lab Med* 1987;111:246–9.
32. Rolston KVI, Uribe-Botero G, Mansell PWA. Bacterial infections in adult patients with the acquired immunodeficiency syndrome (AIDS and AIDS-related complex). *Am J Med* 1987;83:604–5.
33. Gant P, Wong PK, Meyer RD. Pyomyositis in a patient with the

acquired immunodeficiency syndrome. *Arch Intern Med* 1988;148:1608–10.

34. Watts RA, Hofbrand BI, Paton DF, et al. Pyomyositis associated with human immunodeficiency virus infection. *Br Med J* 1987;294:1524–5.

35. Cockerell CJ, Whitlow MA, Webster GF, et al. Epithelioid angiomatosis: a distinct vascular disorder in patients with the acquired immunodeficiency syndrome or AIDS-related complex. *Lancet* 1987;2:654–6.

36. LeBoit P, Berger TG, Egbert BM, et al. Epithelioid haemangioma-like vascular proliferation in AIDS: manifestation of cat scratch disease bacillus infection? *Lancet* 1988;1:960–3.

37. Cockerell CJ, LeBoit PE. Bacillary angiomatosis: a newly characterized, pseudoneoplastic, infectious, cutaneous vascular disorder. *J Am Acad Dermatol* 1990;22:501–12.

37a. Perkocha LA, Geaghan SM, Yen TSB, et al. Clinical and pathological features of bacillary peliosis hepatis in association with human immunodeficiency virus infection. *N Engl J Med* 1990;323:1581–6.

37b. Relman DA, Loutit JS, Schmidt TM, Falkow S, Tompkins LS. The agent of bacillary angiomatosis—an approach to the identification of uncultured pathogens. *N Engl J Med* 1990;323:1573–80.

38. Glover RA, Cockerell CJ. An unusual presentation of syphilis in an HIV infected patient. *Arch Dermatol,* in press.

39. Shylkin D, Tripoli L, Abell E. Lues maligna in a patient with human immunodeficiency virus infection. *Am J Med* 1988;85:425–7.

40. Gregory N, Sanchez M, Buchness MR. The spectrum of syphilis in patients with human immunodeficiency virus infection. *J Am Acad Dermatol* 1990;22:1061–7.

41. Radolf JD, Kaplan RP. Unusual manifestations of secondary syphilis and abnormal humoral immune response to *Treponema pallidum* antigens in a homosexual man with asymptomatic human immunodeficiency virus infection. *J Am Acad Dermatol* 1988;18:423–7.

42. Berry CD, Hoover TM, Colber AC, et al. Neurologic relapse after benzathine penicillin therapy for secondary syphilis in a patient with HIV infection. *N Engl J Med* 1987;316:1587–9.

43. Mohr JA, Griffiths W, Jackson R, et al. Neurosyphilis and penicillin levels in cerebrospinal fluid. *JAMA* 1976;236:2208–9.

44. Hirschmann JV, Chu AC. Skin lesions with disseminated toxoplasmosis in a patient with acquired immunodeficiency syndrome. *Arch Dermatol* 1988;124:1446–7.

45. Coulman CU, Greene I, Archibald RWR. Cutaneous pneumocystosis. *Ann Intern Med* 1987;106:396–8.

46. Schinella RA, Breda SD, Hammerschlag PE. Otic infection due to *Pneumocystis carinii* in an apparently healthy man with antibody to the human immunodeficiency virus. *Ann Intern Med* 1987;106:399–400.

47. Gherman CR, Ward RR, Bassis ML. *Pneumocystis carinii* otitis media and mastoiditis as the initial manifestation of the acquired immunodeficiency syndrome. *Am J Med* 1988;85:250–2.

48. Unger PD, Rosenblum M, Krown SE. Disseminated *Pneumocystis carinii* infection in a patient with acquired immunodeficiency syndrome. *Hum Pathol* 1988;19:113–6.

49. Kwok S, O'Donnell JJ, Wood IS. Retinal cotton wool spots in a patient with *Pneumocystis carinii* infection. *N Engl J Med* 1982;307:184–5.

50. Hennessey NP, Parro EL, Cockerell CJ. Disseminated cutaneous *Pneumocystis carinii* infection in two patients with AIDS. *Arch Dermatol* 1991;127:1699–1701.

51. Sadick N, Kaplan MH, Pahwa SG, et al. Unusual features of scabies complicating human T-lymphotropic virus type III infection. *J Am Acad Dermatol* 1986;15:482–6.

52. Glover R, Young L, Goltz RW. Norwegian scabies in acquired immunodeficiency syndrome. Report of a case resulting in death from associated sepsis. *J Am Acad Dermatol* 1987;16:396–9.

53. Penneys NS. *Skin manifestations of AIDS.* Philadelphia: JB Lippincott, 1990;142.

54. Brown FS, Anderson RH, Burnett JW: Cutaneous tuberculosis. *J Am Acad Dermatol* 1982;6:101–6.

55. Klein RS, Harris CA, Small CB, et al. Oral candidiasis in high risk patients as the initial manifestation of the acquired immunodeficiency syndrome. *N Engl J Med* 1984;311:354–8.

56. Oriba HA, Lo JS, Bergfeld WF. Disseminated cutaneous fungal infections and AIDS. *Cleve Clin J Med* 1990;57:189–91.

57. Rico MJ, Penneys NS. Cutaneous cryptococcosis resembling molluscum contagiosum in a patient with AIDS. *Arch Dermatol* 1985;121:901–2.

58. Hazelhurst JA, Vismer HF. Histoplasmosis presenting with unusual skin lesions in acquired immunodeficiency syndrome (AIDS). *Br J Dermatol* 1985;113:345–8.

59. Kalter DC, Tschen JA, Klima M. Maculopapular rash in a patient with acquired immunodeficiency syndrome. *Arch Dermatol* 1985;121:1455–6,1458–9.

60. Goodman D, Teplitz ED, Wishner A, et al. Prevalence of cutaneous disease in patients with acquired immunodeficiency syndrome (AIDS) or AIDS-related complex. *J Am Acad Dermatol* 1987;17:210–20.

61. Valle SL. Dermatologic findings related to human immunodeficiency virus infection in high risk individuals. *J Am Acad Dermatol* 1987;17:951–61.

62. Mathes BM, Douglass MC. Seborrheic dermatitis in patients with acquired immunodeficiency syndrome. *J Am Acad Dermatol* 1985;13:947–51.

63. Beare JM, Cheeseman EA, MacKenzie DWR. The association between *Candida albicans* and lesions of seborrheic eczema. *Br J Dermatol* 1968;80:675–81.

64. Faergemann J, Frederiksson T. Tinea versicolor with regard to seborrheic dermatitis. *Arch Dermatol* 1979;115:966–8.

65. Leyden JJ, McGinley KJ, Kligman AM. Role of microorganisms in dandruff. *Arch Dermatol* 1976;112:333–8.

66. McGinley KJ, Leyden JJ, Marples RR, et al. Quantitative microbiology of the scalp in non-dandruff, dandruff and seborrheic dermatitis. *J Invest Dermatol* 1975;64:401–5.

67. Soeprono FF, Schinella RA, Cockerell CJ, Comite SL. Seborrheic-like dermatitis of acquired immunodeficiency syndrome. *J Am Acad Dermatol* 1986;14:242–7.

68. Eisenstat BA, Wormser GP. Seborrheic dermatitis and butterfly rash in AIDS [Letter]. *N Engl J Med* 1984;311:189.

69. Johnson TM, Duvic N, Rapini RP, Rios A. AIDS exacerbates psoriasis [Letter]. *N Engl J Med* 1985;313:1415.

70. Lazar AP, Roenigk HH Jr. Acquired immunodeficiency syndrome (AIDS) can exacerbate psoriasis [Letter]. *J Am Acad Dermatol* 1988;18:144.

71. Winchester R, Bernstein DH, Fischer HD, et al. The co-occurrence of Reiter's syndrome and acquired immunodeficiency. *Ann Intern Med* 1987;106:19–26.

72. Lin RY. Reiter's syndrome and human immunodeficiency virus infection. *Dermatologica* 1988;176:39–42.

73. Soeprono FF, Schinella RA. Eosinophilic pustular folliculitis in patients with acquired immunodeficiency syndrome. *J Am Acad Dermatol* 1986;14:1020–2.

74. Jenkins D Jr, Fisher BK, Chalvardjian A, et al. Eosinophilic pustular folliculitis in a patient with AIDS. *Int J Dermatol* 1988;27:34–5.

75. Buchness MR, Lim HW, Hatcher VA, et al. Eosinophilic pustular folliculitis in the acquired immunodeficiency syndrome. *N Engl J Med* 1988;318:1183–6.

76. Valerie K, Delers A, Bruck C, et al. Activation of human immunodeficiency virus type I by DNA damage in human cells. *Nature* 1988;333:78–81.

77. Dahl MV. The immune system in health and disease. In: Moschella SL, Hurley HJ, eds. *Dermatology.* Philadelphia: WB Saunders, 1985;201–8.

78. Gordin FM, Simon GL, Wofsy CD, Mills J. Adverse reactions to trimethoprim-sulfamethoxazole in patients with the acquired immunodeficiency syndrome. *Ann Intern Med* 1984;100:495–9.

79. Cockerell CJ. Non-infectious inflammatory skin diseases in HIV infected individuals. *Clin Dermatol* 1991;9:531–41.

80. Cockerell CJ. Cutaneous signs of AIDS other than Kaposi's sarcoma. In: Friedman-Kien AE, ed. *Color atlas of AIDS* Philadelphia: WB Saunders, 1989;93–124.

81. Cockerell CJ. Pruritus in HIV infected hosts. In: Bernhard JD, ed. *Pruritus.* W.B. Saunders, in press.

82. Schonwetter RS, Nelson EB. Alopecia areata and the acquired immunodeficiency syndrome-related complex [Letter]. *Ann Intern Med* 1986;104:287.

83. Kinchelow T, Schmidt U, Ingato S. Changes in the hair of black patients with AIDS. *J Infect Dis* 1988;157:394–5.

84. Cockerell CJ, Dolan B. Calciphylaxis occurring in the setting of HIV infection. *AJ Am Acad Dermatol,* in press.

85. Young L, Steinman HK. Acquired ichthyosis in a patient with acquired immunodeficiency syndrome and Kaposi's sarcoma. *J Am Acad Dermatol* 1987;16:395–6.

86. Sadick NS, McNutt NS, Kaplan MH. Papulosquamous dermatoses of AIDS. *J Am Acad Dermatol* 1990,22:1270–7.

87. Bakos L, Hampe S, da Rocha HL, et al. Generalized granuloma annulare in a patient with acquired immunodeficiency syndrome (AIDS). *J Am Acad Dermatol* 1987;17:844–5.

88. Lobato MN, Berger TG. Porphyria cutanea tarda associated with the acquired immunodeficiency syndrome. *Arch Dermatol* 1988;124:1009–10.

89. Velji AM. Leukocytoclastic vasculitis associated with positive HTLV-III serologic findings. *JAMA* 1986;256:2196–7.

90. Bang F, Weismann K, Ralfkiaer E, et al. Erythema elevatum diutinum and pre-AIDS. *Acta Dermatovenereol (Stockh)* 1986;66:272–4.

91. Martin A, Cockerell CJ, Berger TG. Pityriasis rubra pilaris in patients infected with HIV. *Br J Dermatol,* in press.

AIDS and Other Manifestations of HIV Infection,
Second Edition, Edited by Gary P. Wormser.
Raven Press, Ltd., New York © 1992.

CHAPTER 31

Ophthalmologic Aspects of HIV Infection

Douglas A. Jabs

Ever since the original description of eye changes in patients with the acquired immunodeficiency syndrome (AIDS) by Holland et al. (1) in 1982, it has become evident that ocular manifestations are seen in the majority of patients with AIDS. Such conditions are generally classified into four areas: (1) a noninfectious microangiopathy, most often seen in the retina, and sometimes called "AIDS retinopathy"; (2) opportunistic ocular infections, particularly cytomegalovirus (CMV) retinitis; (3) conjunctival, eyelid, or orbital involvement by those neoplasms seen in patients with AIDS (e.g., Kaposi's sarcoma and lymphoma); and (4) neuroophthalmic lesions. The retinal microangiopathy is the most frequent ocular manifestation, and CMV retinitis is the most frequent opportunistic intraocular infection. While CMV retinitis was previously a rare disease, with the advent of the AIDS epidemic it has become a major public health problem. Treatment of CMV retinitis is complex and requires cooperation between the ophthalmologist and the infectious disease expert.

AIDS RETINOPATHY

"AIDS retinopathy" is the most frequent form of ocular involvement in patients with AIDS (Table 1). Multiple series (1–16) have reported an abnormal eye exam in 52–100% of patients with AIDS. In the Johns Hopkins series of 200 patients with AIDS (15) retinopathy was present in approximately two-thirds of the patients. Cotton wool spots (Fig. 1) are the most common feature and have been reported in 28–92% of patients with AIDS, with most series reporting that over half of the patients have these lesions. Cotton wool spots are microinfarcts

of the nerve fiber layer of the retina. Ischemia disrupts axonal transport, causing swelling of the axons in the nerve fiber layer, and producing the characteristic white, opaque patches called cotton wool spots. Intraretinal hemorrhages are considerably less frequent and have been reported in 0–54% of patients, with most series reporting their presence in less than 20% of patients. In our series (15), cotton wool spots were present in 64% and intraretinal hemorrhages in 12%. Perivascular sheathing without an infectious retinitis has been reported (3,15) but is uncommon in the United States. Most often perivascular sheathing is seen in association with CMV retinitis or other infections (15). Perivasculitis has been reported to occur in 15% of African patients with AIDS and 60% of African children with AIDS-related complex (ARC) (11,14). The reasons for the difference in perivascular sheathing between these reports from Africa and those from the United States are unclear.

In addition to these ophthalmoscopically visible findings, autopsy and fluorescein angiographic studies have also demonstrated other findings consistent with a widespread microangiopathy. The fluorescein angiographic study by Newsome et al. (8) found microangiopathic changes in all 12 patients studied, including microaneurysms and telangiectatic vessels. The autopsy series by Pepose et al. (10) found ocular involvement in 94% of patients studied and some evidence of retinal microangiopathy in 89%. Histologic findings in the retina have included a loss of pericytes, microaneurysm formation, thickened vascular walls with deposition of periodic acid-Schiff-positive material, and lumenal narrowing (8–10). Ultrastructural studies have shown swelling of the endothelial cells, occlusion of the vascular lumina, and thickening of the vascular basal lamina (17). These vascular lesions result in the microinfarcts producing cotton wool spots.

Although retinopathy is common in patients with AIDS, it is uncommon in patients with asymptomatic

D. A. Jabs: Departments of Ophthalmology and Medicine, The Johns Hopkins University, School of Medicine, Baltimore, Maryland 21205.

TABLE 1. *Retinopathy in patients with AIDS*

Condition	Frequency of occurrence (%)
AIDS retinopathy	66
Cotton wool spots	64
Intraretinal hemorrhages	12
Perivasculitis	<1
Retinal vascular occlusion	1

HIV infection. In our study (15) (Table 2), retinopathy was present in 66% of patients with AIDS, 40% of patients with ARC, 1% of patients with asymptomatic human immunodeficiency virus (HIV) infection, and 0% of non-HIV-infected gay men. These results suggest that the frequency of retinopathy parallels the decline in immune competence. Freeman et al. (16) have also reported that patients with HIV infection and retinopathy have lower CD4+ helper T-cell counts than do patients without retinopathy.

Pathogenesis

The pathogenesis of the AIDS microangiopathy is unknown. Three hypotheses have been proposed, including: (1) immune complex disease; (2) HIV infection of the retinal vascular endothelium; and (3) rheologic abnormalities. Although Kwok et al. (17) reported one case of *Pneumocystis carinii* possibly causing cotton wool spots, multiple other studies have demonstrated no opportunistic infectious organisms associated with cotton wool spots (8–10,15). *Pneumocystis carinii* has not been associated with cotton wool spots in any of the large autopsy series of eyes of patients with AIDS. Thus it is highly unlikely that any opportunistic infection has a direct causal relationship for the microangiopathy.

The earliest hypothesis for the etiology of the microangiopathy was that of circulating immune complexes. Holland et al. (3) noted circulating immune complexes in 10 of 12 patients studied, and Gupta and Licorice (18) found circulating immune complexes in 60% of 10 AIDS patients and 80% of 10 ARC patients. Pepose et al. (10) demonstrated immunoglobulin deposition within arterial walls, supporting this hypothesis. Furthermore, AIDS is characterized by polyclonal B-cell activation and hypergammaglobulinemia (19–20). Other diseases, such as collagen vascular diseases, which also have polyclonal B-cell activation and circulating immune complexes, have an indistinguishable microangiopathy (8). Therefore, immune complex disease seems a possible pathogenic mechanism.

However, alternative hypotheses exist. HIV is known to infect the retinal blood vessels. Pomerantz et al. (21) have been able to culture HIV from the retina of patients with AIDS and have localized HIV proteins to the retinal vascular endothelial cells using immunohistochemical techniques. Shuman et al. (13) have reported electron micrographic evidence of HIV infection of the retina. Since the central nervous system is commonly affected by HIV (22–24), the demonstration of HIV infection in the retina is not surprising. The resulting hypothesis has been that cotton wool spots are a direct consequence of HIV infection of the vascular endothelial cells, in which

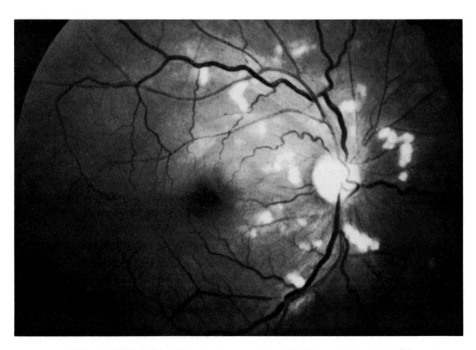

FIG. 1. AIDS retinopathy (cotton wool spots). From Jabs et al. (99).

TABLE 2. *Retinopathy and HIV infection[a]*

Group	No. of patients	Retinopathy (%)
AIDS	200	66
ARC	35	40
Asymptomatic HIV-infected individuals	232	1
Noninfected homosexual men	793	0

Adapted from Jabs et al., (99).
[a] AIDS, acquired immune deficiency syndrome; ARC, AIDS-related complex; HIV, human immunodeficiency virus.

the virus has a toxic effect on the vascular endothelium, producing arteriolar occlusion. An alternative hypothesis is that HIV infection of the vascular endothelial cells may lead to an immune event, resulting in vascular occlusion.

Finally, Engstrom et al. (25) have reported that systemic blood rheologic abnormalities are seen in patients with ocular microangiopathy. However, the etiology of this rheologic abnormality remains unknown. In addition to the microangiopathy seen in the retina, abnormalities of the blood vessels have been reported in the conjunctiva as well (25,26). These abnormalities include vascular occlusion and telangiectatic vessels and suggest a more widespread vascular abnormality.

OPPORTUNISTIC OCULAR INFECTIONS

Multiple opportunistic agents have been documented to infect the eye in patients with AIDS (Table 3). The most common of these is CMV retinitis, but other opportunistic ocular infections include herpes zoster ophthalmicus, *Pneumocystis* choroiditis, varicella-zoster retinitis, and toxoplasmic retinitis.

Cytomegalovirus Retinitis

Epidemiology

CMV retinitis is the most common intraocular infection in patients with AIDS (15). Estimates of the fre-

TABLE 3. *Opportunistic ocular infections in patients with AIDS*

Condition	Frequency of occurrence (%)
Cytomegalovirus retinitis	20–25
Herpes-zoster ophthalmicus	4
Toxoplasmic retinitis	1–2
Pneumocystis carinii choroiditis	<1
Fungal retinitis or endophthalmitis	<1
Infectious keratitis	<1

quency of CMV retinitis in patients with AIDS have varied from 6% to 38% (3–10,15,27,28) with higher estimates coming from surveys of inpatients and autopsy series (10). The variability in these estimates is probably due to a variety of factors, including variability in the patient population studied, underdetection in nonophthalmic series, referral bias in ophthalmic series, and the limitations of retrospective data analysis. Recognizing the potential for ascertainment bias, we (28) have estimated a minimum frequency of 11% among all patients with AIDS seen at the Johns Hopkins Hospital. Our reported frequency among patients seen in the AIDS Ophthalmology Clinic was 29%, and the true frequency is presumably between these two numbers. Reviewing the data from multiple series suggests that approximately 20–25% of patients with AIDS will ultimately develop CMV retinitis at some time during the course of their disease.

While it was initially suggested that CMV retinitis was a preterminal event (3), it has been recognized that CMV retinitis may occur at any time during the course of AIDS (28–30). Holland et al. (30) reported that the median interval from the diagnosis of AIDS to that of CMV retinitis was 9 months, but that the range varied from 0 to 45 months. CMV retinitis has been reported to be the initial AIDS-defining opportunistic infection (28–30). Of patients with CMV retinitis, 11–15% (28,30) will have CMV retinitis present at the time of the initial diagnosis of AIDS; of patients with AIDS, 3% will have CMV retinitis as their initial AIDS-defining opportunistic infection (28). Thus the interval between the diagnosis of AIDS and of CMV retinitis is wide, and CMV retinitis may occur at any time during the course of AIDS.

CMV retinitis is associated with a profound immunodeficiency (9,31). Palestine et al. (9) reported that the average CD4+ T-cell count among patients with CMV retinitis was 20 cells/mm^3. Hoechst et al. (31) reported that the median CD4+ T-cell count in patients with AIDS and CMV retinitis was 37 cells/mm^3, with 94% of the patients having a CD4+ T-cell count of less than 200 cells/mm^3. Because CMV retinitis is associated with profound immunodeficiency, survival after the diagnosis of CMV retinitis is approximately 6–8 months (28,30,32–34) but appears to be increasing (30). Four separate series from different cities (28,30,32,33) reported a median survival of 5–6 months after the diagnosis of CMV retinitis; the most recently reported series by Gross et al. (34) reported a median survival of 8 months. Furthermore, the range of survival after the diagnosis of CMV retinitis is quite wide, with some patients surviving up to 2 years (28,30).

Diagnosis and Natural History

The diagnosis of CMV retinitis can usually be reliably made on ophthalmoscopy by an experienced observer.

CMV retinitis may be asymptomatic, particularly if the lesion is small or anterior, or minimally symptomatic. Often the patient complains only of floaters or a vague sense of blurred vision. For more posteriorly located lesions, the patient often complains of a scotoma or a loss of vision. Ophthalmoscopically, CMV retinitis is described as a necrotic retinitis sometimes admixed with hemorrhage (Fig. 2). The most characteristic feature of CMV retinitis is a yellowish-white area of retinal necrosis with a granular border extending into the surrounding retina. While in the pre-AIDS era CMV retinitis was typically described as hemorrhagic, hemorrhages may or may not be present. The lesions that have extensive necrosis and hemorrhage are often described as "fulminant," while those without hemorrhage are sometimes described as "granular." Occasionally, a very early and small lesion of CMV retinitis may be difficult to distinguish from a cotton wool spot; however, follow-up examination generally reveals the diagnosis, since CMV retinitis will progress and enlarge over time.

Untreated, CMV retinitis is a progressive and potentially blinding disease (28). Cytomegalovirus is a ubiquitous herpes family virus. Approximately 50% of the general population have antibodies to CMV, suggesting previous exposure (35), while essentially 100% of gay men have antibodies to CMV (36). Generally, CMV exists in a latent state. However, when the patient's immune system declines, CMV can reactivate. It is thought that CMV is hematogenously disseminated to the retina, invades the retinal cells, and establishes a productive infection. Over 90% of patients with AIDS and CMV retinitis have positive cultures for CMV from a nonocular

source, such as blood or urine (28). Areas of retina previously infected with CMV show total destruction of the retinal architecture and replacement by a thin gliotic scar (10). Often there is hyperpigmentation of the scarred lesion. The borders of the lesion harbor active CMV, and the retinitis characteristically spreads from the periphery of the lesion outward. This process has sometimes been described as a "brush-fire" lesion. The end stage of this process is a totally destroyed retina, often detached, with no vision. Approximately one-third of patients will present with bilateral ocular involvement (28); of those patients who present with unilateral disease, 60% will ultimately develop bilateral disease unless treated (28). Series on the natural history of CMV retinitis report progression of the disease in virtually 100% of untreated patients with CMV retinitis (28,37).

There are two case reports of the resolution of CMV retinitis after the initiation of zidovudine (also known as azidothymidine or AZT) therapy in patients with AIDS (38,39). Both cases are noteworthy in that they are rare exceptions, that the zidovudine was instituted after the diagnosis of CMV retinitis, and that the lesions were subsequently arrested. In the case report by Guyer et al. (39) with follow-up until the patient's death, ultimate relapse of the retinitis occurred. Furthermore, the patient had progression of the CMV infection and loss of vision prior to the zidovudine-induced arrest of disease.

Treatment

The goal of treatment of CMV retinitis is to arrest the progression of the disease, prevent further spread of in-

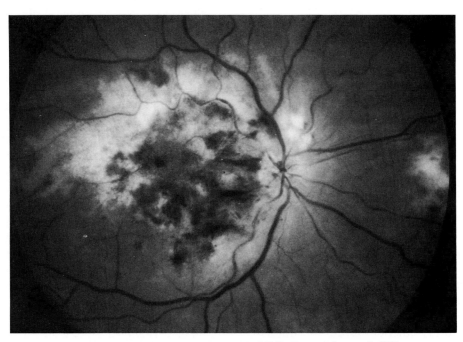

FIG. 2. CMV retinitis in a patient with AIDS. From Jabs et al. (99).

fection in the eye, and maximize visual function. Retina previously infected by CMV is destroyed and will not recover function. In patients successfully treated with an anti-CMV agent, there is arrest of the progression of disease, and the areas of necrotic retinitis will convert to an atrophic and gliotic scar. Patients will be left with a nonprogressive and atrophic lesion (Fig. 3). The clinical picture of treated CMV retinitis in which only an atrophic and gliotic scar can be detected, and there is no evidence of an active process, is often called a complete response or remission.

Two drugs have been reported to be useful in the treatment of CMV retinitis. The first is ganciclovir, which has been approved by the Food and Drug Administration (FDA) for the treatment of CMV retinitis in immunocompromised patients. Ganciclovir (Cytovene) was previously known as 9-(1,3-dihydroxy-2-proproxymethyl) guanine or DHPG. It is a nucleoside analog, which is taken up by the infected cell and triphosphorylated; it then inhibits viral DNA replication and arrests the CMV infection. Autopsy studies of patients treated with ganciclovir (40) have demonstrated the presence of viral DNA at the border of the lesion but have also demonstrated the absence of productive infection or intact virions.

The other drug reported to be efficacious in the treatment of CMV retinitis is foscarnet (Foscavir). Foscarnet is also known as trisodium phosphonoformate hexahydrate. Foscarnet is a pyrophosphate analog, which also inhibits viral DNA replication in the infected cell. Foscarnet was recently FDA approved.

Treatment of CMV retinitis is generally performed in a two-step fashion. Initially high dose of the anti-CMV drug is given to control the infection (induction therapy) and subsequently long-term lower dose therapy is given to prevent relapse (maintenance therapy). The phenomenon of relapse when an antibiotic is discontinued is characteristic of patients with AIDS and occurs in other infections such as *Pneumocystis carinii* pneumonia, cryptococcal meningitis, and toxoplasmosis. For ganciclovir, induction therapy consists of 5 mg/kg every 12 hours intravenously for 14 days (10 mg/kg/day). The other dosing schema previously used for induction was 2.5 mg/kg every 8 hours (7.5 mg/kg/day). Most investigators now use a 14-day induction course, although a 21-day induction course was used in the past; however, there have been no reported differences in efficacy between these two durations of induction.

Because of the high frequency of relapse of CMV retinitis when induction therapy was discontinued, the value of maintenance ganciclovir was appreciated early in the AIDS epidemic. Two dosing schema are recommended for maintenance ganciclovir: either 5 mg/kg/day intravenously once daily (35 mg/kg/week) or 6 mg/kg/day, 5 of 7 days (30 mg/kg/week). Lower doses of maintenance and every-other-day dosing schedules were associated with unacceptably high rates of early relapse.

Maintenance therapy must be continued indefinitely and requires the placement of a permanent indwelling central venous catheter. Because ganciclovir is excreted in the urine, the dose must be adjusted for renal function.

Multiple series have reported the efficacy of ganciclovir for the treatment of CMV retinitis. Response rates have ranged from 80% to 100%, and remission rates from 60% to 80% (27,28,32,33,41–46). In patients treated with ganciclovir, the median time to remission has been reported as 21–38 days (28,33). Prior to the use of maintenance therapy, patients given only induction ganciclovir often achieved remission at 1 month after starting therapy only to suffer relapse of the active retinitis subsequently (41). This lag between the institution of therapy for CMV retinitis and the resolution of the ophthalmoscopic evidence of active disease represents the time required for areas of necrotic retinitis to resolve and leave a scar. When anti-CMV therapy is interrupted for a sufficiently prolonged period of time, relapse is essentially universal. The time to relapse among patients who have had ganciclovir discontinued is approximately 3–4 weeks (28,46). Despite the use of maintenance therapy, CMV patients will often relapse while on maintenance, a phenomenon sometimes called "breakthrough" retinitis. Estimates of the rate of relapse of patients while on maintenance therapy vary from 18% to 50% (28,32, 33,43–46). Gross et al. (34) reported that the cumulative rate of relapse increased over time among patients receiving continuous maintenance therapy, with approximately 35% of patients relapsing by 1 year of treatment. While relapse of retinitis while on maintenance ganciclovir may occasionally be fulminant, it often appears to be a slow "smoldering" intermittent movement of the border, suggesting a partial effect of maintenance ganciclovir. Relapse of retinitis while on maintenance ganciclovir can most often be treated with a second course of induction ganciclovir. While CMV resistance to ganciclovir has been described (47), the usually favorable response to a second course of induction ganciclovir suggests that a major change in susceptibility of CMV is currently an infrequent cause of breakthrough. However, the role of ganciclovir resistance in the future remains to be determined.

The most frequent side effect reported for ganciclovir is granulocytopenia. Other side effects include thrombocytopenia, poorly characterized neurologic side effects, and abnormal liver function tests. Granulocytopenia is often the dose-limiting side effect. Most physicians treating patients with ganciclovir will allow the absolute neutrophil count (ANC) to fall to a level of 500 cells/mm^3 before discontinuing ganciclovir. The granulocytopenia is almost always reversible, and the ANC recovers over several days. Approximately one-third of patients receiving ganciclovir will experience granulocytopenia at some time during the course of their disease (28). Often this

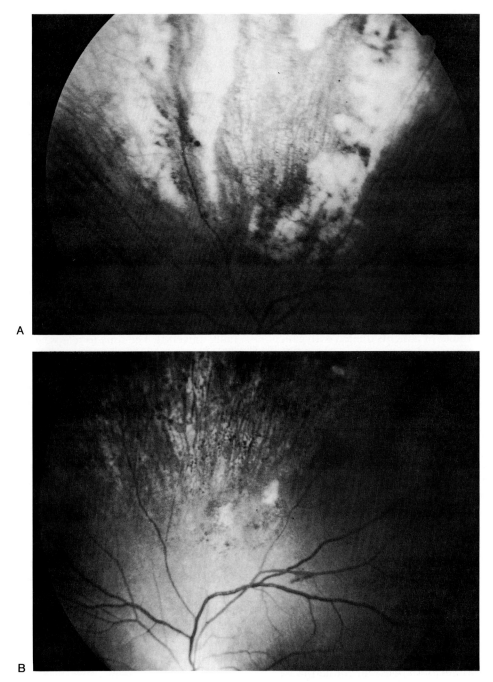

FIG. 3. Successful treatment of CMV retinitis in a patient with AIDS. **A:** CMV retinitis prior to treatment. **B:** Four weeks later, showing resolution of active retinitis. **C:** Six months later, showing continued suppression of CMV retinitis. A and B, from Jabs et al. (44). C, from Jabs (99).

fall in the ANC occurs near or just after the completion of induction therapy, and the ANC will rapidly recover with temporary interruption of therapy. Maintenance therapy may then be started, and the patient will tolerate long-term maintenance. Approximately 16% of patients treated with ganciclovir will be unable to tolerate the drug because of recurrent granulocytopenia (28).

Thrombocytopenia occurs in approximately 10%, and may also limit the dose tolerated. Other side effects rarely lead to discontinuation of therapy. Because of their similar hematologic toxicities, patients on ganciclovir do not tolerate concurrent zidovudine therapy at standard doses (500–600 mg/day) (31). Some investigators will attempt the concurrent use of zidovudine at a

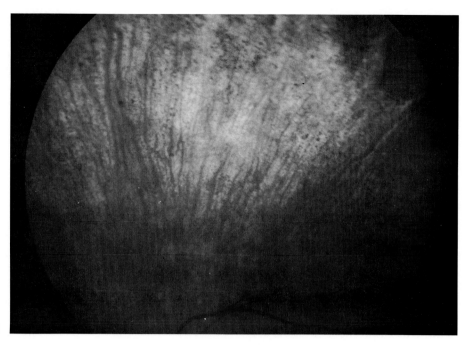

C

FIG. 3. *Continued.*

reduced dose (300 mg/day), but the long-term results of this combination and the number of patients who will tolerate it are unknown.

Foscarnet is a pyrophosphate analog, which also inhibits DNA replication in the virally infected cell. Preliminary studies have demonstrated a similar response rate to ganciclovir, with 80–100% of patients showing some response to the drug and 40–80% achieving a remission (48–50). Foscarnet is also used in a two-step fashion with an initial induction dose of 60 mg/kg/day every 8 hours for 2 weeks and a maintenance dose of 90 mg/kg/day. Jacobson et al. (51) have reported that a maintenance dose of 120 mg/kg/day appears to be more effective than 90 mg/kg/day in preventing relapse. The relative toxicities of these two dosing schema remain unclear at this time.

In contrast to ganciclovir, foscarnet is not marrow toxic. Its primary toxicities are renal, which has been reported to occur in 10–42% of patients treated with foscarnet, and metabolic. The nephrotoxicity is a reversible rise in creatinine. Metabolic problems include abnormalities of calcium, phosphorus, and magnesium. Often supplementation will be required for hypocalcemia or hypomagnesemia. In addition, neurologic events, particularly seizures, have been reported in patients treated with foscarnet. Seizures generally occur in patients who have other reasons for them (e.g., central nervous system toxoplasmosis). While the current hypothesis is that foscarnet may lower the seizure threshold via a metabolic abnormality, this hypothesis remains unproven.

A third method of treatment for CMV retinitis has been the use of intravitreal ganciclovir (52–54). Intravitreal injections are often used in ophthalmology for infectious endophthalmitis at the time of completion of a diagnostic vitrectomy or diagnostic vitreous aspiration. The use of intravitreal injections of ganciclovir attempts to utilize local instillation of ganciclovir into the eye to treat the CMV retinitis and avoid the systemic side effects of this drug. Small series have reported response rates similar to the use of intravenous ganciclovir with similar long-term relapse rates. The treatment is also given in a two-step fashion in which the patient receives an injection of 200 μg of ganciclovir two to three times weekly for 2–3 weeks as induction therapy, followed by maintenance injections one to two times weekly. Local side effects include endophthalmitis and retinal detachments. Because of the logistical difficulties in treating patients with regular intraocular injections, this form of therapy seems best reserved for patients who cannot tolerate intravenous therapy because of the systemic toxicities.

Other Opportunistic Ocular Infections

Ocular Toxoplasmosis

Ocular toxoplasmosis occurs in 1–2% of patients with AIDS. In patients with AIDS, ocular involvement by *Toxoplasma gondii* may be atypical and present with a diffuse necrotizing retinitis. Lesions may be bilateral and multifocal. While the toxoplasmic lesions may occasionally represent the reactivation of congenitally acquired infection, more often they appear to represent newly acquired ocular infection with *Toxoplasma* (55–57). Most lesions respond to treatment with pyrimethamine and sulfadiazine in standard doses. However, long-term maintenance therapy is generally required in order to prevent relapse of the disease. The best maintenance therapy for ocular toxoplasmosis is currently unknown. We have successfully managed patients intolerant of sulfadiazine and pyrimethamine with clindamycin as long-term maintenance.

Other Herpesvirus Infections

Infection of the retina with the varicella-zoster virus has been described (7,58). Clinically, this lesion appears to be identical to the acute retinal necrosis (ARN) syndrome, which is also caused by varicella-zoster, except that it occurs in patients who are HIV infected. The infection is a peripheral necrotizing retinitis, often with multiple scalloped or "thumb print" lesions, which then coalesce. The retinitis has much less hemorrhage than fulminant CMV retinitis. Varicella-zoster retinitis can be managed successfully with intravenous acyclovir at a dose of 500 mg/m² every 8 hours for 10–14 days (59). While long-term maintenance therapy with acyclovir would seem to be appropriate, there are insufficient data available upon which to base a dosing recommendation. Coexistent infection of the retina with herpes simplex and CMV has been described in one histologic case (60).

Fungal Retinitis

Candida retinitis and/or endophthalmitis has been reported in patients with AIDS (5), but occurs in less than 1% of patients with AIDS. A single case report of disseminated bilateral chorioretinitis due to *Histoplasma capsulatum* and a presumed clinical infection of the retina by cryptococcus have been reported (15,61). Cryptococcus has been reported in the choroid more commonly at autopsy (11), but appears to be clinically silent in most cases.

Bacterial Infections

Atypical mycobacterial infection of the choroid has been demonstrated at autopsy (11,15). However, this infection is generally clinically silent, and to the best of our knowledge no reports to date have shown a clinical ocular lesion from atypical mycobacterial infection. Unusual bacterial retinitis has been reported in two patients with AIDS (62). The bacteria were identified morphologically on an endoretinal biopsy specimen but not on culture. Both cases responded to tetracycline therapy.

Pneumocystis carinii *choroiditis*

Pneumocystis carinii choroiditis is a new ocular condition first reported by Rao et al. (63). This disorder is a form of extrapulmonary pneumocystosis and is most often seen in patients treated with aerolized pentamidine as *Pneumocystis* prophylaxis. *Pneumocystis* choroiditis has a striking clinical appearance (Fig. 4), and does respond to systemically administered anti-*Pneumocystis* therapy, such as intravenous trimethoprim/sulfamethoxazole or intravenous pentamidine (64,65). To date,

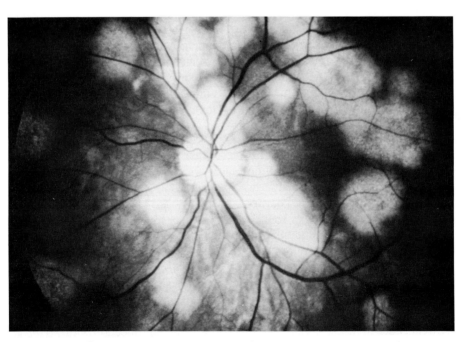

FIG. 4. Pneumocystis choroiditis in a patient with AIDS. From Rao et al. (63).

only case reports have appeared in the literature and the exact frequency of this disorder is unknown. Our own experience so far suggests that it currently occurs in less than 1% of patients with AIDS; however, the incidence and prevalence may well increase over time, particularly with the increasing use of aerosolized pentamidine.

Herpes Zoster Ophthalmicus

Herpes zoster ophthalmicus has been reported to occur in approximately 4% of patients with AIDS and 3% of patients with ARC (15). Ocular complications, including scleritis, iridocyclitis, and sixth nerve palsies, occur in 80% of patients with herpes zoster ophthalmicus and HIV infection. Furthermore, in appropriate populations, herpes zoster ophthalmicus in a young man appears to be a marker for HIV infection (66–68), even without other manifestations of HIV. In immunocompetent patients, herpes zoster ophthalmicus can successfully be treated with oral acyclovir (69). The dose most commonly used is now 800 mg five times daily by mouth. In immunocompromised patients, the initial treatment is often with intravenous acyclovir at a dosage of 500 mg/m² every 8 hours. This form of therapy markedly decreases the incidence of ocular complications. Experience with the use of oral acyclovir in patients with herpes zoster ophthalmicus and HIV infection is limited.

Other Ocular Infections

Other ocular infections reported in patients with AIDS include corneal ulcers (70,71), molluscum conta-giosum (72), microsporidial keratoconjunctivitis (73,74), and ocular syphilis (75–79). Ocular syphilis can occur in patients with any stage of HIV infection, and can cause a uveitis or neuroophthalmic disease. Treatment is with appropriate antibiotics, but in patients with HIV, syphilis may require more aggressive and/or prolonged therapy (79).

OCULAR NEOPLASMS

Ocular involvement by Kaposi's sarcoma has been reported in 2% of patients with AIDS. Of patients with AIDS and Kaposi's sarcoma, 15–22% (15,80) will develop ocular involvement. Either the eyelids or the conjunctiva may be involved. Conjunctival Kaposi's sarcoma (Fig. 5) usually does not require treatment. The lesions grow slowly and do not invade the eye. Furthermore, they do not compromise vision. Eyelid involvement by Kaposi's sarcoma may occasionally require therapy. This need occurs when the lesions are sufficiently large that vision is compromised because of lid edema and/or tumor. If the patient is being treated with systemic chemotherapy, observation for a response to the systemic chemotherapy is appropriate. However, if the eye specifically needs to be treated, then radiation therapy appears to be most effective (80). Surgical resection is generally associated with recurrence. In patients with HIV infection, high-grade lymphoma is an AIDS-defining disorder (81). Orbital involvement by lymphoma has been reported (15,82) but appears to occur in less than 1% of patients with AIDS (15).

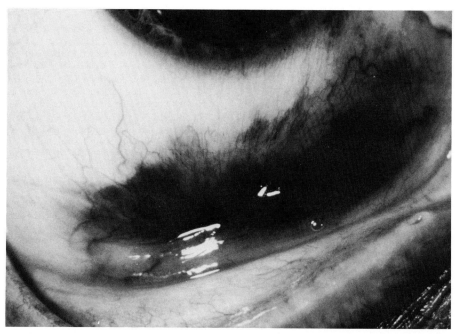

FIG. 5. Kaposi's sarcoma of the conjunctiva in a patient with AIDS. From Jabs et al. (15).

NEUROOPHTHALMIC LESIONS

Neuroophthalmic lesions have been reported in 8% of patients with AIDS (15). These lesions include cranial nerve palsies, papilledema, optic neuropathy, and hemianopsias (15,83–88). The most common etiology for neuroophthalmic lesions is cryptococcal meningitis (15) accounting for 60% of cases. Other causes include herpes zoster ophthalmicus, viral encephalitis, ethambutol toxicity, and CNS lymphoma. Of patients with AIDS and cryptococcal meningitis, one-third will have neuroophthalmic lesions on a careful ophthalmologic examination (15). Subtle ocular motility defects can be detected in patients with AIDS by eye movement recordings using infrared oculography (85,86). These defects include slowed saccades, fixational instability, and abnormal pursuit, and appear to be more directly related to HIV infection than to opportunistic ocular or neurological infections. They may correlate with the severity of the AIDS dementia complex.

HIV AND THE EYE

HIV has been isolated from the tears and conjunctiva of patients with AIDS (89,90), and demonstrated in the cornea of patients with HIV infection (91,92). As such, all potential donors material for corneal transplantation are screened for the presence of HIV infection and all material from donors found to be infected, discarded. HIV has also been isolated from the aqueous and vitreous of patients with HIV infection (93–96). One case of HIV-associated uveitis, which responded to treatment with zidovudine, has been reported (94), but appears to be a very infrequent occurrence. Because of the presence of HIV in the tears of patients, it is recommended that ophthalmologists performing eye exams utilize appropriate universal precautions (97,98).

REFERENCES

1. Holland GN, Gottlieb MS, Yee RD, et al. Ocular disorders associated with a new severe acquired cellular immunodeficiency syndrome. *Am J Ophthalmol* 1982;93:393–402.
2. Newman NM, Mandel MR, Gullett J, et al. Clinical and histologic findings in opportunistic infections. *Arch Ophthalmol* 1983;101:396–401.
3. Holland GN, Pepose JS, Petiti TH, et al. Acquired immune deficiency syndrome. Ocular manifestations. *Ophthalmology* 1983; 90:859–73.
4. Rosenberg PR, Uliss AE, Friedland GH, et al. Acquired immunodeficiency syndrome. Ocular manifestations in ambulatory patients. *Ophthalmology* 1983;90:874–8.
5. Schuman JS, Friedman AH. Retinal manifestations of the acquired immune deficiency syndrome (AIDS): cytomegalovirus, candida albicans, toxoplasmosis, and *Pneumocystis carinii*. *Trans Ophthalmol Soc UK* 1983;103:177–90.
6. Khadem M, Kalish SB, Goldsmith JA, et al. Ophthalmologic findings in acquired immune deficiency syndrome (AIDS). *Arch Ophthalmol* 1984;102:201–6.
7. Freeman WR, Lerner CW, Mines JA, et al. A prospective study of the ophthalmologic findings in the acquired immune deficiency syndrome. *Am J Ophthalmol* 1984;97:133–42.
8. Newsome DA, Green WR, Miller ED, et al. Microvascular aspects of acquired immune deficiency syndrome retinopathy. *Am J Ophthalmol* 1984;98:590–601.
9. Palestine AG, Rodrigues MM, Macher AM, et al. Ophthalmic involvement in acquired immunodeficiency syndrome. *Ophthalmology* 1984;91:1092–9.
10. Pepose JS, Holland GN, Nestor MS, et al. Acquired immune deficiency syndrome. Pathogenic mechanisms of ocular disease. *Ophthalmology* 1985;92:472–84.
11. Kestelyn P, Van de Perre P, Rouvroy D, et al. A prospective study of the ophthalmologic findings in the acquired immune deficiency syndrome in Africa. *Am J Ophthalmol* 1985;100:230–8.
12. Humphry RC, Parkin JM, Marsh RJ. The ophthalmological features of AIDS and AIDS related disorders. *Trans Ophthalmol Soc UK* 1986;105:505–9.
13. Schuman JS, Orellana J, Friedman AH, et al. Acquired immunodeficiency syndrome (AIDS). *Surv Ophthalmol* 1987;31: 384–410.
14. Kestelyn P, Lepage P, Perre PVD. Perivasculitis of the retinal vessels as an important sign in children with AIDS-related complex. *Am J Ophthalmol* 1985;100:614–5.
15. Jabs DA, Green WR, Fox R, Polk BF, Bartlett JG. Ocular manifestations of acquired immune deficiency syndrome. *Ophthalmology* 1989;96:1092–9.
16. Freeman WR, Chen A, Henderly DE, et al. Prevalence and significance of acquired immunodeficiency syndrome-related retinal microvasculopathy. *Am J Ophthalmol* 1989;107:229–335.
17. Kwok S, O'Donnell JJ, Wood IS. Retinal cotton-wood spots in a patient with *Pneumocystis carinii* infection. *N Engl J Med* 1982;307:185.
18. Gupta S, Licorish K. Circulating immune complexes in AIDS. *N Engl J Med* 1984;310:1530–1.
19. Lane HC, Masur H, Edgar LC, et al. Abnormalities of B-cell activation and immunoregulation in patients with the acquired immunodeficiency syndrome. *N Engl J Med* 1983;309:453–8.
20. Schnittman SM, Lane HC, Higgins SE, et al. Direct polyclonal activation of human B lymphocytes by the acquired immune deficiency syndrome virus. *Science* 1986;233:1084–6.
21. Pomerantz RJ, Kuritzkes R, Monte M, et al. Infection of the retina by human immunodeficiency virus type I. *N Engl J Med* 1987;317:1643–7.
22. Shaw GM, Harper ME, Hahn BH, et al. HTLV-III infection in brains of children and adults with AIDS encephalopathy. *Science* 1985;227:177–82.
23. Ho DD, Rota TR, Schooley RT, et al. Isolation of HTLV-III from cerebrospinal fluid and neural tissues of patients with neurologic syndromes related to the acquired immunodeficiency syndrome. *N Engl J Med* 1985;313:1493–7.
24. Koenig S, Gendelman HE, Orenstein JM, et al. Detection of AIDS virus in macrophages in brain tissue from AIDS patients with encephalopathy. *Science* 1986;233:1089–93.
25. Engstrom RE, Holland GN, Hardy D, Meiselman HJ. Abnormal blood rheologic factors in patients with human immunodeficiency virus-associated conjunctival and retinal microvasculopathy. ARVO Abstracts. *Invest Ophthalmol Vis Sci (Suppl)* 1988;29:43 (abst).
26. Teich SA. Conjunctival vascular changes in AIDS and AIDS-related complex. *Am J Ophthalmol* 1987;103:332–3.
27. Jacobson MA, O'Donnell JJ, Porteous D, Brodie HR, Feigal D, Mills J. Retinal and gastrointestinal disease due to cytomegalovirus in patients with the acquired immune deficiency syndrome: prevalence, natural history, and response to ganciclovir therapy. *Q J Med* 1988;67:473–86.
28. Jabs DA, Enger C, Bartlett JG. Cytomegalovirus retinitis and acquired immunodeficiency syndrome. *Arch Ophthalmol* 1989; 107:75–80.
29. Henderly DE, Freeman WR, Smith RE, Causey D, Rao NA. Cytomegalovirus retinitis as the initial manifestation of the acquired immune deficiency syndrome. *Am J Ophthalmol* 1987; 103:316–20.
30. Holland GN, Sison RF, Jatulis DE, et al. Survival of patients with

acquired immune deficiency syndrome after development of cytomegalovirus retinopathy. *Ophthalmology* 1990;97:204–11.

31. Hoechst H, Dieterich D, Bozzette S, et al. Toxicity of combined ganciclovir and zidovudine for cytomegalovirus disease associated with AIDS. *Ann Intern Med* 1990;113:111–7.

32. Henderly DE, Freeman WR, Causey DM, Rao NA. Cytomegalovirus retinitis and response to therapy with ganciclovir. *Ophthalmology* 1987;94:425–34.

33. Orellana J, Teich SA, Friedman AH, Lerebours F, Winterkorn J, Mildvan D. Combined short- and long-term therapy for the treatment of cytomegalovirus retinitis using ganciclovir (BW B759U). *Ophthalmology* 1987;94:831–8.

34. Gross JG, Bozzette SA, Mathews WC et al. Longitudinal study of cytomegalovirus retinitis in acquired immune deficiency syndrome. *Ophthalmology* 1990;97:681–6.

35. Collier AC, Meyers JD, Corey L et al. Cytomegalovirus infection in homosexual men. *Am J Med* 1987;82:593–601.

36. Tange M, Klein EB, Kornfield H, Coope LZ, Greico MH. Cytomegalovirus isolation from healthy homosexual man. *JAMA* 1984;252:1908–10.

37. Holland GN, Buhles WC, Mastre B, Kaplan HJ, UCLA CMV Retinopathy Study Group. A controlled retrospective study of ganciclovir treatment for cytomegalovirus retinopathy. Use of a standardized system for the assessment of disease outcome. *Arch Ophthalmol* 1989;107:1759–66.

38. D'Amico DJ, Sholnik PR, Koslof BR, Pimhsten P, Hirsch MS, Schooley RT. Resolution of cytomegalovirus retinitis with zidovudine therapy. *Arch Ophthalmol* 1988;106:1168–9.

39. Guyer DR, Jabs DA, Brant AM, Beschorner WE, Green WR. Regression of cytomegalovirus retinitis with zidovudine. A clinicopathologic correlation. *Arch Ophthalmol* 1989;107:868–74.

40. Pepose JS, Newman C, Bach MC et al. Pathologic features of cytomegalovirus retinopathy after treatment with the antiviral agent ganciclovir. *Ophthalmology* 1987;94:414–24.

41. Palestine AG, Stevens G, Lane HC, et al. Treatment of cytomegalovirus retinitis with dihydroxy propoxymethyl guanine. *Am J Ophthalmol* 1986;101:95–101.

42. Collaborative DHPG Treatment Study Group. Treatment of serious cytomegalovirus infections with 9-(1,3-dihydroxy-2-propoxymethyl) guanine in patients with AIDS and other immunodeficiencies. *N Engl J Med* 1986;314:801–5.

43. Holland GN, Sidikaro Y, Kreiger AE, et al. Treatment of cytomegalovirus retinopathy with ganciclovir. *Ophthalmology* 1987;94:815–23.

44. Jabs DA, Newman C, de Bustros S, Polk BF. Treatment of cytomegalovirus retinitis with ganciclovir. *Ophthalmology* 1987;94:824–30.

45. Laskin OL, Cederberg DM, Mills J, Eron LJ, Mildvan D, Spector SA. Ganciclovir for the treatment and suppression of serious infections caused by cytomegalovirus. *Am J Med* 1987;83:201–7.

46. Jacobson MA, O'Donnell JJ, Brodie HR, Wofsy C, Mills J. Randomized prospective trial of ganciclovir maintenance therapy for cytomegalovirus retinitis. *J Med Virol* 1988;25:339–49.

47. Erice A, Chou S, Biron KK, Stanat SC, Balfour HH, Jordan MC. Progressive disease due to ganciclovir-resistant cytomegalovirus in immunocompromised patients. *N Engl J Med* 1989;320:291–3.

48. Walmsley SL, Chew E, Read SE, et al. Treatment of cytomegalovirus retinitis with trisodium phosophonoformate hexahydrate (foscarnet). *J Infect Dis* 1988;157:569–72.

49. LaHoang P, Girard B, Robinet TM, et al. Foscarnet in the treatment of cytomegalovirus retinitis in acquired immune deficiency syndrome. *Ophthalmology* 1989;96:864–5.

50. Aweeka F, Gambertoglio J, Mills J, Jacobson J. Pharmacokinetics of intermittently administered intravenous foscarnet in the treatment of acquired immunodeficiency syndrome patients with serious cytomegalovirus retinitis. *Antimicrob Agents Chemother* 1989;33:742–5.

51. Jacobson MA, O'Donnell JJ, Mills J. Foscarnet treatment of cytomegalovirus retinitis in patients with the acquired immunodeficiency syndrome. *Antimicrob Agents Chemother* 1989;33:736–41.

52. Ussery FM, Gibson SR, Conklin RH, Piot DF, Stool EW, Conklin AJ. Intravitreal ganciclovir in the treatment of AIDS-associated cytomegalovirus retinitis. *Ophthalmology* 1988;95:640–8.

53. Cantrill HL, Henry K, Melroe NH, Knobloch WH, Ramsay RC, Balfour HH Jr. Treatment of cytomegalovirus retinitis with intravitreal ganciclovir. Long-term results. *Ophthalmology* 1989;96:367–74.

54. Heinemann MH. Long-term intravitreal ganciclovir therapy for cytomegalovirus retinopathy. *Arch Ophthalmol* 1989;107:1767–72.

55. Parke DW, Font RL. Diffuse toxoplasmic retinochoroiditis in a patient with AIDS. *Arch Ophthalmol* 1986;104:571–5.

56. Wiess A, Margo CE, Ledford DK, et al. Toxoplasmic retinochoroiditis as an initial manifestation of the acquired immune deficiency syndrome. *Am J Ophthalmol* 1987;103:248–9.

57. Holland GN, Engstrom RE, Glasgow BJ, et al. Ocular toxoplasmosis in patients with the acquired immunodeficiency syndrome. *Am J Ophthalmol* 1988;106:653–67.

58. Jabs DA, Schachat AP, Liss R, et al. Presumed varicella zoster retinitis in immunocompromised patients. *Retina* 1987;7:9–13.

59. Blumenkranz MS, Culbertson WW, Clarkson JG, Dix R. Treatment of the acute retinal necrosis syndrome with intravenous acyclovir. *Ophthalmology* 1986;93:296–300.

60. Pepose JS, Hilborne LH, Cancilla PA, Roos RY. Concurrent herpes simplex and cytomegalovirus retinitis and encephalitis in the acquired immune deficiency syndrome (AIDS). *Ophthalmology* 1984;91:1669–77.

61. Macher A, Rodrigues MM, Kaplan W, et al. Disseminated bilateral chorioretinitis due to *Histoplasma capsulatum* in a patient with the acquired immunodeficiency syndrome. *Ophthalmology* 1985;92:1159–64.

62. Davis JL, Nussenblatt RB, Bachman DM, Chan CC, Palestine AG. Endogenous bacterial retinitis in AIDS. *Am J Ophthalmol* 1989;107:613–23.

63. Rao NA, Zimmerman PL, Boyer D, et al. A clinical, histopathologic, and electron microscopic study of *Pneumocystis carinii* choroiditis. *Am J Ophthalmol* 1989;107:218–28.

64. Freeman WR, Gross JG, Labelle J, Oteken K, Katz B, Wiley CA. *Pneumocystis carinii* choroidopathy. A new clinical entity. *Arch Ophthalmol* 1989;107:863–7.

65. Dugel PU, Rao NA, Forster DJ, Chong LP, Frangieh GT, Sattler F. *Pneumocystis carinii* choroiditis after long-term aerosolized pentamidine therapy. *Am J Ophthalmol* 1990;110:113–7.

66. Cole EL, Meisler DM, Calabrese LH, et al. Herpes zoster ophthalmicus and acquired immune deficiency syndrome. *Arch Ophthalmol* 1984;102:1027–9.

67. Sandor EV, Millman A, Croxson S, Mildvan D. Herpes zoster ophthalmicus in patients at risk for the acquired immune deficiency syndrome (AIDS). *Am J Ophthalmol* 1986;101:153–5.

68. Kestelyn P, Stevens AM, Bakkers E, et al. Severe herpes zoster ophthalmicus in young African adults: a marker for HTLV-III seropositivity. *Br J Ophthalmol* 1987;71:806–9.

69. Cobo LM, Foulks GN, Liesegang T, et al. Oral acyclovir in the treatment of acute herpes zoster ophthalmicus. *Ophthalmology* 1986;93:763–70.

70. Santos C, Parker J, Dawson C, Ostler B. Bilateral fungal corneal ulcers in a patient with AIDS-related complex. *Am J Ophthalmol* 1986;102:118–9.

71. Parrish CM, O'Day DM, Hoyle TC. Spontaneous corneal ulcer as an ocular manifestation of AIDS. *Am J Ophthalmol* 1987;104:302–3.

72. Kohn SR. Molluscum contagiosum in patients with acquired immune deficiency syndrome. *Arch Ophthalmol* 1987;105:458.

73. Friedberg DN, Stenson SM, Orenstein JM, Tierno PM, Charles NC. Microsporidial keratoconjunctivitis in acquired immunodeficiency syndrome. *Arch Ophthalmol* 1990;108:504–8.

74. Lowder CY, Meisler DM, McMahon JT, Longworth DL, Rutherford I. Microsporidia infection of the cornea in a man seropositive for human immunodeficiency virus. *Am J Ophthalmol* 1990;109:242–4.

75. Stoumbos VD, Klein ML. Syphilitic retinitis in a patient with acquired immunodeficiency syndrome-related complex. *Am J Ophthalmol* 1987;103:103–4.

76. Passo MS, Rosenbaum JT. Ocular syphilis in patients with human immunodeficiency virus infection. *Am J Ophthalmol* 1988;106:1–5.

77. Carter JB, Hamill RJ, Matoba AY. Bilateral syphilitic optic neuri-

tis in a patient with a positive test for HIV. *Arch Ophthalmol* 1987;105:1485–6.

78. Becerra LI, Ksiazek SM, Savino PJ, et al. Syphilitic uveitis in human immunodeficiency virus-infected and noninfected patients. *Ophthalmology* 1989;96:1727–30.

79. McLeish WM, Pulido JS, Holland S, Culbertson WW, Winward K. The ocular manifestations of syphilis in the human immunodeficiency virus type 1-infected host. *Ophthalmology* 1990;97:196–203.

80. Schuler JD, Holland GN, Miles SA, Miller BJ, Grossman I. Kaposi sarcoma of the conjunctiva and eyelids associated with the acquired immunodeficiency syndrome. *Arch Ophthalmol* 1989;107:858–62.

81. CDC. Revision of the CDC surveillance case definition for the acquired immune deficiency syndrome. *MMWR* 1987;36:1S–15S.

82. Fujikawa LS, Schwartz LK, Rosenbaum EH. Acquired immune deficiency syndrome associated with Burkitt's lymphoma presenting with ocular findings. *Ophthalmology* 1983;90 [Suppl]:50(abst).

83. McArthur J. Neurologic manifestations of AIDS. *Medicine* 1987;66:407–37.

84. Hamed LM, Schatz NJ, Galetta SL. Brainstem ocular motility defects in AIDS. *Am J Ophthalmol* 1988;106:437–42.

85. Nguyen N, Rimmer S, Katz B. Slowed saccades in the acquired immunodeficiency syndrome. *Am J Ophthalmol* 1989;107:356–60.

86. Currie J, Benson E, Ramsden B, Perdices M, Cooper D. Eye movement abnormalities as a predictor of the acquired immunodeficiency syndrome dementia complex. *Arch Neurol* 1988;45:949–53.

87. Slavin ML, Mallin JE, Jacob HS. Isolated homonymous hemianopsia in the acquired immunodeficiency syndrome. *Am J Ophthalmol* 1989;108:198–200.

88. Winward KE, Hamed LM, Glaser JS. The spectrum of optic nerve disease in human immunodeficiency virus infection. *Am J Ophthalmol* 1989;107:373–80.

89. Fujikawa LS, Salahuddin SZ, Ablashi D, et al. HTLV-III in the tears of AIDS patients. *Ophthalmology* 1986;93:1479–81.

90. Fujikawa LS, Salahuddin SZ, Ablashi D, et al. Human T-cell leukemia/lymphotropic virus type III in the conjunctival epithelium of a patient with AIDS. *Am J Ophthalmol* 1985;100:507–9.

91. Salahuddin SZ, Palestine AG, Heck E, et al. Isolation of the human T-cell leukemia/lymphotrophic virus type III form the cornea. *Am J Ophthalmol* 1986;101:149–52.

92. Doro S, Navia BA, Kahn A, et al. Confirmation of HTLV-III virus in cornea. *Am J Ophthalmol* 1986;102:390–1.

93. Kestelyn P, Perre PVD, Goldberger SS. Isolation of the human T-cell leukemia/lymphotrophic virus type III from aqueous humor in two patients with perivasculitis of the retinal vessels. *Int Ophthalmol* 1986;9:247–51.

94. Farrell PL, Heinemann MH, Roberts CW, et al. Response of human immunodeficiency virus-associated uveitis to zidovudine. *Am J Ophthalmol* 1988;106:7–10.

95. Cantrill HL, Henry K, Jackson B, Erice A, Ussery FM, Balfour HH. Recovery of human immunodeficiency virus from ocular tissues in patients with acquired immune deficiency syndrome. *Ophthalmology* 1988;95:1458–62.

96. Srinivasan A, Kalyanaraman S, Dutt K, Butler D, Kaplan HJ. Isolation of HIV-1 from vitreous humor. *Am J Ophthalmol* 1989;108:197–8.

97. CDC. Recommendations for preventing possible transmission of human T-lymphotrophic virus type III/Lymphadenopathy-associated virus from tears. *MMWR* 1985;34:533–4.

98. CDC. Recommendations for prevention of HIV transmission in health-care settings. *MMWR* 1987;36 [Suppl]:15–185.

99. Jabs DA. Ganciclovir treatment of CMV retinitis. In: Spector SA, ed. *Ganciclovir therapy for cytomegalovirus infection*. New York: Marcel Dekker, 1991;91–104.

AIDS and Other Manifestations of HIV Infection,
Second Edition, Edited by Gary P. Wormser.
Raven Press, Ltd., New York © 1992.

CHAPTER 32

Oral Lesions Associated with HIV Infection

John S. Greenspan and Deborah Greenspan

Lesions in the mouth were among the first documented features of the acquired immunodeficiency syndrome (AIDS) (1,2). Their varied nature and common occurrence is reflected in an extensive and growing literature (3–9). Oral candidiasis in non-AIDS patients who were in high-risk categories was shown early in the epidemic to be predictive of AIDS (7,9). With the discovery of hairy leukoplakia (8), it soon became clear that this was also an indicator of human immunodeficiency virus (HIV) infection and the subsequent development of AIDS (10).

In addition to their role in the diagnosis of HIV infection (11,12) and as indicators of the stage and progression of HIV disease, (13) oral lesions are used as clinical correlates of CD4 counts (14), as criteria for entry into clinical trials (15), and as readily studied and accessible models for mucosal abnormalities in HIV infection (16). These lesions cause significant morbidity (17,18), yet many can be treated using fairly simple therapeutic approaches. A thorough oral examination of all patients is thus mandatory, both for purposes of diagnosis and staging of HIV infection and also so that the oral lesions themselves can be treated.

CLASSIFICATION

At least 40 oral manifestations of HIV infection have been recorded, and a detailed classification has been established under the auspices of the European Economic Community (19). However, many of these lesions have

been reported as single cases and may be only coincidentally associated with HIV infection.

The oral lesions most frequently seen and clearly associated with HIV infection are listed in Table 1. For a more complete discussion of the range of oral lesions, see reviews (3–6).

EPIDEMIOLOGY

While there is general agreement that oral lesions are commonly seen in HIV-infected individuals, few well-designed studies involving appropriate and fully characterized populations have been published. Reports include descriptions of otherwise asymptomatic HIV-seropositives [Centers for Disease Control (CDC) group II], those with persistent lymphadenopathy and other manifestations of HIV infection short of full AIDS (CDC groups III and IVA, C2, and E), and patients with AIDS (CDC groups IVC1 and-D). The presence of oral lesions significantly affects the CDC group/category to which cases are assigned (13). The prevalence of oral lesions of any type in these studies ranged from 15% among HIV-seropositive women in Nairobi in 1989 (20), to 54% among patients in all group IV categories in Tanzania in 1987 (11), to even higher percentages in other patient groups (21,22). However, none of those studies represented population-based cohorts, and so all of the numbers reflect positive referral bias.

At the University of California, San Francisco Oral AIDS Center we have examined several cohorts in the San Francisco area beginning in 1987 and in particular have studied the three San Francisco population-based cohorts of homosexual and bisexual men (23). The prevalence of the commonest HIV-associated lesions in these seropositive men (those with AIDS were excluded) ranged from approximately 19% for hairy leukoplakia to 9% for candidiasis to 4% for all other oral lesions. The

J. S. Greenspan: Departments of Oral Biology and Oral Pathology and Stomatology, School of Dentistry; Department of Pathology, School of Medicine; Oral AIDS Center, University of California, San Francisco, California 94143-0512.

D. Greenspan: Departments of Oral Medicine and Stomatology, School of Dentistry and Clinical Director, Oral AIDS Center, University of California, San Francisco, California 94143-0512.

TABLE 1. *Oral lesions in HIV-infected persons*

Fungal	Bacterial
Candidiasis	HIV gingivitis
Pseudomembranous	HIV periodontitis
Erythematous	Necrotizing gingivitis and
Angular cheilitis	stomatitis
Histoplasmosis	*Mycobacterium avium-*
Cryptococcosis	*intracellulare*
	complex
Viral	Neoplastic
Herpes simplex	Kaposi's sarcoma
Hairy leukoplakia	Lymphoma
Herpes zoster	
Warts	
Idiopathic	
Recurrent aphthous ulcers	
Immune thrombocytopenic	
purpura	
HIV salivary gland disease	
Abnormalities of pigmentation	

prevalence of at least one oral lesion was about 30%. The time at which these men acquired HIV infection is variable of course, but most can be assumed to have been infected between 1978 and 1984, with more towards the later period. Our study was performed during 1987–1990 and so most of the subjects would have been seropositive for 3–10 years. The results are, therefore, likely to be reasonably representative of HIV-positive, non-AIDS patients in general.

DIAGNOSTIC CRITERIA

Discussion of the oral manifestations of HIV infection has been marred by a lack of agreement on the definitions of and diagnostic criteria for these lesions. A recent consensus meeting has resulted in a set of agreed definitions and criteria, which can serve as the basis for future epidemiological, clinical, and laboratory studies (24).

FUNGAL LESIONS

Candidiasis (Candidosis)

Candida species are commonly found in the healthy mouth on culture (25) and are even more frequently found in HIV-seropositive patients (26–28). Oral mucosal disease due to this fungus, candidiasis (or candidosis), is seen in association with predisposing factors such as infancy, old age, systemic disease including diabetes, anemia, denture wearing, and many immunosuppressive states including HIV infection.

Oral and esophageal candidiasis were included in the early descriptions of AIDS. Esophageal candidiasis is included in CDC group IV category C1 as a feature of

AIDS, while oral candidiasis is included in group IV category C2.

Oral candidiasis (29) in persons with HIV infection can be of three types, pseudomembranous (thrush), erythematous, and angular cheilitis. Hyperplastic candidiasis (candidal leukoplakia) is only rarely seen in this group of patients.

Pseudomembranous Candidiasis

Pseudomembranous candidiasis presents as white or cream-colored patches on any part of the oral mucosa (Fig. 1). There may be a red change in the adjoining mucosa and the plaques can be removed, sometimes revealing a bleeding surface. There may be soreness, pain, and dysphagia.

Erythematous Candidiasis

The erythematous type shows as red areas of the mucosa (Fig. 2), notably on the palate and dorsal tongue, where papillary atrophy is seen. The lesions are often asymptomatic although soreness and burning may be reported.

Angular Cheilitis

Angular cheilitis is often due to candidal infection and consists of cracks or fissures at the angles of the mouth.

Oral candidiasis is diagnosed by a combination of clinical appearance and simple tests. The best of the latter involves a smear from the lesions in which *Candida* hyphae are demonstrated using potassium hydroxide, periodic acid-Schiff (PAS), or gram stain. Culture is not helpful in diagnosis although it can be used to determine the species involved. Oral candidiasis may or may not be associated with esophageal candidiasis (30–32).

There is a relationship between increased frequency of

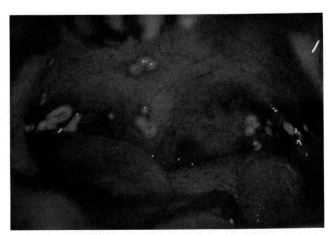

FIG. 1. Pseudomembranous candidiasis.

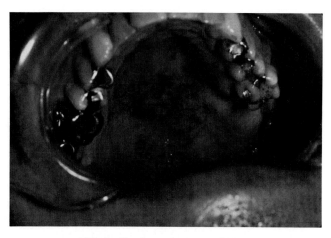

FIG. 2. Erythematous candidiasis.

oral candidiasis in HIV infection and falling CD4 numbers in several studies (14,23). Oral candidiasis is predictive of the development of AIDS in HIV-positive people of all risk groups (7,9). We have recently shown that erythematous candidiasis is of the same significance in this regard as pseudomembranous candidiasis. Erythematous candidiasis is subtle in appearance and may be missed on cursory clinical examination.

The factors determining the transition between the commensal state, with *Candida* present in the mouth as the yeast form, and the mucosal lesion with infection by fungal hyphae are unknown. It does appear that most individuals carry a single strain of *Candida,* as defined by restriction length polymorphism and other criteria, during the course of HIV infection, both when mucosal lesions are absent and when they are present (33,34). The absence of unique or specifically pathogenic strains is evidence for a primary role for defects in host defense mechanisms in the pathogenesis of oral mucosal candidiasis.

Therapy for oral candidiasis, which involves the use of topical or systemic antifungal agents, is indicated to prevent symptoms including pain, burning sensations, soreness, and dysguesia that may occur with any of the clinical presentations. Topical treatment for oral candidiasis includes the use of nystatin, (either as an oral suspension 100,000 units/cc, 5cc orally (swish and swallow) three to four times a day or in the form of pastilles 200,000 units, one to two pastilles dissolved in the mouth five times a day), or clotrimazole oral troches (one 10mg tablet dissolved in the mouth five times a day). If compliance is good, any of these regimens will effectively clear the oral lesions. However, because of the flavor of some of the preparations and the high frequency of administration necessary to be effective, compliance may not be satisfactory. Systemic therapy has the advantage of once daily dosing. However, these drugs may have interactions with several medications that are used in association with HIV infection, and this should be checked before pre-

scribing. Ketoconazole, 200–400 mg/day, should be taken with food. Adverse effects include abnormalities in liver function, occasionally nausea or skin rash and others. Unfortunately, ketoconazole may not be adequately absorbed in people with HIV infection because of hypochlorhydria, or other gastrointestinal problems of HIV infection. Fluconazole does not require gastric acidity for absorption, but it is much more expensive than ketoconazole. The recommended dose is one 100-mg tablet/day. A recent study suggested that fluconazole inhibits candidal adherence to oral epithelial cells (35).

To date there are few data to suggest that *Candida* resistance appears in vivo with any of these antifungal agents, although in vitro resistance has been demonstrated. Rather, lack of efficacy is probably due to poor compliance or poor absorption of the drug. Relapses are common and, once an individual has had two episodes of oral candidiasis, maintenance therapy is advised.

Other Fungal Infections

A few cases of oral histoplasmosis (36–38), geotrichosis (3), cryptococcosis (39,40), and aspergillosis (41) have been reported in HIV-infected patients. Further examples of unusual oral fungal lesions are to be anticipated as the HIV epidemic progresses.

VIRAL LESIONS

Herpes Simplex

Orofacial herpes simplex (HSV) is a fairly common feature of HIV infection (42,43). The lesions may manifest as recurrent intraoral ulcers (43) or (recurrent) herpes labialis. They may be larger and last much longer than in the immunocompetent individual and may be due to either HSV-1 or HSV-2. Topical acyclovir may be useful in herpes labialis but systemic (oral) administration is needed for treatment of the troublesome intraoral lesions. Acyclovir resistant oral and perioral herpes due to HSV2 has been reported in patients with HIV infection (44). The lesions responded to foscarnet (trisodium phosphonoformate hexahydrate).

Varicella-Herpes Zoster

The varicella-zoster virus (VZV) is another human herpesvirus that is frequently the cause of oral lesions in association with HIV infection. Rare cases of chickenpox occur (45), which may respond to high doses of systemic acyclovir.

Herpes zoster, due to reactivation of VZV, may occur early in the clinical course of HIV disease. The development of AIDS has been reported in 23% of such cases in

2 years and 46% in 4 years (46,47). Painful vesicles and ulcers occur in the distribution of one or more branches of the trigeminal nerve. The lesions usually heal, but high-dose acyclovir (4 g/day as tablets, or even intravenous acyclovir, 10mg/kg every 8 hr) is indicated to prevent or treat eye lesions. Postherpetic neuralgia is common.

Warts

In association with HIV infection, oral and labial lesions due to human papillomavirus (HPV) take the form of papilliferous and flat warts (Fig. 3). Many of the former appear to be due to HPV-7, otherwise found only in skin warts in butchers, while oral flat warts in HIV infection (focal epithelial hyperplasia) are associated with HPV-13 and -32 (48,49). Oral warts may be excised surgically or by laser, but recurrence is common.

Hairy Leukoplakia

The white lesion of hairy leukoplakia (HL) (8) is found on the lateral margin (Fig. 4) of the tongue and occasionally elsewhere on the oropharyngeal mucosa (50) of a significant proportion of HIV-seropositive patients of all risk groups (51–54). It occurs in about 19% of persons who are asymptomatic (23), and in higher proportions of patients in CDC group IV, notably those with full AIDS (55).

HL is not found at other mucosal sites (56) but is seen, albeit rarely, in association with non-HIV-induced immunosuppression, such as in renal transplant recipients (57–59), patients receiving cancer chemotherapy (60), cardiac and bone marrow transplant recipients (61,62), and in liver transplant recipients (63). HL in the presence of HIV infection is of itself a criterion for CDC group IV category C2. Many patients with HL, who do not have AIDS, subsequently develop AIDS, often within a relatively short time. In our 1987 study (10), 30% did so within 36 months, while in our subsequent

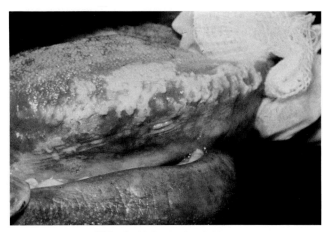

FIG. 4. Hairy leukoplakia.

analysis (64) the probability was 47% by 2 years and 67% by 4 years. However, a few HL patients do not develop AIDS, even after 5 years. Those who do so more rapidly are much more likely to be *Candida* skin test-negative at the time of diagnosis of HL, indicating significant immunosuppression at that time (64). Those with small HL lesions are as likely as those with large lesions to develop AIDS (65).

The HL lesion shows histological features of epithelial thickening, including hyperparakeratosis and acanthosis, as well as prominent and enlarged prickle cells resembling koilocytes (8). At first, we and others considered HPV as a possible etiological agent (8). However, extensive investigations using electron microscopy, immunocytochemistry, and molecular biology have failed to demonstrate the presence of HPV (66,66a). Many of the prickle cells in HL and also some of the more superficial cells contain huge numbers of particles of Epstein-Barr virus (EBV) in fully replicating form (66) (Fig. 5). The presence of EBV is required for the definitive diagnosis of HL (67–70); a convenient noninvasive diagnos-

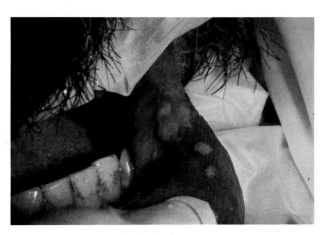

FIG. 3. Oral warts.

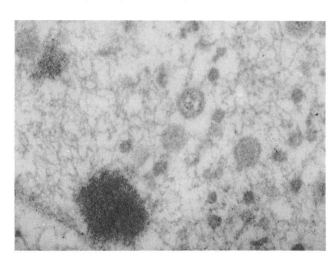

FIG. 5. EBV in the epithelial cells of hairy leukoplakia. Original magnification ×31,320.

tic approach is to examine cells scraped from the lesion (71). The presence of EBV serves to distinguish HL from other lesions with similar clinical or histological appearances (72). EBV appears to be the cause of HL, for its elimination (73,74) results in regression of the lesions, while clinical recurrence is accompanied by renewed EBV activity. The source of EBV infection of the differentiating cells in HL is not known. Three possibilities have been considered: latent EBV infection of the basal cells as a continuing source of infection; salivary EBV continually reinfecting from the oral cavity; or circulating EBV-infected B cells entering from the connective tissue. No EBV DNA has been found in the basal cells, suggesting that latent EBV is not the source (75). It has been suggested that some HL lesions contain defective EBV (76). However, no oncogenic influences of EBV appear to occur, in contrast to the suspected role of the virus in nasopharyngeal carcinoma. No cases of carcinoma arising in HL lesions have been reported and the pattern of keratin differentiation in HL is not suggestive of premalignant potential (77).

The epithelium of the HL lesion contains fewer Langerhans cells than normal (16) and these may be defective, perhaps even infected with HIV (78). This may explain the propensity of EBV to infect this site, although it could also be a consequence rather than a cause of the EBV infection. It has been suggested that the location of the HL lesion is related to the presence of EBV receptors on the lateral margins of the tongue (79).

Therapy for HL is rarely indicated. Indeed, the lesion may spontaneously change in appearance, waxing and waning in extent. A few patients complain of discomfort or dislike the appearance of the lesions. Antifungal therapy should be used to reduce or eliminate superinfection with *Candida,* while systemic acyclovir is occasionally indicated. Although acyclovir is effective, the lesions recur (73). An experimental antiviral agent, desciclovir, has been reported to be effective in eliminating the clinical lesion and all virologic evidence of EBV infection in a controlled study (74). There are case reports of HL disappearing in association with ganciclovir or zidovudine (80–83).

HL must be distinguished from a number of other white lesions of the tongue and oral mucosa, including idiopathic leukoplakia, lichen planus, hyperplastic candidiasis, white sponge nevus, geographic tongue, and lesions due to friction or biting habits (4).

BACTERIAL DISEASES

Unusual oral bacterial infections are seen occasionally in HIV-infected patients, including ones due to Enterobacteriaceae (4,84), mycobacteria (85), and the organism causing bacillary epithelioid angiomatosis (86). However, the most common and dramatic example of bacte-

rial infection is the severe periodontal disease seen in this group of patients.

Periodontal Disease

In association with HIV infection, periodontal diseases (87–91) may present unusual clinical features, notably very rapid progression to destructive disease and poor response to standard therapy.

The forms seen in HIV infection include HIV gingivitis, HIV periodontitis, necrotizing gingivitis, and the more extensive lesion, necrotizing stomatitis.

HIV Gingivitis

HIV gingivitis may be difficult to distinguish from the "conventional" form. A thin red line is seen along the gingival margin of one or more quadrants. There may be spontaneous bleeding and the patient may complain of waking with blood in the mouth. Unlike conventional gingivitis, these signs and symptoms may occur in the absence of plaque and calculus.

Occasionally, acute necrotizing ulcerative gingivitis (ANUG) is seen, with ulceration of the tips of gingival papilla and marginal inflammation, fetid breath, and fever. In HIV infection, this too may occur in a relatively clean mouth and may be localized to a single area.

HIV Periodontitis

HIV periodontitis can be distinguished from "conventional" periodontitis by the rapid and simultaneous loss of both supporting bone and overlying mucosa, leading to exposure of root tissue, and to tooth mobility and even tooth loss (89) (Fig. 6). Because of the type and rapidity of tissue loss, little pocketing is seen. These events are often accompanied by ulceration and necrosis of soft tissue and by complaints of severe pain. Seques-

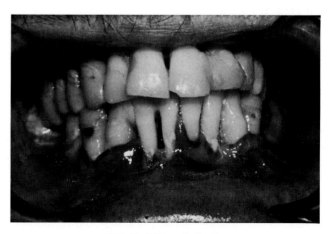

FIG. 6. HIV periodontis.

TABLE 2. *Therapy for HIV-related periodontal diseases*

Condition	Management
HIV gingivitis	Plaque removal
	Chlorhexidine mouth rinse
HIV periodontitis	Plaque removal
	Root planing and curettage
	Irrigation with povidone–iodine
	Antibiotics, chlorhexidine mouth rinse
Necrotizing gingivitis	Débridement
	Povidone–iodine irrigation
	Antibiotics, chlorhexidine mouth rinse
Necrotizing stomatitis	Débridement, including bone sequestra
	Povidone–iodine irrigation, antibiotics
	Chlorhexidine mouth rinse

tration of portions of alveolar bone may occur (necrotizing stomatitis) if the lesion is untreated (17).

Etiology

The causes of this group of lesions are poorly understood. The microorganisms appear to be similar to those seen in conventional periodontal disease and include *Bacteroides intermedius, Porphyromonas gingivalis, Actinobacillus actinomycetemcomitans,* and *Fusobacterium nucleatum. Wolinella recta, Eikenella corrodens,* and even *Candida* are also found (93–95). Polymorphonuclear leukocyte defects related to HIV infection may be involved (96).

Therapy

Treatment for these conditions (97) involves removing necrotic tissue including bony sequestra, root planing and curettage, irrigation of the affected areas with 10% povidone–iodine, and administration of antibiotics such metronidazole, clindamycin, or amoxicillin-clavulamic acid, followed by chlorhexidine mouth rinses (Table 2).

NEOPLASIA

Kaposi's Sarcoma

Oral lesions of Kaposi's sarcoma (KS) were among the first oral features of the epidemic noted (98,99). Oral lesions were the first manifestations of KS in 22% of cases in one series (100). The palate is the most common oral location (Fig. 7) while the gingiva and tongue may also be involved. Salivary gland and cervical lymph node involvement are seen (101,102). Oral KS may present as flat or raised patches of blue, purple, or red color. Yellow stain of the mucosa adjacent to the lesion may be seen. Large nodular lesions may ulcerate and become secondarily infected. Occasionally, oral KS may be covered by

normal colored mucosa (4). The histopathology is the same as that of KS lesions elsewhere (103,104).

Oral KS lesions may be painful and interfere with mastication and swallowing. Visible lesions may be embarrassing to the patient. Small lesions respond well to local therapy, including surgical or laser excision and intralesional chemotherapy, such as vinblastine (105–107). Larger lesions may respond well to external radiation therapy (99). Early lesions should be treated to slow down progress and reduce the morbidity associated, in particular, with secondary infection, which may mimic HIV periodontitis.

Lymphoma

Non-Hodgkin's lymphoma is an increasingly common feature of the AIDS epidemic and may involve the oropharynx (108–111). The oral lesions may precede those at other sites, or be the only lesions and so be the presenting and diagnostic criterion for AIDS.

The lesions can be found anywhere in the mouth as swellings, nodules, or ulcers. They may present a diagnostic challenge and repeated biopsies may be needed.

A case of polymorphic reticulosis in a woman with *Pneumocystis carinii* pneumonia has been reported

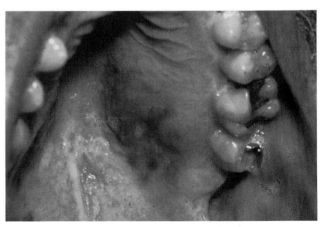

FIG. 7. Kaposi's sarcoma.

(112), but there have been no accounts of oral lesions of AIDS-related Hodgkin's disease.

There is no convincing evidence for an association between oral squamous cell carcinoma and HIV infection. However, as the life expectancy of HIV-infected individuals increases it is possible that oral cancer due to papillomavirus and tobacco may occur.

IDIOPATHIC LESIONS

Recurrent Aphthous Ulcers

There is a slight increase in the prevalence of recurrent aphthous ulcers (RAU) in HIV infection (23) and a dramatic increase in their severity (112) with a shift towards the major variant (113). The major form of RAU (Fig. 8) consists of large (1–2 cm) solitary, occasionally multiple, painful ulcers that may persist for weeks and hamper swallowing and mastication because of pain. The minor form consists of crops of ulcers about 5 mm in diameter, which usually heal more rapidly than the major form, but nevertheless persist much longer than in HIV-negative individuals. Finally, crops of tiny (1–2 mm) ulcers that may coalesce (herpetiform RAU) are also seen. The etiology of RAU is unknown, but the nature and frequency of its association with HIV infection lend support to a role for defects in immune regulation or for the presence of as yet unknown microbiological agents.

These ulcers usually respond to topical steroids, and systemic steroids are rarely indicated (4). In Europe, thalidomide has been used (114).

Very large necrotizing oral ulcers are seen in HIV infection. These may represent major aphthous ulcers further complicated by bacterial infection, or they may be a form of necrotizing stomatitis. They may be associated with similar lesions elsewhere in the gastrointestinal tract (115). They respond to a combination of topical steroids plus antibiotics directed against gram-negative bacteria.

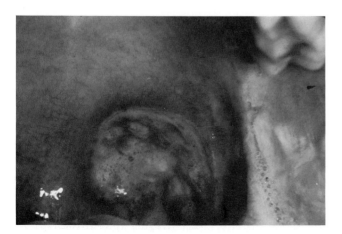

FIG. 8. Major aphthous ulcer.

HIV Salivary Gland Disease

Xerostomia and enlargement of major salivary glands, together or separately, are seen in HIV-infected patients (116–119). There may be a reduced salivary flow rate. Appropriate measures to alleviate symptoms and prevent caries include saliva substitutes, control of sugar intake, fluoride rinses, and fluoride applications.

Initially seen in pediatric AIDS cases (119), salivary gland disease (SGD), notably parotid enlargement, has now been seen in adults of all risk groups. The swelling is bilateral, diffuse, and soft. There may be dry eyes and other features suggestive of Sjögren's syndrome, but significant serological and immunohistochemical differences distinguish HIV SGD from Sjögren's syndrome. HIV SGD may include cases described as branchial cleft cysts or lymphoepithelial cysts of salivary glands (120), and all of these may be the salivary gland expression of the diffuse infiltrative CD8 lymphocytosis syndrome in HIV infection described by Itescu et al. (121). No viral or other microbial causes have been identified, and an association with HLA-DR5 has been suggested (121).

Idiopathic Thrombocytopenia Purpura

Idiopathic thrombocytopenia purpura (ITP) is seen in in HIV infection but oral features are rare. When present (3,4), they consist of small purpuric lesions, large ecchymoses, or spontaneous gingival bleeding.

Hyperpigmentation

Unusual brown pigmentation of the oral mucosa in HIV-infected patients is most commonly associated with zidovudine or ketoconazole therapy. In some cases no obvious predisposing factors other than HIV infection are found (122). A few of these cases may be due to adrenal cortical insufficiency (123).

ORAL PROBLEMS IN PEDIATRIC HIV INFECTION

Oral candidiasis and HIV SGD are common features of pediatric HIV infection (119,124,125). Hairy leukoplakia is occasionally seen (126), while other oral lesions are rare. Caries may be a problem because of neglect and because of the high sugar content of many drug preparations. Oral hygiene instruction and maintenance is essential, while the use of topical fluorides as rinses or gels is recommended.

REFERENCES

1. Gottlieb MS, Schroff R, Schantez HM. *Pneumocystis carinii* pneumonia and mucosal candidiasis in previously healthy homosexual men: evidence of a new acquired cellular immunodeficiency. *N Engl J Med* 1981;305:1425–31.

2. Small CB, Klein RS, Friedland GH, Moll B, Emeson EE, Spigland L. Community-acquired opportunistic infections and defective cellular immunity in heterosexual drug abusers. *Am J Med* 1983;74:433–41.

3. Greenspan D, Greenspan JS, Pindborg JJ, Schiodt M. *AIDS and the dental team.* Copenhagen: Munksgaard, 1986.

4. Greenspan D, Greenspan JS, Pindborg JJ, Schiodt M. *AIDS and the mouth.* Copenhagen: Munksgaard,

5. Scully C, Laskaris G, Pindborg J, Porter SR, Reichart P. Oral manifestations of HIV infection and their management. I. More common lesions. *Oral Surg Oral Med Oral Pathol* 1991;71:158–66.

6. Scully C, Laskaris G, Pindborg J, Porter SR, Reichart P. Oral manifestations of HIV infection and their management. II. More common lesions. *Oral Surg Oral Med Oral Pathol* 1991;71:167–71.

7. Murray HW, Hillman AD, Rubin BY, et al. Patients at risk for AIDS-related opportunistic infections. *N Engl J Med* 1985;313:1504–10.

8. Greenspan D, Greenspan JS, Conant M, Petersen V, Silverman S Jr, DeSouza Y. Oral 'hairy' leucoplakia in male homosexuals: evidence of association with both papillomavirus and a herpesgroup virus. *Lancet* 1984;2:831–4.

9. Klein RS, Harris CA, Small CR, et al. Oral candidiasis in highrisk patients as the initial manifestation of the acquired immunodeficiency syndrome. *N Engl J Med* 1984;311:354–8.

10. Greenspan D, Greenspan JS, Hearst NG, et al. Oral hairy leukoplakia; human immunodeficiency virus status and risk for development of AIDS. *J Infect Dis* 1987;155:475–48.

11. Schiodt M, Bakilana PB, Hiza JF, et al. Oral candidiasis and hairy leukoplakia correlate with HIV infection in Tanzania. *Oral Surg Oral Med Oral Pathol* 1990;69:591–6.

12. Melnick SL, Engel D, Truelove E, et al. Oral mucosal lesions: association with the presence of antibodies to the human immunodeficiency virus. *Oral Surg Oral Med Oral Pathol* 1989;68:37–43.

13. Schulten EAJM, ten Kate RW, van der Waal I. The impact of oral examination on the Centers for Disease Control classification of subjects with human immunodeficiency virus infection. *Arch Intern Med* 1990;150:1259–61.

14. Moss AR, Bacchetti P, Osmond D, et al. Seropositivity for HIV and the development of AIDS or AIDS related condition: three year follow up of the San Francisco General Hospital Cohort. *Br Med J* 1988;296:745–50.

15. Fischl MA, Richman DD, Hansen N, et al. The safety and efficacy of zidovudine (AZT) in the treatment of subjects with mildly symptomatic human immunodeficiency virus type 1 (HIV) infection. *Ann Intern Med* 1990;112:727–37.

16. Daniels TE, Greenspan D, Greenspan JS, et al. Absence of Langerhans' cells in oral hairy leukoplakia, an AIDS-associated lesion. *J Invest Dermatol* 1987;89:178–82.

17. Williams CA, Winkler JR, Grassi M, Murray PA. HIV-associated periodontitis complicated by necrotizing stomatitis. *Oral Surg Oral Med Oral Pathol* 1990;69:351–5.

18. Bach MC, Valenti AJ, Howell DA, Smith TJ. Odynophagia from aphthous ulcers of the pharynx and oesophagus in the acquired immunodeficiency syndrome (AIDS). *Ann Intern Med* 1988;109:338–9.

19. Pindborg JJ. Classification of oral lesions associated with HIV infection. *Oral Surg Oral Med Oral Pathol* 1989;67:292–5.

20. Wanzala P, Manji F, Pindborg JJ, Plummer F. Low prevalence of oral mucosal lesions in HIV-1-seropositive African women. *J Oral Pathol Med* 1989;18:416–8.

21. Ramirez V, Gonzales A, de la Rosa E, et al. Oral lesions in Mexican HIV-infected patients. *J Oral Pathol Med* 1990;19:482–5.

22. Tukutuku K, Muyembe-Tramfun L, Kayembe K, Ntumba M. Oral manifestations of AIDS in a heterosexual population in a Zaire hospital. *J Oral Pathol Med* 1990;19:232–4.

23. Feigal DW, Katz MH, Greenspan D, et al. The prevalence of oral lesions in HIV-infected homosexual and bisexual men: three San Francisco epidemiology cohorts. *AIDS* 1991;5:519–25.

24. Greenspan JS, Barr CE, Sciubba JJ, Winkler JR, U.S.A. Oral AIDS Collaborative Group. Oral manifestations of HIV infection: definitions, diagnostic criteria and principles of therapy. *Oral Surg Oral Med Oral Pathol* 1992;73:142–4.

25. Arendorf TM, Walker DM. The prevalence and intra-oral distribution of *Candida albicans* in man. *Arch Oral Biol* 1980;25:1–10.

26. Torssander J, Morfeldt-Manson L, Biberfeld G, Karlsson A, Putkonen PD, Wasserman J. Oral *Candida albicans* in HIV infection. *Scand J Infect Dis* 1987;19:291–5.

27. Korting HC, Ollert M, Georgii A, Froschl M. In vitro susceptibilities and biotypes of *Candida albicans* isolated from the oral cavities of patients infected with human immunodeficiency virus. *J Clin Microbiol* 1989;26:2626–31.

28. Franker CK, Lucartorto FM, Johnson BS, Jacobson JJ. Characterization of the mycoflora from oral mucosal surfaces of some HIV-infected patients. *Oral Surg Oral Med Oral Pathol* 1990;69:683–7.

29. Samaranayake LP, Homstrup P. Oral candidiasis and human immunodeficiency virus infection. *J Oral Pathol Med* 1989;18:554–64.

30. Tavitian A, Raufman JP, Rosenthal LE. Oral candidiasis as a marker for esophageal candidiasis in the acquired immunodeficiency syndrome. *Ann Intern Med* 1986;104:54–5.

31. Tindal B, Hing M, Edwards P, Barnes T, Mackie A, Cooper DA. Severe clinical manifestations of primary HIV infection. *AIDS* 1989;3:747–9.

32. Connolly GM, Forbes A, Gleeson JA, Gazzard BG. Investigation of upper gastrointestinal symptoms in patients with AIDS. *AIDS* 1989;3:453–6.

33. Stevens DA, Odds FC, Scherer S. Application of DNA typing methods to *Candida albicans* epidemiology and correlations with phenotype. *Rev Infect Dis* 1990;12:258–66.

34. Whelan WL, Kirsch DR, Kwon-Chung KJ, Wahl SM, Smith PD. *Candida albicans* in patients with the acquired immunodeficiency syndrome: absence of a novel or hypervirulent strain. *J Infect Dis* 1990;162:513–8.

35. Darwazeh AMG, Lamey P-J, Lewis MAO, Samaranayake LP. Systemic fluconazole therapy and in vitro adhesion of *Candida albicans* to human buccal epithelial cells. *J Oral Pathol Med* 1991;20:17–9.

36. Werber JL. Histoplasmosis of the head and neck. *Ear Nose Throat J* 1988;67:841–5.

37. Fowler CB, Nelson JF, Henley DW, Smith BR. Acquired immune deficiency syndrome presenting as a palatal perforation. *Oral Surg Oral Med Oral Pathol* 1989;67:313–8.

38. Cohen RP, Kurzrock R. Tongue lesions in the acquired immune deficiency syndrome. *Cutis* 1987;40:406–9.

39. Lynch DP, Naftolin LZ. Oral *Cryptococcus neoformans* infection in AIDS. *Oral Surg Oral Med Oral Pathol* 1987;64:449–53.

40. Glick M, Cohen SG, Cheney RT, Crooks GW, Greenberg MS. Oral manifestations of disseminated *Cryptococcus neoformans* in a patient with acquired immunodeficiency syndrome. *Oral Surg Oral Med Oral Pathol* 1987;64:454–9.

41. Shannon, MT, Sclaroff A, Colm SJ. Invasive aspergillosis of the maxilla in an immunocompromised patient. *Oral Surg Oral Med Oral Pathol* 1990;70:425–7.

42. Silverman S, Migliorati CA, Lozada-Nur F, Greenspan D, Conant M. Oral findings in people with or at risk for AIDS: a study of 375 homosexual males. *J Am Dent Assoc* 1986;112:187–92.

43. Reichart PA, Gelderblom HR, Becker J, Kuntz A. AIDS and the oral cavity: the HIV infection—virology, etiology, origin, immunology, precautions and clinical observations in 110 patients. *Int J Oral Maxillofac Surg* 1987;16:129–53.

44. MacPhail LA, Greenspan D, Schiodt M, et al. Acyclovir-resistant, foscarnet-sensitive oral herpes simplex type 2 lesion in a patient with AIDS. *Oral Surg Oral Med Oral Pathol* 1989;67:427–32.

45. Schiodt M, Rindum J, Bygbert I. Chickenpox with oral manifestations in an AIDS patient. *Dan Dent J* 1987;91:316–9.

46. Melbye M, Grossman RJ, Goedert JJ, Eyster ME, Biggar RJ. Risk of AIDS after herpes zoster. *Lancet* 1987;1:728–31.

47. Colebunders R, Mann J, Francis H, et al. Herpes zoster in African patients: a clinical predictor of human immunodeficiency virus infection. *J Infect Dis* 1988;157:314–8.

48. Greenspan D, de Villiers EM, Greenspan JS, De Souza YG, zur Hausen H. Unusual HPV types in the oral warts in association with HIV infection. *J Oral Pathol* 1988;17:482–7.

49. de Villiers EM. Prevalence of HPV-7 papillomas in the oral mucosa and facial skin of patients with human immunodeficiency virus. *Arch Dermatol* 1989;125:1590.

50. Kabani S, Greenspan D, de Souza Y, Greenspan JS, Cataldo E. Oral hairy leukoplakia with extensive oral mucosal involvement. *Oral Surg Oral Med Oral Pathol* 1989;67:411–5.

51. Reichart PA, Langford A, Gelderblom HR, Pohle H-D, Becker J, Wolf H. Oral hairy leukoplakia: observations in 95 cases and review of the literature. *J Oral Pathol Med* 1989;18:410–5.

52. Rindum JL, Schiodt M, Pindborg JJ, Scheibel E. Oral hairy leukoplakia in three hemophiliacs with human immunodeficiency virus infection. *Oral Surg Oral Med Oral Pathol* 1987;63:437–40.

53. Ficarra G, Barone R, Gaglioti D. Oral hairy leukoplakia among HIV-positive intravenous drug abusers: a clinico-pathologic and ultrastructural study. *Oral Surg Oral Med Oral Pathol* 1988;65:421–6.

54. Barone R, Ficarra G, Gaglioti D, Orsi A, Mazzotta F. Prevalence of oral lesions among HIV-infected intravenous drug abusers and other risk groups. *Oral Surg Oral Med Oral Pathol* 1990;69:169–73.

55. Schiodt M, Bygberg I, Bakilana P, et al. Oral manifestations of AIDS in Tanzania. *J Dent Res* 1988;67:201.

56. Hollander H, Greenspan D, Stringari S, Greenspan J, Schiodt M. Hairy leukoplakia and the acquired immunodeficiency syndrome. *Ann Intern Med* 1986;104:892.

57. Itin P, Rufli I, Rudlinser R, et al. Oral hairy leukoplakia in a HIV-negative renal transplant patient: a marker for immunosuppression. *Dermatologica* 1988;17:126–8.

58. Greenspan D, Greenspan JS, De Souza YG, Levy JA, Ungar AM. Oral hairy leukoplakia in an HIV-negative renal transplant recipient. *J Oral Pathol Med* 1989;18:32–4.

59. MacLeod RI, Long RQ, Soames JV, Ward MK. Oral hairy leukoplakia in an HIV-negative renal transplant patient. *Br Dent J* 1990;169:208–9.

60. Syrjanen S, Laine P, Happoinen RP, Niemela M. Oral hairy leukoplakia is not a specific sign of HIV infection but related to suppression in general. *J Oral Pathol Med* 1989;18:28–31.

61. Epstein JB, Priddy RW, Sherlock CH. Hairy leukoplakia-like lesions in immunosuppressed patients following bone marrow transplantation. *Transplantation* 1988;46:462–4.

62. Epstein JB, Sherlock CH, Greenspan JS. Hairy leukoplakia-like lesions following bone marrow transplantation [Letter]. *AIDS* 1991;5:101–2.

63. Reggiani M, Paulizzi P. Hairy leukoplakia in liver transplant patients. *Acta Derm Venerol (Stockh)* 1990;70:87–8.

64. Greenspan D, Greenspan JS, Overby G, et al. Risk factors for rapid progression from hairy leukoplakia to AIDS: a nested case-control study. *J Acquired Immune Deficiency Syndrome* 1991;4:652–8.

65. Schiodt M, Greenspan D, Daniels TE, Greenspan JS. Clinical and histologic spectrum of oral hairy leukoplakia. *Oral Surg Oral Med Oral Pathol* 1987;64:716–20.

66. Greenspan JS, Greenspan D, Lennette ET, et al. Replication of Epstein-Barr virus within the epithelial cells of "hairy" leukoplakia, an AIDS-associated lesion. *N Engl J Med* 1985;313:1564–71.

67. Greenspan JS, Greenspan D. Oral hairy leukoplakia: diagnosis and management. *Oral Surg Oral Med Oral Pathol* 1989;67:396–403.

68. Greenspan D, Greenspan JS. The significance of oral hairy leukoplakia. *Oral Surg Oral Med Oral Pathol* 1992;73:151–4.

69. De Souza YG, Greenspan D, Felton JR, Hartzog GA, Hammer M, Greenspan JS. Localization of Epstein-Barr virus DNA in the epithelial cells of oral hairy leukoplakia using in-situ hybridization on tissue sections. *N Engl J Med* 1989;320:1559–60.

70. Loning T, Henke RP, Reichart P, Becker J. In situ hybridization to detect Epstein-Barr virus DNA in oral tissues of HIV-infected patients. *Virchows Arch [A]* 1987;412:127–33.

71. De Souza Y, Freese UK, Greenspan D, Greenspan JS. Diagnosis of EBV infection in hairy leukoplakia using nucleic acid hybrid-

ization and noninvasive techniques. *J Clin Microbiol* 1990;28:2775–8.

72. Green TL, Greenspan JS, Greenspan D, DeSouza YG. Oral lesions mimicking hairy leukoplakia: a diagnostic dilemma. *Oral Surg Oral Med Oral Pathol* 1989;67:522–6.

73. Resnick L, Herbst JHS, Ablashi DV, et al. Regression of oral hairy leukoplakia after orally administered acyclovir therapy. *JAMA* 1988;259:384–8.

74. Greenspan D, De Souza Y, Conant MA, et al. Efficacy of desciclovir in the treatment of Epstein-Barr virus infection in oral hairy leukoplakia. *J Acquired Immune Deficiency Syndrome* 1990;3:571–8.

75. Young LS, Lau R, Rowe M, et al. Differentiation-associated expression of the Epstein-Barr virus BZLF1 transactivator protein in oral hairy leukoplakia. *J Virol* [in press].

76. Patton DF, Shirley P, Raab-Traub N, Resnick L, Sixbey JW. Defective viral DNA in Epstein-Barr virus-associated oral hairy leukoplakia. *J Virol* 1990;64:397–400.

77. Williams DM, Leigh IM, Greenspan D, Greenspan JS. Altered patterns of keratin expression in oral hairy leukoplakia: prognostic implications. *J Oral Pathol Med* 1991;20:167–71.

78. Riccardi R, Pimpinelli N, Ficarra G, et al. Morphology and membrane antigens of nonlymphoid accessory cells in oral hairy leukoplakia. *Hum Pathol* 1990;21:897–904.

79. Corso B, Eversole LR, Hutt-Fletcher L. Hairy leukoplakia: Epstein-Barr virus receptors on oral keratinocyte plasma membranes. *Oral Surg Oral Med Oral Pathol* 1989;67:416–21.

80. Newman C, Polk BF. Resolution of hairy leukoplakia during therapy with 9-(1,3-dihydroxy-2-propoxymethyl) guanine (DHPG). *Ann Intern Med* 1987;107:348–50.

81. Brockmeyer NH, Kreuzfelder E, Mertins L, Kaecke D, Boos M. Zidovudine therapy of asymptomatic HIV-1-infected patients and combined zidovudine-acyclovir therapy of HIV-1-infected patients with oral hairy leukoplakia. *J Invest Dermatol* 1989;92:647.

82. Kessler HA, Benson CA, Urbanski P. Regression of oral hairy leukoplakia during treatment with azidothymidine. *Ann Intern Med* 1988;148:2496–7.

83. Phelan JA, Klein RS. Resolution of oral hairy leukoplakia during treatment with azidothymidine. *Oral Surg Oral Med Oral Pathol* 1988;65:717–20.

84. Schmidt-Westhausen A, Fehrenbach FJ, Reichart PA. Oral enterobacteriaceae in patients with HIV infection. *J Oral Pathol Med* 1990;19:229–31.

85. Fowler CB, Nelson JF, Henley DW, Smith BR. Acquired immune deficiency syndrome presenting as a palatal perforation. *Oral Surg Oral Med Oral Pathol* 1989;67:313–8.

86. Cockrell CJ, Whitlow MA, Webster GF, Friedman-Kien AE. Epithelioid angiomatosis: a distinct vascular disorder in patients with the acquired immunodeficiency syndrome or AIDS-related complex. *Lancet* 1987;2:654–6.

87. Winkler JR, Murray PA. Periodontal disease: a potential intraoral expression of AIDS may be rapidly progressive periodontitis. *Calif Dent Assoc J* 1987;15:20–4.

88. Winkler JR, Grassi M, Murray PA. Clinical description and etiology of HIV-associated periodontal diseases. In: Robertson PB, Greenspan JS, eds. *Perspectives on oral manifestations of AIDS: diagnosis and management of HIV-associated infections,* Littleton, MA: PSG, 1988;49–70.

89. Winkler JR, Murray PA, Grassi M, Hammerle C. Diagnosis and management of HIV-associated periodontal lesions. *J Am Dent Assoc* 1989;119[Suppl]:S25–34.

90. Rosenstein DI, Eigner TL, Levin MP, Chiodo GT. Rapidly progressive periodontal disease associated with HIV infection: report of case. *J Am Dent Assoc* 1989;118:313–4.

91. Pindborg JJ, Thorn JJ, Schiodt M, Gamb J, Black FT. Acute necrotizing gingivitis in an AIDS patient. *Dan Dent J* 1986;90:450–3.

92. Murray PA, Grassi M, Winkler JR. The microbiology of HIV-associated periodontal lesions. *J Clin Periodontol* 1989;16:636–42.

93. Murray PA, Winkler JR, Sadkowski L, et al. Microbiology of HIV-associated gingivitis and periodontitis. In: Robertson PB, Greenspan JS, eds. *Perspectives on oral manifestations of AIDS:*

diagnosis and management of HIV-associated infections. Littleton, MA: PSG, 1988;105–18.

94. Zambon JJ, Reynolds HS, Genco RJ. Studies of the subgingival microflora in patients with acquired immunodeficiency syndrome. *J Periodontol* 1990;61:699–704.

95. Vaccaro K, Murray P, Peros W, et al. Evaluation of HIV virus associated periodontitis using DNA probe hybridization analysis. *J Dent Res* 1988;67:75.

96. Ryder MI, Winkler JR, Weintreb RN. Elevated phagocytosis, oxidative burst and F action formation in PMNs from individuals with intraoral manifestations of HIV infection. *J Acquired Immune Deficiency Syndrome* 1988;1:346–53.

97. Grassi M, Williams CA, Winkler JR, Murray PA. Management of HIV-associated periodontal diseases. In: Robertson PB, Greenspan JS, eds. *Perspectives on oral manifestations of AIDS: diagnosis and management of HIV-associated infections.* Littleton, MA: PSG, 1988;119–30.

98. Lozada F, Silverman S, Conant M. New outbreak of oral tumours, malignancies and infectious disease strikes young male homosexuals. *Calif Dent Assoc J* 1982;10:39–42.

99. Lozada F, Silverman S, Migliorati CA, Conant MA, Volberding PA. Oral manifestations of tumors and opportunistic infections in the acquired immunodeficiency syndrome (AIDS): findings in 53 homosexual men with Kaposi's sarcoma. *Oral Surg Oral Med Oral Pathol* 1983;56:491–4.

100. Ficarra G, Berson AM, Silverman S, et al. Kaposi's sarcoma of the oral cavity: a study of 134 patients with a review of the pathogenesis, epidemiology, clinical aspects, and treatment. *Oral Surg Oral Med Oral Pathol* 1988;66:543–50.

101. Petow CA, Steis R, Longo DL. Kaposi's sarcoma in the head and neck in the acquired immune deficiency syndrome. *Otololaryngol Head Neck Surg* 1983;92:255.

102. Yeh CK, Fox PC, Fox CH, Travis WD, Lane HC, Baum BJ. Kaposi's sarcoma of the parotid gland in acquired immunodeficiency syndrome. *Oral Surg Oral Med Oral Pathol* 1989;67:308–12.

103. Green TL, Beckstead JH, Lozada-Nur F, Silverman S, Hansen LS. Histopathologic spectrum of oral Kaposi's sarcoma. *Oral Surg Oral Med Oral Pathol* 1984;58:306–14.

104. Lummerman H, Freedman PD, Kerpel SM, Phelan JA. Oral Kaposi's sarcoma: a clinicopathologic study of 23 homosexual and bisexual men from the New York metropolitan area. *Oral Surg Oral Med Oral Pathol* 1988;65:711–6.

105. Epstein JB, Scully C. Intralesional vinblastine for oral Kaposi's sarcoma in HIV infection. *Lancet* 1989;2:1100–1.

106. Epstein JB, Lozada-Nur F, McLeod A, Spinelli J. Oral Kaposi's sarcoma in acquired immunodeficiency syndrome. *Cancer* 1989;64:2424–30.

107. Ficarra G, Person AM, Silverman S, et al. Kaposi's sarcoma of the oral cavity: a study of 134 patients with a review of the pathogenesis, epidemiology, clinical aspects, and treatment. *Oral Surg Oral Med Oral Pathol* 1988;66:543–50.

108. Ziegler JL, Drew WL, Miner RC, et al. Outbreak of Burkitt's-like lymphoma in homosexual men. *Lancet* 1982;2:631–3.

109. Ziegler JL, Beckstead JA, Volberding PA, et al. Non-Hodgkin's lymphoma in 90 homosexual men: relation to generalized lymphadenopathy and the acquired immunodeficiency syndrome. *N Engl J Med* 1984;311:565–70.

110. Kaugars GE, Burns JC. Non-Hodgkin's lymphoma of the oral cavity associated with AIDS. *Oral Surg Oral Med Oral Pathol* 1989;67:433–6.

111. Green TL, Eversole LR. Oral lymphomas in HIV-infected patients: association with Epstein-Barr virus DNA. *Oral Surg Oral Med Oral Pathol* 1989;67:437–42.

112. Najjar T, Gadol C. Khan MY. Immune deficiency with polymorphic reticulosis. *Oral Surg Oral Med Oral Pathol* 1989;67:322–6.

113. MacPhail LA, Greenspan D, Feigal DW, Lennette ET, Greenspan JS. Recurrent aphthous ulcers in association with HIV infection: major variant more common and associated with T-cell subset alterations. *Oral Surg Oral Med Oral Pathol* 1991; 71:678–83.

114. Youle M, Clarbour J, Farthing C, et al. Treatment of resistant aphthous ulceration with thalidomide in patients positive for HIV antibody. *Br Med J* 1989;298:432.

115. Akula SK, Creticos CM, Weldon-Linne CM. Gangrenous stomatitis in AIDS. *Lancet* 1989;1:955.

116. Schiodt M, Greenspan D, Daniels TE, et al. Parotid gland enlargement and xerostomia associated with labial sialadenitis in HIV-infected patients. *J Autoimmun* 1989;2:415–25.

117. Schiodt M, Greenspan D, Levy J, et al. Does HIV cause salivary gland disease? *AIDS* 1989;3:819–22.

118. Ulirsch RC, Jaffe ES. Sjögren's syndrome-like illness associated with the acquired immunodeficiency syndrome-related complex. *Hum Pathol* 1987;18:1063–8.

119. Pawha S, Fikrig S, Kaplan M, et al. Expression of HTLV-III infection in a pediatric population. *Adv Exp Med Biol* 1985;187: 45–51.

120. Finfer MD, Schinella RA, Rothstein SG, Persky MS. Cystic parotid lesions in patients at risk for the acquired immunodeficiency syndrome. *Arch Otolaryngol Head Neck Surg* 1988;144: 1290–4.

121. Itescu S, Brancato LJ, Buxbaum J, et al. A diffuse infiltrative CD8 lymphocytosis syndrome in human immunodeficiency virus (HIV) infection: a host immune response associated with HLA-DR5. *Ann Intern Med* 1990;112:3–10.

122. Langford A, Pohle HD, Gelderblom H, Zhang X, Reichart PA. Oral hyperpigmentation in HIV-infected patients. *Oral Surg Oral Med Oral Pathol* 1989;67:301–7.

123. Porter SR, Glover S, Scully C. Oral hyperpigmentation secondary to adrenocortical suppression in a patient with AIDS. *Oral Surg Oral Med Oral Pathol* 1990;70:59–61.

124. Leggott PJ, Robertson PB, Greenspan D, et al. Oral manifestations of primary and acquired immunodeficiency diseases in children. *Pediatr Dent* 1987;9:89–104.

125. Rubinstein A, Sicklick M, Gupta A, et al. Acquired immunodeficiency with reversed T4/T8 ratio in infants born to promiscuous and drug-addicted mothers. *JAMA* 1983;249:2350–7.

126. Greenspan JS, Mastrucci T, Leggott P, Greenspan D, Scott GW, De Souza Y. Hairy leukoplakia in a child. *AIDS* 1988;2:143.

AIDS and Other Manifestations of HIV Infection,
Second Edition, Edited by Gary P. Wormser.
Raven Press, Ltd., New York © 1992.

CHAPTER 33

General Pathology of HIV Infection

James L. Finley, Vijay V. Joshi, and James S. A. Neill

Since the initial cases of what was subsequently labeled as acquired immunodeficiency syndrome (AIDS) (1,2), pathologic diagnosis of the major indicator diseases [opportunistic infections and neoplastic disorders according to the Centers for Disease Control (CDC) definition of AIDS (3)] has played a major role in the recognition of the syndrome. In addition to the diagnosis of known lesions, new or previously undescribed lesions were also recognized in biopsy material (e.g., pulmonary lymphoid lesions in children with AIDS, bacillary angiomatosis of skin). The same was true for autopsy studies on fatal cases of AIDS that extended the clinical spectrum by demonstrating involvement of clinically unsuspected organs in opportunistic infections and neoplastic disorders. Familiarity with the clinical spectrum and dissemination of information regarding the various clinicopathologic findings had led to a plateau with respect to new or unsuspected pathologic observations about the infectious and neoplastic complications in AIDS. However, with longer patient survival due to effective prophylactic and supportive therapy, we have begun to identify and study a variety of processes for which the pathogenesis is obscure, though clearly associated with human immunodeficiency virus (HIV) infection (i.e., nephropathy, cardiomyopathy, arteriopathy, etc.). We are also seeing examples of tissue damage associated with toxic reactions to different drugs, with diagnostic and therapeutic procedures, and with the chronic debilitating disease process of AIDS. Thus, we broadly classify pathologic lesions seen in patients with AIDS into three major categories (4): (1) primary lesions directly due to HIV infection itself (lymphoreticular system and brain); (2) associated lesions due to direct or indirect sequelae of HIV infection (opportunistic infection due to defective cell-mediated immunity, iatrogenic lesions, lesions asso-

ciated with chronic debilitating disease); and (3) lesions of undetermined pathogenesis (cardiomyopathy, nephropathy, arteriopathy, etc.). Finally, it is recognized that many lesions are the result of more than one pathogenetic mechanism and are modified by attempts to influence the disease process with chemotherapy or immunotherapy.

Most pathology reviews of this subject have employed either an organ systems approach or have concentrated on specific infections and neoplasms. As the pathology of diseases associated with AIDS represents a broad spectrum of lesions affecting virtually all tissues and organs, we have endeavored to integrate both approaches to avoid redundancy and stress important clinicopathologic correlations.

The first sections in this chapter address the diagnosis of AIDS-related opportunistic infections in cytology and biopsy material by the use of both conventional and the more recently described immunologic and molecular methods. This is followed by an overview of important aspects of opportunistic infections in these patients, common neoplasms, and some of the poorly understood complications of the disease. Neuropathology of HIV infection, which is described in a separate chapter, is excluded. The pathology of AIDS in children emphasizes characteristic lesions of this age group and highlights important similarities and differences as compared with adults. The chapter concludes with a discussion of the risks of nosocomial transmission of HIV and recommendations to laboratory personnel on procedures to prevent mucosal and parenteral exposure to infectious agents.

GENERAL ASPECTS OF PATHOLOGY OF AIDS

Because of the profound deficiency in cell-mediated immunity, the pathologic lesions related to infections in AIDS patients have certain unusual features. Thus the

J. L. Finley, V. V. Joshi, and J. S. A. Neill: Department of Pathology and Laboratory Medicine, East Carolina University School of Medicine, Greenville, North Carolina 27858-4354.

lesions tend to be larger than usual (e.g., molluscum contagiosum of skin); the inflammatory reaction is minimal or absent (e.g., cryptococcosis); granuloma formation is indistinct or absent [e.g., *Mycobacterium avium-intracellulare* (MAI) infection]; they contain large numbers of organisms (e.g., MAI); infection with two or more organisms may involve the same site [e.g., *Pneumocystis carinii,* cryptococcal and cytomegalovirus (CMV) pneumonitis]; necrotizing lesions may be present (e.g., CMV lesions in gastrointestinal tract or adrenal glands); and wide dissemination of organisms (e.g., *Pneumocystis carinii* infection) may occur. Concerning neoplastic lesions, the malignant lymphomas are usually of high grade and occur more frequently in extranodal sites. Similarly, HIV-related Kaposi's sarcoma is clinically distinct from the endemic form and often shows wide cutaneous dissemination, early visceral spread, and incomplete brief response to therapy.

DIAGNOSIS OF AIDS-RELATED OPPORTUNISTIC INFECTIONS

Opportunistic infections are the most common initial manifestation of AIDS, and the etiologic diagnosis of these infections is generally made through examination of tissue biopsies or through cytologic techniques. Many of these organisms either cannot be cultured (e.g., *Pneumocystis carinii*) or require several days for positive culture results. Therefore, morphologic identification of the etiologic agents of infections is of prime importance in these patients. Besides the routine histologic procedures, immunologic and molecular biologic methods can be used as ancillary diagnostic techniques.

Cytologic Specimens and Techniques for Diagnosis of Infectious Diseases

The rapidity with which a diagnosis can be rendered is one of the major strengths of cytologic techniques. Respiratory specimens (bronchial washings, brushings, transtracheal aspirates, and bronchoalveolar lavage), fine-needle aspiration biopsies, cerebrospinal fluid, effusions, and gastrointestinal brushings are the principle sources of material for diagnostic cytologic studies in these patients. The more common respiratory cytopreparatory methods include the Saccomanno technique, cytocentrifugation, and membrane filtration. Most specimens are received in the fixed state due to their infectious nature, but fresh material gives laboratory personnel greater flexibility if ancillary techniques including immunocytochemistry and in situ hybridization are to be employed. From cerebrospinal fluid and effusions, slides are prepared from cytocentrifuged material or membrane preparations. For gastrointestinal brushings, direct smears are usually employed. Attention to the pre-

cautions outlined later in this chapter make the cytopreparatory techniques safe.

Fine-needle aspiration biopsy (FNAB) has assumed an important role in the diagnosis of opportunistic infections and neoplasms in AIDS patients. Aspiration biopsy of superficial lesions is easily performed using a 22-gauge needle attached to a 20-ml syringe. Percutaneous FNAB of deep lesions are generally performed by a radiologist using a 22-gauge Chiba needle employing ultrasound, computerized tomography (CT), or fluoroscopic guidance. Smears are prepared by spreading the material over a small area with another slide (similar to the preparation of a bone marrow aspirate) and are air-dried and alcohol-fixed. The rapid staining and interpretation of air-dried smears using a modified Wright-Giemsa stain (Diff-Quik) determines the adequacy of a specimen and can often provide prompt information to clinicians, in addition to identifying those cases requiring more material for ancillary studies such as immunohistochemistry, electron microscopy, flow cytometry, and in situ hybridization. FNAB is also an excellent source of material for bacterial, fungal, or viral cultures. Alcohol-fixed smears are stained by a modified Papanicolaou technique.

From the sources described above, a variety of special stains are selectively employed to detect microbiologic organisms. These include Gomori's methenamine silver (GMS) for fungi, *Nocardia,* and *Pneumocystis carinii;* periodic acid-Schiff (PAS) for fungi; mucicarmine to demonstrate the capsule of cryptococcus; modified Ziehl-Neelsen, Fite, or Kinyoun for mycobacteria; Brown-Brenn and Brown-Hoff for bacteria; Giemsa for certain protozoans; and Dieterle for *Legionella.*

Calcofluor white, a nonspecific fluorochrome with affinity for chitin and cellulose, has been used to delineate fungal elements and cysts of acanthamoeba in clinical specimens (5,6). While not widely utilized, fluorescence microscopy performed on Papanicolaou-stained material can identify several genera of fungi such as aspergillus, blastomyces, histoplasma, cryptococcus, and coccidioides that demonstrate autofluorescence (7). The choice of fixatives or unfixed material employed for immunocytochemistry, immunofluorescence, and DNA probe studies for microbiologic organisms must be tailored to the particular antibody or probe.

Surgical Biopsy Specimens

The most common surgical biopsy specimens for diagnosis of infections and neoplasms in AIDS patients are those from lung, lymph nodes, alimentary tract, skin, liver, bone marrow, and brain. The proper handling of this material is dependent on the disease process suspected. Frozen section examination plays a pivotal role by allowing the pathologist to triage the specimen for appropriate diagnostic studies in a timely and cost-effective manner similar to that provided by an immediate examination of an FNAB specimen. Recognition of an infectious process in a frozen section of lung or lymph node would prompt submitting tissue for appropriate microbiologic cultures, molecular biology studies, and preparing touch imprints or frozen sections for histochemical stains. If a neoplastic process were suggested, routine light microscopy could be supplemented with immunocytochemical studies, cytogenetics, and flow cytometry.

Immunologic and Molecular Biologic Procedures in the Diagnosis of Infectious Agents

When traditional methods fail to establish an unequivocal diagnosis, newer immunologic and molecular biologic procedures may improve recovery rates and detect fastidious organisms. These include immunoperoxidase and immunofluorescence methods, RNA/DNA hybridization techniques, and the polymerase chain reaction. Commercially available polyclonal and monoclonal antibodies can be used to detect a variety of antigens and infectious agents including many fungi, viruses, bacteria, and protozoa (8). DNA/RNA hybridization techniques identify specific microbial DNA or RNA sequences in tissue sections, smears, or clinical specimens. Commercially available probes useful in AIDS include those to Epstein-Barr virus, cytomegalovirus, mycobacteria, legionella, campylobacter, herpes simplex virus, and HIV (8–13). The polymerase chain reaction results in the rapid replication of target DNA sequences providing a dramatic improvement in sensitivity. Because of the extreme sensitivity of this technique, control studies are essential and specimen/reagent contamination must be meticulously avoided. A wide variety of infectious agents, including mycobacterium, cytomegalovirus, Epstein-Barr virus, and HIV have been detected using this method (14–17). A case of HIV infection occurring in 1959 was identified by using this technique on the DNA extracted from paraffin blocks of autopsy tissues in a 25-year-old sailor (18).

IMPORTANT OPPORTUNISTIC INFECTIONS IN AIDS PATIENTS

Parasitic Infections

Pneumocystis carinii

Pneumocystis carinii (PC) pneumonia is an important indicator of severe immunodeficiency due to HIV infection and is a criterion for the diagnosis of AIDS as defined by the Centers for Disease Control (CDC) (3). Approximately 60% of patients with AIDS reported to the CDC present with PC pneumonia as their initial opportunistic infection (19). While PC infections are most com-

monly confined to the lungs, an increasing number of patients with extrapulmonary spread, including widely disseminated disease, are being reported (20–24).

Although traditionally classified as a sporozoan protozoal parasite, the taxonomy is unresolved, as ribosomal RNA sequencing and some ultrastructural studies have suggested an association with fastidious fungi (25,26). The organism's natural reservoir and life cycle are poorly understood. Current studies support four stages in the life cycle: precyst, cyst, sporozoites within cysts, and freestanding trophozoites (26,27). The cyst, presumed to be the proliferative form, contains up to eight small nucleated structures termed *sporozoites.* After rupture of the cyst wall, sporozoites are released and mature into trophozoites, the vegetative form. Large trophozoites develop into precysts, which undergo further maturation to cysts containing sporozoites.

PC has been recovered from a large number of animal species and humans (28). Serologic investigations in humans imply that many infections are acquired early in childhood (29) and disease develops through reactivation of latent infection. Alternatively, de novo infections probably also occur and transmission is by the aerosol route (30,31).

Diagnosis

Pulmonary specimens including induced sputum, bronchial washings and brushings, bronchoalveolar lavage, FNAB, transtracheal aspirate, transbronchial biopsy, and open lung biopsy are used for diagnosis. However, with the recognition of disseminated pneumocystosis, FNAB and surgical biopsies of tissues from a variety of sites are also employed. In our experience and from a number of studies, bronchoalveolar lavage has shown the greatest sensitivity in the diagnosis of lung infections when compared with other noninvasive methods. Bedrossian (32), in reviewing 17 studies comparing various techniques, reported yields of 83% for transbronchial biopsy, 82% for bronchoalveolar lavage, and 53% for washing and brushing cytology. When bronchoalveolar lavage is combined with other methods such as bronchial washings and brushings, diagnostic yields approach 100%. Open lung biopsy and transbronchial biopsy remain the gold standard but are rarely necessary to secure a diagnosis. Spontaneous and induced sputum appear to yield the worst results as compared with other methods. CT-guided FNAB is usually reserved for focal or cavitary lung lesions (33) but may also have a role in the evaluation of pediatric patients (34).

Staining Methods

While the Grocott or GMS stains are the most commonly used methods, Gram-Weigert, PAS, and toluidine blue also detect the cyst wall. Sporozoites and trophozoites are best demonstrated with Diff-Quik, cresyl violet, Giemsa, May-Grunwald-Giemsa, PAS, and Wright-Giemsa stains (35–37). The cyst wall stains can be used to evaluate tissue sections, imprints, and cytology specimens, whereas the trophozoite/sporozoite stains are applicable only on imprints and cytology specimens. We utilize the GMS stain with a microwave modification and have found this to be the single best method as it can be rapidly performed and has the advantage of staining other pathogens such as fungi, bacteria, and the cytoplasmic inclusions of cytomegalovirus (38). With this stain, cyst forms are spherical, crescentic, or cup-shaped and measure 5–7 μm in diameter. Single or paired capsule dots correspond to the internal capsular thickening seen ultrastructurally. Ghali et al. (39) have shown fluorescence of the cysts in Papanicolaou-stained material when it is examined under UV light.

Other methodologies for the detection of PC in cytology specimens and tissue biopsies include immunofluorescence and immunoperoxidase techniques (40–42). Genomic DNA fragments of PC have been used as probes in the Southern blot technique and ribosomal RNA sequences employed as probes for in situ hybridization (25,43). Recently attempts have been made to detect PC by DNA amplification (44). While the antibody and probe techniques have been shown to be specific, demonstrating little or no crossreactivity with common fungi, bacteria, or parasites, they offer few advantages over traditional staining methods.

Histopathologic Features

As compared with the human sporadic and endemic forms, the AIDS-associated PC lung infections generally show less interstitial widening and lymphoplasmacytic infiltrate and more atypical features (45). The pattern of reaction also differs from that described in animal models in which cortisone and a low protein diet are used for immunosuppression (46). The characteristic and specific feature is a foamy refractile intraalveolar exudate in which variable numbers of organisms are demonstrated with the cyst wall stains (Fig. 1). This is accompanied not infrequently by nonspecific features including diffuse alveolar damage with hyaline membrane formation, hyperplasia and atypia of type II pneumocytes, and sparse septal inflammation. Less common manifestations include epithelioid granulomas, giant cell formation, necrotizing bronchopneumonia, interstitial fibrosis, a desquamative interstitial (DIP)-like pneumonitis, and cavitary lesions showing central necrosis (33,47–53). In a recent study of 123 lung biopsies from 76 AIDS patients with PC pneumonitis, Travis et al. (47) additionally noted (in a small percentage of patients) parenchymal cysts, interstitial microcalcifications, vasculitis, and vascular permeation by PC; the latter finding was also described by Liu et al. (50) and was suggested as a possible mechanism for dissemination. The characteristic alveolar infiltrate was not present in 19% of PC-positive biopsies, emphasizing the importance of performing special stains in the absence of typical features (47). Concomitant polymicrobial infections with a variety of viruses, fungi, and bacteria are common.

Extrapulmonary Spread

An increasing number of extrapulmonary infections, including widely disseminated disease, are being reported (20–24). Approximately 25 cases of extrapulmonary PC infections have been described to date, most occurring in patients with AIDS. In a study by Telzak et al. (21), 2.5% of 161 patients with AIDS showed evi-

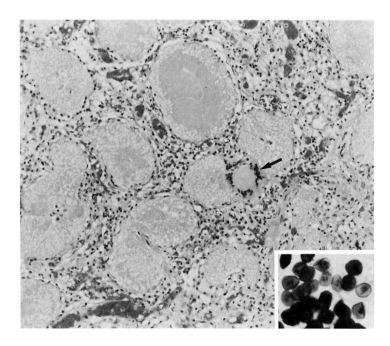

FIG. 1. *Pneumocystis carinii* pneumonitis characterized by foamy alveolar exudate and mild interstitial mononuclear cell infiltrate. Giant cell reaction (*arrow*) is an unusual feature. Hematoxylin and eosin, ×100. **Inset:** GMS stain demonstrating cup-shaped and spherical cysts with dot-like or double comma-shaped capsule thickenings. Gomori's methenamine silver, ×1000.

dence of extrapulmonary PC infection. The most common extrapulmonary site of spread is lymph node; however, involvement of bone marrow, spleen, liver, GI tract, pancreas, palate, pericardium, thymus, central nervous system, and eye has also been reported. These patterns suggest lymphatic and hematogenous spread, but the risk factors for dissemination are not well understood. Rarely, patients with AIDS may present with extrapulmonary disease without a documented lung infection (21). Sites of involvement in this setting have included spleen, thyroid, external auditory canal, and middle ear.

The histopathology of extrapulmonary PC infections is generally similar to that described in typical pulmonary disease. Frothy eosinophilic exudates containing numerous cysts and trophozoites are usually associated with necrosis and scant inflammatory infiltrates.

Toxoplasma gondii

Transmission of *Toxoplasma gondii* (TG) to humans occurs primarily by ingesting oocysts from cat feces or by eating meat that contains tissue cysts (54). When the oocysts are ingested by secondary hosts (possibly all mammals), the organisms excyst, cross the bowel wall, and invade cells of many organs. Before immunity develops, they divide rapidly, giving rise to tachyzoites in a pseudocyst that eventually fills the cell, ruptures it, and enters contiguous cells. In chronic and latent infections, bradyzoites develop slowly and form within true cysts.

Toxoplasmosis is the most common opportunistic infection of the central nervous system in AIDS, occurring in at least 10% of AIDS patients overall and is the presenting (index) infection in about 5% of cases (55). The overall incidence of clinical toxoplasmosis among AIDS patients with neurological disease is about 30% and it is particularly common in Haitian patients with AIDS (56). Toxoplasmosis appears to represent reactivation of latent infection rather than primary infection, as serologic studies have shown detectable toxoplasma IgG antibodies in patients several months prior to the development of clinical disease (57).

Chorioretinitis is an infrequent manifestation, but may appear associated with or independent of encephalitis (58). Extraneural toxoplasmosis has been reported in the heart, lungs, testis, and skin of AIDS patients with concurrent central nervous system (CNS) disease (59–62). In autopsy studies, the organisms have been detected in many other organs, including stomach, adrenals, skeletal muscle, and pancreas, but infections in these sites are usually of little clinical significance (63,64).

Diagnosis and Histopathology

The primary method of diagnosing toxoplasmosis is by demonstrating the tachyzoites and cysts in clinical specimens including fluids, smears, and tissue biopsies. While serologic studies are considered reliable in the normal host, in the immunocompromised individual they play a limited role in establishing the diagnosis of acute infection. Even with severe toxoplasmosis, it is unusual for AIDS patients to demonstrate positive IgM titers or appropriate fourfold increases in IgG titers (63). However, the absence of antibodies against TG is strong evidence against a diagnosis of toxoplasmosis (65). Methods to detect TG antigens [dot-blot and enzyme-linked immunosorbent assay (ELISA)] are under investigation and may prove more reliable than antibody tests (66,67).

TG can be grown in cell culture media or in mice but recovery may require long time periods and these methods are generally considered too lengthy for routine diagnosis (68). Since TG are rarely demonstrable in bronchoalveolar lavage fluid and cerebrospinal fluid, diagnosis is usually made by tissue biopsy. TG recovered in fluids, tissue imprints, and histologic sections show the characteristic crescentic or oval tachyzoites, pseudocysts, and true cysts. In Giemsa- or Wright-stained material, the tachyzoite cytoplasm stains blue and the eccentric nucleus dark red. The organisms are small, measuring 3–4 μm in length and 1–2 μm in width. They are generally broader at the end containing the nucleus. The cysts are more variable in size, measuring up to 40 μm in diameter and contain numerous tightly aggregated bradyzoites surrounded by a thin eosinophilic membrane that is weakly positive with silver and PAS stains (Fig. 2). Bradyzoites within cysts contain amylopectin and are strongly PAS-positive. The lack of a kinetoplast and distinct nucleus differentiates TG from leishmania and *Trypanosoma cruzi* (69).

The gross and microscopic pathology of TG infection, which is described in another chapter devoted to the central nervous system pathology of HIV infection, will be

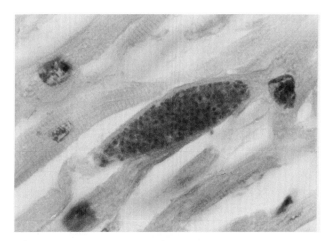

FIG. 2. Chronic myocardial infection with *Toxoplasma gondii.* Elongated cyst contains numerous tightly aggregated bradyzoites unassociated with inflammation. Hematoxylin and eosin, ×1,000.

only briefly reviewed here since TG can produce lesions outside the CNS. In the brain, the principal microscopic features are a diffuse meningoencephalitis or a focal necrotizing encephalitis with associated arteritis and thrombosis (70,71). Tachyzoites and cysts can be demonstrated in the brain tissue surrounding the areas of necrosis although organisms may not be seen in over 50% of cases.

Ocular toxoplasmosis often produces a granulomatous inflammatory reaction of the retina and choroid, which is in part related to a hypersensitivity reaction. There may be retinal necrosis with hemorrhage and vascular thrombosis. The parasites may be numerous or difficult to demonstrate (72).

Toxoplasma pneumonitis shows a variable histology often consisting of an interstitial and intraalveolar infiltration by mononuclear cells of a focal or diffuse nature. Abundant tachyzoites are usually demonstrable (59).

Involvement of many other organs such as heart, liver, adrenal gland, and stomach has been documented in AIDS patients with these lesions usually showing focal necrosis and variable numbers of organisms and inflammatory cells (63,64). Rarely, tachyzoites can be found in peripheral blood smears (Fig. 3).

Cryptosporidia and Other Protozoa

Cryptosporidium, a parasite taxonomically related to *Toxoplasma, Isospora,* and *Plasmodium* species, has be-

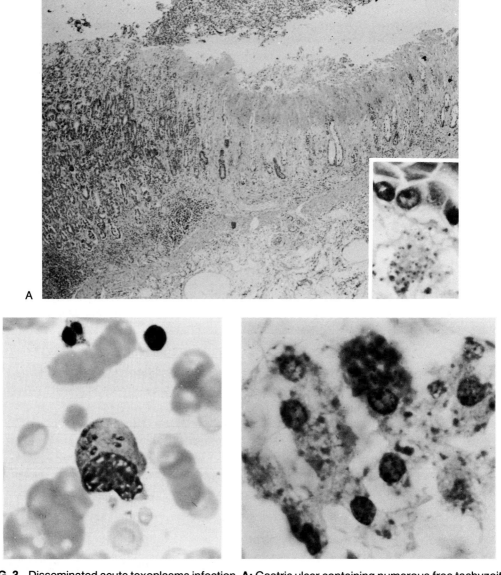

FIG. 3. Disseminated acute toxoplasma infection. **A:** Gastric ulcer containing numerous free tachyzoites within lamina propria (**inset**). Hematoxylin and eosin, ×100. Inset: hematoxylin and eosin, ×400. **B,C:** Tachyzoites within peripheral blood mononuclear cells and cells of adrenal cortex. B, hematoxylin and eosin, ×630; C, hematoxylin and eosin, ×400.

come recognized as a common cause of enteritis in the immunocompromised host (73–77). The life cycle of *Cryptosporidium* is similar to other coccidia in that asexual and sexual stages lead to production of oocysts that are released into the gastrointestinal tract and discharged in the feces. The organism gains access to humans through inhalation or ingestion and thus can be sexually transmitted through the oral–fecal route (78,79). As the oocysts are resistant to most common disinfectants, strict handwashing and enteric precautions are necessary to prevent nosocomial transmission.

In the United States, cryptosporidia are responsible for about 4% of diarrheal illnesses in AIDS patients reported to the CDC, while in African patients with enteropathic AIDS, they are implicated in up to 48% of cases (74,80). These infections can involve the entire gastrointestinal tract from esophagus to rectum (73,81). Less common sites of infection include gallbladder, pancreas, biliary and pancreatic ducts, and the respiratory tract (76,77,82,83). The biliary and pulmonary forms have been described almost exclusively in the immunocompromised host.

The diagnosis of cryptosporidiosis is usually based on fecal examination or small intestinal biopsy, but in our experience, the parasite can also be recognized in cytology preparations of small intestinal aspirates or brushings (84) (Fig. 4). The organisms are readily detected in stool by a Kinyoun modified acid-fast stain in which 4–5 μm bright red oocysts are present in background fecal material (85,86). The acid-fastness allows differentiation from yeast (86). As oocyst excretion can be sporadic, multiple stool examinations are sometimes necessary. In infections shedding low numbers of organisms, concentrating techniques such as Sheather's sucrose or zinc sulfate flotation improve rates of detection. A specific and sensitive direct immunofluorescence method has been described and can be used on smears and paraffin-embedded tissue sections (87).

In small intestinal mucosal biopsies, histologic changes do not correlate well with the degree of infection or clinical symptoms. Small intestinal villi exhibit mild atrophy and a nonspecific increase in lamina propria chronic inflammation. The diagnostic feature in hematoxylin and eosin-stained sections is the presence of basophilic organisms located along the brush border or within parasitophorous vacuoles (75) (Fig. 5). The organisms are best demonstrated with the Giemsa or Gram stains and are inconsistently positive with the Kinyoun acid-fast stain in tissue sections (75,88). Cryptosporidia are differentiated from isospora by their smaller size and location along the brush border.

Cryptosporidial infections of the gallbladder and extrahepatic biliary tree are observed in up to 10% of AIDS patients and present as acalculous and rarely gangrenous cholecystitis (76). The gallbladder shows luminal exudates and ulceration, and as in other sites, the organisms are visible lining the mucosa. Liver biopsies reveal pericholangitis and organisms attached to the epithelium of large bile ducts (83). Respiratory tract infections are less well characterized and probably result from aspiration of gastroduodenal material. Cryptosporidia are demonstrated lining bronchiolar epithelium associated with mild chronic inflammation (77). About one-third of patients with cryptosporidiosis have other gastrointestinal pathogens including herpes, candida, cytomegalovirus, mycobacterium, giardia, *Entamoeba histolytica,* shigella, and salmonella (89).

Isospora belli, a protozoan related to the *Cryptosporidium* species, is an uncommon pathogen in AIDS patients in the United States but is present in up to 45% of Haitian patients with AIDS (90,91). The clinical manifestations closely resemble those of cryptosporidial infection, most commonly chronic or relapsing enteritis (91,92). The diagnosis is made by demonstrating the oocysts in stool or duodenal aspirates with the Kinyoun

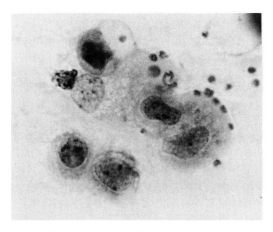

FIG. 4. Small intestinal brushing cytology demonstrating loosely cohesive group of epithelial cells with cryptosporidia aligned along luminal surface. Diff-Quik, ×630.

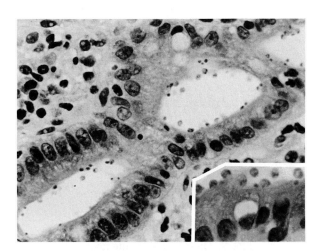

FIG. 5. Concomitant gastric mucosal biopsy with cryptosporidium along surface of epithelium. Hematoxylin and eosin, ×250. **Inset:** hematoxylin and eosin, ×1,000.

acid-fast or auramine–rhodamine stains (91,93). Concentration methods similar to those described for *Cryptosporidium* enhance recovery and identification (91). In small intestinal mucosal biopsies, the organisms are seen in an intracellular location within clear vacuoles (93). Giemsa and PAS stains with diastase pretreatment enhance the ability to identify the organism (94). In gastrointestinal infection, *isospora* may disseminate to regional lymph nodes and rarely to extraintestinal lymph nodes (lymphadenopathic isosporiasis) (91,94).

Only a limited number of human microsporidial infections have been recognized in AIDS patients, usually associated with gastrointestinal involvement (95–98). The role of these organisms (usually *Enterocytozoan bieneusi* or *Encephalitozoan cuniculi*) in the pathogenesis of diarrhea is unclear as patients often have concomitant infections with other better characterized enteric and systemic pathogens. The predominant clinical manifestations of microsporidial infections are weight loss and chronic diarrhea (96). Small intestinal biopsy is currently the best method to demonstrate the organisms (97). They appear as small refractile bodies in a supranuclear location in epithelial cells of the villi. While difficult to visualize in hematoxylin and eosin-stained sections, some species are variably Gram- and Giemsa-positive and acid-fast (99). Electron microscopy has been used diagnostically and ultrastructural characteristics allow species identification (98). These organisms have also been reported to infect other tissues including liver, peritoneum, eye, and skeletal muscle (95).

Other protozoan parasites including leishmania, *Giardia lamblia, Blastocystis hominis,* and a large coccidian-like oocyte, possibly a blue-green algae related to a chlorella species, have also been infrequently reported to cause enteric infections in AIDS (100–103).

Fungal Infections

Fungal infections have been recognized as important AIDS-related opportunistic infections dating from early clinical reports. Initially, mucosal candidiasis and cryptococcosis were identified as the most prominent AIDS-related opportunistic pathogens while histoplasmosis and coccidioidomycosis were recognized much less frequently. While this trend still holds true today, in certain endemic locations, histoplasmosis and coccidioidomycosis are now being diagnosed with increasing frequency. Other fungi reported less commonly in these patients include aspergillus, sporothrix, alternaria, zygomycetes, and the superficial/deep dermatophytes.

Detection

As fungal serologic tests, with the exception of cryptococcal antigen testing, are generally not useful in making a specific diagnosis of fungal infections and culture methods may require extended periods of time, direct microscopic examination of clinical specimens plays an important role in the management of AIDS patients providing prompt and useful information to clinicians.

In our laboratory, specimens from biopsy sites and cytology preparations from fluids, smears, or FNAB are initially stained with the Papanicolaou technique, and a modified Wright-Giemsa (Diff-Quik) stain. We have found the GMS and PAS stains in combination with calcofluor-white to be the best general purpose fungal stains. In the microbiology laboratory, prompt handling of freshly collected specimens and the use of a battery of enriched culture media with and without antibiotics are essential for recovering pathogenic fungi. Table 1 outlines the characteristic morphologic features of fungi seen in clinical specimens discussed in this section.

Candida

Candida is a genus of yeast that is a well-recognized cause of mucocutaneous and invasive disease in patients with AIDS. Oral and esophageal candidiasis, the most common fungal infections in HIV-positive patients, are often the first indications of advancing immune dysfunction (104,105).

Oral candidiasis occurs as four distinct clinical variants: (1) pseudomembranous; (2) erythematous; (3) hyperplastic; and (4) angular cheilitis (106,107). The pseudomembranous type is the most frequent variant and presents as small yellow patches often on the tongue and buccal mucosa. Scrapings of these lesions contain epithelial cells mixed with necrotic debris, inflammatory exudate, and fungi consisting of yeast and pseudohyphae (Fig. 6).

Gastrointestinal candidiasis most frequently involves the esophagus but is also commonly seen in the stomach and to a lesser extent the small and large intestine (108). In AIDS patients, esophageal candidiasis almost always coexists with oral candidiasis (109). The diagnosis is made by esophagoscopy, in which the characteristic white patches overlay inflamed mucosa, and by endoscopic biopsy, which demonstrates spores and pseudohyphae within the epithelium or submucosa (Fig. 7). As candida is a normal commensal organism in the esophagus and mouth, positive culture alone from biopsy specimens is not definitive evidence of infection.

While oral and esophageal candidiasis are extremely common in patients with AIDS, systemic candida infections are less frequently encountered. Recently, however, because of the more widespread use of indwelling catheters and parenteral hyperalimentation, increasing numbers of reports of candidemia have appeared. Depending upon the cause and mechanism of entry, candidemia may spontaneously resolve, or the patient may

TABLE 1. *Summary of characteristic features of fungi in tissues and smears*

Organism	Size range (μm)	Characteristic morphologic features
Candida spp.	2.5–5 (yeast) 5–10 (pseudohyphae)	Yeast exhibit single buds (blastoconidia) and are oval to round Pseudohyphae have linear chains of blastoconidia with "pinched" separations Rarely true hyphae with septation
Cryptococcus neoformans	2–15	Yeast (blastoconidia) are characteristically variable in size Yeast usually spherical but can be oval or elliptical with "pinched-off" buds Polysaccharide capsule demonstrated with mucicarmine stain or by India ink preparation (rarely capsule-deficient strains) Rarely pseudohyphae in exudates or CSF
Histoplasma capsulatum	2–5	Small oval to round yeast with budding found within histiocytes, giant cells, or neutrophils Less size variability than cryptococcus
Coccidioides immitis	1–5 (endospores) 5–30 (immature spherules) 30–200 (mature spherules)	Spherules vary in size Mature spherules contain spores that stain with GMS and PAS[a] Immature spherule walls are strongly PAS positive Endospores resemble *H. capsulatum* but show no evidence of budding

[a] GMS, Gomori's methenamine silver stain; PAS, periodic acid-Schiff stain.

succumb to overwhelming sepsis or develop visceral candidiasis. Widespread visceral dissemination usually involves the central nervous system, kidneys, heart, bone, skin, and lung (Fig. 8) (110–113). Unusual cutaneous presentations of mixed infections include coexistent candida within lesions of molluscum contagiosum and candida with herpes simplex (114).

Cryptococcus

Cryptococcosis is the fourth most common infection in AIDS patients after pneumocystis, cytomegalovirus, and mycobacterial disease (115). This life-threatening opportunistic infection is observed in between 5% and 10% of AIDS patients in the United States and has three major clinical presentations of disease: CNS, pulmonary, and disseminated infection (116). As many as 10–20% of

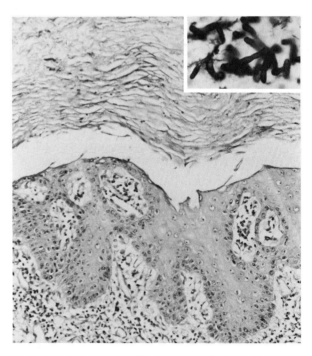

FIG. 7. Candida esophagitis, hyperplastic type. Hyperkeratotic layer above epithelium contains numerous yeast and pseudohyphae. Hematoxylin and eosin, ×200. **Inset:** GMS stain demonstrating pseudohyphae and budding yeast. Gomori's methenamine silver, ×400.

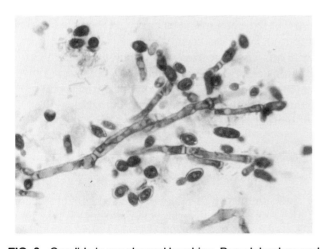

FIG. 6. Candida in esophageal brushing. Pseudohyphae and budding yeast differentiate this from other fungi. Papanicolaou, ×400.

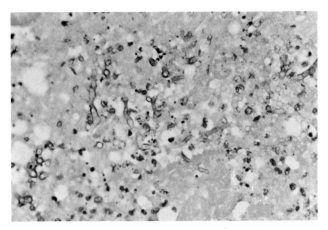

FIG. 8. Necrotizing candida pneumonitis. Pseudohyphae admixed with fibrin and inflammatory cells in destroyed lung parenchyma. Hematoxylin and eosin, ×250.

patients with cryptococcosis have cutaneous involvement (papules, pustules, nodules, infiltrative plaques, ulcers, bullae, and cellulitis) as a component of disseminated disease, although there are rare reports of isolated cutaneous infection in the absence of systemic involvement (117). The vesicular and ulcerative forms may be mistaken for a herpetic infection or pyoderma gangrenosum, respectively, while the umbilicated papules may resemble molluscum contagiosum (118,119). Rarely, cutaneous lesions can clinically mimic Kaposi's sarcoma (120). Disseminated infections frequently involve lung, lymph node, adrenal gland, skin, and kidney (121,122). Unusual manifestations of systemic infections include myocarditis, massive peripheral and mediastinal lymphadenopathy mimicking malignant lymphoma, isolated pleural effusion, and biliary tract obstruction secondary to cryptococcal lymphadenitis (123–126). Simultaneous infections with other opportunistic organisms including *Pneumocystis carinii* in the lung and toxoplasma in the brain have been found in up to 13% of cases (116,122, 127). Cryptococcus has also been reported within lesions of Kaposi's sarcoma (128).

Diagnosis

The diagnosis of cryptococcosis requires isolation of the organism from body fluids, biopsy demonstration of the encapsulated yeast, or detection of the polysaccharide capsular antigen in serum or cerebrospinal fluid (CSF).

In cytology specimens such as CSF, bronchial washings and lavage, and joint fluid, the diagnosis is made by identifying the 4–6 μm in diameter yeast with double refractile cell walls, a distinctly outlined capsule, and narrow based budding. Organisms are highlighted by the PAS or methenamine silver stains. The mucicarmine stain, specific for the mucopolysaccharide capsule, and

the characteristic variability in size, distinguish cryptococcus from other fungi.

The India ink method, in which nigrosin or India ink is added to CSF (or other body fluid) and examined by light microscopy, is a commonly used technique to detect cryptococcus. While the method is simple, the test suffers from poor sensitivity and requires strict attention to criteria for identification, as encapsulated forms of *Klebsiella pneumoniae, Rhodotorula, Candida,* and *Prototheca* can be confused with cryptococcus. It is preferable to utilize routine cytologic stains supplemented by methenamine silver, PAS, and Mayer's mucicarmine stains to establish the diagnosis.

Although not unique to AIDS patients, recent reports have suggested that poorly encapsulated or capsule-deficient strains may be more commonly isolated from AIDS patients (129,130). Capsule-deficient strains can be presumptively identified by demonstrating the melanin-like substance in the cell wall with a Fontana-Masson stain (131).

The reaction to cryptococcus in the skin has been classified as gelatinous or granulomatous, but both reaction patterns may be seen in the same lesion. The gelatinous type shows numerous organisms surrounded by abundant capsular polysaccharide and little inflammation (Fig. 9). The granulomatous lesion shows fewer cryptococci, predominantly in an intracellular location with greater inflammation consisting primarily of lymphocytes, histiocytes, and occasional giant cells (132).

In transbronchial lung biopsies, a variety of histopathologic abnormalities can be seen. Most commonly, fungi are present in an interstitial location with a minimal accompanying inflammatory infiltrate (Fig. 10). There may also be alveolar invasion and rarely vascular invasion (122). The organisms often coexist with other pathogens including pneumocystis and cytomegalovirus.

Infections by cryptococcus have been demonstrated in a variety of other sites, particularly lymph node, bone marrow, adrenal gland, and kidney. The inflammatory response to infection can be quite variable, ranging from absent to florid. As cryptococcus elaborates no known exotoxins, tissue necrosis is minimal and inflammatory reactions are usually sparse. Occasionally, some inflammatory cells of mixed types accompany the proliferating organisms, but well-formed granulomas are generally not present (121–133).

Endemic Mycoses—Histoplasmosis and Coccidioidomycosis

The endemic mycoses are designated as such because of their characteristic geographic ranges. While these pathogens can produce disease in normal individuals, they generally do not cause progressive disseminated infections in hosts with intact cellular immunity. However, patients with AIDS who live in or have traveled to

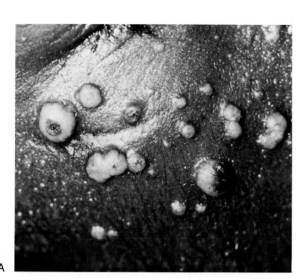

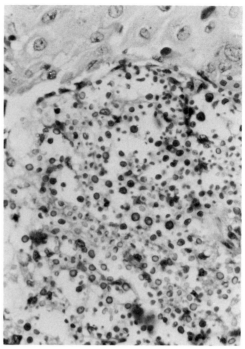

A

B

FIG. 9. A: Cryptococcus of skin: multiple umbilicated nodules involving the face. **B:** Skin biopsy demonstrating gelatinous dermal reaction. Numerous organisms surrounded by abundant capsular material with a paucity of inflammation. PAS, ×250.

endemic areas are at an increased risk for disseminated multisystem disease. Major organisms in this group include *Histoplasma capsulatum, Coccidioides immitis,* and *Blastomyces dermatitidis.*

Histoplasma capsulatum

Histoplasma capsulatum, a dimorphic fungus, exists in soil contaminated by bird feces. The major endemic

area is the central United States and most normal persons living in that region show skin test evidence of past infection (134,135). Reactivation of latent infections and newly acquired primary infection are both important modes of acquiring disease in immunocompromised patients. As expected, the frequency of histoplasmosis in AIDS patients shows marked geographic variability. In highly endemic regions, *H. capsulatum* has been reported in up to 27% of AIDS patients, while

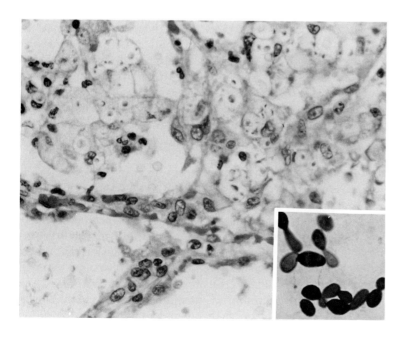

FIG. 10. *Cryptococcus neoformans* in lung. Organisms within alveoli and interstitium demonstrate characteristic variability in size, surrounding clear zones occupied by mucopolysaccharide material and narrow based budding (**inset**). Hematoxylin and eosin, ×250. Inset: Gomori's methenamine silver, ×1,000.

in some autopsy series from nonendemic areas, the infection is documented very rarely (136,137). The clinical manifestations, including high fever, maculopapular rash or necrotic papules, hepatomegaly, splenomegaly, lymphadenopathy, anemia, and pulmonary infiltrates, reflect a disseminated process.

Diagnosis. The diagnosis is made by the identification or culture of the fungus in clinical specimens and tissue biopsies. Because of the disseminated nature of the infection in AIDS patients, a variety of specimens including bone marrow, blood, respiratory specimens (lavage, washings, and bronchial biopsy), CSF, lymph node, and skin can be diagnostically useful (Figs. 11 and 12). Culture of bone marrow specimens is highly sensitive, but because of the organism's slow growth, up to 6 weeks may be required for identification (138). Positive cultures from peripheral blood have been reported in about 40% of published cases in AIDS patients, with the lysis centrifugation technique being the most sensitive method to detect the organism (136,138–140). Occasionally, yeast will be identified in Wright-stained peripheral blood or buffy coat smears (141).

Biopsy of focal sites of disease such as skin, lymph nodes, or liver will reveal the typical 2–5 μm oval to round budding yeast in clusters within histiocytes. Special stains including methenamine silver or PAS are usually necessary to visualize the organisms because of their small size. Bone marrow biopsy is particularly useful and positive in most cases of disseminated disease. Four patterns of involvement are recognized in marrow biopsies: (1) no evidence of infection (positive culture without morphologic abnormality); (2) discrete granulomas; (3) lymphohistiocytic aggregates; and (4) diffuse macrophage infiltration. Organisms are found within

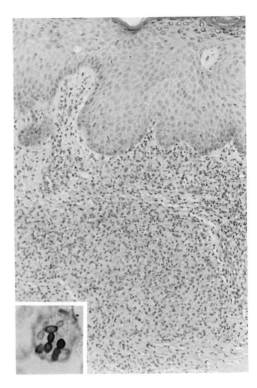

FIG. 12. Cutaneous histoplasmosis. Dermal infiltrate of histiocytes and poorly formed granulomas containing numerous yeast in an intracellular location (**inset**). Hematoxylin and eosin, ×200. Inset: Gomori's methenamine silver, ×400.

and outside of macrophages. Other common findings reported, which are probably unrelated to infection with this organism, include megaloblastoid erythropoiesis and dysplastic myeloid and megakaryocytic maturation (142).

Coccidioides immitis

Coccidioidomycosis, a systemic mycosis endemic to arid regions of North and South America, is becoming recognized as a significant cause of morbidity and mortality in AIDS patients, particularly in endemic regions (143). Symptomatic disease may occur from reactivation of latent infection or by progressive primary infection (144). The immunocompromised host is prone to develop severe pulmonary and widely disseminated disease (145).

Diagnosis. The diagnosis of coccidioidomycosis is made by serologic methods, skin testing, microbiologic culture, and identification of the endosporulating spherules in body fluids or tissue biopsies. The most effective method for diagnosis is evaluation of respiratory tract specimens (bronchial washings, bronchoalveolar lavage, and transbronchial biopsy) using culture and special stains including Grocott's or GMS and PAS. In tissue sections, *C. immitis* is identified as large spherules measuring 30–60 μm in diameter containing endospores 2–5

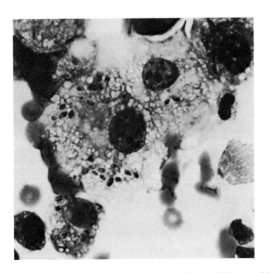

FIG. 11. *Histoplasma capsulatum* in bronchial washing. Small oval to round yeast are primarily within macrophages. Narrow based budding, intracellular location, and absence of cup-shaped organisms differentiates this from *Pneumocystis carinii.* Papanicolaou, ×1,000.

μm in diameter. Because of the large spherule size, they are often visualized in routine hematoxylin and eosin-stained sections. The inflammatory response to the organisms in lung biopsies usually consists of poorly formed granulomas and lymphohistiocytic aggregates with few multinucleated giant cells (Fig. 13). Older lesions may show areas of organizing pneumonitis. AIDS patients show greater numbers of spherules compared with non-AIDS patients, and the fungus often coexists with other opportunistic pathogens including *Pneumocystis carinii,* cytomegalovirus, and *M. avium-intracellulare* (145). In keeping with the disseminated nature of the infection, organisms have also been cultured or identified histologically in lymph node, liver, spleen, bone marrow, kidney, skin, and blood (143,145–148).

Other Fungi

While considerably less common than candida, cryptococcus, histoplasma, and coccidioides, a variety of other fungi have infrequently been described in AIDS patients. These include *Sporothrix schenckii* (149,150), aspergillus (151,152), alternaria (153), and *Blastomyces dermatitidis* (154).

Bacterial Infections

Mycobacteria

Up to 50% of AIDS patients will develop a mycobacterial infection at some stage of their disease (155). The pathogenicity of mycobacteria is modulated by the host's immune response to determine the type and extent of infection (156). About 10% of the isolates are *Mycobacterium tuberculosis* (MTB) and the remaining are nontuberculous mycobacteria (NTM), which include MAI, *M. kansasii,* and *M. scrofulaceum* (157). In-

fections with other mycobacteria, especially *M. gordonae, M. xenopi,* and *M. fortuitum,* are also being recognized with increasing frequency (158,159).

Nontuberculous Mycobacteria

As environmental saprophytes, the organisms gain access through the aerosol route or drinking water and may temporarily colonize the nasopharynx or intestinal mucosa (160). In immunodeficient individuals, once established, these opportunistic pathogens can extensively disseminate and proliferate to enormous numbers before causing overt disease (gastrointestinal, pulmonary, soft tissue, and systemic lesions are seen in these infections) (161). NTM infections may be clinically silent, the diagnosis being made incidentally in a lymph node biopsy, in endoscopic biopsy of gastrointestinal tract, or at autopsy. When clinical manifestations occur they may be nonspecific (fever, weight loss, anorexia, abdominal pain, etc.).

Tuberculous Mycobacteria

MTB among patients with AIDS is seen most frequently in those groups with historically high rates of infection (intravenous drug users, Haitians, Hispanics, and blacks) and tends to occur early in the course of HIV infection, often in a disseminated (miliary) extrapulmonary form (162).

A case of disseminated *M. bovis* infection following bacille Calmette-Guérin (BCG) vaccination highlights the importance of not using this vaccine in individuals with HIV infection (163).

Histopathologic Diagnosis

Although microbiologic culture is required for precise species identification, rapid diagnosis of mycobacterial

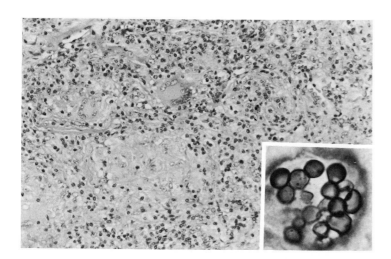

FIG. 13. Lung biopsy with *Coccidioides immitis.* Diffuse granulomatous reaction with giant cells. **Inset:** Endosporulating spherule diagnostic for *C. immitis.* Hematoxylin and eosin, ×100. Inset: Gomori's methenamine silver, ×400.

infections rests on morphologic demonstration of the organisms in cytologic preparations and tissue sections. Gastrointestinal tract, lymph nodes, lung, liver, and bone marrow are the most common biopsy specimens. The cellular response to the organisms is variable and includes well- or poorly formed granulomas, lymphohistiocytic reactions, histoid pattern, and paucity of immune response.

MAI Infections

In endoscopic biopsies of the small intestine, MAI infections show villous atrophy with diffuse infiltration of the lamina propria by foamy or granular histiocytes (Fig. 14). Necrosis is unusual, and granulomas are generally not present or are poorly formed. Acid-fast bacilli (AFB) stains demonstrating the abundant beaded or magenta rods within these histiocytes differentiate this lesion from Whipple's disease, which can have similar clinical and histologic features and from intestinal *Corynebacterium equi* infection (164,165). Focal involvement of gastric or colonic mucosa may be overlooked, and special stains are appropriate even in the absence of an obvious infiltrate.

Lymph node involvement with NTM can take several forms. The cortex and part of the medulla are replaced by sheets of histiocytes containing many organisms. Granulomas, necrosis, fibrosis, and calcification are usually absent. An unusual spindle cell proliferation, described by Wood and similar to the histoid reaction of lepromatous leprosy, may suggest a connective tissue tumor or Kaposi's sarcoma, but special stains demonstrate abundant bacilli within the spindle cells (166) (Fig. 15).

In the lungs, NTM infections manifest minimal tissue response. In the interstitium, rare clusters of histiocytes containing numerous organisms associated with minimal chronic inflammation are often the only evidence of infection. Special stains may demonstrate abundant organisms throughout the interstitium in the absence of reaction.

Hepatic involvement by MAI is seen in about 70% of liver biopsies in patients with systemic MAI infection and has been reported in up to as many as 83% of patients coming to autopsy (167,168). The histologic appearance can be deceptively bland, ranging from widely dispersed histiocytes to focal granuloma-like collections lacking necrosis and giant cells. AFB stains show numerous organisms within histiocytes and rarely within Kupffer cells (169). Occasionally organisms are cultured from biopsies demonstrating no tissue reaction (170).

Bone marrow involvement by mycobacteria manifests as lymphohistiocytic aggregates to poorly formed granulomas that tend to be very small and focal in distribution. AFB stains demonstrate organisms within granulomas and also within more widely dispersed histiocytes (171). As formic acid decalcification may interfere with AFB stains, EDTA decalcification solutions are recommended since it is desirable to perform acid-fast stains routinely on bone marrow biopsies from HIV-infected patients (172).

The fluorescent stain auramine–rhodamine can be used on cytology preparations and adapted to tissue sections to facilitate the demonstration of mycobacteria. This method requires less time to screen the slides as it can be read at lower magnification and has been shown to be about twice as sensitive as the Ziehl-Neelsen stain in demonstrating AFB in lymph node biopsies (173).

Monoclonal antibodies to mycobacterial antigens, DNA hybridization probes, and the polymerase chain reaction are methods under investigation with the aim to shorten recovery time, improve sensitivity and specific-

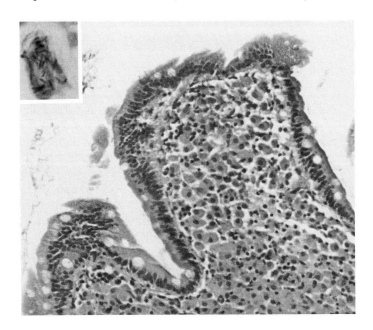

FIG. 14. MAI enteritis. Small intestinal biopsy demonstrating blunting and expansion of villi with a histiocytic infiltrate in the lamina propria. Inset shows large numbers of acid-fast bacilli within histiocytes. The differential diagnosis includes Whipple's disease and infection by *Corynebacterium equi*. Hematoxylin and eosin, ×200. Inset: Ziehl-Neelsen, ×1,000.

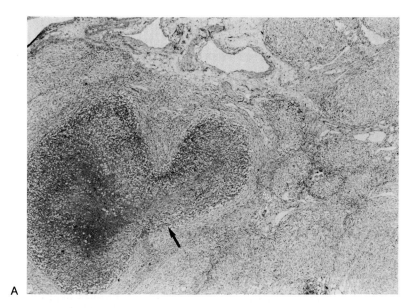

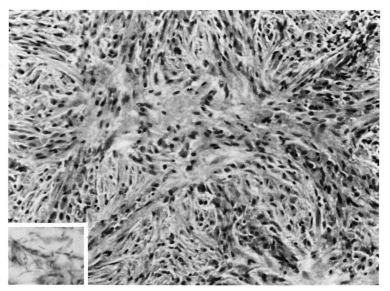

FIG. 15. Necrotizing lymphadenitis and "histoid" reaction. **A:** Atypical MAI infection of lymphoid tissue. Culture-proven MAI infection demonstrating unusual feature of zonal necrosis (*arrow*). Hematoxylin and eosin, ×25. **B:** Histoid reaction with spindle-shaped histiocytes arranged in interlacing fascicles. Hematoxylin and eosin, ×250. Inset: Ziehl-Neelsen stain showing acid-fast bacilli within spindle cells. Ziehl-Neelsen, ×1,000.

ity, and allow direct identification from patient material (174–176).

MTB Infections

HIV-associated MTB infections of any site generally present a more variable tissue response, ranging from well-formed granulomata to loose clusters of histiocytes with lesser numbers of organisms than are seen in NTM infections. However, in our experience, MTB infections in AIDS patients cannot be reliably distinguished from MAI infections solely on the basis of morphologic features such as necrosis, type of inflammatory response, presence of granulomas, or numbers of organisms. In the lungs, miliary patterns are common and typical necrotizing cavitary lesions infrequent (177). Dual pulmonary infections with MTB and MAI have been reported (178).

Involvement of other organs shows similar histologic features.

In summary, the tissue reactions to mycobacterial infections are few and depend on factors such as the inherent virulence of the particular mycobacterial species, degree of immunodeficiency when the infection occurs, the length of time the lesion is present prior to biopsy, and the influence of concomitant or prior chemotherapeutic agents. Because of this histologic variability and differences in the response and treatment of NTM and MTB, stains to demonstrate the bacteria should always be supplemented with methods to culture the organisms and determine chemotherapeutic sensitivities.

Other Bacteria

Infections with a variety of bacteria such as *Streptococcus pneumoniae, Haemophilus influenzae, Staphylococ-*

cus aureus, Neisseria meningitidis, salmonella, shigella, campylobacter, and *Treponema pallidum* are important causes of morbidity and mortality in HIV-infected children and adults (179–195). The multiplicity of immunologic defects of cellular and humoral types presumably predisposes these patients to persistent infections and bacteremia (196). In addition, chemotherapeutic and antineoplastic agents used to treat opportunistic infections and neoplasms may cause neutropenia, further compromising their immune status. These infections often show atypical presentations including multiple infections with more than one organism and high relapse rates despite appropriate antibiotic therapy. Infections with *Streptococcus pneumoniae* and *Haemophilus influenzae* are particularly frequent in children with AIDS and the latter organism is responsible for about 10% of pneumonias in adult AIDS patients (179,183,184). Important enteric pathogens in HIV-infected patients include salmonella, campylobacter, and shigella. Salmonellosis may present initially as acute gastroenteritis or less commonly as bacteremia. Salmonella infections often have a severe clinical course with bacteremia in up to 45% of AIDS patients and show a tendency to relapse following antibiotic therapy (181,182,185). Cultures of blood and stool usually confirm the diagnosis, but salmonella may be recovered from many sources including brain, bone marrow, urine, and spleen. Campylobacter species have been recognized as important pathogens in the general population as well as in homosexual men and immunocompromised patients. Most infections in AIDS patients are associated with gastroenteritis while bacteremia and cholecystitis are infrequently reported (189,190). *Shigella flexneri* is the most common species isolated from AIDS patients with shigella gastroenteritis (186–188). Bacteremia is infrequently seen and the diagnosis is principally made by culture of stool.

A number of studies have suggested that HIV infection may be associated with rapid progression of secondary syphilis or tertiary neurosyphilis, even following appropriate antibiotic therapy (191,192). Unusual clinical presentations, atypical serologic responses after appropriate treatment and false-negative serologic tests make the diagnosis of syphilis in HIV-infected patients difficult (193,195,197). Darkfield examination or direct fluorescent antibody staining of scrapings or exudates from suspicious primary lesions will help to establish the diagnosis even with negative rapid plasma reagin (RPR) or Venereal Disease Research Laboratory (VDRL) serologic studies. Silver stains such as the Steiner or Warthin-Starry stains can be performed on tissue biopsies but in the author's experience are difficult to interpret (198). Overall, the diagnosis of syphilis can be problematic in HIV-infected patients, and many clinicians will presumptively treat patients for early syphilis and closely monitor serial serologic tests to detect delayed antibody response.

Bacterial infections are seen more commonly at autopsy than in biopsy specimens. Few pathologic studies, however, describe the microscopic features of pure bacterial enteric infections uncomplicated by the more common pathogens seen in AIDS patients. In typical enteric infections by most of these organisms, the initial phase is an invasion of the epithelium with propagation of the bacterial in epithelial cells followed by entry into the lamina propria. The subsequent reaction is acute and pyogenic with superficial mucosal necrosis and pseudomembrane formation beginning as a focal process and in severe infections becoming confluent. Organisms can be demonstrated within epithelial cells, lamina propria, and adherent membranes by Gram, Giemsa, and silver stains. Microbiologic culture will confirm the species of the enteropathic bacteria. This typical reaction pattern is modified by the host's ability to mount an immunologic response depending on the degree of immune suppression. Dissemination to other organs will result in necrotizing lesions associated with scant inflammatory infiltrates and an abundance of organisms, particularly in neutropenic patients.

Viral Infections

Cytomegalovirus

Cytomegalovirus (CMV) is a common opportunistic pathogen found in cytology and biopsy specimens from AIDS patients surpassed in frequency only by pneumocystis and MAI (199,200). Nearly all AIDS patients have serologic evidence of prior exposure, suggesting these infections almost always represent reactivation and dissemination of latent virus (201).

The gastrointestinal tract is a common site of CMV infection in AIDS. Colitis is the most frequent clinical presentation of enteric disease and lesions appear as focal or diffuse areas of ulceration and hemorrhage commonly involving the more distal colon (199). Intestinal perforation may occur. Multiple biopsies are usually required to establish a diagnosis. Esophageal involvement results in ulceration predominantly involving the distal portion (202). In the stomach, CMV appears as a nonspecific gastritis with focal ulceration or as a submucosal mass (203). Other alimentary tract sites less commonly involved include the duodenum, pancreas, biliary tree, and gallbladder (204). In patients with AIDS, CMV pneumonitis is not a well-characterized syndrome and is frequently found to coexist with other opportunistic pulmonary pathogens, especially *Pneumocystis carinii* (205). The histopathologic findings reported in lung biopsies or autopsy tissues from AIDS patients with CMV pneumonitis range from focal and mild interstitial pneumonitis to severe diffuse alveolar damage with necrosis. Infections in a variety of other organs including brain, lymph nodes, skin, endocrine organs (especially adrenal gland), genitourinary system, liver, and heart have also been described (206,207).

Diagnosis

The most widely utilized method of diagnosing active CMV infection is by demonstrating the characteristic inclusion bodies in biopsies or cytology specimens. The significance of a positive CMV culture in the absence of clinical or pathologic evidence of tissue injury or viral cytopathic effects remains unclear. The identification of infection based on the presence of cytopathic changes, while specific, is a relatively insensitive technique. The diagnostic accuracy in biopsy material can be enhanced by immunohistochemical stains for CMV early and late antigens and in situ hybridization for CMV nucleic acids (208,209). Recently the polymerase chain reaction has been used to demonstrate CMV DNA in clinical specimens and paraffin-embedded tissues. However, the presence of CMV DNA does not necessarily indicate active disease as the virus is latent in a very high proportion of the HIV-infected population (210).

Cells actively infected by CMV show characteristic cytologic changes including cellular and nuclear enlargement, acidophilic intranuclear inclusions, and granular basophilic cytoplasmic inclusions (Fig. 16A). Gomori's methenamine silver and PAS stain the viral glycoproteins of the cytoplasmic inclusions because of their high carbohydrate content (38). Mesenchymal cells, especially endothelium, are preferentially involved, while epithelial cell involvement is seen less frequently (Fig. 16B). CMV infections display wide variability in the degree of associated inflammation, necrosis, and tissue damage, which ranges from focal and mild to extensive with organ perforation (211). Rarely, CMV vasculitis is associated with severe infections (212).

Herpes Simplex and Varicella-Zoster

Primary infections with herpes simplex virus (HSV) are unusual in adults with AIDS because of the high rates of previous infection. However, these patients are prone to severe recurrent infections, which show delayed healing, prolonged virus shedding, and frequent relapses (213,214). HSV produces oral, labial, genital, and anal

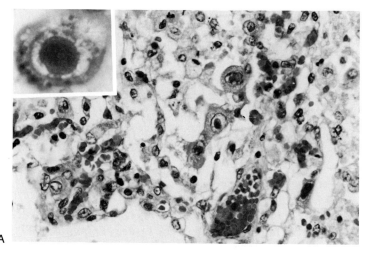

A

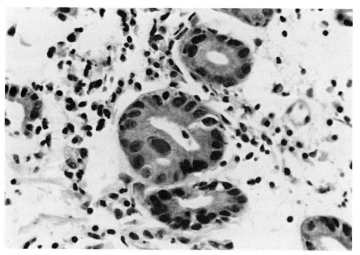

B

FIG. 16. Cytomegalovirus pneumonitis and gastritis. **A:** Pneumocytes showing cytomegaly and large intranuclear inclusions. Hematoxylin and eosin, ×200. **Inset:** Nuclear and prominent cytoplasmic inclusions. Hematoxylin and eosin, ×1,000. **B:** Gastric biopsy with cytomegalic inclusion in epithelial cell. Hematoxylin and eosin, ×250.

lesions, esophagitis, pneumonitis, and encephalitis, while the lesions of varicella-zoster (HZ) occur in a dermatomal distribution or show extensive cutaneous dissemination (215). During recurrences, patients may develop visceral disease (216). In most studies from western countries, cases reported in association with HIV infection usually have disease progression to AIDS prior to the onset of disseminated HZ infection (214). In African patients, HZ is highly predictive of HIV infection; in one study 91% of African patients with HZ were HIV-seropositive (217).

Diagnosis

Serologic tests for herpes antibody are rarely useful in AIDS patients because antibody formation occurs late in primary infection and is usually unchanged during recurrent infection. Definitive diagnosis requires demonstrating viral cytopathic effects in cytology specimens or surgical biopsies, culturing the virus from tissues, or detecting viral antigens. Cultures of fresh vesicles show high recovery rates whereas specimens from crusted lesions are usually negative. Biopsy specimens or swabs from vesicles are inoculated onto tissue monolayers capable of supporting virus growth. Viral cytopathic changes or staining of the monolayer with specific monoclonal antibodies permit rapid identification usually within 4–5 days (218).

Cytologic preparations from scrapings of fresh vesicles provide a rapid and inexpensive method to identify virally infected cells but are a relatively insensitive technique and cannot differentiate HSV types 1 and 2 from varicella-zoster infections. This procedure (Tzanck preparation) consists of unroofing a fresh vesicle and gently scraping the base of the lesion. The scrapings are transferred to a glass slide and stained with any of the routine cytologic methods (usually Wright-Giemsa or Papanicolaou). Typical viral cytopathic changes include nuclear enlargement and multinucleation with nuclear molding. The nuclear features consist of a diffuse homogenization giving the chromatin a "ground glass" appearance (Fig. 17). Alternatively, nuclei may contain prominent eosinophilic inclusions surrounded by a clear halo and prominent nuclear membrane.

Tissue biopsies of skin or mucosal lesions show vesicle formation or ulceration with dermal or submucosal necrosis and inflammation. The virally transformed cells described previously are frequently seen at the margins of the ulcer (Fig. 18). In contrast to CMV, HSV preferentially infects squamous epithelial cells whereas CMV shows a propensity for mesenchymal and endothelial cells. HSV-infected cells do not show marked cytomegaly or produce the intracytoplasmic inclusions seen in CMV-infected cells. The diagnosis in smears and in tissue sections can be confirmed by immunoperoxidase

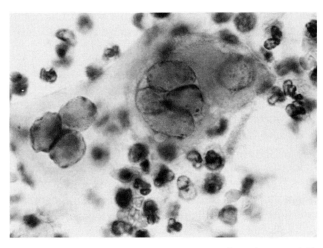

FIG. 17. Tzanck preparation demonstrating characteristic viral changes of herpes infection. Epithelial cells show multinucleation, nuclear molding, and "ground glass" nuclear chromatin. Diff-Quik, ×400.

methods to identify viral proteins or by in situ hybridization techniques that demonstrate HSV DNA (219,220).

Herpes simplex and varicella-zoster viral pneumonitis are often antedated by oral or labial lesions. Histologically, this type of viral pneumonitis usually produces parenchymal necrosis, lymphohistiocytic inflammatory infiltrates, multinucleated giant cells, and intranuclear inclusions. There may be associated necrotizing tracheobronchitis.

Evidence of disseminated herpetic infections can be detected in many visceral organs and lymph nodes. Biopsies from these sites show necrotizing changes with scattered virally transformed cells.

Other Viruses

A number of other viral infections have been described in patients with AIDS. Epstein-Barr virus (EBV), another member of the herpes virus group, is endemic in humans and serologic studies show it to be a frequent latent infection in AIDS patients. There is considerable evidence associating EBV with malignancies including lymphoma and nasopharyngeal carcinoma (221–223). Oral hairy leukoplakia, a benign papillomatous epithelial proliferation usually involving the tongue or buccal mucosa and described predominantly in AIDS patients, has been shown to contain EBV DNA sequences in most cases (224). Some children with AIDS develop a lymphocytic interstitial pneumonitis also shown to contain EBV capsid antigen and viral DNA (222). Infections with this virus can be demonstrated using DNA probes and serologic techniques (222,225,226). Histopathologic features of acute EBV infections of lymph nodes show characteristic but nonspecific hyperplastic patterns and are sometimes confused with Hodgkin's disease (227).

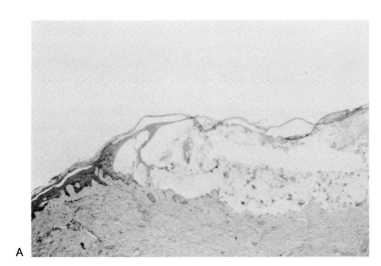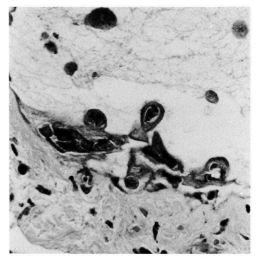

FIG. 18. Persistent herpes skin infection. **A:** Multiloculated intraepidermal vesicle. Hematoxylin and eosin, ×40. **B:** Higher magnification showing acantholysis and multinucleated giant cells. Hematoxylin and eosin, ×400.

Other viral diseases described in AIDS or AIDS-related complex include the pox virus associated with molluscum contagiosum and human papillomavirus associated with verruca vulgaris and cervical/vaginal neoplasia (228,229). Molluscum contagiosum may be generalized and severe in patients with AIDS and can clinically mimic cutaneous cryptococcosis (119). Lesions of condyloma accuminata may be large and extensive in patients with AIDS, and one study has suggested a high prevalence of cervical and vaginal cytologic abnormalities of squamous epithelium in HIV-infected women (229). Progressive multifocal leukoencephalopathy caused by a papovavirus is described in a separate chapter.

NEOPLASMS ASSOCIATED WITH HIV

Kaposi's Sarcoma

Kaposi's sarcoma (KS), the most common neoplasm occurring in association with AIDS, is recognized clinically in approximately 25% of patients at some point during their illness and has been reported in between 50% and 95% of AIDS patients at autopsy (152,230,231). Epidemiologic studies have shown the highest prevalence to be in white male homosexuals with AIDS (232).

AIDS-associated KS differs from the classical form seen in elderly individuals of Mediterranean or Jewish extraction in the sites of involvement (arms, oral cavity, trunk, and face rather than of lower extremities) and appearance (multicentric pink to violet patches, infiltrated plaques, or small angiomatoid nodules in contrast to purple macules, papules, or nodules). Although these characteristics enable a clinical diagnosis to be made, a biopsy diagnosis, particularly of early lesions, is recom-

mended. Most AIDS patients with KS have cutaneous and visceral involvement, but between 5% and 29% show visceral involvement in the absence of cutaneous lesions (233,234). In autopsy studies, many organs have been reported to be involved; however, lymph nodes, gastrointestinal tract, and lung are the most frequent sites of extracutaneous disease (152,233). Most patients with KS die as a result of opportunistic infections and only rarely as a direct consequence of their tumors (233,235).

The histogenesis and pathogenesis of KS have been extensively studied but are poorly understood. The proposed cell of origin has included most cells of mesodermal origin, but recent research has focused on the vascular (capillary) endothelium, lymphatic endothelium, or a combination of both (236–239). Many investigators favor a lymphatic origin of the tumor (238–240). Immunohistochemical comparisons between the AIDS-related KS and sporadic KS have shown no significant differences between these two forms despite the marked clinical dissimilarities (239,241). The presence of angioproliferative changes of nonlesional skin from AIDS patients, diploid DNA content, multicentric nature, and occasional reversibility have led some investigators to hypothesize that KS is a reactive proliferation rather than a true sarcoma (242). Some epidemiologic and demographic findings suggest that an infectious agent may be important in the development of the tumor. While cytomegalovirus has been most often implicated, at present the etiologic role of viruses in the pathogenesis of KS has yet to be established (243).

Clinical Characteristics

Cutaneous lesions are often first recognized on the face, oral cavity (especially hard palate), arms, and soles of feet, and can be quite subtle (244,245). They may present as asymptomatic pigmented pink to violaceous macules, papules or small angiomatoid nodules being mistaken for hemangioma, pyogenic granuloma, dermatofibroma, melanoma, molluscum contagiosum, or lichen planus (246,247). Gastrointestinal KS may cause bleeding, obstruction, and perforation, but is more commonly asymptomatic (235,248,249). Pulmonary involvement can result in cough, shortness of breath, hemoptysis, and respiratory failure as a consequence of intraalveolar hemorrhage, tracheal and bronchial obstruction, and hemorrhagic pleural effusions (250,251). Lymph node KS can be seen in a high proportion of cases with estimates varying from 30% to 95% (231). As lymph node enlargement from a variety of causes is commonly encountered in patients with AIDS, confirmation of lymphadenopathic KS requires excisional biopsy.

Diagnosis

Any cutaneous or mucous membrane pigmented lesion in a member of a high-risk group for HIV infection should raise the suspicion of KS and prompt tissue biopsy to establish a histological diagnosis. In small biopsy specimens of early skin lesions, it may be necessary to examine multiple levels, and the diagnosis of patch KS should be made cautiously in the presence of healed ulceration or at sites of previous trauma (252). Gastrointestinal tract lesions can be seen with or without cutaneous disease and usually present as either small red macules with associated submucosal hemorrhage or violaceous nodules involving the stomach and duodenum most commonly (249). Endoscopic biopsies will sometimes yield diagnostic material, although yields tend to be low because of the submucosal location of these lesions (249). Pulmonary KS occurs in between 20% and 50% of cases and clinically can be difficult to distinguish from opportunistic infections, especially *Pneumocystis carinii,* as both can have similar symptoms and show diffuse interstitial infiltrates. The bronchoscopic appearance is that of multiple discrete raised red to violaceous mucosal plaques of the trachea or bronchial tree. KS is usually confirmed by bronchoscopy without biopsy, but involvement of the parenchyma in the absence of bronchial disease may require an open lung biopsy for confirmation (250). Bone marrow involvement has rarely been reported in core biopsies (253). Fine-needle aspiration biopsies from a variety of sites infrequently yield diagnostic material (254).

Histopathology

The histopathologic appearance of AIDS-associated KS in the skin does not differ significantly from the clas-

sical, endemic, and allograft-associated types despite the marked differences in clinical behavior between these groups. Two microscopic features are seen in the lesions: vascular spaces and spindle cells. The basic histologic patterns as described by Ackerman (255) include the patch, plaque, and nodular types, although mixed patterns are commonly observed. In the early patch stage, anastomosing thin-walled vascular spaces with irregular outlines involve the upper dermis and dissect collagen bundles (256). The lining endothelial cells display little nuclear atypia, and luminal erythrocytes are infrequent. These lesions, resembling granulation tissue, reaction to trauma, or areas of recently healed ulceration, can be quite subtle and difficult to diagnose. Thin-walled anastomosing angulated and irregularly outlined vascular spaces admixed with spindle cells are the hallmark of the plaque lesion (Fig. 19A). Nodular lesions contain a predominance of spindle-shaped cells, usually in well-defined aggregates that involve the dermis but may extend into the subcutaneous tissue (Fig. 19B). Vascular slits containing erythrocytes and hemosiderin deposits between the spindle cells help distinguish KS from other sarcomas. The spindle cells frequently show erythrophagocytosis and may contain eosinophilic inclusions, the latter shown ultrastructurally to represent lysosomal residual bodies (257). In the late stages, the histologic picture may resemble fibrosarcoma with minimal nuclear atypia and occasional mitotic figures. Features said to be useful in differentiating KS from other vasoproliferative lesions include the promontory sign and the angiomatoid lesion. The former is a proliferation of jagged irregular endothelial lined spaces arising around a normal dermal vessel, while the latter is a collection of small vascular spaces lined by prominent "hobnail" endothelial cells surrounded by small numbers of proliferating spindle cells (252).

Differential Diagnosis

A number of recent reports have described cutaneous nonneoplastic angiomatous lesions in AIDS patients that may be mistaken clinically and histologically for KS (258–260). These lesions usually present as erythematous papules, dome-shaped papules and nodules, or more deeply located circumscribed tumors. Their microscopic features resemble pyogenic granuloma, lobular capillary hemangioma, and epithelioid (histiocytoid) hemangioma. In most instances, organisms similar to the cat-scratch disease bacilli have been suggested as the causative agent. However, in two separate reports, cytomegalovirus and Epstein-Barr virus DNA have also been identified in these lesions (260,261). Bacteria can be demonstrated in the lesions within endothelial cells and neutrophilic aggregates by the Warthin-Starry silver stain and electron microscopy. A specific antiserum devel-

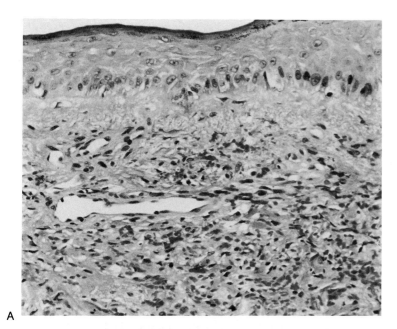

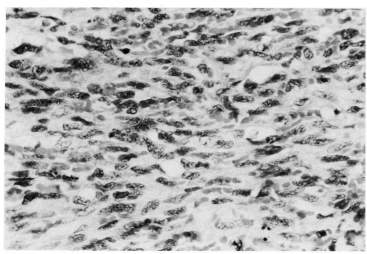

FIG. 19. Cutaneous Kaposi's sarcoma. **A:** Vascular spaces and spindle cells characterize the plaque lesion. Hematoxylin and eosin, ×100. **B:** Late stage lesion with predominantly spindle cell proliferation and extravasated erythrocytes. Hematoxylin and eosin, ×200.

oped against the cat-scratch disease bacillus stains the organism using an immunoperoxidase method (262). The term *bacillary angiomatosis* (BA) has been proposed for this pseudoneoplastic lesion (258). The presence of neutrophils, granular debris, and clumps of bacteria in the absence of spindle cells, bizarrely shaped vascular channels, and eosinophilic inclusions helps to distinguish BA from KS. The microscopic features of BA resemble the cutaneous form of bartonellosis—"verruga peruana"—a benign cutaneous vascular proliferation associated with systemic infections with *Bartonella bacilliformis* (263). Table 2 highlights the important histologic features of BA and KS. Also included in the differential diagnosis are angiosarcoma, pyogenic granuloma, and hemangioma. Angiosarcomas generally exhibit greater endothelial atypia and poor circumscription. Hemangioma and pyogenic granuloma are usually more circumscribed and lack the neutrophilic debris, and bac-

teria are not demonstrable. Accurate diagnosis of BA is important as treatment with erythromycin, doxycycline, and some antimycobacterial agents has resulted in complete and rapid resolution of the lesions (264).

Extracutaneous KS

The histopathology of lymphadenopathic KS is that of a focal or diffuse expansion of the sinuses by a vascular and spindle cell proliferation that may progress to the classic nodular pattern. The subcapsular sinusoids, medulla, and T-cell zones are usually involved first, with eventual involvement of germinal centers. Eosinophilic globules can be found in macrophages or spindle cells. The lesions may coexist with infectious processes, malignant lymphoma, and the various reactive patterns described in AIDS-associated lymphadenopathy. The

TABLE 2. *Histologic features of bacillary angiomatosis and Kaposi's sarcoma*

Histologic feature	Bacillary angiomatosis	Kaposi's sarcoma
Circumscription	Good	Poor
Lobular capillary proliferation	Present	Absent
Endothelial cell shape	Polygonal	Spindled
Protuberant endothelial cells	Present	Absent
Nuclear atypia	Present, nuclei vesicular, never hypochromatic	Sometimes, but usually nodular stage
Smooth muscle around vessels	Absent	Absent
Vascular spaces	Round	Slitlike, bizarre
Hyaline globules	Absent	Present
Neutrophils	Numerous, with debris	Absent unless ulcerated
Eosinophils	Absent	Absent
Granular material (bacteria)	Present in most cases on H & E	Absent
Stromal edema	Present	Absent
Immunophenotype (FVIIIRAg/UEA)[a]	+/+	−/+

Adapted from LeBoit et al. (258).
[a] Factor VIII-related antigen/*Ulex europaeus* lectin.

main entity in the differential diagnosis of early node involvement is nodal angiomatosis.

AIDS-associated bronchopulmonary KS may be the first site of involvement recognized, but more commonly the diagnosis has been established by prior skin or oral biopsy. KS grows first along lymphatic pathways and involves intralobular septae and pleura, and forms distinct proliferations around bronchi and pulmonary vessels (250). The lesions consist predominantly of spindle cells and, to a lesser extent, small vascular lumina and variable inflammation that grow in a diffuse fashion rather than as nodules (265).

Endoscopic biopsies of the gastrointestinal tract can show diffuse mucosal plaque-like involvement or polypoid proliferations whose histologic appearance is similar to that described in the skin. The tumors usually first involve the submucosa, but later intramucosal lesions also occur (Fig. 20). Involvement of the muscularis propria is uncommon (249).

Involvement of other organs including liver, spleen, heart, adrenal gland, and kidney is seen less frequently (265,266). The lesions can present as distinct parenchymal nodules or infiltrate along preexisting lymphatic and vascular pathways. Microscopically, the classic mixture of spindle cells and vascular spaces are recapitulated regardless of the site of involvement.

Malignant Lymphoma and Lymphadenopathy

AIDS-associated malignant lymphomas may be preceded by multifocal lymph node enlargement termed *persistent generalized lymphadenopathy* (PGL) (267, 268). PGL is defined by the CDC as palpable lymphade-

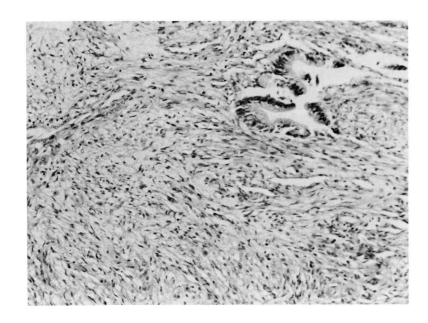

FIG. 20. Kaposi's sarcoma involving the stomach. The lamina propria is extensively infiltrated by a spindle cell proliferation with few vascular spaces. Residual gland is seen in upper right. Hematoxylin and eosin, ×100.

nopathy (≥1.0 cm) at two or more extrainguinal sites persisting for more than 3 months in the absence of a concurrent illness or conditions other than HIV infection to explain the findings (269). Biopsies of lymph nodes from patients with PGL show three characteristic, although nonspecific, histopathologic patterns of reaction (270,271). These patterns have been shown to correlate with the progression of immune dysfunction and the clinical course (272–274).

Histologic Patterns Seen in Lymphadenopathy

In florid follicular hyperplasia (type I or A pattern), the normal architecture is altered by a marked proliferation of irregularly shaped follicles in the cortex and medulla. The follicles may show confluence and attenuation of the mantle zones. The germinal centers contain a mixture of cell types, including large and small lymphocytes, immunoblasts, tingible body macrophages, nuclear debris, and numerous mitoses (Fig. 21). Invagination of mantle zone lymphocytes into the germinal centers—termed *follicular lysis* results in islands of large transformed germinal center lymphocytes and disruption of follicles. Interfollicular zones show a prominent vasculature with a mixture of small lymphocytes, immunoblasts, plasma cells, and histiocytes. Neutrophilic aggregates and multinucleated giant cells similar to the Warthin-Finkeldey giant cells of measles are frequently observed. Changes resembling dermatopathic lymphadenitis and prominent histiocytic proliferation with erythrophagocytosis may also be seen.

Lymphoid depletion (type III or pattern C) shows atrophic "burned out" follicles with depletion of lymphocytes, absent or vestigial germinal centers, and promi-

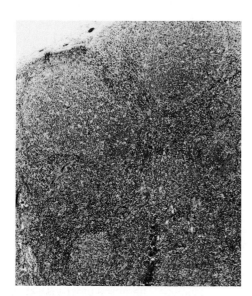

FIG. 21. Lymph node biopsy demonstrating marked follicular and interfollicular hyperplasia (type I pattern). Hematoxylin and eosin, ×40.

nent vasculature. Interfollicular zones show loss of lymphocytes and excessive vascularization. Sinuses are dilated and usually contain numerous histiocytes, some of which show erythrophagocytosis. Multinucleated giant cells may also be seen. This pattern, which has the worst prognosis, is associated with the shortest intervals of progression to AIDS and the shortest patient survivals.

Mixed or intermediate patterns of reaction (type II or pattern B) include features of both florid hyperplasia and lymphoid depletion. This pattern is strongly associated with the impending development of AIDS (270,271).

At the present time lymph node biopsy is rarely done in HIV-infected patients with PGL. It is selectively performed to diagnose treatable opportunistic infections, lymphadenopathic Kaposi's sarcoma, and malignant lymphoma.

Malignant Lymphoma

Non-Hodgkin's lymphoma (NHL) is the second most common neoplasm associated with AIDS. Most cases have been reported in homosexual men and intravenous drug users, although lymphomas can occur in individuals belonging to any AIDS risk group. PGL precedes the development of NHL in about one-third of patients (267,268). Most AIDS-associated NHL present with widely disseminated disease usually involving extranodal sites, particularly gastrointestinal tract, central nervous system, liver, bone marrow, and skin. These tumors belong to three aggressive histopathologic subtypes: small cell noncleaved; large cell immunoblastic, and large cell noncleaved types (Fig. 22) (275). However, a variety of low- and intermediate-grade lymphomas have also been reported and are listed later in this section.

About 95% of AIDS-associated NHL are of B-cell origin, many of which express surface immunoglobulins, B-cell restricted antigens, immunoglobulin and c-myc gene rearrangements, and chromosomal translocations (276). HIV does not appear to be directly involved in malignant transformation, as HIV DNA sequences have not been found in the genome of these neoplastic lymphoid cells (277). AIDS-associated NHL shares features with Epstein-Barr virus-induced African Burkitt's lymphoma and B-cell NHL seen in other immunodeficiency states including multiple clonal B-cell expansions and c-myc gene rearrangement and translocation (278,279). However, only about one-third of AIDS-associated NHL have detectable Epstein-Barr virus DNA sequences or proteins (276,280).

Hodgkin's malignant lymphoma has been described in HIV-positive individuals, and, like AIDS-associated NHL, the majority of patients present with extensive disseminated disease that often involves extranodal sites,

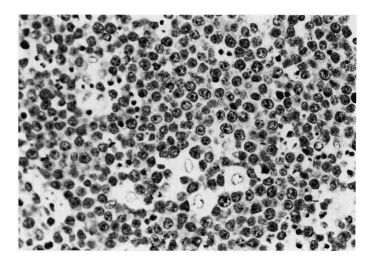

FIG. 22. AIDS-associated small noncleaved cell lymphoma involving lymph node. The presence of benign histiocytes within tumor imparts a "starry sky" appearance. Hematoxylin and eosin, ×250.

including bone marrow, liver, skin, and soft tissues. In contrast with classic Hodgkin's disease, most patients with AIDS-associated Hodgkin's disease have an aggressive clinical course and a rapidly fatal outcome. The distribution of histopathologic categories includes mixed cellularity, nodular sclerosis, and lymphocyte-depleted types (Fig. 23) (275,281,282).

Other Malignancies

Many other hematopoietic and nonhematopoietic neoplasms have been reported in HIV-positive individuals (Table 3) (229,283–314). While the occurrence of many of these tumors is probably coincidental, some investigators believe tumor development is facilitated by the immunosuppression of HIV infection (315). These include low-grade B-cell NHL, T-cell leukemias and lymphomas, plasmacytomas, acute lymphoblastic leukemia, multiple myelomas, squamous cell carcinomas of several sites, adenocarcinomas of pancreas and colon, malignant melanomas, metastasizing basal cell carcinomas, thymomas, mesenchymal tumors including fibrosarcomas, liposarcomas, leiomyosarcomas, leiomyomas, and angiolipomas, and germ cell tumors including seminomas and embryonal carcinomas. Anorectal carcinomas and squamous cell carcinomas of the oral cavity are the most frequently reported malignancies after Kaposi's sarcoma and malignant lymphomas (283,284). Some of the squamous neoplasms have been associated with infections by human papillomavirus (287,315,316).

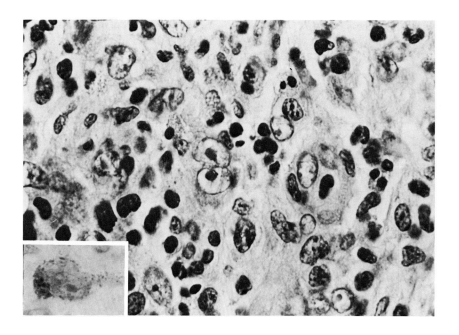

FIG. 23. AIDS-associated mixed cellularity Hodgkin's disease. Polymorphous infiltrate including the presence of Reed-Sternberg cell. Hematoxylin and eosin, ×200. **Inset:** Leu M-1 (CD-15) immunoperoxidase stain of atypical mononuclear variant. Avidin-biotin complex, hematoxylin counterstain, ×1,000.

TABLE 3. *Neoplastic disorders reported in association with HIV infection*

Disorder	Reference
Kaposi's sarcoma	
Non-Hodgkin's lymphoma[a]	275,276,280,289,292,296,297,315
Hodgkin's lymphoma	281,282
Squamous cell carcinoma of anorectum, head and neck, cervix and vagina, conjunctiva, skin, and lung	229,283,284,287,290,295,303,310,315
T-cell leukemia	275,313
Plasmacytoma	311
Multiple myeloma	312
Acute myelogenous leukemia/myelodysplasia	286
Adenocarcinoma of pancreas, stomach, and colon	302,307,313
Malignant melanoma/eruptive dysplastic nevi	288,293,294
Metastasizing basal cell carcinoma	301
Thymoma	309
Mesenchymal tumors including liposarcoma, leiomyosarcoma, fibrosarcoma, leiomyoma, and angiolipoma	298,305,308,314
Germ cell tumors including seminoma and embryonal carcinoma	291,304,306

[a] These lymphomas are commonly of the B-cell phenotype; however, lymphomas of the T-cell phenotype have also been observed.

POORLY UNDERSTOOD COMPLICATIONS OF AIDS

Cardiac Pathology

Early reports of cardiac pathology in autopsy studies focused on opportunistic infections and neoplasms involving the heart, and later reports focused on other cardiac lesions. Clinical studies subsequently established the presence of cardiac dysfunction in patients with HIV infection in the absence of opportunistic infection (317). The incidence of symptomatic heart disease in AIDS patients is estimated to be approximately 7% (318).

Infectious and neoplastic involvement is usually seen in the setting of systemic disease. The findings of cardiac disease unrelated to opportunistic infections and neoplasia emerged in a report of dilated cardiomyopathy in 1986 (319). Since that report several patterns of cardiac dysfunction in AIDS patients have been described that may be grouped into pericardial effusions and tamponade, dilated cardiomyopathy, heart failure without ventricular dilatation, refractory ventricular tachycardia, sudden death, and systemic thromboembolic disease (318).

Pericardial effusions are frequently detected in AIDS patients (320,321). Most often these effusions, which may result in cardiac tamponade, are seen in association with opportunistic infections (e.g., toxoplasmosis, cytomegalovirus infection) and malignancies (e.g., Kaposi's sarcoma, malignant lymphoma) (62,322). When cardiac tamponade is present, infectious or neoplastic involvement is found in 88% of the reported cases.

AIDS-related dilated cardiomyopathy (DCM) has been associated with ventricular dilatation and idiopathic myocarditis. Ventricular dilatation may involve the left or right ventricles. Isolated right ventricular dilatation usually reflects severe pulmonary disease. The myocardium grossly appears normal in thickness, flaccid, and pale. Enlargement of valvular annuli is seen in biventricular dilatation. Cardiac hypertrophy (heart weight > 400 g) is usually absent. Microscopic findings with the exclusion of cases with myocarditis include enlarged myocyte nuclei with bizarre shapes, lipochrome pigment deposits, variable interstitial fibrosis, and edema (319,323). Myocyte fiber loss is variable.

Myocarditis, defined as myocyte degeneration or necrosis associated with adjacent inflammatory infiltrates, has been observed in some cases of dilated cardiomyopathy, ventricular tachycardia and sudden death, and pericardial effusions (323). Clinical symptoms were seen in 58% of the cases that were detected at autopsy (324). Idiopathic myocarditis was detected by endomyocardial biopsy in a patient with refractory ventricular tachycardia (325). The cause of myocarditis in HIV infection remains obscure in the majority of cases (323). No correlation has been found between therapy and the occurrence of myocarditis (323,324). Viral-induced injury either directly or by activation of latent viral infections by immunosuppression has been proposed.

Nonbacterial thrombotic endocarditis (NBTE) is usually a right-sided, asymptomatic finding at autopsy. The vegetations are small masses of fibrin and blood that collect on the valve leaflets along the lines of closure. Either side of the heart may be affected. The vegetations resemble the lesions seen in acute rheumatic endocarditis. These lesions are commonly seen in chronic debilitating conditions such as metastatic cancer, renal failure, or chronic sepsis. Their presence in AIDS patients probably reflects the underlying severe illness. Involvement of all four cardiac valves has been reported. Complications are rare, but one patient with cerebral infarctions has been reported (322).

Other cardiac lesions such as the accumulation of lipochrome pigment, myofibrillar loss, and attenuation of myofibers have been reported (62,323). The significance of these findings is not well understood at this time.

HIV-Associated Enteropathy

Diarrhea, weight loss, and malabsorption have been recognized as major manifestations of HIV infection and may precede the AIDS-related complex (ARC) or AIDS stage of HIV infection (326). Mucosal injury may result from immunosuppression leading to the development of opportunistic infections or AIDS-associated malignancies. Some of the opportunistic infections, such as cryptosporidiosis, are primary for the gastrointestinal tract (75,161,168,327). Alternatively, evidence for direct mucosal injury by HIV itself has been recognized as HIV-associated enteropathy (328).

HIV-associated enteropathy has been postulated in those patients who do not have a demonstrable specific infectious agent. HIV antigen and virus have been demonstrated in the lamina propria of intestinal biopsies (329,330). Diarrhea and malabsorption have been documented in 29% of patients who are HIV-seropositive but have negative stool cultures and other examinations for the infectious agents common to AIDS patients (331). Duodenal mucosal biopsies in these patients may show nonspecific changes of mucosal atrophy, normal crypt depth, and decreased mitotic activity (329). Jejunal biopsies have demonstrated an increase in intraepithelial lymphocytes over control subjects (331). Rectal biopsy findings include focal epithelial cell degeneration (apoptosis) with intranuclear viral inclusions (328). Electron microscopy studies demonstrate contact between intraepithelial lymphocytes and apoptotic cells, which suggests a cell-mediated immune response. Apoptosis is not a typical feature of infectious enteritides, but has been observed in acute graft-versus-host disease of the colon following bone marrow transplantation. It has been postulated that viral infection induces changes in the cell membranes that trigger a host response and apoptosis (328). In those patients with diarrhea the changes seen are most pronounced. Mucosal atrophy, crypt hyperplasia, and lymphoplasmacytic infiltration of the lamina propria are not specific for HIV enteropathy. Similar changes may be seen in other enteric infections (332).

Damage to autonomic nerve bundles in the jejunal mucosal lamina propria has been described and is similar to that reported in laxative abuse, diabetic autonomic neuropathy, inflammatory bowel disease, and amyloidosis (333).

The carrier rate for enteric pathogens increases for the population of HIV-infected patients with AIDS. In these patients with diarrhea and malabsorption, one-third will be found to have a treatable infection, which underscores the importance of searching for enteric pathogens.

Renal Pathology

The renal manifestations of HIV infection may be the result of indirect or direct mechanisms (334–336). These include acute tubular necrosis, allergic interstitial nephritis (AIN), immune complex-associated glomerulonephritis, and focal segmental glomerulosclerosis.

Acute tubular necrosis is not usually directly attributable to HIV but secondarily follows episodes of hypovolemic shock and sepsis, or to exposure to radiocontrast agents. Acute interstitial nephritis or acute tubular necrosis may be the result of therapy with trimethoprim–sulfamethoxazole, gentamicin, pentamidine, acyclovir, and amphotericin B. Biopsies are infrequently performed in the typical clinical setting of AIN but may reveal interstitial edema, epithelial damage, and inflammatory infiltrates. Eosinophils may be present in variable numbers. Toxic or ischemic injuries occur in a clinical setting, which likewise infrequently leads to a biopsy. The histopathologic findings at biopsy include low flattened tubular epithelium with sloughing, loss of brush border, dilatation of tubules, mild interstitial edema, and sparse cellular infiltrates. The acute renal failure experienced by these patients often contributes to their death because of underlying serious illness.

Immune complex-mediated glomerulonephritis has been reported in sporadic cases, often related to various infectious diseases in these patients. Mesangial proliferation and diffuse proliferative glomerulonephritis have been described (337,338). Immunoglobulins and complement proteins are usually seen in the mesangial areas and along capillary loops by immunofluorescence.

Fluid and electrolyte abnormalities are frequently seen in these critically ill patients, with hyponatremia being one of the most common. Gastrointestinal fluid loss, before hospital admission, is the etiology of the hyponatremia in 40% of patients with AIDS. Mortality in hospitalized hyponatremic patients with AIDS is twice as high as in normonatremic patients (339).

HIV-Associated Nephropathy

In 1984, Rao and associates (340) recognized a renal disorder characterized by heavy proteinuria and progression to renal failure in AIDS patients. Since then, HIV-associated nephropathy has been recognized in many medical centers but has been controversial for several reasons (339). Initially, the lesion was described in AIDS patients with a high proportion of drug abuse cases. Controversy was spawned because some centers, notably those in San Francisco (341), did not see this lesion with

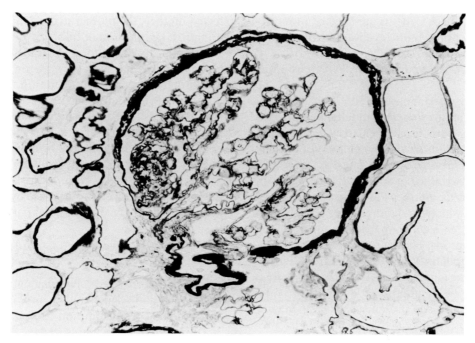

FIG. 24. Biopsy specimen from a patient with AIDS nephropathy. The glomerulus is segmentally sclerosed. Gomori's methenamine-silver, ×200.

the same frequency. Later, this renal lesion was shown to be present in children with AIDS, which strengthened the argument for a primary causal relationship (342). A second controversial point was whether this lesion was secondary to immunological changes that accompany AIDS or was just associated with HIV infection. Again, recently the lesion has been described in patients with HIV infection, but no manifestation of AIDS (343). So,

in spite of initial controversies, acceptance of HIV nephropathy is generally agreed as valid.

The clinical features of HIV-associated nephropathy have the following characteristics. The lesion may be found in asymptomatic, HIV-positive patients or in patients with ARC and AIDS. Males are more frequently affected than females, with variations in incidence in different geographic areas (i.e., high in New York City, low

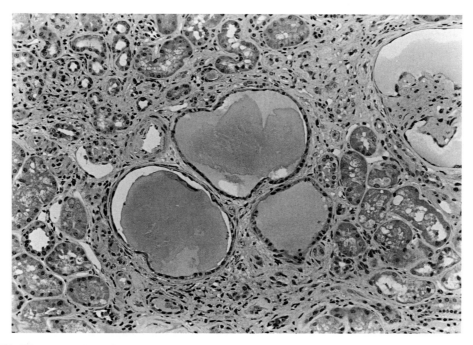

FIG. 25. Biopsy specimen from a patients with AIDS nephropathy. The interstitium is fibrotic and dilated tubules are present. Hematoxylin and eosin, ×200.

in San Francisco). Black patients are affected more frequently than white. Proteinuria is always present and is usually heavy. The course is usually marked by early and rapidly progressive azotemia. Mild hypertension is present.

Morphologic manifestations of HIV-associated nephropathy are found in glomeruli, tubules, and interstitium. The kidneys are usually enlarged. Progressive changes may be seen in the affected glomeruli. Initially the epithelial cells become swollen and the underlying capillary loops are wrinkled or collapsed. Occasional intraluminal foam cells are seen. In the more advanced lesions the capillary loops are completely collapsed, with expansion of the mesangial matrix–basement membrane material (Fig. 24). Plasma proteins may accumulate within the capillary loops (hyalinosis). In far advanced lesions more glomeruli are involved and there is complete capillary obliteration.

Microcystic dilation and proteinaceous casts may be found in the tubules. Interstitial fibrosis and tubular atrophy are seen as the glomerular lesion advances (Fig. 25). Interstitial infiltrates containing lymphocytes, histiocytes, and plasma cells are present.

Ultrastructural studies demonstrate a diffuse effacement of epithelial foot processes and detachment of cells from the basement membranes. Inclusions of tubuloreticular bodies are almost always present in the vascular endothelium. Cytoplasmic inclusions of parallel stacks and cylindrical confronting cisternae, also known as test tube- and ring-shaped forms, have been described. Immunofluorescence studies demonstrated C_3, C1q, and IgM in the sclerotic segments. Granular deposits of these proteins may also be seen in mesangial areas. In vitro hybridization techniques have now demonstrated proviral HIV DNA in the tubular and glomerular epithelial cells.

PATHOLOGY OF AIDS IN CHILDREN

Since the first published series of AIDS in children (344,345), over 2,000 cases have been reported to the CDC. Pediatric AIDS cases constitute about 1.5% of total AIDS cases.

There are basic similarities between pediatric and adult AIDS in major clinical features and pathologic lesions. However, pediatric AIDS is different with respect to mode of transmission, frequency, and types of certain clinical features, immunologic abnormalities, and pathologic lesions. These differences will be highlighted, and the pathologic lesions that occur more frequently or predominantly in children and perinatal pathology of HIV infection will be described in this section.

Mode of Transmission

There are two major modes of transmission (346): (1) transplacental/perinatal transmission from an HIV infected mother (the mother may or may not have symptomatic HIV infection or full-blown AIDS); and (2) parenteral transmission through transfusion of infected blood or blood products (e.g., factor VIII). Of the two, the former is by far more common. Transmission can occur prenatally, during delivery, and possibly postnatally via breast milk. Of these, transplacental transmission with prenatal intrauterine exposure seems to present the greatest risk. The risk estimates of transmission of HIV from infected mothers to their infants vary from 25% to 35%. The most common risk factor for HIV in the mother is intravenous drug use by herself and/or by her male heterosexual or bisexual partners.

Clinical Features and Immunologic Abnormalities

Failure to thrive, fever, lymphadenopathy, respiratory symptoms and signs, and neurologic abnormalities are among the most common clinical features (344,345, 347). Immunologic features include both T- and B-cell abnormalities such as cutaneous anergy, low absolute T-helper cell counts, reversed T-helper/suppressor cell ratio, lack of response to mitogens, and polyclonal hypergammaglobulinemia.

Pathologic Lesions

All the lesions described in adults occur in children with AIDS. Although these lesions occur with different frequency, lesions of lymphoreticular, central nervous, respiratory and digestive systems, and heart and kidneys have all been reported in pediatric AIDS cases as have various infections and malignancies (4,348). The following lesions are seen predominantly, or at least more frequently, in children with AIDS: (1) thymic lesions (primary lesions), (2) pulmonary lymphoid lesions (associated lesions), (3) systemic lymphoproliferative disorder (associated lesions), and (4) arteriopathy (lesion of undetermined pathogenesis). Most of these lesions occur in adults but are rare or uncommon in them.

The lesions in the thymus and lungs and those related to the systemic lymphoproliferative disorder and arteriopathy in children will be discussed and compared with those occurring in adults. Similarities, differences, and frequency of these lesions in adults with AIDS will also be described.

Lesions of the Thymus

Three types of lesions have been noted in biopsy and autopsy specimens of the thymus (4,348).

1. Precocious involution is characterized by marked depletion to virtual absence of lymphocytes, loss of corticomedullary differentiation, and microcystic dilatation of Hassall's corpuscles (HC), which are present

in normal numbers. Hyalinization of the cortex and medulla is present in some cases at autopsy. The location, configuration, and blood vessels of the thymus are normal. These features resemble age and stress-related involutionary changes but occur prematurely and are out of proportion to the severity of stress. There is marked reduction in weight of the thymus often to less than 1 g.

2. Dysinvolution (Fig. 26) is characterized by all the features noted above except that HC are virtually absent. Rare HC can be demonstrated in an occasional lobule by studying step serial sections of the thymus. These features, particularly the virtual absence of HC, resemble the dysplastic thymus seen in certain congenital immune deficiency syndromes—hence the term *dysinvolution.*

3. Thymitis is characterized by one of the following features: lymphoid follicles with germinal centers in the medulla, focal or diffuse lymphomononuclear, or lymphoplasmacytic infiltrate disrupting the normal architecture of the thymus or multinucleated giant cells in the medulla.

The etiology and precise target cell in thymic injury are not known. However, it is possible that thymic epithelial cells may be directly injured by HIV since: (1) HIV has been isolated from a thymic biopsy specimen in one of our cases and from the thymus of a 20-week-old fetus, and (2) simian immunodeficiency virus (SIV) has been demonstrated by immunoperoxidase staining in the thymic epithelial cells in rhesus monkeys with an AIDS-like disease complex (4).

It is of interest to note that severe involutionary changes with thymic epithelial injury have been reported in adults with AIDS (349). Thymic enlargement with thymitis characterized by presence of lymphoid follicles with germinal centers and vascularized lymphoid follicles in the medulla resembling those seen in Castleman's disease has been observed in an adult with AIDS (350). Thymic injury in AIDS thus may lead to defective T-cell differentiation and maturation and contribute to the immune deficiency in AIDS both in children and adults.

Lesions of the Lungs

Pulmonary lesions associated with the frequently observed respiratory symptoms and signs in children with AIDS are listed in Table 4. The lesions related to pulmonary opportunistic and pathogenic bacterial infections are the same as in adults. The pulmonary lymphoid lesions including the systemic lymphoproliferative disorder are seen much less frequently in adults.

Lymphoid Lesions

These are of two types: pulmonary lymphoid hyperplasia/lymphoid interstitial pneumonitis complex (PLH/LIP complex) (3,351) and polyclonal polymorphic B-cell lymphoproliferative disorder (PBLD), which is a systemic disorder with prominent pulmonary involvement, and will be described separately in the next section. Peribronchiolar lymphoid nodules commonly with germinal centers characterize PLH (Fig. 27). The

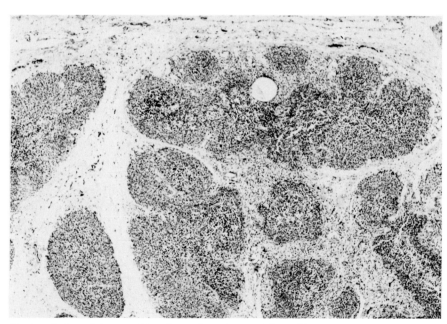

FIG. 26. Dysinvolution of thymus. Note loss of corticomedullary differentiation, lymphocytic depletion of both cortex and medulla, and markedly reduced number of Hassall's corpuscles, only one of which is present in one of the lobules. Hematoxylin and eosin, ×20.

TABLE 4. *Comparison of pulmonary lesions in children and adults with AIDS*

Type of lesion	Children	Adults
PLH/LIP complex	Commonest pulmonary lesion	Uncommon
DIP	May represent response around other pulmonary lesions	Not reported
Bacterial pneumonia	More common; severe necrotizing lesions	Less common
Opportunistic infections	Relatively less common	More common
Lymphoproliferative disorder (PBLD)	Part of systemic involvment, intermediate between benign and malignant	Rare
Malignant lymphoma	Rare	Rare
Kaposi's sarcoma	Not reported	Part of systemic involvement
Diffuse alveolar damage (DAD)	Common	Common
NIP	Not reported	Rare, ? related to PLH/LIP spectrum
LB	Not reported	Rare, ? related to PLH/LIP spectrum

DIP, desquamative interstitial pneumonitis; LB, lymphocytic bronchiolitis; NIP, nonspecific interstitial pneumonitis; PBLD, polyclonal polymorphic B-cell lymphoproliferative disorder; PLH/LIP complex, pulmonary lymphoid hyperplasia/lymphoid interstitial pneumonitis complex.

lymphoid nodules are composed of mature and immature lymphoid cells of the germinal center with plasma cells at the periphery. Diffuse infiltration of the alveolar septa by mature and immature lymphoid cells, plasmacytoid lymphocytes, and plasma cells with occasional Russell bodies characterize LIP (Fig. 28). Nodular aggregates of lymphoid cells are seen in some foci. There is no involvement of blood vessels or destruction of bronchi. No viral inclusions are seen. Special stains for fungi, acid-fast bacilli, and *Pneumocystis carinii* are negative. Immunoperoxidase stains for κ and λ light chains of immunoglobulins show that the pulmonary lymphoid infiltrates are polyclonal.

With experience of larger numbers of cases, the overlap between PLH and LIP as evidenced by (1) variable degrees of alveolar septal infiltration in cases that could otherwise be labeled as PLH, (2) presence of peribronchiolar lymphoid nodules in cases that could be labeled as LIP, and (3) gradual transition between (1) and (2) became more evident and of more common occurrence. Therefore, it was recommended that these lesions be designated as PLH/LIP complex (351).

Besides B cells, demonstrated by routine histologic methods and by immunoperoxidase stain for light chains, T cells are also present in the lesions of PLH/LIP complex shown by cell marker studies on bronchoalveo-

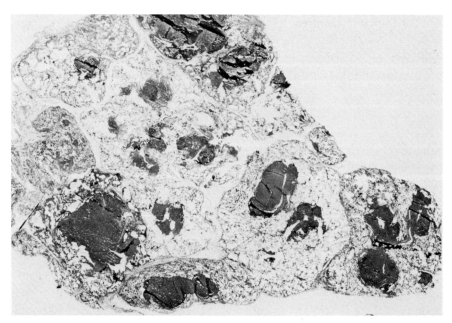

FIG. 27. Lung biopsy specimen showing lymphoid nodules around bronchioles. Note slight extension of lymphoid infiltrate into adjacent alveolar septa and germinal centers vaguely discernible at this magnification (PLH/LIP complex). Hematoxylin and eosin, ×10.

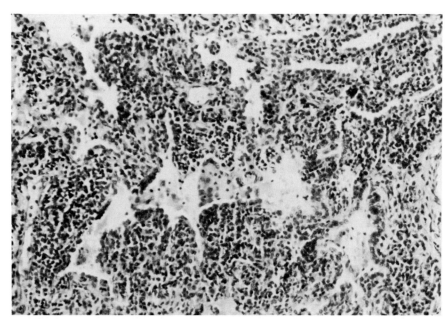

FIG. 28. Lung biopsy specimen showing dense infiltration of alveolar septa by lymphoid cells (PLH/LIP complex). Hematoxylin and eosin, ×100.

lar lavage fluid or lung biopsy tissue. T8 cells predominate in the T-cell population.

PLH/LIP complex has been described in adults with AIDS (53). It occurs much less frequently. However, the recent study by Guillon et al. (352) indicates that PLH/ LIP complex diagnosed by lymphocytosis in bronchoalveolar lavage fluid is more common in adults than generally thought. The lesion in adults has been labeled as LIP or lymphocytic alveolitis. Although detailed descriptions and illustrations are lacking, it is apparent from the limited accounts (53,352) that the lesion in adults represents PLH/LIP complex similar to that in children.

Although the pathogenesis of pulmonary lymphoid lesions is not yet established with certainty, there is evidence to suggest that both EBV and HIV may be etiologically related (4,353).

Diffuse Alveolar Damage

Diffuse alveolar damage (DAD) is seen in both biopsy and autopsy specimens. The exudative phase is characterized by hyaline membrane formation, interstitial and alveolar edema, mild mixed interstitial inflammatory infiltrate, and focal intraalveolar hemorrhage (Fig. 29). In the proliferative phase there is cuboidal metaplasia of alveolar epithelium, interstitial fibroblastic proliferation, and interstitial edema.

A variety of pathogenetic factors, which include oxygen toxicity, pulmonary infections, sepsis, and shock relate to DAD. One or more of these factors are operative in individual cases, and DAD may obscure the infectious nature of the lesion. In adults, DAD related to similar factors is seen. However, in some cases of adult AIDS

features of DAD with proliferative changes in the lung biopsy are present without any demonstrable pathogenetic factors (354).

In addition to these lesions occurring in children and adults, two inflammatory lesions, nonspecific interstitial pneumonitis (NIP) (355) and lymphocytic bronchiolitis (LB) (356), have been described in isolated cases of AIDS in symptomatic adults. In NIP histologic features are essentially those of a combination of exudative and proliferative phases of DAD and consist of alveolar edema, fibrin deposition, hyaline membranes, interstitial inflammation, and loose and dense interstitial fibrosis. The lesion is labeled NIP, presumably because the inflammatory component is more prominent. In a later article on this subject published by the same group, the inflammatory component of the lesion was apparently more prominent (356a). In most instances NIP is seen in association with or following other pulmonary lesions, such as KS, drug reactions, drug abuse, or PC pneumonitis and shows prominent fibroproliferative changes. However, in a minority of the patients no associated factor or other pulmonary lesion is found. In this latter group NIP is characterized by interstitial lymphoid cell aggregates and absence of loose or dense interstitial fibrosis. Hyaline membranes are seen in some cases. The condition with only interstitial lymphocytic infiltrate without hyaline membranes has also been described in adults with AIDS having no respiratory symptoms or signs. The importance of recognition of NIP is related to similarities between clinical features of NIP and pulmonary opportunistic infections, particularly PC pneumonitis.

LB has been reported in only one case (356). It is characterized by an intense infiltration of the wall of terminal

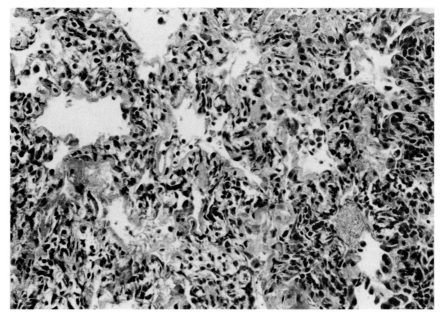

FIG. 29. Lung biopsy showing diffuse alveolar damage. Note the hyaline membranes and alveolar septal inflammatory infiltrate. The alveolus in the lower right corner contains foamy exudate (Gomori's methenamine silver stain revealed *Pneumocystis carinii*). Hematoxylin and eosin, ×400.

and respiratory bronchioles by lymphocytes and plasma cells. An increased number of T8 suppressor cells was found in a bronchoalveolar lavage specimen.

Both NIP and LB need to be characterized further with detailed description and illustration of pathologic features. It is possible that NIP and LB in adults are less severe variants of the PLH/LIP complex described above in children.

Systemic Lymphoproliferative Disorder

In four children with AIDS a systemic lymphoproliferative disorder with prominent involvement of lungs and less severe involvement of liver, spleen, kidneys, other extranodal sites, and lymph nodes was seen (4) (Figs. 30 and 31). There was no involvement of the brain.

Histologically, the cellular infiltrates in the various organs mentioned above and in skin, skeletal muscle, and salivary glands were polymorphic and consisted of an admixture of lymphocytes, plasma cells, plasmacytoid lymphocytes, and immature lymphoid cells or immunoblasts. The polyclonal nature of the lymphoid infiltrates was demonstrated by the presence of both κ and λ light chain immunoglobulins in paraffin sections of different organs stained by an immunoperoxidase method. In the kidneys and spleen, vascular invasion by the cellular infiltrate was noted. It appears that this lymphoproliferative disorder is distinctive and it has been designated polyclonal polymorphic B-cell lymphoproliferative disorder (PBLD). It is considered to be intermediate between a benign and a full-fledged malignant lymphoproliferation. In two cases PBLD appeared to represent a progression of PLH/LIP complex, while in other cases it seemed to arise de novo.

A spectrum of lymphoproliferation (follicular hyperplasia of lymph nodes, PLH/LIP complex, lymphoid hyperplasia of GI tract, lymphoid follicles in the thymus, and nodal and extranodal malignant lymphoma) similar to that in children can also be proposed for adults with

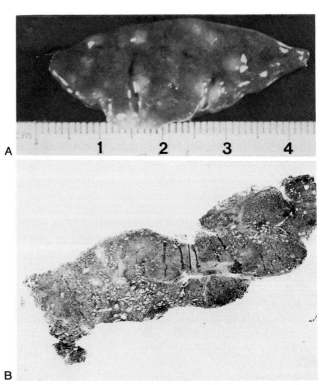

FIG. 30. Polyclonal polymorphic B-cell lymphoproliferative disorder (PBLD) involving the lung. **A:** Subpleural grayish-white nodules seen on gross examination. **B:** Whole mount of histologic section from the same lung. Note multinodular involvement. Hematoxylin and eosin, ×5.

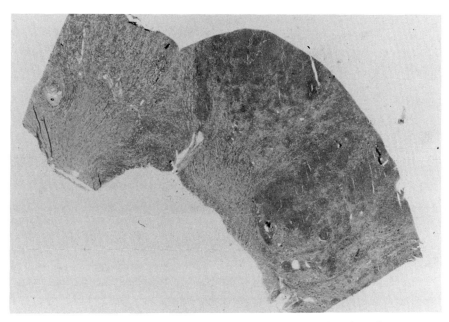

FIG. 31. PBLD involving kidney. Hematoxylin and eosin, ×5.

AIDS. Thus, the following lymphoid lesions described in adults may belong to such a spectrum: follicular hyperplasia of lymph nodes, adenoidal hypertrophy (357), PLH/LIP complex, EBV-related lymphoproliferative disorder (358) similar to PBLD in children, and nodal and extranodal malignant lymphoma.

Arteriopathy

The lesion designated as arteriopathy is seen in small and medium-sized arteries of different organs (heart, lungs, kidneys, spleen, intestine, brain) (4). It is characterized by intimal fibrosis, fragmentation of elastic fibers in the media, fibrosis, and calcification of internal elastic lamina and media with variable luminal narrowing (Fig. 32). (Vasculitis seen only in the brain in association with progressive HIV encephalopathy is not considered as part of the arteriopathy described here.) In one case fatal

outcome resulted from aneurysms of the right coronary artery with thrombosis (Fig. 33) and myocardial infarction. Aneurysm formation of cerebral arteries has been reported in another case.

The pathogenesis of arteriopathy is not clear. Arteriopathy is therefore included under the category of lesions of undetermined pathogenesis. However, it is possible that repeated bacterial and opportunistic infections secondary to immunodeficiency may result in increased exposure to endogenous and exogenous elastases. Elastic tissue damage, which is a striking feature of the arterial lesions, may be related to such an increased and repeated exposure.

The arteriopathy seen in children with AIDS appears to be distinctive. Similar arterial lesions have not been reported to occur in adults with AIDS, although we have seen similar fibrocalcific lesions of the media of small and medium-sized arteries of the thyroid, mesentery,

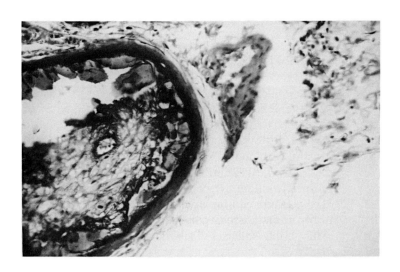

FIG. 32. Arteriopathy characterized by intimal fibrosis with calcification and fibrosis of media of an artery. Note the markedly narrowed lumen. Hematoxylin and eosin, ×25.

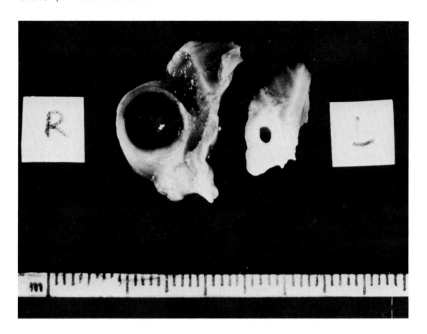

FIG. 33. Gross photograph of both coronaries. Note the aneurysmal dilatation with thrombotic occlusion of the lumen of the right coronary artery.

and kidney in a 30-year-old male intravenous drug user who died of AIDS.

Perinatal Pathology

Transplacental/perinatal transmission is by far the most common route of transmission of HIV to children. HIV was isolated from amniotic fluid, thymus, lungs, spleen, and brain of a 15- and a 20-week-old fetus, but pathologic description of the various fetal tissues and placenta was not given (359). Jauniaux et al. (360) studied 49 placentas, 7 fetuses, and 2 stillbirths from Central African and European HIV-positive women with or without fully developed AIDS. No villitis was noted, but, irrespective of gestational age, the villi were coarse, cellular, and hypovascularized, and the intervillous spaces were narrow with fibrin deposition and calcification. There was a high incidence (43%) of chorioamnionitis, which was unrelated to HIV. The fetuses did not show any histologic lesions in the viscera. The two stillbirths had pneumonia (associated with chorioamnionitis) and nodular peribronchiolar and alveolar septal lymphocytic aggregates in the lungs. Ultrastructural studies in 13 placentas revealed isolated retrovirus-like particles with some morphologic similarities to HIV (100 nM in size, dense central or eccentric core) in the syncytiotrophoblast, fibroblasts, and endothelial cells in villous capillaries and free membranes. These observations do not lend themselves to definitive conclusions. Systematic prospective virologic, immunologic, and pathologic studies of placenta, abortuses, and stillborn fetuses of HIV-positive mothers with and without full-blown AIDS are needed to confirm the observations outlined above. Such studies on a larger number of pregnant women in various stages of HIV infection would also provide data regarding timing of HIV infection(s) of the fetus, the cell types and tissues of the fetus infected by HIV, and the relationship of severity of HIV infection in the mother to that in the fetus.

Perinatal transmission, i.e., transmission shortly before, during, or shortly after the process of birth, has also been implicated but is probably far less common than intrauterine transplacental transmission. Findings in cervical biopsy tissue of four HIV-positive women described by Pomerantz et al. (361) and isolation of HIV from vaginal and cervical secretions reported by Wofsy et al. (362) support the possibility of perinatal transmission to the neonate (and also of heterosexual transmission of HIV). The findings described by Pomerantz et al. (361) were as follows: chronic cervicitis characterized by mononuclear cell infiltration and lymphoid aggregates in the mucosa and/or submucosa, isolation of HIV from cervical biopsy tissue, and demonstration of HIV antigens in the monocytes, endothelial cells, and lymphocytes in the cervical biopsy.

PATHOLOGY OF AIDS IN AFRICAN PATIENTS

The epidemiology and clinical spectrum of AIDS in Africa differs markedly from that in the United States and western European countries (363). Heterosexual activity, a history of prostitution or sexual contact with prostitutes, blood transfusion, the use of unsterilized needles in medical facilities, and vertical transmission from mother to infant are considered the primary modes of HIV transmission in African countries (364). Published histopathologic studies of AIDS in Africa are meager as a result of inadequacies of laboratory facilities in these developing countries. Limited investigations have shown the pathologic lesions to be similar to those described in western patients. However, the following differences in the frequencies and types of opportunistic infections and other lesions have been noted between these two groups (103,365): (1) MTB infections are more common, (2) MAI infections are infrequent, (3) *Cryptosporidium* and *Isospora belli* are frequently found in endoscopic biopsies, (4) PC pneumonitis is infrequent, (5) a generalized, pruritic, maculopapular dermatosis is seen in about 50% of patients as the initial disease presentation, and (6) growth retardation and chronic diarrhea are more frequently seen in African children with AIDS (103,366).

There are few studies comparing HIV-associated Kaposi's sarcoma and malignant lymphoma in African and western patients.

PREVENTING HIV TRANSMISSION IN THE CLINICAL LABORATORY

Occupational transmission of HIV to health care workers by sharps injuries or mucocutaneous contact is well reported (367–374).

Microbiologic or other specimens requiring manipulation during processing are handled under a laminar flow hood to control aerosol dispersion. Mechanical pipetting devices are routinely used and mouth pipetting strictly forbidden. Specimens requiring centrifugation should be capped and placed in a centrifuge with a sealed dome. Accidental spillage of a specimen is promptly cleaned with a suitable disinfectant solution (375–378).

All laboratory work areas should be cleaned and sanitized at the end of each shift or at least daily using an appropriate chemical disinfectant such as 0.5% sodium hypochlorite (1:10 dilution of household bleach). Specimens leaking from their containers are discarded if specimen replacement is possible. Otherwise, the outside of the container is appropriately disinfected.

Tissue sent from the operating room for frozen section studies should be placed in leak-proof containers during transport and handled with latex or vinyl gloves to prevent inadvertent skin contamination. During cryostat cutting of specimens, the use of tissue-freezing aerosol is discouraged to prevent aerosolization. The cryostat and all cutting areas exposed to blood or body fluids should be decontaminated at frequent intervals with an appropriate germicide. Face shields or a face mask and goggles should be routinely worn during the gross examination and cutting of surgical specimens.

Autopsy Procedures

Currently, there is no documentation of an autopsy assistant or pathologist having contracted AIDS or sero-converting as a result of performing an autopsy on a patient with AIDS (379).

The autopsy recommendations of the National Committee for Clinical Laboratory Standards are for total-body barrier protection with water repellent protective clothing. This includes a hood that covers the hair, face shield, or safety goggles with mask to cover the nose and mouth, as well as water-protective boots, double surgical gloves, and, in certain instances, heavy overgloves (380). Aerosols generated by an oscillating electric saw (Stryker) can be minimized by the use of a plastic bag over the head and neck of the corpse and shielding the spray by keeping wet towels immediately adjacent to the blade. A circulating assistant outside the work area should be designated to perform tasks such as answering telephones and pages and obtaining supplies. Some institutions, including ours, have elected to perform autopsies in special "isolation" rooms.

Following the autopsy, the closed body is washed with a detergent solution and then with dilute sodium hypochlorite, rinsed with water, and placed into a body bag. Tables, instruments, and floors are washed with a detergent to remove dried blood and fluids, and then decontaminated with a dilute solution of household bleach or other effective germicides. The prosector and assistant should discard all disposable materials into a specially marked bag for incineration. Reusable materials are cleaned and disinfected or autoclaved. Adequate washing or shower facilities should be available in the vicinity of the autopsy suite.

Recommendations for preventing nosocomial acquired HIV are designed to minimize the risk of mucosal or percutaneous exposure to potentially infectious materials. This can be accomplished through the establishment of departmental protocols developed from the known scientific, clinical, and epidemiologic information about HIV and its associated diseases. Special attention to inservice training of laboratory workers on the hazards posed by all specimens should diminish the risk of acquiring HIV in the clinical laboratory setting.

ACKNOWLEDGMENTS

The authors wish to thank Drs. Jan Silverman and John Christie for their assistance. Special thanks are extended to Ms. Tricia Robbins for typing the manuscript.

REFERENCES

1. Gottlieb MS, Schroff R, Schanker HM, et al. *Pneumocystis carinii* pneumonia and mucosal candidiasis in previously healthy homosexual men: evidence of a new acquired cellular immunodeficiency. *N Engl J Med* 1981;305:1425–31.
2. Masur H, Michelis MA, Greene JB, et al. An outbreak of community-acquired *Pneumocystis carinii* pneumonia: initial manifestation of cellular immune dysfunction. *N Engl J Med* 1981;305:1431–8.

3. CDC. Revision of the CDC surveillance case definition for acquired immunodeficiency syndrome. *MMWR* 1987;36:3S–25S.

4. Joshi VV. Pathology of AIDS in children. *Pathol Annu* 1989;24:356–81.

5. Hageage GJ, Harrington GJ. Use of calcofluor while in clinical mycology. *Lab Med* 1984;15:109–12.

6. Marines HM, Osato MG, Fout RL. The value of calcofluor white in the diagnosis of mycotic and *Acanthamoeba* infections of the eye and ocular adnexa. *Ophthalmology* 1987;94:23–6.

7. Graham AR. Fungal autofluorescence with ultraviolet illumination. *Am J Clin Pathol* 1983;79:231–4.

8. *Linscott's directory of immunological and biologic reagents.* Mill Valley, CA: Linscott's, 1988.

9. Singer RH, Lawrence JB, Villnave C. Optimization of in situ hybridization using isotopic and nonisotopic detection methods. *Biotechnics* 1986;4:230–50.

10. Brigati DJ, Myerson D, Leary JJ, et al. Detection of viral genomes in cultured cells and paraffin embedded tissue sections using biotin-labeled hybridization probes. *Virology* 1983;126:32–50.

11. Peterson EM, Lu R, Floyd C, Nakasone A, Friedly G, de la Maza LM. Direct identification of *Mycobacterium tuberculosis, mycobacterium avium,* and *mycobacterium intracellulare* from amplified primary cultures in BACTEC media using DNA probes. *J Clin Microbiol* 1989;27:1543–7.

12. Tenover FC. Diagnostic DNA probes for infectious diseases. *Clin Microbiol Rev* 1988;1:82–101.

13. Edelstein PH. Evaluation of the Gen-Probe DNA probe for detection of legionella in culture. *J Clin Microbiol* 1986;23:484–4.

14. Hermans PW, Schuitema AR, Van Soolingen D, et al. Specific detection of *Mycobacterium tuberculosis* complex strains by polymerase chain reaction. *J Clin Microbiol* 1990;28:1204–13.

15. Shibata D, Martin WJ, Appleman MD, Causey DM, Leedom JM, Arnheim N. Detection of cytomegalovirus DNA in peripheral blood of patients infected with human immunodeficiency virus. *J Infect Dis* 1988;158:1185–92.

16. Myers JL, Peiper SC, Katzenstein AL. Pulmonary involvement in infectious mononucleosis: histopathologic features and detection of Epstein-Barr virus-related sequences. *Mod Pathol* 1989;2:444–8.

17. Rayfield M, De Cock K, Heyward W, et al. Mixed human immunodeficiency virus (HIV) infection in an individual: demonstration of both HIV type 1 and 2 proviral sequences by using polymerase chain reaction. *J Infect Dis* 1988;158:1170–6.

18. Corbitt G, Bailey AS, Williams G. HIV infection in Manchester, 1959. *Lancet* 1990;336:51.

19. Murray JF, Felton CP, Garay SM, et al. Pulmonary complications of the acquired immunodeficiency syndrome. Report of a National Heart, Lung, and Blood Institute workshop. *N Engl J Med* 1984;310:1682–8.

20. Unger PD, Rosenblum M, Krown SE. Disseminated *Pneumocystis carinii* infection in a patient with acquired immunodeficiency syndrome. *Hum Pathol* 1988;19:113–6.

21. Telzak EE, Cote RJ, Gold JW, Campbell SW, Armstrong D. Extrapulmonary *Pneumocystis carinii* infections. *Rev Infect Dis* 1990;12:380–6.

22. Luna MA, Cleary KR. Spectrum of pathologic manifestations of *Pneumocystis carinii* pneumonia in patients with neoplastic diseases. *Semin Diagn Pathol* 1989;6:262–72.

23. Carter TR, Cooper PH, Petri WA, et al. *Pneumocystis carinii* infection of the small intestine in a patient with acquired immunodeficiency syndrome. *Am J Clin Pathol* 1988;89:679–83.

24. Schinella RA, Breda SD, Hammerschlag PE. Otic infection due to *Pneumocystis carinii* in an apparently healthy man with antibody to the human immunodeficiency virus. *Ann Intern Med* 1987;106:399–400.

25. Edman JC, Kovacs JA, Masur H, Santi DV, Elwood HJ, Sogin ML. Ribosomal RNA sequence shows *Pneumocystis carinii* to be a member of the fungi. *Nature* 1988;334:519–22.

26. Campbell WG. Ultrastructure of *Pneumocystis* in human lung: life cycle of human pneumocystosis. *Arch Pathol* 1972;93:312–24.

27. Cushion MT, Ruffolo JJ, Walzer PD. Analysis of the developmental stages of *Pneumocystis carinii,* in vitro. *Lab Invest* 1988;58:324–31.

28. Esterly JA. *Pneumocystis carinii* in lungs of adults at autopsy. *Am Rev Respir Dis* 1988;97:935–7.

29. Pifer LL, Hughes WT, Stagno S, Woods D. *Pneumocystis carinii* infection: evidence for high prevalence in normal and immunocompromised children. *Pediatrics* 1978;61:35–41.

30. Millard PR, Heryet AR. Observations favouring *Pneumocystis carinii* pneumonia as a primary infection: a monoclonal antibody study on paraffin sections. *J Pathol* 1988;154:365–70.

31. Hughes WT. Natural mode of acquisition for de novo infection with *Pneumocystis carinii. J Infect Dis* 1982;145:842–48.

32. Bedrossian CWM, Mason MR, Gupta PK. Rapid cytologic diagnosis of *Pneumocystis:* a comparison of effective techniques. *Semin Diagn Pathol* 1989;6:245–61.

33. Hartz JW, Geisinger KR, Scharyj M, Muss HB. Granulomatous pneumocystosis presenting as a solitary pulmonary nodule. *Arch Pathol Lab Med* 1985;109:466–69.

34. Chaudhary S, Hughes WT, Feldman S, et al. Percutaneous transthoracic needle aspiration of the lung: diagnosing *Pneumocystis carinii* pneumonitis. *Am J Dis Child* 1977;131:902–5.

35. Grocott RG. A stain for fungi in tissue sections and smears using Gomori's methenamine silver nitrate technique. *Am J Clin Pathol* 1955;25:975–9.

36. Chalvardjian AM, Grawe LA. A new procedure for the identification of *Pneumocystis carinii* cysts in tissue sections and smears. *J Clin Pathol* 1963;16:383–4.

37. Kim HK, Hughes WT. Comparison of methods for identification of *Pneumocystis carinii* in pulmonary aspirates. *Am J Clin Pathol* 1973;60:462–6.

38. Gorelkin L, Chandler FW, Ewing EP. Staining qualities of cytomegalovirus inclusions in the lungs of patients with the acquired immunodeficiency syndrome. *Hum Pathol* 1986;17:926–9.

39. Ghali VS, Garcia RL, Skolom J. Fluorescence of *Pneumocystis carinii* in Papanicolaou smears. *Hum Pathol* 1984;15:907–9.

40. Kovacs JA, Ng VL, Masur H, et al. Diagnosis of *Pneumocystis carinii* pneumonia: improved detection in sputum with use of monoclonal antibodies. *N Engl J Med* 1988;318:589–93.

41. Linder J, Radio SJ. Immunohistochemistry of *Pneumocystis carinii. Semin Diagn Pathol* 1989;6:238–44.

42. Cartun RW, Lachman MF, Pedersen CA, et al. Immunocytochemical identification of *Pneumocystis carinii* in formalin-fixed, paraffin-embedded tissues with monoclonal antibodies 2G2. *Mod Pathol* 1989;2:16A.

43. Tanabe K, Fuchimoto M, Egawa K, Nakamura Y. Use of *Pneumocystis carinii* genomic DNA clones for DNA hybridization analysis of infected human lungs. *J Infect Dis* 1988;157:593–6.

44. Wakefield AE, Pixley FJ, Banerji S, et al. Detection of *Pneumocystis carinii* with DNA amplification. *Lancet* 1990;336:451–3.

45. Gal AA, Koss MN, Strigle S, Angritt P. *Pneumocystis carinii* infection in acquired immunodeficiency syndrome. *Semin Diagn Pathol* 1989;6:287–99.

46. Lanken PN, Minda M, Pietra GG, Fishman AP. Alveolar response to experimental *Pneumocystis carinii* pneumonia in the rat. *Am J Pathol* 1980;99:561–88.

47. Travis WD, Pittaluga S, Lipschik GY, et al. Atypical pathologic manifestations of *Pneumocystis carinii* pneumonia in the acquired immune deficiency syndrome. Review of 123 lung biopsies from 76 patients with emphasis on cysts, vascular invasion, vasculitis, and granulomas. *Am J Surg Pathol* 1990;14:615–25.

48. Eng RHK, Bishburg E, Smith SM. Evidence for destruction of lung tissues regarding *Pneumocystis carinii* infection. *Arch Intern Med* 1987;147:746–9.

49. Saldana MJ, Mones JM. Cavitation and other atypical manifestations of *Pneumocystis carinii* pneumonia. *Semin Diagn Pathol* 1989;6:273–86.

50. Liu YC, Tomashefski JF Jr, Tomford JW, Green H. Necrotizing *Pneumocystis carinii* vasculitis associated with lung necrosis and cavitation in a patient with acquired immunodeficiency syndrome. *Arch Pathol Lab Med* 1989;113:494–7.

51. Nash G, Fligiel S. Pathologic features of the lung in the acquired immune deficiency syndrome (AIDS): an autopsy study of seventeen homosexual males. *Am J Clin Pathol* 1984;81:6–12.

52. Askin FB, Katzenstein AL. Pneumocystis infection masquerading as diffuse alveolar damage: a potential source of diagnostic error. *Chest* 1981;79:420–2.

53. Marchevsky A, Rosen MJ, Chrystal G, et al. Pulmonary complications of the acquired immunodeficiency syndrome: a clinicopathologic study of 70 cases. *Hum Pathol* 1985;16:659–70.
54. Frenkel JK. Toxoplasmosis: parasite life cycle, pathology, and immunology. In: Hammond DM, ed. *The coccidia.* Baltimore: University Park Press, 1973;343–410.
55. Holliman RE. Toxoplasmosis and the acquired immune deficiency syndrome. *J Infect* 1988;16:121–8.
56. Levy RM, Bredesen DF, Rosenblum ML. Neurological manifestations of the acquired immunodeficiency syndrome (AIDS): experience at UCSF and review of the literature. *J Neurosurg* 1985;62:475–95.
57. Navia BA, Petito CK, Gold JWM, Cho ES, Jordan BD, Price RW. Cerebral toxoplasmosis complicating the acquired immune deficiency syndrome: clinical and neuropathological findings in 27 patients. *Ann Neurol* 1986;19:224–38.
58. Weiss A, Margo CE, Ledford DK, Lockey RF, Brinser JH. Toxoplasmic retinochoroiditis as an initial manifestation of the acquired immune deficiency syndrome. *J Ophthalmol* 1986;101:248–9.
59. Catterall JR, Hofflin JM, Remington JS. Pulmonary toxoplasmosis. *Am Rev Respir Dis* 1986;133:704–5.
60. Nistal M, Santan A, Paniaqua R, Palacios J. Testicular toxoplasmosis in two men with the acquired immunodeficiency syndrome. *Arch Pathol Lab Med* 1986;110:744–6.
61. Leyva WH, Santa Cruz DJ. Cutaneous toxoplasmosis. *J Am Acad Dermatol* 1986;14:600–5.
62. Roldan EO, Moskowitz L, Hensley GT. Pathology of the heart in acquired immunodeficiency syndrome. *Arch Pathol Lab Med* 1987;111:943–6.
63. Luft BJ, Conley F, Remington JS. Outbreak of central nervous system toxoplasmosis in Western Europe and North America. *Lancet* 1983;1:781–4.
64. Mobley K, Rotterdam H, Lerner CW, et al. Autopsy findings in the acquired immunodeficiency syndrome. *Pathol Annu* 1985;20:45–65.
65. Wanke C, Tuazon CU, Kovacs A, et al. Toxoplasma encephalitis in patients with acquired immune deficiency syndrome: diagnosis and response to therapy. *Am J Trop Med Hyg* 1987;36:509–16.
66. Knapen F van, Panggabean SO, Leusden J van. Demonstration of *Toxoplasma* antigen containing complexes in active toxoplasmosis. *J Clin Microbiol* 1985;22:645–50.
67. Brooks RG, Sharma SD, Remington JS. Detection of *Toxoplasma gondii* antigens by a dot-immunobinding technique. *J Clin Microbiol* 1985;21:113–6.
68. Hofflin JM, Remington JS. Tissue culture isolation of *Toxoplasma* from blood of a patient with AIDS. *Arch Intern Med* 1985;145:925–6.
69. Frenkel JK. *Fascicle on pathology of tropical and extraordinary diseases,* vol 1. Washington, DC: AFIP, 1976;284–300.
70. Huang TE, Chou SM. Occlusive hypertrophic arteritis as the cause of discrete necrosis in CNS toxoplasmosis in AIDS. *Hum Pathol* 1988;19:1210–4.
71. Sharer LR, Kapila R. Neuropathologic observations in acquired immunodeficiency syndrome (AIDS). *Acta Neuropathol* 1985;66:188–98.
72. Holland GN, Engstrom RE, Glasgow BJ, et al. Ocular toxoplasmosis in patients with the acquired immunodeficiency syndrome. *Am J Ophthalmol* 1988;106:653–67.
73. Kazlow PG, Kumudini S, Benkov KJ, Dische R, LeLeiko NS. Esophageal cryptosporidiosis in a child with acquired immune deficiency syndrome. *Gastroenterology* 1986;91:1301–3.
74. CDC. Cryptosporidiosis: assessment of chemotherapy of males with acquired immune deficiency syndrome (AIDS). *MMWR* 1982;31:589–92.
75. Guarda LA, Stein SA, Cleary KA, et al. Human cryptosporidiosis in the acquired immune deficiency syndrome. *Arch Pathol Lab Med* 1983;107:562–6.
76. Hinnant K, Schwartz A, Rotterdam H, et al. Cytomegaloviral and cryptosporidial cholecystitis in two patients with AIDS. *Am J Surg Pathol* 1989;13:57–60.
77. Brady EM, Margolis ML, Korzeniowski OM. Pulmonary cryptosporidiosis in acquired immune deficiency syndrome. *JAMA* 1984;252:89–90.
78. Blagburn BL, Current WL. Accidental infection of a researcher with human cryptosporidium [Letter]. *J Infect Dis* 1983;148:772–3.
79. Hojlyng N, Holten-Andersen W, Jepsen S. Cryptosporidiosis: a case of airborne transmission. *Lancet* 1987;2:271–2.
80. Sewankambo N, Mugerwa RD, Goodgame R, et al. Enteropathic AIDS in Uganda. An endoscopic, histological and microbiological study. *AIDS* 1987;1:9–13.
81. Grigolato PG, Villanacci V, Mangiarini MG, Cadeo GP, Casari S, Ravelli P. Cryptosporidium of human large intestine in HIV. Report of a case examined under light and electron microscope study. *Pathologica* 1989;81:47–56.
82. Pitlik SD, Fainstein V, Garza D, et al. Human cryptosporidiosis: spectrum of disease. Report of six cases and review of the literature. *Arch Intern Med* 1983;143:2269–76.
83. Gross TL, Wheat J, Bartlett M, O'Connor W. AIDS and multiple system involvement with *Cryptosporidium. Am J Gastroenterol* 1986;81:456–8.
84. Silverman JF, Levine J, Finley JL, et al. Small intestinal brushing cytology in the diagnosis of cryptosporidiosis in AIDS. *Diagn Cytopathol* 1990;6:193–6.
85. Ma P, Sve R. Three step stool examination for cryptosporidiosis in 10 homosexual men with protracted watery diarrhea. *J Infect Dis* 1983;147:824–8.
86. Henricksen SA, Pohlenz JFL. Staining of cryptosporidia by a modified Ziehl-Neelsen technique. *Acta Vet Scand* 1981;22:594–6.
87. Sterling CR, Arrowood MJ. Detection of *Cryptosporidium* sp. infections using a direct immunofluorescent assay. *Pediatr Infect Dis* 1986;5:S139–42.
88. Soave R, Danner RL, Honig CL, et al. Cryptosporidiosis in homosexual men. *Ann Intern Med* 1984;110:504–11.
89. Wolfson JS, Richter JM, Waldron MA, et al. Cryptosporidiosis in immunocompetent patients. *N Engl J Med* 1985;312:1278–82.
90. Sun T. Opportunistic parasitic infections in patients with acquired immunodeficiency syndrome. *Pathol Annu* 1988;23:1–32.
91. Ma P, Kaufman D, Montana J. *Isospora belli* diarrheal infection in homosexual men. *AIDS Res* 1984;1:327–8.
92. DeHovitz JA, Pape JW, Boncy M, Johnson WD Jr. Clinical manifestations and therapy of *Isospora belli* infection in patients with acquired immunodeficiency syndrome. *N Engl J Med* 1986;315:87–90.
93. Current WL, Owen RL. Cryptosporidiosis and microsporidiosis. In: Farthing MJG, Keusch GT, eds. *Enteric infections: mechanisms, manifestations and management.* London: Chapman & Hill, 1989;223–49.
94. Restrepo C, Macher AM, Radany EH. Disseminated extraintestinal isosporiasis in a patient with acquired immune deficiency syndrome. *Am J Clin Pathol* 1987;87:536–42.
95. Canning EU, Hollister WS. *Enterocytozoon bieneusi* (Microspora): prevalence and pathogenecity in AIDS patients. *Trans R Soc Trop Med Hyg* 1990;84:181–6.
96. Modigliani R, Bories C, le Charpentier Y, et al. Diarrhea and malabsorption in acquired immune deficiency syndrome: a study of four cases with special emphasis on opportunistic protozoan infections. *Gut* 1985;26:179–87.
97. Rijpstra AC, Canning EU, van Ketel RJ, et al. Use of light microscopy to diagnose small-intestinal microsporidiosis in patients with AIDS. *J Infect Dis* 1988;157:827–31.
98. Gourley WK, Swedo JL. Intestinal infection by microsporidia *Enterocytozoon bieneusi* of patients with AIDS: an ultrastructural study of the use of human mitochondria by a protozoan. *Lab Invest* 1988;58:35A.
99. Zender HO, Arrigoni E, Ecker J, et al. A case of *Encephalitozoon cuniculi* peritonitis in a patient with AIDS. *Am J Clin Pathol* 1989;92:352–6.
100. Llibre JM, Tor J, Manterola JM, Carbonell C, Foz M. *Blastocystis hominis* chronic diarrhea in AIDS patients. *Lancet* 1989;1:221.
101. Datry A, Similowski T, Jais P, et al. AIDS associated leishmaniasis: an unusual gastroduodenal presentation. *Trans R Soc Trop Med Hyg* 1990;84:239–40.

102. Long E, Ebrahimzadeh A, White EH, Swisher B, Callaway CS. Alga associated with diarrhea in patients with acquired immunodeficiency syndrome and in travelers. *J Clin Microbiol* 1990;28:1101–9.

103. Colebunders R, Lusakumuni K, Nelston AM, et al. Persistent diarrhea in Zairian AIDS patients: an endoscopic and histologic study. *Gut* 1988;29:1687–91.

104. CDC. Revision of the case definition of acquired immunodeficiency syndrome for national reporting—United States. *MMWR* 1985;34:373–5.

105. Klein RS, Harris CA, Small CB, et al. Oral candidiasis in high risk patients as the initial manifestation of the acquired immunodeficiency syndrome. *N Engl J Med* 1984;311:354–7.

106. Samaranayake LP, Holmstrup P. Oral candidiasis and human immunodeficiency virus infection. *J Oral Pathol Med* 1989;18:554–64.

107. Goodwin AM. Oral manifestations of AIDS: an overview. *Dent Hyg* 1987;61:304–8.

108. Trier JS, Bjorkman DJ. Esophageal, gastric, and intestinal candidiasis. *Am J Med* 1984;77:39–43.

109. Tavitian A, Raufman JP, Rosenthal LE. Oral candidiasis as a marker of esophageal candidiasis in the acquired immunodeficiency syndrome. *Ann Intern Med* 1986;104:54–5.

110. Whimbey E, Gold JWM, Polsky B, et al. Bacteremia and fungemia in patients with the acquired immunodeficiency syndrome. *Ann Intern Med* 1986;104:511–4.

111. Colligan PJ, Sorrell TC. Disseminated candidiasis: evidence of a distinctive syndrome in heroin abusers. *Br Med J* 1983;287:861–2.

112. Levy RM, Bredesen DE, Rosenblum ML. Opportunistic central nervous system pathology in patients with AIDS. *Ann Neurol* 1988;23:7S–11S.

113. Ehni WF, Ellison RT III. Spontaneous *Candida albicans* meningitis in a patient with the acquired immune deficiency syndrome. *Am J Med* 1987;83:806–7.

114. Pierard GE. Unusual candidosis superimposed to pox and herpes-virus infections in a patient with AIDS. *Ann Pathol* 1986;6:225–7.

115. Diamond RD. *Cryptococcus neoformans,* In: Mandel GL, Douglas RG, Bennett JE, eds. *Principles and practice of infectious diseases.* New York: Churchill Livingstone, 1990;1980–1989.

116. Chuck SL, Sande MA. Infections with *Cryptococcus neoformans* in the acquired immunodeficiency syndrome. *N Engl J Med* 1989;321:794–9.

117. Sussman EJ, MacMahon F, Wright D, et al. Cutaneous cryptococcosis without evidence of systemic involvement. *J Am Acad Dermatol* 1984;11:371–4.

118. Massa MC, Doyle JA. Cutaneous cryptococcosis simulating pyoderma gangrenosum. *J Am Acad Dermatol* 1981;5:32–6.

119. Concus AP, Helfand RF, Imber MJ, et al. Cutaneous cryptococcosis mimicking molluscum contagiosum in a patient with AIDS. *J Infect Dis* 1988;158:897–8.

120. Jones C, Orengo I, Rosen T, et al. Cutaneous cryptococcosis simulating Kaposi's sarcoma in the acquired immunodeficiency syndrome. *Cutis* 1990;45:163–7.

121. Kovacs JA, Kovacs AA, Polis M, et al. Cryptococcosis in the acquired immunodeficiency syndrome. *Ann Intern Med* 1985;103:533–8.

122. Gal AA, Koss MN, Hawkins J, et al. The pathology of pulmonary cryptococcal infection in the acquired immunodeficiency syndrome. *Arch Pathol Lab Med* 1986;110:502–7.

123. Lafont A, Wolff M, Marche C, et al. Overwhelming myocarditis due to *Cryptococcus neoformans* in an AIDS patient. *Lancet* 1987;2:1145–6.

124. Newman TG, Soni A, Acaron S, et al. Pleural cryptococcosis in the acquired immune deficiency syndrome. *Chest* 1987;91:459–61.

125. Torres RA. Cryptococcal mediastinitis mimicking lymphoma in the acquired immune deficiency syndrome. *Am J Med* 1987;88:1004–5.

126. Markowitz SM, Kerkering TM, Gervin AS. Biliary obstruction and cholestasis in AIDS: case report. *Va Med* 1990;117:114–6.

127. Bahls F, Sumi SM. Cryptococcal meningitis and cerebral toxoplasmosis in a patient with acquired immune deficiency syndrome. *J Neurol Neurosurg Psychiatry* 1986;49:328–40.

128. Sofman MS, Heilman ER. Simultaneous occurrence of Kaposi's sarcoma and cryptococcus within a cutaneous lesion in a patient with acquired immunodeficiency syndrome. *Arch Dermatol* 1990;126:683–4.

129. Bottone EJ, Wormser GP. Capsule-deficient cryptococci in AIDS. *Lancet* 1985;2:553.

130. Bottone EJ, Wormser GP. Poorly encapsulated *Cryptococcus neoformans* from patients with AIDS. II. Correlation of capsule size observed directly in cerebrospinal fluid with that after animal passage. *AIDS Res* 1986;2:219–25.

131. Ro JY, Lee SS, Ayala AG. Advantage of Fontana-Masson stain in capsule-deficient cryptococcal infection. *Arch Pathol Lab Med* 1987;111:53–7.

132. Chu AC, Hay RJ, MacDonald DM. Cutaneous cryptococcosis. *Br J Dermatol* 1980;103:95–100.

133. Eng RHK, Bishburg E, Smith SM. Cryptococcal infections in patients with acquired immune deficiency syndrome. *Am J Med* 1986;81:19–23.

134. Ajello L. Relationship of *Histoplasma capsulatum* to avian habitats. *Public Health Rep* 1964;79:266–72.

135. Edwards LB, Acquaviva FA, Livesay VT, Cross FW, Palmer CE. An atlas of sensitivity to tuberculin, PPD-B and histoplasmin in the United States. *Am Rev Respir Dis* 1969;99:1–18.

136. Wheat JL, Slama TG, Zeckel ML. Histoplasmosis in the acquired immunodeficiency syndrome. *Am J Med* 1985;78:203–10.

137. Wheat LJ, Connolly-Stringfield PA, Baker RL, et al. Disseminated histoplasmosis in the acquired immune deficiency syndrome: clinical findings, diagnosis and treatment, and review of the literature. *Medicine* 1990;69:361–74.

138. Johnson PC, Sarosi GA, Septimus EJ, et al. Progressive disseminated histoplasmosis in patients with the acquired immune deficiency syndrome: a report of 12 cases and a literature review. *Semin Respir Infect* 1986;1:1–9.

139. Bonner JR, Alexander J, Dismukes WE, et al. Disseminated histoplasmosis in patients with the acquired immune deficiency syndrome. *Arch Intern Med* 1984;199:2178–81.

140. Mandell W, Goldberg DM, Neu HC. Histoplasmosis in patients with the acquired immune deficiency syndrome. *Am J Med* 1986;81:974–8.

141. Henochowicz S, Sahovic E, Pistole M, Rodrigues M, Macher A. Histoplasma diagnosed on peripheral blood smear from a patient with AIDS. *JAMA* 1985;253(21):3148.

142. Kurtin PJ, McKinsey DS, Gupta MR, et al. Histoplasmosis in patients with acquired immunodeficiency syndrome. Hematologic and bone marrow manifestations. *Am J Clin Pathol* 1990;93:367–72.

143. Fish DG, Ampel NM, Galgiani JN, et al. Coccidioidomycosis during human immunodeficiency virus infection. A review of 77 patients. *Medicine* 1990;69:384–98.

144. Bronnimann DA, Adam RD, Galgiani JN, et al. Coccidioidomycosis in patients with the acquired immunodeficiency syndrome. *Ann Intern Med* 1987;106:372–9.

145. Graham AR, Sobonya RE, Bronnimann DA, et al. Quantitative pathology of coccidioidomycosis in acquired immunodeficiency syndrome. *Hum Pathol* 1988;19:800–6.

146. Prichard JG, Sorotzkin RA, James RE III. Cutaneous manifestations of disseminated coccidioidomycosis in the acquired immunodeficiency syndrome. *Cutis* 1987;39:203–5.

147. Ampel NM, Ryan KJ, Carry PJ, et al. Fungemia due to *Coccidioides immitis.* An analysis of 16 episodes in 15 patients and a review of the literature. *Medicine* 1986;65:312–21.

148. Abrams DI, Robia M, Blumenfeld W, et al. Disseminated coccidioidomycosis in AIDS. *N Engl J Med* 1984;310:986–7.

149. Lipstein-Kresch E, Isenberg HD, Singer C, et al. Disseminated *Sporothrix schenckii* infection with arthritis in a patient with acquired immunodeficiency syndrome. *J Rheumatol* 1985;12:805–8.

150. Shaw JC, Levinson W, Montanaro A. Sporotrichosis in the acquired immunodeficiency syndrome. *J Am Acad Dermatol* 1989;21:1145–7.

151. Woods GL, Goldsmith JC. Aspergillus infection of the central nervous system in patients with acquired immunodeficiency syndrome. *Arch Neurol* 1990;47:181–4.

152. Niedt GW, Schinella RA. Acquired immunodeficiency syn-

drome. Clinicopathologic study of 56 autopsies. *Arch Pathol Lab Med* 1985;109:727–34.

153. Wiest PM, Wiese K, Jacobs MR, et al. *Alternaria* infection in a patient with acquired immunodeficiency syndrome: case report and review of invasive *Alternaria* infections. *Rev Infect Dis* 1987;9:799–803.

154. Leoung G, Mills J. *Opportunistic infections in patients with the acquired immunodeficiency syndrome.* New York: Marcel Dekker, 1989;311.

155. Collins FN. *M. avium complex* infections and development of AIDS: causal opportunist or causal cofactor? *Int J Leprosy* 1986;54:458–74.

156. Dannenberg AM. Chemical and enzymatic host factors in resistance to tuberculosis. *Microbiol Ser* 1984;15:721–60.

157. Collins FM. Mycobacterial disease, immunosuppression and AIDS. *Clin Microbiol Rev Vol* 1989;2:360–77.

158. Good RC. Opportunistic pathogens in the genus mycobacterium. *Ann Rev Microbiol* 1986;39:347–69.

159. Brady MT, Marcon MJ, Maddux H. Broviac catheter-related infection due to *Mycobacterium fortuitum* in a patient with acquired immunodeficiency syndrome. *Pediatr Infect Dis J* 1987;6:492–4.

160. Parker BC, Ford MA, Gruft H, et al. Epidemiology of infection by nontuberculous mycobacteria. IV. Preferential aerosolization of *M. intracellulare* from natural waters. *Am Rev Respir Dis* 1983;128:652–6.

161. Hawkins CC, Gold JWM, Whimby E, et al. *Mycobacterium avium complex* infection in patients with the acquired immunodeficiency syndrome. *Ann Intern Med* 1986;105:184–8.

162. Pitchenik AE, Fertel D, Bloch AB. Pulmonary effects of AIDS. Mycobacterial disease: epidemiology, diagnosis, treatment, and prevention. *Clin Chest Med* 1988;9:425–41.

163. CDC. Disseminated *Mycobacterium bovis* infection from BCG vaccination of a patient with AIDS. *MMWR* 1985;34:227–8.

164. Gillin JS, Urmacher C, West R, et al. Disseminated *M. avium intracellulare* infection in acquired immunodeficiency syndrome mimicking Whipple's disease. *Gastroenterology* 1983;85:1187–91.

165. Wang HH, Tollerud D, Danar D, et al. Another Whipple-like disease in AIDS? *N Engl J Med* 1986;314:1577–8.

166. Wood C, Nikoloff BJ, Todes-Taylor NR. Pseudotumor resulting from atypical mycobacterial infection: a histoid variety of *Mycobacterium avium-intracellulare* complex infection. *Am J Clin Pathol* 1985;83:524–7.

167. Schneiderman DJ, Arenson DJ, Cello JP, et al. Hepatic disease in patients with the acquired immune deficiency syndrome (AIDS). *Hepatology* 1987;7:925–30.

168. Klatt EC, Jensen DF, Meyer PR. Pathology of *Mycobacterium avium-intracellulare* infection in acquired immunodeficiency syndrome. *Hum Pathol* 1987;18:709–14.

169. Lebovics E, Thung SN, Schaffner F, et al. The liver in the acquired immunodeficiency syndrome: a clinical and histologic study. *Hepatology* 1985;5:293–8.

170. Nakanuma Y, Liew CT, Peters RL, et al. Pathologic features of the liver in acquired immune deficiency syndrome (AIDS). *Liver* 1986;6:158–66.

171. Osborne BM, Guarda LA, Butler JJ. Bone marrow biopsies in patients with the acquired immunodeficiency syndrome. *Hum Pathol* 1984;15:1048–53.

172. Anderson G, Coup AJ. Effect of decalcifying agents on the staining of *Mycobacterium tuberculosis*. *J Clin Pathol* 1975;28:744–5.

173. Sommers HM, Good RC. Mycobacterium. In: Lennette EH, Balows A, Hausler WJ Jr, Shadomy HJ, eds. *Manual of clinical microbiology*, 4th ed. Washington, DC: American Society for Microbiology, 1985;216–48.

174. Body BA, Warren NG, Spicer A, et al. Use of Gen-probe and Bactec for rapid isolation and identification of mycobacteria correlation of probe results with growth index. *Am J Clin Pathol* 1990;93:415–20.

175. Humphrey DM, Weiner MH. Mycobacterial antigen detection by immunohistochemistry in pulmonary tuberculosis. *Hum Pathol* 1987;18:701–8.

176. Ellner PD, Kiehn TE, Cammarata R, Hosmer M. Rapid detection and identification of pathogenic mycobacteria by combining radiometric and nucleic acid probe methods. *J Clin Microbiol* 1988;26:1349–52.

177. Pitchenik E, Rubinson A. The radiographic appearance of tuberculosis in patients with AIDS and pre-AIDS. *Am Rev Respir Dis* 1985;131:393–6.

178. Ducanson FP, Hewlett D, Maayan S, et al. *Mycobacterium tuberculosis* infection in the acquired immunodeficiency syndrome. A review of 14 patients. *Tubercule* 1986;67:295–302.

179. Polsky B, Gold JWM, Whimbey E, et al. Bacterial pneumonia in patients with the acquired immunodeficiency syndrome. *Ann Intern Med* 1986;104:38–41.

180. Garbowit DL, Alsip AG, Griffin FM. *Hemophilus influenzae* bacteremia in a patient with immunodeficiency caused by HTLV-III. *N Engl J Med* 1986;314:56.

181. Jacobs JL, Gold JWM, Murray HW, et al. Salmonella infections in patients with acquired immunodeficiency syndrome. *Ann Intern Med* 1985;102:186–9.

182. Celum CL, Chaisson RE, Rutherford GW, et al. Incidence of salmonellosis in patients with AIDS. *J Infect Dis* 1987;157:998–1002.

183. Krasinski K, Borkowsky W, Bonk S, et al. Bacterial infections in human immunodeficiency virus-infected children. *Pediatr Infect Dis J* 1988;7:323–8.

184. Bernstein LJ, Krieger BZ, Novick B, et al. Bacterial infection in the acquired immunodeficiency syndrome of children. *Pediatr Infect Dis* 1985;4:472–5.

185. Fischl MA, Dickinson GM, Sinave C, et al. Salmonella bacteremia as a manifestation of acquired immunodeficiency syndrome. *Arch Intern Med* 1985;146:113–5.

186. Smith PD, Lane HC, Gill VJ, et al. Intestinal infections in patients with the acquired immunodeficiency syndrome (AIDS): etiology and response to therapy. *Ann Intern Med* 1988;108:328–33.

187. Mandell W, Neu HC. Shigella bacteremia in patients with the acquired immune deficiency. *JAMA* 1986;255:3116–7.

188. Baskin DH, Lax JD, Barenberg D. Shigella bacteremia in patients with the acquired immune deficiency. *Am J Gastroenterol* 1987;82:338–41.

189. Dworkin B, Wormser GP, Abdoo RA, et al. Persistence of multiply antibiotic-resistant *Campylobacter jejuni* in a patient with the acquired immune deficiency syndrome. *Am J Med* 1986;80:965–70.

190. Wheeler AP, Gregg CR. Campylobacter bacteremia, cholecystitis, and the acquired immunodeficiency syndrome. *Ann Intern Med* 1986;105:804.

191. Johns DR, Tierney M, Felsenstein D. Alteration in the natural history of neurosyphilis by concurrent infection with the human immunodeficiency virus. *N Engl J Med* 1987;316:1569–72.

192. Berry CD, Hooten TM, Collier AC, et al. Neurologic relapse after benzathine penicillin therapy for secondary syphilis in a patient with HIV infection. *N Engl J Med* 1987;316:1587–9.

193. Hicks CB, Benson PM, Lupton GP, et al. Seronegative secondary syphilis in a patient infected with the human immunodeficiency virus (HIV) with Kaposi's sarcoma. A diagnostic dilemma. *Ann Intern Med* 1987;107:492–5.

194. Zaidman GW. Neurosyphilis and retrobulbar neuritis in a patient with AIDS. *Ann Ophthalmol* 1986;18:260–1.

195. Radolph JD, Kaplan RP. Unusual manifestations of secondary syphilis and abnormal humoral immune response to *Treponema pallidum* antigens in a homosexual man with asymptomatic human immunodeficiency virus infection. *J Am Acad Dermatol* 1988;18:423–8.

196. Lane HC, Masur H, Edgar LC, et al. Abnormalities of B-cell activation and immunoregulation in patients with the acquired immunodeficiency syndrome. *N Engl J Med* 1983;309:453–8.

197. Zambrano W, Perez GM, Smith JL. Acute syphilitic blindness in AIDS. *J Clin Neuro Ophthalmol* 1987;7:1–5.

198. Swisher BL. Modified Steiner procedure for microwave staining of spirochetes and nonfilamentous bacteria. *J Histotechnol* 1987;10:241–3.

199. Rotterdam H. Tissue diagnosis of selected AIDS-related opportunistic infections. *Am J Surg Pathol* 1987;11:3–15.

200. Reichert CM, O'Leary TJ, Levens DL, et al. Autopsy pathology

in the acquired immune deficiency syndrome. *Am J Pathol* 1983;12:357–82.

201. Gold JW. Clinical spectrum of infections in patients with HTLV-III-associated disease. *Cancer Res* 1985;45:4652S–4S.

202. Villar LA, Massanari RM, Mitros FA. Cytomegalovirus infection with acute erosive esophagitis. *Am J Med* 1984;76:924–8.

203. Elta G, Turnage R, Eckhauser FE, et al. A submucosal antral mass caused by cytomegalovirus infection in a patient with acquired immunodeficiency syndrome. *Am J Gastroenterol* 1986;82:714–7.

204. Galloway PG. Widespread cytomegalovirus infection involving the gastrointestinal tract, biliary tree, and gallbladder in an immunocompromised patient [Letter]. *Gastroenterology* 1984;87:1407.

205. Klatt EC, Shibata D. Cytomegalovirus infection in the acquired immunodeficiency syndrome: clinical and autopsy findings. *Arch Pathol Lab Med* 1988;112:540–4.

206. Morgello S, Cho ES, Nielsen S, et al. Cytomegalovirus encephalitis in patients with acquired immunodeficiency syndrome: an autopsy study of 30 cases and a review of the literature. *Hum Pathol* 1987;18:289–97.

207. Klatt EC. Diagnostic findings in patients with acquired immune deficiency syndrome. *J Acquired Immune Deficiency Syndrome* 1988;1:459–65.

208. Keh WC, Garber MA. In situ hybridization for cytomegalovirus DNA in AIDS patients. *Am J Pathol* 1988;131:490–6.

209. Robey SS, Gage WR, Kuhajda FP. Comparison of immunoperoxidase and DNA in situ hybridization techniques in the diagnosis of cytomegalovirus colitis. *Am J Clin Pathol* 1988;89:666–71.

210. Seto E, Yen TSB. Detection of cytomegalovirus infection by means of DNA isolated from paraffin-embedded tissues and dot hybridization. *Am J Pathol* 1987;127:409–13.

211. Frank D, Raicht RF. Intestinal perforation associated with cytomegalovirus infection in patients with acquired immune deficiency syndrome. *Am J Gastroenterol* 1984;79:201–5.

212. Goodman D, Porter D. Cytomegalovirus vasculitis with fatal colonic hemorrhage. *Arch Pathol* 1973;96:281–4.

213. Armstrong D, Gold JWM, Dryjanski BJ, et al. Treatment of infections in patients with the acquired immunodeficiency syndrome. *Ann Intern Med* 1985;103:738–43.

214. Qunnan GV, Masur H, Rook AH, et al. Herpes virus infections in the acquired immune deficiency syndrome. *JAMA* 1984;252:72–7.

215. Cohen PR, Beltrani VP, Grossman ME. Disseminated herpes zoster in patients with human immunodeficiency virus infection. *Am J Med* 1988;84:1076–80.

216. Weller TH. Varicella and herpes zoster. Changing concepts of the natural history, control, and importance of a not-so-benign virus. *N Engl J Med* 1983;309:1362–8, 1434–40.

217. Colebunders R, Mann JM, Francis H, et al. Herpes zoster in African patients: a clinical predictor of human immunodeficiency virus infection. *J Infect Dis* 1988;157:314–8.

218. Pruneda RC, Almanza I. Centrifugation-shell vial technique for rapid detection of herpes simplex virus cytopathic effect in Vero cells. *J Clin Microbiol* 1987;25:423–4.

219. Burns J, Redfern DRM, Esiri MM, et al. Human and viral gene detection in routine paraffin embedded tissue by in situ hybridization with biotinylated probes: Viral localization in herpes encephalitis. *J Clin Pathol* 1986;39:1066–73.

220. Landry ML, Zibello TA, Hsiung GD. Comparison of in situ hybridization and immunologic staining with cytopathology for detection and identification of herpes simplex virus infection in cultured cells. *J Clin Microbiol* 1986;24:968–71.

221. Hochberg FH, Miller G, Schooley RT, et al. Central nervous system lymphoma related to Epstein-Barr virus. *N Engl J Med* 1983;309:745–8.

222. Andiman W, Gradoville L, Heston L, et al. Use of cloned probes to detect Epstein-Barr viral DNA in tissue of patients with neoplastic and lymphoproliferative diseases. *J Infect Dis* 1983;148:967–77.

223. Raab-Traub N, Flynn K, Pearson G, et al. The differentiated form of nasopharyngeal carcinoma contains Epstein-Barr virus DNA. *Int J Cancer* 1987;39:25–9.

224. Eversole LR, Stone CE, Beckman AM. Detection of EBV and HPV DNA sequences in oral "hairy" leukoplakia by in situ hybridization. *J Med Virol* 1988;26:271–7.

225. Greenspan JS, Greenspan D, Lennette ET, et al. Replication of Epstein-Barr virus within the epithelial cells of oral "hairy" leukoplakia, an AIDS-associated lesion. *N Engl J Med* 1985;313:1564–71.

226. Sumaya CV. Serological testing for Epstein-Barr virus—developments in interpretation. *J Infect Dis* 1985;151:984–7.

227. Salvador AH, Harrison EG Jr, Kyle RA. Lymphadenopathy due to infectious mononucleosis: its confusion with malignant lymphoma. *Cancer* 1971;27:1029–40.

228. Goodman DS, Teplitz ED, Wishner A, et al. Prevalence of cutaneous disease in patients with acquired immunodeficiency syndrome (AIDS) or AIDS-related complex. *J Am Acad Dermatol* 1987;17:210–20.

229. Schrager LK, Friedland GH, Maude D, et al. Cervical and vaginal squamous cell abnormalities in women infected with human immunodeficiency virus. *J Acquired Immune Deficiency Syndrome* 1989;2:570–5.

230. Ficarra G, Berson AM, Silverman S, et al. Kaposi's sarcoma of the oral cavity: a study of 134 patients with a review of the pathogenesis, epidemiology, clinical aspects, and treatment. *Oral Surg Oral Med Oral Pathol* 1988;66:543–50.

231. Moskowitz EB, Hensley CT, Gould EW, et al. Frequency and anatomic distribution of lymphadenopathic Kaposi's sarcoma in AIDS. *Hum Pathol* 1985;16:447–56.

232. Curran JW, Morgan WM, Hardy AM, et al. Epidemiology of AIDS: current status and future prospectives. *Science* 1985;229:1352–7.

233. Lemlich G, Schwan L, Lebwohl M. Kaposi sarcoma and AIDS. Postmortem findings in twenty-four cases. *J Am Acad Dermatol* 1987;16:319–25.

234. Longo DL, Steis RG, Lane HC, et al. Malignancies in the AIDS patient: natural history, treatment strategies and preliminary results. In: Selikoff IJ, Teirstein AS, Hirschman SZ, eds. *Acquired immune deficiency syndrome. Ann NY Acad Sci* 1984;437:421–9.

235. Steis RG, Longo DL. Clinical, biologic, and therapeutic aspects of malignancies associated with the acquired immunodeficiency syndrome. Part I. *Ann Allergy* 1988;60:310–4.

236. Dictor M, Anderson C. Lymphaticovenous differentiation in Kaposi's sarcoma. *Am J Pathol* 1988;130:411–7.

237. Scully P, Steinman H, Kennedy C, Trueblood K, Frisman D, Voland J. Aids-related Kaposi's sarcoma displays differential expression of endothelial surface antigens. *Am J Pathol* 1988;130:244–51.

238. Beckstead JH, Wood GS, Fletcher V. Evidence for the origin of Kaposi's sarcoma from lymphatic endothelium. *Am J Pathol* 1985;119:294–300.

239. Jones RR, Spaull J, Spry C, Jones EW. Histogenesis of Kaposi's sarcoma in patients with and without acquired immune deficiency syndrome (AIDS). *J Clin Pathol* 1986;39:742–9.

240. Dorfman RF. Kaposi's sarcoma: evidence supporting its origin from the lymphatic system. *Lymphology* 1988;21:45–52.

241. Werner S, Hofschneider PH, Roth WK. Cells derived from sporadic and AIDS-related Kaposi's sarcoma reveal identical cytochemical and molecular properties in vitro. *Cancer* 1989;43:1137–44.

242. Auerbach HE, Brooks JJ. Kaposi's sarcoma: neoplasia or hyperplasia? *Surg Pathol* 1989;2:19–28.

243. Grody WW, Lewin KJ, Naeim F. Detection of cytomegalovirus DNA in classic and epidemic Kaposi's sarcoma by in situ hybridization. *Hum Pathol* 1988;19:524–8.

244. Kory WP, Rico MJ, Gould E, Penneys NS. Dermatopathologic findings in patients with acquired immunodeficiency syndrome. *South Med J* 1987;80:1529–32.

245. Fisher BK, Warner LC. Cutaneous manifestations of the acquired immunodeficiency syndrome. *Int J Dermatol* 1987;26:615–30.

246. Farthing CF, Brown SE, Staughton RCD. *A colour atlas of AIDS.* London: Wolfe Medical Publications Ltd, 1986;24–37.

247. Blumenfield W, Egbert BM, Sagebiel RW. Differential diagnosis of Kaposi's sarcoma. *Arch Pathol Lab Med* 1985;109:123–7.

248. Safai B, Johnson KG, Myskowski PL, et al. The natural history of

Kaposi's sarcoma in the acquired immunodeficiency syndrome. *Ann Intern Med* 1985;103:744–50.

249. Friedman SL, Wright TL, Altman DF. Gastrointestinal Kaposi sarcoma in patients with AIDS: endoscopic and autopsy findings. *Gastroenterology* 1985;89:102–8.

250. Fouret PJ, Touboul JL, Mayaud CM, Akoun GM, Roland J. Pulmonary Kaposi's sarcoma in patients with acquired immune deficiency syndrome: a clinicopathological study. *Thorax* 1987;42:262–8.

251. Kaplan LD, Hopewell PC, Jaffe H, Goodman PC, Bottles K, Volberding PA. Kaposi's sarcoma involving the lung in patients with the acquired immunodeficiency syndrome. *J Acquired Immune Deficiency Syndrome* 1988;1:23–30.

252. Francis ND, Parkin JM, Weber J, Boylston AW. Kaposi's sarcoma in acquired immune deficiency syndrome (AIDS). *J Clin Pathol* 1986;39:469–74.

253. Little BJ, Spivak JL, Quinn TC, Mann RB. Case report: Kaposi's sarcoma with bone marrow involvement: occurrence in a patient with the acquired immunodeficiency syndrome. *Am J Med Sci* 1986;292:44–6.

254. Bottles K, McPhaul LW, Volberding P. Fine-needle aspiration biopsy of patients with the acquired immunodeficiency syndrome (AIDS): experience in an outpatient clinic. *Ann Intern Med* 1988;108:42–5.

255. Ackerman AB. Subtle clues to diagnosis by conventional microscopy. The patch stage of Kaposi's sarcoma. *Am J Dermatopathol* 1979;1:165–72.

256. Niedt GW, Myskowski PL, Urmacher C, Niedzwiecki D, Chapman D, Safai B. Histology of early lesions of AIDS-associated Kaposi's sarcoma. *Mod Pathol* 1990;3:64–70.

257. Niemi M, Mustakallic KK. The fine structure of the spindle cell in Kaposi's sarcoma. *Arch Pathol Microbiol Scand* 1965;63:567–75.

258. LeBoit PE, Berger TG, Egbert BM, Beckstead JH, Yen TS B, Stoler MH. Bacillary angiomatosis; the histopathology and differential diagnosis of a pseudoneoplastic infection in patients with human immunodeficiency virus disease. *Am J Surg Pathol* 1989;13:909–20.

259. Cockerell CJ, Webster GF, Whitlow MA, et al. Epithelial angiomatosis: a distinct vascular disorder in patients with AIDS or AIDS related complex. *Lancet* 1987;2:654–6.

260. Abrams J, Farhood A. Infection-associated vascular lesions in acquired immunodeficiency syndrome patients. *Hum Pathol* 1989;20:1025–6.

261. Guarner J, Unger ER. Association of Epstein-Barr virus in epithelioid angiomatosis of AIDS patients. *Am J Surg Pathol* 1990;14:956–60.

262. LeBoit PE, Bergen TG, Egbert BM, et al. Epithelioid hemangioma-like vascular proliferations in AIDS. Manifestations of cat-scratch disease bacillus or infection? *Lancet* 1988;1:960–3.

263. Arias-Stella J, Lieberman PH, Erlandson RA, et al. Histology, immunocytochemistry and ultrastructure of verruga in Carrion's disease. *Am J Surg Pathol* 1986;10:595–610.

264. Koehler JE, LeBoit PE, Egbert BM, Berger TG. Cutaneous vascular lesions and disseminated cat-scratch disease in patients with the acquired immunodeficiency syndrome (AIDS) and AIDS-related complex. *Ann Intern Med* 1988;109:449–55.

265. Templeton AC. Pathology of Kaposi's sarcoma. In: Ziegler JL, Dorfman RF, eds. *Kaposi's sarcoma.* New York: Marcel Dekker, Inc., 1988;55–60.

266. Lewis W. AIDS: Cardiac findings from 115 autopsies. *Prog Cardiovasc Dis* 1989;32:207–15.

267. Purtillo DT, Linder J, Volsky DJ. Acquired immune deficiency syndrome (AIDS). *Clin Lab Med* 1986;6:3–26.

268. Mathur-Wagh U, Enlow RW, Spigland I, et al. Longitudinal study of persistent generalized lymphadenopathy in homosexual men: relation to acquired immunodeficiency syndrome. *Lancet* 1984;1:1033–8.

269. CDC. Current trends: classification system for human T lymphotropic virus type III/lymphadenopathy associated virus infections. *MMWR* 1986;35:334–9.

270. Ioachim HL. Biopsy diagnosis in human immunodeficiency virus infection and acquired immunodeficiency syndrome. *Arch Pathol Lab Med* 1990;114:284–94.

271. Burns BF, Wood GS, Dorfman RF. The varied histopathology of lymphadenopathy in the homosexual male. *Am J Surg Pathol* 1985;9:287–97.

272. Brynes RK, Ewing EP, Joshi VV, et al. The histopathology of HIV infection: an overview. In: Rotterdam H, Sommers SC, Raez P, Meyer PR, eds. *Progress in AIDS pathology.* New York: Field & Wood Medical Publishers Inc, 1989;1–28.

273. Ioachim HL, Cronin W, Roy M, Maya M. Persistent lymphadenitis in individuals at high risk for HIV infection: clinicopathologic correlations and longterm follow-up in 79 cases. *Am J Clin Pathol* 1990;93:208–18.

274. Chadburn A, Metroka C, Mouradian J. Progressive lymph node histology and its prognostic value in patients with acquired immunodeficiency syndrome and AIDS-related complex. *Hum Pathol* 1989;20:579–87.

275. Knowles DM, Chamulak GA, Subar M, et al. Lymphoid neoplasia associated with the acquired immunodeficiency syndrome (AIDS): the New York Medical Center experience with 105 patients (1981–1986). *Ann Intern Med* 1988;108:744–53.

276. Subar M, Neri A, Inghirami G, et al. Frequent c-myc oncogene activation and infrequent presence of Epstein-Barr virus genome in AIDS-associated lymphoma. *Blood* 1988;72:667–71.

277. Pelicci PG, Knowles DM, Arlin Z, et al. Multiple monoclonal B-cell expansions and c-myc oncogene rearrangements in AIDS-related lymphoproliferative disorders, implications for lymphogenesis. *J Exp Med* 1986;164:2049–60.

278. Cleary ML, Sklar J. Lymphoproliferative disorders in cardiac recipients are multiclonal lymphoma. *Lancet* 1984;2:489–93.

279. Shearer WT, Ritz J, Finegold M, et al. Epstein-Barr virus associated B-cells proliferations of diverse clonal origins after bone marrow transplantation in a 12 year old patient with severe combined immunodeficiency. *N Engl J Med* 1985;312:1151–9.

280. Knowles DM, Chamulak GA, Subar M. Clinicopathologic, immunophenotypic, and molecular genetic analysis of AIDS-associated lymphoid neoplasia: clinical and biologic implications. *Pathol Annu* 1988;23:33–67.

281. Unger PD, Strauchen JA. Hodgkin's disease in AIDS complex patients. Report of four cases and tissue immunologic marker studies. *Cancer* 1986;58:821–5.

282. Scheib RG, Siegel RS. Atypical Hodgkin's disease and the acquired immunodeficiency syndrome. *Ann Intern Med* 1985;102:554.

283. Cooper HS, Patchefsky AS, Marks G. Cloacogenic carcinoma of the anorectum in homosexual men: an observation of four cases. *Dis Colon Rectum* 1979;22:557–8.

284. Conant MA, Volberding P, Fletcher V, Fletcher V, Lozada FI, Silverman S Jr. Squamous cell carcinoma in sexual partner of Kaposi's sarcoma patient. *Lancet* 1982;1:286.

285. Hiddemann W. What's new in malignant tumors in acquired immunodeficiency disorders? *Pathol Res Pract* 1989;185:930–4.

286. Napoli VM, Stein SF, Spira TJ, et al. Myelodysplasia progressing to acute myeloblastic leukemia in an HTLV-III virus-positive homosexual man with AIDS-related complex. *Am J Clin Pathol* 1986;86:788–91.

287. Howard LC, Paterson-Brown S, Weber JN, et al. Squamous carcinoma of the anus in young homosexual men with T helper cell depletion. *Genitourin Med* 1986;62:393–5.

288. Krause W, Mittag H, Gieler U, et al. A case of malignant melanoma in AIDS-related complex. *Arch Dermatol* 1987;123:867–8.

289. Nasr SA, Brynes RK, Garrison CP, et al. Peripheral T-cell lymphoma in a patient with acquired immune deficiency syndrome. *Cancer* 1988;61:947–51.

290. Palefsky JM, Gonzales J, Greenblatt RM, et al. Anal intraepithelial neoplasia and anal papillomavirus infection among homosexual males with group IV HIV disease. *JAMA* 1990;263:2911–6.

291. Szypula G, Sen P, Tan KL, et al. Unusual presentation: testicular seminoma. *NJ Med* 1989;86:295–7.

292. Srivastava BI, Getchell JP, Stoll HL Jr. HTLV-III antibodies in a patient with mycosis fungoides. *J Med* 1986;17:57–63.

293. Gupta S, Imam A. Malignant melanoma in a homosexual man with HTLV-III/LAV exposure. *Am J Med* 1987;82:1027–30.

294. Duvic M, Lowe L, Rapini RP, et al. Eruptive dysplastic nevi associated with human immunodeficiency virus infection. *Arch Dermatol* 1989;125:397–401.

295. Winward KE, Curtin VT. Conjunctival squamous cell carcinoma in a patient with human immunodeficiency virus infection. *Am J Ophthalmol* 1989;107:554–5.

296. Ruff P, Bagg A, Papadopoulos K. Precursor T-cell lymphoma associated with human immunodeficiency virus type 1 (HIV-1) infection. *Cancer* 1989;64:39–42.

297. Longacre TA, Foucar K, Koster F, Burgdorf W. Atypical cutaneous lymphoproliferative disorder resembling mycosis fungoides in AIDS. Report of a case with concurrent Kaposi's sarcoma. *Am J Dermatopathol* 1989;11:451–6.

298. Chadwick EG, Connor EJ, Guerra-Hanson IC, et al. Tumors of smooth-muscle origin in HIV-infected children. *JAMA* 1990; 263:3182–4.

299. Mittal K, Neri A, Feiner H, et al. Lymphomatoid granulomatosis in the acquired immunodeficiency syndrome. Evidence of Epstein-Barr virus infection and B-cell clonal selection without myc rearrangement. *Cancer* 1990;65:1345–9.

300. Slazink L, Stall JR, Mathews CR. Basal cell carcinoma in a man with acquired immunodeficiency syndrome. *J Am Acad Dermatol* 1984;11:140–1.

301. Sitz KV, Keppen M, Johnson DF. Metastatic basal cell carcinoma in acquired immunodeficiency syndrome-related complex. *JAMA* 1987;257:340–3.

302. Ravalli S, Chabon AB, Khan AA. Gastrointestinal neoplasia in young HIV antibody-positive patients. *Am J Clin Pathol* 1989;91:458–61.

303. Irwin LE, Begandy MK, Moore TM. Adenosquamous carcinoma of the lung and the acquired immunodeficiency syndrome [Letter]. *Ann Intern Med* 1984;100:158.

304. Logothetis CJ, Newell GR, Samuels ML. Testicular cancer in homosexual men with cellular immunodeficiency: report of two cases. *J Urol* 1985;133:484–6.

305. Ninane J, Moulin D, Latinne D, et al. AIDS in two African children—one with fibrosarcoma of the liver. *Eur J Pediatr* 1985;144:385–90.

306. Tessler AN, Catanese A. AIDS and germ cell tumors of the testis. *Urology* 1987;30:203–4.

307. Cappell MS, Yao F, Cho KC. Colonic adenocarcinoma associated with the acquired immune deficiency syndrome. *Cancer* 1988;62:616–9.

308. Grieger TA, Carl M, Liebert HP, Cotelingam JD, Wagner KF. Mediastinal liposarcoma in a patient infected with the human immunodeficiency virus. *Am J Med* 1988;84:366.

309. Bluff DD, Greenberg SD, Leong P, et al. Thymoma, *Pneumocystis carinii* pneumonia, and AIDS. *NY State J Med* 1988;88: 276–7.

310. Alhashimi MM, Krasnow SH, Johnston-Early A, Cohen MH. Squamous cell carcinoma of the epiglottis in a homosexual man at risk for AIDS. *JAMA* 1985;253:2366.

311. Israel AM, Koziner B, Straus DJ. Plasmacytoma and the acquired immunodeficiency syndrome. *Ann Intern Med* 1983; 99:635–6.

312. Vandermolen LA, Fehir KM, Rice L. Multiple myeloma in a homosexual man with chronic lymphadenopathy. *Arch Intern Med* 1985;145:745–6.

313. Kaplan MH, Susin M, Pahwa SG, et al. Neoplastic complications of HTLV-III infection: lymphomas and solid tumors. *Am J Med* 1987;82:389–96.

314. Weldon-Linne CM, Rhone DP, Blatt D, Moore D, et al. Angiolipomas in homosexual men [Letter]. *N Engl J Med* 1984;310: 1193–4.

315. Levine AM. Non-Hodgkin's lymphomas and other malignancies in the acquired immune deficiency syndrome. *Semin Oncol* 1987;14:34–9.

316. Frazer IH, Medley G, Crapper RM, et al. Association between anorectal dysplasia, human papillomavirus, and human immunodeficiency virus infection in homosexual men. *Lancet* 1986;2: 657–60.

317. Levy WS, Simon GL, Rios JC, Ross AM. Prevalence of cardiac abnormalities in human immunodeficiency virus infection. *Am J Cardiol* 1989;63:86–9.

318. Anderson DW, Virmani R. Emerging patterns of heart disease in human immunodeficiency virus infection. *Hum Pathol* 1990; 21:253–9.

319. Cohen IS, Anderson DW, Virmani R, et al. Congestive cardiomyopathy in association with the acquired immunodeficiency syndrome. *N Engl J Med* 1986;315:628–30.

320. Monsuez J-J, Kinney EL, Vittecoq D, et al. Comparison among acquired immune deficiency syndrome patients with and without clinical evidence of cardiac disease. *Am J Cardiol* 1988;62: 1311–3.

321. Fink L, Reichek N, Sutton MG. Cardiac abnormalities in acquired immune deficiency syndrome. *Am J Cardiol* 1984;54: 1161–3.

322. Cammarosano C, Lewis W. Cardiac lesions in acquired immune deficiency syndrome (AIDS). *J Am Coll Cardiol* 1985;5:703–6.

323. Anderson DW, Virmani R, Reilly JM, et al. Prevalent myocarditis at necropsy in the acquired immunodeficiency syndrome. *J Am Coll Cardiol* 1988;11:792–9.

324. Reilly JM, Cunnion RE, Anderson DW, et al. Frequency of myocarditis, left ventricular dysfunction and ventricular tachycardia in the acquired immune deficiency syndrome. *Am J Cardiol* 1988;62:789–93.

325. Levy WS, Varghese J, Anderson DW, et al. Myocarditis diagnosed by endomyocardial biopsy in human immunodeficiency virus infection with cardiac dysfunction. *Am J Cardiol* 1988;62:658–9.

326. Gottlieb MS, Groopman JE, Weinstein WM, et al. The acquired immunodeficiency syndrome. *Ann Intern Med* 1983;99:208–20.

327. Current WL, Reese NC, Ernst JV, Bailey WS, Heyman MB, Weinstein WM. Human cryptosporidiosis in immunocompetent and immunodeficient persons. Studies of an outbreak and experimental transmission. *N Engl J Med* 1983;308:1252–7.

328. Kotler DP, Goetz HP, Lange M, Klein EB, Holt PR. Enteropathy associated with the acquired immunodeficiency syndrome. *Ann Intern Med* 1984;101:421–8.

329. Ullrich R, Zeitz M, Heise W, L'age M, Hoffken G, Riecken EO. Small intestinal structure and function in patients infected with human immunodeficiency virus (HIV): evidence for HIV-induced enteropathy. *Ann Intern Med* 1989;111:15–21.

330. Nelson JA, Wiley CA, Reynolds-Kohler C, Reese CE, Margaretten W, Levy JA. Human immunodeficiency virus detected in bowel epithelium from patients with gastrointestinal symptoms. *Lancet* 1988;1:259–62.

331. Batman PA, Miller AR, Forster SM, Harris JR, Pinching AJ, Griffin GE. Jejunal enteropathy associated with human immunodeficiency virus infection: Quantitative histology. *J Clin Pathol* 1989;42:275–81.

332. Kotler DP, Francisco A, Clayton F, Scholes JV, Orenstein JM. Small intestinal injury and parasitic disease in AIDS. *Ann Intern Med* 1990;113:444–9.

333. Griffin GE, Miller A, Batman P, et al. Damage to jejunal intrinsic autonomic nerves in HIV infection. *AIDS* 1988;2:379–82.

334. Rao TKS, Freidman EA, Nicastri AD. The types of renal disease in the acquired immunodeficiency syndrome. *N Engl J Med* 1987;316:1062–8.

335. Gardenwartz MH, Lerner CW, Seligson GR, et al. Renal disease in patients with AIDS: a clinicopathologic study. *Clin Nephrol* 1984;21:197–204.

336. Bourgoignie JJ, Meneses R, Ortiz C, Jaffe D, Pardo V. The clinical spectrum of renal disease associated with human immunodeficiency virus. *Am J Kidney Dis* 1988;12:131–7.

337. Dabbs DL, Kendrick PW, Harris LS. Proliferative glomerulonephritis with immune deposits in the acquired immunodeficiency syndrome. *Kidney Int* 1986;29:272(abst).

338. Appel R, Neill JSA. HIV-associated steroid responsive nephrotic syndrome. *Ann Intern Med* 1990;113:892–3.

339. Glassrock RJ, Cohen AH, Danovitch G, Parsa KP. Human immunodeficiency virus (HIV) infection and the kidney. *Ann Intern Med* 1990;112:35–49.

340. Rao TKS, Filippone EJ, Nicastri AD, et al. Associated focal and segmental glomerulosclerosis in the acquired immunodeficiency syndrome. *N Engl J Med* 1984;310:669–73.

341. Humphreys MH, Schoenfeld PY. Renal complications in patients with the acquired immune deficiency syndrome (AIDS). *Am J Nephrol* 1987;7:1–7.

342. Strauss J, Abitol C, Zilleruelo G, et al. Renal disease in children

with the acquired immunodeficiency syndrome. *N Engl J Med* 1989;321:625–30.

343. Pardo V, Jaffe D, Roth D, Hensley G, Fischl M, Bourgoigne JJ. Nephrotic syndrome with focal and segmental glomerular sclerosis (FSS) as a prodrome of AIDS: report of seven patients. *Kidney Int* 1986;29:288(abst).

344. Oleske J, Minnefor A, Cooper R Jr, et al. Immune deficiency syndrome in children. *JAMA* 1983;29:2345–9.

345. Rubinstein A, Sicklick M, Gupta A, et al. Acquired immunodeficiency with reversed T4/T8 ratios in infants born to promiscuous and drug-addicted mothers. *JAMA* 1983;249:2350–6.

346. Oxtoby MJ. Perinatally acquired HIV infection. In: Pizzo PA, Wilfert CM, eds. *Pediatric AIDS.* Baltimore: Williams & Wilkins, 1990;3–21.

347. Rubinstein A. Pediatric AIDS. *Curr Probl Pediatr* 1986;16:361–409.

348. Joshi VV, Oleske J, Minnefor AB, et al. Pathology of suspected acquired immune deficiency syndrome in children: a study of eight cases. *Pediatr Pathol* 1984;2:71–87.

349. Savino W, Dardenne M, Marche C, et al. Thymic epithelium in AIDS. An immunohistologic study. *Am J Pathol* 1986;122:302–7.

350. Karmarkar S. Personal communication, 1988.

351. Joshi VV, Oleske J. Pulmonary lesions in children with the acquired immunodeficiency syndrome: a reappraisal based on data in additional cases and follow-up study of previously reported cases. *Hum Pathol* 1986;17:641–2.

352. Guillon JM, Autran B, Denis M, et al. Human immunodeficiency virus related lymphocytic alveolitis. *Chest* 1988;94:1264–70.

353. Andiman WA, Eastman R, Martin K, et al. Opportunistic lymphoproliferations associated with Epstein-Barr viral DNA in infants and children with AIDS. *Lancet* 1985;2:1390–3.

354. Ramaswamy G, Jagadha V, Tchertkoff V. Diffuse alveolar damage and interstitial fibrosis in acquired immunodeficiency syndrome patients without concurrent pulmonary infection. *Arch Pathol Lab Med* 1985;109:408–12.

355. Ognibene FP, Masur H, Rogers P, et al. Nonspecific interstitial pneumonitis without evidence of *Pneumocystis carinii* in asymptomatic patients infected with human immunodeficiency virus (HIV). *Ann Intern Med* 1988;109:874–9.

356. Ettensohn DB, Mayer KH, Kessimian N, et al. Lymphocytic bronchiolitis associated with HIV infection. *Chest* 1988;93:201–2.

356a. Ognibene FP, Masur H, Rogers P, Travis WD, et al. Nonspecific interstitial pneumonitis without evidence of *Pneumocystis carinii* in asymptomatic patients with human immunodeficiency virus (HIV). *Ann Intern Med* 1988;109:874–9.

357. Olsen WL, Jeffrey RB Jr, Sooy CD, et al. Lesions of the head and neck in patients with AIDS: CT and MR findings. *AJR* 1988;151:785–90.

358. Beissner RS, Rapport ES, Diaz JA. Fatal case of Epstein-Barr virus-induced lymphoproliferative disorder associated with a human immunodeficiency virus infection. *Arch Pathol Lab Med* 1987;111:250–3.

359. Sprecher S, Soumenkoff G, Puissant F, et al. Vertical transmission of HIV in 15-week fetus. *Lancet* 1986;2:288–9.

360. Jauniaux E, Nessmann C, Imbert C, et al. Morphologic aspects of placenta in HIV pregnancies. *Placenta* 1988;9:633–42.

361. Pomerantz RJ, de-la-Monte SM, Donegan SP, et al. Human immunodeficiency virus (HIV) infection of the uterine cervix. *Ann Intern Med* 1988;108:321–7.

362. Wofsy CB, Cohen JB, Hauer LB. Isolation of AIDS-associated retrovirus from genital secretions of women with antibodies to the virus. *Lancet* 1986;1:527–9.

363. Quinn TC, Mann JM, Curran JW, et al. AIDS in Africa: an epidemiologic paradigm. *Science* 1986;234:955–63.

364. Hardy DB. Cultural practices contributing to the transmission of human immunodeficiency virus in Africa. *Rev Infect Dis* 1987;9:1109–19.

365. Wamukota W, Lucas SB. Morbid anatomy of AIDS in Uganda. *J Pathol* 1986;149:245A.

366. Lepage P, Van de Perre P. Clinical manifestations in infants and children. *Baillieres Clin Trop Communicable Dis* 1988;3:89–101.

367. Gerberding JL. Transmission of HIV in health care workers. In: *The AIDS knowledge base.* The Medical Publishing Group, 1990;1.2.8–1.2.9.

368. Marcus R. Surveillance of health care workers exposed to blood from patients infected with the human immunodeficiency virus. *N Engl J Med* 1988;319:1118–23.

369. Occupational exposure to blood borne pathogens: proposed role and notice of hearings (29 CFS 1910). *Federal Register.* 1989 May 30; 54:23042–139.

370. CDC. Recommendations for prevention of HIV transmission in health care settings. *MMWR* 1987;258:1S–18S.

371. CDC. Update: universal precautions for prevention of transmission of human immunodeficiency virus, hepatitis B virus, and other blood borne pathogens in health care settings. *MMWR* 1988;37:377–88.

372. Garner JS, Simmon BD. Guidelines for isolation precautions in hospitals. *Infect Control* 1983;4:275–325.

373. McCray E. Cooperative needle stick group. Occupational risks of the acquired immunodeficiency syndrome among health care workers. *N Engl J Med* 1986;314:1127–32.

374. Tierno PM. Preventing acquisition of human immunodeficiency virus in the laboratory: safe handling of AIDS specimens. *Lab Med* 1986;17:696–8.

375. Martin LS, MacDougal JS, Loskoski SL. Disinfection and inactivation of the human T lymphotropic virus type III/lymphadenopathy-associated virus. *J Infect Dis* 1985;152:400–3.

376. Spire B, Barre-Sinoussi F, Montagnier L, Chermann JC. Inactivation of lymphadenopathy associated virus by chemical disinfectants. *Lancet* 1984;2:899–901.

377. Resnick L, Veren S, Salahuddin SZ, Tondreau S, Markham PD. Stability and inactivation of HTLV-III/LAV under clinical and laboratory environments. *JAMA* 1986;255:1887–191.

378. Kaplan JC, Crawford DC, Durno AG, et al. Inactivation of human immunodeficiency virus by betadine. *Infect Control* 1987;8:412–4.

379. Geller SA. The autopsy in acquired immunodeficiency syndrome. *Arch Pathol Lab Med* 1990;114:324–9.

380. National Committee for Clinical Laboratory Standards. *Protection of laboratory workers: tentative guidelines.* Villanova PA: National Committee for Clinical Laboratory Standards, 1989. National Committee for Clinical Laboratory Standards document M29-T.

AIDS and Other Manifestations of HIV Infection,
Second Edition, Edited by Gary P. Wormser.
Raven Press, Ltd., New York © 1992.

CHAPTER 34

Pathology of the Nervous System in HIV-Infected Patients

Ana Sotrel and Pratik Multani

Neurological and neuropathological abnormalities in AIDS are diverse and very common. Of 376 autopsied AIDS cases, compiled from five published autopsy series (1), 78% had various forms of neuropathology that range from the most common HIV-related conditions to a wide spectrum of other diseases, including viral, fungal, parasitic, and bacterial opportunistic infections, and neoplastic, lymphoproliferative, and vascular disorders (1).

In this chapter, we attempt to elaborate on the pathogenetic and pathological aspects of a number of clinicopathological entities that affect the brain, spinal cord, meninges, peripheral nerves, and skeletal muscles of HIV-infected patients (Table 1).

AIDS-DEMENTIA COMPLEX: SUBACUTE HIV ENCEPHALOPATHY

This is a novel, progressive disease of the central nervous system (CNS), pathogenetically related to HIV. It has been extensively studied and reported in the literature under different names, most often as encephalitis or encephalomyelitis (2–6), encephalitis with multinucleated cells (MNCs) (6,7), and AIDS-dementia complex (8–11). AIDS-dementia complex represents a clinical term for a disease that may be a manifestation of varied pathological processes caused not only by HIV but also by cytomegalovirus (CMV) (12) or by dual infection with HIV and CMV (13,14), which sometimes target the same cell (15,16). JC virus is another often mentioned copathogen of HIV (17,18) that, together with CMV, has been implicated as a "cofactor" in the pathogenesis of

AIDS-dementia complex, acting as the instigator of an immunological reaction, which in turn provokes invasion of the CNS by monocytes that are infected by HIV (11).

In their subclassification of AIDS-dementia complex, taking into consideration the clinical presentation, pathological findings, and detectability of HIV in the CNS, Price et al. (10) have outlined three principal categories: (a) Patients with AIDS and overtly progressive dementia, presence of MNCs in the brain, damage of hemispheral white matter, and detectable HIV in CNS tissue. About 25% of all autopsied cases of AIDS belong to this subgroup. (b) AIDS patients with mild dementia and postmortem pathology characterized by diffuse hemispheral attenuation of myelin without MNC. Although HIV infection of brain tissue can be demonstrated in only 15% of cases in this category, as many as 50% of all autopsied patients with AIDS belong to this clinicopathological subset of cases. (c) Of the remaining 25% of autopsied patients with AIDS who have no clinical signs of dementia and no pathological changes in the brain, 5% will have demonstrable HIV infection in brain tissue (10). This essentially implies that about 45% of all AIDS patients have detectable HIV infection of the brain; only 25% of these have MNCs in the brain tissue (considered to be histologically pathognomonic of HIV infection), whereas as many as 75% of all AIDS cases have mild to severe, clinically detectable dementia at the time of death. Thus our previously proposed designations (1) of "AIDS-dementia complex," as the best clinical term for a progressive dementing illness, and of "HIV encephalopathy," as the most accurate pathological and virological term applicable to all those patients with AIDS whose autopsied or biopsied brain tissue contains HIV and/or

A. Sotrel and P. Multani: Department of Pathology, Beth Israel Hospital, Boston, Massachusetts 02215.

TABLE 1. *Clinicopathologic correlation of various central and peripheral nervous system and skeletal muscle disorders associated with AIDS*

Progressive dementing illness ("subcortical") with global brain atrophy (CT)
  HIV encephalopathy
  (?) Cytomegalovirus encephalitis
  Both
Spinal cord and/or spinal root disorders
  Vacuolar myelopathy
  Herpes simplex virus type II (±) cytomegalovirus myelitis
  Cytomegalovirus polyradiculitis
  (?) HIV-related polyradiculopathy
  Vasculitis
Single or multiple brain lesions (CT) with and without mass effect, focal neurologic signs (±), generalized neurologic symptoms
  Toxoplasmosis
  Primary brain lymphoma
  Mycobacterial abscess
  Bacterial abscess
  Infarcts (embolic, vasculitic)
  Amoebic necrotizing–hemorrhagic lesions
Multifocal, mostly subcortical hypodensities (CT) with focal neurologic signs (±), global neurologic symptoms
  Progressive multifocal leukoencephalopathy
  Varicella zoster virus demyelinating encephalopathy
  HIV-encephalopathy
  Acute multiple sclerosis-like lesions
Meningitis–ventriculitis
  Cryptococcal
  Bacterial
  (?) HIV-related
  Cytomegalovirus ventriculitis
Neuropathy
  Immunologic
  (?) HIV-related
  Other
Myopathies
  Inflammatory
  Nemaline rod
  Mitochondrial

Adapted from ref. 1.

the characteristic MNCs, regardless of the clinical presentation or other associated pathologies in the CNS, seem to be appropriate (2–33).

Radiological Findings

CT scan usually demonstrates *ex vacuo,* sulcal, and ventricular enlargement (Fig. 1), probably due to a global wasting of the brain tissue rather than just cortical atrophy (8). The white matter damage is visualized as focal or more diffuse "hypoattenuation" (34). Magnetic resonance imaging (MRI) is more sensitive in detecting myelin damage (8), which is usually presented as focal or diffuse hyperintensity on T2-weighted MR images (34).

Metabolic studies indicate that a majority of patients with AIDS-dementia complex have an increased general metabolism in the basal ganglia and thalami in early

stages of the disease and normal cortical metabolism, whereas in more advanced stages, a more diffuse cortico–subcortical hypometabolism supersedes (35).

Pathological Findings in HIV Encephalopathy

Gross findings at the time of autopsy are nonspecific and quite repetitive in that the most advanced cases of the disease have marked fibrous thickening of leptomeninges, widening of sulci, predominantly frontal, and diffuse enlargement of the ventricular system. Occasionally, diffuse or focal white matter damage may also be discernible (36).

Microscopic Features

Even though HIV encephalopathy seems to be directly related to HIV infection of the brain, the absence of any microscopically demonstrable cytopathic effect on neurons, oligodendroglia, or astrocytes is one of the salient features of all histological variants of the disease. In addition, at least four repetitive types of pathological change can be detected.

HIV Encephalopathy with Focal Microglial Infiltrates and Multinucleated Cells (MNCs)

This is the only histologically distinctive and virologically consistently positive form of HIV encephalopathy. The typical lesion consists of an ill-defined, irregular conglomerate of microglia and other unidentifiable, small, rounded, darkly staining nuclei (these are referred to as microglial nodules by others, but, for reasons indicated, we choose to distinguish the two lesions) (Fig. 2). In more typical viral encephalitides, microglial nodules appear as small tightly packed clusters of microglia drawn to an infected and injured cell. In contrast, similar lesions in HIV encephalopathy range from a few haphazardly disposed microglial cells to very large, irregular cellular infiltrates that contain not only microglia but also macrophages and one or more multinucleated cells. MNCs are usually devoid of discernible cytoplasm, containing only a tightly drawn pile of numerous, unusually small, overlapping dark nuclei that resemble those of neighboring microglia (Fig. 2A). An occasional microglial conglomerate is present in the neocortex, limbic system, and spinal cord, but most of them are located in the hemispheral white matter, brain stem, and deep gray structures, particularly the basal ganglia. The microglial infiltrates are often situated in the immediate vicinity of a blood vessel wall, occasionally encircling a small vessel.

Although HIV infection can be demonstrated in microglial cells and macrophages, in addition to MNCs, the presence of these cell types in brain tissue does not neces-

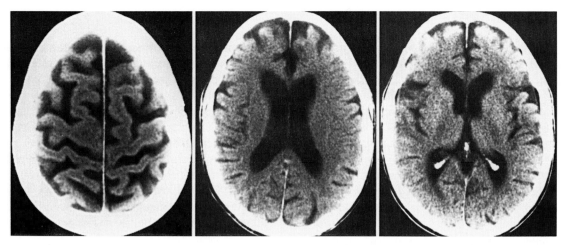

FIG. 1. A 61-year-old man with clinically progressive AIDS-dementia complex and pathologically proven HIV encephalopathy. CT scan without contrast material shows marked *ex vacuo* widening of sulci and fissures as well as diffuse, symmetrical ventricular enlargement.

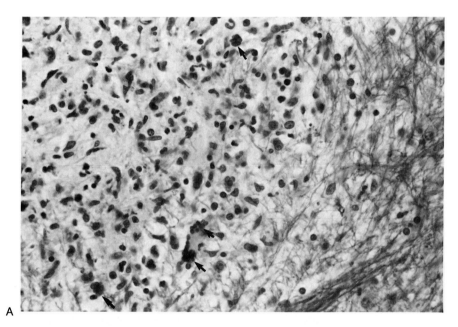

A

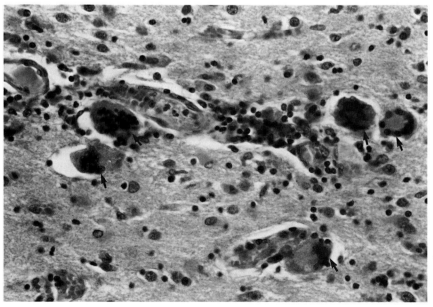

B

FIG. 2. HIV encephalopathy (H&E, LFB*). The most typical histological features. **A:** An area of myelin loss containing a large loose conglomerate of microglial and other mononuclear cells. Characteristically, clusters of unusually small, darkly staining nuclei (*arrows*), which appear as if they were drawn together by a magnet, represent the pathognomonic multinucleated cells (MNCs). Myelinated axons (on the right) outside the lesion appear intact (×400). **B:** MNCs (*arrows*), the pathognomonic histological sign of HIV encephalopathy, are shown here in another typical location—adjacent to blood vessel walls and scanty perivascular lymphocytic infiltrates (×400).

---

* Most tissue sections used in this chapter were stained with a combination of hematoxylin and eosin (H&E) and Luxol fast blue (LFB) (for myelin).

sarily denote HIV infection (37). This may occur in some cases of primary CMV encephalitis and progressive multifocal leukoencephalopathy. This should caution against pathological diagnosis of HIV encephalopathy solely on the bases of the presence of microglial nodules (38), single microglial cells, macrophages, or astrocytes, even when other infectious agents cannot be identified. On the other hand, systematic immunocytochemical staining, with different HIV-specific antibodies, of a large number of autopsied or biopsied brains from AIDS patients demonstrated that 65–73% of all specimens contained HIV-positive cells of the monocyte–microglial cell lineage (37). Forty-six percent of these cases had HIV pathognomonic pathology (the presence of MNCs), and in 10% of cases, single, scattered microglial cells stained positively for HIV, despite the absence of any other microscopically identifiable pathology (37). Dual infection of the CNS or even a single cell by both CMV and HIV has been observed in a number of cases (13–16), raising the speculation that CMV may indeed play a role in the pathogenesis of HIV encephalopathy. Moreover, a fairly large percentage of otherwise rare AIDS patients with progressive multifocal leukoencephalopathy also acquire HIV infection of the CNS, as if somehow brain damage inflicted by JC virus "recruits" HIV-infected macrophages into the region of primary tissue destruction (17,18,37). Budka's findings indicate that there may be more to this propensity of the HIV virus to coinfect the CNS with JCV than a simple "recruitment," because such coinfection with other opportunistic organisms seems to be very rare (37).

There is now ample evidence that HIV infection of single microglial cells and macrophages occurs in cases of HIV encephalopathy without MNCs (10,37). With rare exceptions (38), MNCs (Fig. 2B) can always be shown to harbor HIV particles and/or HIV antigen. Electron microscopy has revealed both viral particles and budding of virions from the plasma membranes of MNCs as well as other cell types (see below) (39–42). Based on ultrastructural evidence (42), it has been suggested that MNCs in the brain may be formed under the well-known cytopathic influence of HIV which *in vitro* induces fusion of infected T cells (43) as well as brain-derived microglia (43). MNCs also contain HIV-RNA based on studies using *in situ* hybridization techniques on formalin-fixed tissue obtained from autopsied patients with HIV encephalopathy (40,44). With rare exceptions (38), MNCs in isopentane-frozen brain tissue can be shown to possess an HIV antigen that reacts with a mouse monoclonal antibody against a structural HIV protein (45), and immunocytochemical studies of formalin-fixed, paraffin-embedded brain tissue have demonstrated the presence of HIV antigen within MNCs (6,37,46). Budka, using four commercially available antibodies, directed toward HIV p24, HIV p17, HIV gp41, or HIV gp120, found that MNCs invariably stain with at

least one of them, thus confirming the previous notion that they can be regarded as a histological hallmark of HIV infection of the brain (37,46).

Based on the results of immunohistochemical studies with a wide variety of cell-specific markers, and on ultrastructural examination, the cell of origin of MNCs seems to be microglia (6,46,47) and less likely monocyte-derived macrophages (39–41,45). In human brain-derived tissue cultures, microglial cells, once infected with HIV, first cluster and then fuse into MNC forms, thus creating a replica of microglial-multinucleated cellular conglomerates that are so often seen in the brains of patients with HIV encephalopathy (43).

In addition to microglial conglomerates, hemispheral white matter in HIV encephalopathy usually shows minimal to moderate, focal or diffuse myelin damage; scattered, scanty perivascular collections of mononuclear cells and/or macrophages; occasional isolated MNCs; and more or less diffuse reactive astrocytosis. Focal hyperplasia of oligodendroglial cells, without viral inclusions, may also be present. Astrocytes and oligodendroglia have never been unequivocally shown to be infected by HIV.

Axons are relatively well preserved, although minimal axonal loss and presence of axonal spheroids serve as subtle signs that HIV encephalopathy is not a strictly demyelinating disorder.

Vessels in the affected white matter and basal ganglia may show hyperplasia of the endothelial lining, overall thickening of the vessel walls, and perivascular collections of macrophages with an occasional MNC (48, and *personal observations*). In some cases, this could be a response to cryptic CMV infection of endothelial cells (49,50) or to HIV infection itself (45,46). However, the presence of HIV antigen in the endothelium of these vessels cannot always be demonstrated (37,48), and endothelial cells are not susceptible to infection by HIV *in vitro* (11). A few adults and most children with HIV encephalopathy also develop various degrees of bilateral striatal mineralizing vasculopathy (Fig. 3), which occasionally extends to the periventricular and deep hemispheral white matter (42). The pathogenesis of this distinctive vascular change is only speculative (1). Direct CMV, HIV, or, less likely, rubella infection of vessel walls has been proposed, as well as intramural deposition of immune complexes following a transient, regional breakdown of the blood–brain barrier (1). While the basal ganglia in children with extensive mineralizing angiopathy invariably show various forms of parenchymal damage, consisting of astrocytic scars and small infarct-like lesions, the relationship between regional vasculopathy and consequent white matter damage is more difficult to prove; however, the possibility of an increase in vascular permeability, resulting from vessel wall injury, may be implicated in the pathogenesis of leukoencephalopathy (48). For a more detailed review of HIV encepha-

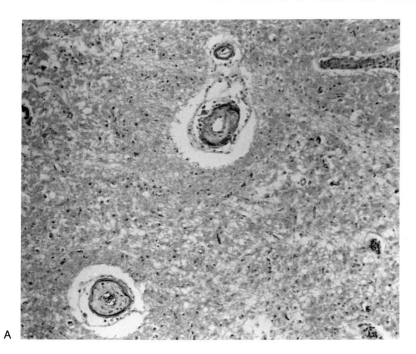

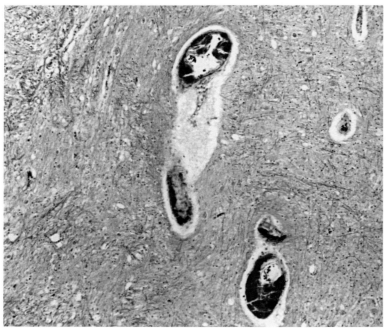

FIG. 3. HIV encephalopathy in a child with *in utero* acquired infection and characteristic mineralizing vasculopathy in the basal ganglia (H&E/LFB). **A:** Concentric fibrous thickening of vessel walls with narrowing of lumen and subtle mineralization along the abluminal border of the wall. Surrounding brain parenchyma shows neuronal loss, cystic degeneration of neuropil, and gliosis (×200). **B:** Diffuse or multifocal, subendothelial "bumpy-lumpy" deposits of mineralized material in the walls of other vessels within the basal ganglia of the same specimen (×200).

lopathy and other neurological complications of AIDS in children, please see Kozlowski et al. (48A).

Multifocal Leukoencephalopathy

Occasionally (1,51,52), the subcortical white matter of one or more adjacent gyri contains multiple, grossly discernible (1), punched-out foci of a grey discoloration due to myelin loss, minimal to marked axonal damage, accumulation of macrophages, and scanty perivascular microglial and mononuclear-macrophage infiltrates with a

conspicuous absence of typical HIV-related MNCs, although multinucleated macrophages may be present. These lesions are, upon gross brain inspection, indistinguishable from progressive multifocal leukoencephalopathy or varicella zoster virus (VZV) encephalitis (1); yet microscopically and/or ultrastructurally, the presence of either JCV or VZV cannot be demonstrated. These may be smaller variants of multiple sclerosis-like lesions that have been noted to occur in patients with HIV infection (53,54; *personal unpublished data*). Some of these patients present with clinical, radiological (Fig. 4A), and immunological findings typical of classical multiple scle-

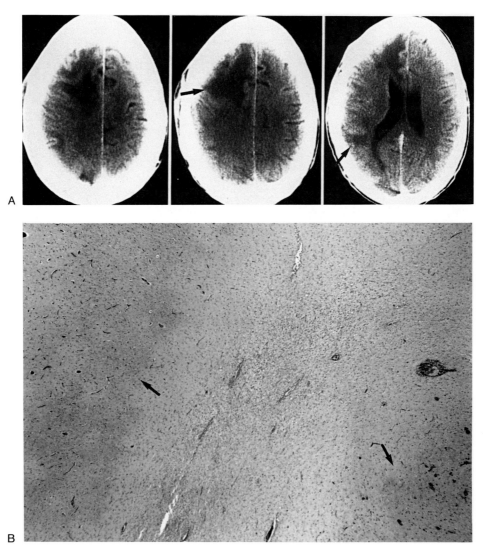

FIG. 4. A 44-year-old man with AIDS. **A:** CT scan with contrast material shows large, frontal and temporal, hypodense, nonenhancing lesions that are well defined, produce no mass effect, and are confined to the subcortical and deep white matter. **B:** Biopsy of the temporal lobe lesion (H&E/LFB) shows intact cortex (*arrows*) and complete myelin loss in the subcortical white matter (×25). **C:** A close-up view of the demyelinated white matter shows multifocal perivascular lymphocytic infiltrates, microcystic degeneration of tissue, almost total loss and atrophy of oligodendroglia, and a profusion of reactive astrocytes and macrophages (×200). **D:** Ultrastructurally, the white matter lesion shows a perivascular macrophage loaded with membrane-bound cytoplasmic inclusions (*arrows*) that are morphologically identical to those observed in non-AIDS-related multiple sclerosis (MS) cases (×10,000).

rosis (MS) (54), while others have focal neurological signs, headache, and multiple large, hypodense, nonenhancing lesions by CAT scan (53). Histologically, the gray matter is intact, and all lesions present with typically well-defined areas of myelin loss, profusion of macrophages, astrocytosis (Fig. 4B), and scanty perivascular mononuclear infiltrates (Fig. 4C). This process raises the question of an HIV-mediated demyelinating illness, which in most other aspects resembles acute forms of multiple sclerosis (54). HIV-specific immunocytochemistry, however, has failed to disclose the presence of HIV within the lesion (53). Likewise, in one case of AIDS-

associated acute MS, we could not find HIV particles by electron microscopy. It is of some interest to mention that ultrastructural findings in this case were identical (Fig. 4D) to those in non-HIV-related cases of acute MS (55,56).

Diffuse Bilateral Leukoencephalopathy with Severe Myelin and Axonal Damage

This is a very rare form of HIV-related encephalopathy, histologically characterized by an almost total, bilat-

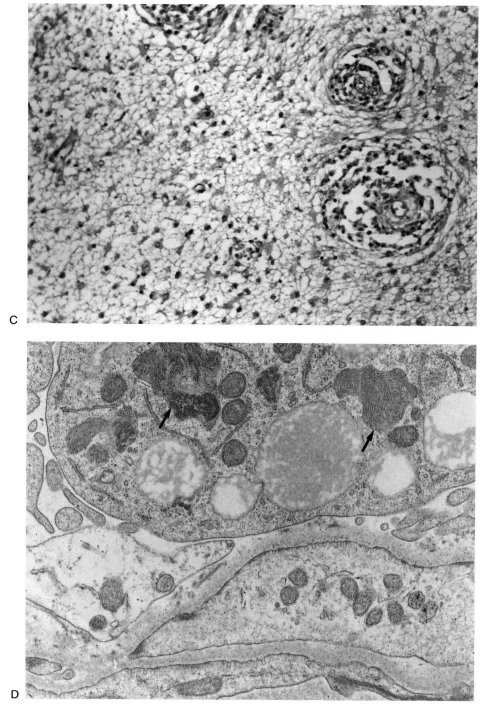

FIG. 4. *Continued.*

erally symmetrical degeneration of myelin sheaths in the cerebral hemispheres (1,36). We have only seen one such case (1) in which, in addition to bilateral hemispheral myelin loss, there were exuberant perivascular inflammatory infiltrates (Fig. 5A), a multitude of scattered MNCs (Fig. 5B,C), diffuse reactive astrocytosis, and proliferation of macrophages. All pathological changes were most severe in the deep and periventricular white matter, whereas the subcortical parts were better preserved.

Diffuse, Subtle, Nonspecific Pathological Changes with Brain Atrophy

According to some authors, 50% of all AIDS patients with mild to moderate dementia have very subtle nonspecific pathological changes characterized by minimal diffuse attenuation of hemispheral myelin and astrocytosis. HIV infection can be demonstrated in 15% of these cases (10). Some consider such "subcortical leukoencephalop-

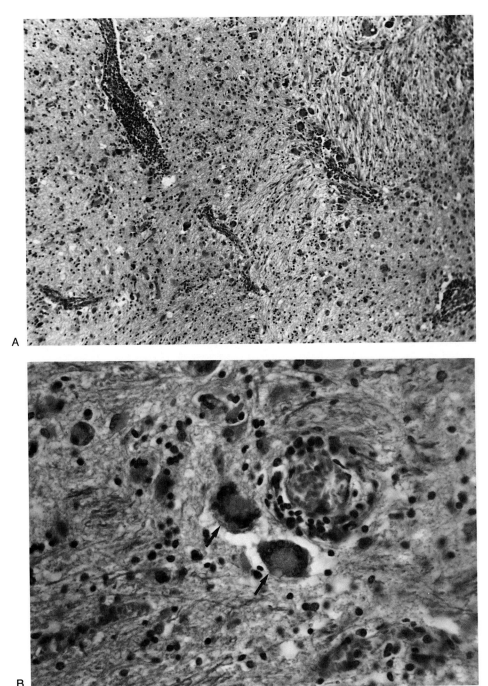

FIG. 5. HIV leukoencephalopathy, diffuse, inflammatory, bilaterally symmetrical variant (H&E/LFB). **A:** Hemispheral white matter shows total loss of myelin, perivascular lymphocytic infiltrates, relative preservation of oligodendroglia and axons, and a profusion of reactive astrocytes and macrophages, many of which are multinucleated (×100). **B:** Typical MNCs located in the vicinity of a scanty, perivascular lymphocytic infiltrate (×400). **C:** A single MNC with minute overlapping nuclei amid a small mononuclear infiltrate in the partially demyelinated subcortical white matter (×400).

athy," characterized by various degrees of symmetrical white matter pallor and diffuse reactive astrocytosis, to be the most consistent correlate of AIDS-dementia complex (57). However, similar pathological findings in the CNS can be present in HIV-positive, clinically asymptomatic individuals (58). We have studied postmortem-

obtained brains from two AIDS patients (a 51-year-old homosexual man and a 36-year-old IV drug user) who had no recorded clinical history of dementia or any other neurological problems. Yet at autopsy, both patients had subtle, diffuse telencephalic myelin pallor with minimal to moderate astrocytosis in addition to grossly observed,

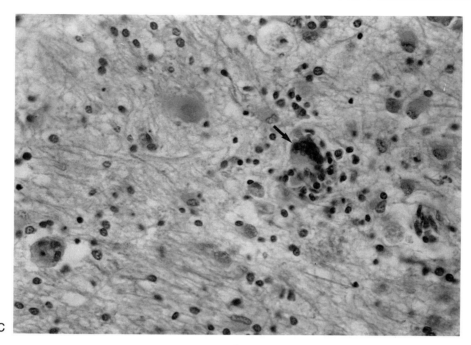

C

FIG. 5. *Continued.*

strikingly symmetrical cortical atrophy confined to the dorsolateral prefrontal cortex. Both had mild to moderate fibrous thickening of the leptomeninges over the dorsal-frontoparietal aspects of the hemispheres and focal loss of the ependymal lining with an astrocytic response. The IV drug user also had diffuse ventricular enlargement. Sections from the grossly atrophic prefrontal cortex showed barely discernible neuronal loss, minimal astrocytic reaction, and an occasional microglial cell. Ongoing neuronal degeneration could not be seen. Neither case showed any other specific pathologic finding in the 17–20 brain sections available for the light microscopic study.

Pathology of the Cerebral Cortex

The two aforementioned cases provide evidence that lobar cortical atrophy can take place in the absence of either more advanced white matter disease or any other more typical histological signs of HIV infection.

In a recent morphometric study (59) of grossly and histologically "normal" orbitofrontal cortex obtained at autopsy from 18 "unselected" patients with AIDS and variable neurological–neuropathological findings, it was shown that neuronal density in AIDS cases was 18% lower than that of normal controls. Although 71% of these brains tested positive for HIV antigen, only eight patients had "dementing" symptoms, and only four cases had histologically typical HIV encephalopathy with MNCs. This indicates that patients with AIDS who have a spectrum of CNS pathologies may indeed have significant cortical neuronal loss, which occurs independently of all other more specific pathological processes (59). In a similar morphometric analysis of frontal, temporal, and parietal cortices obtained at autopsy from 12 patients with histologically proven HIV encephalopathy with MNCs (plus six HIV-seropositive, neurologically normal patients and 14 normal controls), it was demonstrated that patients with HIV encephalopathy have a 30–50% reduction in the number of large cortical neurons and a consequent 20% reduction in cortical thickness (60).

Some studies suggest that, judging by the number of reactive cells, microglia, and astrocytes, the cortical pathology in many AIDS cases may parallel that of the white matter (61).

Finally, AIDS-dementia complex can also be a manifestation of "polyodystrophy" (62). This condition is reported far more frequently by European investigators (63). Pathologically, there is striking, extensive cortical pathology characterized by focal necrosis, neuronal loss, perivascular accumulation of macrophages and MNCs, and reactive astrocytosis. Both macrophages and MNCs are positive for HIV antigen when stained with monoclonal anti-p24 antibodies. In our laboratory, with more than 100 autopsied and carefully studied brains from patients with AIDS, we have yet to see a single case of such "polyodystrophy."

PATHOGENESIS OF BRAIN DAMAGE IN HIV-RELATED ENCEPHALOPATHIES

The presence of HIV-infected MNCs, microglia, and macrophages in brain tissue represents only one line of evidence that HIV may be causally related to AIDS encephalopathy (37). The virus has also been isolated from brain tissue and cerebrospinal fluid (CSF) (28,29). A far greater amount of HIV antigen is present in brains of patients with encephalopathy than in blood, lymph nodes, or bone marrow (64), suggesting active viral replication in the CNS. HIV antigen can be demonstrated in the CSF of asymptomatic HIV-seropositive individuals, and in the course of progressive encephalopathy, its CSF accumulation is greater than that in serum (65,66). Neurologically symptomatic patients with HIV encephalopathy have oligoclonal bands in CSF and an increased rate of IgG synthesis, indicative of an intra-blood–brain barrier response to the viral infection with production of HIV-specific IgG (27,66).

Despite unequivocal evidence that HIV infects the CNS, replicates in it, and elicits an immune response, the actual mechanism of extensive and diverse tissue damage remains elusive. The fact that HIV invades the brain in such a large number of cases suggested dual tropism of the virus, possibly from similarities in surface membrane determinants of T lymphocytes and brain cells (64), yet there is no convincing evidence to date that the virus is truly "neurotropic."

CD4 molecules serve as a receptor for HIV on all human cells, and the CNS has been shown to contain messenger RNA corresponding to such a molecule (67). This suggests that there is at least a theoretical possibility for HIV neurotropism. However, in spite of the observation that low-grade HIV infection can take place even in CD4− cells, astrocytes do not become any more susceptible to in vitro HIV infection with increasing levels of the CD4 gene. Even when these cells were rendered CD4+, they still failed to form syncytia in tissue culture incubated with the virus (68). Furthermore, in tissue cultures of human brain-derived astrocytes and microglia exposed to various strains of HIV-1 and HIV-2, only microglia became infected, whereas astrocytes remained infection-free after 3 weeks of coincubation with the virus (43).

As for evidence of in vivo infection of neural elements, there were a few early reports of HIV infection of astrocytes, "neuroglia," axons, and even some neurons in the brains of AIDS patients (6,41,45,46,49). However, most subsequent studies employing in situ hybridization and double-labeling immunohistochemistry have failed to demonstrate the presence of HIV in any cells of neuroectodermal origin (11,70). In a study of HIV cell tropism in formalin-fixed brain tissue from 69 patients with AIDS, Budka could not demonstrate any positive glial or neuronal elements (37). Even the cerebral endothelium may not be susceptible to HIV infection. By using double-labeling anti-FVIII and HIV-specific antibodies, Budka concluded that seemingly HIV-positive "endothelial" cells are probably pericytes or perivascular microglia (37). Ultrastructural studies of brain tissue from AIDS patients and brain lesions not necessarily related to direct HIV infection of the CNS show that endothelial cells contain nonspecific tubuloreticular inclusions, and that mononuclear cells can contain confronting cylindrical cisterns, both of which occur in other viral and immunological disorders, as well as in AIDS (71,72). Although nonspecific, these cytoplasmic inclusions may nevertheless be indicative of HIV infection. Gyorkey et al. (73,74) adamantly insist that they demonstrated ultrastructural evidence of budding HIV virions from the endoplasmic reticulum of "degenerating oligodendroglial and astroglial cells" in the white matter biopsies of five AIDS patients. This was categorically disputed by at least two other investigators (75,76), both of whom stated that the infected cells were microglia or macrophages and not oligodendroglia.

The absence of in vivo HIV-infected neural cells casts doubt on the neurotropism of the virus, and the apparent inability of others (37) to confirm a previous finding of primary HIV infection of the cerebral endothelium (45,46) opens up even the question of the route of viral entry into the CNS.

Passive transport of virus across an intact blood–brain barrier as a "passenger" in an infected white blood cell seems to occur during CNS infection by a variety of neurotropic viruses, including herpes, measles, polio, visna, and canine distemper virus (77,78), without concomitant infection of endothelial cells (79). Infected monocytes serve as a traveling "sanctuary," which allows the virus to replicate without causing cell destruction, maintains low antigenic expression that prevents immunological detection, and, most importantly, such an intact monocyte–virus package becomes a "Trojan horse," which is presented to the brain (11,80,81). Once the virus is introduced into the CNS, secondary in situ infection of other monocytes and microglia may ensue (10), which explains the large number of infected cells in the CNS.

A similar mechanism of viral persistence and transport seems to operate in visna (78), a retrovirus from the lentivirus subfamily that causes encephalitis in Icelandic sheep, an inflammatory and demyelinating disease of white matter, which in many ways resembles HIV encephalopathy in humans and, to a certain extent, multiple sclerosis. Visna virus and HIV have other similarities (82,83); most importantly, they are both prone to mutation and production of new antigenic variants (84–86). Such newly formed strains of the virus may differ from the original virus in cytotoxicity, virulence (87), or cellular tropism (84). Distinctive cellular tropism by different HIV variants has been demonstrated in vivo (87) and in vitro (86). Likewise, in primary cultures of brain-derived glial cells, microglia could be infected with a macrophage-adapted HIV-1 viral strain but not with a T lymphocyte-adapted HIV-1 isolate or HIV-2 strains (43).

Despite apparent similarities between visna virus and HIV, there are some differences, the most important of which is that visna infection does not alter the immune system of the host (81,88,89). The healthy immune system in visna plays an important role in the development of CNS pathology, which is characterized by exuberant inflammation of white matter in the acute stages of the disease and, later, myelin loss. Experimentally immunosuppressed animals, whose circulating T lymphocytes are reduced, fail to develop the inflammatory leukoencephalopathy, despite the presence of virus in brain tissue (88), indicating that the brunt of brain damage in visna is immunologically mediated via mechanisms similar, but not identical, to those employed in experimental allergic encephalitis (EAE) (90). Our observation of at least one case of HIV encephalopathy with profuse inflammatory response and complete bilateral, symmetrical myelin destruction indicates that immunologically mediated mechanisms of myelin damage may indeed be operating in AIDS patients, especially in those with relatively well-preserved cellular immunity. On the other hand, the profound alteration in immune response in AIDS patients may provide an explanation for the very subtle pathological changes, found in a large number of HIV-infected brains, consisting only of myelin attenuation and astrocytosis and almost devoid of either inflammatory cells or macrophages. Thus the seemingly paradoxical idea that at least some patients with HIV encephalopathy may actually benefit from corticosteroid or ACTH therapy, as do patients with postinfectious encephalomyelitis and those with multiple sclerosis, may not be so paradoxical after all (91).

In an outline of a possible pathogenetic model of AIDS-dementia complex, assuming that this is a "single entity" with HIV being the "driving force" behind all cases, Price et al. (22) postulate that various HIV strains trigger an immune response that is both virus-specific and host genetic make-up-specific. In this model the interplay between the particular viral strain and the patient's specific genetic control, as well as individual variability in the degree or type of immune response, determines the nature of the CNS pathology. Price et al. believe that the immunopathological response in AIDS patients is likely to involve cytokines, which induce brain damage based on the principle of an "innocent bystander," rather than through a true autoimmune reaction directed against self-antigens. Thus one could speculate that myelin and, to a lesser extent, neuronal destruction in HIV encephalopathy could be executed by macrophages attracted to the CNS by infected microglia and other peripheral monocyte-derived cells. Macrophages would release monokines or proteolytic enzymes that may have myelinolytic properties or be directly toxic to various vital cellular elements such as glia and neurons. Macrophages could also "mistakenly" initiate destruction of myelin rather than that of virus-infected

cellular elements to which they responded in the first place. Either way, myelin sheaths and nerve cells are injured not as primary targets but as "innocent bystanders" (11,22,92,93).

At least one monokine, tumor necrosis factor-α (TNF-α), has been shown *in vitro* to be capable of inducing disintegration of oligodendroglia with resultant myelin loss (94). In the *in vitro* environment, HIV-1 can induce secretion of cytokines, such as TNF-α and TNF-β, by blood mononuclear cells as well as by CD4+ T lymphocytes. Most interestingly, once released, TNF-α dramatically increases HIV-related fusion of infected cells, an effect that can be inhibited by the addition of anticytokine antibodies (95). These antibodies also suppress replication of the virus (95). It has also been suggested that infected resident microglia in the CNS may be capable of releasing TNF *in vivo*, which could directly induce brain damage. In theory, HIV-induced production and release of cytokines into the bloodstream could indirectly cause diffuse damage of the CNS and/or spinal cord and possibly explain those cases of CNS disease in which there is no demonstrable virus, or provide an etiology of vacuolar myelopathy in which evidence for a direct etiologic role for HIV is unconvincing (see below) (22,96).

Another theoretically applicable mechanism of HIV-related brain tissue injury would be that of virus-induced malfunction of latently infected cells. In the case of oligodendroglia, this would imply an inability to maintain or regenerate myelin. Such "premature senescence" or virus-induced alteration of "higher cellular functions" occurs in lymphocytic choriomeningitis, in which infection of the murine anterior pituitary selectively inhibits production of growth hormone (97). Similarly, it has been shown that at least one retrovirus, known to cause lower motor neuron disease and spongiform myeloencephalopathy in mice, infects nerve cells abortively in such a way that its presence cannot be detected by ordinary means. It is postulated that intracellular accumulation of viral products due to aberrant protein synthesis could interfere with neuronal function and lead to altered cellular metabolism and eventual, slowly evolving cell destruction (98). A similar mechanism of undetectable, abortive infection of neurons and glia could take place in HIV infection of the CNS in AIDS (98).

Some evidence suggests that neurologic dysfunction in HIV infection may be directly caused by components of the virus. Viral envelope glycoprotein (gp120) purified from HIV isolates can induce neuronal damage and disintegration in hippocampal cultures from fetal mice. Thus, it has been postulated that, in human brains, gp120 shed from HIV contained in white matter macrophages could exhibit its toxic effect on neurons in cortex at a distance and that actual physical contact between the two would not be necessary for neuronal destruction to take place (99). Dreyer et al. (100) have taken this line of reasoning one step further in demonstrating that gp120 damages and destroys retinal and hippocampal neurons in cultures by first elevating levels of intracellular free calcium. Both Ca^{2+} entry and cell injury could be blocked by the Ca^{2+} channel antagonist, nimodipine. The authors believe this to be a potential mechanism of gp120 neurotoxicity. Despite skepticism expressed by others (101), they suggested that this drug, presently used in prevention of brain damage related to subarachnoid hemorrhage, may prove beneficial in the treatment of neurological and psychiatric problems caused by HIV in humans with AIDS (100).

For an exhaustive review of all aspects of HIV-associated diseases of the CNS, including nomenclature, pathology, pathogenesis, and clinical presentation, please see *Brain Pathology* 1991;1:143–212. Treatment issues are discussed by Broder et al. (102) and others (91, 103–106).

VACUOLAR MYELOPATHY

Vacuolar myelopathy is a novel, progressive disease with a prevalence among AIDS patients of approximately 25% based on autopsy series (107). The condition involves noninflammatory, spongiform degeneration of the white matter tracts. It most commonly accompanies AIDS-dementia complex (107,108), but it has also been seen in HIV-infected patients in association with toxoplasmosis (109) or CMV infection (13). Clinically, the disorder presents with symmetrical lower extremity motor and sensory dysfunction, including ataxia, spasticity, and paresthesias. Incontinence is also common. The course is subacute and progressive, developing over weeks to months (107,108,110). Laboratory studies yield little information. The CSF is usually normal, as are serum B_{12} and folic acid levels (107,110,111).

Affected spinal cords appear normal on gross examination, but light microscopic studies reveal striking white matter vacuolation with no evidence of inflammation or any other cellular reaction. Closer examination of vacuolated regions reveals that intramyelinic swellings give the spinal cord its spongiform appearance. Axons themselves show no significant pathology but are disrupted in regions of advanced vacuolar change. The vacuolar change is more pronounced in the posterolateral zones of gracile, cuneate, and corticospinal tracts with relative sparing of the anterior columns (Fig. 6A,B). There is no strict predilection for particular spinal tracts, and in advanced cases, the entire white matter can be affected. The gray matter is spared. The lower thoracic and lumbar levels are most affected (107,110), and electrophysiological studies suggest that the vacuolar process then spreads rostrally (112). These findings, both clinical and pathologic, resemble subacute combined degeneration associated with vitamin B_{12} deficiency, which has led

some researchers to propose a metabolic/nutritional basis for vacuolar myelopathy (96,107,110).

Although no etiology has yet been determined, much effort has gone into trying to demonstrate HIV antigens or productive infection in the spinal cord, using immunohistochemical and molecular genetic techniques. Several groups have reported localizing HIV antigens to areas of vacuolar change through the use of labeled monoclonal antibodies; however, positive staining is usually limited to macrophages and multinucleated cells (111,113), which are not an integral part of the diffuse pathology; rather, they are quite rare and very segmental in distribution. Detection of HIV-1 RNA via *in situ* hybridization in regions of vacuolar change was also confined to macrophages and multinucleated cells (114,115). Although these findings suggest that HIV-1 can establish productive infection in the spinal cord and may cause pathology in a manner analogous to the HIV-related MNC encephalopathy (111,114,115), the extreme paucity of MNCs and macrophages in the spinal cord and the overwhelming diffuse nature of the spongiform change make HIV a very unlikely causative agent for vacuolar myelopathy (22). Furthermore, others report no association between vacuolar myelopathy and productive HIV-1 infection of the spinal cord (96).

The dissimilarity to the white matter disease seen in HIV encephalopathy also argues against a simple extrapolation from HIV MNC encephalopathy to vacuolar myelopathy. The striking symmetry of the vacuolar change and the pathologic resemblance to subacute combined degeneration have led some to suggest a systemic insult. This could be due to a cytokine that may act via the bloodstream to derail the metabolic processes in spinal cord tissue (see above) (22). The pathology of vacuolar myelopathy, with its lack of cellular reaction and striking symmetry of the spongiform change, seems more typical of a metabolic-toxic process rather than a primary infectious one.

Nevertheless, biologically distinctive forms of HIV, with different cellular tropisms and different pathogenetic capabilities, should be considered as a possible cause of the spongiform degeneration (84). Another interesting possibility is coinfection of the spinal cord with human T-lymphotropic virus type I (HTLV-I). HTLV-I has been implicated in chronic progressive myelopathies, including tropical spastic paraparesis (116–118) and familial spastic paraparesis (119). One case report described a patient with a lower extremity motor myelopathy syndrome and serologic evidence of HIV-1 and HTLV-I coinfection. The authors suggested that the primary cause of the myelopathy may have been the HTLV-I infection. Prednisolone therapy in this case resulted in improvement of weakness (120). Other researchers, however, have found no evidence of HTLV-I infection in a series of autopsied AIDS patients with vacuolar myelopathy (96,121).

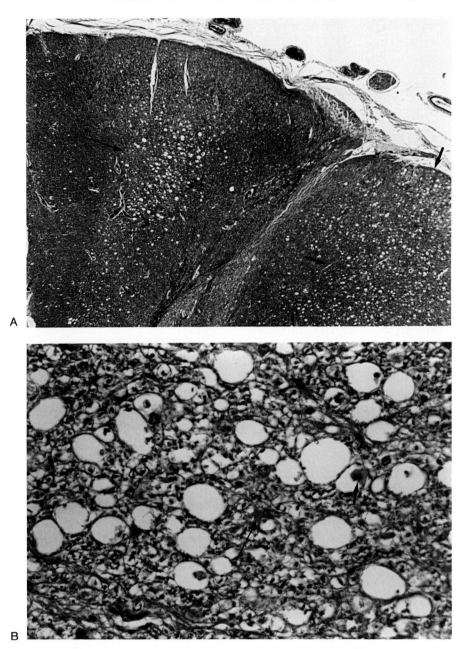

FIG. 6. Vacuolar myelopathy (H&E/LFB). **A:** A low-power view of the affected dorsal and lateral white matter columns of the cervical spinal cord. Spongy change is most apparent in the cuneate (*long arrow*), dorsal spinocerebellar and corticospinal tracts (*short arrows*). **B:** Higher magnification shows round, empty intramyelinic vacuoles of various sizes with an occasional macrophage (*arrow*) and very modest astrocytic response (*long arrow*) (×400).

PERIPHERAL NEUROPATHY

The prevalence of peripheral neuropathies in AIDS patients ranges from 16 to 26%, based on autopsy (3,4) as well as clinical studies (122,123). Many feel this figure to be an underestimate (123,124). One study claimed that 52% of patients with AIDS or AIDS-related complex (ARC) had clinical neuropathic syndromes and that 95% had histopathologic evidence of neuropathy (125).

Clearly, the prevalence is greater than was reported in earlier series, but an actual figure remains elusive.

Dalakas et al. (122) have identified six clinical and pathophysiological subtypes: (a) acute inflammatory demyelinating polyneuropathy (AIDP); (b) chronic inflammatory demyelinating polyneuropathy (CIDP); (c) mononeuritis multiplex (MM); (d) distal symmetrical polyneuropathy (DSPN); (e) sensory ataxic neuropathy due to ganglionitis; and (f) progressive inflammatory polyradiculoneuropathy. Some of these subtypes tend to be associated only with certain phases of HIV infection, be they initial seroconversion or full-blown AIDS. They also differ with respect to prognosis and therapy, indicating that these subdivisions of peripheral neuropathies have important clinical implications and are not just an exercise in nosology.

The first two subtypes, AIDP and CIDP, have similar histologic pictures, showing segmental demyelination with endoneurial inflammatory infiltrates (122,124). The clinical picture is one of symmetric proximal and distal weakness, mild sensory dysfunction, and areflexia (123). In some patients, the process is acute and is indistinguishable from Guillain-Barré syndrome occurring in HIV-seronegative individuals. In others, the progression is more subacute or chronic, evolving over 1 or 2 months (122). In both subtypes, however, the CSF shows increased protein as well as pleocytosis, a feature unique to inflammatory demyelinating polyneuropathies (IDP) associated with HIV (122–124,126). Also, HIV antigens can, in some cases, be found in CSF or in sural nerve biopsies (122).

These acute and chronic IDPs are the predominant subtypes found in the asymptomatic, HIV-seropositive population (122–124,127). In several cases, AIDP has occurred concurrently with HIV seroconversion (128, 129). The prognosis is good. Most patients either remit spontaneously or respond to corticosteroids and/or plasmapheresis (122–124,130,131). The prevalence of peripheral neuropathy in asymptomatic HIV-seropositive patients may be higher than reported; one group reported subclinical deficits in 35% of such patients, based on nerve conduction studies (132).

The AIDS-related complex population develops an even broader range of neuropathy. The IDP subtypes comprise about 38% of cases and have good prognoses, although not as good as IDP developing in asymptomatic HIV-seropositive patients (124). Cases of mononeuritis multiplex (MM) and distal symmetrical polyneuropathy (DSPN) in the ARC patient population comprise about 29% and 24% of cases, respectively (124).

The MM subtype typically presents with multiple sensory and/or motor deficits of spinal, cranial, and/or peripheral nerves, such as paresthesias, weakness, and hyporeflexia (122,133). On histologic examination of sural nerve biopsies, there is multifocal axonal degeneration and endoneurial mononuclear infiltrates. Sometimes, necrotizing vasculitis may be present, as well as multifocal infarct-like lesions. CSF analysis reveals increased protein and pleocytosis. The process may resolve spontaneously or progress to a DSPN-like picture, as nerve lesions become confluent (122,134,135).

Patients with DSPN present with sensory symptoms, including painful, often debilitating dysesthesias of the lower extremities and, to a lesser extent, the upper extremities, absent ankle jerks, and minimal muscle weakness (122–124,136). Besides being seen in ARC patients, DSPN is the predominant neuropathy associated with AIDS (131), comprising 80% of cases (124). One report claims that clinical and electrophysiological evidence of a milder form of DSPN exists in 35% of AIDS patients (137). CSF is usually normal (123,124), but electrophysiological studies demonstrate signs of dying-back axonopathy and muscle denervation (122,123,130,136).

On histologic examination of sural nerve biopsies, there is significant axonal loss with scanty inflammation (122,123,127). One autopsy study reported selective degeneration of the gracile tract in all four of their cases. These were patients with AIDS who had lower extremity dysesthesias and hyporeflexia (138). The prognosis is said to be poor with little hope of spontaneous remission (122,123). In some cases, improvement occurred with zidovudine treatment (139–141), but therapy is generally limited to symptomatic treatment with tricyclic antidepressants and control of neuropathic pain (131, 136,137).

Sensory ataxic neuropathy has a clinical picture resembling the ataxic neuropathy associated with HTLV-I infection (122). In some instances, evidence of coinfection with HTLV-I has been found, and treatment with corticosteroids was successful (120,142); however, other reports claim no evidence of HTLV-I infection and no response to steroid therapy (122). Sural nerve biopsy shows loss of large myelinated fibers with no inflammation. At autopsy, dorsal root ganglia and proximal dorsal roots reveal neuronal loss with inflammatory infiltrates (122).

Finally, patients with progressive inflammatory polyradiculopathy present with a lower extremity, often asymmetrical, flaccid paraparesis, with sphincter dysfunction, areflexia, and hypoesthesias. The condition may be due to CMV infection. CSF contains increased protein and pleocytosis. Sural nerve biopsy reveals demyelination and perivascular inflammation. Unlike the IDPs, this subtype is seen mainly in patients with AIDS and has a relentless, progressive course. At autopsy, the proximal dorsal and ventral roots show extensive myelin and axon loss with mononuclear inflammatory infiltrates (49,122,124,143). In addition, typical CMV inclusions can be seen in Schwann cells and endothelial cells of the endoneurial thin-walled vessels (49).

The pathogenesis of these various peripheral neuropathies and radiculopathies remains undefined. Autoimmune mechanisms have been postulated for the IDP subtypes, based on the similarity of AIDP to typical Guillain-Barré syndrome, in non-HIV-infected patients, as well as the response of both AIDP and CIDP to corticosteroids and plasmapheresis. That these conditions tend to occur in patients with early HIV infection (when their immune status is not yet fully compromised) further supports an immune-mediated etiology (122,124,137, 144). Another possibility is that direct HIV infection of nerve elements may be eliciting an immune response (122,124,125). HIV has been isolated from peripheral nerve (29,126), although its presence does not necessarily imply an etiologic role for the virus.

The DSPN subtype is less likely to involve an autoimmune process, since it tends to occur in patients with more pronounced immunosuppression than is seen in patients with IDP. Again, direct HIV or CMV infection has been postulated (122,124,131,137,145,146).

One group has proposed that the peripheral neuropathies seen in both AIDS and ARC patients are different expressions of the same disease process (125). This premise is that the basic lesion is a sensorimotor polyneuropathy with demyelination, axonal degeneration, inflammation, and positive HIV cultures from peripheral nerve. ARC patients tend to follow a subacute course, labeled CIDP, while AIDS patients have a more chronic course, labeled DSPN. Despite this clinical difference, they claim to find no other valid or reliable distinctions, based on electrophysiological, histopathological, and immunological analysis. Through immunohistochemical staining techniques, a predominance of CD8+T lymphocytes and Leu M3+ macrophages has been observed in the inflammatory infiltrates; and when compared to control nerve tissue, there is increased staining for class I major histocompatibility complex (MHC) antigens as well as for class II MHC antigens. Thus it has been postulated that either HIV infection of Schwann cells elicits a T-cell-mediated immune attack against the infected cells, or that T cells destroy myelin and/or axons due to sensitization caused by viral infection of the nerves (i.e., an autoimmune response).

The pathogenesis of MM and sensory ataxic neuropathy also remains obscure. A vasculitis has been seen in some cases of the former (124), while HTLV-I coinfection has been found in a few cases of the latter (120,142). The polyradiculopathy subtype, on the other hand, has been strongly associated with CMV infection of Schwann cells and local, endoneurial CMV vasculitis (49,122,124,143).

SKELETAL MUSCLE DISORDERS ASSOCIATED WITH HIV INFECTION

At least 15% and perhaps as many as 50% of HIV-seropositive individuals have or will develop some form of myopathy (122), either during the asymptomatic stages of HIV infection or in the course of AIDS (122). Inflammatory myopathy, akin to that of idiopathic polymyositis occurring in HIV-negative adults, is by far the most common condition (122,147–150). Other disorders of skeletal muscle associated with HIV infection include nemaline rod myopathy (122,151,152), mitochondrial myopathy (153,153a), myositis with MNCs (154), drug-induced myopathy (155,156), pyomyositis (157), type II atrophy (122), and amyotrophic lateral sclerosis (ALS)-like syndrome (122,158).

The electromyogram (EMG) is a useful tool for the detection of skeletal muscle involvement in all diffuse myopathies, which, with certain precautions as outlined by Dalakas and Pezeshkpour (122), can safely be done for HIV-infected patients.

Polymyositis in AIDS presents clinically with diffuse proximal muscle weakness, an increase in CPK, and myopathic EMG findings (148). Pathologically, most specimens show segmental/coagulative necrosis of single muscle fibers, accumulation of macrophages, and endomysial or angiocentric inflammatory infiltrates. Occasionally, inflammatory infiltrates may contain MNCs in their midst (154). In some cases of otherwise typical inflammatory myopathy, nemaline rods can be found (148), and electron microscopy may reveal a loss of thick filaments (149). Although polymyositis may very well be causally related to HIV infection (147), direct invasion of muscle fibers by HIV has not been demonstrated immunocytochemically (147), by *in situ* hybridization (122,148,149) or by electron microscopy (149). On the other hand, at least one HIV- and HTLV-I-seropositive patient with polymyositis was shown to harbor HTLV-I nucleic acid and antigen within atrophic muscle fibers. The same tests and electron microscopy failed to disclose direct HIV infection of the muscle (149). In a comparative viral and immunological study of biopsies of muscle tissue obtained from 19 HIV-seropositive and five HIV-seronegative polymyositis patients, it was concluded that the inflammatory and necrotizing change in both groups was due to a "T cell-mediated and major histocompatibility class (MHC) I-restricted immune mechanism" (147).

HIV-associated polymyositis may have a self-limited clinical course (148,154), or it may respond to treatment with corticosteroids (148,150), plasmapheresis (150), or zidovudine (122,150).

Nemaline rod myopathy in HIV-infected individuals may occur as an isolated condition without inflammation. It is characterized by progressive proximal weakness, wasting, myopathic EMG, and a profusion of nemaline rods within atrophic type I fibers (151,152). As in some cases of polymyositis combined with nemaline rods (149), muscle fibers in HIV-related nemaline rod myopathy also show selective loss of thick filaments (152). Furthermore, these patients also respond to treatment with steroids and plasmapheresis, suggesting that nemaline rod myopathy in HIV-seropositive individuals may actually be a form of polymyositis with minimal or absent inflammation and necrosis (152). Cases with unequivocal features of inflammation and an abundance of nemaline rods affirm this notion (148). Attempts to isolate HIV from affected muscle tissue have failed (152). Likewise, the presence of virus within muscle fibers could not be shown either by *in situ* hybridization (151,152) or by electron microscopy (152).

Mitochondrial (153,153a) and *necrotizing myopathy* (155,156) associated with AIDS appears to be due to a total dose-dependent toxicity of zidovudine (153a). According to some studies, 15% of zidovudine-treated patients show signs of myopathy as evidenced by an increased CPK level (153). More than one-third of muscle biopsies obtained from zidovudine-treated patients with peripheral neuromuscular symptoms show structural changes usually associated with mitochondrial myopathy (153a). These changes include the presence of ragged red fibers (4–30% of fibers) on modified trichrome-stained sections of muscle tissue and an abnormal ultrastructure of the mitochondria (153,153a). In addition, various degrees of muscle fiber necrosis and vacuolar degeneration may be present, as well as scanty interstitial inflammatory infiltrates. At the ultrastructural level, all muscle biopsies show loss of myofilaments and the presence of cytoplasmic bodies, and some fibers contain an occasional nemaline rod (153a). Most interestingly, biochemical studies also demonstrate abnormalities in mitochondrial enzymes, primarily a decline in respiratory chain capacity (153a). Patients with mitochondrial myopathy respond to treatment with prednisone and nonsteroidal anti-inflammatory agents, as well as to the cessation of zidovudine therapy (153,153a).

Amyotrophic lateral sclerosis (ALS)-like syndrome has been observed in some HIV-positive cases (122,158). This is clinically characterized by the presence of fasciculations, diffuse, symmetrical muscle weakness and wasting, and a moderate increase in CPK (158). The muscle tissue shows signs of neurogenic atrophy as well as myopathic changes, focal inflammation, and "dying back" of intramuscular nerve twigs. The nature of the spinal cord pathology is nonspecific and at best uncertain, described vaguely as consisting of recent hemorrhages and increased vascularity in the anterior horns and patchy axonal degeneration in the spinal white matter, ventral spinal roots, and peripheral nerves. Anterior horn cells, primary motor cortex, and corticospinal tracts—anatomical sites characteristically diseased in classical ALS—are said to be well preserved (158).

Pyomyositis designates a focal bacterial infection of a skeletal muscle, resulting in the formation of an abscess, which in turn causes painful local swelling and fever (157). Without treatment, this can lead to septicemia and blood-borne dissemination of the infectious process to other organs.

TOXOPLASMOSIS

Toxoplasmosis is the most common opportunistic infection of the CNS associated with AIDS (1,3,4,159–185) and the most common cause of mass lesions detectable by cranial CT scan (109,162) (see Fig. 8A). The prevalence of toxoplasmosis among patients with AIDS is highest in Haitians (61%) (162), and least common among hemophiliacs (163). The causative organism is *Toxoplasma gondii*, an obligate intracellular parasite that belongs to coccidian protozoa (164,165). Actively infected human brain tissue contains organisms in the form of single tachyzoite-trophozoites, cysts with many bradyzoites, and pseudocysts, representing recently infected brain cells filled with newly formed single organisms (Fig. 7A). Encysted organisms reside in skeletal muscle, heart, and brains of latently infected humans, lambs, and pigs, whereas oöcysts, that contain sporozoites, are found in the feces of infected domestic cats (165–167). Latent infection of humans is common, but the rate of infection is variable, ranging from a relatively low figure of 11% to an unusually high one of 93%, depending on climate, geographic location, and meat-consuming habits (168).

Tachyzoites represent the active form of the organism, which is always present in brain tissue of untreated patients with toxoplasmosis. In tissue, they appear as ovoid or elongated structures, about 4–7 μm long and 2–4 μm wide, with small nuclei (169). It is often stated that they cannot be readily discerned by light microscopy "even with special stains" (170), but our experience has always been that in brain tissue stained with combined H&E and Luxol fast blue (LFB), single organisms can be recognized without difficulty, if the observer is vigilant and familiar with their morphology. Ultrastructurally, their appearance is highly typical (169–173), characterized by a crescent or teardrop-shaped, double membrane-bound structure containing a nucleus with prominent nucleolus, saccular, sausage-like profiles (rhoptries), near the apical end, numerous ribosomes, mitochondria, glycogen granules, endoplasmic reticulum, and Golgi apparatus. Encysted forms of the organism can readily be recognized in infected brain tissue stained with H&E. Cysts are rounded encapsulated structures that range in size between 20 and 100 μm and contain slowly multiplying bradyzoites (Fig. 7B).

Invasion of brain cells by tachyzoites occurs by active penetration of the cell membrane (173) or via a mechanism of "parasite-stimulated phagocytosis," which operates on the cells that naturally possess phagocytic properties as well as those that do not (172). All cellular constituents of the brain are vulnerable to *Toxoplasma* infection, including glia, neurons, and endothelial cells. Once within a cell, the parasite starts the process of endodyogenous multiplication (172), which in immunosuppressed individuals evolves freely and rapidly and ends in mechanical destruction of the infected cell (171). Cells without phagocytic properties and those with vital processes that can easily be altered disintegrate much sooner (174).

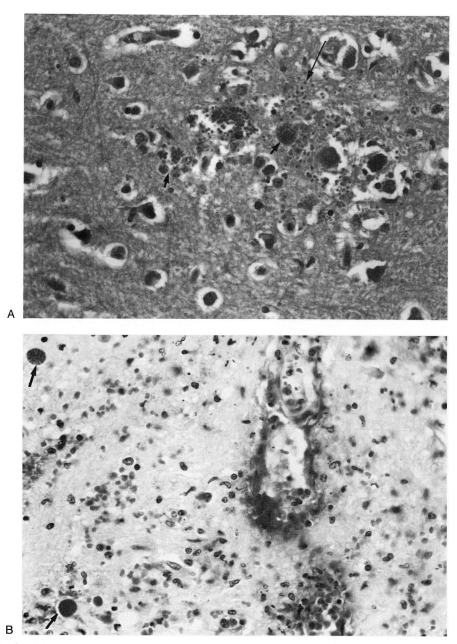

FIG. 7. CNS toxoplasmosis (H&E/LFB). **A:** Single organisms—tachyzoites (*long arrow*) and ill-defined pseudocysts (*short arrows*)—which often assume the shape of the infected cells (×400). **B:** *Toxoplasma* cysts (*arrows*) appear as well-defined, round, encapsulated structures containing minute bradyzoites. A thin-walled vessel shows fibrinoid necrosis of the wall (×400).

In addition to this principal mechanism of tissue damage via primary destruction of infected cells, CNS toxoplasmosis can indirectly cause massive necrosis of viable brain tissue through necrotizing, thrombo-occlusive parenchymal vasculitis (Fig. 7B), initiated by direct *Toxoplasma* infection of arterial walls (175) or by intramural deposits of immune complexes (174). *Toxoplasma* antigen and free tachyzoites have been demonstrated in the walls of arteries situated at the edge of necrotic brain tissue (175), and necrotizing thrombotic vasculitis can be visualized within areas of brain tissue necrosis, but

vasculitis is rarely seen as a primary, isolated phenomenon in CNS toxoplasmosis.

Pathologic Diagnosis of CNS Toxoplasmosis

Brain biopsy is the only way to make an unequivocal diagnosis of CNS toxoplasmosis and to rule out other diseases, with similar CT–MRI presentation, as well as to determine if HIV or other concomitant infections are also present (186–189). Brain biopsy involves some risk of complications, but it also has some advantages. Biopsy tissue must be handled in a way that will allow other more sophisticated diagnostic methods to be utilized, if routine histology produces negative results. Laboratory methods that are useful in diagnosis of CNS toxoplasmosis include the following. (a) Electron microscopy of tachyzoites shows a highly characteristic image of the organism that may be difficult to detect at the light microscopic level (170). (b) Direct immunofluorescence staining with *Toxoplasma*-specific antibodies of smears of diseased brain tissue demonstrates tachyzoites, intra-cellular parasites, and the encysted organisms (190). (c) The peroxidase–antiperoxidase immunohistochemical method can be used on formalin-fixed, paraffin-embedded tissue (191). (d) *Toxoplasma* nucleic acid can be demonstrated in infected brain tissue by the polymerase chain reaction (PCR) (192).

Grossly, at autopsy, recent brain lesions resemble a nonhemorrhagic infarction and appear as ill-defined areas of softening, swelling, and dusky discoloration. Lesions in more advanced stages of organization usually appear as well-defined, yellow-tan foci of tissue necrosis

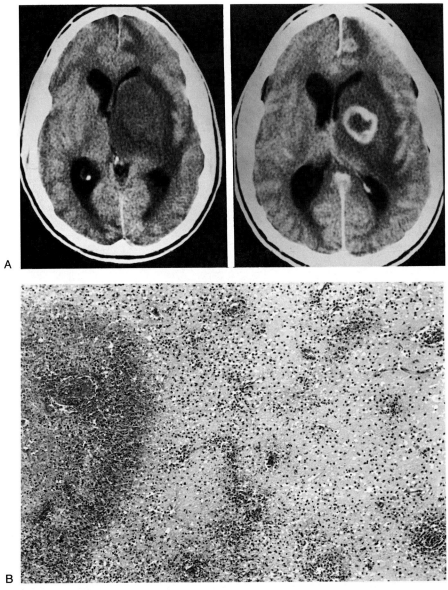

FIG. 8. CNS toxoplasmosis. A 32-year-old patient with AIDS. **A:** CT scan before (**left**) and after contrast injection, showing hypodense space-occupying lesions with edema of the surrounding tissue in the right frontal lobe and basal ganglia. Both lesions show typical diffuse or ring enhancement with contrast material (**right**). **B:** Typical pathohistology of a ring-enhancing lesion (H&E/LFB). Central (*left*) region of coagulative necrosis is encircled (*right*) by numerous damaged or newly formed vessels, perivascular inflammatory infiltrates as well as clustered and diffusely proliferating microglia intermingled with *T. gondii* (×100).

of variable sizes, or as small pseudocysts with ragged margins. *Toxoplasma* lesions are often multifocal, most frequently occupying various parts of the cortex, subcortical white matter, or deep periventricular gray structures; brain stem and cerebellar involvement are less common but not unusual. Lobar brain edema, anatomically related to the lesions, and generalized brain swelling are common.

By light microscopy, small or large areas of recent coagulative necrosis elicit little or no cellular reaction. Tachyzoites, as well as cysts and pseudocysts, may be numerous in untreated patients. When a cellular reaction becomes apparent, it consists of clustered or diffusely spread microglia and perivascular lymphocytic infiltrates, along the edges of the necrotic center (Fig. 8B). Blood vessels in the viable tissue band surrounding the necrotic center show various signs of vasculitis consisting of intramural inflammatory infiltrates, hyperplasia of endothelium, and fibrinoid necrosis of vessel walls, with or without thrombotic obliteration of their lumina (Fig. 9).

It appears that focal lesions result from centrifugal expansion of *Toxoplasma*-induced tissue damage, which along its pathway elicits microglial and inflammatory

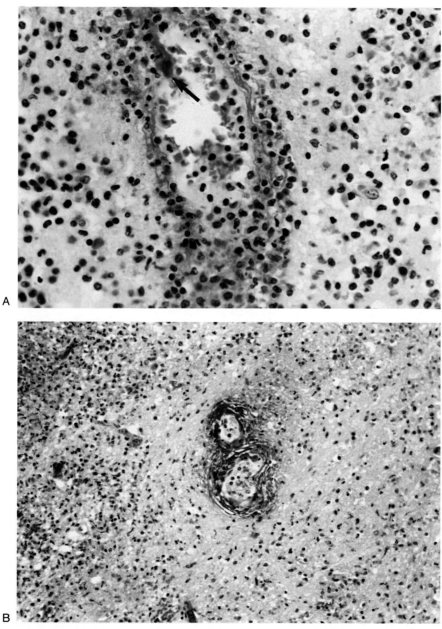

FIG. 9. CNS toxoplasmosis, vascular injury within an active lesion (H&E/LFB). **A:** Transmural inflammatory infiltrate with incipient thrombosis (*arrow*) (×400). **B:** Fibrinoid necrosis of blood vessel walls (×200).

infiltrates. Ischemic tissue injury due to thrombo-occlusive vasculitis greatly contributes to the extent of parenchymal necrosis.

Old and treated lesions are devoid of single organisms and pseudocysts but rare encysted bradyzoites may still be present. The central part of these lesions is usually loaded with macrophages and surrounding brain tissue contains numerous newly formed vessels, inflammatory cells and reactive astrocytes. Contrary to the often misused term of "*Toxoplasma* abscesses," these lesions are never encased in a solid capsule of granulation and connective tissue nor do they contain pus.

In most untreated cases of CNS toxoplasmosis associated with AIDS, in addition to the above-described focal lesions, there is usually a more extensive, albeit subtle, "meningoencephalitic" component of the disease. This is characterized by a focal or more diffuse microglial response to parasitic infection of single cells. Perivascular lymphocytic infiltrates and hypertrophic astrocytes are also present. Leptomeningeal lesions are rare. When

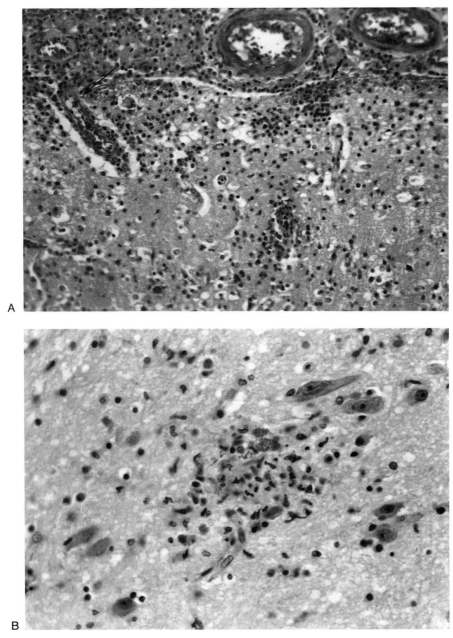

FIG. 10. CNS toxoplasmosis, meningoencephalitic component (H&E/LFB). **A:** Inflammatory infiltrate from the subarachnoidal space expands into the underlying cortex via the perivascular spaces (*long arrow*) or by direct invasion of pia and the adjacent molecular layer (*short arrow*) (×200). **B:** A microglial nodule is formed around *Toxoplasma* pseudocysts and single organisms (×400).

present, they consist of minimal to moderate focal lymphocytic infiltrates (Fig. 10).

CRYPTOCOCCOSIS

Cryptococcal infections of the nervous system are a major complication of AIDS, ranking third in frequency behind HIV and *T. gondii* as a cause of neurologic disease. The prevalence of CNS cryptococcal infections ranges from 3 to 12%, according to different autopsy series (7,193). It may be the first manifestation of AIDS (194–198). Meningitis is the most common form of CNS cryptococcal infection, but parenchymal as well as disseminated systemic infections are also possible.

Clinically, many patients do not present with the classic signs and symptoms of meningitis; rather, nonspecific complaints of fever, headache, and malaise are often the only symptoms of cryptococcal meningitis (194,195,197).

Radiologic examination is usually normal or reveals nonspecific findings such as diffuse atrophy or ventricu-

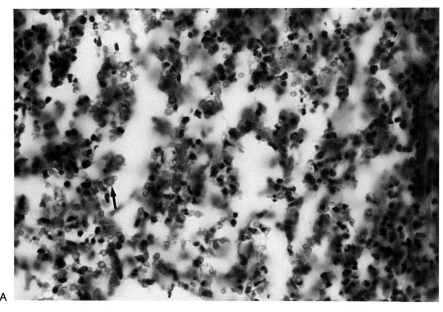

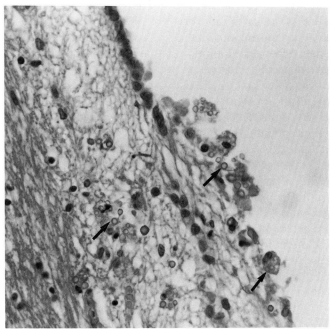

FIG. 11. Cryptococcal meningitis and ventriculitis (Mucicarmine stain). **A:** Numerous organisms (*arrow*) are intermixed with the subarachnoidal inflammatory exudate (×400). **B:** A wall of a ventricle with disrupted ependymal lining and numerous free and intracytoplasmic (*arrows*) cryptococci. There is no reactive cellular response (×400).

lar enlargement (199). In some cases, solid or ring-enhancing mass lesions can be identified, corresponding to a focus of parenchymal infection, often called a cryptococcoma (196,199).

At autopsy, there may be no grossly apparent signs of meningitis, especially since many AIDS patients mount little or no inflammatory response to the infection. The presence of numerous organisms in the subarachnoid space, however, can make infected brains feel quite "slippery." Parenchymal lesions consist of multiple irregular pseudocysts filled with a colorless mucoid material.

Microscopic examination of H&E sections reveals numerous faintly staining organisms within the subarachnoid space as well as within the pseudocysts and along the wall of the ventricular system. Mucicarmine stains can highlight the cryptococci (Fig. 11). Sometimes there can be a marked inflammatory reaction to leptomeningeal infection, possibly even with granuloma formation (193). The parenchymal lesions, however, lack any cellular response, despite the abundance of organisms.

HERPES VIRUS INFECTIONS

Herpes Simplex Virus

HSV-1 is the most common cause of sporadic encephalitis in previously healthy adults. The disease is initiated either through a *de novo* infection of the brain or by activation of a latent infection of the trigeminal ganglia (200).

The patient typically presents with fever and headache, along with signs suggestive of temporal and/or frontal lobe involvement: behavioral abnormalities, hallucinations, aphasia, and personality changes. Examination of CSF usually reveals increased protein and pleocytosis; however, the virus itself can rarely be isolated. EEG abnormalities localized to temporal and/or frontal lobes and a similar distribution of CT abnormalities both provide strong evidence for HSV-1 encephalitis.

The predominant pathologic finding is that of multifocal or massive necrosis and hemorrhage of the orbitofrontal and temporal lobes (200). The tissue reveals intranuclear viral inclusions within neurons and oligodendroglia, as well as meningeal and parenchymal inflammatory infiltrates and microglial nodules. Immunohistochemical methods can be used to confirm the presence of viral antigen. Culture of the tissue will also yield virus.

Classic HSV-1 encephalitis has not been seen in the setting of AIDS. Several AIDS patients with a combined CNS infection by CMV and HSV-1 have been reported. These patients developed a diffuse necrotizing ventriculoencephalitis in which both CMV and HSV-1 antigens could be demonstrated through immunocytochemical techniques (12,201). This has important therapeutic implications, given that acyclovir effectively treats only HSV-1 but not CMV.

Herpes Simplex Virus-2

HSV-2 infection is primarily associated with genital herpes. The virus is sexually transmitted and establishes a latent infection of the sacral ganglia. The virus can then spread to the genital area and cause recurrent herpetic lesions.

HSV-2 encephalitis, a severe, diffuse necrotizing and hemorrhagic disease of the CNS, primarily affects newborn children who acquire the virus from mothers with genital lesions during delivery. Healthy immunocompetent adults can very rarely develop HSV-2 encephalitis (202). Cases of encephalitis have been reported, however, in adults with either a post-transplant or a congenital immunodeficiency state (203,204).

HSV-2 infections in AIDS patients most commonly present as an ascending necrotizing myelitis. Coinfection with CMV that localizes to the sites of HSV-2 infection can be demonstrated (205,206).

Several cases of HSV-2 encephalitis in AIDS patients have been reported (207,208). The clinical presentation in two of the patients closely resembled that of HSV-1 encephalitis, based on EEG and CT abnormalities localized to a temporal lobe (207). The pathology was also similar, consisting of hemorrhagic and necrotizing lesions with viral inclusions.

Herpes (Varicella) Zoster Virus (VZV)

VZV is the etiologic agent of chickenpox (varicella) in children and shingles (zoster) in adults. After initial infection, the virus establishes a latent state within dorsal root ganglia. Reactivation can then occur many years later, producing a vesicular eruption confined to one of more contiguous sensory dermatomes. Zoster can develop in normal immunocompetent adults, but elderly and immunosuppressed patients develop it with greater frequency and have the added risk of dissemination and encephalitis. The most common CNS complication of zoster, however, is a local necrotizing ganglionitis, which can extend centrally, producing a myelitis and/or a bulbitis.

Approximately 2% of AIDS patients develop VZV encephalitis, based on autopsy studies (7). The disease presents as a leukoencephalitis in which there is prominent, multifocal subcortical and/or spinal cord demyelination and necrosis. The clinical picture is one of progressive mental deterioration with confusion and memory deficits and focal signs such as hemiparesis. CSF cultures usually fail to yield VZV, and the routine parameters are nonspecific. CT studies are equally unhelpful, although they may show white matter attenuation with expanding, nonenhancing or poorly enhancing lesions as the disease progresses (209,210). The first symptoms can occur months after an episode of zoster and can lead to death within a few months (209,210), although a case of a chronic VZV leukoencephalitis lasting 18 months has been reported (211).

The pathology reveals a multifocal process within the white matter of the brain and/or spinal cord. The individual lesions are well-defined gray-yellow areas up to 0.5 cm in diameter that may have undergone cavitation. On light microscopy, there is a central zone of necrosis with peripheral demyelination. Glial cells and occasional neurons within this demyelinated zone contain Cowdry type A intranuclear inclusions, which stain positively for VZV-specific antigens (7,210,211).

A VZV vasculopathy has also been described. The patient usually presents with a contralateral hemiparesis several weeks following an episode of ophthalmic zoster (212). A recent case report presented evidence of intraneuronal and transsynaptic anterograde spread of the virus through the visual system in an AIDS patient who had herpes zoster ophthalmicus and a subsequent encephalitis (213). The vasculopathy, however, need not follow a clinically apparent episode of ophthalmic zoster. The pathology consists of a thrombo-occlusive vasculopathy that can affect the circle of Willis and its proximal branches as well as leptomeningeal arteries. The vessels show thrombosis and marked, concentric, intimal smooth muscle and fibroblast proliferation without evidence of active vasculitis, fibrinoid necrosis, or a granulomatous process (Fig. 18B). VZV antigens can be identified within these proliferative regions (212,214) (Fig. 18C). This condition can coexist with VZV leukoencephalitis (214) and has been described in AIDS patients (7,214). The actual frequency of VZV vasculopathy may be higher than reported, since infarcts by CT scan are often misinterpreted as CNS toxoplasmosis or lymphoma and CNS angiography is rarely done in AIDS patients; in addition, staining of thrombosed vessels with VZV-specific antibodies is rarely performed at autopsy examination.

Epstein-Barr Virus (EBV)

EBV has a high prevalence in the general population, with a seropositivity rate of 50% by young adulthood in the United States (202). The virus is a known cause of infectious mononucleosis and has been implicated in Burkitt's lymphoma; however, most infections are asymptomatic and result in latent infection of B lymphocytes.

CNS complications secondary to EBV infection have not been described in AIDS patients. One case report implicated EBV infection as an etiologic agent in an AIDS patient's primary brain lymphoma (215).

Cytomegalovirus

CMV infection of the nervous system has a broad range of clinical and pathologic manifestations, including asymptomatic encephalitis with multiple microglial nodules, progressive dementia possibly due to superimposed HIV encephalopathy, necrotizing ventriculitis, vasculitis, and cauda equina syndrome with necrotizing and inflammatory polyradiculopathy. The majority of CMV infections in immunocompetent hosts are asymptomatic, and, by mid-adulthood, 60–80% of people in the United States have been infected with the virus (216). The prevalence of CMV seropositivity among homosexual men has been reported to be even higher, with one study finding a 94% seroprevalence rate among gay men compared to only 54% among heterosexual men (217).

As with other viruses of the herpes group, CMV establishes a latent infection in its host. It has not been demonstrated, however, that it can latently infect the central or peripheral nervous system. Reactivation or systemic dissemination is rare in normal immunocompetent persons, although there have been a few case reports of CMV encephalitis and/or polyneuropathy in previously normal adults (218,219). A defective immune system, especially depressed cell-mediated immunity as seen in organ-transplant recipients and AIDS patients, makes systemic CMV infection almost a rule (216,220).

CMV infection of the brain in AIDS patients occurs in 16–28% of cases, based on autopsy studies (7,12,193, 221). Patients with CMV encephalitis almost always have signs of systemic CMV infection (12). Coinfection with other organisms is not uncommon, and *Toxoplasma gondii* and HSV-2 lead the list (12,206,221). One autopsy series of AIDS patients with CMV encephalitis reported an interesting association with primary cerebral lymphoma, five of their 31 cases showing this pathology (13).

The clinical manifestations of CMV encephalitis can vary from a normal neurologic exam to a confusional state, memory impairment, dementia, and new onset seizures (12,221). One study of six AIDS patients with autopsy-confirmed progressive CMV encephalitis reported that patients began having CNS symptoms 8 days to 3 months prior to admission and died within 6 days to 8 weeks (221). Whether the subacute course for CMV encephalitis in this study is due solely to the CMV infection or is, perhaps, superimposed on the subtle pathology of HIV encephalopathy cannot be determined. A case can be made, however, that CMV encephalitis in the setting of AIDS runs a more rapid course than in other immunocompromised hosts. Beyond the global encephalopathic changes described above, CMV infection can also give rise to focal peripheral deficits of pain and weakness, usually attributable to a polyradiculopathy (12,49,143,206,222,223) or a dorsal root ganglionitis (224).

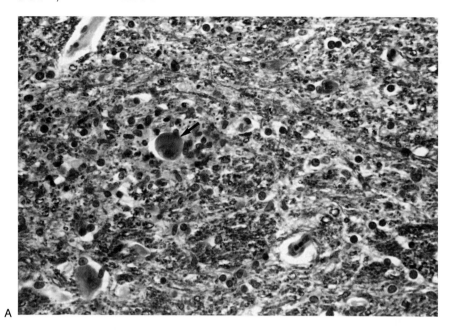

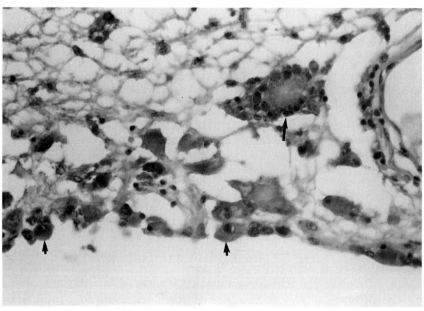

FIG. 12. Pathological changes in CNS related to CMV infection (H&E/LFB). **A:** Typical "cytomegalic" enlargement of the infected neural cell (*arrow*), which is surrounded by a small microglial nodule. The cell contains a large intranuclear viral inclusion (×400). **B:** CMV ventriculitis. Disruption of the ependymal lining, cytomegalic enlargement of the infected ependymal cells (*arrows*), and extensive damage of the subependymal tissue, which contains inflammatory cells, reactive and infected astrocytes, and a multinucleated giant cell (*arrow*) (×400). **C:** CMV vasculitis. Infected endothelial cells of a small parenchymal vessel harbor typical intranuclear inclusions (*arrow*). Nearby brain tissue (*upper left*) is clearly necrotic and vacuolated (recent infarction) (×400).

The CT scan is not very specific for CMV disease. Some cortical atrophy and mild *ex vacuo* hydrocephalus can be seen, as well as periventricular enhancement and focal white matter hypodensity. With the exception of periventricular hypodensity and enhancement, which is usually due to CMV ventriculitis, other findings are not specific, nor are they very sensitive, since the CT tends to underestimate the degree of CMV involvement. There is some optimism regarding MRI studies, which can better assess diffuse CNS disease (13,193,221).

Examination of the CSF is often normal and yields negative viral cultures. Some pleocytosis and increased protein can be found in cases of necrotizing polyradiculopathy (49,143,206).

The pathology of CMV infection is as varied as are its clinical manifestations. The most common CMV-associated lesion is the microglial nodule, a tightly packed, discrete collection of microglia and macrophages, often seen in deep gray structures and cortex, limbic system, and, to a lesser extent, white matter (Fig. 12A). These microglial nodules need to be distinguished from the looser, ill-defined aggregates of microglia with occasional MNCs that are associated with HIV infection. The next most common manifestation of CMV infection is the classic augmentation of the infected cell, harboring intranuclear and intracytoplasmic inclusions (Fig. 12A). Infected neurons, glia, and endothelial cells can exist isolated in the brain parenchyma, without asso-

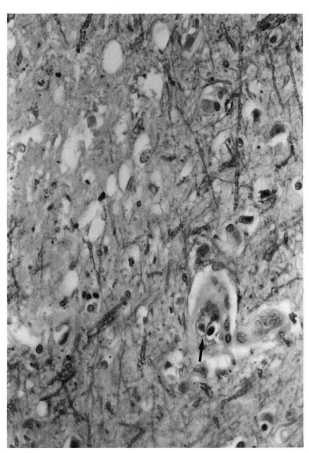

C

FIG. 12. *Continued.*

ciated inflammatory cells, usually in the basal ganglia, brain stem, and cortical gray matter (12,225). Whether such lesions, along with the microglial nodules, can sufficiently account for all the clinical features of CMV encephalitis has been called into question. The possibility of combined CMV and HIV infection, acting either directly or indirectly through systemic toxic mediators, has also been proposed (225).

More aggressive pathology can be seen in the form of focal parenchymal necrosis. Such lesions are discrete and contain many macrophages and cells with CMV inclusions but lack an inflammatory reaction (12). Related to this pathology is a necrotizing ventriculitis. CMV has a predilection for ependymal surfaces, sometimes resulting in a periventricular distribution of a wide band of tissue necrosis with an accumulation of macrophages and giant cells (12,13,193) (Fig. 12B). In one patient, it was reported that periaqueductal necrosis contributed to the development of an obstructive hydrocephalus (13).

A vasculitis has also been observed, secondary to CMV infection of endothelial cells (Fig. 12C) (13,49, 205; *personal observations*). Necrotizing polyradiculopathy due to CMV is characterized by focal hemorrhage, inflammatory infiltrates, axonal and myelin degeneration, vasculitis, and a widespread infection of Schwann cells within the spinal roots (12,226).

PROGRESSIVE MULTIFOCAL LEUKOENCEPHALOPATHY (PML)

Clinical Observations

Progressive multifocal leukoencephalopathy (PML) is a rare, viral, opportunistic infection of the oligodendroglial cells that leads to a progressive, fatal white matter disease. Prior to the emergence of AIDS, those most commonly affected by PML were patients with lymphoproliferative disorders (227), organ transplant recipients, patients on immunosuppressive drugs, and elderly patients with chronic debilitating diseases (227,228). The disease is extremely rare in childhood and among immunocompetent individuals (229,230).

Two percent to 4% of all autopsied patients with AIDS have PML as the main neurological disease (7,231), although superimposed HIV infection seems to occur in the course of PML more often than with any other AIDS-related CNS disorder (17,18), with the possible exception of CMV encephalitis (13–16). The pathology, clinical course, and severity of AIDS-related PML do not substantially differ from PML occurring in other immunosuppressive disorders (232,233). Clinically, PML patients have focal neurological signs that reflect involvement of the hemispheral white matter and the major supratentorial and infratentorial white matter tracts (234,235). Although some patients were said to have memory problems, overt dementia does not seem to occur (234,235). In the fully developed disease, radiological findings are characterized by frontoparietal or cerebellar white matter hypodensities, which produce no mass effect and no enhancement with contrast (Fig. 13) (228,231,236–239). However, "clinical-CT scan dissociation" is a common diagnostic problem (231), because the CT scan may be negative at presentation in the face of numerous neurological signs (228,234,236,238), or the anatomical distribution of CT scan lesions does not fully explain the patient's symptomatology (231). Survival among AIDS patients with PML usually ranges from 1 to 4 months (240).

The Causative Organism

Although the disease was first recognized as a distinct entity in 1958 (241), it was not until 1965 (242), when viral particles were ultrastructurally visualized within the oligodendroglial nuclei, that PML became known as an infectious disease. The virus was first isolated from diseased brain tissue obtained from a PML patient whose initials, JC, were used as its designation (243). The virus is now classified as a member of the large family of papovaviruses, and the most important human pathogen in the polyoma subgroup, which JC virus shares with human BK virus (BKV) and Simian vacuolated virus 40

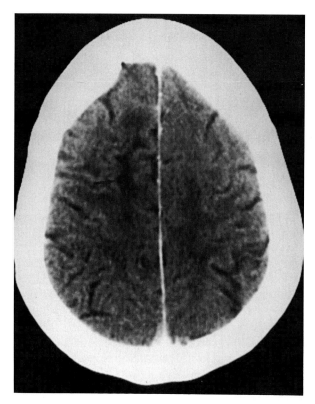

FIG. 13. A 36-year-old man with progressive multifocal leuko-encephalopathy (PML). CT scan, after contrast injection, shows a large frontal, subcortical, hypodense lesion. There is no enhancement or mass effect.

(SV40) (244,245). While 75–80% of adults are seropositive for JCV and BKV, SV40 naturally infects only rhesus monkeys (244), and the alleged isolation of this virus from two cases of human PML (246) is now considered to have resulted from contamination with the monkey kidney cell line (233,244). For all practical purposes, JC virus has been the only one subsequently isolated from all humans with PML, including AIDS patients (233,244).

JC is a small DNA virus with a singular propensity to induce a dual cytopathic effect. (a) It infects productively the permissive oligodendroglia in human brains and human-derived cultures of fetal glial cells. Nuclei of such massively infected cells at first grow in size, accommodating the actively replicating virus that can be visualized by light microscopy as amphophilic inclusions (Fig. 14A). Very early in the course of infection, the functions of oligodendroglial cells are impaired (247) and soon thereafter they disintegrate during the process of virus-induced cytolysis. (b) Abortive infection of nonpermissive cells, such as astrocytes in human brains, leads to an excessive uncontrollable growth of infected cells in the face of near absence of viral replication and incomplete antigenic expression (244). This results in the formation of persistently infected, bizarre tumorlike astrocytes (Fig. 14B), containing a few difficult-to-detect viral parti-

cles (248). These cells seem to be less common in PML cases associated with AIDS (232), but their presence in demyelinating lesions is almost as characteristic of PML as is that of enlarged oligodendroglial nuclei harboring viral inclusions. A few non-AIDS PML patients with more prolonged survival and a relatively intact immune system have developed multifocal malignant astrocytomas within the virus-induced demyelinating white matter lesions (249). In laboratory animals, JCV expresses only its oncogenic properties and is known to induce a wide variety of malignant tumors ranging from gliomas and medulloblastomas to pineoloblastomas (244,245).

Not until recently was it known that oligodendroglia and astrocytes in the CNS of normal elderly individuals can be latently infected by JC virus (250). This finding is potentially interesting, but it needs to be confirmed by other methods and in other age groups, especially in light of the fact that Telenti et al. (251) could not detect JC viral DNA in control brains by using a far more sensitive technique, the polymerase chain reaction (PCR), which amplifies specific nucleic acid sequences. Meanwhile, the prevailing wisdom holds that immunosuppression or debilitating illness helps activate the virus, which latently resides in the kidneys, and that the CNS invariably becomes infected via blood-borne dissemination of the organism from the primary site of infection (233).

The virus is selectively neurotropic, and once within the CNS, it infects oligodendroglia and, to a lesser extent, astrocytes. However, there are several interesting aspects of JCV infection and PML, which cannot be readily explained. For instance, the disease is very rare, even among immunosuppressed individuals, in spite of the extremely high rate of 75–80% of latent infection in adults (227,244). Second, the immune system of some patients with relentlessly progressive PML was able to successfully fight off other infections but not JCV (252). Finally, most patients with PML do not produce intra-blood–brain barrier JCV-specific antibodies, nor do their serum titers increase during active infection (227). These observations and some *in vitro* conducted tests (253) suggest that patients with PML may have a specific defect in their immune system that prevents them from responding to JCV at the time when they are capable of mounting an adequate reaction to mitogens and other viruses.

Pathology of PML

Typically, lesions of PML in the early stages of development occupy the subcortical white matter. Smaller lesions can be grossly visualized on formalin-fixed sliced brain as slightly sunken well-defined demyelinated grayish-tan spots, which stand out in sharp contrast to the surrounding healthy white matter. In more advanced stages of the disease, these lesions expand and coalesce

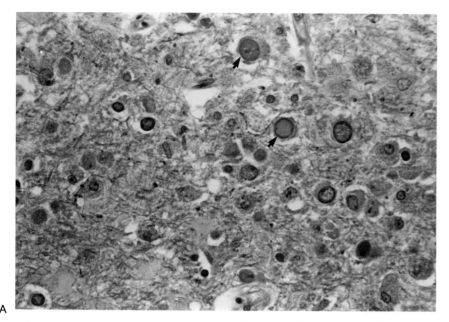

A

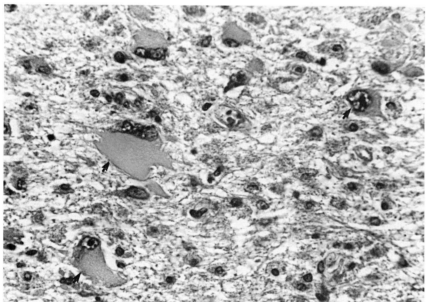

B

FIG. 14. Characteristic cytopathic features of JC virus in PML (H&E/LFB). **A:** Greatly augmented nuclei of the productively infected oligodendroglial cells (*arrows*) contain viral inclusions (×400). **B:** Abortively infected astrocytes (*arrows*) have large, bizarre, tumorlike nuclei and abundant cytoplasm but no viral inclusions (×400).

with similar demyelinating foci in their vicinity, thus forming larger zones of softening and gray discoloration with scalloped margins. At times, the white matter of an entire lobe can be demyelinated and occasionally even replaced by a multiloculated cystic lesion. By light microscopy, an active PML lesion is pathognomonic of the disease (Fig. 15A). It features a central region of myelin loss and its active degradation by macrophages. Axons are relatively spared. Reactive astrocytes with abundant eosinophilic cytoplasm are usually present in all lesions. Astrocytes with cytological features of tumor cells having one or more large, bizarre nuclei, may or may not be present. They seem to be less frequent in PML associated with AIDS than in other PML cases (232), but their presence in a demyelinating lesion is highly characteristic of

PML. At the periphery of the demyelinated zone, there is usually vacuolar degeneration of myelin and greatly enlarged (i.e., four- to fivefold) oligodendroglial nuclei containing amphophilic viral inclusions that intermix with the remaining specks of chromatin. Such inclusions cannot be seen in any other cell kind, but infected astrocytes may contain single viral particles detectable by electron microscopy. Inflammatory infiltrates of any kind and microglial reaction may be completely absent, but they are said to be more common in AIDS-related PML lesions than in other immunosuppressed patients (232). The disease progresses by centrifugal expansion of the individual lesions and their ultimate fusion into ever so larger areas of demyelination (Fig. 15B). Larger lesions, especially those that involve the entire lobe, are more

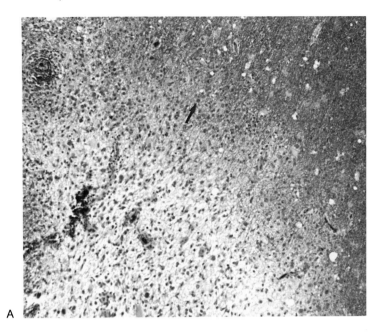

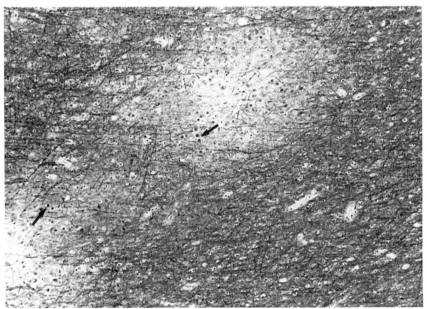

FIG. 15. Typical histopathological features of PML lesions (H&E/LFB). **A:** The center of an advanced lesion (*lower left*) shows total loss of myelin, severe reduction in number of oligodendroglia, reactive and infected astrocytes, and macrophages. The margin of the lesion (*upper right*) is ill-defined. It contains partially demyelinated axons and enlarged, infected oligodendroglia (*arrow*) (×100). **B:** Multiple adjacent foci of demyelination contain numerous infected oligodendroglia along their margins (*arrows*), resulting in a progressive myelin damage and eventual fusion of the neighboring lesions.

necrotizing, rather than strictly demyelinating in character, and with age they tend to transform into multilocular cystic spaces.

With these pathological characteristics in mind, diagnostic biopsies should include the smallest lesions visualized by MRI or seemingly healthy tissue from the edge of a larger lesion that is most likely to contain the pathognomonic JC-infected oligodendroglia. Even though CT and MRI findings are quite typical of PML, in the absence of any specific CSF findings, brain biopsy is usually the only way of establishing the diagnosis. In all typical cases of PML, a pathologist can make the diagnosis based on the histological appearance of the lesion, if the tissue sample adequately represents the lesion.

In addition, the presence of JCV in the biopsy or au-

topsy tissue samples can be demonstrated in the following ways: (a) *Viral cultures* of JC are rarely done because of the slow growth of the virus and the requirement of human-derived fetal glial cells as the culture medium (243). (b) *Electron microscopy* of massively infected oligodendroglia usually reveals JC virions, which come in conglomerates of ovoid or hexagonal single electron dense particles with lighter centers, or they may be arranged in bundles of filamentous profiles. The more common hexagonal virions usually measure 20–40 nm in diameter, double the size of filamentous particles (242). (c) *Indirect immunofluorescence* can be performed on frozen tissue by using JCV, SV40, and BK virus-specific antisera (227). (d) The peroxidase–antiperoxidase method is very practical because it can detect viral antigen in formalin-fixed and paraffin- or Epon-embedded tissue (247). (e) *In situ* hybridization and polymerase chain reaction (PCR) techniques can detect JC viral DNA and common papova viral capsid protein in formalin-fixed, paraffin-embedded autopsied and biopsied tissue (250,251).

NEUROSYPHILIS IN AIDS

Homosexual men are at a high risk for acquiring both syphilis and HIV infection. In the past 10 years, at least 40 HIV-positive individuals were reported to have had either asymptomatic neurosyphilis or signs of meningitis and cranial nerve abnormalities, as well as occlusive meningeal arteriopathy and cerebral infarcts (254).

About 1.5% of patients hospitalized for AIDS may also have neurosyphilis (255). In almost one-half of all cases, neurosyphilis and HIV infection were diagnosed at the same time, and in 40% of cases neurosyphilis developed despite previous treatment for treponemal infection outside the CNS (254). There is some evidence that impaired cellular immunity, altered function of macrophages, and decreased production of specific immunoglobulins by B cells in HIV-infected patients may modify the usual clinical course of syphilis (256,257). For instance, some HIV-positive homosexual men have developed meningovascular syphilis within months following the primary treponemal infection (258), whereas such a complication in non-AIDS cases usually takes from 5 to 12 years to occur (256). Furthermore, there has been at least one case report (257) of a concomitant, untreated

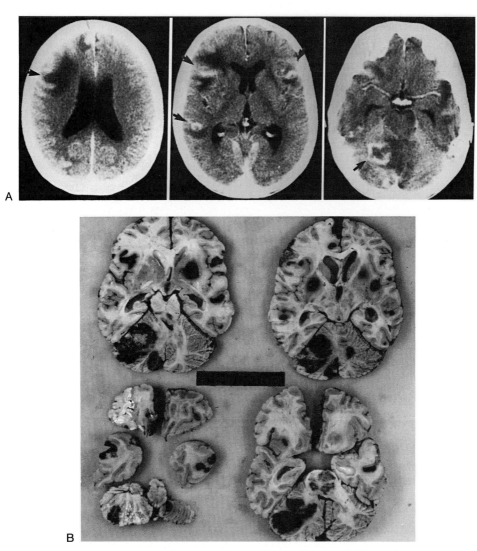

FIG. 16. A 39-year-old man with AIDS and amoebic CNS vasculitis, cerebritis, and hemorrhagic infarcts. **A:** CT scan, after contrast injection, shows multifocal supratentorial and cerebellar lesions (*arrows*) with a variable degree and patterns of enhancement and surrounding edema. Of note is a considerable ventricular enlargement, which was shown postmortem to be due to a severe cryptococcal infection of the arachnoidal villi. **B:** Autopsied, formalin-fixed brain shows numerous hemorrhagic infarcts.

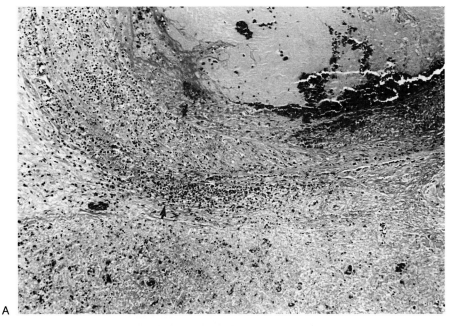

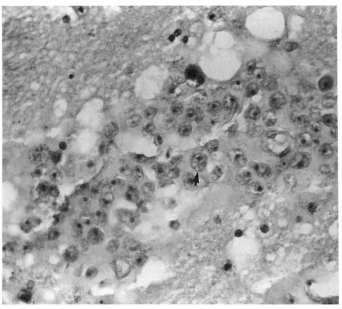

FIG. 17. Amoebic vasculitis and cerebritis (H&E/LFB). **A:** A segment of the wall of a medium-sized subarachnoidal artery showing necrosis and inflammatory infiltrates (between *arrows*). The lumen is thrombosed, and underlying brain tissue shows hemorrhagic necrosis (×100). **B:** Numerous amoebic organisms are present within swollen and necrotic brain tissue (*arrow*) (×400). **C:** The same organisms are permeating a wall of a parenchymal artery (×400).

infection with both HIV and *Treponema pallidum* that led not only to a relatively rapid development of neurosyphilis, but also to an unusually virulent meningitis, necrotizing and endarteriopathic occlusive vasculitis of the large branches of the circle of Willis, and multifocal cerebritis. The appearance of such grave (257) and unpredictable (255) complications of syphilis in HIV-positive individuals has led some to recommend both more aggressive treatment of the initial treponemal infection and "maintenance" therapy for a prolonged period of time (256). Thus AIDS patients, with their un-

ending propensity to unusual CNS complications, may be teaching the medical community yet another lesson, which is that an adequate immune response to *Treponema* may be as important as antibiotic treatment, and that in patients with altered immunity, previously established rules of treatment may have to be changed (259). In addition, both CSF testing and sound clinical expertise need to be employed in diagnosing neurosyphilis in these patients, because the Venereal Disease Research Laboratory Test (VDRL) on CSF, although very specific, has a level of sensitivity of only 27% (260).

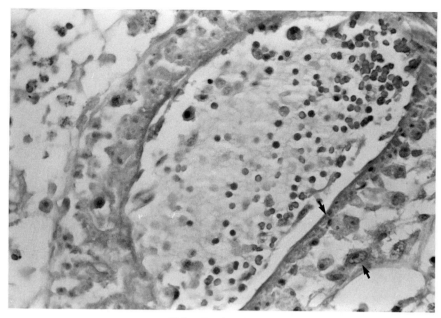

FIG. 17. *Continued.*

Clinically, most patients with neurosyphilis have signs of meningitis with CSF pleocytosis and increased protein. Focal neurological signs are sometimes due to CT scan demonstrable cerebral infarcts, and at other times, they are present in spite of a normal CT scan. Ophthalmological problems are common, as is an abnormal mental status. Seizures and cranial nerve signs may also be related to meningovascular syphilis, whereas general paresis seems to be quite rare (255).

CEREBROVASCULAR COMPLICATIONS OF AIDS

About 8% of adult patients with AIDS have autopsy-proven infarcts or recent hemorrhages due to embolization from mural thrombi related to marantic endocarditis or primary cardiac disease, bleeding diathesis, or thrombo-occlusive vasculitis (261). Cerebral vasculitis and transient or permanent ischemic brain damage may occur in the course of infections due to CMV, mycobacteria, fungi, toxoplasma, or amoebas (Figs. 16 and 17) (Table 2) (262). However, primary, isolated vasculitis also occurs in about 1.5% of AIDS cases (262). The pathogenesis of some AIDS-associated necrotizing vasculitides is uncertain (263,264), but at least two causative agents have been unequivocally linked with endarteriopathic vasculitis of the large branches of the circle of Willis, as listed next.

1. *Varicella zoster virus (VZV)-associated arteritis* occurring in AIDS patients is clinically and pathologically indistinguishable from that occurring in non-AIDS patients following ophthalmic infection (212; *personal observation*). Vasculitis caused by VZV usually affects the large vessels at the base of the brain and their branches within the Sylvian or interhemispheric fissure. Grossly, segments of the affected vessel walls are circumferentially thickened and whitish (Fig. 18A), their lumina are severely narrowed, sometimes thrombosed or recanalized. Microscopically, the most striking and most repetitive feature is an exuberant subendothelial proliferation of smooth muscle cells and fibroblasts, sparing of internal elastica and media, and a surprising absence of vessel wall necrosis, inflammation, granulomatous change, or signs of repair (Fig. 18B). Smaller subarachnoidal arterial branches may also be involved, whereas intraparenchymal vessels and veins are conspicuously well preserved. Special stains with VZV-specific antibodies reveal viral antigen within some cells of the media, intima, and along the internal elastic lamina, but not within the endothelium (Fig. 18C) (265). Vascular

TABLE 2. *Rare CNS complications of AIDS*

Neuropathologic findings	Reference
Mycobacterial abscess	290, 291
Escherichia coli meningitis	291, 292
Nocardial abscess	293, 294
Whipple's disease	295
Candidiasis	7
Aspergillosis	291, 297
Histoplasmosis	7, 296, 298
Cysticercosis	291
Amoebic encephalitis	299
Central pontine myelinolysis	294, 296
Mineralizing necrosis of pontocerebellar fibers	296
Lymphomatoid granulomatosis	296
Kaposi's sarcoma	292, 300
Wernicke's encephalopathy	301

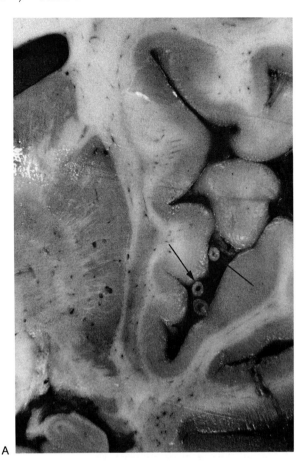

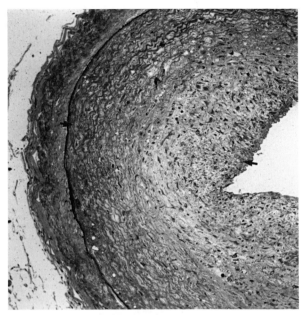

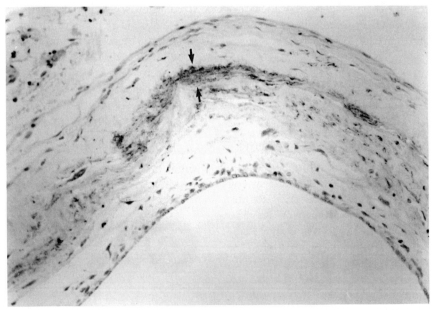

FIG. 18. VZV vasculopathy. **A:** Formalin-fixed brain, cut in a CT scan plane. Branches of middle cerebral artery (Sylvian fissure) show concentrically thickened walls and narrowing of lumena. **B:** A branch of the middle cerebral artery showing (from *left* to *right*) an intact media and internal elastic lamina. The salient histological feature is a thick subendothelial (between *arrows*) deposit of fibroblasts, smooth muscle cells, collagen, and macrophages (Toluidine blue stain applied to a 2-μm thick Epon-embedded tissue section (×100). **C:** A segment of the diseased vessel wall stained with immunoperoxidase-labeled VZV-specific antibody. The highest concentration of the positive staining is present along the inner part of the media (between *arrows*) and, to a lesser extent, within single cells of the newly formed subendothelial cellular deposit (×200).

changes are not typically accompanied by meningitis or encephalitis. The histology of the cerebral infarcts reveals no signs of inflammation or viral inclusions.

In a single case report of an HIV-positive patient with a similar gross pathology in multiple proximal branches of the circle of Willis, light microscopy also disclosed the presence of multinucleated cells along the internal elastic lamina. The patient had no history of herpes zoster, and the fluorescent antibody membrane antigen test for VZV in the CSF was negative. The authors speculated that HIV could be the cause of such a vasculitis (266).

2. *Syphilitic vasculitis* can grossly, and to a certain extent microscopically, resemble VZV vasculopathy (257), but this type of vasculitis is also associated with necrosis and fibrosis of the vessel wall, inflammation, and meningitis. In the best-documented case report of meningovascular syphilis occurring in an untreated HIV-positive Haitian man, the cerebral angiogram was described as being identical to that of Moyamoya disease, characteristically showing numerous narrowings of all parts of the circle of Willis. Treponemas as well as HIV were shown in the walls of the diseased vessels (257).

PRIMARY BRAIN LYMPHOMA

Lymphoma in AIDS patients almost always presents as extranodal disease with primary CNS involvement in

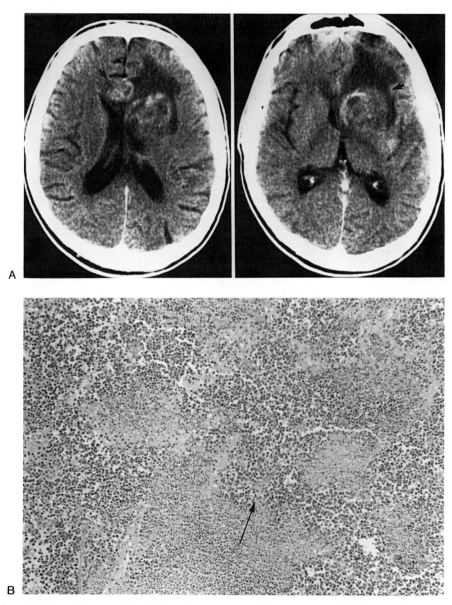

FIG. 19. A 37-year-old man with AIDS and a primary brain lymphoma. **A:** CT scan, after contrast injection, shows bilateral mass lesions with patchy enhancement and surrounding edema. **B:** Histologically, these lesions represent densely cellular tumor in which regions of viable tissue (*long arrow*) appear intermixed with areas of necrosis (H&E/LFB) (×100).

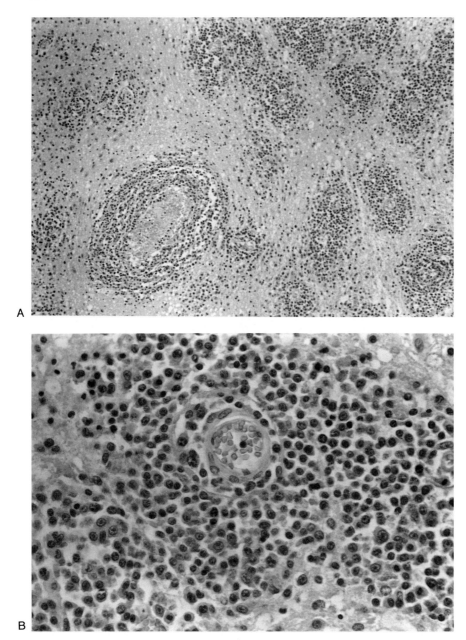

FIG. 20. Primary brain lymphoma (H&E/LFB). **A:** A viable peripheral zone of an expanding tumor mass often consists of numerous thin-walled, "leaky" vessels cuffed by dense tumorous infiltrates (×100). **B:** Typical cytology of a mixed cell type PBL (×400). **C:** Reticulin stain of PBL shows individual tumor cells or small clusters of cells encased by reticulin fibers (Reticulin stain) (×400).

about 23% of cases (267,268). The overall prevalence of primary brain lymphoma (PBL) associated with AIDS is up to 6% based on autopsy series (4,7,193,269). In non-immunosuppressed patients, PBL comprises only 1% of all non-Hodgkin's lymphomas (270), suggesting some role for the immune system in the pathogenesis of PBL. Also, whereas the frequency of opportunistic infections in AIDS patients varies among different high-risk groups and geographical regions, the prevalence of PBL does not (271). Thus AIDS follows the pattern of other acquired and congenital immunosuppressed states, which all confer a significantly increased risk of developing non-Hodgkin's lymphomas (NHLs) (272–275).

Theories to explain the discrepancy in prevalence of NHLs between immunocompetent and immunosuppressed states implicate either a deficiency in immunoregulation or chronic infection with a virus associated with oncogenesis, such as EBV (220,274). In one study, the authors detected EBV sequences in four cases of PBL in immunocompromised patients but not in four other cases in immunocompetent patients. The authors argued that this strong association implicates EBV sequences in the pathogenesis of PBLs in immunocompromised patients (276). Chronic B-cell stimulation secondary to EBV and/or HIV infection, in the setting of the T-cell dysregulation seen in AIDS, can lead to poly-

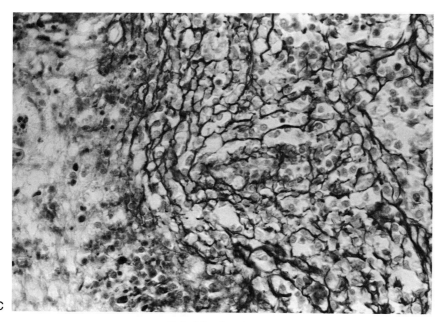

C

FIG. 20. *Continued.*

clonal B-cell proliferation. This lymphoproliferative state, in which many B cells are undergoing immunoglobulin gene rearrangements, increases the probability that aberrant rearrangements (i.e., translocations) may occur, especially rearrangements that alter the expression of the c-*myc* oncogene (277) and result in neoplastic transformation.

Another study found a significant association between systemic and CNS infection by CMV and PBL in AIDS patients compared to both non-AIDS patients with PBL and AIDS patients without PBL. The authors again suggest that viral infections in immunocompromised patients may provide a lymphoproliferative stimulus that predisposes to the development of malignant lymphoma (278).

The disproportionately high rate of primary lymphomatous involvement of the CNS also needs explanation. To the extent that reduced immunoregulation is involved in lymphoma pathogenesis, the lymphoproliferative stimuli of EBV or other viral infections may be more potent in "immunoprivileged" sites such as the brain, when compared to extraneural sites (274,279).

The clinical presentation of PBLs is variable. Signs of increased intracranial pressure and focal neurological deficits, such as hemiparesis, aphasia, and cranial nerve palsies, are common, as are memory impairment, confusion, and seizures (270,280,281). CSF usually contains increased protein, decreased glucose, pleocytosis, and tumor cells in 20% of tested cases. One study of CSF cytology in non-AIDS patients with PBL found tumor cells in 28% and pleocytosis in 58% of tested cases (282).

Neuroradiologic studies in non-AIDS patients with PBL reveal hypodense lesions on CT scans with variable patterns of enhancement after injection of contrast (270). Some researchers make a distinction between the CT image of gray and white matter lesions. Gray matter

lesions are clearly defined, hypodense images that produce little edema or mass effect and diffusely enhance with contrast. White matter lesions, on the other hand, are poorly defined, variably dense images with marked edema and mass effect and heterogeneous enhancement with contrast (283).

The CT findings in AIDS patients with PBL are more variable. Most patients have images similar to those described above for non-AIDS patients (3,280) (Fig. 19A). A lesion with ring enhancement after contrast can also be observed (280,281,284), as can a normal CT image (3,280,281).

The MRI scan in AIDS patients usually shows a slightly hypointense lesion on T1-weighted images and a slightly hyperintense lesion on proton density and T2-weighted images. There is mild edema and some mass effect. The lesions are often multiple and less than 2 cm in diameter (285).

Tumors that are less necrotic and therefore that have viable vasculature at the core of the lesion appear homogeneously enhancing after contrast. Similarly, lesions with multifocal necrosis (Fig. 19B) would exhibit heterogeneous, patchy enhancement (Fig. 19A). The pathologic correlate of ring-enhancing lesions is usually a large area of central necrosis with a peripheral zone of numerous, newly formed blood vessels cuffed by many viable tumor cells (Fig. 20A). Normal CT images, on the other hand, correspond to a diffusely infiltrative, perivascular, inflammatory-like pattern of tumor growth (284).

On gross examination, PBLs that have little necrosis can be difficult to distinguish from normal brain parenchyma, appearing as areas of grayish discoloration, granularity, and softening. Diffusely infiltrating tumors are virtually impossible to recognize grossly. More necrotic tumors are better distinguished, having a yellow-tan core and a grayish periphery that merges with the normal parenchyma. Necrotizing toxoplasmosis lesions can have a similar gross appearance, which also makes them difficult to distinguish from PBLs through radiologic studies (3,280,281). Lymphomatous involvement tends to be multicentric (280) and supratentorial.

Immunohistologic examination of PBLs shows that they are almost uniformly of B-cell origin (267,268, 278,280). When PBLs are classified according to the working formulation for NHLs, most tumors fall into the intermediate and high-grade categories. In one autopsy series of 15 cases of PBL from AIDS patients, seven were large cell lymphomas, six were mixed cellularity, one was small cleaved cell, and one was unclassifiable. Nine of the cases had significant perivascular lymphoplasmacytoid infiltrates at the periphery of, or remote from, the tumor masses. The six mixed cellularity (Fig. 20B) cases also contained a prominent population of medium-sized cells that could not be classified according to the working formulation (278). Three other studies of AIDS patients with PBL reported a similar preponderance of the more aggressive subtypes of NHL (267,268,280). Most malignant PBLs stain positively with reticulin stains (Fig. 20C).

A recent study has shown that whole brain radiotherapy significantly increases the survival of AIDS patients with PBL. While the nontreated patients had a mean survival of 42 days after the first appearance of symptoms, treated patients had a mean survival of 134 days. Moreover, patients in the untreated group died from progression of the PBL, while the patients in the treated group died of opportunistic infections. The authors therefore recommend that patients suspected of having PBL should undergo biopsy, so that immediate radiotherapy can be started on those patients shown to have lymphoma (286).

In contrast to PBL, secondary lymphomatous involvement of the CNS mainly involves infiltration of the leptomeninges, paraspinal–epidural compartment, cranial nerves, and spinal roots. One study found that 66% of systemic lymphomas in AIDS patients secondarily involve the CNS (287), but systemic lymphoma itself is rare, occurring in only about 3% of AIDS patients (3,4,7,193).

Finally, an increased risk of developing one other lymphoproliferative disorder—namely, lymphomatoid granulomatosis (LG)—has been associated with AIDS. One study reported three patients with angiocentric pleomorphic mononuclear cell infiltrates and vascular thrombosis and infarction, which the authors called LG. In two of the cases, however, the authors also claimed to find PBL (288). Whether one can reliably diagnose LG in the background of PBL is questionable, given that PBL can mimic many of the features said to characterize LG, such as infiltration of vessels, multifocality, necrosis, and mixed cellular infiltrate (289). More work needs to be done to characterize and define LG before a reliable assessment can be made concerning the prevalence of LG in the AIDS population.

Table 2 provides a list of some rare neuropathological findings in AIDS.

REFERENCES

1. Sotrel A. The nervous system. In: Harawi SJ, O'Hara CJ, eds. *Pathology and pathophysiology of AIDS and HIV-related diseases.* London: Chapman and Hall Medical; 1989;206–68.
2. de la Monte SM, Ho DD, Schooley RT, et al. Subacute encephalomyelitis of AIDS and its relation to HTLV-III infection. *Neurology* 1987;37:562–9.
3. Levy RM, Bredesen DE, Rosenblum ML. Neurological manifestations of AIDS: experience at UCSF and review of the literature. *J Neurosurg* 1985;62:475–95.
4. Snider WD, Simpson DM, Nielsen S, et al. Neurological complications of AIDS: analysis of 50 patients. *Ann Neurol* 1983;14: 403–18.
5. Gabuzda DH, Hirsch MS. Neurologic manifestations of infection with human immunodeficiency virus. Clinical features and pathogenesis. *Ann Intern Med* 1987;107:383–91.
6. Vazeux R, Brousse N, Jarry A, et al. AIDS subacute encephalitis. Identification of HIV-infected cells. *Am J Pathol* 1987;126: 403–10.
7. Petito CK, Cho ES, Lemann W, et al. Neuropathology of AIDS: an autopsy review. *J Neuropathol Exp Neurol* 1986;45:635–46.
8. Navia BA, Jordan BD, Price RW. The AIDS dementia complex. I. Clinical features. *Ann Neurol* 1986;19:517–26.
9. Navia BA, Cho ES, Petito CK, et al. The AIDS dementia complex. II. Neuropathology. *Ann Neurol* 1986;19:525–35.
10. Price RW, Brew B, Sidtis J, Rosenblum M, Scheck AC, Cleary P. The brain in AIDS: central nervous system HIV-1 infection and AIDS dementia complex. *Science* 1988;239:586–92.
11. Ho DD, Bredesen DE, Vinters HV, Daar ES. The acquired immunodeficiency syndrome (AIDS) dementia complex. *Ann Intern Med* 1989;111:400–10.
12. Morgello S, Cho ES, Nielsen S, et al. CMV encephalitis in patients with AIDS: an autopsy study of 30 cases and a review of the literature. *Hum Pathol* 1987;18:289–97.
13. Vinters HV, Kwok MK, Ho HW, et al. Cytomegalovirus in the nervous system of patients with the acquired immune deficiency syndrome. *Brain* 1989;112:245–68.
14. Wiley CA, Nelson JA. Role of human immunodeficiency virus and cytomegalovirus in AIDS encephalitis. *Am J Pathol* 1988;133:73–81.
15. Nelson JA, Reynolds-Kohler C, Oldstone MB, Wiley CA. HIV and CMV coinfect brain cells in patients with AIDS. *Virology* 1988;165:286–90.
16. Bélec L, Gray F, Mikol J, et al. Cytomegalovirus (CMV) encephalomyeloradiculitis and human immunodeficiency virus (HIV) encephalitis: presence of HIV and CMV co-infected multinucleated giant cells. *Acta Neuropathol (Berl)* 1990;81:99–104.
17. Vazeux R, Cumont M, Girard PM, et al. Severe encephalitis resulting from coinfections with HIV and JC virus. *Neurology* 1990;40:944–8.
18. Wiley CA, Grafe M, Kennedy C, Nelson JA. Human immunodeficiency virus (HIV) and JC virus in acquired immune deficiency syndrome (AIDS) patients with progressive multifocal leukoencephalopathy. *Acta Neuropathol (Berl)* 1988;76:338–46.
19. Cummings JL, Benson FD. Subcortical dementia. Review of an emerging concept. *Arch Neurol* 1984;41:874–9.
20. Wong MC, Suite ND, Labar DR. Seizures in human immunodeficiency virus infection. *Arch Neurol* 1990;47:640–2.
21. Mirra SS, Anand R, Spira TJ. HTLV-III/LAV infection of the central nervous system in a 57-year-old man with progressive dementia of unknown cause (letter). *N Engl J Med* 1986;314: 1191–2.
22. Price RW, Brew BJ, Rosenblum M. The AIDS dementia complex and HIV-1 brain infection: a pathogenetic model of virus-immune interaction. In: Waksman BH, ed. *Immunologic mecha-*

nisms in neurologic and psychiatric disease. New York: Raven Press; 1990:269–90.

23. Maj M. Organic mental disorders in HIV-1 infection. *AIDS* 1990;4:831–40.

24. Meeting Report: World Health Organization consultation on the neuropsychiatric aspects of HIV-1 infection, Geneva, 11–13 January 1990. *AIDS* 1990;4:935–6.

25. Hollander H. Cerebrospinal fluid normalities and abnormalities in individuals infected with human immunodeficiency virus. *J Infect Dis* 1988;158:855–8.

26. Koralnik IJ, Beaumanoir A, Häusler R, et al. A controlled study of early neurologic abnormalities in men with asymptomatic human immunodeficiency virus infection. *N Engl J Med* 1990;323:864–70.

27. Resnick L, Di Marzo-Veronese F, Schupbach J, et al. Intra blood–brain barrier synthesis of HTLV-III specific IgG in patients with neurologic symptoms associated with AIDS or ARC. *N Engl J Med* 1985;313:1498–504.

28. Levy JA, Shimabukuro J, Hollander H, et al. Isolation of AIDS-associated retroviruses from cerebrospinal fluid and brain of patients with neurological symptoms. *Lancet* 1985;2:586–8.

29. Ho DD, Rota TR, Schooley RT, et al. Isolation of HTLV-III from cerebrospinal fluid and neural tissues of patients with neurologic syndromes related to AIDS. *N Engl J Med* 1985;313:1493–7.

30. Marshall DW, Brey RL, Cahill WT, Houk RW, Zajac RA, Boswell RN. Spectrum of cerebrospinal fluid findings in various stages of human immunodeficiency virus infection. *Arch Neurol* 1988;45:954–8.

31. McArthur JC, Cohen BA, Farzedegan H, et al. Cerebrospinal fluid abnormalities in homosexual men with and without neuropsychiatric findings. *Ann Neurol* 1988;23(suppl):S34–7.

32. Hollander H, Levy JA. Neurologic abnormalities and recovery of human immunodeficiency virus from cerebrospinal fluid. *Ann Intern Med* 1987;106:692–5.

33. Brew BJ, Bhalla RB, Fleisher M, et al. Cerebrospinal fluid β_2 microglobulin in patients infected with human immunodeficiency virus. *Neurology* 1989;39:830–4.

34. Chrysikopoulos HS, Press GA, Grafa MR, Hesselink JR, Wiley CA. Encephalitis caused by human immunodeficiency virus: CT and MR imaging manifestations with clinical and pathologic correlation. *Radiology* 1990;175:185–91.

35. Rottenberg DA, Moeller JR, Strother SC, et al. The metabolic pathology of the AIDS dementia complex. *Ann Neurol* 1987;22:700–6.

36. Kleihues P, Lang W, Burger PC, et al. Progressive diffuse leukoencephalopathy in patients with AIDS. *Acta Neuropathol (Berl)* 1985;68:333–9.

37. Budka H. Human immunodeficiency virus (HIV) envelope and core proteins in CNS tissues of patients with the acquired immune deficiency syndrome (AIDS). *Acta Neuropathol (Berl)* 1990;79:611–9.

38. Gabuzda DH, Ho DD, de la Monte SM, et al. Immunohistochemical identification of HTLV-III antigen in brains of patients with AIDS. *Ann Neurol* 1986;20:289–95.

39. Epstein LG, Sharer LR, Cho ES, et al. HTLV-III/LAV-like retrovirus particles in the brains of patients with AIDS encephalopathy. *AIDS Res* 1984/1985;1:447–54.

40. Koenig S, Gendelman HE, Orenstein JM, et al. Detection of AIDS virus in macrophages in brain tissue from AIDS patients with encephalopathy. *Science* 1986;233:1089–93.

41. Meyenhofer MF, Epstein LG, Cho ES, et al. Ultrastructural morphology and intracellular production of HIV in brain. *J Neuropathol Exp Neurol* 1987;46:474–84.

42. Sharer LR, Epstein LG, Cho ES, et al. Pathologic features of AIDS encephalopathy in children: evidence for LAV/HTLV-III infection of brain. *Hum Pathol* 1986;17:271–84.

43. Watkins BA, Dorn HH, Kelly WB, et al. Specific tropism of HIV-1 for microglial cells in primary human brain cultures. *Science* 1990;249:549–53.

44. Stoler MH, Eskin TA, Benn S, et al. HTLV-III infection of the central nervous system: a preliminary *in situ* analysis. *JAMA* 1986;256:2360–4.

45. Pumarola-Sune T, Navia BA, Cordon-Cardo C, et al. HIV anti-

gen in the brains of patients with the AIDS dementia complex. *Ann Neurol* 1987;21:490–6.

46. Budka H. Multinucleated giant cells in brain: a hallmark of AIDS. *Acta Neuropathol (Berl)* 1986;69:253–8.

47. Dickson DW. Multinucleated cells in AIDS encephalopathy. Origin from endogenous microglia? *Arch Pathol Lab Med* 1986;110:967–8.

48. Smith TW, DeGirolami U, Hénin D, Bolgert F, Hauw J-J. Human immunodeficiency virus (HIV) leukoencephalopathy and the microcirculation. *J Neuropathol Exp Neurol* 1990;49:357–70.

48a. Kozlowski PB, Sher JH, Dickson DW, Sharer L, Cho E-S, Kanzer MD. Central nervous system in children with AIDS—a multicenter study. *J Neuropathol Exp Neurol* 1990;49:350.

49. Eidelberg D, Sotrel A, Vogel H, et al. Progressive polyradiculopathy in AIDS. *Neurology* 1986;36:912–6.

50. Hawley DA, Schaffer JF, Schulz DM, et al. CMV encephalitis in AIDS. *Am J Clin Pathol* 1983;80:874–7.

51. Guarda LA, Luna MA, Smith LJ Jr, et al. AIDS: postmortem findings. *Am J Clin Pathol* 1984;81:549–57.

52. Rhodes RH. Histopathology of the central nervous system in AIDS. *Hum Pathol* 1987;18:636–43.

53. Gray F, Chimelli L, Mohr M, Clavelou P, Scaravilli F, Poirier J. Fulminating multiple sclerosis-like leukoencephalopathy revealing human immunodeficiency virus infection. *Neurology* 1991;41:105–9.

54. Berger JR, Sheremata WA, Resnick L, Atherton S, Fletcher MA, Norenberg M. Multiple sclerosis-like illness occurring with human immunodeficiency virus infection. *Neurology* 1989;39:324–9.

55. Sotrel A, Herbert J, Kuban K, Ronthal M. Acute pseudotumoral demyelinating disorder in children and young adults: Schilder's disease or a variant of multiple sclerosis? *J Neuropathol Exp Neurol* 1984;43:319.

56. Sotrel A. On the dual nature and lack of specificity of intracytoplasmic inclusions in a case of adult onset orthochromatic leukodystrophy. *J Neuropathol Exp Neurol* 1988;47:490–1.

57. Rostad SW, Sumi SM, Shaw CM, Olson K, McDougall JK. Human immunodeficiency virus (HIV) infection in brains with AIDS-related leukoencephalopathy. *AIDS Res Hum Retroviruses* 1987;3:363–73.

58. Lenhardt TM, Super MA, Wiley CA. Neuropathological changes in an asymptomatic HIV seropositive man. *Ann Neurol* 1988;23:209–10.

59. Ketzler S, Weis S, Haug H, Budka H. Loss of neurons in the frontal cortex in AIDS brains. *Acta Neuropathol (Berl)* 1990;80:92–4.

60. Wiley CA, Masliah E, Morey M, et al. Neocortical damage during HIV infection. *Ann Neurol* 1991;29:651–7.

61. Ciardi A, Sinclair E, Scaravilli F, Harcourt-Webster NJ, Lucas S. The involvement of the cerebral cortex in human immunodeficiency virus encephalopathy: a morphological and immunohistochemical study. *Acta Neuropathol (Berl)* 1990;81:51–9.

62. Clague CPT, Ostrowski MA, Deck JHN, Harnish DG, Colley EA, Stead RH. Severe diffuse necrotizing cortical encephalopathy in acquired immune deficiency syndrome (AIDS): an immunocytochemical and ultrastructural study. *J Neuropathol Exp Neurol* 1988;47:346.

63. Budka H, Costanzi G, Cristina S, et al. Brain pathology induced by infection with the human immunodeficiency virus (HIV). A histological, immunocytochemical, and electron microscopical study of 100 autopsy cases. *Acta Neuropathol (Berl)* 1987;75:185–98.

64. Shaw GM, Harper ME, Hahn BH, et al. HTLV-III infection in brains of children and adults with AIDS encephalopathy. *Science* 1985;227:177–81.

65. Goudsmit J, Wolters EC, Bakker M, et al. Intrathecal synthesis of antibodies to HTLV-III in patients without AIDS or ARC. *Br Med J* 1986;292:1231–4.

66. Goudsmit J, Paul DA, Lange JMA, et al. Expression of HIV-Ag in serum and cerebrospinal fluid during acute and chronic infection. *Lancet* 1986;1:177–80.

67. Maddon PJ, Dalgleish AG, McDougal JS, Clapham PR, Weiss RA, Axel R. The T4 gene encodes the AIDS virus receptor and is

expressed in the immune system and the brain. *Cell* 1986;47:
333–48.

68. Chesebro B, Buller R, Portis J, Wehrly K. Failure of human immunodeficiency virus entry and infection in CD4-positive human brain and skin cells. *J Virol* 1990;64:215–21.

69. Kato T, Dembitzer HM, Hirano A, et al. HTLV III-like particles within a cell process surrounded by a myelin sheath in an AIDS brain. *Acta Neuropathol (Berl)* 1987;73:306–8.

70. Kure K, Lyman WD, Weidenheim KM, Dickson DW. Cellular localization of an HIV-1 antigen in subacute AIDS encephalitis using an improved double-labeling immunohistochemical method. *Am J Pathol* 1990;136:1085–92.

71. Lee S, Harris C, Hirschfeld A, Dickson DW. Case report. Cytomembranous inclusions in the brain of a patient with the acquired immunodeficiency syndrome. *Acta Neuropathol (Berl)* 1988;76:101–6.

72. Sidhu GS, Stahl RE, el-Sadr W, Cassai ND, Forrester EM, Zolla-Pazner S. The acquired immunodeficiency syndrome: an ultrastructural study. *Hum Pathol* 1985;16:377–86.

73. Gyorkey F, Melnick JL, Gyorkey P. Human immunodeficiency virus in brain biopsies of patients with AIDS and progressive encephalopathy. *J Infect Dis* 1987;155:870–6.

74. Gyorkey F, Melnick JL, Gyorkey P. Human immunodeficiency virus in glial cells: reply [letter]. *J Infect Dis* 1988;157:205.

75. Budka H, Lassmann H. Human immunodeficiency virus in glial cells? [letter] *J Infect Dis* 1988;157:203.

76. Sharer LR, Prineas JW. Human immunodeficiency virus in glial cells, continued [letter]. *J Infect Dis* 1988;157:204.

77. Koestner A. Animal model: distemper-associated demyelinating encephalomyelitis. *Am J Pathol* 1975;78:361–4.

78. Peluso R, Haase A, Stowring L, et al. A Trojan horse mechanism for the spread of visna virus in monocytes. *Virology* 1985;147:231–6.

79. Summers BA, Greisen HA, Appel MJG. Possible initiation of viral encephalomyelitis in dogs by migrating lymphocytes infected with distemper virus. *Lancet* 1978;2:187–9.

80. Ho DD, Pomerantz RJ, Kaplan JC. Pathogenesis of infection with HIV. *N Engl J Med* 1987;317:278–86.

81. Haase AT. Pathogenesis of lentivirus infections. *Nature* 1986; 322:130–6.

82. Sonigo P, Alizon M, Staskus K, et al. Nucleotide sequences of the visna lentivirus: relationship to the AIDS virus. *Cell* 1985;42: 369–82.

83. Gonda MA, Wong-Staal F, Gallo RC, et al. Sequence homology and morphologic similarity of HTLV-III and visna virus, a pathogenic lentivirus. *Science* 1985;227:173–7.

84. Koyanagi Y, Miles S, Mitsuyasu RT, et al. Dual infection of the central nervous system by AIDS viruses with distinct cellular tropisms. *Science* 1987;236:819–22.

85. Lutley R, Petursson G, Palsson PA, et al. Antigenic drift in visna: virus variation during long term infection of Icelandic sheep. *J Gen Virol* 1983;64:1433–40.

86. Gendelman HE, Baca LM, Husayni H, et al. Macrophage–HIV interaction: viral isolation and target cell tropism. *AIDS* 1990;4:221–8.

87. Cheng-Mayer C, Seto D, Tateno M, Levy JA. Biologic features of HIV-1 that correlate with virulence in the host. *Science* 1988;240:80–2.

88. Nathanson N, Pantich H, Palsson PA, et al. Pathogenesis of visna. II. Effect of immunosuppression upon early central nervous system lesions. *Lab Invest* 1976;35:444–51.

89. Petursson G, Nathanson N, Georgsson G, et al. Pathogenesis of visna. I. Sequential virologic, serologic and pathologic studies. *Lab Invest* 1976;35:402–12.

90. Pantich H, Petursson G, Georgsson G, et al. Pathogenesis of visna. III. Immune responses to CNS antigens in experimental allergic encephalomyelitis and visna. *Lab Invest* 1976;35:452–60.

91. Poser CM. White matter lesions of AIDS encephalomyelitis. *Lancet* 1990;336:757–8.

92. Johnson RT. Selective vulnerability of neural cells to viral infections. *Brain* 1980;103:447–72.

93. Wisniewski HM. Immunopathology of demyelination in autoimmune diseases and virus infections. *Br Med Bull* 1977;33:54–9.

94. Selmaj KW, Raine CS. Tumor necrosis factor mediates myelin

95. Vyakarnam A, McKeating J, Meager A, Beverley PC. Tumour necrosis factors (α,β) induced by HIV-1 in peripheral blood mononuclear cells potentiate virus replication. *AIDS* 1990;4: 21–7.

96. Rosenblum M, Scheck AC, Cronin K, et al. Dissociation of AIDS-related vacuolar myelopathy and productive HIV-1 infection of the spinal cord. *Neurology* 1989;39:892–6.

97. Oldstone MBA, Sinha YN, Blount P, et al. Virus-induced alterations in homeostasis: alterations in differentiated functions of infected cells *in vivo. Science* 1982;218:1125–7.

98. Sharpe AH, Hunter JJ, Chassler P, Jaenisch R. Role of abortive retroviral infection of neurons in spongiform CNS degeneration. *Nature* 1990;346:181–3.

99. Brenneman DE, Westbrook GL, Fitzgerald SP, et al. Neuronal cell killing by the envelope protein of HIV and its prevention by vasoactive intestinal peptide. *Nature* 1988;335:639–42.

100. Dreyer EB, Kaiser PK, Offermann JT, Lipton SA. HIV-1 coat protein neurotoxicity prevented by calcium channel antagonists. *Science* 1990;248:364–7.

101. Gibbons A. Is AIDS dementia due to increases in calcium? *Science* 1990;248:303.

102. Broder S, Mitsuya H, Yarchoan R, Pavlakis GN. NIH conference. Antiretroviral therapy in AIDS. *Ann Intern Med* 1990;113:604–18.

103. Yarchoan R, Berg G, Brouwers P, et al. Response of human-immunodeficiency-virus-associated neurological disease to 3'-azido-3'-deoxythymidine. *Lancet* 1987;1:132–5.

104. Schmitt FA, Bigley JW, McKinnis R, Logue PE, Evans RW, Drucker JL. Neuropsychological outcome of zidovudine (AZT) treatment of patients with AIDS and AIDS-related complex. *N Engl J Med* 1988;319:1573–8.

105. Portgies P, de Gans J, Lange MA, et al. Declining incidence of AIDS dementia complex after introduction of zidovudine treatment. *Br Med J* 1989;299:299–321.

106. Routy JP, Blanc AP, Rodriguez E, et al. Intrathecal zidovudine for AIDS dementia [letter]. *Lancet* 1990;336:248.

107. Petito CK, Navia BA, Cho E-S, Jordan BD, George DC, Price RW. Vacuolar myelopathy pathologically resembling subacute combined degeneration in patients with the acquired immunodeficiency syndrome. *N Engl J Med* 1985;312:874–9.

108. Horoupian DS, Pick P, Spigland I, et al. Acquired immune deficiency syndrome and multiple tract degeneration in a homosexual man. *Ann Neurol* 1984;15:502–5.

109. Navia BA, Petito CK, Gold JW, Cho ES, Jordan BD, Price RW. Cerebral toxoplasmosis complicating the acquired immune deficiency syndrome: clinical and neuropathological findings in 27 patients. *Ann Neurol* 1986;19:224–38.

110. Goldstick L, Mandybur TI, Bode R. Spinal cord degeneration in AIDS. *Neurology* 1985;35:103–6.

111. Budka H, Maier H, Pohl P. Human immunodeficiency virus in vacuolar myelopathy of the acquired immunodeficiency syndrome. *N Engl J Med* 1988;319:1667–8.

112. Smith T, Jakobsen J, Trojaborg W. Myelopathy and HIV infection. *AIDS* 1990;4:589–91.

113. Rhodes RH, Ward JM, Cowan RP, Moore PT. Immunohistochemical localization of human immunodeficiency viral antigens in formalin-fixed spinal cords with AIDS myelopathy. *Clin Neuropathol* 1989;8:22–7.

114. Eilbott DJ, Peress N, Burger H, et al. Human immunodeficiency virus type 1 in spinal cords of acquired immunodeficiency syndrome patients with myelopathy: expression and replication in macrophages. *Proc Natl Acad Sci USA* 1989;86:3337–41.

115. Weiser B, Peress N, La Neve D, Eilbott DJ, Seidman R, Burger H. Human immunodeficiency virus type 1 expression in the central nervous system correlates directly with extent of disease. *Proc Natl Acad Sci USA* 1990;87:3997–4001.

116. Johnson RT, McArthur JC. Editorial: myelopathies and retroviral infections. *Ann Neurol* 1987;21:113–6.

117. Román GC. Retrovirus-associated myelopathies. *Arch Neurol* 1987;44:659–63.

118. Bhagavati S, Ehrlich G, Kula RW, et al. Detection of human T-cell lymphoma/leukemia virus type I DNA and antigen in spi-

and oligodendrocyte damage in vitro. *Ann Neurol* 1988;23: 339–46.

nal fluid and blood of patients with chronic progressive myelopathy. *N Engl J Med* 1988;318:1141–7.

119. Salazar-Grueso EF, Holzer TJ, Gutierrez RA, et al. Familial spastic paraparesis syndrome associated with HTLV-I infection. *N Engl J Med* 1990;323:732–7.

120. Aboulafia DM, Saxton EH, Koga H, Diagne A, Rosenblatt JD. A patient with progressive myelopathy and antibodies to human T-cell leukemia virus type I and human immunodeficiency virus type 1 in serum and cerebrospinal fluid. *Arch Neurol* 1990;47: 477–9.

121. Brew BJ, Hardy W, Zuckerman E, et al. AIDS-related vacuolar myelopathy is not associated with coinfection by human T-lymphotropic virus type I. *Ann Neurol* 1989;26:679–81.

122. Dalakas MC, Pezeshkpour GH. Neuromuscular diseases associated with human immunodeficiency virus infection. *Ann Neurol* 1988;23(suppl):S38–48.

123. Leger JM, Bouche P, Bolgert F, et al. The spectrum of polyneuroathies in patients infected with HIV. *J Neurol Neurosurg Psychiatry* 1989;52:1369–74.

124. Parry GJ. Peripheral neuropathies associated with human immunodeficiency virus infection. *Ann Neurol* 1988;23(suppl):S49–53.

125. de la Monte SM, Gabuzda DH, Ho DD, et al. Peripheral neuropathy in the acquired immunodeficiency syndrome. *Ann Neurol* 1988;23:485–92.

126. Cornblath DR, McArthur JC, Kennedy PG, Witte AS, Griffin JW. Inflammatory demyelinating peripheral neuropathies associated with human T-cell lymphotropic virus type III infection. *Ann Neurol* 1987;21:32–40.

127. Chaunu MP, Ratinahirana H, Raphael M, et al. The spectrum of changes on 20 nerve biopsies in patients with HIV infection. *Muscle Nerve* 1989;12:452–59.

128. Piette AM, Tusseau F, Vignon D, et al. Acute neuropathy coincident with seroconversion for anti-LAV/HTLV-III. *Lancet* 1986;1:852.

129. Vendrell J, Heredia C, Pujol M, Vidal J, Blesa R, Graus F. Guillain-Barré syndrome associated with seroconversion for anti-HTLV-III. *Neurology* 1987;37:544.

130. Miller RG, Parry GJ, Pfaeffl W, Lang W, Lippert R, Kiprov D. The spectrum of peripheral neuropathy associated with ARC and AIDS. *Muscle Nerve* 1988;11:857–63.

131. Cornblath DR. Treatment of the neuromuscular complications of human immunodeficiency virus infection. *Ann Neurol* 1988;23(suppl):S88–91.

132. Chavanet P, Solary E, Giroud M, et al. Infraclinical neuropathies related to immunodeficiency virus infection associated with higher T-helper cell count. *J Acquired Immune Deficiency Syndrome* 1989;2:564–9.

133. Lipkin WI, Parry G, Kiprov D, Abrams D. Inflammatory neuropathy in homosexual men with lymphadenopathy. *Neurology* 1985;35:1479–83.

134. Said G, Lacroix-Ciaudo C, Fujimura H, Blas C, Faux N. The peripheral neuropathy of necrotizing arteritis: a clinicopathological study. *Ann Neurol* 1988;23:461–5.

135. Lange DJ, Britton CB, Younger DS, Hays AP. The neuromuscular manifestations of human immunodeficiency virus infections. *Arch Neurol* 1988;45:1084–88.

136. Cornblath DR, McArthur JC. Predominantly sensory neuropathy in patients with AIDS and AIDS-related complex. *Neurology* 1988;38:794–6.

137. So YT, Holtzman DM, Abrams DI, Olney RK. Peripheral neuropathy associated with acquired immunodeficiency syndrome. Prevalence and clinical features from a population-based survey. *Arch Neurol* 1988;45:945–8.

138. Rance NE, McArthur JC, Cornblath DR, Landstrom DL, Griffin JW, Price DL. Gracile tract degeneration in patients with sensory neuropathy and AIDS. *Neurology* 1988;38:265–71.

139. Yarchoan R, Berg G, Brouwers P, et al. Response of human-immunodeficiency-virus-associated neurological disease to 3'-azido-3'-deoxythymidine. *Lancet* 1987;1:132–5.

140. Yarchoan R, Thomas RV, Grafman J, et al. Long-term administration of 3'-azido-2',3'-dideoxythymidine to patients with AIDS-related neurological disease. *Ann Neurol* 1988;23(suppl):S82–7.

141. Dalakas MC, Yarchoan R, Spitzer R, Elder G, Sever JL. Treatment of human immunodeficiency virus-related polyneurop-

142. McArthur JC, Griffin JW, Cornblath DR, et al. Steroid-responsive myeloneuropathy in a man dually infected with HIV-1 and HTLV-1. *Neurology* 1990;40:938–44.

143. Behar R, Wiley C, McCutchan JA. Cytomegalovirus polyradiculoneuropathy in acquired immune deficiency syndrome. *Neurology* 1987;37:557–61.

144. Elder GA, Sever JL. AIDS and neurological disorders: an overview. *Ann Neurol* 1988;23(suppl):S4–6.

145. Robert ME, Geraghty JJ III, Miles SA, Cornford ME, Vinters HV. Severe neuropathy in a patient with acquired immune deficiency syndrome (AIDS). Evidence for widespread cytomegalovirus infection of peripheral nerve and human immunodeficiency virus-like immunoreactivity of anterior horn cells. *Acta Neuropathol (Berl)* 1989;79:255–61.

146. Fuller GN, Jacobs JM, Guiloff RJ. Association of painful peripheral neuropathy in AIDS with cytomegalovirus infection. *Lancet* 1989;2:937–41.

147. Illa I, Nath A, Dalakas M. Immunocytochemical and virological characteristics of HIV-associated inflammatory myopathies: similarities with seronegative polymyositis. *Ann Neurol* 1991;29:474–81.

148. Simpson DM, Bender AN. Human immunodeficiency virus-associated myopathy: analysis of 11 patients. *Ann Neurol* 1988;24:79–84.

149. Wiley CA, Nerenberg M, Cros D, Soto-Aguilar MC. HTLV-I polymyositis in a patient also infected with the human immunodeficiency virus. *N Engl J Med* 1989;320:992–5.

150. Dalakas M, Wichman A, Sever J. AIDS and the nervous system. *JAMA* 1989;261:2396–9.

151. Dalakas MC, Pezeshkpour GH, Flaherty M. Progressive nemaline (rod) myopathy associated with HIV infection. *N Engl J Med* 1987;317:1602–3.

152. Gonzales MF, Olney RK, SO YT, et al. Subacute structural myopathy associated with human immunodeficiency virus infection. *Arch Neurol* 1988;45:585–7.

153. Dalakas MC, Illa I, Pezeshkpour GH, Laukaitis JP, Cohen B, Griffin JL. Mitochondrial myopathy caused by long-term zidovudine therapy. *N Engl J Med* 1990;322:1098–105.

153a. Illa I, Nath A, Dalakas M. Immunocytochemical and virological characteristics of HIV-associated inflammatory myopathies: similarities with seronegative polymyositis. *Ann Neurol* 1991;29: 474–81.

154. Bailey RO, Turok DI, Jaufmann BP, Singh JK. Myositis and acquired immunodeficiency syndrome. *Hum Pathol* 1987;18: 749–51.

155. Gorard DA, Henry K, Guiloff RI. Necrotising myopathy and zidovudine [letter]. *Lancet* 1988;1:1050.

156. Panegyres PK, Tan N, Kakulas BA, Armstrong JA, Hollingsworth P. [Letter]. *Lancet* 1988;1:1050–1.

157. Balachandran T, McLean KA. Pyomyositis associated with AIDS. *AIDS* 1990;4:471.

158. Verma RK, Ziegler DK, Kepes JJ. HIV-related neuromuscular syndrome simulating motor neuron disease. *Neurology* 1990; 40:544–6.

159. Gray F, Gherardi R, Scaravilli F. The neuropathology of the acquired immune deficiency syndrome (AIDS). A review. *Brain* 1988;111(pt 2):245–66.

160. Hirano A. Neuropathology of AIDS: Montefiore experience. *Rinsho Shinkeigaku* 1989;29:1546–7.

161. Lang W, Miklossy J, Deruaz JP, et al. Neuropathology of the acquired immune deficiency syndrome (AIDS): a report of 135 consecutive autopsy cases from Switzerland. *Acta Neuropathol (Berl)* 1989;77:379–90.

162. Donovan Post JM, Kursunoglu SJ, Hensley GT, et al. Cranial CT in AIDS: spectrum of diseases and optimal contrast enhancement technique. *Am J Roentgenol* 1985;145:929–40.

163. Esiri MM, Scaravilli F, Millard PR, Harcourt Webster JN. Neuropathology of HIV infection in haemophiliacs: comparative necropsy study. *Br Med J* 1989;299:1312–5.

164. Feldman HA. Toxoplasmosis (concluded). *N Engl J Med* 1968;279:1431–7.

165. Remington JS, McLeod R. Toxoplasmosis. In: Braude AI, et al, eds. *Infectious diseases and medical microbiology, 2nd ed.* Philadelphia: Saunders; 1986:1521–35.

166. Krick JA, Remington JS. Current concepts in parasitology. Toxoplasmosis in the adult—an overview. *N Engl J Med* 1978;298:550–3.

167. Ryning FW, McLeod R, Maddox JC, et al. Probable transmission of *Toxoplasma gondii* by organ transplantation. *Ann Intern Med* 1979;90:47–9.

168. Feldman HA. Toxoplasmosis. *N Engl J Med* 1968;279:1370–5.

169. Yermakov V, Raskid R, Vuletin JC, et al. Disseminated toxoplasmosis. *Arch Pathol Lab Med* 1982;106:524–8.

170. Tang TT, Harb JM, Dunne MW, et al. Cerebral toxoplasmosis in an immunocompromised host. A precise and rapid diagnosis by electron microscopy. *Am J Clin Pathol* 1986;85:104–10.

171. Ghatak NR, Sawyer DR. A morphologic study of opportunistic cerebral toxoplasmosis. *Acta Neuropathol (Berl)* 1978;42:217–21.

172. Jones TC, Yeh S, Hirsch JG. The interaction between *Toxoplasma gondii* and mammalian cells. I. Mechanism of entry and intracellular fate of the parasite. *J Exp Med* 1972;136:1157–72.

173. Powell HC, Gibbs CJ Jr, Lorenzo AM, et al. Toxoplasmosis of the central nervous system in the adult. Electron microscopic observations. *Acta Neuropathol (Berl)* 1978;41:211–6.

174. Frenkel JK. Pathology and pathogenesis of congenital toxoplasmosis. *Bull NY Acad Med* 1974;50:182–91.

175. Huang TE, Chou SM. Occlusive hypertrophic arteritis as the cause of discrete necrosis in CNS toxoplasmosis in the acquired immunodeficiency syndrome. *Hum Pathol* 1988;19:1210–4.

176. Wong B, Gold JWM, Brown AE, et al. Central nervous system toxoplasmosis in homosexual men and parenteral drug abusers. *Ann Intern Med* 1984;100:36–42.

177. Wery D, Lemort M, Catteau A, Hermans P, Blumeck N, Jeanmart L. Computed tomography aspects of cerebral toxoplasmosis in AIDS. *J Belge Radiol* 1990;73:162–72.

178. Townsend JJ, Wolinsky JS, Baringer RJ, et al. Acquired toxoplasmosis. A neglected cause of treatable nervous system disease. *Arch Neurol* 1975;32:335–43.

179. Carrazana EJ, Rossitch E Jr, Schachter S. Cerebral toxoplasmosis masquerading as herpes encephalitis in a patient with the acquired immunodeficiency syndrome. *Am J Med* 1989;86:730–2.

180. Gray F, Gherardi R, Wingate E, et al. Diffuse "encephalitic" cerebral toxoplasmosis in AIDS. Report of four cases. *J Neurol* 1989;236:273–7.

181. Levy RM, Mills CM, Posin JP, Moore SG, Rosenblum ML, Bredesen DE. The efficacy and clinical impact of brain imaging in neurologically symptomatic AIDS patients: a prospective CT/MRI study. *J Acquired Immune Deficiency Syndrome* 1990;3:461–71.

182. Nolla-Salas J, Ricart C, D'Olhaberriague L, Gali F, Lamarca J. Hydrocephalus: an unusual CT presentation of cerebral toxoplasmosis in a patient with acquired immunodeficiency syndrome. *Eur Neurol* 1987;27:130–2.

183. Hakes TB, Armstrong D. Toxoplasmosis. Problems in diagnosis and treatment. *Cancer* 1983;52:1535–40.

184. Bishburg E, Eng RHK, Slim J, Perez G, Johnson E. Brain lesions in patients with acquired immunodeficiency syndrome. *Arch Intern Med* 1989;149:941–3.

185. Montgomery H, Adam A, Dollery CT, et al. Cerebral mass lesions in patients with AIDS. Role and timing of cerebral biopsy. *Br Med J* 1990;301:226–8.

186. Leport C, Bastuji-Garin S, Perronne C, et al. An open study of the pyrimethamine–clindamycin combination in AIDS patients with brain toxoplasmosis. *J Infect Dis* 1989;160:557–8.

187. Cohn JA, McMeeking A, Cohen W, Jacobs J, Holzman RS. Evaluation of the policy of empiric treatment of suspected *Toxoplasma* encephalitis in patients with the acquired immunodeficiency syndrome. *Am J Med* 1989;86:521–7.

188. Kure K, Harris C, Morin LS, Dickson DW. Solitary midbrain toxoplasmosis and olivary hypertrophy in a patient with acquired immunodeficiency syndrome. *Clin Neuropathol* 1989;8:35–40.

189. Bahls F, Sumi SM. Cryptococcal meningitis and cerebral toxoplasmosis in a patient with acquired immune deficiency syndrome. *J Neurol Neurosurg Psychiatry* 1986;49:328–30.

190. Sun T, Greenspan J, Tenebaum M. Diagnosis of toxoplasmosis using fluorescein-labeled antitoxoplasma monoclonal antibodies. *Am J Surg Pathol* 1986;10:312–6.

191. Conley FK, Jenkins KA, Remington JS. *Toxoplasma gondii* infection of the central nervous system. Use of peroxidase and antiperoxidase method to demonstrate toxoplasma in formalin fixed, paraffin embedded tissue sections. *Hum Pathol* 1981;12:690–8.

192. Holliman RE, Johnson JD, Savva D. Diagnosis of cerebral toxoplasmosis in association with AIDS using the polymerase chain reaction. *Scand J Infect Dis* 1990;22:243–4.

193. Anders KH, Guerra WF, Tomiyasu U, Verity MA, Vinters HV. The neuropathology of AIDS. UCLA experience and review. *Am J Pathol* 1986;124:537–58.

194. Kovacs JA, Kovacs AA, Polis M, et al. Cryptococcosis in the acquired immunodeficiency syndrome. *Ann Intern Med* 1985;103:533–8.

195. Chuck SL, Sande MA. Infections with *Cryptococcus neoformans* in the acquired immunodeficiency syndrome. *N Engl J Med* 1989;321:794–9.

196. Zuger A, Louie E, Holzman RS, Simberkoff MS, Rahal JJ. Cryptococcal disease in patients with the acquired immunodeficiency syndrome. *Ann Intern Med* 1986;104:234–40.

197. Dismukes WE. Cryptococcal meningitis in patients with AIDS. *J Infect Dis* 1988;157:624–8.

198. Eng RHK, Bishburg E, Smith SM, Kapila R. Cryptococcal infections in patients with acquired immune deficiency syndrome. *Am J Med* 1986;81:19–23.

199. Popovich MJ, Arthur RH, Helmer E. CT of intracranial cryptococcosis. *Am J Roentgenol* 1990;154:603–6.

200. Davis LE, Johnson RT. An explanation for the localization of herpes simplex encephalitis? *Ann Neurol* 1979;5:2–5.

201. Laskin OL, Stahl-Bayliss CM, Morgello S. Concomitant herpes simplex virus type 1 and cytomegalovirus ventriculoencephalitis in acquired immunodeficiency syndrome. *Arch Neurol* 1987;44:843–7.

202. Johnson RT. *Viral infections of the nervous system.* New York: Raven Press; 1982.

203. Linneman CC Jr, First MR, Alvira MM, et al. Herpes virus hominis type II meningoencephalitis following renal transplantation. *Am J Med* 1976;61:703–8.

204. Sutton AL, Smithwick EM, Seligman SJ, Kim DS. Fatal disseminated herpesvirus hominis type 2 infection in an adult with associated thymic dysplasia. *Am J Med* 1974;56:545–53.

205. Britton CB, Mesa-Tejada R, Fenoglio CM, Hays AP, Garvey GG, Miller JR. A new complication of AIDS: thoracic myelitis caused by herpes simplex virus. *Neurology* 1985;35:1071–4.

206. Tucker T, Dix RD, Katzen C, Davis RL, Schmidley JW. Cytomegalovirus and herpes simplex virus ascending myelitis in a patient with acquired immune deficiency syndrome. *Ann Neurol* 1985;18:74–9.

207. Dix RD, Waitzman DM, Follansbee S, et al. Herpes simplex virus type 2 encephalitis in two homosexual men with persistent lymphadenopathy. *Ann Neurol* 1985;17:203–6.

208. Gateley A, Gander RM, Johnson PC, Kit S, Otsuka H, Kohl S. Herpes simplex virus type 2 meningoencephalitis resistant to acyclovir in a patient with AIDS. *J Infect Dis* 1990;161:711–5.

209. Horten B, Price RW, Jimenez D. Multifocal varicella-zoster virus leukoencephalitis temporally remote from herpes zoster. *Ann Neurol* 1981;9:251–66.

210. Ryder JW, Croen K, Kleinschmidt-DeMasters BK, Ostrove JM, Straus SE, Cohn DL. Progressive encephalitis three months after resolution of cutaneous zoster in a patient with AIDS. *Ann Neurol* 1986;19:182–8.

211. Gilden DH, Murray RS, Wellish M, Kleinschmidt-DeMasters BK, Vafai A. Chronic progressive varicella-zoster virus encephalitis in an AIDS patient. *Neurology* 1988;38:1150–3.

212. Eidelberg D, Sotrel A, Horoupian DS, Neumann PE, Pumarola-Sune T, Price RW. Thrombotic cerebral vasculopathy associated with herpes zoster. *Ann Neurol* 1986;19:7–14.

213. Rostad SW, Olson K, McDougall J, Shaw C-M, Alvord Jr EC. Transsynaptic spread of varicella zoster virus through the visual system: a mechanism of viral dissemination in the central nervous system. *Hum Pathol* 1989;20:174–9.

214. Morgello S, Block GA, Price RW, Petito CK. Varicella-zoster virus leukoencephalitis and cerebral vasculopathy. *Arch Pathol Lab Med* 1988;112:173-7.

215. Rosenberg NL, Hochberg FH, Miller G, Kleinschmidt-DeMasters BK. Primary central nervous system lymphoma related to Epstein-Barr virus in a patient with acquired immune deficiency syndrome. *Ann Neurol* 1986;20:98-102.

216. Bale JF Jr. Human cytomegalovirus infection and disorders of the nervous system. *Arch Neurol* 1984;41:310-20.

217. Drew WL, Mintz L, Miner RC, Sands M, Ketterer B. Prevalence of cytomegalovirus infection in homosexual men. *J Infect Dis* 1981;143:188-92.

218. Duchowny M, Caplan L, Siber G. Cytomegalovirus infection of the adult nervous system. *Ann Neurol* 1979;5:458-61.

219. Phillips CA, Fanning WL, Gump DW, Phillips CF. Cytomegalovirus encephalitis in immunologically normal adults. Successful treatment with vidarabine. *JAMA* 1977;238:2299-300.

220. Fauci AS, Macher AM, Longo DL, et al. NIH conference. Acquired immunodeficiency syndrome: epidemiologic, clinical, immunologic, and therapeutic considerations. *Ann Intern Med* 1984;100:92-106.

221. Donovan Post MJ, Hensley GT, Moskowitz LB, Fischl M. Cytomegalic inclusion virus encephalitis in patients with AIDS: CT, clinical, and pathologic correlation. *Am J Roentgenol* 1986;146:1229-34.

222. Grafe MR, Wiley CA. Spinal cord and peripheral nerve pathology in AIDS: the roles of cytomegalovirus and human immunodeficiency virus. *Ann Neurol* 1989;25:561-6.

223. Moskowitz LB, Gregorios JB, Hensley GT, Berger JR. Cytomegalovirus. Induced demyelination associated with acquired immune deficiency syndrome. *Arch Pathol Lab Med* 1984;108:873-7.

224. Fuller GN, Jacobs JM, Guiloff RJ. Association of painful peripheral neuropathy in AIDS with cytomegalovirus infection. *Lancet* 1989;2:937-41.

225. Wiley CA, Nelson JA. Role of human immunodeficiency virus and cytomegalovirus in AIDS encephalitis. *Am J Pathol* 1988;133:73-81.

226. Mahieux F, Gray F, Fenelon G, et al. Acute myeloradiculitis due to cytomegalovirus as the initial manifestation of AIDS. *J Neurol Neurosurg Psychiatry* 1989;52:270-4.

227. Padgett BL, Walker DL. Virologic and serologic studies of PML. *Prog Clin Biol Res* 1983;105:107-17.

228. Jakobsen J, Diemer NH, Gaub J, et al. PML in a patient without other clinical manifestations of AIDS. *Acta Neurol Scand* 1987;75:209-13.

229. Faris AA, Martinez JA. Primary PML. A CNS disease caused by a slow virus. *Arch Neurol* 1972;27:357-60.

230. Rockwell D, Ruben FL, Winkelstein A, et al. Absence of immune deficiencies in a case of PML. *Am J Med* 1976;61:433-6.

231. Krupp LB, Lipton RB, Swerdlow ML, et al. PML: clinical and radiographic features. *Ann Neurol* 1985;17:344-9.

232. Aksamit AJ, Gendelman HE, Orenstein JM, Pezeshkpour GH. AIDS-associated progressive multifocal leukoencephalopathy (PML): comparison to non-AIDS PML with *in situ* hybridization and immunohistochemistry. *Neurology* 1990;40:1073-8.

233. Lipton HL. Is JC virus latent in brain? *Ann Neurol* 1991;29:433-4.

234. Bedri J, Weinstein W, De Gregorio P, et al. PML in AIDS [letter]. *N Engl J Med* 1983;309:492-3.

235. Blum LW, Chambers RA, Schwartzman RJ, et al. PML in AIDS. *Arch Neurol* 1985;42:137-9.

236. Bernick C, Gregorios JB. PML in a patient with AIDS. *Arch Neurol* 1984;41:780-2.

237. Elkin CM, Leon E, Grenell SL, et al. Intracranial lesions in AIDS. Radiological (computed tomographic) features. *JAMA* 1985;253:393-6.

238. Levy JD, Cottingham KL, Campbell RJ, et al. PML and magnetic resonance imaging. *Ann Neurol* 1986;19:399-401.

239. Whelan MA, Kricheff II, Handler M, et al. AIDS: cerebral computed tomographic manifestations. *Radiology* 1983;149:477-84.

240. Speelman JD, ter Schegget J, Bots GThAM, et al. PML in a case of AIDS. *Clin Neurol Neurosurg* 1985;87:27-33.

241. Astrom KE, Mancall EL, Richardson EP Jr. PML. *Brain* 1958;81:93-111.

242. ZuRhein GM, Chou SM. Particles resembling papovavirus in human cerebral demyelinating disease. *Science* 1965;148:1477-9.

243. Padgett BL, ZuRhein GM, Walker DL, et al. Cultivation of papova-like virus from human brain with PML. *Lancet* 1971;1:1257-60.

244. Oxman MN, Howley PM. Papovaviruses. In: Braude AI, et al, eds. *Infectious diseases and medical microbiology, 2nd ed.* Philadelphia: Saunders; 1986:482-506.

245. Walker DL. PML: an opportunistic viral infection of the central nervous system. In: Vinken PJ, et al, eds. *Handbook of clinical neurology.* Amsterdam: North-Holland; 1978:307-29.

246. Weiner LP, Herndon RM, Narayan O, et al. Isolation of virus related to SV40 from patients with PML. *N Engl J Med* 1972;286:385-90.

247. Itoyama Y, Webster H de F, Sternberger NH, et al. Distribution of papova-virus, myelin-associated glycoprotein, and myelin basic protein in PML lesions. *Ann Neurol* 1982;11:396-407.

248. Mazlo M, Tariska I. Are astrocytes infected in PML? *Acta Neuropathol (Berl)* 1982;56:45-51.

249. Castaigne P, Rondot P, Escourolle R, et al. Leucoencephalopathie multifocale progressive et 'gliomes' multiples. *Rev Neurol (Paris)* 1974;130:379-92.

250. Mori M, Kurata H, Tajima M, Shimada H. JC virus detection by *in situ* hybridization in brain tissue from elderly patients. *Ann Neurol* 1991;29:428-32.

251. Telenti A, Aksamit AJ Jr, Proper J, Smith TF. Detection of JC virus DNA by polymerase chain reaction in patients with progressive multifocal leukoencephalopathy. *J Infect Dis* 1990;162:858-61.

252. Knight A, O'Brien P, Osoba D. "Spontaneous" PML. Immunologic aspects. *Ann Intern Med* 1972;77:229-33.

253. Willoughby E, Price RW, Padgett BL, et al. PML: *in vitro* cell-mediated immune responses to mitogens and JC virus. *Neurology* 1980;30:256-62.

254. Musher DM, Hamill RJ, Baughn RE. Effect of human immunodeficiency virus (HIV) infection on the course of syphilis and on the response to treatment. *Ann Intern Med* 1990;113:872-81.

255. Katz DA, Berger JR. Neurosyphilis in acquired immunodeficiency syndrome. *Arch Neurol* 1989;46:895-8.

256. Johns DR, Tierney M, Felsenstein D. Alteration in the natural history of neurosyphilis by concurrent infection with the human immunodeficiency virus. *N Engl J Med* 1987;316:1569-72.

257. Morgello S, Laufer H. Quaternary neurosyphilis in a Haitian man with human immunodeficiency virus infection. *Hum Pathol* 1989;20:808-11.

258. Berry CD, Hooton TM, Collier AC, Lukehart SA. Neurologic relapse after benzathine penicillin therapy for secondary syphilis in a patient with HIV infection. *N Engl J Med* 1987;316:1587-9.

259. Tramont EC. Syphilis in the AIDS era. *N Engl J Med* 1987;316:1600-1.

260. Davis LE, Schmitt JW. Clinical significance of cerebrospinal fluid tests for neurosyphilis. *Ann Neurol* 1989;25:50-5.

261. Berger JR, Harris JO, Gregorios J, Norenberg M. Cerebrovascular disease in AIDS: a case-control study. *AIDS* 1990;4:239-44.

262. Engstrom JW, Lowenstein DH, Bredesen DE. Cerebral infarctions and transient neurologic deficits associated with acquired immunodeficiency syndrome. *Am J Med* 1989;86:528-32.

263. Vinters HV, Guerra WF, Eppolito L, Keith PE III. Necrotizing vasculitis of the nervous system in a patient with AIDS-related complex. *Neuropathol Appl Neurobiol* 1988;14:417-24.

264. Scaravilli F, Daniel SE, Harcourt Webster N, Guiloff RJ. Chronic basal meningitis and vasculitis in acquired immunodeficiency syndrome. A possible role for human immunodeficiency virus. *Arch Pathol Lab Med* 1989;113:192-5.

265. Stillman IE, Rosenblum ML, Sotrel A. Thrombosing CNS vasculopathy associated with herpes zoster virus in AIDS. *Hum Pathol,* (in press).

266. Yankner BA, Skolnik PR, Shoukimas GM, Gabuzda DH, Sobel RA, Ho DD. Cerebral granulomatous angiitis associated with iso-

lation of human T-lymphotropic virus type III from the central nervous system. *Ann Neurol* 1986;20:362–4.

267. Di Carlo EF, Amberson JB, Metroka CE, Ballard P, Moore A, Mouradian JA. Malignant lymphomas and the acquired immunodeficiency syndrome. Evaluation of 30 cases using a working formulation. *Arch Pathol Lab Med* 1986;110:1012–6.

268. Ziegler JL, Beckstead JA, Volberding PA, et al. Non-Hodgkin's lymphoma in 90 homosexual men. Relation to generalized lymphadenopathy and the acquired immunodeficiency syndrome. *N Engl J Med* 1984;311:565–70.

269. Moskowitz LB, Hensley GT, Chan JC, Gregorios J, Conley FK. The neuropathology of acquired immune deficiency syndrome. *Arch Pathol Lab Med* 1984;108:867–72.

270. Woodman R, Shin K, Pineo G. Primary non-Hodgkin's lymphoma of the brain. A review. *Medicine (Baltimore)* 1985;64:425–30.

271. Levy RM, Janssen RS, Bush TJ, Rosenblum ML. Neuroepidemiology of acquired immunodeficiency syndrome. *J Acquired Immune Deficiency Syndrome* 1988;1:31–40.

272. Hanto DW, Frizzera G, Purtilo DT, et al. Clinical spectrum of lymphoproliferative disorders in renal transplant recipients and evidence for the role of Epstein-Barr virus. *Cancer Res* 1981;41:4253–61.

273. Louie S, Schwartz RS. Immunodeficiency and the pathogenesis of lymphoma and leukemia. *Semin Hematol* 1978;15:117–38.

274. Penn I. Depressed immunity and the development of cancer. *Clin Exp Immunol* 1981;46:459–74.

275. Schneck SA, Penn I. *De-novo* brain tumours in renal-transplant recipients. *Lancet* 1971;2:983–6.

276. Bashir RM, Harris NL, Hochberg FH, Singer RM. Detection of Epstein-Barr virus in CNS lymphomas by *in-situ* hybridization. *Neurology* 1989;39:813–7.

277. Freter CE. Acquired immunodeficiency syndrome-associated lymphomas. *J Natl Cancer Inst Monogr* 1990;10:45–54.

278. Morgello S, Petito CK, Mouradian JA. Central nervous system lymphoma in the acquired immunodeficiency syndrome. *Clin Neuropathol* 1990;9:205–15.

279. Kay HEM. Immunosuppression and the risk of brain lymphoma. *N Engl J Med* 1983;308:1099–100.

280. So YT, Beckstead JH, Davis RL. Primary central nervous system lymphoma in acquired immune deficiency syndrome: a clinical and pathological study. *Ann Neurol* 1986;20:566–72.

281. Levy RM, Bredesen DE. Central nervous system dysfunction in acquired immunodeficiency syndrome. *J Acquired Immune Deficiency Syndrome* 1988;1:41–64.

282. Jellinger K, Radaskiewicz TH, Slowik F. Primary malignant lymphomas of the central nervous system in man. *Acta Neuropathol [Suppl] (Berl)* 1975; VI:95–102.

283. Thomas M, MacPherson P. Computed tomography of intracranial lymphoma. *Clin Radiol* 1982;33:331–6.

284. Lee Y-Y, Bruner JM, Van Tassel P, Libshitz HI. Primary central nervous system lymphoma: CT and pathologic correlation. *Am J Roentgenol* 1986;147:747–52.

285. Schwaighofer BW, Hesselink JR, Press GA, Wolf RL, Healy ME, Berthoty DP. Primary intracranial CNS lymphoma: MR manifestations. *Am J Neuroradiol* 1989;10:725–9.

286. Baumgartner JE, Rachlin JR, Beckstead JH, et al. Primary central nervous system lymphomas: natural history and response to radiation therapy in 55 patients with acquired immunodeficiency syndrome. *J Neurosurg* 1990;73:206–11.

287. Loureiro C, Gill PS, Meyer PR, Rhodes R, Rarick MU, Levine AM. Autopsy findings in AIDS-related lymphoma. *Cancer* 1988;62:735–9.

288. Anders KH, Latta H, Chang BS, Tomiyasu U, Quddusi AS, Vinters HV. Lymphomatoid granulomatosis and malignant lymphoma of the central nervous system in the acquired immunodeficiency syndrome. *Hum Pathol* 1989;20:326–34.

289. Colby TV. Editorial: central nervous system lymphomatoid granulomatosis in AIDS? *Hum Pathol* 1989;20:301–2.

290. Fischl MA, Pitchenik AE, Spira TJ. Tuberculous brain abscess and toxoplasma encephalitis in a patient with AIDS. *JAMA* 1985;253:3428–30.

291. Moskowitz LB, Hensley GT, Chan JC, et al. The neuropathology of AIDS. *Arch Pathol Lab Med* 1984;108:867–72.

292. Welch K, Finkbeiner W, Alpers CE, et al. Autopsy findings in the AIDS. *JAMA* 1984;252:1152–9.

293. Adair JC, Beck AC, Apfelbaum RI, et al. Nocardial cerebral abscess in the AIDS. *Arch Neurol* 1987;44:548–50.

294. Sharer LR, Kapila R. Neuropathologic observation in AIDS. *Acta Neuropathol* 1985;66:188–98.

295. Jankovic J. Whipple's disease of the CNS in AIDS [letter]. *N Engl J Med* 1986;315:1029–30.

296. Anders KH, Wayne GF, Tomiyasu U, et al. The neuropathology of AIDS. UCLA experience and review. *Am J Pathol* 1986;124:537–58.

297. Brocheriou C, Badillet G, Gluckman E, et al. Mycotic infection in immunosuppressed patients. An anatomopathologic study. *Ann Pathol* 1990;10:99–108.

298. Wheat LJ, Batteiger BE, Sathapatayavongs D. *Histoplasma capsulatum* infections of the central nervous system. A clinical review. *Medicine (Baltimore)* 1990;69:244–60.

299. Gardner HAR, Martinez AJ, Visvesvara GS, Sotrel A. Granulomatous amebic encephalitis in an AIDS patient. *Neurology* 1991;41:1193–5.

300. Ariza A, Kim JH. Kaposi's sarcoma of the dura mater. *Hum Pathol* 1988;19:1461–3.

301. Soffer D, Zirkin H, Alkan M, Berginer VM. Wernicke's encephalopathy in acquired immune deficiency syndrome (AIDS): a case report. *Clin Neuropathol* 1989;8:192–4.

AIDS and Other Manifestations of HIV Infection,
Second Edition, Edited by Gary P. Wormser.
Raven Press, Ltd., New York © 1992.

CHAPTER 35

Infection Control Considerations in HIV Infection

Jerome I. Tokars and William J. Martone

The primary modes of transmission of human immunodeficiency virus (HIV), the virus that causes acquired immunodeficiency syndrome (AIDS), are sexual contact, exposure to infected blood or blood components, and perinatal transmission from mother to neonate (1). HIV has been isolated from blood and a number of other body fluids, including semen, vaginal secretions, saliva, tears, breast milk, cerebrospinal fluid, amniotic fluid, bronchoalveolar-lavage fluid, and urine (2–16). However, epidemiologic evidence has implicated only blood, semen, vaginal secretions, and breast milk in transmission (1,2). Among persons living in the same household with persons infected with HIV, transmission of HIV has occurred only to direct sexual contacts of infected persons and to neonates of infected mothers; transmission of HIV through ordinary social or occupational contact with HIV-infected persons or through air, water, or food has not been demonstrated (17–21). The mode of transmission of HIV is similar to that of hepatitis B virus, although the potential for hepatitis B virus transmission is greater (22).

In the health-care setting, blood is the single most important source of HIV, and transmission has been documented only after exposure to blood, bloody pleural fluid, or culture medium containing concentrated virus (22–25). Percutaneous inoculation has been the route of infection in most instances of nosocomial HIV transmission; however, transmission by contact with mucous membranes and possibly by contact with an open wound or nonintact (e.g., chapped, abraded, weeping, or dermatitic) skin has also been reported (22,26–28).

This chapter outlines infection control measures to prevent nosocomial transmission of bloodborne pathogens such as HIV and of other pathogens that occur frequently in HIV-infected patients. Precautions designed to prevent transmission of bloodborne pathogens, referred to as "universal precautions," should be applied to all patients (21,22,29). Prevention of transmission of other pathogens require precautions specific either to the disease ("disease-specific") or to the transmission category ("category-specific") (30).

DISINFECTION, STERILIZATION, AND ENVIRONMENTAL HYGIENE

An important infection control issue is whether routine sterilization and disinfection procedures are adequate for preventing HIV transmission. A number of laboratory studies using various experimental conditions and assays for viral inactivation suggest that HIV does not possess unusual resistance properties (31–36). In these studies, HIV was inactivated by many chemical germicides at concentrations below those commonly used. In one study, HIV was rapidly inactivated by drying, but continued to be detectable after 1–3 days (31). However, in this study, HIV was used in a concentration of 10,000,000 tissue culture infective doses (TCID) per milliliter, a much higher concentration than that estimated to be present in the blood of HIV-infected persons (60–7000 TCID per milliliter) (4). Studies performed at the Centers for Disease Control (CDC) have shown that HIV is reduced in concentration by 1–2 logs (90–99%) within several hours when allowed to dry (21). Instruments, devices, or other items contaminated with blood or other body fluids from persons infected with HIV may be disinfected and sterilized according to standard procedures (21).

J. I. Tokars and W. J. Martone: Hospital Infections Program, Center for Infectious Diseases, Centers for Disease Control, Atlanta, Georgia 30333.

Critical, Semicritical, and Noncritical Items

The rationale for cleaning, disinfection, and sterilization can be more readily understood if medical devices, equipment, and surgical materials are divided into three general categories: critical items (e.g., surgical instruments, cardiac catheters, and implants), which are introduced directly into the bloodstream or into normally sterile areas of the body; semicritical items (e.g., flexible and rigid fiberoptic endoscopes, endotracheal tubes, anesthesia breathing circuits, and cystoscopes), which come in contact with intact mucous membranes but do not ordinarily penetrate body surfaces; and noncritical items (e.g., crutches, bedboards, and blood pressure cuffs), which do not ordinarily touch the patient or touch only intact skin (37).

Disinfection and Sterilization

Disinfection and sterilization procedures for critical, semicritical, and noncritical items and for environmental surfaces are presented in the CDC Guideline for Handwashing and Hospital Environmental Control, 1985, and are summarized in Table 1 (37). It is important that all items and surfaces be cleaned to remove debris prior to disinfection or sterilization.

Chemical germicides classified as sterilants or disinfectants are regulated and registered by the Environmental Protection Agency (EPA) (38). The EPA requires testing under specific and standardized protocols of chemical germicides formulated as general disinfectants, hospital disinfectants, and disinfectants applied to other environments (38). EPA-registered tuberculocidal "hospital grade" disinfectants will inactivate HIV. The EPA has also approved a standard testing protocol that allows manufacturers to claim that a product inactivates HIV specifically. When using chemical germicides, the manufacturer's instructions for use, length of treatment, and specifications for compatibility of the medical device with chemical germicides should be followed. Information on specific label claims of commercial germicides can be obtained by writing to the Disinfectants Branch, Office of Pesticides, Environmental Protection Agency, 401 M Street, S.W., Washington, DC 20460.

Cleaning and Decontaminating of Spills of Blood and Body Fluids

When spills of blood or body fluids occur in the patient-care setting, visible material should first be removed and then the area disinfected. With large spills of cultured or concentrated infectious agents in the laboratory, the contaminated area should be flooded with a liquid germicide before cleaning, then disinfected with fresh germicidal chemical. In both patient-care and laboratory settings, gloves should be worn during the cleaning and decontaminating procedures. Disinfection can be accomplished with chemical germicides that are approved for use as "hospital disinfectants" and are tuberculocidal when used at recommended dilutions, or with a 1:100 solution of household bleach (21,37).

Housekeeping

Environmental surfaces such as walls and floors are not associated with transmission of infections to patients or health-care workers. Therefore extraordinary efforts to disinfect or sterilize these environmental surfaces are not necessary. However, cleaning and removal of soil should be done routinely. Disinfectant-detergent formulations registered by the EPA can be used for cleaning environmental surfaces, but the actual physical removal of microorganisms by scrubbing is probably at least as important as any antimicrobial effect of the cleaning agent used. Therefore cost, safety, and acceptability by housekeepers can be the main criteria for selecting any such registered agent. The manufacturers' instructions for appropriate use should be followed (21,37).

Laundry

Although soiled linen is a source of large numbers of certain pathogenic microorganisms, the risk of actual disease transmission is negligible. Rather than rigid procedures and specifications, hygienic and common-sense storage and processing of clean and soiled linen are recommended. Soiled linen should be handled as little as possible and with minimum agitation to prevent gross microbial contamination of the air and of persons handling the linen. All soiled linen should be bagged at the location where it was used. Linen soiled with blood or body fluids should be placed and transported in bags that prevent leakage (21).

Infective Waste

No epidemiologic evidence suggests that most hospital waste is any more infective than residential waste or that improper disposal of hospital waste has caused disease in the community. However, it appears prudent to take special precautions in disposal of blood specimens or blood products and waste from microbiology and pathology laboratories. Such waste should either be incinerated or autoclaved before disposal in a sanitary landfill. Bulk blood, suctioned fluids, excretions, and secretions may be carefully poured down a drain connected to a sanitary sewer. Sanitary sewers may also be used to dispose of other infectious wastes capable of being ground and

TABLE 1. *Disinfection and sterilization procedures*[a]

Sterilization

Destroys: All forms of microbial life, including high numbers of bacterial spores.
Methods: Steam under pressure (autoclave), gas (ethylene oxide), dry heat or immersion in EPA-approved chemical "sterilant"[b] for prolonged period of time (e.g., 6–10 hr) or according to manufacturers' instructions. *Note:* Liquid chemical "sterilants" should be used *only* on those instruments that are impossible to sterilize or disinfect with heat. After use and before sterilization, surgical instruments should be decontaminated with a chemical germicide rather than just rinsed with water.
Use: Critical items.[c] Disposable invasive equipment eliminates the need to reprocess critical items.

High-level disinfection

Destroys: All forms of microbial life *except* high numbers of bacterial spores.
Methods: Hot-water pasteurization (80–100°C, 30 min) or exposure to an EPA-registered "sterilant"[b] chemical as above, except for a short exposure time (10–45 min or as directed by the manufacturer).
Use: Semicritical items.[c]

Intermediate-level disinfection

Destroys: *Mycobacterium tuberculosis,* vegetative bacteria, most viruses (including hepatitis B and HIV), and most fungi; does *not* kill bacterial spores.
Methods: EPA-registered "hospital disinfectant"[b] chemical germicides that have a label claim for tuberculocidal activity; commercially available hard-surface germicides or solutions containing at least 500 ppm free available chlorine (a 1:100 dilution of common household bleach—approximately $\frac{1}{4}$ cup bleach per gallon of tap water).
Use: Noncritical[c] items that have been visibly contaminated with blood.

Low-level disinfection

Destroys: Most bacteria, some viruses, some fungi, but *not Mycobacterium tuberculosis* or bacterial spores.
Methods: EPA-registered "hospital disinfectants"[b] *without* a label claim for tuberculocidal activity.
Use: Noncritical[c] items or surfaces *without* visible blood contamination.

Environmental disinfection

Methods: Any cleaner or disinfectant agent that is intended for environmental use.
Use: Environmental surfaces such as floors, woodwork, and countertops that have become soiled but *not* contaminated with visible blood.

[a] *Important:* To ensure the effectiveness of any sterilization or disinfection process, items and surfaces must first be cleaned of all visible soil.
[b] The manufacturer's instructions for use, length of treatment, and specifications for compatibility of the medical device with chemical germicides should be followed.
[c] See text for definition of critical, semicritical, and noncritical items.

flushed into the sewer (21,37). In all cases, appropriate local and state regulations should be followed.

Sharp items should be considered as potentially infectious and should be handled and disposed of with extraordinary care to prevent accidental injuries (see Prevention of Percutaneous Injury below).

UNIVERSAL PRECAUTIONS

In 1987, CDC developed the strategy of "universal blood and body fluid precautions" to address concerns regarding transmission of HIV in the health-care setting (21). This concept, now referred to simply as universal precautions, stresses that *all patients should be assumed to be infectious for HIV and other bloodborne pathogens.* Such an approach is necessary because patients with bloodborne infection cannot always be identified by history, physical examination, or readily available laboratory tests (21,22). Implementation of universal precautions for all patients eliminates the need for use of the isolation category "Blood and Body Fluid Precautions" previously recommended by CDC (21). The basic components of universal precautions are (a) barrier precautions to prevent contact with blood and infectious fluids, (b) handwashing, and (c) prevention of percutaneous injuries (e.g., needlesticks, cuts from sharp objects). Hepatitis B vaccination is also stressed as an important measure in prevention of bloodborne disease.

Fluids to Which Universal Precautions Apply

Universal precautions apply to (a) blood, which is the single most important source of HIV, hepatitis B, and other bloodborne pathogens in the occupational setting; (b) visibly bloody fluids; (c) semen and vaginal secretions, which have been implicated in the sexual (but not occupational) transmission of hepatitis B and HIV; (d) fluids for which the risk of transmission of hepatitis B and HIV is undetermined, including amniotic, pericardial, peritoneal, pleural, synovial, and cerebrospinal fluids; (e) laboratory specimens that contain hepatitis B or HIV (e.g., suspensions of concentrated virus); and (f) saliva in the dental setting, where contamination with blood is likely. Universal precautions do not apply to feces, nasal secretions, sputum, sweat, tears, urine, and vomitus, since these fluids have not been associated with transmission of hepatitis B or HIV (21,22,29).

Saliva positive for hepatitis B surface antigen (HBsAg) has been shown to be infectious when injected into experimental animals and in human bite exposures, but not through contamination of musical instruments or cardioresuscitation dummies used by hepatitis B carriers (39–43). In addition, epidemiologic studies of nonsexual household contacts of HIV-infected patients, including several small series in which HIV transmission failed to occur after bites or after percutaneous inoculation or contamination of cuts and open wounds with saliva, suggest that the potential for salivary transmission of HIV is remote (1,17,19,20,28). A case of possible HIV transmission after a human bite has been reported. However, the bite did not break the skin or result in bleeding and the date of seroconversion is unknown, so the role of the bite and of saliva in transmission is unclear (44). Universal precautions do not apply to saliva, except in the dental setting, where saliva is predictably contaminated with blood (29).

Barrier Precautions

Barrier precautions, such as gloves, masks, protective eyewear, and gowns, should be used to protect the health-care worker's skin and mucous membranes from contact with fluids to which universal precautions apply. Barrier precautions appropriate to the situation should be employed whenever such contact is anticipated (21).

Gloves should be worn when touching (a) blood and other fluids to which universal precautions apply, (b) items or surfaces contaminated with such fluids, (c) a patient's mucous membrane, or (d) a patient's body tissues. Gloves should be changed and hands washed after contact with each patient (21).

Medical gloves include those marketed as sterile surgical or nonsterile examination gloves made of vinyl or latex (29). There have been conflicting reports that latex gloves are superior to vinyl gloves in integrity and ability to exclude virus (45–48). It is unknown whether such differences, if substantiated, would be of practical importance as long as the glove is intact during use. Thus the type of gloves selected should be appropriate for the task being performed. Medical gloves should be discarded after use and not be washed or disinfected for reuse, because washing with surfactants may cause enhanced penetration of liquids through undetected holes in the gloves ("wicking"), and disinfecting agents may cause deterioration (29).

During phlebotomy, gloves reduce the chance of blood contact with skin but cannot prevent penetrating injuries such as needlesticks. Gloves should be made available to health-care workers performing phlebotomy and should be used if the health-care worker has breaks in his/her skin, is performing a finger or heel stick on an infant or child, is being trained in phlebotomy, or is working in other situations where the worker judges that hand contamination may occur. In other circumstances, the decision on glove use during phlebotomy should be based on (a) the prevalence of infection with bloodborne pathogens in the patient population, (b) the skill and technique of the worker, (c) the frequency with which the worker performs phlebotomy, and (d) any circumstances of the phlebotomy that may increase the risk of hand contamination, such as phlebotomy on an uncooperative patient or in an emergency situation (29).

Masks and protective eyewear or face shields should be worn during procedures (i.e., endotracheal intubation, bronchoscopy, and endoscopy) that are likely to generate splashes of blood or fluids to which universal precautions apply, and during many common dental procedures. Precautions during other procedures should be determined on an individual basis. Gowns or aprons should be worn during procedures that are likely to generate splashes of blood or other potentially infective sources (21).

Efficacy of Universal Precautions

Use of universal precautions has been shown to reduce the number of blood contacts. After implementation of universal precautions, the mean number of contacts with blood or body fluids decreased from 5.07 to 2.66 exposures per month among physicians at two acute-care hospitals, and from 35.8 to 18.1 per year among workers at the Clinical Center, National Institutes of Health (49,50). A study in emergency rooms revealed that use of gloves was associated with a reduction in the adjusted blood contact rate from 11.2 to 1.3 per 100 procedures (51).

Handwashing

Handwashing is the single most important procedure for preventing nosocomial infections (37). Universal precautions dictate that hands and other skin surfaces should be washed immediately and thoroughly if contaminated with blood or other body fluids to which universal precautions apply (21).

For general infection control purposes, hands should be washed (a) after taking care of a patient(s), even if gloves are used; (b) after touching excretions (i.e., feces and urine) or secretions (e.g., from wounds or skin infections) and before touching any patient again; (c) after touching materials soiled with excretions or secretions; (d) before performing invasive procedures, touching wounds, or touching immunocompromised patients; and (e) immediately after gloves are removed, even if the gloves appear to be intact (37). When handwashing facilities are not available, a waterless antiseptic hand cleanser may be used according to the manufacturer's recommendations (22).

Prevention of Percutaneous Injury

Among occupational exposures, percutaneous injuries, such as needlesticks and cuts from sharp instruments and objects, have been most frequently implicated in occupational transmission of bloodborne pathogens (22,26,27). Precautions to prevent such injuries must therefore be implemented by all health-care workers during procedures, when cleaning used instruments, during disposal of used needles, and when handling sharp instruments after procedures. To prevent needlestick injuries, needles should not be recapped, purposely bent or broken by hand, removed from disposable syringes, or otherwise manipulated by hand. After they are used, disposable syringes and needles, scalpel blades, and other sharp items should be placed in puncture-resistant containers for disposal; the puncture-resistant containers should be located as close as practical to the use area. Large-bore reusable needles should be placed in a puncture-resistant container for transport to the reprocessing area (21).

A study at a university hospital revealed that one-third of all needlesticks were related to recapping and that devices requiring disassembly had the highest rates of injury, suggesting the need for continued education of health-care workers as well as for development of devices providing for safer covering of contaminated sharps (e.g., self-sheathing needles) and disassembling of devices (52–54).

Resuscitation Equipment

Although saliva has not been implicated in HIV transmission, the need for mouth-to-mouth resuscitation should be minimized by placing mouthpieces, resuscitation bags, or other ventilation devices in areas where the need for resuscitation is predictable (21).

Health-Care Workers with Nonintact Skin

Health-care workers with exudative lesions or weeping dermatitis should refrain from all direct patient care and from handling patient-care equipment until the condition resolves (21).

Serologic Testing

For the medical benefit of the patients, routine voluntary HIV counseling and testing should be considered in hospitalized patients in age groups deemed to have a high prevalence of HIV infection (55). The utility of routine HIV serologic testing of patients as an infection control measure to protect health-care workers is unknown; drawbacks include the unavailability of results in some emergency or outpatient settings and the inability to detect HIV antibody in some recently infected patients (21). In addition, it is uncertain whether health-care workers who are using universal precautions can further reduce their risk of exposure to blood and body fluids even if they know that a patient is HIV-infected.

Personnel in some hospitals have advocated serologic testing of patients in settings in which exposure of health-care workers to large amounts of patients' blood may be anticipated. Specific patients for whom serologic testing has been advocated include those undergoing major operative procedures and those undergoing treatment in critical-care units, especially if they have conditions involving uncontrolled bleeding. Decisions regarding the need to establish testing programs for patients should be made by physicians or individual institutions. In addition, when deemed appropriate, testing of individual patients may be performed on agreement between the patient and the physician providing care (21).

In addition to the universal precautions recommended for all patients, certain additional precautions during the care of HIV-infected patients undergoing major surgical operations have been proposed by personnel in some hospitals. For example, surgical procedures on an HIV-infected patient might be altered so that hand-to-hand passing of sharp instruments would be eliminated; stapling instruments rather than hand-suturing equipment might be used to perform tissue approximation; electrocautery devices rather than scalpels might be used as cutting instruments; and, even though uncomfortable, gowns that totally prevent seepage of blood onto the skin of members of the operative team might be worn. While such modifications might further minimize the risk of HIV infection for members of the operative team, some of these techniques could result in prolongation of operative time and could potentially have an adverse effect on the patient (21). Observational studies done in operating rooms to date have not demonstrated that fewer blood exposures occur during surgical procedures performed on patients known to be HIV seropositive (56–58).

Testing programs, if developed, should include the following: (a) obtaining consent for testing; (b) informing patients of test results, and providing counseling for seropositive patients by properly trained persons; (c) assuring that confidentiality safeguards are in place to limit knowledge of test results to those directly involved in the care of infected patients or as required by law; (d) assuring that identification of infected patients will not result in denial of needed care or in provision of suboptimal care; (e) and evaluating prospectively (i) the efficacy of the program in reducing the incidence of parenteral, mucous membrane, or significant cutaneous exposures of health-care workers to the blood or other body fluids of HIV-infected patients and (ii) the effect of modified procedures on patients (21). In all cases, local and state regulations regarding confidentiality and reporting of HIV test results and patient-care information should be observed.

Among 561 hospitals responding to a survey in 1989, 83% had formal written policies about HIV testing. Among hospitals with written policies, 78% required pretest informed consent and 75% required that seropositive patients be informed of their result; 56% required that test results appear in patient records, and 38% required a review of treatment plans for patients with positive HIV test results (59).

In a voluntary HIV screening program at a large private hospital, 51% of 8868 admitted patients not previously known to be HIV-infected consented to HIV screening (60). Twelve seropositive patients were found (seroprevalence rate 0.26%), 10 of whom were known to

be in a high-risk group at the time of admission. The authors concluded that although the testing program may have benefited patients, there was no evidence that it reduced the risk of nosocomial HIV transmission. The potential efficacy of screening programs as an infection control measure might depend in part on the HIV seroprevalence among hospital inpatients not known to be HIV positive, which is highly variable among hospitals (61,62).

The Role of the Occupational Safety and Health Administration

CDC recommendations for universal precautions are guidelines that should be interpreted according to local policies and needs. Statutory authority to regulate health-care facilities and other workplaces to protect the health of workers rests with the Occupational Safety and Health Administration (OSHA) (63). OSHA is in the process of developing regulations, termed a "standard," regarding protection of health-care workers from occupational exposure to bloodborne pathogens (64). A proposed OSHA standard, based in part on OSHA's interpretation of available CDC guidelines, has been published (65). Until this standard is finalized, OSHA has elected to interpret certain CDC guidelines (including provisions of universal precautions) as enforceable under existing regulations and the "general duty clause" of the Occupational Safety and Health Act, which requires employers to provide a workplace "free from recognized hazards that are causing or are likely to cause death or serious physical harm" (66). A compliance instruction, including OSHA's interpretation of existing CDC guidelines, has been sent to all OSHA field inspectors (67).

Department of Labor and Department of Health and Human Services Joint Advisory Notice

Detailed recommendations for employer responsibilities in protecting workers from acquisition of bloodborne disease in the workplace have been published in the Department of Labor and Department of Health and Human Services Joint Advisory Notice (68). General responsibilities can be summarized as a series of steps:

1. Work activities should be categorized as Class I (direct contact with blood or other fluids to which universal precautions apply); Class II (activity performed without blood exposure but exposure may occur in emergency); or Class III (task/activity does not entail predictable or unpredictable exposure to blood). Personal protective equipment should be available for

Class I or II activities and should always be worn for Class I activities.

2. Standard operating procedures for all activities having the potential for exposure should be developed. These procedures should incorporate universal precautions, as well as recommended methods for disinfection, decontamination, and disposal of infective waste.
3. Initial and periodic worker education programs should be provided to potentially exposed workers.
4. Procedures to ensure and monitor compliance with standard operating procedures should be implemented.
5. The employer should, whenever possible, identify devices and other approaches to modify the work environment in ways that will reduce exposure risk (22,68).

In addition to these general responsibilities, the employer has the specific responsibility to make available to the worker a program of medical management, including hepatitis B vaccination, management of occupational exposures to blood and body fluids, documentation of exposures and reporting in accordance with state and federal laws, and management of hepatitis B- or HIV-infected workers (22,68). The Public Health Service has provided guidelines on management of occupational HIV exposures, including considerations regarding zidovudine postexposure use (69).

Blood or Tissue Aerosols

Aerosols are inspirable airborne particles less than approximately 100 μm in diameter and should be distinguished from larger, noninspirable droplets or spatter. Aerosols are not known to present a risk of transmission of HIV, hepatitis B virus, or other bloodborne pathogens in the health-care setting. In studies conducted in dental operatories and hemodialysis centers, hepatitis B virus could not be detected in the air during the treatment of infected patients, including during procedures known to generate aerosols (70–72). This suggests that detection of HIV in aerosols in clinical settings would also be uncommon, since the concentration of HIV in blood is generally lower than that of hepatitis B virus (4). Detection of HIV in an artificially produced aerosol in a laboratory experiment would not necessarily mean that HIV-containing aerosols are produced in clinical settings or that HIV is transmissible by aerosol in a clinical setting (73). CDC is sponsoring research to assess the potential for aerosolization of blood and tissue during various surgical procedures and the possible resulting hazards to surgical personnel. At this time, however, the possibility that HIV may be transmitted via aerosolized blood remains theoretical.

Body Substance Isolation

An alternate system of infection control in the health-care setting, body substance isolation, has been proposed (74). Unlike universal precautions, which apply only to fluids that may transmit HIV and certain other bloodborne pathogens, body substance isolation includes precautions to prevent contact with all body substances, including blood, secretions, and other moist body substances (feces, urine, sputum, saliva, wound drainage, and other body fluids) (63,74). Gloves and other barrier precautions are used for anticipated contact with any of these body substances, or with mucous membranes or nonintact skin. Hands are washed only when visibly soiled. Additional measures, such as private rooms, are used for patients with infections transmitted by the airborne route (74).

The fact that handwashing is not routinely required when gloves are changed between patients is a theoretical disadvantage of body substance isolation (75). Only a few reports have addressed the efficacy of body substance isolation, and this issue requires further study (76–78).

PRECAUTIONS FOR INFECTIOUS DISEASES OCCURRING WITH HIGH FREQUENCY IN HIV-INFECTED PATIENTS

Universal precautions, which should be followed during care of all patients, are designed to prevent transmission of bloodborne pathogens. When patients are known or suspected to be infected with pathogens transmitted by other than the bloodborne route, additional precautions should be followed. CDC guidelines provide two alternate approaches for such precautions: (a) disease-specific guidelines, which are designed to prevent transmission of specific diseases (e.g., salmonellosis and pertussis), and (b) category-specific guidelines, which can be used for groups of diseases with similar modes of transmission (e.g., enteric and respiratory diseases)(30).

Table 2 lists category-specific isolation precautions for many microorganisms that commonly infect AIDS patients. Appropriate precautions will prevent transmission of these microorganisms in health-care settings. Detailed instructions for both disease-specific and category-specific precautions are outlined in the "CDC Guideline for Isolation Precautions in Hospitals" (30).

Private Versus Multiple-Bed Rooms for HIV-Infected Patients

A private room is not necessary for patients infected with HIV unless the patient's hygiene is poor or the pres-

TABLE 2. *Category-specific isolation precautions for microorganisms causing opportunistic infections in patients with AIDS*

Microorganism	Syndrome	Precautions
Bacteria		
Mycobacteria, nontuberculous (atypical)	Pulmonary	None
	Wound	Drainage/secretion
Mycobacterium tuberculosis	Extrapulmonary, draining lesion	Drainage/secretion
	Extrapulmonary, meningitis	None
	Pulmonary	Tuberculosis
Nocardia asteroides	Draining lesions	None
	Other	None
Salmonella species	Gastroenteritis	Enteric
	Bacteremia	Enteric[a]
Listeria monocytogenes	Infection at any site	None
Legionella species	Pneumonias, cellulitis	None
Streptococcus pneumoniae	Pneumonia	None
Haemophilus influenzae	Adults	None
	Infant/children	Respiratory
Staphylococcus aureus	Skin, wound, or burn infection	
	Major	Contact
	Minor or limited	Drainage/secretion
	Pneumonia or draining lung abscess	Contact
Shigella species	Gastroenteritis	Enteric
	Bacteremia	Enteric[a]
Viruses		
Cytomegalovirus	Infection at any site	Pregnant personnel may need special counseling
Herpes simplex	Encephalitis	None
	Mucocutaneous, disseminated or primary, severe (skin, oral, and genital)	Contact
	Mucocutaneous, recurrent (skin, oral, and genital)	Drainage/secretion
Herpes zoster (varicella zoster)	Localized in immunocompromised patient, or disseminated	Strict
Epstein-Barr	Infectious mononucleosis	None
Adenoviruses	Respiratory infection in infants and young children	Contact
Parasites		
Pneumocystis carinii	Pneumonia	None
Toxoplasma gondii	Encephalitis, brain abscess	None
Cryptosporidium species	Gastroenteritis	Enteric
Fungi		
Candida species	Infection at any site, including mucocutaneous (thrush, moniliasis)	None
Cryptococcus neoformans	Infection at any site	None
Histoplasma capsulatum	Infection at any site	None
Aspergillus species	Infection at any site	None

[a] Unless stool culture negative.

ence of other infections makes a private room necessary (e.g., infection with *Mycobacterium tuberculosis*). However, if HIV-infected patients or other immunosuppressed patients are placed in the same room, cross-infection with opportunistic pathogens may occur. If intensive care unit (ICU) care is required, HIV-infected patients without infections requiring a private room may be placed in an open ICU. Otherwise, an isolation room is desirable (30).

Tuberculosis

Transmission of tuberculosis in the health-care setting has been well documented (79,80). Concern about nosocomial transmission of tuberculosis has been heightened by recent outbreaks in health-care settings, including outbreaks involving multidrug-resistant strains of *M. tuberculosis* in HIV-infected patients (81–83).

Nosocomial transmission of tuberculosis is most

likely to occur from patients with unrecognized pulmonary or laryngeal tuberculosis who are not on effective antituberculous therapy and have not been placed in tuberculous (acid-fast bacilli [AFB]) isolation. Recognition of tuberculosis in HIV-infected persons may be delayed because of impaired response to tuberculin skin testing, atypical clinical or radiographic presentations, simultaneous occurrence of other pulmonary infections, low sensitivity of sputum smears for detecting AFB, and overgrowth of cultures with *Mycobacterium avium* complex among patients with dual infections (83).

The prevention of tuberculosis transmission in health-care settings is based on the following principles; when inadequate attention is given to any of these principles, the probability of tuberculosis transmission increases (83).

1. Generation of infectious airborne particles (droplet nuclei) should be prevented by early identification and treatment of persons with tuberculosis infection and active tuberculosis.
2. Spread of infectious droplet nuclei into the general air circulation should be prevented by applying source-control methods. In hospitals and other inpatient facilities, any patient known or suspected to have infectious tuberculosis should be placed in AFB isolation in a private room. Recommendations for ventilation of rooms used for AFB isolation have been published (84,85). Infectious patients should cover all coughs and sneezes with a tissue. Booths should be used for sputum induction or administration of aerosolized medications (e.g., aerosolized pentamidine).
3. When air is contaminated with infectious droplet nuclei, the number of such nuclei should be reduced by ventilation. Ventilation standards for indoor air quality have been published (84,85). Ventilation may be supplemented by other approaches, such as use of high-efficiency particulate air (HEPA) filtration or germicidal ultraviolet irradiation.
4. To protect both health-care workers and patients, each health-care facility should conduct surveillance for tuberculosis and tuberculosis infection.

Cytomegalovirus

Many patients with AIDS are infected with and excrete cytomegalovirus (CMV)(86). Although CMV has been found in nearly all body fluids and secretions, transmission usually results only from close intimate contact. In health-care facilities, transmission has been documented to occur from patient to patient, but not from patient to health-care worker (87,88). A practical approach to reducing the risk of infection with CMV among health-care workers is to stress careful handwashing after all patient contacts and to avoid contact with materials that are potentially infective. Because of risk to the fetus, all pregnant patient-care personnel should at least be counseled about precautions for preventing acquisition of CMV (30). Other measures, such as serologic screening of pregnant personnel, with reassignment of those susceptible, are controversial (89).

Pneumocystis carinii

Pneumocystis carinii is usually thought to be ubiquitous, and CDC guidelines do not recommend isolation of patients infected with this organism (30,90). However, clusters of *Pneumocystis carinii* infection have been noted in immunosuppressed persons, and a cluster in elderly immunocompetent patients has recently been reported (91–93). Such reports have led some authors to recommend isolation of patients infected with this organism (90–92).

PRECAUTIONS FOR SPECIFIC SETTINGS

Dental and Oral Surgical Procedures

Most microorganisms known to be human pathogens have been isolated from oral secretions (94). General infection-control precautions and disinfection and sterilization procedures for dentistry have been described (95).

Blood, saliva, and gingival fluid from all dental patients should be considered potential sources of blood-borne pathogens requiring universal precautions. In addition to wearing gloves for contact with oral mucous membranes of all patients, dental workers should wear surgical masks and protective eyewear or chin-length plastic face-shields during procedures in which splashing or splattering of blood, saliva, or gingival fluids is likely. Rubber dams, high-speed evacuation, and proper patient positioning, when appropriate, should be used to minimize generation of droplets and spatter (21).

Hemodialysis and Peritoneal Dialysis

Patients infected with HIV may occasionally require hemodialysis or peritoneal dialysis. An HIV serosurvey among hemodialysis patients at 28 dialysis centers found that 0.98% (13/1328) were HIV-infected (96). HIV-infected patients can be dialyzed in hospital-based or free-standing dialysis units using conventional infection-control precautions (97). Universal precautions should be used when dialyzing all patients. Procedures for disinfecting the fluid pathways of the hemodialysis machine are targeted to control bacterial contamination and need not be changed for dialyzing patients infected with HIV (21).

When HIV-infected patients receive peritoneal dialysis, peritoneal dialysis bags and other disposable items can be disposed of in the same fashion as other solid waste (37). Bags containing peritoneal dialysis fluid should be handled with care, but extraordinary precautions are not needed. Disposable gloves should be worn when handling bags containing peritoneal dialysis fluid. In the home environment, the peritoneal dialysis fluid can be carefully poured down a toilet. The empty bag should be wrapped securely in an impervious plastic bag or double bagged and discarded in the conventional trash system.

Surgical Procedures

Surgical personnel should routinely use barrier precautions, such as gloves, masks, and gowns or aprons; protective eyewear or face shields should be used during procedures likely to cause splashes or droplets of blood and body fluids, or to generate bone chips (21). Observational studies have reported percutaneous injuries such as needlesticks and cuts during 1.3–6.9% of surgical procedures, and blood contacts of any type (percutaneous injuries, blood–skin contacts, and blood–mucous membrane contacts) during 6.4–46.6% of procedures (56–58). Because many blood contacts are caused by perforations in surgical gloves, use of two pairs of gloves ("double-gloving") has been suggested (58). Use of instruments, such as a forceps, to manipulate suture needles may help minimize the number of percutaneous injuries during surgery (57). Careful adherence to guidelines will help to minimize blood contacts during surgery, but innovative approaches to this problem may also be required.

Laboratories

Universal precautions should be observed when handling specimens of blood, other fluids to which universal precautions apply, and tissues from all patients. Specimens should be placed in secure containers for transport. Laboratory workers processing blood and body fluid specimens should wear gloves, and a mask and protective eyewear should be worn if generation of droplets or splashes is likely. Mouth pipetting should not be done, and use of needles and syringes should be limited to situations in which there is no alternative. After completion of laboratory activities, protective clothing should be removed and hands washed (21).

Postmortem Care

Universal precautions should be followed during postmortem procedures on all patients. In addition, gloves, masks, protective eyewear, gowns, and waterproof aprons should be worn, and instruments and surfaces that become contaminated during the procedure should be disinfected with an appropriate chemical germicide (21).

OTHER INFECTION CONTROL CONSIDERATIONS

Pregnant Health-Care Workers

Pregnant health-care workers are not known to be at greater risk of contracting HIV infection than health-care workers who are not pregnant; however, if a health-care worker develops HIV infection during pregnancy, the infant is at risk of infection from perinatal transmission. Therefore pregnant health-care workers should be especially familiar with and strictly adhere to precautions to minimize the risk of HIV transmission (21).

Immunosuppressed Health-Care Workers

Health-care workers with defective immune systems are not known to be at greater risk of acquiring HIV infection than workers with normal immune systems. However, they may have an increased risk of acquiring or experiencing serious complications from other infectious diseases. Of particular concern is the risk of severe infection following exposure to patients infected with HIV who may be infected with microorganisms that are easily transmitted if appropriate precautions are not adhered to (e.g., *M. tuberculosis*). Health-care workers with defective immune systems should be counseled about the potential risk associated with taking care of patients with transmissible infections and should follow existing recommendations for infection control to minimize their risk of exposure to other infectious agents (98,99).

Blood and Blood Products

The risk of acquiring HIV infection from transfusion of blood and blood products has been significantly reduced by voluntary deferral of blood donation by those with HIV risk factors and screening of donated blood for HIV since 1985 (100). The risk from screened blood has been estimated by statistical models to be 1:38,000–1:153,000 per unit, and by prospective studies to be approximately 1:36,000–1:42,000 per unit (100–104).

Strategies that have been suggested to minimize the risk include increased use of blood from female donors, use of blood from a smaller group of donors who make frequent donations and consequently have been repeatedly tested for HIV, transfusion of fewer units, and, in any one patient, use of blood from as small a number of donors as possible (100,105).

Factor concentrates that have been heat-treated or otherwise treated to reduce the risk of transmission of infectious agents are available for treatment of persons with hemophilia. Instances of HIV seroconversion associated with the use of heat-treated products are now rare; the rate of HIV seroconversion among those using such products appears to be less than 1 per 1000 persons per year (106,107).

Two types of hepatitis B vaccines are licensed in the United States: recombinant vaccine produced in yeast cultures and vaccine derived from human plasma. Although plasma-derived vaccines have not been associated with disease transmission, they are no longer produced in the United States, and their use is now limited to hemodialysis patients, other immunocompromised hosts, and persons with known allergy to yeast (69,108–112).

Transmission of HIV has not been associated with use of immune globulin preparations (108,109,113).

CONCLUSION

Health-care institutions should develop educational programs regarding the epidemiology of HIV and precautions recommended to prevent transmission of bloodborne infection. Universal precautions, a set of precautions to prevent transmission of HIV and other bloodborne pathogens, should be followed during care of all patients. Additional disease-specific or category-specific precautions should be used if patients have infectious diseases transmitted by nonbloodborne routes. Adherence to routine procedures for disinfection, sterilization, and environmental hygiene is adequate during care of persons with HIV infection.

ACKNOWLEDGMENTS

We gratefully acknowledge the assistance of David M. Bell, M.D., Mary E. Chamberland, M.D., M.P.H., Martin S. Favero, Ph.D., and Julie Garner, R.N., M.S., Hospital Infections Program, Center for Infectious Diseases, CDC, in preparation of this chapter.

REFERENCES

1. Curran JW, Jaffe HW, Hardy AM, Morgan WM, Selik RM, Dondero TJ. Epidemiology of HIV infection and AIDS in the United States. *Science* 1988;239:610–6.
2. Oxtoby MJ. Human immunodeficiency virus and other viruses in human milk: placing the issues in broader perspective. *Pediatr Infect Dis J* 1988;7:825–35.
3. Barre-Sinoussi F, Chermann JC, Rey F, et al. Isolation of a T-lymphotrophic retrovirus from a patient at risk for acquired immune deficiency syndrome (AIDS). *Science* 1983;220:868–71.
4. Ho DD, Moudgil T, Alam M. Quantitation of human immunodeficiency virus type 1 in the blood of infected persons. *N Engl J Med* 1989;321:1621–5.
5. Zagury D, Bernard J, Leibowitch J, et al. HTLV-III in cells cultured from semen of two patients with AIDS. *Science* 1984;226:449–51.
6. Vogt MW, Witt DJ, Craven DE, et al. Isolation of HTLV-III/LAV from cervical secretions of women at risk for AIDS. *Lancet* 1986;1:525–7.
7. Wofsy CB, Cohen JB, Hauer LB, et al. Isolation of AIDS-associated retrovirus from genital secretions of women with antibodies to the virus. *Lancet* 1986;1:527–9.
8. Ho DD, Byington RE, Schooley RT, et al. Infrequency of isolation of HTLV-III virus from saliva in AIDS [letter]. *N Engl J Med* 1985;313:1606.
9. Thiry L, Sprecher-Goldberger S, Jonckheer T, et al. Isolation of AIDS virus from cell-free breast milk of three healthy virus carriers [letter]. *Lancet* 1985;2:891–2.
10. Levy JA, Kaminshy LS, Morrow WJW, et al. Infection by the retrovirus associated with the acquired immunodeficiency syndrome. Clinical, biological, and molecular features. *Ann Intern Med* 1985;103:694–9.
11. Fujikawa LS, Salahuddin SZ, Palestine AG, et al. Isolation of human T-lymphotropic virus type III from the tears of a patient with the acquired immunodeficiency syndrome. *Lancet* 1985;2:529–30.
12. Ho DD, Rota TR, Schooley RT, et al. Isolation of HTLV-III from cerebrospinal fluid and neural tissues of patients with neurologic syndromes related to the acquired immunodeficiency syndrome. *N Engl J Med* 1985;313:1493–7.
13. Levy JA, Shimabukuro J, Hollander H, et al. Isolation of AIDS associated retrovirus from cerebrospinal fluid and brain of patients with neurological symptoms. *Lancet* 1985;2:586–8.
14. Ziza JM, Brun-Vezinet F, Venet A, et al. Lymphadenopathy-associated virus isolated from bronchoalveolar lavage fluid in AIDS-related complex with lymphoid interstitial pneumonitis [letter]. *N Engl J Med* 1985;313:183.
15. Mundy DC, Schinazi RF, Gerber AR, et al. Human immunodeficiency virus isolated from amniotic fluid. *Lancet* 1987;2:459–60.
16. Groopman JE, Salahuddin SZ, Sarngadharan MG, et al. HTLV-III in saliva of people with AIDS-related complex and healthy homosexual men at risk for AIDS. *Science* 1984;226:447–9.
17. Lifson AR. Do alternate modes for transmission of human immunodeficiency virus exist? *JAMA* 1988;259:1353–6.
18. Gershon RM, Vlahov D, Nelson KE. The risk of transmission of HIV-1 through non-percutaneous, non-sexual modes—a review. *AIDS* 1990;4:645–50.
19. Friedland GH, Saltzman BR, Rogers MF. Lack of transmission of HTLV-III/LAV infection to household contacts of patients with AIDS or AIDS-related complex with oral candidiasis. *N Engl J Med* 1986;314:344–9.
20. Jason JM, McDougal JS, Dixon G, et al. HTLV-III/LAV antibody and immune status of household contacts and sexual partners of persons with hemophilia. *JAMA* 1986;255:212–5.
21. CDC. Recommendations for prevention of HIV transmission in health-care settings. *MMWR* 1987;36(suppl 2S).
22. CDC. Guidelines for prevention of transmission of human immunodeficiency virus and hepatitis B virus to health-care and public-safety workers. *MMWR* 1989;38(2S):95–110.
23. Weiss SH, Goedert JJ, Gartner S, et al. Risk of human immunodeficiency virus (HIV-1) infection among laboratory workers. *Science* 1988;239:68–71.
24. Oksenhendler E, Harzic M, Le Roux JM, Rabian C, Clauvel JP. HIV infection with seroconversion after a superficial needlestick injury to the finger [letter]. *N Engl J Med* 1986;315:582.
25. CDC. Occupationally acquired human immunodeficiency virus

infections in laboratories producing virus concentrates in large quantities: conclusions and recommendations of an expert team convened by the Director of the National Institutes of Health (NIH). *MMWR* 1988;37(S-4):19–22.

26. Marcus R, CDC Cooperative Needlestick Surveillance Group. Surveillance of health care workers exposed to blood from patients infected with the human immunodeficiency virus. *N Engl J Med* 1988;319:1118–23.

27. Henderson DK, Fahey BJ, Willy M, et al. Risk for occupational transmission of human immunodeficiency virus type 1 (HIV-1) associated with clinical exposures. *Ann Intern Med* 1990;113: 740–6.

28. CDC. Update: human immunodeficiency virus infections in health-care workers exposed to blood of infected patients. *MMWR* 1987;36:285–9.

29. CDC. Update: universal precautions for prevention of transmission of human immunodeficiency virus, hepatitis B virus, and other bloodborne pathogens in health-care setting. *MMWR* 1988;37:377–382,387–8.

30. Garner JS, Simmons BP. Guideline for isolation precautions in hospitals. *Infect Control* 1983;4:245–325.

31. Resnick L, Veren K, Salahuddin SZ, Tondrequ S, Markham PD. Stability and inactivation of HTLV-III/LAV under clinical and laboratory environments. *JAMA* 1986;255:1887–91.

32. Martin LS, McDougal JS, Loskoski SL. Disinfection and inactivation of the human T lymphotropic virus type III/lymphadenopathy-associated virus. *J Infect Dis* 1985;152:400–3.

33. Spire B, Barre-Sinousi F, Montagnier L, Chermann JC. Inactivation of lymphadenopathy associated virus by chemical disinfectants. *Lancet* 1984;2:899–901.

34. Hanson PJV, Gor D, Jeffries DJ, Collins JV. Chemical inactivation of HIV on surfaces. *Br Med J* 1989;298:862–4.

35. Prince DL, Prince RN, Prince HN. Inactivation of human immunodeficiency virus type 1 and herpes simplex virus type 2 by commercial hospital disinfectants. *Chemical Times Trends* 1990;13–54.

36. Hanson PJV, Gor D, Jeffries DJ, Collins JV. Elimination of high titre HIV from fibreoptic endoscopes. *Gut* 1990;31:657–9.

37. Garner JS, Favero MS. *Guidelines for handwashing and hospital environmental control, 1985.* Publication No. 99-1117. Atlanta: Centers for Disease Control; 1985.

38. Favero M. Principles of sterilization and disinfection. *Infect Anesth* 1989;7:941–9.

39. Cancio-Bello TP, de Medina M, Shorey J, Valledor MD, Schiff ER. An institutional outbreak of hepatitis B related to a human biting carrier. *J Infect Dis* 1982;146:652–6.

40. MacQuarrie MB, Forghani B, Wolochow DW. Hepatitis B transmitted by a human bite. *JAMA* 1974;230:723–4.

41. Scott RM, Snitbhan R, Bancroft WH, Alter HJ, Tingpalapong M. Experimental transmission of hepatitis B virus by semen and saliva. *J Infect Dis* 1980;142:67–71.

42. Glaser JB, Nadler JP. Hepatitis B virus in a cardiopulmonary resuscitation training course: risk of transmission from a surface antigen-positive participant. *Arch Intern Med* 1985;145:1653–5.

43. Osterholm MT, Bravo ER, Croson JT, et al. Lack of transmission of viral hepatitis type B after oral exposure to HBsAg-positive saliva. *Br Med J* 1979;2:1263–4.

44. Wahn V, Kramer HH, Voit T, Bruster HT, Scrampical B, Scheid A. Horizontal transmission of HIV infection between two siblings [letter]. *Lancet* 1986;2:694.

45. Korniewicz DM, Laughon BE, Butz A, Larson E. Integrity of vinyl and latex procedure gloves. *Nurs Res* 1989;38:144–6.

46. Klein RC, Party E, Gershey EL. Virus penetration of examination gloves. *BioTechniques* 1990;9:196–9.

47. Zbitnew A, Greer K, Heise-Qualtiere J, Conly J. Vinyl versus latex gloves as barriers to transmission of viruses in the health-care setting. *J Acquired Immune Deficiency Syndrome* 1989;2:201–4.

48. Dalgleish AG, Malkovshy M. Surgical gloves as a mechanical barrier against human immunodeficiency viruses. *Br J Surg* 1988;75:171–2.

49. Wong ES, Stotka JL, Chinchilli VM, Williams DS, Stuart CG, Markowitz SM. Are universal precautions effective in reducing the number of occupational exposures among health care workers? *JAMA* 1991;265:1123–8.

50. Fahey BA, Koziol DE, Banks SM, Henderson DK. Frequency of nonparenteral occupational exposures to blood and body fluids before and after universal precautions training. *Am J Med* 1991;90:145–53.

51. Marcus R, Bell DM, Culver DH, Cooperative Emergency Department Study Group. Contact with blood of patients infected with HIV among emergency care providers (ECPs). 6th International Conference on AIDS, San Francisco, June 1990; ThC604(abst).

52. Jagger J, Hunt EH, Brand-Elnaggar J, Pearson RD. Rates of needlestick injury caused by various devices in a university hospital. *N Engl J Med* 1988;319:284–8.

53. Jagger J, Hunt EH, Pearson RD. Sharp object injuries in the hospital: causes and strategies for prevention. *Am J Infect Control* 1990;18:227–31.

54. Jagger J, Hunt EH, Pearson RD. Recapping used needles: is it worse than the alternative? *J Infect Dis* 1990;162:784–5.

55. CDC. Public health service guidelines for counseling and antibody testing to prevent HIV infection and AIDS. *MMWR* 1987;36:509–15.

56. Panlilio AL, Foy DR, Edwards JR, et al. Blood contacts during surgical procedures. *JAMA* 1991;265:1533–7.

57. Tokars JI, Marcus R, Culver DH, Bell DM, Cooperative Study Group. Blood contacts during surgical procedures. 30th Interscience Conference on Antimicrobial Agents and Chemotherapy, Atlanta, GA, Oct 21–24, 1990; Abst 958.

58. Gerberding JL, Littell C, Tarkington A, Brown A, Schecter WP. Risk of exposure of surgical personnel to patients' blood during surgery at San Francisco General Hospital. *N Engl J Med* 1990;322:1788–93.

59. Lewis CE, Montgomery K. The HIV-testing policies of US hospitals. *JAMA* 1990;264:2764–7.

60. Harris RL, Boisaubin EV, Salyer PD, Semands DF. Evaluation of a hospital admission HIV antibody voluntary screening program. *Infect Control Hosp Epidemiol* 1990;11:628–34.

61. St Louis ME, Rauch KJ, Peterson LR, et al. Seroprevalence rates of human immunodeficiency virus infection at sentinel hospitals in the United States. *N Engl J Med* 1990;323:213–8.

62. Gordin FM, Gibert C, Hawley HP, Willoughby A. Prevalence of human immunodeficiency virus and hepatitis B virus in unselected hospital admissions: implications for mandatory testing and universal precautions. *J Infect Dis* 1990;161:14–7.

63. Bell DM. Human immunodeficiency virus infection in health-care workers: occupational risk and prevention. In: Gostin LO, ed. *AIDS and the health care system.* New Haven: Yale University Press; 1990:120.

64. Occupational Safety and Health Administration. Occupational exposure to hepatitis B virus and human immunodeficiency virus; advance notice of proposed rule-making. *Fed Reg* 1987;52:45438–41.

65. Occupational Safety and Health Administration. Occupational exposure to bloodborne pathogens; proposed rule and notice of hearing. *Fed Reg* 1989;54:23042–139.

66. 29 CFR 1910.132. 1910.22 (a)(1) and (a)(2); 1910.141 (a)(4)(i) and (ii); 1910.145 (f); Occupational Safety and Health Act of 1970, Public Law 91-596. Sec 5(a)(1).

67. Occupational Safety and Health Administration. Enforcement procedures for occupational exposure to hepatitis B virus (HBV) and human immunodeficiency virus (HIV). OSHA Instruction CPL 2.244A. Washington, DC, Aug 15, 1988.

68. US Department of Labor, US Department of Health and Human Services. Joint Advisory Notice: protection against occupational exposure to hepatitis B virus (HBV) and human immunodeficiency virus (HIV). *Fed Reg* 1987;52:41818–24.

69. CDC. Public health service statement on management of occupational exposure to human immunodeficiency virus, including considerations regarding zidovudine postexposure use. *MMWR* 1990;39(RR-1).

70. Petersen NJ, Bond WW, Favero MS. Air sampling for hepatitis B surface antigen in a dental operatory. *J Am Dental Assoc* 1979;99:465–7.

71. Petersen NJ, Bond WW, Marshall JH, Favero JS, Raij L. An air

sampling technique for hepatitis B surface antigen. *Health Lab Sci* 1976;13:233-7.

72. Petersen NJ. An assessment of the airborne route in hepatitis B transmission. *Ann NY Acad Sci* 1980;353:157-66.

73. Johnson GK, Robinson WS. Human immunodeficiency virus-1 (HIV-1) in the vapors of surgical power instruments. *J Med Virol* 1990;33:47-50.

74. Lynch P, Jackson MM, Cummings MJ, Stamm WE. Rethinking the role of isolation practices in the prevention of nosocomial infections. *Ann Intern Med* 1987;107:243-6.

75. Garner JS, Hughes JM. Options for isolation precautions. *Ann Intern Med* 1987;107:248-50.

76. Lynch P, Cummings MJ, Roberts PL, Herriott MJ, Yates B, Stamm WE. Implementing and evaluating a system of generic infection precautions: body substance isolation. *Am J Infect Control* 1990;18:1-12.

77. Jackson MM, Gilchrist E, Hartley S, et al. An evaluation of the body substance isolation (BSI) system by questionnaire and observation. 3rd International Conference on Nosocomial Infections, Atlanta, Aug 3, 1990; Abst C/4.

78. Weinstein SA, Kotilaninen HR, Avato JL, Gantz NM. A comparison study of universal precautions and body substance isolation. 3rd International Conference on Nosocomial Infections, Atlanta, Aug 3, 1990; Abst C/5.

79. Catanzaro A. Nosocomial tuberculosis. *Am Rev Respir Dis* 1982;125:559-62.

80. Hutton MD, Stead WW, Cauthen GM, Bloch AB, Ewing WM. Nosocomial transmission of tuberculosis associated with a draining abscess. *J Infect Dis* 1990;161:286-95.

81. CDC. Nosocomial transmission of multidrug-resistant tuberculosis to health care workers and HIV-infected patients in an urban hospital—Florida. *MMWR* 1990;39:718-22.

82. Di Perri G, Cruciani M, Danzi MC, et al. Nosocomial epidemic of active tuberculosis among HIV-infected patients. *Lancet* 1989;2:1502-4.

83. CDC. Guidelines for preventing the transmission of tuberculosis in health-care settings, with special focus on HIV-related issues. *MMWR* 1990;39(RR-17).

84. American Society of Heating, Refrigerating and Air Conditioning Engineers. *1987 ASHRAE handbook: heating, ventilating, and air-conditioning systems and applications.* Atlanta, GA: American Society of Heating, Refrigerating, and Air Conditioning Engineers; 1987:23.1-23.12.

85. Health Resources and Services Administration. *Guidelines for construction and equipment of hospital and medical facilities.* Rockville, MD: US Department of Health and Human Services, Public Health Service; 1984: PHS publication (HRSA)84-14500.

86. Jacobson MA, Mills J. Serious cytomegalovirus disease in the acquired immunodeficiency syndrome (AIDS). *Ann Intern Med* 1988;108:585-94.

87. Adler SP. Nosocomial transmission of cytomegalovirus. *Pediatr Infect Dis* 1986;5:239-46.

88. Brady MT. Cytomegalovirus infections: occupational risk for health professionals. *Am J Infect Control* 1986;14:197-203.

89. Onorato IM, Morens DM, Martone WJ, Stansfield SK. Epidemiology of cytomegalovirus infections: recommendations for prevention and control. *Rev Infect Dis* 1985;7:474-97.

90. Walzer PD. *Pneumocystis carinii*—new clinical spectrum? *N Engl J Med* 1991;324:263-5.

91. Giron JA, Martinez S, Walzer PD. Should inpatients with *Pneumocystis carinii* be isolated? *Lancet* 1982;2:46.

92. Haron E, Bodey GP, Luna MA, Dekmezian R, Elting L. Has the incidence of *Pneumocystis carinii* pneumonia in cancer patients increased with the AIDS epidemic? *Lancet* 1988;2:904-5.

93. Jacobs J, Libby DM, Winters RA, et al. A cluster of *Pneumocystis carinii* pneumonia in adults without predisposing illnesses. *N Engl J Med* 1991;324:246-50.

94. Cottone JA, Terezhalmy GT, Molinari JA. Rationale for practical infection control in dentistry. In: *Practical infection control in dentistry.* Malvern, PA: Lea & Febiger; 1991:71-9.

95. CDC. Recommended infection-control practices for dentistry. *MMWR* 1986;35:237-42.

96. Marcus R, Favero MS, Banerjee S, et al. HIV prevalence and incidence among patients undergoing chronic hemodialysis. *Am J Med* 1991;90:614-9.

97. Favero MS. Dialysis associated diseases and their control. In: Bennett JV, Brachman PS, eds. *Hospital infections,* 2nd ed. Boston: Little, Brown; 1985:267-84.

98. CDC. Recommendations for preventing transmission of infection with human T-lymphotropic virus type III/lymphadenopathy-associated virus in the workplace. *MMWR* 1985;34:681-95.

99. Williams WW. Guidelines for infection control in hospital personnel. *Infect Control* 1983;4:245-325.

100. Cumming PD, Wallace EL, Schorr JB, Dodd RY. Exposure of patients to human immunodeficiency virus through the transfusion of blood components that test antibody-negative. *N Engl J Med* 1989;321:941-6.

101. Cohen ND, Munoz A, Reitz BA, et al. Transmission of retroviruses by transfusion of screened blood in patients undergoing cardiac surgery. *N Engl J Med* 1989;320:1172-6.

102. Donahue JG, Nelson KE, Munoz A, et al. Transmission of HIV by transfusion of screened blood [letter]. *N Engl J Med* 1990;320:1709.

103. Busch M, Eble B, Heilbron D, Vyas G. Risk associated with transfusion of HIV-antibody-negative blood [letter]. *N Engl J Med* 1990;322:850-1.

104. Ward JW, Holmberg SD, Allen JR, et al. Transmission of human immunodeficiency virus (HIV) by blood transfusion screened as negative for HIV antibody. *N Engl J Med* 1988;318:473-8.

105. Menitove JE. The decreasing risk of transfusion-associated AIDS. *N Engl J Med* 1989;321:966-8.

106. CDC. Safety of therapeutic products used for hemophilia patients. *MMWR* 1988;37:441-3.

107. Remis RS, O'Shaughnessy MV, Tsoukas C, et al. HIV transmission to patients with hemophilia by heat-treated, donor-screened factor concentrate. *Can Med Assoc J* 1990;142:1247-54.

108. Tedder RS, Uttley A, Cheingsong-Popov R. Safety of immunoglobulin preparations containing anti-HTLV-III [letter]. *Lancet* 1985;1:815.

109. Steele DR. HTLV-III antibodies in human immune-globulin [letter]. *JAMA* 1986;255:609.

110. Wells MA, Wittek A, Marcus-Sekura C, et al. Chemical and physical inactivation of human T-lymphotropic virus, type III (HTLV-III). *Transfusion* 1986;26:110-30.

111. CDC. The safety of hepatitis B virus vaccine. *MMWR* 1983;32:134-6.

112. Francis DP, Feorino PM, McDougal S, et al. The safety of hepatitis B vaccine: inactivation of the AIDS virus during routine vaccine manufacture. *JAMA* 1986;256:869-72.

113. CDC. Safety of therapeutic immune globulin preparations with respect to transmission of human T-lymphotropic virus type III/lymphadenopathy-associated virus infection. *MMWR* 1986;35:231-3.

AIDS and Other Manifestations of HIV Infection,
Second Edition, Edited by Gary P. Wormser.
Raven Press, Ltd., New York © 1992.

CHAPTER 36

Occupational Issues Related to the HIV Epidemic

Stanley H. Weiss

HISTORICAL OVERVIEW

The unusual occurrence of Kaposi's sarcoma and *Pneumocystis carinii* pneumonia in a small number of homosexual men led to the initial clinical recognition of the acquired immunodeficiency syndrome (AIDS) epidemic a decade ago (1–6). The theory that a transmissible infectious agent was the cause of AIDS (7) and also bloodborne was fueled by cases of AIDS in intravenous drug users and subsequently among hemophiliacs and blood transfusion recipients (8–10). The first occupational guidelines were based on our acquired experience with hepatitis B, known to be a highly infectious bloodborne pathogen. In 1982 these guidelines were formulated and widely disseminated (11). In 1983 these guidelines were reiterated (12,13), highlighting the potential risk of parenteral exposure and the recognition that the epidemic undoubtedly was spread by bloodborne as well as sexual routes. Although occupational issues are certainly of concern to persons outside the health-care and laboratory settings, there is a paucity of specific data from other professions and settings. Since degree of risk may be inferred from the studies conducted within the health-care field, this chapter deals only with the medical setting.

Reassurances concerning the apparent adequacy of the 1983 occupational guidelines were based primarily on the concordance of three types of data. (a) Several prospective surveillance studies of health-care workers with documented parenteral or mucous membrane exposures to potentially infectious body fluids of AIDS patients were in progress. No worker had developed symptoms suggestive of AIDS (14,15). (b) There was no statistically significant increase in the number of AIDS cases in the Centers for Disease Control (CDC) surveillance statistics for health-care workers, when compared to the frequency of these jobs among the U.S. workforce. (c) No study had revealed any risk to be associated with either airborne exposure or casual contact.

The isolation and culturing of the human immunodeficiency virus type 1 (HIV-1) in 1984 (16,17) enabled the development of reliable serological screening for HIV, which became available in 1985 (18,19). Use of a test for HIV antibody helped to establish a convincing etiologic connection between HIV and AIDS (20,21). These discoveries subsequently led to the realization that the magnitude of the epidemic was far greater than had been imagined, with the number of AIDS cases dwarfed by the number of persons infected with HIV (18).

This meant that in the United States transmission of HIV had silently occurred during the 1970s with continued spread in the 1980s. Thus, in the early years of the epidemic, health-care and laboratory workers were unknowingly in routine contact with a great many patients infected with HIV beyond those recognized to have AIDS, as well as with their body fluids. In retrospect, it is remarkable how few workers took even the most limited of precautions during the early 1980s. Those rare workers who heavily garbed, in an effort to protect themselves, engaged in such practices only with patients identified as having AIDS, unaware of the many patients with whom they failed to take precautions. Needlestick injuries in the medical setting were documented (15).

The mainstay of HIV diagnosis is testing for antibodies ("seropositivity") (see Weiss, Laboratory Detection of Human Retroviruses). HIV seropositivity is believed to indicate chronic, persistent infection and does not connote protection. In the "window" period before anti-

S. H. Weiss: Division of Infectious Disease Epidemiology, Department of Preventive Medicine and Community Health, University of Medicine and Dentistry of New Jersey, New Jersey Medical School, Newark, New Jersey 07107.

body becomes detectable but after exposure and infection with HIV, other tests may occasionally be positive. However, latent infection not detectable by antibody tests is unusual (22,23).

By early 1985 there were some clues that HIV infection was a chronic disease with long latency (18). The demonstration of a long incubation period between first acquiring HIV and developing AIDS or other severe clinical sequelae involved the use of both prospective epidemiologic data and tests for the causative agent (24). It was at least theoretically possible that many health-care workers might have (unknowingly) become infected with HIV and feel and look perfectly well; the initial studies of occupational risk could conceivably have failed to detect widespread transmission.

It was therefore quite reassuring in January 1985 when two groups found HIV antibody to be absent serologically in a combined total of 273 persons drawn from institutions and laboratories where AIDS and HIV, respectively, were routinely encountered (20,25).

The CDC subsequently reported on 40 health-care workers, representing persons who had specific potential HIV exposures. These exposures included 29 needlestick injuries, 5 cuts, 5 mucosal exposures, and 5 skin exposures (26). No worker was seropositive, with a median follow-up period of 8 months. Additionally, T-cell subsets were normal and HIV clinical sequelae were absent among over 200 workers followed prospectively (26). This reinforced the message that the initial Public Health Service (PHS) guidelines for AIDS had been reasonable initial measures. These data, however, still did not exclude the statistical possibility of a substantial public health risk (27), since needlestick transmission rates for HIV exceeding 1% were within the 95% upper confidence bounds given the still limited observation base. The transmission by a needlestick injury from an AIDS patient of hepatitis B virus (HBV) *without* transmission of HIV (28) suggested that transmission of HBV was more likely compared to HIV (29). These findings supported the tendency to offer reassurances to a somewhat nervous workforce, but also tended to instill a sense of complacency in many institutions. The limitations of the data were largely ignored by the medical community.

In late 1984 a nurse in Great Britain became infected with HIV as a consequence of accidental inoculation of fresh blood from an arterial blood gas syringe in an intensive care unit setting (30). The source patient was known to have AIDS. Health-care workers could no longer deny that they were at some risk for occupational acquisition of HIV.

Needlestick transmission was next documented in a cross-sectional study of high-risk workers in early 1985 (29), conducted before commercial availability of HIV antibody tests. One of 42 (2.4%) persons who had reported parenteral exposure to patients with AIDS was HIV seropositive, without any other risk after thorough

investigation. Two other seropositive health-care workers with nosocomial parenteral exposure were also reported (29). Since negative data from other studies do not enter the denominator, first positive reports not infrequently overestimate the magnitude of risk. Since several other large studies had not yet observed any unexplained HIV infection or seroconversions among exposed workers (31,32), many investigators initially felt that the risk to workers had been grossly overplayed.

Documentation of HIV transmission to health-care and laboratory workers by multiple investigators around the world has since occurred (33–39), leading to general acknowledgment that HIV risk must be considered in the workplace. This apparent change in viewpoint has led some physicians, particularly surgeons at high risk of percutaneous injury, to feel they had been misled and betrayed by earlier advice and reassurances. Some have retreated from active clinical practice because of their concerns and attracted national publicity in doing so.

There have been a limited number of clusters of HBV transmission from dentists and surgeons to patients (40), including very rare instances of recurrent HBV transmission despite attempts to improve the professional's infection control techniques. Until recently, such risks from professionals to patients were not perceived as a major issue. No such clusters of HBV transmission were reported from 1987 through 1991.

Nevertheless, given the theoretical possibility that HIV might be transmitted to a patient and recurrent inquiries to the New Jersey Board of Medical Examiners for advice, a multidisciplinary conference was convened in 1990 (41). Interest has subsequently been heightened by the CDC investigation of the practice of a dentist in Florida (42).

There has been a public outcry for regulation. There is a desire to only tolerate absolutely zero risk in the medical-care setting. This reflects, in part, the Hippocratic axiom to "first do no harm." Such self-regulation was historically important, particularly in antiquity, to minimize unwarranted commercial gain from the innocent and ill. Medical historians have commented that it was not until the turn of this century that patients had a better than even chance of benefiting from their encounter with a physician! Thus, historically, there was good reason for the fears of patients beyond simple denial of illness. Given the great possibility for good that modern medicine brings, it is not clear now how to best balance the failure to do good that arises from inaction while avoiding any chance of harm, against the possibility of harm itself. The cries of AIDS activists for unproven drugs speaks to their desire to have input into their own care, but perhaps also to increased willingness of patients to take some risks that the medical community has traditionally striven to protect patients against.

As we struggle to protect patients and health-care providers and to render appropriate care despite limited resources, compromises shall occur that may have long-standing impact on the delivery of health-care services. The quantitative risks and costs are being weighed by the medical community. Some medical economists and clinicians have suggested that the financial burden of some of the possible new guidelines for physicians and the medical workplace may be exorbitant (43). Given the reality of fixed budgets (or diminishing resources), some programs otherwise viewed by the medical establishment as higher priority may have to be sacrificed to comply with mandatory regulations. Public policy is likely to continue to evolve rapidly over the next year. In many institutions, surveys are in progress to assess, document, and summarize the implications of some of the proposed measures. It is unclear how lawyers, politicians, and others will ultimately weigh such data.

This chapter places the magnitude of risks to workers and to patients in perspective and outlines key medical issues involved in the development of institutional policies. Periodic policy review at individual institutions by a multidisciplinary committee will be useful. Members of the committee might include an epidemiologist knowledgeable about nosocomial risks, an infectious diseases expert knowledgeable about HIV, administrative and legal staff representatives, a bioethicist, and a patient advocate.

OCCUPATIONAL RISK TO THE WORKER

Anecdotal case reports are important in describing modes of transmission but cannot be used to calculate the magnitude of risk. HIV transmission to health-care workers has resulted from several types of HIV exposure: contaminated hollow-bore needles with parenteral injury, cuts, mucosal splashes, and skin contact. Similarly, persons rendering home health care are at risk (44,45). The limited number of documented transmissions precludes much further generalization. However, some cases of transmission associated with needlestick injuries appear to have involved only limited blood infusion or relatively superficial injury. Although HIV has been detected in many body fluids (21,46), epidemiologic evidence has demonstrated transmission only in association with blood, semen, cervicovaginal secretions, and breast milk. The importance, if any, of saliva is less clear. In the dental setting, saliva is invariably contaminated with blood and thus viewed as infectious. One case report has suggested HIV transmission by a human bite (47). Since skin was not broken, neither temporal seroconversion information nor viral strain comparison data were available, and no other cases of transmission by bite have been reported; transmission by bite remains uncertain. Similarly, one report of female-to-male HIV transmission implicating saliva exposure during fellatio (48) has been questioned (49). Thus saliva alone has generally not been included among the list of body fluids for which universal precautions should apply.

The risk of HIV transmission is thought to be related to the mode and dose of exposure, although the data are too sparse to substantiate this. Measures of HIV infectivity have not been defined. Specimens with high p24 antigen titers might, for example, pose special risk. Host susceptibility factors to HIV remain an area of investigation. It is also possible that some HIV strains may have altered virulence (49a). These issues may help explain the lack, so far, of a clear relationship between magnitude of blood exposure and risk of transmission to workers. However, given that virtually all recipients of blood transfusions derived from HIV-seropositive donors become HIV infected, exposure dose must have some effect on risk.

Within an individual patient infected with HIV, the titer of HIV may vary over the course of infection, so that a given person's infectiousness likely varies considerably over time. Limited data suggest that during the "window" before seroconversion plasma HIV titers, and hence the potential for infection, may be particularly high (50). This situation would be particularly risky if clinical precautions were taken only for patients with known, documented infection. Some occupational exposures to blood and body fluids occur where the HIV status of the source patient is unknown, and many such patients may refuse HIV testing even in the setting where a worker has been exposed (51). Thus there is considerable rationale behind the concept of "universal precautions" (52–54), especially in regions where the seroconversion incidence remains high. Institutions need to develop policies to deal with these situations, which balance the worker's right to a safe workplace against the privacy rights of an individual.

The many epidemiologic studies of occupational transmission risk provide numerators for cases of work-related acquisition and denominators for persons-exposed and specific exposures. Within these studies, persons who have had parenteral exposure have the greatest risk: about 0.3–0.5% per parenteral exposure (55). The risk associated with working with highly concentrated HIV is of the same magnitude (39).

The observed risk in prospective studies associated with mucosal membrane and cutaneous HIV exposures is zero (56). The limited number of persons in the denominator of these studies, however, still leads to wide statistical confidence limits concerning the specific level of risk. For example, an article summarizing 14 surveys totaling 757 persons with potential HIV exposure through nonpercutaneous, nonsexual modes of contact found no documented case of transmission, with a 95% upper confidence bound of 0.4% (57). Nevertheless, the existence of anecdotal cases shows that such exposure can sometimes lead to transmission (56). While it can sometimes be difficult to pinpoint the precise mode of

HIV acquisition (56), the evolving tools of molecular epidemiology hold promise for verification (39,49a), as well as for elimination, of a suspected origin of transmission (49). The interpretation of these research tests remains uncertain, given the newness of the techniques and applications, and the very limited control data (57a).

UNIVERSAL PRECAUTIONS

The initial CDC recommendations called for blood and body fluid precautions when a patient was known or suspected to be infected with bloodborne pathogens (13). In 1987 the CDC called for precautions to be consistently used all the time, regardless of the apparent bloodborne infection status of a given patient (58). These "universal precautions" are intended to prevent parenteral, mucous membrane, and nonintact skin exposures of health-care workers to bloodborne pathogens. Since it was acknowledged that available medical and laboratory data might not always identify those persons and specimens with bloodborne pathogens, universal precautions in effect eliminate the "need to know." The recommendations were further clarified in 1988, with the emphasis that blood was the single most important source of exposure in the occupational setting (52). In part, this clarification was a response to the practical issues of daily patient care. Barrier precautions and handwashing are among the mainstays of universal precautions (Tokars and Martone, Infection Control Considerations in HIV Infection).

The estimated prevalence of HIV within the United States, projected from mathematical models, is about 1 million persons. There is wide geographic variation in HIV seroprevalence. In some hospitals, for example public hospitals in San Francisco, New York City, or Newark, a very high proportion of patients are infected (59). In such locations a person of unknown HIV status has a high probability of seropositivity, as highlighted by a study of emergency room patients in Baltimore (60). The incidence of new infections (community seroconversion rates) may also be sufficiently high that HIV seronegativity cannot be relied on to rule out HIV infection. The implementation of "universal precautions" for blood and body fluids, once controversial in such settings, is now commonly accepted. Nevertheless, many professionals still express the desire to "know" their patient's status. The gap between the positions of infection control specialists and the average worker is even wider in settings of lower HIV seroprevalence.

The success of universal precautions is limited (61–68). Gloves do not prevent needlestick or other penetrating sharps injuries (69–73) and gloves certainly can tear (73). The quality of disposable (and of sterile) gloves can be variable (74,75). Latex gloves appear preferable to vinyl (70,74,76,77), with rates of perforation in latex gloves generally lower than those made from polyvinyl chloride.

During a surgical operation, when an overt sharps injury occurs, the aseptic barrier is broken and except under emergency circumstances the injured worker leaves the operating field and returns upon the reestablishment of asepsis. Thus the primary risk in these circumstances is generally from patient to worker. Inapparent barrier breakdown, however, appears to be common (78,79). If a single glove is worn, surveys have found frequent gross contamination of the hands (80). With double gloving, such gross contamination is greatly reduced (80). Many surgeons now also include a thin cloth glove between the two latex gloves, in an effort to impede minor needlestick injuries.

One study found that over half of needlestick injuries occurred to the index finger of the nondominant hand (81). Thus the addition of reinforcement to this portion of the glove or the routine use of a thimble-equivalent could dramatically reduce occupational exposures. Various safety devices to guard against needlesticks have also been marketed (82). Thus there is ample margin for continued refinement and improvement toward injury reduction, which would protect both patient and worker.

Universal precautions are expensive, both for materials (such as gloves) as well as the educational effort required. Studies that assess efficacy are mixed in their results (54,68,78,79,83–90) and the effort may not be cost effective (91). Adherence to guidelines may be greater when employee compliance is monitored. Institutions may find it useful to work with employee unions to effect meaningful changes that enhance workplace safety.

POSTEXPOSURE PROPHYLAXIS

The time period immediately following an occupational exposure is a difficult one both for the exposed worker and his/her physician or occupational health service. The low statistical risk of acquisition of a deadly infection provides limited comfort. It is helpful to have a comprehensive program in place to deal with the anticipated accidental exposures (33,92,93).

The Burroughs-Wellcome company initially sponsored a randomized trial offering zidovudine to workers exposed to HIV (94). Given the low risk of seroconversion, it was unlikely that a sufficient sample size could ever have been accrued for this clinical trial to prove efficacy. Furthermore, the ready availability of the FDA approved drug (zidovudine), worker apprehensions, and the delay in drug access through the trial led few to enroll. The trial was abandoned after very limited enrollment.

Evidence from animal studies suggesting that zidovudine might be useful (95–97) prompted the Public Health Service (PHS) to formulate guidelines concerning postexposure prophylaxis (98). Zidovudine does have some toxicity in this setting (99,100). Recent data, on otherwise healthy workers given a limited course of zidovudine, found a worker whose neutrophil declined to 500/mm^3 (101), a level at which serious infections might occur. There is also concern about the potential for delayed mutagenicity or carcinogenicity. Embryonic toxicity in mice at high AZT doses has been demonstrated (102). The PHS judgment that it could "not make a recommendation for or against the use of zidovudine for this [postexposure prophylaxis] purpose because of the limitations of current knowledge" (98) still remains. In the absence of demonstration of high clinical efficacy in the postexposure setting, some clinicians have questioned the wisdom of administration. Since some laboratory data suggest that administration of zidovudine within an hour or two may be requisite to achieve a substantial likelihood of prophylactic efficacy (103), mechanisms for rapid decision making and initiation of therapy are important if zidovudine is to be given at all.

A decision analysis study, concerning the issue of postexposure prophylaxis for needlestick exposures to HIV, concluded that even a very low zidovudine efficacy (of 3–8%) might warrant its use (104). On the other hand, subsequent laboratory data suggest a limitation to its usefulness (103,105,106). Zidovudine benefits do not clearly outweigh the risks after exposure to blood of unknown serologic status, or if there is a delay in starting therapy (104). Furthermore, several documented instances of seroconversion in which prophylactic zidovudine was given, and sometimes initiated extremely rapidly, demonstrate it is not 100% efficacious (107–112). Thus whether or not to administer zidovudine or other postexposure therapy will depend on individual circumstances, including the nature of the exposure, documentation of the likelihood that the source was infected with HIV and any surrogate measures of infective titer, the risk-taking perceptions of the exposed worker, and the availability of alternative experimental therapy. Some workers may reasonably decide to "take their chances." Others who have a particularly high risk of seroconversion (e.g., an inoculation with a substantial amount of blood) might decide to try highly experimental combination chemotherapy in consultation with an infectious disease expert, rather than zidovudine alone.

All exposed persons must be counseled regarding the risks of transmission to others, particularly sexual partners, and the need for follow-up. Until there are, at the least, animal studies that demonstrate the efficacy of therapy for protection in the postexposure situation, if not human clinical trials, postexposure therapy must be considered experimental.

RISK TO THE PATIENT

The provisional guidelines published in 1989 by the Occupational Safety and Health Administration (OSHA) regulating the health-care environment in the post-"universal precautions" era are oriented toward the protection of both worker and patient (113), and permanent regulations were released in December 1991 (113a).

The cumulative HIV risk to the provider, such as trauma surgeons in regions of high HIV prevalence, may be substantial. Injuries remain commonplace (79,114). With widespread publicity concerning the CDC investigation of a dental practice in Florida (42,57a,115,116), much attention has now focused on a related issue: the potential for transmission of HIV from health-care workers to their patients and the risk of acquisition related to the health-care environment.

In previous studies, no evidence of risk of AIDS or HIV transmission to patients was found (117–121). Several other ongoing investigations have not so far revealed any evidence of transmission.

In the Florida investigation, several patients who had a history of invasive dental procedures were found to be HIV seropositive. Molecular studies suggested the possibility of transmission from the dentist, who died with AIDS, based on the degree of strain similarity. However, limited data on the degree of homology within epidemiologic clusters exist (42,57a). Some studies suggest extremely little variation in such clusters (122–124)—raising the possibility that the changes observed by the CDC may be in excess of that associated with immediate (direct or indirect) transmission. Also, the period from first dental visit to AIDS in one person (patient A) was less than 2 years. This would be an exceptionally short latency period, raising the question of possible earlier acquisition from an unidentified source outside the dental practice.

Investigations of the Florida dental practice indicate general (although not absolute) compliance with the CDC recommendations for infection control in dentistry (125), and the CDC has not concluded how transmission might have taken place. This is problematic, since the public health implications of transmission to patient(s) via a direct blood–blood transfer versus an indirect route (e.g., faulty decontamination) differ considerably.

Mathematical models of direct transmission suggest a very low risk even with invasive procedures (126–128). When the HIV status of a surgeon is unknown, the overall likelihood of reverse HIV transmission (to the patient) is about 1 chance in 21 million hours of surgery, with an upper bound 95% risk of 1 in 4 million (128). If the surgeon were known to be HIV seropositive, the estimate is 1 chance in 83,000 hours of surgery. These risks are of about the same magnitude as fatal injury to the patient on the way to the hospital (128). This would imply limited need to restrict the work of persons infected with HIV.

A meeting held by the CDC in February 1991 explored many related issues (43). Should the practices of HIV-infected surgeons and dentists engaged in invasive procedures be restricted? What procedures are "invasive" or "exposure-prone"? Who, if anyone, and under what conditions, should be tested for HIV? The guidelines from the CDC issued in July 1991 concerning these matters (129) focus on several of these key issues but have left many questions unresolved.

Spurred by public apprehensions, new studies looking back at several thousand former patients of health-care workers known to be HIV seropositive are in progress. It has been suggested that these look-back ventures may not be worth the cost (130) and perhaps should only be conducted when there is a clearly identifiable risk of transmission (130). Preliminary but unpublished accounts of these new studies have not documented HIV transmission from workers to any patients. These preliminary data have led some medical groups to reappraise the scientific rationale of the new CDC recommendations (43) and to recommend that implementation of policy decisions should await further data. Other groups have seized on these issues, using them as a surrogate for mobilizing public reaction amid longstanding fears, with the debate becoming increasingly charged and politicized. Further attention to the improvement of workplace safety, which offers bilateral enhancement of protection, remains critical.

OTHER WORKPLACE TRANSMISSION ISSUES

The immune system impairment that results from infection with HIV leads to an inability to control certain infectious organisms, including pathogens such as *Mycobacterium tuberculosis* (131–135). This organism has been associated with secondary transmission within urban communities as well as in hospitals, since *M. tuberculosis* (unlike HIV) can be highly infectious through aerosol transmission routes (136). Close-contact spread has been compounded by the crack cocaine epidemic (137), the existence of anergy in HIV-infected persons (leading to delay in diagnosis of infection with *M. tuberculosis*) (138–140), and reduced physician prescription of isoniazid prophylaxis (due to hepatotoxicity concerns) during the 1980s (141–143). In addition, multiply-drug-resistant strains of *M. tuberculosis* have been described, particularly in HIV-seropositive prisoners and intravenous drug users (144,145). One death of a health-care worker, who had an underlying malignancy and worked in close contact with infected prisoners, has been attributed to occupational acquisition of multiply-drug-resistant tuberculosis (145). These issues have im-

portant ramifications regarding the implementation of respiratory precautions, as well as the design and adequacy of ventilation systems in many types of medical institutions. Some buildings are clearly inadequate in terms of the availability of private rooms and of respiratory isolation (145a,b), and the cost would be great to correct these deficiencies.

Infections by classic pyogenic pathogens also occur in HIV-infected persons (146,147), including pneumococcal infections (148). Recent reports of antibiotic-resistant strains in some common bacteria (149) suggest a possible future problem regarding nosocomial spread of these agents. The possibility of nosocomial spread of *Pneumocystis carinii* has been raised (150–153).

Nosocomial outbreaks of other highly infectious agents, such as measles (154), have also been described. A high clinical index of suspicion and adherence to infection control guidelines can be expected to minimize these problems.

SUMMARY

The perception of degree of risk can vary markedly from actual risk. About 5% of the cases of AIDS and HIV infection in the United States have occurred in health-care workers, a percentage that has remained stable over time. Nearly all these infections are related to life-style factors, not occupational risk. The risk to patients appears to be very much smaller but has received even more publicity. Apprehension exists concerning the future framework of our medical-care delivery system and who will care for whom (155,156). The sensitive handling of legitimate fears and the balancing of conflicting risks will be a challenging task in the decades ahead.

REFERENCES

1. CDC. *Pneumocystis* pneumonia—Los Angeles. *MMWR* 1981; 30:250–2.
2. CDC. Kaposi's sarcoma and *Pneumocystis* pneumonia among homosexual men—New York City and California. *MMWR* 1981;30:305–8.
3. Gottlieb MS, Schroff R, Schanker HM, et al. *Pneumocystis carinii* pneumonia and mucosal candidiasis in previously healthy homosexual men: evidence of a new acquired cellular immunodeficiency. *N Engl J Med* 1981;305:1425–31.
4. Masur H, Michelis MA, Greene JB, et al. An outbreak of community-acquired *Pneumocystis carinii* pneumonia: initial manifestation of cellular immune dysfunction. *N Engl J Med* 1981;305:1431–8.
5. Siegal FP, Lopez C, Hammer GS, et al. Severe acquired immunodeficiency in male homosexuals, manifested by chronic perianal ulcerative herpes simplex lesions. *N Engl J Med* 1981;305:1439–44.
6. Masur H, Michelis MA, Wormser GP, et al. Opportunistic infection in previously healthy women: initial manifestation of a community-acquired cellular immunodeficiency. *Ann Intern Med* 1982;97:533–9.
7. CDC. A cluster of Kaposi's sarcoma and *Pneumocystis carinii* pneumonia among homosexual male residents of Los Angeles and Orange counties, California. *MMWR* 1982;31:305–7.

8. CDC. Possible transfusion-associated acquired immune deficiency syndrome (AIDS)—California. *MMWR* 1982;31:652–4.
9. Ammann AJ, Wara DW, Dritz S, et al. Acquired immunodeficiency in an infant: possible transmission by means of blood products. *Lancet* 1983;1:956–8.
10. Oleske J, Minnefor A, Cooper R Jr, et al. Immune deficiency syndrome in children. *JAMA* 1983;249:2345–9.
11. CDC. Acquired immune deficiency syndrome (AIDS): precautions for clinical and laboratory staffs. *MMWR* 1982;31:577–80.
12. CDC. An evaluation of the acquired immunodeficiency syndrome (AIDS) reported in health care personnel—United States. *MMWR* 1983;32:358–60.
13. Garner JS, Simmons BP. Guideline for isolation precautions in hospitals. *Infect Control* 1983;4:245–53.
14. CDC. Prospective evaluation of health-care workers exposed via parenteral or mucous-membrane routes to blood and body fluids of patients with acquired immunodeficiency syndrome. *MMWR* 1984;33:181–2.
15. Wormser GP, Joline C, Duncanson F, Cunningham-Rundles S. Needle-stick injuries during the care of patients with AIDS. *N Engl J Med* 1984;310:1461–2.
16. Gallo RC, Salahuddin SZ, Popovic M, et al. Frequent detection and isolation of cytopathic retroviruses (HTLV-III) from patients with AIDS and at risk for AIDS. *Science* 1984;224:500–3.
17. Sarngadharan MG, Popovic M, Bruch L, Schupbach J, Gallo RC. Antibodies reactive with human T-lymphotropic retroviruses (HTLV-III) in the serum of patients with AIDS. *Science* 1984;224:506–8.
18. Landesman SH, Ginzburg HM, Weiss SH. The AIDS epidemic. *N Engl J Med* 1985;312:521–5.
19. CDC. Results of human T-lymphotropic virus type III test kits reported from blood collection centers—United States, April 22–May 19, 1985. *MMWR* 1985;34:375–6.
20. Weiss SH, Goedert JJ, Sarngadharan MG, et al. Screening test for HTLV-III (AIDS agent) antibodies: specificity, sensitivity, and applications. *JAMA* 1985;253:221–5.
21. Melbye M. The natural history of human T lymphotropic virus-III infection: the cause of AIDS. *Br Med J* 1986;292:5–12.
22. Shoebridge GI, Gatenby PA, Nightingale BN, et al. Polymerase chain reaction testing of HIV-1 seronegative at-risk individuals. *Lancet* 1990;336:180–1.
23. Wormser GP, Joline C, Bittker S, Forseter G, Kwok S, Sninsky JJ. Polymerase chain reaction for seronegative health care workers with parenteral exposure to HIV-infected patients. *N Engl J Med* 1989;321:1681–2.
24. Goedert JJ, Biggar RJ, Weiss SH, et al. Three-year incidence of AIDS in five cohorts of HTLV-III-infected risk group members. *Science* 1986;231:992–5.
25. Hirsch MS, Wormser GP, Schooley RT, et al. Risk of nosocomial infection with human T-cell lymphotropic virus III (HTLV-III). *N Engl J Med* 1985;312:1–4.
26. CDC. Update: prospective evaluation of health-care workers exposed via the parenteral or mucous-membrane route to blood or body fluids from patients with acquired immunodeficiency syndrome—United States. *MMWR* 1985;34:101–3.
27. DeBeau CE. Risk of transmission of HTLV-III by needlestick. *N Engl J Med* 1985;312:1128–9.
28. Gerberding JL, Hopewell PC, Kamingky LS, Sande MA. Transmission of hepatitis B without transmission of AIDS by accidental needlestick. *N Engl J Med* 1985;312:56.
29. Weiss SH, Saxinger WC, Rechtman D, et al. HTLV-III infection among health care workers: association with needle-stick injuries. *JAMA* 1985;254:2089–93.
30. Anonymous. Needlestick transmission of HTLV-III from a patient infected in Africa. *Lancet* 1984;2:1376–7.
31. Gerberding JL, Bryant-LeBlanc CE, Nelson K, et al. Risk of transmitting the human immunodeficiency virus, cytomegalovirus and hepatitis B virus to health care workers exposed to patients with AIDS and AIDS-related conditions. *J Infect Dis* 1987;156:1–8.
32. Henderson DK, Saah AJ, Zak BJ, et al. Risk of nosocomial infection with human T-cell lymphotropic virus type III/lymphadenopathy-associated virus in a large cohort of intensively exposed health care workers. *Ann Intern Med* 1986;104:644–7.

33. Henderson DK, Gerberding JL. Prophylactic zidovudine after occupational exposure to the human immunodeficiency virus: an interim analysis. *J Infect Dis* 1989;160:321–7.
34. Ippolito G, Cadrobbi P, Carosi G, et al. Risk of HIV transmission among health care workers: a multicentre study. *Scand J Infect Dis* 1990;22:245–6.
35. McCray E, The Cooperative Needlestick Surveillance Group. Occupational risk of the acquired immunodeficiency syndrome among health care workers. *N Engl J Med* 1986;314:1127–32.
36. Raub W. Risk of occupational transmission of human immunodeficiency virus evaluated. *JAMA* 1991;265:706.
37. Klein RS, Phelan JA, Freeman K, et al. Low occupational risk of human immunodeficiency virus among dental professionals. *N Engl J Med* 1988;318:86–90.
38. Weiss SH, Biggar RJ. The epidemiology of human retrovirus-associated illnesses. *Mt Sinai J Med* 1986;53:579–91.
39. Weiss SH, Goedert JJ, Gartner S, et al. Risk of human immunodeficiency virus (HIV-1) infection among laboratory workers. *Science* 1988;239:68–71.
40. Anonymous. Two deaths blamed on outbreak: hepatitis B cases traced to Indiana dentist. *Am Med News* 1985;March 1.
41. Price DM. What should we do about HIV-positive health professionals? *Arch Intern Med* 1991;151:658–9.
42. CDC. Possible transmission of human immunodeficiency virus to a patient during an invasive dental procedure. *MMWR* 1990;39:489–92.
43. CDC. Open meeting on the risks of transmission of bloodborne pathogens to patients during invasive procedures: February 21–22, 1991. Atlanta, GA: US Department of Health and Human Services; 1991:1–488.
44. Grint P, McEvoy M. Two associated cases of the acquired immune deficiency syndrome (AIDS). *Communicable Disease Rep* 1985;42:4.
45. CDC. Apparent transmission of human T-lymphotropic virus type III/lymphadenopathy-associated virus from a child to a mother providing health care. *MMWR* 1986;35:76–9.
46. Van de Perre P, De Clercq A, Cogniaux-Leclerc J, Nzaramba D Butzler J-P, Sprecher-Goldberger S. Detection of HIV p17 antigen in lymphocytes but not epithelial cells from cervicovaginal secretions of women seropositive for HIV: implications for heterosexual transmission of the virus. *Genitourin Med* 1988;64:30–3.
47. Wahn V, Kramer HH, Voit T, Bruster HT, Scrampical B, Scheid A. Horizontal transmission of HIV infection between two siblings. *Lancet* 1986;2:694.
48. US Department of Labor, US Department of Health and Human Services. Joint advisory notice: protection against occupational exposure to hepatitis B virus (HBV) and human immunodeficiency virus (HIV). *Fed Reg* 1987;52:41818–24.
49. Weiss SH. Unusual modes of HIV transmission. *N Engl J Med* 1989;321:1476.
49a. Wolinsky SM, Wike CM, Korber BTM, et al. Selective transmission of human immunodeficiency virus type-1 variants from mothers to infants. *Science* 1992;255:1134–1137.
50. Daar ES, Moudgil T, Meyer RD, Ho DD. Transient high levels of viremia in patients with primary human immunodeficiency virus type 1 infection. *N Engl J Med* 1991;324:961–4.
51. Miller PJ, Farr BM. A study of the rate of postexposure human immunodeficiency virus testing in a hospital requiring written informed consent. *J Occup Med* 1989;31:524–7.
52. CDC. Update: universal precautions for prevention of transmission of human immunodeficiency virus, hepatitis B virus, and other bloodborne pathogens in health-care settings. *MMWR* 1988;37:377–382, 387–8.
53. Hughes JM. Universal precautions: CDC perspective. In: Becker CE, ed. *Occupational medicine: state of the art review. Occupational HIV infection: risks and risk reduction*, Vol. 4. Philadelphia: Hanley and Belfus, Inc., 1989:13–20.
54. Klein RS. Universal precautions for preventing occupational exposures to human immunodeficiency virus type 1. *Am J Med* 1991;90:141–4.
55. Marcus R, The Cooperative Needlestick Surveillance Group. Surveillance of health care workers exposed to blood from patients infected with human immunodeficiency virus. *N Engl J Med* 1988;319:1118–23.

56. CDC. Update: acquired immunodeficiency syndrome and human immunodeficiency virus infection among health-care workers. *MMWR* 1988;37:229–39.

57. Gershon RRM, Vlahov D, Nelson KE. The risk of transmission of HIV-1 through non-percutaneous, non-sexual modes—a review. *AIDS* 1990;4:645–50.

57a. Palca J. The case of the Florida dentist. *Science* 1992;255:392–4.

58. CDC. Recommendations for prevention of HIV transmission in health-care settings. *MMWR* 1987;36(suppl 2S):1S–18S.

59. Lombardo JM, Kloser PC, Pawel BR, Trost RC, Kapila R, St Louis ME. Anonymous human immunodeficiency virus surveillance and clinically directed testing in a Newark, NJ, hospital. *Arch Intern Med* 1991;151:965–8.

60. Kelen GD. Human immunodeficiency virus and the emergency department: risks and risk protection for health care providers. *Ann Emerg Med* 1990;19:242–8.

61. Linn LS, Kahn KL, Leake B. Physicians' perceptions about increased glove-wearing in response to risk of HIV infection. *Infect Control Hosp Epidemiol* 1990;11:248–54.

62. Korniewicz DM, Laughon BE, Cyr HW, Lytle CD, Larson E. Leakage of virus through used vinyl and latex examination gloves. *J Clin Microbiol* 1990;28:787–8.

63. Dalgleish AG, Malkovsky M. Surgical gloves as a mechanical barrier against human immunodeficiency viruses. *Br J Surg* 1988;75:171–2.

64. DeGroot-Kosolcharoen J. Pandemonium over gloves: use and abuse. *Am J Infect Control* 1991;19:225–7.

65. Kaczmarek RG, Moore RM Jr, McCrohan J, et al. Glove use by health care workers: results of a tristate investigation. *Am J Infect Control* 1991;19:228–32.

66. Stringer B, Smith JA, Scharf S, Valentine A, Walker MM. A study of the use of gloves in a large teaching hospital. *Am J Infect Control* 1991;19:233–6.

67. Timmerman T, Lawlar E, Reinhardt B. Health care facilities in a rural state: an examination of infection control policies. *Am J Infect Control* 1991;19:250–3.

68. Jagger J, Hunt EH, Pearson RD. Recapping used needles: is it worse than the alternative? *J Infect Dis* 1990;162:784–5.

69. Jagger J, Pearson RD. Universal precautions: still missing the point on needlesticks. *Infect Control Hosp Epidemiol* 1991;12:211–3.

70. Dashner FD, Habel H. HIV prophylaxis with punctured gloves? *Infect Control Hosp Epidemiol* 1988;9:184–6.

71. Eckersley JRT, Williamson DM. Glove punctures in an orthopaedic trauma unit. *Injury* 1990;21:177–8.

72. Tokars J, Bell D, Marcus R, et al. Percutaneous injuries during surgical procedures. 7th International Conference on AIDS, Florence, Italy, 1991;2:83(abst).

73. Wright JG, McGeer AJ, Chyatte D, Ransohoff DF. Mechanisms of glove tears and sharp injuries among surgical personnel. *JAMA* 1991;266:1668–71.

74. Kotilainen HR, Brinker JP, Avato JL, Gantz NM. Latex and vinyl examination gloves: quality control procedures and implications for health care workers. *Arch Intern Med* 1989;149:2749–53.

75. Makulowich GS. FDA establishes new quality standards for gloves. *AIDS Patient Care* 1991;5:143–5.

76. Zbitnew A, Greer K, Heise-Qualtiere J, Conly J. Vinyl versus latex gloves as barriers to transmission of viruses in the health care setting. *J Acquired Immune Deficiency Syndrome* 1989;2:201–4.

77. DeGroot-Kosolcharoen J, Jones JM. Permeability of latex and vinyl gloves to water and blood. *Am J Infect Control* 1989;17:196–201.

78. Mendelson MH, Short LJ, Dong JT, Solomon J, Meyers BR, Hirschman SZ. Analysis of sharps injuries at an 1100 bed teaching medical center: priorities for injury reducing devices. 31st Interscience Conference on Antimicrobial Agents and Chemotherapy, Chicago, Illinois 1991;261.

79. Kneer C, Sinnott J, Shaw K. Percutaneous and mucocutaneous exposure of third year medical students to blood and blood-tinged body fluids. 31st Interscience Conference on Antimicrobial Agents and Chemotherapy, Chicago, Illinois, 1991;261.

80. Tokars JI, Bell DM, Marcus R, et al. Glove use and blood–hand contacts (BHCs) during surgical procedures. 31st Interscience Conference on Antimicrobial Agents and Chemotherapy, Chicago, Illinois, 1991;261.

81. Lowenfels AB, Wormser GP, Jain R. Frequency of puncture injuries in surgeons and estimated risk of HIV infection. *Arch Surg* 1989;124:1284–6.

82. Nixon AD, Law R, Officer JA, Cleland JF, Goldwater PN. Simple device to prevent accidental needle-prick injuries. *Lancet* 1986;1:888–9.

83. Bowman AM, Nicholas TJ. Improving compliance with universal blood and body fluid precautions in a rural medical center. *J Nurs Qual Assur* 1990;5:73–81.

84. Fahey BJ, Koziol DE, Banks SM, Henderson DK. Frequency of nonparenteral occupational exposures to blood and body fluids before and after universal precautions training. *Am J Med* 1991;90:145–53.

85. Francioli P, Saghafi L, Raselli P. Exposure of health care workers (HCW) to blood during various procedures: results of two surveys before and after the implementation of universal precautions (UP). 6th International Conference on AIDS, San Francisco, 1990;1:275(abst).

86. Kelen GD, DiGiovanna TA, Celentano DD, et al. Adherence to universal (barrier) precautions during interventions on critically ill and injured emergency department patients. *J Acquired Immune Deficiency Syndrome* 1990;3:987–94.

87. Linnemann CC, Cannon C, DeRonde M, Lanphear B. Effect of educational programs, rigid sharps containers, and universal precautions on reported needlestick injuries in health care workers. *Infect Control Hosp Epidemiol* 1991;12:214–9.

88. LeF Porteous MJ. Operating practices of and precautions taken by orthopaedic surgeons to avoid infection with HIV and hepatitis B virus during surgery. *Br Med J* 1990;301:167–9.

89. Wong ES, Stotka JL, Chinchilli VM, Williams DS, Stuart CG, Markowitz SM. Are universal precautions effective in reducing the number of occupational exposures among health care workers: a prospective study of physicians on a medical service. *JAMA* 1991;265:1123–8.

90. Short LJ, Mendelson MH, Rosa M, Fallick N, Hirschman SZ. Economic implications of accidental needlestick injuries at a large urban hospital. 31st Interscience Conference on Antimicrobial Agents and Chemotherapy, Chicago, Illinois, 1991;261.

91. Stock SR, Gafni A, Bloch RF. Universal precautions to prevent HIV transmission to health care workers: an economic analysis. *Can Med Assoc J* 1990;142:937–46.

92. Gerberding J. Post-HIV exposure management: the San Francisco General Hospital experience. *AIDS Patient Care* 1990;4(Oct):22–4.

93. Sowa PE, Miller D. Administrative response to issues of health-care worker safety and HIV exposure. *Occup Med* 1989;4 (suppl):45–50.

94. LaFon SW, Lehrman SN, Barry DW. Prophylactically administered retrovir in health care workers potentially exposed to the human immunodeficiency virus. *J Infect Dis* 1988;158:503.

95. Ruprecht RM, O'Brien LG, Rossoni LD, Nusinoff-Lehram S. Suppression of mouse viraemia and retroviral disease by 3'-azido-3'-deoxythymidine. *Nature* 1986;323:467–9.

96. Tavaras L, Roneker C, Johnston K, Nusinoff-Lehman S, deNoronha F. 3'-azido-3'-deoxythymidine in feline leukemia virus-infected cats: a model for therapy and prophylaxis of AIDS. *Cancer Res* 1987;47:3190–4.

97. McCune JM, Namikawa R, Shih C-C, Rabin L, Kaneshima H. Suppression of HIV infection in AZT-treated SCID-hu mice. *Science* 1990;247:564–6.

98. CDC. Public health service statement on management of occupational exposure to human immunodeficiency virus, including considerations regarding zidovudine postexposure use. *MMWR* 1990;39:1–14.

99. Puro V, Ippolito G, The Italian Study Group on Occupational Risk of HIV Infection. AZT prophylaxis after occupational exposure to HIV in health care workers. 7th International Conference on AIDS, Florence, Italy, 1991;2:425(abst).

100. Puro V, Ippolito G. Zidovudine in post-exposure prophylaxis of health-care workers. *Lancet* 1990;335:1166–7.

101. Gerberding JL, Fahrner R, Berkvam G, Thibault K. Zidovudine postexposure chemoprophylaxis for health care workers exposed to human immunodeficiency virus at San Francisco General. 31st Interscience Conference on Antimicrobial Agents and Chemotherapy, Chicago, Illinois, 1991;55.

102. Toltzis P, Marx CM, Kleinman N, Levine EM, Schmidt EV. Zidovudine-associated embryonic toxicity in mice. *J Infect Dis* 1991;163:1212–8.

103. Shih C-C, Kaneshima H, Rabin L, et al. Postexposure prophylaxis with zidovudine suppresses human immunodeficiency virus type 1 infection in SCID-hu mice in a time-dependent manner. *J Infect Dis* 1991;163:625–7.

104. Sacks HS, Rose DN. Zidovudine prophylaxis for needlestick exposure to human immunodeficiency virus: a decision analysis. *J Gen Intern Med* 1990;5:132–7.

105. Miller RA. Zidovudine prophylaxis following exposure to human immunodeficiency virus. *J Gen Intern Med* 1990;5:265–7.

106. Gerberding JL, Marx P, Gould R, Joye S, Lackner A. Simian model of retrovirus chemoprophylaxis with constant infusion zidovudine ± interferon-alpha. 31st Interscience Conference on Antimicrobial Agents Chemotherapy, Chicago, Illinois, 1991;261.

107. Lange JMA, Boucher CAB, Hollak CEM, et al. Failure of zidovudine prophylaxis after accidental exposure to HIV-1. *N Engl J Med* 1990;322:1375–7.

108. Miller RA. Failure of zidovudine prophylaxis after exposure to HIV-1. *N Engl J Med* 1990;323:915–6.

109. Bernard N, Boulley A-M, Perol R, Rouzioux C, Foch CM-C. Failure of zidovudine prophylaxis after exposure to HIV-1. *N Engl J Med* 1990;323:916.

110. Lange JMA, Hollak CEM, Reiss P. Failure of zidovudine prophylaxis after exposure to HIV-1. *N Engl J Med* 1990;323:916.

111. Durand E, Jeunne CL, Hugues F-C. Failure of prophylactic zidovudine after suicidal self-inoculation of HIV-infected blood. *N Engl J Med* 1991;324:1062.

112. Fazely F, Haseltine WA, Rodger RF, Ruprecht RM. Postexposure chemoprophylaxis with ZDV or ZDV combined with interferon-alpha: failure after inoculating rhesus monkeys with a high dose of SIV. *J Acquired Immune Deficiency Syndrome* 1991;4:1093–7.

113. Occupational Safety and Health Administration. The proposed standard for bloodborne pathogens, 29 CFR 1910.1030. *Fed Reg* 1989;54:23134–9.

113a. Occupational Safety and Health Administration, Occupational exposure to bloodborne pathogens; final rule. *Fed Reg* 1991;56:64004–182.

114. Gerberding JL, Littell C, Tarkington A, Brown A, Schecter WP. Risk of exposure of surgical personnel to patients' blood during surgery at San Francisco General Hospital. *N Engl J Med* 1990;322:1788–93.

115. CDC. Update: transmission of HIV infection during an invasive dental procedure—Florida. *MMWR* 1991;40:21–33.

116. CDC. Update: transmission of HIV infection during invasive dental procedures—Florida. *MMWR* 1991;40:377–81.

117. Armstrong FP, Miner JC, Wolfe WH. Investigation of a health care worker with symptomatic human immunodeficiency virus infection: an epidemiologic approach. *Milit Med* 1987;152:414–8.

118. Mishu B, Schaffner W, Horan JM, Wood LH, Hutcheson RH, McNabb PC. A surgeon with AIDS: lack of evidence of transmission to patients. *JAMA* 1990;264:467–70.

119. Mishu B, Schaffner W. A surgeon with AIDS. *JAMA* 1990;264:3147–8.

120. Sacks JJ. AIDS in a surgeon. *N Engl J Med* 1985;313:1017–8.

121. Porter JD, Cruickshank JG, Gentle PH, Robinson RG, Gill ON. Management of patients treated by surgeon with HIV infection. *Lancet* 1990;335:113–4.

122. McNeary T, Westervelt P, Thielan BJ, et al. Limited sequence heterogenicity among biologically distinct human immunodeficiency virus type I isolates from individuals involved in a clustered infectious outbreak. *Proc Natl Acad Sci USA* 1990;87:1917–21.

123. Kleim JP, Ackermann A, Brackmann HH, Gahr M, Schneweis KE. Epidemiologically closely related viruses from hemophilia B

124. Cichutek K, Norley S, Linde R, et al. Lack of HIV-1 V3 region sequence diversity in two haemophiliac patients infected with a putative biologic clone of HIV-1. *AIDS* 1991;5:1185–7.

125. CDC. Recommended infection-control practices for dentistry. *MMWR* 1986;35:237–42.

126. Bell DM, Martone WJ, Culver DH, et al. Risk of endemic HIV and hepatitis B virus (HBV) transmission to patients during invasive procedures. 7th International Conference on AIDS, Florence, Italy, 1991;1:37(abst).

127. Lowenfels AB, Wormser GP. Transmission of HIV infection from surgeon to patient: estimating the risk. 7th International Conference on AIDS, Florence, Italy, 1991;1:37(abst).

128. Lowenfels AB, Wormser G. Risk of transmission of HIV from surgeon to patient. *N Engl J Med* 1991;325:888–9.

129. CDC. Recommendations for preventing transmission of human immunodeficiency virus and hepatitis B virus to patients during exposure-prone invasive procedures. *MMWR* 1991;40(RR-8):1–9.

130. Danila RN, MacDonald KL, Rhame FS, et al. A look-back investigation of patients of an HIV-infected physician: public health implications. *N Engl J Med* 1991;325:1406–11.

131. Goedert JJ, Weiss SH, Biggar RJ, et al. Lesser AIDS and tuberculosis. *Lancet* 1985;2:52.

132. CDC. Tuberculosis—United States, 1985—and the possible impact of human T-lymphotropic virus type III/lymphadenopathy-associated virus infection. *MMWR* 1986;35:74–6.

133. Sunderam G, McDonald RJ, Maniatis T, Oleske J, Kapila R, Reichman LB. Tuberculosis as a manifestation of the acquired immunodeficiency syndrome (AIDS). *JAMA* 1986;256:362–6.

134. Klein NC, Duncanson FP, Lenox TH, Pitta A, Cohen SC, Wormser GP. Use of mycobacterial smears in the diagnosis of pulmonary tuberculosis in AIDS/ARC patients. *Chest* 1989;95:1190–2.

135. Selwyn PA, Hartel D, Lewis VA, et al. A prospective study of the risk of tuberculosis among intravenous drug users with human immunodeficiency virus infections. *N Engl J Med* 1989;320:545–50.

136. DiPerri G, Cruciani M, Danzi MC, et al. Nosocomial epidemic of active tuberculosis among HIV-infected patients. *Lancet* 1989;2:1502–4.

137. CDC. Crack cocaine use among persons with tuberculosis—Contra Costa County, California, 1987–1990. *MMWR* 1991;40:485–9.

138. CDC. Purified protein derivative (PPD)-tuberculin anergy and HIV infection: guidelines for anergy testing and management of anergic persons at risk of tuberculosis. *MMWR* 1991;40:27–33.

139. Barnes PF, Bloch AB, Davidson PT, Snider DE Jr. Tuberculosis in patients with human immunodeficiency virus infection. *N Engl J Med* 1991;324:1644–50.

140. CDC. Tuberculosis outbreaks among persons in a residential facility for HIV-infected persons—San Francisco. *MMWR* 1991;40:649–52.

141. Colice GL. Decision analysis, public health policy, and isoniazid chemoprophylaxis for young adult tuberculin skin reactors. *Arch Intern Med* 1990;150:2517–22.

142. Steele MA, Burk RF, DesPrez RM. Toxic hepatitis with isoniazid and rifampin. A meta-analysis. *Chest* 1991;99:465–71.

143. Moulding T. Decision analysis, public health policy, and isoniazid chemoprophylaxis for young adult tuberculin skin reactors. *Arch Intern Med* 1991;151:2101–5.

144. CDC. Transmission of multidrug-resistant tuberculosis from an HIV-positive client in a residential substance-abuse treatment facility—Michigan. *MMWR* 1991;40:129–31.

145. CDC. Nosocomial transmission of multidrug-resistant tuberculosis among HIV-infected persons—Florida and New York, 1988–1991. *MMWR* 1991;40:585–91.

145a. CDC. Tuberculosis outbreaks among persons in a residential facility for HIV-infected persons—San Francisco. *MMWR* 1991;40:649–52.

145b. CDC. Tuberculosis among residents of shelters for the homeless—Ohio, 1990. *MMWR* 1991;40:869–77.

146. Robert-Guroff M, Weiss SH, Giron JA, et al. Prevalence of anti-

patients display high homology in two hypervariable regions of the HIV-1 *env* gene. *AIDS Res Hum Retroviruses* 1991;7:417–21.

bodies to HTLV-I, -II, and -III in intravenous drug abusers from an AIDS endemic region. *JAMA* 1986;255:3133–7.

147. Schrager LK. Bacterial infections in AIDS patients. *AIDS* 1988;2(suppl 1):S183–9.

148. Selwyn PA, Feingold AR, Hartel D, et al. Increased risk of bacterial pneumonia in HIV-infected intravenous drug users without AIDS. *AIDS* 1988;2:267–72.

149. Gellert G, Bock BV, Meyers H, Robertson C, Ehling LR. Penicillin-resistant pneumococcal meningitis in an HIV-infected man. *N Engl J Med* 1991;325:1047–8.

150. Jacobs JL, Libby DM, Winter RA, et al. A cluster of *Pneumocystis carinii* pneumonia in adults without predisposing illnesses. *N Engl J Med* 1991;324:246–50.

151. Jacobs JL, Libby DM, Hartmen BJ, Laurence J. *Pneumocystis carinii* pneumonia in adults without predisposing illnesses. *N Engl J Med* 1991;325:1314–5.

152. Haron E, Bodey GP, Luna MA, Dekmezian R, Elting L. Has the incidence of *Pneumocystis carinii* pneumonia in cancer patients increased with the AIDS epidemic. *Lancet* 1988;2:904–5.

153. Walzer PD. *Pneumocystis carinii*—new clinical spectrum? *N Engl J Med* 1991;324:263–5.

154. Oleske JM. Epidemiology and clinical aspects of HIV infection of children. American Public Health Association 119th Annual Meeting and Exhibit, Nov 13, 1991;195(abst).

155. O'Connor TW. Do patients have the right to infect their doctor? *Aust NZ J Surg* 1990;60:157–62.

156. Zuger A, Miles SH. Physicians, AIDS, and occupation risk: historic traditions and ethical obligations. *JAMA* 1987;258:1924–8.

AIDS and Other Manifestations of HIV Infection,
Second Edition, Edited by Gary P. Wormser.
Raven Press, Ltd., New York © 1992.

CHAPTER 37

Antiretroviral Chemotherapy

Robert T. Schooley

Antiretroviral chemotherapy is at a crossroads on the 10th anniversary of the initial description of the acquired immunodeficiency syndrome (AIDS). Over the past decade, the etiologic agent for AIDS, human immunodeficiency virus type-1 (HIV-1), has been isolated, and multiple isolates have been sequenced. Much has been learned at the molecular level about replicative and regulatory mechanisms of HIV-1. This knowledge, coupled with a deepening appreciation of HIV pathogenesis, has led to an increasing array of potential approaches to therapeutic intervention. At this writing, two antiretroviral drugs have been approved by the Food and Drug Administration. Another is likely to be approved before the end of 1992. The expansion of treatment IND programs, the increasing availability of drugs from "underground" sources, and the trend toward more widespread application of combination chemotherapy have added further complexity to management of the antiretroviral aspects of therapeutic regimens for individuals with HIV infection. This chapter outlines a reasonable current approach to antiretroviral chemotherapy and provides insight into the directions likely to be followed by the field over the next several years.

RATIONAL DESIGN OF ANTIRETROVIRAL CHEMOTHERAPEUTIC AGENTS

The rational development of antiretroviral chemotherapeutic compounds is based on the development of agents that are directed at aspects of the viral replicative cycle that are not shared by the host. In the case of HIV-1, additional complexity is added by the wide variety of cell types in which the virus replicates, artifacts that are introduced by the *in vitro* cultivation of the virus in continuous cell lines, and the highly error-prone process of

reverse transcription. The high rate of errors introduced into the replicative process results in major strain diversity at the population level and in a propensity in individual patients for the emergence of strains with reduced susceptibility to antiretroviral agents following prolonged exposure to antiviral drugs. Finally, HIV-1 poses unique problems of drug delivery, both in terms of general pharmacokinetic principles, which must take into account the probable need for the continuous maintenance of therapeutic levels of drug and the need for penetration of the central nervous system, and in terms of the intracellular site of action for many of the currently contemplated agents.

The initial step in replication of HIV-1 involves its use of the CD4 molecule as its major ligand for interaction of the viral envelope glycoprotein, gp120, with susceptible cells (1–3). This high-affinity interaction, which accounts for much of the selectivity of the virus for cells of the CD4 surface phenotype, has led to several major efforts directed at interfering with gp120–CD4 binding. Approaches directed at interfering with the gp120–CD4 interaction must now take into account the recently developed data, which indicate that alternative modes of entry into the cell may also be available to the virus, including involving the compound galactosyl ceramide in the case of the central nervous system (4).

After gaining entry into a susceptible cell, the virus is confronted with the problem of converting its genetic information, which is contained in two identical strands of single-stranded RNA, into double-stranded DNA. This conversion requires reverse transcription of the viral genomic RNA in the hostile milieu of the cellular cytoplasm. This reverse transcription is mediated by an RNA-dependent DNA polymerase known as reverse transcriptase. This enzyme has, so far, served as the major target of antiretroviral drug development. Inhibition of reverse transcription is the mechanism of action for all the nucleoside analogs currently approved or in development (zidovudine, dideoxyinosine, dideoxycytidine, and

R. T. Schooley: Infectious Disease Division, University of Colorado Health Sciences Center, Denver, Colorado 80262.

d4T), as well as for the new class of allosteric inhibitors, which have been called "TIBO" derivatives after the prototype compound of one of the members of this group (5). TIBO derivatives include the initially described Janssen drugs, as well as more recently described agents developed by Boehringer Ingelheim (BI-RG 587), Merck (L-697,661), and Upjohn (not yet named).

The double-stranded DNA that results from reverse transcription may exist in a free form within the cytoplasm of the cell for several days, or it may be integrated into the host cell DNA. Cellular activation favors integration, which is catalyzed by another viral enzyme termed integrase. Systems have been developed to screen for inhibitors of integrase activity, but no compounds have yet emerged from these screening attempts into later stages of drug development (6). After integration, the virus may remain within the host cell in latent form for long periods of time. Viral transcription is controlled by the long terminal repeat (LTR) sequence of the virus. Activation of the viral LTR sequence is, like integration, favored by cellular activation. HIV-1 has evolved a complex regulatory strategy to control its replication. This regulatory process includes several HIV-1 gene products that interact to control splicing and intracellular trafficking of viral RNA. *Tat* is an 86-kd protein that binds to a short segment of viral messenger RNAs (7,8). *Tat* binding segments of viral messenger RNAs, which are termed the trans-acting responsive (TAR) region, are located in the 5' end of all HIV-1 messenger RNAs. Binding of these segments by *tat* protein enhances the efficiency of viral replication by several thousandfold. Strategies for screening for *tat* inhibition have been developed by several laboratories. One group has synthesized a series of *tat* inhibitors, which entered clinical trials in late 1991.

Rev is another regulatory gene of HIV-1 which plays a critical role in determining the success of the virus in production of its structural genes, especially the viral envelope (9). *Rev* encodes a protein which binds to messenger RNA encoding the viral envelope and which is required for efficient translation of the viral envelope mRNA. No prototypic drugs have yet been developed that inhibit the action of the *rev* protein, but it is clear that both *tat* and *rev* will receive increasing attention as potential targets of both chemotherapeutic and genetic approaches to antiretroviral therapy.

Several other viral genes including *nef, vif, vpu,* and *vpr* with regulatory properties or properties affecting efficiency of cell-to-cell transmission of HIV have also been identified (10). At this point several investigative groups are attempting to delineate in more detail the function of these genes using molecular biological approaches. The recent demonstration of the importance of *nef* in determining the clinical virulence of simian immunodeficiency virus type 1 suggests that interference with the function of the *nef* gene product might pose an excellent target for antiretroviral drug development (11).

Translation of the viral gag–pol messenger RNA results in a large fusion polyprotein that must be cleaved into separate gag and pol proteins. This cleavage is mediated by a viral proteinase, which is located within the polyprotein near the gag–pol junction (12). This proteinase activity, which cleaves the large gag–pol fusion polyprotein into the polymerase component and into four separate gag polypeptides, is essential for the production of viral structural proteins that are capable of being assembled into infectious viral particles. Several groups have developed compounds that are capable of inhibiting the viral proteinase with a high degree of selectivity (13–16).

The envelope glycoprotein of HIV-1 is heavily glycosylated by cellular glycosidation enzymes. Inhibition of this process results in a significant reduction in viral infectivity (17,18). This approach has been demonstrated to be extremely effective *in vitro,* but because the target for such inhibition is cellular, rather than viral, in origin, clinical trials have not yet been reported which have demonstrated antiviral activity in the absence of unacceptable toxicity.

After synthesis of viral structural proteins has occurred, viral genomic RNA is packaged with the structural elements of the virus at the cell membrane. Viral packaging is a complex process that is dependent on the recognition of specific sequences within the RNA. Inhibition of this recognition process has been put forward as a potential antiviral strategy, but a practical means of achieving this goal has not yet been developed. Inhibition of packaging has also been hypothesized to be one of the sites of action of interferon-α, although it is not yet clear whether this is the primary mechanism by which interferons mediate antiretroviral activity (19). Evidence has been developed that the *vif* gene product plays a role in maintaining integrity of the viral particle and thus increasing the infectivity of the free viral particle (20).

Thus many potential steps in the viral replicative cycle have been identified that might serve as excellent candidates for the rational development of effective antiretroviral agents. This chapter focuses primarily on approaches that have progressed to clinical trials, namely, inhibition of binding or entry, reverse transcription, viral proteinase activity, glycosylation, and packaging.

INHIBITORS OF REVERSE TRANSCRIPTION

Up to now, the greatest success in the development of antiretroviral drugs has been derived from agents directed at inhibiting reverse transcription. The prototype drug in this class, zidovudine (AZT, Retrovir), made its debut as an antineoplastic agent in the 1960s and was resurrected as an antiretroviral drug in 1985. Zidovudine is capable of inhibiting HIV replication in cell lines at concentrations in the range of 0.1 μm. Zidovudine and the other nucleoside analogs currently in development as antiretroviral agents serve as competitive inhibitors of reverse transcription (Table 1). In each case these nucleoside analogs are taken up by cells susceptible to HIV infection and phosphorylated by kinases of the host cell to triphosphate derivatives of the parent compound. These nucleotides are incorporated by the reverse transcriptase enzyme as the viral RNA template is used to construct complementary DNA (Fig. 1). This incorporation prevents further elongation of the DNA and terminates reverse transcription. Thus, because such agents serve primarily to protect susceptible cells from initial infection with HIV, these agents have no effect on previously infected cells.

Zidovudine

Demonstration of Efficacy

Zidovudine was initially found to have antiretroviral activity against murine retroviruses in the 1960s (21). Broder and his colleagues noted that zidovudine also had activity against HIV-1 in tissue culture and initiated a small phase I escalating dose tolerance trial of zidovudine in individuals with advanced HIV infection in 1985 (22–24). This trial demonstrated that the drug could be tolerated in doses of up to 15–20 mg/kg/day, but that hematologic toxicity limited further dose escalation. Several subjects in the trial exhibited transient increases in the number of CD4 cells circulating in the peripheral blood.

Based on these results, a placebo-controlled trial was designed that subsequently enrolled 282 subjects with

TABLE 1. *Selected antiretroviral agents classified by putative mechanism of action*

A. Inhibitors of binding or entry
  1. Recombinant soluble CD4
  2. CD4/immunoglobulin conjugates
  3. Dextran sulfate
  4. Carbomethoxycarbonyl-pyrolyl-phenalanine esters (CPFs)
B. Reverse transcriptase inhibitors
  1. Nucleoside analogs
    a. Zidovudine (AZT, Retrovir)
    b. Dideoxycytidine (ddC)
    c. Dideoxyinosine (ddI, Didanosine)
    d. 3'-Deoxythymidin-2'-ene (d4T)
  2. Non-nucleoside analogs
    a. Tetrahydro-imidazol (4-5 1-j,k) (1,4) benzodiazepin-2-(1H)-one ("TIBO")
    b. Dipyridodiazepinone (BI-RG-587)
    c. Other pyridinone derivatives (L-697, 661)
    d. Foscarnet (Foscavir)
C. TAT inhibitors
D. Proteinase inhibitors
E. Glycosylation inhibitors
  1. Castanospermine
  2. *l*-deoxynojirimycin (*N*-butyl-DNJ)
F. Interferons

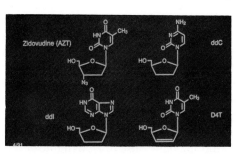

FIG. 1. Comparison of chemical structures of four nucleoside analog reverse transcriptase inhibitors: zidovudine (AZT), dideoxycytidine (ddC), dideoxyinosine (ddI), and 3'-deoxythymidin-2'-ene (d4T).

AIDS or advanced AIDS-related complex (ARC) (25). This trial chose the maximally tolerated zidovudine dose that had been determined with the phase I trial (1500 mg/day). This study was terminated by a Data Safety and Monitoring Board after 4 months when it became apparent that there was a significant excess in morbidity and mortality in study participants receiving placebo. In addition, the trial demonstrated a transient increase in CD4 cells in the peripheral blood of zidovudine recipients, as well as increases in Karnofsky scores and weight. Subsequently, when it became possible to quantitate HIV-1 p24 antigen in serum, an antiviral effect was also demonstrated among the zidovudine recipients in this study (26).

The initial placebo-controlled trial of zidovudine also exhibited significant toxicity. The major dose limiting toxicity was hematologic (28). Forty-five percent of study participants receiving zidovudine experienced hematologic toxicity; more than 30% of zidovudine recipients required transfusions. In addition to hematologic toxicity, zidovudine recipients were more likely to experience fatigue, anorexia, and mild to moderate headaches (27). This study resulted in approval of zidovudine by the Food and Drug Administration in July 1987, for individuals with AIDS or with symptoms of HIV infection and less than 200 CD4 cells/mm^3 in the peripheral blood. The participants in the initial placebo-controlled trial were offered the option to remain under observation on zidovudine. Almost all of the initial drug and placebo recipients opted to do so (28). Placebo recipients experienced a transient rise in CD4 cells and a decrease in the rate of HIV-related opportunistic infections at the time of zidovudine initiation. Survival of the study subjects after 21 months was roughly 60%. Additional long-term experience was generated from the expanded access IND program, which was initiated shortly after completion of the placebo-controlled trial (29).

Dose Modification and Extension to Earlier Stages of HIV Infection

The past 4 years have witnessed a host of clinical trials that have provided a better understanding of optimal dosing for zidovudine and that have extended its use to earlier phases of the illness. Shortly after the completion of the initial placebo-controlled trial, the NIH initiated the AIDS Clinical Trials Group (ACTG) network. Among the first studies of this program were three that provided important insights into both dosing of zidovudine and the utility of antiretroviral chemotherapy at earlier stages in the disease process. ACTG 002 compared a 1200-mg daily dose of zidovudine to a regimen that included a 6-week "induction" phase of 1500 mg daily followed by 100 mg every 4 hr (30). This study demonstrated that the higher dose of zidovudine conferred no advantages in terms of survival or prevention of recurrent *Pneumocystis carinii* pneumonia. Those receiving the lower daily dose of zidovudine were able to be maintained on zidovudine therapy for a significantly longer period of time than those randomized to the 1200-mg daily dose arm. On the basis of this trial and a subsequent dose-finding study in patients in earlier stages of the disease process (ACTG 019), the highest recommended daily dose of zidovudine was reduced to 500–600 mg daily. The zidovudine experience of selecting an excessive dose of zidovudine for large-scale clinical trials after limited phase I studies was the result of a dose-finding process based on the oncology model. When zidovudine was initially introduced into clinical trials, no technique was available for quantitating the antiretroviral effect of the drug *in vivo*. The zidovudine dose chosen for the initial placebo-controlled efficacy study was chosen on the basis of the maximal tolerated dose rather than on the basis of that required to demonstrate antiretroviral activity. This mistake, which was subsequently repeated with dideoxycytidine (ddC), resulted in significant excess toxicity in the phase I/II trials and greatly decreased the rate at which the drug was clinically accepted. More recently, a small pilot study conducted by Collier and her colleagues has demonstrated that serum levels of HIV-1 p24 antigen can be suppressed by as little as 300 mg of zidovudine daily (31). This study has been widely misquoted to indicate that equal clinical efficacy has been demonstrated at this dose of zidovudine as with the currently accepted 500–600-mg daily dose. It is important to emphasize that the Collier study was conducted with the primary goal of determining the dose of zidovudine that would be just below that which would decrease serum HIV-1 p24 antigen. This dose of zidovudine would subsequently be used in studies designed to examine whether synergistic interactions could be demonstrated between zidovudine and other antiretroviral agents. Participation in the Collier study was restricted by the FDA to individuals with more than 200 CD4 cells/mm³ and serum HIV-1 p24 antigen levels of more than 70 pg/ml. In this highly selected patient population, which included less than 70 participants, serum HIV p24 antigen levels were suppressed as effectively by 300 mg of zidovudine daily as by doses of up to 1200 mg daily. The study did not examine clinical

endpoints or include individuals with more advanced disease. At this point it is premature to conclude that the 300-mg daily dose of zidovudine used in the Collier study is equivalent to the currently recommended 500–600-mg daily dose in terms of clinical efficacy.

Two large-scale studies examined the role of zidovudine in individuals with less advanced disease (32,33). ACTG 016 enrolled 711 participants who had one or two early signs of HIV infection. These study participants were stratified into a group with more than 500 CD4 cells/mm³ at entry and a second group with 200–500 CD4 cells/mm³ and randomized to receive either 1200 mg of zidovudine daily or a placebo. This study was terminated when it was determined that study participants receiving placebo entering the trial with less than 500 CD4 cells/mm³ progressed to AIDS or late AIDS-related complex at roughly three times the rate of those receiving zidovudine. Too few individuals entered the study with more than 500 CD4 cells/mm³ to detect differences in the progression rate in this stratum of study participants.

A parallel study was also conducted that recruited 3200 asymptomatic HIV-infected individuals (33). This study had a similar design in that participants were randomized to receive zidovudine or placebo. In this study, however, individuals were stratified into a group with less than 200 CD4 cells/mm³ at entry, another with 200–500 CD4 cells/mm³, and a final group with more than 500 CD4 cells/mm³. Participants in each CD4 cell stratum were then randomized to received a placebo or one of two daily doses of zidovudine (500 or 1500 mg daily). This study demonstrated that zidovudine at either dose level decreased by half the rate of clinical progression to AIDS or advanced ARC among trial participants entering the study with less than 500 CD4 cells/mm³. In addition, zidovudine recipients experienced increases in the number of CD4 cells in the peripheral blood and a significant decrease in serum HIV-1 p24 antigen compared to the placebo recipients. Hematologic toxicity was significantly more likely (12%) in the 1500-mg daily dose group than in those receiving 500 mg daily (3%). On the basis of these data, the study was terminated for those who had entered the trial with less than 500 CD4 cells/mm³; these participants were offered zidovudine at 500 mg daily. Because there was no demonstrable difference in the clinical progression rate for those entering the study with more than 500 CD4 cells/mm³, these individuals remained on study in an effort to determine whether zidovudine decreased the rate at which CD4 cells reached 500/mm³. Because of the decreased hematologic toxicity of the 500-mg daily dose of drug, the 1500-mg/day-arm participants were reduced to 500 mg of zidovudine daily for the continuation phase of the study.

Taken together, these three studies established the current dosing regimen and patient populations for whom zidovudine is indicated. After completion of these studies, the recommended daily dose was decreased to

500–600 mg, and it was recommended that the use of the drug be extended to HIV-infected individuals with 500 or fewer CD4 cells/mm³, regardless of the presence of symptoms or signs of HIV infection. The ongoing continuation of ACTG 019 should provide insights as to whether antiretroviral chemotherapy will be useful in even earlier stages of the disease process. At this writing, one of the practical effects of the earlier use of zidovudine is that the rate of progression of HIV-associated morbidity has slowed. Thus, the rate of new AIDS cases previously projected by epidemiologic modeling has not been achieved (34,35). This new case rate deficit has been further increased by the widespread adoption of primary *Pneumocystis* prophylaxis (36) and has prompted a recent redefinition of AIDS for epidemiologic purposes (37).

Effects of Zidovudine on Other Manifestations of HIV Infection

Zidovudine has also been demonstrated to exhibit beneficial effects on several other complications of HIV infection. At the time the initial efficacy trials were being conducted, there was great concern that zidovudine might have positive effects on viral replication in the periphery, and thus lead to immune restoration and morbidity reduction, but yet that it would achieve insufficient levels in the central nervous system to reduce the impact of the virus there. This has not proved to be the case. In the initial placebo-controlled trial of zidovudine (26), an analysis of neuropsychological function demonstrated an improvement in cognitive function among zidovudine recipients (38). A more recently completed double-blinded randomized study of zidovudine in individuals with HIV encephalopathy as the major clinical manifestation of HIV infection has also demonstrated benefits of zidovudine in this setting (ACTG 005). This study indicated a slightly more beneficial effect with dosing of zidovudine as high as 2 g/day, but the number of individuals in each of the dosing arms of this study is insufficient to recommend this dose of zidovudine on a routine basis for AIDS-dementia complex. Indeed, as zidovudine has achieved wider use in the early phases of the disease process, epidemiologic surveys have indicated a decrease in the incidence of the AIDS-dementia complex (39).

Thrombocytopenia is commonly encountered in the setting of HIV infection (40). HIV-associated thrombocytopenia may be encountered in AIDS, or it may be the presenting manifestation of the illness in an individual who otherwise has no HIV-related symptoms (41). The mechanism(s) by which HIV causes thrombocytopenia remains to be fully elucidated. The two mechanisms that have received the most attention are direct involvement of platelet precursors in HIV-infected individuals (42) and an immune-based mechanism by which immune complexes bind to platelets and enhance clearance by the reticuloendothelial system (43,44). A number of approaches to the management of HIV-associated thrombocytopenia including corticosteroids (40,45), immune globulin (45), and splenectomy (40) have been used. Zidovudine has also been shown to be useful in the management of HIV-related thrombocytopenia in both open label (46–49) and crossover-designed studies (50).

Zidovudine has not proved useful as a primary therapy for Kaposi's sarcoma (51,52), despite anecdotal reports of regression of Kaposi's sarcoma with its use (53). Zidovudine has been combined with interferon-α in several clinical trials of the efficacy of this combination in the management of Kaposi's sarcoma (54,55). In this setting, hematologic toxicity may require dose reduction of the zidovudine to 300 mg daily, but in these trials individuals tolerating zidovudine and interferon-α frequently demonstrated both antitumor effects and rises in CD4 cells in the peripheral blood.

Zidovudine is not efficacious in the management of HIV-associated lymphoma and may complicate the hematologic toxicity of combination chemotherapy. A recent report from the National Cancer Institute raised concerns that prolonged nucleoside analog therapy for HIV infection might contribute to the development of non-Hodgkin's lymphoma (56). A much larger retrospective analysis has not confirmed this observation (57) and suggests a more likely alternative possibility, namely, that prolonged survival associated with antiretroviral chemotherapy and more effective management of HIV-associated opportunistic infections allows the development of lymphoma in individuals who previously would have succumbed to other HIV-related complications.

As noted earlier, zidovudine has been shown to decrease the incidence of HIV-associated opportunistic infections in several placebo-controlled trials (26,32,33). Anecdotal reports have noted the occurrence of temporary remissions of several HIV-associated opportunistic infections including cytomegalovirus retinitis (58), hairy leukoplakia (59,60), molluscum contagiosum (61), cryptosporidiosis (62), and progressive multifocal leukoencephalopathy (63). It is likely that these benefits are mediated in individual cases by partial restoration of pathogen-specific immune responses, although the drug itself has been demonstrated to have efficacy in a murine *E. coli* or *Salmonella dublin* model (64). Another setting in which reversal of the HIV-associated immune dysfunction by zidovudine has been of demonstrated utility is in the management of HIV-associated psoriasis (65,66).

Zidovudine in Children and Special Patient Populations

Zidovudine has also undergone extensive investigation in pediatric populations (67–70). These studies, which have included both continuous intravenous (67) and oral administration (68,69), have demonstrated similar effects of the drug on disease manifestations, immunologic function, and virologic activity (71) as that seen in adult populations. Because HIV infection has a particularly heavy impact on the neurologic and physical development in children, several of these studies have focused on the effects of zidovudine on neuropsychometric testing, CNS glucose metabolism (67,68), or physical growth (69). These studies have demonstrated both the utility of zidovudine in terms of these measures of HIV-associated morbidity and the suitability of these parameters in the assessment of efficacy of antiretroviral chemotherapy in clinical trials involving children.

A recently completed study of zidovudine among individuals with early HIV infection was reported by VA investigators to the Antiviral Advisory Panel to the Food and Drug Administration (72). The study design was altered several times during the trial due to the expanding clinical indications for zidovudine that resulted from ACTG studies 016 and 019, which were completed while the VA study was still underway. These design changes altered the initial objectives of the study and required that the final analysis compare early to late administration of zidovudine. This study revealed a decrease in the rate of occurrence of AIDS-defining opportunistic infections among zidovudine recipients, but a post hoc analysis revealed an apparent increase in the death rate of black and Hispanic study participants who received early zidovudine therapy. The apparent increase, however, included a significant number of deaths unrelated to AIDS, such as suicides and motor vehicle accidents. A much more extensive analysis of the survival experience of the HIV-infected population of Maryland between 1983 and 1989 has revealed survival benefits among minority group members who were treated with zidovudine (73). In this analysis, non-Hispanic whites had a more prolonged survival than minority group members, but this difference appeared to be primarily related to access to medical care. Thus, at this point, there is no evidence that there is a cultural difference in the responsiveness to antiretroviral chemotherapy.

Zidovudine Toxicity

The major dose-limiting toxicity of zidovudine is suppression of bone marrow function (27,32,33). Bone marrow toxicity is a function both of the stage of disease and the zidovudine dose. Dose-limiting anemia or granulocytopenia is unusual in asymptomatic individuals receiving 500 mg of zidovudine daily. In this setting, discontinuation of the drug or dose reduction is required in less than 3% of individuals (33). Hematologic toxicity in individuals with AIDS or late ARC taking 1200–1500 mg daily may occur in over one-third of cases (27).

As experience with granulocytopenia in the setting of HIV infection has accumulated, it has become clear that bacterial sepsis attributable to granulocytopenia is seen less frequently than might be expected from the experiences with cytotoxic chemotherapy. Thus it is often reasonable to tolerate granulocyte counts of 500–750/mm^3 in the setting of HIV infection. Zidovudine-related bone marrow toxicity is almost always reversible (74). Management of an initial bout of granulocytopenia is approached by withholding the drug temporarily and resuming therapy at a lower dose (generally 300 mg daily). In individuals in whom the granulocyte count does not recover over the course of 7–10 days, consideration should be given to other possible causes for the granulocytopenia, including other drugs or involvement of the bone marrow with an infectious organism such as *Mycobacterium avium-intracellulare.*

If the granulocytopenia recurs after resumption of reduced dose zidovudine, alternative antiviral agents such as dideoxyinosine (ddI) or dideoxycytidine (ddC) should be considered. At this writing, ddI has been approved by the FDA and is available through an expanded use Investigational New Drug (IND) program. It is likely that ddC will be approved for zidovudine-intolerant individuals before the end of 1992.

If the granulocytopenia persists despite replacement of zidovudine with ddC or ddI, another option involves the use of granulocyte monocyte–colony stimulating factor (GM-CSF)(75–77) or granulocyte colony stimulating factor (G-CSF) (78). Although both GM-CSF and G-CSF stimulate production of granulocytes, G-CSF is generally better tolerated than GM-CSF and does not have the theoretical concern that has been raised about stimulation of HIV-1 replication with GM-CSF (79).

Zidovudine administration is associated with macrocytosis in virtually all individuals who take the drug for more than 6 weeks; this has been used as an indicator of compliance in blinded controlled trials of zidovudine (33). Anemia, like granulocytopenia, is a dose-related toxicity that occurs more frequently in individuals with more advanced disease. If anemia is encountered in the setting of zidovudine therapy, other causes of anemia, such as hemolysis or bone marrow suppression from other drugs or infection involving the marrow, should be ruled out. If dose reduction of zidovudine to 300 mg daily does not lead to stabilization of the hematocrit at an acceptable level, substitution of ddI or ddC should be considered. Erythropoietin is preferable to transfusions for those who are not able to maintain an acceptable hematocrit (80).

In addition to bone marrow toxicity, zidovudine is also associated with several subjective complaints. In the initial randomized placebo-controlled trial of zidovudine, anorexia, mild to moderate headaches, and insomnia were reported significantly more frequently by zidovudine recipients than by those receiving placebo. In practice, anorexia and headache are the subjective complaints that most frequently trouble patients to the extent that discontinuation of the drug is contemplated. In most cases these symptoms subside despite continuation of the drug over the first 2–3 weeks of therapy. In situations in which anorexia, nausea, or headache are particularly troublesome, symptomatic relief may be offered with antiemetics, aspirin, or nonsteroidal anti-inflammatory agents.

Zidovudine is rarely associated with confusion or more serious alteration of consciousness (81–83). The mechanism for this complication of zidovudine therapy has not been delineated, but it is more frequently seen in individuals with underlying CNS dysfunction or in individuals who are taking other drugs with CNS effects. A final toxicity that has been reported with zidovudine is a myositis-like syndrome (28,84) that is associated with muscle tenderness and wasting. It has been hypothesized that this complication of zidovudine therapy is a manifestation of inhibitory effects of zidovudine on mitochondrial DNA polymerase (85).

Drug Interactions

Zidovudine undergoes glucuronidation in the liver. Zidovudine and zidovudine glucuronide are both excreted by the kidney. The hepatic metabolism of zidovudine coupled with an apparent increased rate of hematologic toxicity in zidovudine recipients who also received acetaminophen in controlled trials (27) raised concerns about adverse interactions between acetaminophen and zidovudine. This was not confirmed in a subsequent study (86). The major adverse drug interactions involve zidovudine and other agents that suppress the bone marrow such as interferons (54,55), ganciclovir (87–89), or cytotoxic chemotherapeutic agents.

Decreased Susceptibility of HIV-1 Isolates to Zidovudine

Over the past 2 years it has become apparent that prolonged therapy with zidovudine is associated with an increased rate of isolation of HIV-1 with decreased *in vitro* susceptibility to zidovudine (90). This was first demonstrated by Richman and colleagues, who obtained serial viral isolates from participants in the initial placebo-controlled study of zidovudine (25,27). A subsequent *in vitro* analysis revealed a progressive decrease in zidovudine susceptibility in isolates of HIV-1 obtained 12–18 months after initiation of zidovudine therapy. Isolates obtained from two trial participants after this period of therapy were 100–1000-fold less susceptible to zidovudine in an *in vitro* plaque-forming assay than were isolates obtained prior to the initiation of therapy. Subsequent studies revealed that the decreased susceptibility to zidovudine is associated with the stepwise appearance

of mutations of four amino acids of the reverse transcriptase enzyme (91). Isolates of HIV-1 with reduced susceptibility to zidovudine exhibit cross-resistance to 3'-azido-2',3'-dideoxyuridine (AZdu), but not to non-azido group containing nucleoside analog antiretroviral drugs, such as ddC, ddI, or d4T, or to drugs with other mechanisms of antiretroviral activity (92). Other investigative groups have confirmed and extended these findings (93–95), and a polymerase-chain-reaction-based assay for detection of genotypic changes in *pol* associated with the resistant phenotype has been developed (95). Recently, isolates of HIV-1 that exhibit decreased susceptibility to dideoxyinosine have been obtained from patients receiving ddI (96,97). ddI resistance has been detected primarily among isolates obtained from individuals who were first treated for a prolonged period with zidovudine, after which ddI was administered as monotherapy. In one of these reports, the ddI resistance was associated with an amino acid change in the viral reverse transcriptase at a position remote from those that conferred zidovudine resistance. The change related to ddI resistance was associated with restoration of susceptibility to zidovudine (97). It has been demonstrated that the rate at which isolates with decreased *in vitro* zidovudine susceptibility emerge is a function of disease stage (98). This is presumably a reflection of increased viral load in individuals with more advanced immunodeficiency (99–101).

The clinical significance of the emergence of viral isolates with reduced *in vitro* susceptibility to zidovudine is unclear. It has not yet been possible to relate *in vitro* susceptibility of HIV-1 to progressive clinical disease. It is not clear whether this difficulty is a reflection of a true lack of relationship between susceptibility to antiretroviral drugs and disease progression or is merely due to imprecision in quantitating progression of clinical disease. Several large-scale randomized clinical trials are currently underway which should help address this issue. At present, however, there are no data to support the routine use of *in vitro* susceptibility testing in the management of individual patients, or to arbitrarily change antiretroviral agents after individuals have been treated for a specific period of time.

Use of Zidovudine Following Nosocomial Exposure

Transmission of HIV-1 to health-care workers after percutaneous or mucosal exposure to virus-containing material is infrequent (102,103). The administration of zidovudine has been recommended after "significant" nosocomial exposure to HIV-1 (104). Such recommendations have been made despite several anecdotal reports of the failure of postexposure prophylaxis to prevent infection (105–107), and the absence of animal model data that administration of drug after viral exposure prevents infection (108). Prevention of infection by administering therapy after exposure is a formidable task. The therapeutic agents currently available merely prevent infection of uninfected cells and must be present in the cytoplasm as triphosphate derivatives of the parent compound at the time of reverse transcription. In addition, many hospitalized patients from whom the infectious virus might have arisen are likely to be in the later stages of infection and thus to have had extensive zidovudine experience. Therefore it is possible that prophylaxis will be compromised by the fact that the transmitted virus will exhibit less susceptibility to the agent used for prophylaxis. Nonetheless, it is prudent to offer zidovudine after significant nosocomial exposure for several reasons. First, anecdotal reports of transmission following postexposure treatment with zidovudine do not address whether the incidence of infection is decreased by prophylaxis. Second, it is possible that, while early therapy might not prevent infection, a decrease in the early burst of viral replication in the setting of primary infection might be of benefit to the host (109,110). Finally, and perhaps most important, the establishment of a comprehensive postexposure counseling and testing service is essential from the standpoint of employee support and of risk management.

Dideoxycytidine (ddC)

Dideoxycytidine (ddC) is another nucleoside analog with potent and selective antiretroviral activity (111). The agent is roughly tenfold more active against HIV-1 *in vitro* than is zidovudine. As with the case with zidovudine, ddC must be phosphorylated intracellularly by cellular kinases (112). Preclinical studies with ddC revealed that the drug exhibited significantly less hematopoietic toxicity than zidovudine. These findings prompted an escalating dose tolerance trial of ddC, which revealed that the drug exhibited antiviral effects in vivo, as ascertained by decreases in the serum HIV-1 p24 antigen levels, however, significant dose-related toxicities were encountered (113,114). These included painful peripheral neuropathy, oral ulcerations, a cutaneous eruption, and thrombocytopenia (Table 2). A larger multicenter dose-ranging study was subsequently completed that further refined the relationships among ddC dosage, effects on

surrogate markers for antiviral activity, and toxicity (115). This study revealed that daily doses of ddC in the range of 0.005–0.01 mg/kg/day were required for suppression of serum HIV-1 p24 antigen. Peripheral neuropathy was encountered in all patients receiving 0.01 mg/kg/day; the neuropathy was so severe at doses of 0.03 mg/kg/day that discontinuation of medication was frequently required at this dose level. Fewer patients receiving 0.005 mg/kg/day or less required dose modification. Thus this study confirmed the smaller pilot efficacy study conducted at the National Cancer Institute but documented an extremely limited therapeutic index for ddC.

The neuropathy associated with ddC may be relatively sudden in onset and may be extremely severe (116). Nonetheless, it is almost always reversible if the drug is discontinued promptly. Patients usually note the bilaterally symmetrical onset of painful paresthesias, which are burning in character. These paresthesias may progress to be almost incapacitating if drug administration is continued and may progress to motor involvement. This toxicity, which has proved to be dose-limiting very near the threshold for demonstration of efficacy using surrogate virologic markers, has raised the strong probability that therapeutic uses of ddC will be reserved primarily for combination chemotherapy (117,118) or for salvage therapy for individuals who are failing or intolerant of other forms of therapy (119).

Dideoxyinosine (ddI)

Dideoxyinosine (ddI) is another nucleoside analog with antiretroviral activity *in vitro,* which followed zidovudine and ddC into clinical trials in 1988 (120). ddI administration was associated with decreases in viral HIV-1 p24 antigen, decreased proviral HIV-1 DNA in peripheral blood mononuclear cells, and increased numbers of CD4 cells in the initial dose-finding studies (120–123). ddI administration was associated with increases in the serum uric acid level but exhibited no significant bone marrow toxicity. The major dose-limiting toxicities associated with ddI administration were pancreatitis and a peripheral neuropathy similar to that seen in the ddC experience. ddI has a serum half-life of 30–90 min, but

TABLE 2. *Pharmacologic characteristics and toxicities of nucleoside analog reverse transcriptase inhibitors*

Agent	Terminal serum $T_{1/2}$	Intracellular triphosphate $T_{1/2}$	Major toxicities
Zidovudine (AZT, Retrovir)	45–60 min	3 hr	Granulocytopenia, anemia, nausea, headaches, confusion, myositis
Dideoxyinosine (ddI, Didanosine)	65–75 min	12 hr	Pancreatitis, peripheral neuropathy, nausea, diarrhea, confusion
Dideoxycytidine (ddC)	35–40 min	3 hr	Peripheral neuropathy, stomatitis, cutaneous eruption, thrombocytopenia, pancreatitis

the intracellular half-life of the active metabolite of ddI, dideoxyadenosine triphosphate, is several hours (Table 2) (124,125). The prolonged intracellular half-life of ddI has prompted the 8 to 12 hr dosing regimen that has been used in most of the phase II/III clinical trials. Indeed, considerations of the issue of the half-life of the active intracellular metabolite from the standpoint of ddI pharmacokinetics has led to reconsideration of zidovudine dosing. Many American practitioners have altered zidovudine prescribing practices to follow the European 8-hr dosing regimen.

ddI was approved by the Food and Drug Administration for individuals who are intolerant of zidovudine or who are exhibiting disease progression despite zidovudine therapy. The extensive clinical experience that has been gained with ddI both in long-term clinical trials (126) and in the expanded access treatment IND program has revealed that the major toxicity to ddI requiring discontinuation of therapy is pancreatitis, which can be associated with death (127). The experience in pediatric populations is very similar to that in adults in terms of both efficacy and toxicity (128–130). In the expanded access program, pancreatitis associated with ddI was much more frequently encountered in individuals with prior pancreatitis or with clinical or immunologic evidence of advanced disease. Neuropathy is also reported with ddI and may be rapidly encountered in individuals who have experienced ddC-associated neuropathy (129). Other reported toxicities of ddI include encephalopathy, seizures (128), optic neuritis (131), hypokalemia, and hepatitis (132).

The final niche for ddI has not yet been determined. It is clear that favorable clinical and immunologic responses may be seen in individuals who appear to be exhibiting advancing disease on zidovudine (133). ddI exhibits antiviral synergy *in vitro* with zidovudine (134), dipyridamole (135), ribavirin (136), and CD4 *Pseudomonas* exotoxin (137). Pilot clinical trials of the combined use of ddI and zidovudine have revealed no adverse interactions between the two agents (138). It is likely that the drug will initially be used in individuals who are intolerant of or clinically failing on zidovudine therapy, or in combination with other antiretroviral agents. Two large-scale clinical trials currently underway within the ACTG network (ACTG 116, ACTG 117) should establish the proper use of ddI as monotherapy in individuals who have not been treated with other therapy, or who have not exhibited drug intolerance or disease progression on zidovudine therapy.

3'-Deoxythymidin-2'-ene (d4T)

3'-Deoxythymidin-2'-ene (d4T) is entering phase II/III studies at this writing. This agent exhibits significant antiretroviral activity *in vitro* (139–141) and is less cyto- toxic to bone marrow progenitor cells *in vitro* than is zidovudine (142). Preliminary clinical trial experience has revealed that peripheral neuropathy and hepatitis may be associated with administration of d4T, but much more extensive trials will be required to determine the full therapeutic and toxicity profiles of d4T.

Non-nucleoside-Based Reverse Transcriptase Inhibitors

Several investigative groups have independently discovered a series of compounds that exhibit potent inhibitory activity against the HIV-1, but not the HIV-2, reverse transcriptase enzyme (5,143,144). The agents have been referred to as "TIBO" drugs, after the abbreviation for the initially described drug in this class: tetrahydroimidazol (4-5 1-jk) (1,4) benzodiazepin-2-(1H)-one. These compounds are superficially quite dissimilar in terms of structure but appear to exert antiretroviral activity by the same allosteric mechanism of action. Each group of agents is extremely selective for HIV-1. The agents exhibit activity against clinical strains of HIV-1, including those that show reduced zidovudine susceptibility (145). TIBO drugs exhibit synergistic antiretroviral activity with nucleoside analog antiretroviral agents (146). These drugs have entered clinical trials, but reports of safety, tolerance, and efficacy have not yet appeared.

Foscarnet (phosphonoformate, PFA) is a pyrophosphase analog that exhibits activity against both retroviruses and herpes group viruses, including cytomegalovirus (147,148). The antiretroviral activity is mediated by inhibition of reverse transcriptase activity (149) and is demonstrable *in vitro* at concentrations of drug in serum which are attainable following intravenous administration (150,151). Although suppression of serum HIV-1 p24 antigen has been demonstrated in clinical trials (152,153), this activity has required intravenous administration of the drug. The poor absorption of foscarnet after oral administration (154) limits its potential clinical utility except in selected settings.

INHIBITORS OF VIRAL ENTRY

Binding of HIV-1 to the CD4 molecule plays a central role in viral entry (1–3). This feature of the virus–host interaction has led to the development of several strategies designed to inhibit this event. Several groups independently demonstrated that the N-terminal region of the CD4 molecule produced by recombinant DNA technology is a potent inhibitor of HIV-1 replication in vitro (155–159). The demonstration of in vitro antiretroviral activity led to two escalating dose tolerance trials of recombinant soluble CD4, (rsCD4) (160,161). Each trial demonstrated that rsCD4 was well tolerated in doses of up to 1 mg/kg/day and could be administered by the intramuscular, subcutaneous, or intravenous route. Although serum levels of rsCD4 approached concentrations of the agent that were capable of inhibiting the LAI strain of HIV-1 *in vitro,* evidence of biologic activity of the compound *in vivo* was lacking (160,161). This apparent discrepancy led to a reevaluation of the *in vitro* activity of receptor-based therapies against HIV-1 (162). These studies revealed that clinical isolates of HIV-1 are 100–1000-fold less sensitive to rsCD4 and other CD4-directed therapeutic agents than are isolates of HIV-1, which have been propagated for prolonged periods *in vitro* in T-cell lines. This major difference in susceptibility of clinical isolates of HIV-1 to rsCD4 has dampened enthusiasm for this drug as an agent that will be used alone in the therapy of HIV-1.

Several modifications to the rsCD4 molecule have been undertaken in an effort to confer better pharmacokinetic properties (163,164) or to change the basic therapeutic approach to use CD4–gp120 binding as a tool to target toxins to HIV-1 infected cells (165–167). Fusion of the N-terminal region of CD4 to the Fc portion of IgG (163), or of IgM (164), results in significant prolongation of the serum half-life of the molecule. These fusion molecules are, however, no more active against clinical isolates of HIV-1 than is the parent rsCD4 molecule (162). To date, the only evidence of *in vivo* activity with the IgG–CD4 fusion molecule includes a rise in the platelet count exhibited by HIV-1-infected patients treated with IgG–CD4 (168). Another approach that has been demonstrated to have antiviral activity *in vitro* is the fusion of CD4 to *Pseudomonas* exotoxin (165) or ricin (166). Each approach has demonstrated that these fusion molecules are able to kill cells exhibiting the HIV-1 gp120 molecule on the surface selectively, but the approach fails to take into account that most HIV-1-infected cells *in vivo* do not express HIV antigens (99). When cells do express HIV-1 antigens *in vivo,* they become targets for attack by the virus-specific host immune response (169,170). In addition, toxin-based therapies employed in the treatment of malignancy have revealed that these molecules have inherent toxicity and that antibodies to the foreign protein emerge with ongoing therapy. These practical problems, coupled with the fact that most HIV-1-infected cells *in vivo* do not express viral antigen at any given point in time, greatly temper enthusiasm for this therapeutic approach.

Other receptor-based approaches have included AL721 (171), dextran sulfate (172), and the newly described carbomethoxycarbonyl-pyrolyl-phenalanine esters (CPFs) (173). AL721 underwent a period of interest and was available on the underground market for several years based on a single report of *in vitro* antiretroviral activity (171). Subsequent efforts to confirm these *in vitro* observations in several laboratories were unsuccessful. Dextran sulfate and other high molecular weight polyanions interfere with absorption of DNA and RNA viruses to target cells (172,174,175). On the basis of these observations, a phase I trial of oral dextran sulfate was initiated by the NIAID AIDS Clinical Trials Group in 1988 (176). This study revealed that administration of the compound was associated with gastrointestinal complaints and hepatic transaminase elevations and failed to demonstrate any evidence of biologic activity *in vivo.* This lack of activity is likely due to the absence of significant gastrointestinal absorption of dextran sulfate.

Finberg and colleagues have developed a class of compounds termed CPFs, which are small phenylalanine-containing peptides (173). These compounds are based on a mutational analysis of CD4, which emphasized the likely importance of the binding of the Phe[43] of CD4 to HIV-1 gp120. This class of compounds exhibits potent antiretroviral activity *in vitro* but is highly hydrophobic. The impact of the hydrophobicity in the potential clinical utility of these compounds remains to be determined.

PROTEINASE INHIBITORS AND OTHER MODIFIERS OF POST-TRANSLATIONAL PRODUCTS

As noted earlier, the HIV-1 gag–pol fusion polyprotein is cleaved by a viral proteinase (protease) that is contained within the gag–pol polyprotein (12). The viral protease enzyme has been expressed in *E. coli* and found to be a dimeric aspartic protease (177,178). The definition of structure–activity relationships for the viral protease (179,180) has greatly enhanced insights into mechanisms of action of this enzyme, and into directed approaches to the development of inhibitors. Several investigative groups have developed prototypic compounds that inhibit the HIV-1 protease and that exhibit significant antiretroviral activity *in vitro* (13–16). HIV-1 protease inhibitors entered phase I clinical studies in 1991.

The envelope glycoprotein of HIV-1 undergoes extensive glycosylation by cellular enzymes (17,18). Several compounds, including castanospermine and l-deoxynojirimycin (*N*-butyl-DNJ), have been demonstrated to inhibit glycosylation of HIV-1 *in vitro,* which causes a decrease in viral infectivity (17,18,181,182). *N*-butyl DNJ has entered phase I clinical trials, but no reports of *in vivo* activity or toxicity have emerged.

The mechanism(s) of action of interferon against HIV-1 has been postulated to involve packaging of the virus. Interferon-α, -β, and -γ are active *in vitro* against HIV-1 in concentrations that can be achieved pharmacologically (19,183). Interferon-α has been studied extensively in the context of therapy for Kaposi's sarcoma (184,185). An early study of interferon-α in late-stage patients with HIV-1 infection demonstrated neither beneficial clinical nor immunologic effects (186), but two more recent studies with higher doses of interferon-α in patients with Kaposi's sarcoma have demonstrated antiviral activity of interferon-α among individuals who also exhibited an antitumor response (187,188). The demonstration of synergistic antiviral activity *in vitro* between interferon-α and zidovudine (189), ddC (190), or foscarnet (191) has stimulated the design of several ongoing studies of interferon in conjunction with other antiretroviral agents. Results of these trials should be available over the next 12–24 months.

COMBINATION ANTIRETROVIRAL CHEMOTHERAPY

Over the past several years, increasing attention has been directed toward combination chemotherapy. This approach is attractive for several conceptual reasons. The first is the possibility that concurrent use of two or more antiretroviral agents will exhibit increased antiviral activity. Second, the demonstration of emergence of resistant strains of HIV-1 following prolonged monotherapy with zidovudine (90,93–95) or ddI (96,97) has greatly increased interest in the use of combination chemotherapy as a means to retard the development of resistance to antiviral agents. Third, reduction in the dose-related toxicities associated with currently used agents (28,113,115,125,126) would be desirable if equivalent antiviral activity could be demonstrated with lower doses of antiretroviral agents. Finally, pharmacokinetic considerations such as issues related to tissue tropism, serum half-life, or CNS penetration might suggest combination regimens that would exhibit increased effectiveness over single-agent regimens.

As the number of antiretroviral agents grows, the number of possible combinations of antiretroviral drugs will also proliferate exponentially, especially as combinations of three or more drugs are considered (192). The planning of antiretroviral regimens should rest on firm rationale and *in vitro* data. Although it has been suggested that combination regimens might be optimal if different steps in the viral life cycle are targeted, in fact, combinations of reverse transcriptase inhibitors such as zidovudine and ddI (193) or zidovudine and L-697,661 (145) may also exhibit considerable additive or synergistic antiretroviral activity. It is also important to emphasize that some combinations of antiretroviral agents are antagonistic, as has been demonstrated with zidovudine and ribavirin (194).

Clinical trials of combination chemotherapy may include either sequential (195) or concurrent (138, 196–198) designs. In general, selection of agents with nonoverlapping toxicities should permit concurrent, rather than sequential, administration of antiretroviral drugs. Combinations of zidovudine and ddC (138) and zidovudine and ddI (196) have been shown to be well tolerated in phase I/II clinical trials and to exhibit evi-

dence of *in vivo* activity as manifested by decreases in serum HIV-1 p24 antigen and increases in circulating CD4 cells. The clinical investigation of combination regimens from the standpoint of clinical endpoints is a resource-intensive endeavor that will require careful planning over the next several years.

SUMMARY

At present, two antiretroviral drugs (zidovudine and ddI) have been approved by the FDA. Over the past several years, clinical studies have resulted in a decrease in the recommended dose of zidovudine to 500–600 mg/day and have demonstrated its clinical utility in HIV-infected individuals at earlier stages of the disease process. These trials have outlined the long-term toxicity profile of zidovudine and have begun to provide insights into problems related to the emergence of drug-resistant isolates. Two additional nucleoside analog reverse transcriptase inhibitors (ddC and ddI) have demonstrated beneficial effects on surrogate markers of viral replication. ddI was approved by the FDA in October 1991; ddC is likely to be approved by the FDA within the next 6–12 months. An array of additional antiretroviral agents with several other mechanisms of action entered phase I/II clinical trials in 1991. The availability of these agents, coupled with an increased understanding of the resistance problem of HIV-1 to antiretroviral drugs, will increase the momentum that is developing toward the widespread application of combination antiretroviral chemotherapy.

REFERENCES

1. Klatzmann D, Champagne E, Chamaret S, et al. T-lymphocyte T4 molecule behaves as the receptor for human retrovirus LAV. *Nature* 1984;312:767–8.
2. Dalgleish AG, Beverley PC, Clapham PR, Crawford DH, Greaves MF, Weiss RA. The CD4 (T4) antigen is an essential component of the receptor for the AIDS retrovirus. *Nature* 1984;312:763–7.
3. McDougal JS, Kennedy MS, Sligh JM, Cort SP, Mawle A, Nicholson JK. Binding of HTLV-III/LAV to T4+ T cells by a complex of the 110K viral protein and the T4 molecule. *Science* 1986;231:382–5.
4. Harouse JM, Bhat S, Spitalnik SL, et al. Inhibition of entry of HIV-1 in neural cell lines by antibodies against galactosyl ceramide. *Science* 1991;253:320–3.
5. Pauwels R, Andires K, Desmyter J, et al. Potent and selective inhibition of HIV-1 replication *in vitro* by a novel series of TIBO derivatives. *Nature* 1990;343:470–4.
6. Bushman FD, Fujimara T, Cragie R. Retroviral DNA integration directed by HIV integration protein *in vitro. Science* 1990;249:1555–8.
7. Dayton AI, Sodroski JG, Rosen CA, Goh WE, Haseltine WA. The *trans*-activator gene of the human T cell lymphotropic virus type III is required for replication. *Cell* 1986;44:941–7.
8. Sadaie MR, Benter T, Wong-Stahl F. Site directed mutagenesis of two *trans*-regulatory genes (*tat*-III, *trs*) of HIV-1. *Science* 1988;239:910–13.
9. Feinberg MB, Jarrett F, Aldovini A, Gallo RC, Wong-Stahl F. HTLV III expression and production involve complex regulation at the levels of splicing and translation of viral RNA. *Cell* 1986;46:807–17.

10. Haseltine WA. Development of antiviral drugs for the treatment of AIDS: strategies and prospects. *J AIDS* 1989;2:311–34.
11. Kestler HW, Ringler DJ, Mori K, et al. Importance of the *nef* gene for maintenance of high virus loads and for development of AIDS. *Cell* 1991;65:651–62.
12. Kohl NE, Emini EA, Schleif WA, et al. Active human immunodeficiency virus protease is required for viral infectivity. *Proc Natl Acad Sci USA* 1988;85:4686–90.
13. Kotler M, Katz RA, Danho W, Leis J, Skalka AM. Synthetic peptides as substrates and inhibitors of a retroviral protease. *Proc Natl Acad Sci USA* 1988;85:4185–89.
14. Erickson J, Neidhart PJ, VanDrie J, et al. Design, activity, and 2.8Å crystal structure of a C_2 symmetric inhibitor complexed to HIV-1 protease. *Science* 1990;249:527–33.
15. Navia MA, Fitzgerald PM, McKeever BM, et al. Three-dimensional structure of aspartyl protease from human immunodeficiency virus HIV-1. *Nature* 1989;337:615–20.
16. Grinde B, Hungnes O, Tjotta E. The proteinase inhibitor pepstatin A inhibits formation of reverse transcriptase in H9 cells infected with human immunodeficiency virus-1. *AIDS Res Hum Retroviruses* 1989;5:269–74.
17. Walker BD, Kowalski M, Goh WC, et al. Inhibition of human immunodeficiency virus syncytium formation and virus replication by castanospermine. *Proc Natl Acad Sci USA* 1987;84: 8120–4.
18. Gruters RA, Neejfes JJ, Tersmette M, et al. Interference with HIV-induced syncytium formation and viral infectivity by inhibitors of trimming glucosidase. *Nature* 1987;330:74–7.
19. Ho DD, Hartshorn KL, Rota TR, et al. Recombinant human interferon alpha-A suppresses HTLV-III replication *in vitro*. *Lancet* 1985;1:602–4.
20. Fischer AG, Ensoli B, Ivanott L, et al. The *sor* gene of HIV-1 is required for efficient virus transmission *in vitro*. *Science* 1987;237:888–93.
21. Ostertag W, Roesler G, Krieg CJ, et al. Induction of endogenous virus and of thymidine kinase by bromodeoxyuridine in cell cultures transformed by Friend virus. *Proc Natl Acad Sci USA* 1974;71:4980–5.
22. Mitsuya H, Weinhold KJ, Furman PA, et al. 3'-Azido-3'-deoxythymidine (BW A509U): an antiviral agent that inhibits the infectivity and cytopathic effect of human T-lymphotropic virus type III/lymphadenopathy-associated virus *in vitro*. *Proc Natl Acad Sci USA* 1985;82:7096–100.
23. Yarchoan R, Weinhold K, Lyerly HK, et al. Administration of 3'-azido-3'-deoxythymidine, an inhibitor of HTLV-III/LAV replication, to patients with AIDS or AIDS-related complex. *Lancet* 1986;1:575–80.
24. Yarchoan R, Brouwers P, Spitzer AR, et al. Response of human immunodeficiency virus-associated neurological disease to 3'-azido-3'-deoxythymidine. *Lancet* 1987;1:132–5.
25. Fischl MA, Richman DD, Grieco MH, et al. The efficacy of azidothymidine (AZT) in the treatment of patients with AIDS and AIDS-related complex. A double-blind, placebo-controlled trial. *N Engl J Med* 1987;317:185–91.
26. Chaisson RE, Leuther MD, Allain JP, Nusinoff-Lehrman S, Boone GS, Feigal D, Volberding P. Effect of zidovudine on serum human immunodeficiency virus core antigen levels. Results from a placebo-controlled trial. *Arch Intern Med* 1988;148:2151–3.
27. Richmann DD, Fischl MA, Grieco MH, et al. The toxicity of azidothymidine (AZT) in the treatment of patients with AIDS and AIDS-related complex. A double-blind, placebo-controlled trial. *N Eng J Med* 1987;317:192–7.
28. Fischl MA, Richman DD, Grieco MH, et al. Prolonged zidovudine therapy in patients with AIDS and advanced AIDS-related complex. *JAMA* 1990;262:2405–10.
29. Creagh-Kirk T, Doi P, Andrews E, Nusinoff-Lehrman S, Tilson H, Hoth D, Barry DW. Survival experience among patients with AIDS receiving zidovudine. Follow-up of patients in a compassionate plea program. *JAMA* 1988;260:3009–15.
30. Fischl MA, Parker CB, Pettinelli C, et al. The efficacy and safety of a lower daily dose of zidovudine in the treatment of patients with AIDS-associated *Pneumocystis carinii* pneumonia: a randomized controlled trial. *N Engl J Med* 1990;323:1009–14.

31. Collier AC, Bozzette S, Coombs RW, et al. A pilot study of low-dose zidovudine in human immunodeficiency virus infection. *N Engl J Med* 1990;323:1015–21.
32. Fischl MA, Richman DD, Hansen N, et al. The safety and efficacy of zidovudine (AZT) in the treatment of patients with mildly symptomatic HIV infection: a double-blind, placebo-controlled trial. *Ann Intern Med* 1990;112:727–37.
33. Volberding PA, Lagakos SW, Koch MA, et al. Safety and efficacy of zidovudine in asymptomatic HIV infected individuals with less than 500 CD4+ cells/mm3. *N Eng J Med* 1990;322:941–9.
34. Gail MH, Rosenberg PS, Goedert JJ. Therapy may explain recent deficits in AIDS incidence. *J Acquired Immune Deficiency Syndrome* 1990;3:296–306.
35. Rosenberg PS, Gail MH, Schrager LK, et al. National AIDS incidence trends and the extent of zidovudine therapy in selected demographic and transmission groups. *J Acquired Immune Deficiency Syndrome* 1991;4:392–401.
36. Centers for Disease Control. Guidelines for prophylaxis against *Pneumocystis carinii* pneumonia for persons infected with human immunodeficiency virus. *MMWR* 1989;38(supplS-5):1–5.
37. Centers for Disease Control. Human immunodeficiency virus (HIV) infection codes and new codes for Kaposi's sarcoma. Official authorized addenda, ICS-9-CM. *MMWR* 1991;40(RR9):1–19.
38. Schmitt FA, Bigley JW, McKinnis R, Logue PE, Evans RW, Drucker JL. Neuropsychological outcome of zidovudine (AZT) treatment of patients with AIDS and AIDS-related complex. *N Engl J Med* 1988;319:1573–8.
39. Portegies P, de Gans J, Lange JM, et al. Declining incidence of AIDS dementia complex after introduction of zidovudine treatment. *BMJ* 1989;299:819–21.
40. Walsh C, Krigel R, Lennette E, Karpatkin S. Thrombocytopenia in homosexual patients. Prognosis, response to therapy, and prevalence of antibody to the retrovirus associated with the acquired immunodeficiency syndrome. *Ann Intern Med* 1985;103:542–5.
41. Holzman RS, Walsh CM, Karpatkin S. Risk for the acquired immunodeficiency syndrome among thrombocytopenic and nonthrombocytopenic homosexual men seropositive for the human immunodeficiency virus. *Ann Intern Med* 1987;106:383–6.
42. Zucker-Franklin D, Termin CS, Cooper MC. Structural changes in the megakaryocyte of patients infected with the human immunodeficiency virus (HIV-1). *Am J Pathol* 1989;134:1295–303.
43. Yu JR, Lennette ET, Karpatkin S. Anti-F(ab')2 antibodies in thrombocytopenic patients at risk for acquired immunodeficiency syndrome. *J Clin Invest* 1986;77:1756–61.
44. Sthoenger D, Nardi M, Travis S, Karpatkin M, Karpatkin S. Micromethod for demonstrating increased platelet surface immunoglobulin G: findings in acute, chronic and human immunodeficiency virus-1-related immunologic thrombocytopenias. *Am J Hematol* 1990;34:275–82.
45. Beard J, Savidge GF. High-dose intravenous immunoglobulin and splenectomy for the treatment of HIV-related immune thrombocytopenia in patients with severe haemophilia. *Br J Haematol* 1988;68:303–6.
46. Hymes KB, Greene JB, Karpatkin S. The effect of azidothymidine on HIV-related thrombocytopenia. *N Engl J Med* 1988;318:516–7.
47. Oksenhendler E, Bierling P, Ferchal F, Clauvel JP, Seligmann M. Zidovudine for thrombocytopenic purpura related to human immunodeficiency virus (HIV) infection. *Ann Intern Med* 1989; 110(5):365–8.
48. Montaner JS, Le T, Fanning M, et al. The effect of zidovudine on platelet count in HIV-infected individuals. *J Acquired Immune Deficiency Syndrome* 1990;3:565–70.
49. Pena JM, Arnalich F, Barbado FJ, Dominguez A, Mostaza J, Valencia ME, Vazquez JJ. Successful zidovudine therapy for HIV-related severe thrombocytopenia. Report of sustained remission. *Acta Haematol (Basel)* 1990;83:86–8.
50. The Swiss Group for Clinical Studies on the Acquired Immunodeficiency Syndrome (AIDS). Zidovudine for the treatment of thrombocytopenia associated with human immunodeficiency virus (HIV). A prospective study. *Ann Intern Med* 1988;109: 718–21.
51. Lane HV, Falloon J, Walker RE,. et al. Zidovudine in patients

with human immunodeficiency virus (HIV) infection and Kaposi sarcoma. A phase II randomized, placebo-controlled trial. *Ann Intern Med* 1989;111:41–50.

52. de Wit R, Reiss P, Bakker PJ, Lange JM, Danner SA, Veenhof KH. Lack of activity of zidovudine in AIDS-associated Kaposi's sarcoma. *AIDS* 1989;3:847–50.

53. Langford A, Ruf B, Kunze R, Pohle HD, Reichart P. Regression of oral Kaposi's sarcoma in a case of AIDS on zidovudine (AZT). *Br J Dermatol* 1989;120:709–13.

54. Kovacs JA, Deyton L, Davey R, et al. Combined zidovudine and interferon-alpha therapy in patients with Kaposi's sarcoma and the acquired immunodeficiency syndrome (AIDS). *Ann Intern Med* 1989;111:280–7.

55. Fischl MA, Uttamchandani RB, Resnick L, et al. A phase I study of recombinant human interferon-alpha 2a or human lymphoblastoid interferon-alpha n1 and concomitant zidovudine in patients with AIDS-related Kaposi's sarcoma. *J Acquired Immune Deficiency Syndrome* 1991;4:1–10.

56. Pluda JM, Yarchoan R, Jaffe ES, et al. Development of non-Hodgkin's lymphoma in a cohort of patients with severe human immunodeficiency virus (HIV) infection on long-term antiretroviral therapy. *Ann Intern Med* 1990;113:276–82.

57. Moore RD, Kessler H, Richman DD, Flexner C, Chaisson RE. Non-Hodgkin's lymphoma in patients with advanced HIV infection treated with zidovudine. *JAMA* 1991;265:2208–11.

58. D'Amico DJ, Skolnik PR, Kosloff BR, et al. Resolution of cytomegalovirus retinitis with zidovudine therapy. *Arch Opthalmol* 1988;106:1168–9.

59. Kessler HA, Benson CA, Urbanski P. Regression of oral hairy leukoplakia during zidovudine therapy. *Arch Intern Med* 1988;148:2496–7.

60. Brockmeyer NH, Kreuzfelder E, Mertins L, Daecke C, Goos M. Zidovudine therapy of asymptomatic HIV-1-infected patients and combined zidovudine-acyclovir therapy of HIV-1-infected patients with oral hairy leukoplakia. *J Invest Dermatol* 1989;92:647.

61. Betiloch I, Pinazo I, Mestre F, Altes J, Villalonga C. Molluscum contagiosum in human immunodeficiency virus infection: response to zidovudine. *Int J Dermatol* 1989;28:351–2.

62. Greenberg RE, Mir R, Bank S, Siegal FP. Resolution of intestinal cryptosporidiosis after treatment of AIDS with AZT. *Gastroenterology* 1989;97:1327–30.

63. Conway B, Halliday WC, Brunham RC. Human immunodeficiency virus-associated progressive multifocal leukoencephalopathy: apparent response to 3'-azido-3'-deoxythymidine. *Rev Infect Dis* 1990;12:479–82.

64. Keith BR, White G, Wilson HR. *In vivo* efficacy of zidovudine (3'-azido-3'-deoxythymidine) in experimental gram-negative-bacterial infections. *Antimicrob Agents Chemother* 1989;33:479–83.

65. Diaz F, del Hoyo M, Serrano S. Zidovudine treatment of psoriasis associated with acquired immunodeficiency syndrome. *J Am Acad Dermatol* 1990;22:146–7.

66. Kaplan MH, Sadick NS, Wieder J, Farber BF, Neidt GW. Antipsoriatic effects of zidovudine in human immunodeficiency virus-associated psoriasis. *J Am Acad Dermatol* 1989;20:76–82.

67. Brouwers P, Moss H, Wolters P, Eddy J, Balis F, Poplack DG, Pizzo PA. Effect of continuous-infusion zidovudine therapy on neuropsychologic functioning in children with symptomatic human immunodeficiency virus infection. *J Pediatr* 1990;117:980–5.

68. Brunetti A, Berg G, Di Chiro G, et al. Reversal of brain metabolic abnormalities following treatment of AIDS dementia complex with 3'-azido-2',3'-dideoxythymidine (AZT, zidovudine): a PET-FDG study. *J Nucl Med* 1989;30:581–90.

69. McKinney RE Jr, Maha MA, Connor EM, et al. A multicenter trial of oral zidovudine in children with advanced human immunodeficiency virus disease. The Protocol 043 Study Group. *N Engl J Med* 1991;324:1018–25.

70. Pizzo PA. Treatment of human immunodeficiency virus-infected infants and young children with dideoxynucleosides. *Am J Med* 1991;88:168–98.

71. Parks WP, Parks ES, Fischl MA, et al. HIV-1 inhibition by azidothymidine in a concurrently randomized placebo-controlled trial. *J Acquired Immune Deficiency Syndrome* 1988;1:125–30.

72. Hamilton JD, Hartigan PM, Simberkoff MS, et al. A controlled trial of early versus late treatment with zidovudine in symptomatic human immunodeficiency virus infection. Results of the Veterans Affairs Cooperative Study. *N Eng J Med* 1992;326:437–43.

73. Moore RD, Hidalgo J, Sugland BW, Chaisson RE. Zidovudine and the natural history of the acquired immunodeficiency syndrome. *N Engl J Med* 1991;324:1412–6.

74. Goldsmith JC, Irvine W. Reversible agranulocytosis related to azidothymidine therapy. *Am J Hematol* 1989;30:264–5.

75. Groopman JE, Mitsuyasu RT, DeLeo MJ, Oette DH, Golde DW. Effect of recombinant human granulocyte-macrophage colony-stimulating factor on myelopoiesis in the acquired immunodeficiency syndrome. *N Engl J Med* 1987;317:593–8.

76. Pluda JM, Yarchoan R, Smith PD, et al. Subcutaneous recombinant granulocyte-macrophage colony-stimulating factor used as a single agent and in an alternating regimen with azidothymidine in leukopenic patients with severe human immunodeficiency virus infection. *Blood* 1990;76:463–72.

77. Israel RJ, Levine JD. Granulocyte-macrophage colony-stimulating factor and azidothymidine in patients with acquired immunodeficiency syndrome. *Blood* 1991;77:2085–7.

78. Miles SA, Mitsuyasu RT, Moreno J, Baldwin G, Alton NK, Souza L, Glaspy JA. Combined therapy with recombinant granulocyte colony-stimulating factor and erythropoietin decreases hematologic toxicity from zidovudine. *Blood* 1991;77:2109–17.

79. Folks TM, Justement J, Kinter A, Dinarello CA, Fauci AS. Cytokine-induced expression of HIV-1 in a chronically infected promonocyte cell line. *Science* 1987;238:800–2.

80. Fischl M, Galpin JE, Levine JD, et al. Recombinant human erythropoietin for patients with AIDS treated with zidovudine. *N Engl J Med* 1990;322:1488–93.

81. Allworth AM, Kemp RJ. A case of acute encephalopathy caused by the human immunodeficiency virus apparently responsive to zidovudine. *Med J Aust* 1989;151:285–6.

82. Saracchini S, Vaccher E, Covezzi E, Tortorici G, Carbone A, Tirelli U. Lethal neurotoxicity associated to azidothymidine therapy. *J Neurol Neurosurg Psychiatry* 1989;52:544–5.

83. Riedel RR, Clarenbach P, Reetz KP. Coma during azidothymidine therapy for AIDS. *J Neurol* 1989;236:185.

84. Bessen LJ, Greene JB, Louie E, Seitzman P, Weinberg H. Severe polymyositis-like syndrome associated with zidovudine therapy of AIDS and ARC. *N Engl J Med* 1988;318:708.

85. Dalakas MC, Illa I, Pezeshkpour GH, et al. Mitochondrial myopathy caused by long-term zidovudine therapy. *N Engl J Med* 1990;322:1089–105.

86. Steffe EM, King JH, Inciard JF, et al. The effect of acetaminophen on zidovudine metabolism in HIV-infected patients. *J AIDS* 1990;3:691–94.

87. Collaborative DHPG Treatment Study Group. Treatment of serious cytomegalovirus infections with 9-(1,3-dihydroxy-2-propoxymethyl) guanine in patients with AIDS and other immunodeficiencies *N Engl J Med* 1986;314:801–5.

88. Hochster H, Dieterich D, Bozzette S, et al. Toxicity of combined ganciclovir (DHPG) and zidovudine (AZT) with the therapy of AIDS-related CMV disease: results of a NIAID AIDS Clinical Trials Group Phase I Study (ACTG 004). *Ann Intern Med* 1990;113:111–7.

89. Causey D. Concomitant ganciclovir and zidovudine treatment of cytomegalovirus retinitis in patients with HIV infection: an approach to treatment. *J Acquired Immune Deficiency Syndrome* 1991;4:S16–21.

90. Larder BA, Darby G, Richman DD. HIV with reduced sensitivity to zidovudine isolated during prolonged therapy. *Science* 1989;243:1731–4.

91. Larder BA, Kemp SD. Multiple mutations in HIV-1 reverse transcriptase confer high-level resistance to zidovudine (AZT). *Science* 1989;246:1155–8.

92. Larder BA, Chesebro B, Richman DD. Susceptibilities of zidovudine-susceptible and -resistant human immunodeficiency virus isolates to antiviral agents determined by using a quantitative

plaque reduction assay. *Antimicrob Agents Chemother* 1990; 34:436–41.

93. Land S, Treloar G, McPhee D, et al. Decreased *in vitro* susceptibility to zidovudine of HIV isolates obtained from patients with AIDS. *J Infect Dis* 1990;161:326–9.

94. Rooke R, Tremblay M, Soudeyns H, et al. Isolation of drug-resistant variants of HIV-1 from patients on long-term zidovudine therapy. *AIDS* 1989;3:411–5.

95. Boucher CAB, Tersmette M, Lange J, et al. Zidovudine sensitivity of human immunodeficiency viruses from high-risk, symptom-free individuals during therapy. *Lancet* 1990;336:585–90.

96. Japour AJ, Chatis PA, Eigenrauch HA, Crumpacker CS. Detection of human immunodeficiency virus type 1 clinical isolates with reduced sensitivity to zidovudine and dideoxyinosine by RNA–RNA hybridization. *Proc Natl Acad Sci USA* 1991; 88:3092–6.

97. St Clair MH, Martin JL, Tudor-Williams G, et al. A single mutation in HIV-1 reverse transcriptase confers dideoxyinosine resistance and collateral sensitivity to zidovudine. *Science* 1991;253:1557–9.

98. Richman DD, Grimes JM, Lagakos SW. Effect of stage of disease and drug dose on zidovudine susceptibilities of isolates of human immunodeficiency virus. *J Acquired Immune Deficiency Syndrome* 1990;3:743–6.

99. Ho DD, Moudgil T, Alam M. Quantitation of human immunodeficiency virus type 1 in the blood of infected persons. *N Engl J Med* 1989;321:1621–5.

100. Coombs RW, Collier AC, Allain J-P, et al. Plasma viremia in human immunodeficiency virus infection. *N Engl J Med* 1989;321:1626–31.

101. Schnittman SM, Greenhouse JJ, Psallidopoulos MC, et al. Increasing viral burden in CD4+ T cells from patients with human immunodeficiency virus (HIV) infection reflects rapidly progressive immunosuppression and clinical disease. *Ann Intern Med* 1990;113:438–43.

102. Hirsch MS, Wormser G, Schooley RT, et al. Risk of nosocomial infection with human T-lymphotropic virus-III. *N Engl J Med* 1985;312:1–4.

103. Friedland GH, Klein RS. Transmission of the human immunodeficiency virus. *N Engl J Med* 1987;317:1125–35.

104. Public Health Service statement on management of occupational exposure to human immunodeficiency virus, including considerations regarding zidovudine postexposure use. *MMWR* 1990;39(RR 1):1–14.

105. Miller RA. Failure of zidovudine prophylaxis after exposure to HIV-1. *N Engl J Med* 1990;323:915–6.

106. Lange JM, Boucher CA, Hollak CE, et al. Failure of zidovudine prophylaxis after accidental exposure to HIV-1. *N Engl J Med* 1990;322:1375–7.

107. Looke DF, Grove DI. Failed prophylactic zidovudine after needlestick injury. *Lancet* 1990;335:1280.

108. Ruprecht RM, Chou TC, Chipty F, Sosa MG, Mullaney S, O'Brien L, Rosas D. Interferon-alpha and 3'-azido-3'-deoxythymidine are highly synergistic in mice and prevent viremia after acute retrovirus exposure. *J Acquired Immune Deficiency Syndrome* 1990;3:591–600.

109. Clark SJ, Saag MS, Decker WD, et al. High titers of cytopathic virus in plasma of patients with symptomatic primary HIV-1 infection. *N Engl J Med* 1991;324:954–60.

110. Daar ES, Moudgil T, Meyer RD, Ho DD. Transient high level of viremia in patients with primary human immunodeficiency virus type 1 infection. *N Engl J Med* 1991;324:961–4.

111. Balzarini J, Pauwels R, Herdewijn P, et al. Potent and selective anti-HTLV-III/LAV activity of 2',3'-dideoxycytidinene, the 2',3'-unsaturated derivative of 2',3'-dideoxycytidine. *Biochem Biophys Res Commun* 1986;140:735–42.

112. Broder S. Pharmacodynamics of 2',3'-dideoxycytidine: an inhibitor of human immunodeficiency virus. *Am J Med* 1990;88: 2S–7S.

113. Yarchoan R, Perno CF, Thomas RV, et al. Phase I studies of 2',3'-dideoxycytidine in severe human immunodeficiency virus infection as a single agent and alternating with zidovudine (AZT). *Lancet* 1988;1:76–81.

114. McNeely MC, Yarchoan R, Broder S, Lawley TJ. Dermatologic complications associated with administration of 2',3'-dideoxycytidine in patients with human immunodeficiency virus infection. *J Am Acad Dermatol* 1989;21:1213–7.

115. Merigan TC, Skowron G, Bozzette SA, Richman D, Uttamchandani R, Schooley R. Circulating p24 antigen levels and responses to dideoxycytidine in human immunodeficiency virus (HIV) infections. A phase I and II study. *Ann Intern Med* 1989;110: 189–94.

116. Dubinsky RM, Yarchoan R, Dalakas M, Broder S. Reversible axonal neuropathy from the treatment of AIDS and related disorders with 2',3'-dideoxycytidine (ddC). *Muscle Nerve* 1989;12: 856–60.

117. Vogt MW, Durno AG, Chou TC, et al. Synergistic interaction of 2',3'-dideoxycytidine and recombinant interferon-α-A on replication of human immunodeficiency virus type 1. *J Infect Dis* 1988;158:378–85.

118. Pizzo PA, Butler K, Balis F, et al. Dideoxycytidine alone and in an alternating schedule with zidovudine in children with symptomatic human immunodeficiency virus infection. *J Pediatr* 1990;117:799–808.

119. Bozette SA, Richman DD. Salvage therapy for zidovudine-intolerant HIV-infected patients with alternating and intermittent regimens of zidovudine and dideoxycytidine. *Am J Med* 1990;88: 24S–26.

120. Yarchoan R, Mitsuya H, Thomas RV, et al. *In vivo* activity against HIV and favorable toxicity profile of 2',3'-dideoxyinosine. *Science* 1989;245:412–5.

121. Aoki S, Yarchoan R, Thomas RV, et al. Quantitative analysis of HIV-1 proviral DNA in peripheral blood mononuclear cells from patients with AIDS or ARC: decrease of proviral DNA content following treatment with 2',3'-dideoxyinosine (ddI). *AIDS Res Hum Retroviruses* 1990;6:1331–9.

122. Lambert JS, Seidlin M, Reichman RC, et al. 2',3'-Dideoxyinosine (ddI) in patients with the acquired immunodeficiency syndrome or AIDS-related complex. A phase I trial. *N Engl J Med* 1990;322:1333–40.

123. Cooley TP, Kunches LM, Saunders CA, et al. Once-daily administration of 2',3'-dideoxyinosine (ddI) in patients with the acquired immunodeficiency syndrome or AIDS-related complex. Results of a phase I trial. *N Engl J Med* 1990;322:1340–5.

124. Hartman NR, Yarchoan R, Pluda JM, et al. Pharmacokinetics of 2',3'-dideoxyinosine in patients with severe human immunodeficiency virus infection. *Clin Pharmacol Ther* 1990;47:647–54.

125. Knupp CA, Shyu WC, Dolin R, et al. Pharmacokinetics of didanosine in patients with acquired immunodeficiency syndrome or acquired immunodeficiency syndrome-related complex. *Clin Pharmacol Ther* 1991;49:523–35.

126. Yarchoan R, Pluda JM, Thomas RV, et al. Long-term toxicity/activity profile of 2',3'-dideoxyinosine in AIDS or AIDS-related complex. *Lancet* 1990;336:526–9.

127. Bouvet E, Casalino E, Prevost MH, Vachon F. Fatal case of 2',3'-dideoxyinosine-associated pancreatitis. *Lancet* 1990;336:1515.

128. Butler KM, Husson RN, Balis FM, et al. Dideoxyinosine in children with symptomatic human immunodeficiency virus infection. *N Engl J Med* 1991;324:137–44.

129. LeLacheur SF, Simon GL. Exacerbation of dideoxycytidine-induced neuropathy with dideoxyinosine. *J Acquired Immune Deficiency Syndrome* 1991;4:538–9.

130. Yarchoan R, Mitsuya H, Pluda JM, et al. The National Cancer Institute Phase I study of 2',3'-dideoxyinosine administration in adults with AIDS or AIDS-related complex: analysis of activity and toxicity profiles. *Rev Infect Dis* 1990;12:S522–33.

131. Lafeuillade A, Aubert L, Chaffanjon P, Quilichini R. Optic neuritis associated with dideoxyinosine. *Lancet* 1991;337:615–6.

132. Lai KK, Gang DL, Zawacki JK, Cooley TP. Fulminant hepatic failure associated with 2',3'-dideoxyinosine (ddI). *Ann Intern Med* 1991;115:283–4.

133. Bach MC. Clinical response to dideoxyinosine in patients with HIV infection resistant to zidovudine. *N Engl J Med* 1990;323:275.

134. Hayashi S, Fine RL, Chou TC, Currens MJ, Broder S, Mitsuya H. *In vitro* inhibition of the infectivity and replication of human immunodeficiency virus type 1 by combination of antiretroviral

2',3'-dideoxynucleosides and virus-binding inhibitors. *Antimicrob Agents Chemother* 1990;34:82–8.

135. Weinstein JN, Bunow B, Weislow OS, Schinazi RF, Wahl SM, Wahl LM, Szebeni J. Synergistic drug combinations in AIDS therapy: dipyridamole/3'-azido-3'-deoxythymidine in particular and principles of analysis in general. *Ann NY Acad Sci* 1990;616:367–84.

136. Balzarini J, Naesens L, Robins MJ, de Clercq E. Potentiating effects of ribavirin on the *in vitro* and *in vivo* antiretrovirus activities of 2',3'-dideoxyinosine and 2',3'-dideoxy-2,6-diaminopurine riboside. *J Acquired Immune Deficiency Syndrome* 1990;3: 1140–7.

137. Ashorn P, Moss B, Weinstein JN, et al. Elimination of infectious human immunodeficiency virus from human T-cell cultures by synergistic action of CD4-*Pseudomonas* exotoxin and reverse transcriptase inhibitors. *Proc Natl Acad Sci USA* 1990;87: 8889–93.

138. Meng TC, Fischl MA, Boota AM, et al. A phase III study of combination therapy with zidovudine and dideoxycytidine in subjects with advanced human immunodeficiency virus (HIV) disease. *Ann Intern Med* 1992;116:13–20.

139. Balzarini J, Kang G-J, Dalal D, et al. The anti-HTLV-III (anti-HIV) and cytotoxic activity of 2',3'-didehydro-2',3'-dideoxyribonucleosides: a comparison with their parental 2',3'-dideoxyribonucleosides. *Mol Pharmacol* 1987;32:162–7.

140. Hamamoto Y, Nakashima H, Matsui T, et al. Inhibitory effect of 2',3'-didehydro-2',3'-dideoxynucleosides on infectivity, cytopathic effects, and replication of human immunodeficiency virus. *Antimicrob Agents Chemother* 1987;31:907–10.

141. Baba M, Pauwels R, Herdewijn P, et al. Both 2',3'-dideoxythymidine and its 2',3'-unsaturated derivative (2',3'-dideoxythymidinene) are potent and selective inhibitors of human immunodeficiency virus *in vitro*. *Biochem Biophys Res Commun* 1987;142: 128–34.

142. Sommadossi J-P, Carlisle R. Toxicity of 3'-azido-3'-deoxythymidine and 9-(1,3-dihydroxy-2-propoxymethyl) guanine for normal human hematopoietic progenitor cells *in vitro*. *Antimicrob Agents Chemother* 1987;31:452–5.

143. Merluzzi VJ, Hargrave KD, Labadia M, et al. Inhibition of HIV-1 replication by a nonnucleoside reverse transcriptase inhibitor. *Science* 1990;250:1411–3.

144. Nunberg JH, Schleif WA, Boots EJ, et al. Viral resistance to HIV-1 specific pyridinone reverse transcriptase inhibitors. *J Virol* 1991;65:4887–92.

145. Koup RA, Merluzzi VJ, Hargrave KD, Adams J, Grozinger K, Eckner RJ, Sullivan JL. Inhibition of human immunodeficiency virus type 1 (HIV-1) replication by the dipyridodiazepinone BI-RG-587. *J Infect Dis* 1991;163:966–70.

146. Goldman ME, Nunberg JH, O'Brien JA, et al. Pyridinone derivatives. Specific HIV-1 reverse transcriptase inhibitors with antiviral activity. *Proc Natl Acad Sci USA* 1991;88:6863–7.

147. Oberg B. Antiviral effects of phophonoformate (PFA, foscarnet sodium). *Pharmacol Ther* 1983;19:387–415.

148. Walmsley SL, Chew E, Fanning MM, Read SE, Velend H, Salit I, Rachlis A. Treatment of cytomegalovirus retinitis with trisodium phosphonoformate hexahydrate (foscarnet). *J Infect Dis* 1988;157:569–72.

149. Sundquist B, Oberg B. Phosphonoformate inhibits reverse transcriptase. *J Gen Virol* 1979;45:273–81.

150. Sandstrom EG, Kaplan JC, Byington RE, Hirsch MS. Inhibition of human T-cell lymphotropic virus type III *in vitro* by phosphonoformate. *Lancet* 1985;1:1480–2.

151. Sarin PS, Taguchi Y, Sun D, et al. Inhibition of HTLV-III/LAV replication by foscarnet. *Biochem Biophys Res Commun* 1985;34:4075–80.

152. Bergadahl S, Sonnerborg A, Larsson A, Strannegard O. Declining levels of HIV p24 antigen in serum during treatment with foscarnet. *Lancet* 1988;1:1052.

153. Jacobson MA, Crowe S, Levy J, et al. Effect of foscarnet therapy on infection with human immunodeficiency virus in patients with AIDS. *J Infect Dis* 1988;158:862–5.

154. Sjovall J, Karlsson A, Ogenstad S, Sandstrom E, Saarimaki M. Pharmacokinetics and absorption of foscarnet after intravenous and oral administration to patients with human immunodeficiency virus. *Clin Pharmacol Ther* 1988;44:65–73.

155. Smith DH, Byrn RA, Marsters SA, et al. Blocking of HIV-1 infectivity by a soluble, secreted form of the CD4 antigen. *Science* 1987;238:1704–7.

156. Fisher RA, Bertonis JM, Meier W, et al. HIV infection is blocked *in vitro* by recombinant soluble CD4. *Nature* 1988;331:76–8.

157. Hussey RE, Richardson NE, Kowalski M, et al. A soluble CD4 protein selectively inhibits HIV replication and syncytium formation. *Nature* 1988;331:78–81.

158. Deen KC, McDougal JS, Inacker R, et al. A soluble form of CD4 (T4) protein inhibits AIDS virus infection. *Nature* 1988;331: 82–4.

159. Traunecker A, Luke W, Karjalainen K. Soluble CD4 molecules neutralize human immunodeficiency virus type 1. *Nature* 1988;331:84–6.

160. Schooley RT, Merigan TC, Gaut P, et al. Recombinant soluble CD4 therapy in patients with the acquired immunodeficiency syndrome (AIDS) and AIDS-related complex. *Ann Intern Med* 1990;112:247–53.

161. Kahn JO, Allan JD, Hodges TL, et al. The safety and tolerance of recombinant soluble CD4 (rsCD4) in subjects with the acquired immunodeficiency syndrome (AIDS) and AIDS-related complex: a phase 1 study. *Ann Intern Med* 1990;112:254–61.

162. Daar ES, Li XL, Moudgil T, Ho DD. High concentrations of recombinant soluble CD4 are required to neutralize primary human immunodeficiency virus type 1 isolates. *Proc Natl Acad Sci USA* 1990;87:6574–8.

163. Capon DJ, Chamow SM, Mordenti J, et al. Designing CD4 immunoadhesins for AIDS therapy. *Nature* 1989;337:525–31.

164. Traunecker A, Schneider J, Kiefer H, Karjalainen K. Highly efficient neutralization of HIV with recombinant CD4-immunoglobulin molecules. *Nature* 1989;339:68–70.

165. Chaudhary VK, Mizukami T, Fuerst TR, et al. Selective killing of HIV-infected cells by recombinant human CD4-*Pseudomonas* exotoxin hybrid protein. *Nature* 1988;335:369–72.

166. Till MA, Ghetie V, Gregory T, et al. HIV-infected cells are killed by rCD4-ricin A chain. *Science* 1988;242:1166–8.

167. Berger EA, Clouse KA, Chaudhary VK, et al. CD4-*Pseudomonas* exotoxin hybrid protein blocks the spread of human immunodeficiency virus infection *in vitro* and is active against cells expressing the envelope glycoproteins from diverse primate immunodeficiency retroviruses. *Proc Natl Acad Sci USA* 1989;86:9539–43.

168. Kahn J, Hassner A, Arri C, et al. A phase I study of recombinant CD4 human immunoglobulin-G (rCD4-IgG) in patients with HIV-associated immune thrombocytopenic purpura. *7th International Conference on AIDS, Florence, Italy* June 1991; abst.

169. Walker BD, Moss B, Paradis TJ, et al. Detection of HIV-specific cytotoxic cells in seropositive individuals. *Nature* 1987;328: 345–8.

170. Blumberg RS, Hartshorn KL, Paradis TJ, et al. Antibody dependent cell mediated cytotoxicity (ADCC) against cells infected with the human immunodeficiency virus. *J Infect Dis* 1987;156:878–84.

171. Sarin PS, Gallo RC, Scheer DI, et al. Effects of a novel compound (AL 721) on HTLV-III infectivity *in vitro*. *N Engl J Med* 1991;313:1289–90.

172. Ueno R, Kuno S. Dextran sulphate, a potent anti-HIV agent *in vitro* having synergism with zidovudine. *Lancet* 1987;2:796–7.

173. Finberg RW, Diamond DC, Mitchell DB, et al. Prevention of HIV-1 infection and preservation of CD4 function by the binding of CPFs to gp120. *Science* 1990;249:287–91.

174. De Somer P, De Clercq E, Billian A, Schonne E, Claesen M. Antiviral activity of polyacrylic acid and polymethacrylic acid. *J Virol* 1968;2:88–93.

175. De Clercq E. Chemotherapeutic approaches to the treatment of acquired immune deficiency syndrome (AIDS). *J Med Chem* 1986;29:1561–9.

176. Abrams DI, Kuno S, Wong R, et al. Oral dextran sulphate (UA001) in the treatment of the acquired immunodeficiency syndrome (AIDS) and AIDS-related complex. *Ann Intern Med* 1989;110:183–8.

177. Meek TD, Dayton BD, Metcalf BW, et al. Human immunodefi-

ciency virus 1 protease expressed in *Escherichia coli* behaves as a dimeric aspartic protease. *Proc Natl Acad Sci USA* 1989;86: 1841–5.

178. Darke PL, Leu CT, Davis LJ, et al. Human immunodeficiency virus protease. *J Biol Chem* 1989;264:2307–12.

179. Pearl LH, Taylor WR. A structural model for the retroviral proteases. *Nature* 1987;329:351–4.

180. Wlodawer A, Miller M, Jaskolski M, et al. Conserved folding in retroviral proteases: crystal structure of a synthetic HIV-1 protease. *Science* 1989;245:616–21.

181. Karpas A, Fleet GW, Dwek RA, et al. Aminosugar derivatives as potential anti-human immunodeficiency virus agents. *Proc Natl Acad Sci USA* 1988;85:9229–33.

182. Bollen M, Stalmans W. The antiglycogenolytic action of 1-deoxynojirimycin results from a specific inhibition of the alpha-1,6-glucosidase activity of the debranching enzyme. *Eur J Biochem* 1989;181:775–80.

183. Hartshorn KL, Neumeyer D, Vogt MW, Schooley RT, Hirsch MS. Activity of interferons alpha, beta and gamma against human immunodeficiency virus replication *in vitro*. *AIDS Res Hum Retroviruses* 1987;3:125–33.

184. Groopman JE, Gottlieb MS, Goodman J, et al. Recombinant α-2 interferon therapy for Kaposi's sarcoma associated with the acquired immunodeficiency syndrome. *Ann Intern Med* 1984; 100:671–6.

185. Krown SD, Real FX, Cunningham-Rundles S, et al. Preliminary observations on the effect of recombinant leukocyte A interferon in homosexual men with Kaposi's sarcoma. *N Engl J Med* 1983;308:1071–6.

186. Interferon Alpha Study Group. A randomized placebo-controlled trial of recombinant human interferon alpha 2a in patients with AIDS. *J AIDS* 1988;1:111–8.

187. Lane CH, Feinberg J, Davey V, et al. Antiretroviral effects of interferon-α in AIDS-associated Kaposi's sarcoma. *Lancet* 1988;1:1218–22.

188. deWit R, Boucher CAB, Veenhof KHN, Schattenkerk JKME, Bakker PJM, Danner SA. Clinical and virological effects of high-dose recombinant interferon-α in disseminated AIDS-related Kaposi's sarcoma. *Lancet* 1988;1:1214–7.

189. Hartshorn KL, Vogt MW, Chou TC, et al. Synergistic inhibition of human immunodeficiency virus *in vitro* by azidothymidine and recombinant alpha A interferon. *Antimicrob Agents Chemother* 1987;31:168–72.

190. Vogt MW, Durno AG, Chou T-C, et al. Synergistic interaction of 2′,3′-dideoxycytidine (ddCyd) and recombinant interferon alpha-A (-IFN-alpha-A) on HIV-I replication. *J Infect Dis* 1988;158: 378–85.

191. Hartshorn KL, Sandstrom EF, Neumeyer D, et al. Synergistic inhibition of human T-cell lymphotropic virus type III replication *in vitro* by phosphonoformate and recombinant alpha-A interferon. *Antimicrob Agents Chemother* 1986;30:189–91.

192. Johnson VA, Barlow MA, Merrill DP, Chou TC, Hirsch MS. Three-drug synergistic inhibition of HIV-1 replication *in vitro* by zidovudine, recombinant soluble CD4, and recombinant interferon-alpha A. *J Infect Dis* 1990;161:1059–67.

193. Eron JJ, Hirsch MS, Merrill DP, Chou T-C, Johnson VA. Synergistic inhibition of HIV-1 by the combination of zidovudine (AZT) and 2′,3′-dideoxycytidine (ddC) *in vitro*. *7th International Conference on AIDS, Florence, Italy,* June 1991; abst.

194. Vogt MW, Hartshorn KL, Furman PA, et al. Ribavirin antagonizes anti-HIV effect of azidothymidine (AZT) by phosphorylation inhibition. *Science* 1987;235:1376–9.

195. Skowron G, Merigan TC. Alternating and intermittent regimens of zidovudine (3′-azido-3′ deoxythymidine) and dideoxycytidine (2′,3′-dideoxycytidine) in the treatment of patients with acquired immunodeficiency syndrome (AIDS) and AIDS-related complex. *Am J Med* 1990;88:20S–3.

196. Collier AC, Fischl MA, Kaplan LD, et al. Effect of combination therapy with zidovudine (ZDV) and didanosine (ddI) on surrogate markers. *7th International Conference on AIDS, Florence, Italy,Italy,* June 1991st.

197. Fischl MA, Uttamchandani RB, Resnick L, et al. A phase I study of recombinant human interferon-α_{2a} or human lymphoblastoid interferon-α_{n1} and concomitant zidovudine in patients with AIDS-related Kaposi's sarcoma. *J AIDS* 1991;4:1–10.

AIDS and Other Manifestations of HIV Infection,
Second Edition, Edited by Gary P. Wormser.
Raven Press, Ltd., New York © 1992.

CHAPTER 38

Immunotherapy for AIDS

Status and Prospects

Steven Specter and John W. Hadden

Human immunodeficiency virus (HIV) infection and the subsequent development of the acquired immunodeficiency syndrome (AIDS) have been a major focus of attention of the medical and lay community during this past decade. HIV has been under intensive study, regarding virus biology and pathogenesis, since its description in 1983 (1,2). Progress in studying this virus has been remarkable; however, we still do not have a complete understanding of the pathogenesis of HIV. The virus attains latency in lymphocytes and probably macrophages and then active multiplication of the virus ultimately leads to AIDS. The incubation period for this progression is now described as having a 50% incidence of 10 years. Very little is understood about the factors or cofactors that are involved in viral reactivation and the evolution of clinical disease during this lengthy interval. A variety of viruses can reactivate HIV (3), and a role for *Mycoplasma* has been suggested (4,5). In addition, reports exist that suggest that the use of narcotic drugs may serve as a cofactor in the etiology of AIDS (6), and there is evidence that indicates that immune stimulation can activate HIV (7). However, there is still no hard evidence that progression from HIV-seropositive to overt AIDS involves one or another of these cofactors.

Antiviral chemotherapy has yielded some beneficial effects but results to date clearly show that such therapy is only palliative and temporary (8–11). The most successful drug to date has been zidovudine (azidothymidine—AZT), which has slowed the progression of HIV infection to AIDS, has reduced the symptoms of AIDS,

and has prolonged the life of AIDS patients. Use of zidovudine has not resulted in total prevention of breakthrough opportunistic infections, and drug-resistant strains of HIV have emerged. Further development of antivirals for AIDS has mostly employed nucleoside analogs, although other approaches have included enzyme inhibitors and monoclonal antibodies bound to microbial toxins.

Vaccine development for HIV is still in its early stages. Candidate vaccines include whole inactivated virus, inactivated virus from which a single component has been removed, purified envelope glycoproteins, core proteins, and polypeptide sequences from such proteins (12–16). Interestingly, vaccine trials are also being performed for therapeutic effect in HIV-seropositive asymptomatic individuals. The latter is a unique role for vaccines to date. It is likely that postexposure vaccination alone will not provide full protection against subsequent disease. Thus, as for immunotherapy using immunostimulants, this form of therapy will have to be designed to maintain latency of the virus but may only prove successful when used in conjunction with antiviral agents such as AZT. At present, there is no licensed vaccine in the United States for immunization against any known latent virus, although promising vaccines are in trial for several of the herpes group viruses. It is still too early in the study of these vaccines to determine their effectiveness with regard to prevention of recurrent infection caused by latent virus. It is noteworthy, however, that one experimental herpes simplex virus vaccine, which successfully protected healthy monkeys, failed to protect against lethal infection when tested in immunocompromised monkeys. By analogy, vaccines for HIV may not be effective in preventing virus reactivation or AIDS. Clearly, a better understanding of the pathogenesis of HIV and

S. Specter and J. W. Hadden: Department of Medical Microbiology and Immunology and Immunopharmacology Program, University of South Florida College of Medicine, Tampa, Florida 33612.

greater insight into the role of immune responses in controlling latency are needed.

Existing limitations of antiviral drugs and vaccine strategies suggest that other approaches are necessary, at least for the next several years, if we are to devise better ways to limit morbidity and mortality in HIV-infected individuals. An important approach may be the use of immune therapy either in place of antivirals or, more likely, as an adjunct to antiviral therapy.

To optimize immunotherapy it is necessary to understand the role of the immune system in controlling HIV infection and progression of disease. The most likely candidates for such control are neutralizing antibodies, antibody-dependent cellular cytotoxicity (ADCC), cytotoxic T lymphocytes (Tc), natural killer (NK) cells, and macrophages (17,18). Drug intervention to maintain effective levels of responsive elements, as, for example, through growth factors to maintain granulocyte, macrophage, or lymphocyte numbers, is an integral part of the immunotherapeutic approach. In approaching the problem of developing effective immunotherapy for AIDS, we must realize that the HIV-infected host does initially develop both humoral and cell-mediated immunity to the virus. What then changes that results in expression of HIV and precipitation of frank disease? This aspect of the pathogenesis of AIDS is poorly understood. However, the more important question is: How do we reverse this phenomenon and restore protective immunity?

IMMUNOTHERAPY OF AIDS

Early predictions regarding the effectiveness of immunotherapeutic approaches to treating AIDS were consistently negative (19–21). More recent reviews of collected studies document the accuracy of these early predictions and the frustration to date with attempts at immunotherapy (8,19,22,23). Clearly, immunotherapy alone has not been successful in reversing the immunodeficiency of AIDS. This has led increasingly to the use of immunotherapy in combination with AZT (24).

Serum Therapy

Passive transfer of antibodies is the most widely used and oldest form of immunotherapy. Thus it has received serious consideration for therapy of AIDS patients. Sera from patients with high titers of neutralizing antibodies against HIV were treated to inactivate the virus and then administered to AIDS patients (25,26). Preliminary results from treatment of 16 patients suggested that therapy reduced p24 antigenemia, increased the CD4+ lymphocyte count, and improved the clinical condition of some patients. However, these studies need to be reexamined after a longer follow-up to determine the true effectiveness of such therapy.

Pediatric AIDS patients have been treated with intravenous immunoglobulin (IVIG). This has been useful for decreasing morbidity due to bacterial infections and measles (27). The effectiveness of this therapy in conjunction with AZT is under evaluation in 250 patients in a NIH-sponsored multicenter phase III trial (8). IVIG also has been reported anecdotally to improve the clinical course of AIDS and AIDS-related complex (ARC) in adults. Thus a multicenter trial has been undertaken to compare IVIG alone versus IVIG plus AZT in adults with ARC and AIDS (28). If benefits should be documented from this approach, it will be necessary to determine if the IVIG treatment had any direct effect on HIV (i.e., were HIV neutralizing antibodies involved) or whether it proved effective via prevention of opportunistic infections, or both.

Adoptive Transfer of Lymphocytes

Bone marrow transplantation, which is a widely used treatment for severe combined immunodeficiency (SCID), certain forms of leukemia, and more recently a variety of other clinical entities, has now been used to treat AIDS patients. Most reports indicate that this therapeutic approach is unsuccessful. However, one recent report of bone marrow transplantation in combination with AZT claimed successful eradication of the virus (29). These results must be interpreted cautiously, as noted in a recent *Oncology Times* article (March 1990) in which Anthony Fauci and others expressed "serious reservations" and termed the conclusions "premature."

Interferon (IFN) and Interferon Inducers

IFN-α and IFN-γ are capable of modulating immune responses via their ability to stimulate lymphocytes, macrophages, and NK cells, while depressing lymphocyte proliferation and secretion of cytokines. They have the potential additional benefit of inhibiting viral replication. IFN-α has been effective therapy for Kaposi's sarcoma (KS) in AIDS patients. Abrams et al. (8) report a 20–40% major response rate using IFN alone; notably, this is improved to greater than 60% when IFN is used in combination with AZT. Although the IFN–AZT combination does not diminish the immunodeficiency of HIV infection, neither is it immunosuppressive, as are standard combinations of cytotoxic chemotherapeutic agents. It is possible that IFN may also decrease the incidence of certain opportunistic viral infections through its well recognized antiviral properties. Two IFN-α preparations have been licensed by the Food and Drug Administration (FDA) for use in patients with Kaposi's sarcoma.

Two reports using IFN-α indicate that treatment of patients with HIV infection leads to a reduction in recoverable HIV from blood, lowers p24 antigenemia, and reduces opportunistic infections (30,31). These studies were performed using high-dose parenterally administered IFN and patients frequently experienced a "flu-like" syndrome. More recently, Cummins and co-workers have indicated that daily low-dose 2 IU/kg IFN-α administered orally to each of 40 HIV-infected patients (38 symptomatic and 2 asymptomatic) in Kenya resulted in an increase in CD4+ lymphocytes, an increase in weight, and alleviation of clinical symptoms (32). These findings require confirmation. Other clinical studies involving IFN are in progress looking at IFN-α used in combination with AZT, interleukin-2 (IL-2), or diethyldithiocarbamate (DTC—Imuthiol).

Additionally, phase I trials have been conducted examining IFN-γ for treatment of 16 HIV-infected patients with Kaposi's sarcoma (22). These studies used either intramuscular or continuous intravenous infusion of IFN at doses ranging from 0.001 to 1.0 mg/M^2. The doses were all reasonably well tolerated with side effects typical of IFN administration (e.g., fever, malaise). No effect was seen on either the Kaposi's sarcoma, the lymphoblastogenic responses by patient lymphocytes, or HLA-DR expression; however, natural killer cell function increased at an IFN dose of 0.1 mg/M^2 and monocyte-mediated killing increased at a dose of 1.0 mg/M^2. At the higher concentration, NK activity was suppressed. It is anticipated that this protocol is undergoing further evaluation.

Ampligen

Ampligen is a polynucleotide derivative of polyinosinic:polcytidylic acid (poly I:C, a potent IFN inducer) with spaced uridines that serve as RNase cleavage sites. While ampligen is capable of inducing IFN and enhancing NK cell activity, it lacks the toxicity of poly I:C and other related derivatives (33). In an initial double-blind multicenter phase II clinical trial, lack of activity resulted in cessation of the study. However, retrospective examination of the data suggested that the method of drug storage was an important variable in patient response. Patients treated with ampligen stored in glass fared better than those treated with drug stored in plastic containers (34). Thus pilot studies are ongoing to evaluate whether glass-stored ampligen is beneficial.

Interleukin-2

Interleukin-2 (IL-2) initially appeared to be ineffective in the treatment of patients with AIDS. However, Lane (35) reported that persistent intravenous infusion of high concentrations of IL-2 resulted in a lymphocytosis without any increase in virus recovery. Side effects included a "flu-like" syndrome, fluid retention, and an increase in

bacterial infections (36). There are currently a number of phase I clinical trials using IL-2 in combination with AZT (reviewed in ref. 8). These protocols are examining different routes (iv and subcutaneous), doses, and frequencies (continuous versus weekly) of IL-2 administration. IL-2 in combination with AZT has also been studied by Schwartz et al. (37). Preliminary data have indicated an increase in CD4+ lymphocyte and total leukocyte counts, active cellular cytotoxicity against virus (HIV and EBV)-infected and NK cell targets, and enhanced skin test reactivity, with no signs of drug toxicity or drug antagonism. Virus infection, as measured by p24 levels or recovery of HIV in culture remained stable during therapy. More extensive investigation of this combination is warranted.

Growth and Differentiation Factors

In addition to IL-2, other factors involved in the growth and differentiation of blood cells are being investigated in combination therapy with AZT, principally with the aim of preventing or ameliorating cytopenias. Granulocyte/macrophage colony stimulating factor (GM-CSF) has been utilized (38,39) to reduce the frequency or severity of the granulocytopenia that often complicates AZT therapy. Kimura et al. (40) demonstrated that GM-CSF could elevate neutrophil counts in neutropenic AIDS or ARC patients using 100–200 μg/M^2/day given for 1 week or longer. However, patients required 300 μg/M^2 to maintain the increased neutrophil counts if they were receiving 400 mg or more of AZT per day. GM-CSF had no effect on either total CD4+ cell count or on the CD4/CD8 ratio.

Erythropoietin has been studied as a component of combination therapy (41). Recombinant human erythropoietin 100 IU/kg administered iv 3 times/week was used to treat 29 AIDS patients receiving AZT therapy, in a randomized double-blind protocol that included 34 placebo-treated controls. After 2–3 months the investigators noted a reduction in the red blood cell transfusion requirement in the erythropoietin-treated group and an increase in hematocrit. Those who responded had a baseline serum erythropoietin level of less than 500 mU/ml; patients with levels in excess of this did not respond. This study was subsequently criticized (42) since AZT doses were high (750 mg/day) at the beginning of the study but were lowered thereafter. This intervention could have contributed to the improved hematologic profile. Thus additional studies are needed to confirm the findings.

Thymic Hormones

Thymic hormones have been evaluated for anti-HIV effects in several small studies. Thymopentin, a pentapeptide comprising part of the active site of thymopoietin, has been investigated by Barcellini et al. (43). A dose of 50 mg of thymopentin given subcutaneously three times weekly for 3 weeks resulted in increases in CD4 counts, IgG production, and lymphocyte proliferation in response to pokeweed mitogen in eight HIV-infected pre-AIDS patients as compared to eight uninfected controls. This trial was extended to 12 months with 29 patients and 11 controls (44) and similar benefits were again observed. This has been followed by a blinded multicenter trial (45) involving 47 thymopentin-treated asymptomatic HIV-seropositives and ARC patients not receiving AZT and 44 placebo-treated controls. At the time of this writing, four controls had progressed to AIDS, compared to none of the thymopentin-treated patients. Treated patients with entry CD4 counts above 400/mm^3 maintained those levels while controls showed reductions in these counts. There was no increase in p24 or β_2-microglobulin levels in thymopentin-treated patients. These studies are being continued and additional ones using thymopentin in combination with AZT are planned.

Thymic humoral factor, a chemically defined peptide from bovine thymus, has been used in a controlled trial in 14 asymptomatic HIV-infected patients (46). Five out of seven treated patients showed an increase in CD4 cell count versus none out of seven controls. Phase I trials are progressing with this hormone. Additional thymic hormones have been examined for beneficial effects in AIDS, but thymulin, thymosin-α_1, and thymostimulin (TP-1) are no longer being clinically evaluated.

Transfer Factor

Transfer factor (TF) is a dialyzed extract from peripheral blood leukocytes. This dialysate is believed to contain factors that can transfer both specific immune responses (delayed hypersensitivity) and nonspecific host responses. While the structure of any single transfer factor has not been identified, TF is believed to contain inosine and amino acids. Hadden (19) has previously reported that TF has thymomimetic properties, which the author suggests might be attributed to the inosine moiety. TF preparations were used to treat nine anergic HIV-infected patients on a weekly basis for 4 weeks (47). Skin test responses returned in 6/7 patients, as did *in vitro* mitogen responses, and CD4 lymphocyte counts improved. Kirkpatrick et al. (*personal communication*) have treated seven patients with TF preparations from other mixtures of leukocytes from several donors or a highly purified preparation derived from *Candida*-sensitized donors. Those treated with the mixed leukocyte preparation had no response, while two AIDS patients with esophageal candidiasis who were treated with the purified TF preparation responded clinically and re-

gained skin test responsiveness to *Candida* antigen. No toxicity was reported using TF from either source.

ImReg-1

ImReg-1 is another dialyzed leukocyte extract shown by Gottlieb et al. (48) to have immunostimulatory activity. The small peptides Tyr-Gly and Try-Gly-Gly are believed to be the active components (49). Intracutaneous injection with tetanus toxoid leads to enhanced dermal skin reactions and *in vitro* treatment of lymphocytes leads to increased lymphokine release. Gottlieb et al. (48) led a multicenter clinical trial using ImReg-1 to treat 93 ARC patients twice weekly (48 nontreated controls were included). Progression to a clinically defined endpoint (4.3% ImReg versus 25% control) or to AIDS (3% versus 17%) was significantly reduced. Marginal improvements in CD4+ cell counts and clinical symptoms were also recorded. No toxicity was observed. Thus a larger confirmatory trial is under consideration.

Isoprinosine

Isoprinosine, like TF, is an inosine-containing compound with thymomimetic activity. This compound has been demonstrated to induce T lymphocyte differentiation and stimulate T cell function both *in vitro* and *in vivo* (see ref. 19). Early controlled trials in HIV-infected patients with CD4+ cell counts greater than 500/mm^3 demonstrated increased NK cell activity and increased CD4+ cell counts with a reduction in clinical symptoms and infrequency of conversion of ARC to AIDS (50–52). Disappointing results both clinically and immunologically, however, were obtained in a multicenter trial involving nearly 700 HIV-infected, symptomatic patients with CD4+ cell counts of less than 400/mm^3 (8). In contrast, a Scandinavian trial of 866 ARC patients with a mean CD4+ count of about 425/mm^3 demonstrated a significant reduction in the conversion of ARC to AIDS (4% untreated versus 0.5% treated) during a 6-month period (53,54). In a similar trial conducted in Italy with 553 asymptomatic HIV-infected patients, DeSimone et al. (55,56) reported no new opportunistic infections in the isoprinosine-treated patients, while untreated controls reported 12 such infections. Several immunologic parameters improved in the treated group as compared to controls. These studies suggest that isoprinosine therapy in pre-AIDS patients with CD4+ counts greater than 400/mm^3 provides beneficial effects, at least transiently. Longer evaluation periods are needed to determine if the effects of such treatment are lasting. Unfortunately, the loss of patent rights by the pharmaceutical company supporting these trials has resulted in failure to apply for licensing of this drug.

Pursuit of additional inosine derivatives has been a focus of our laboratory and second-generation drugs relative to isoprinosine will soon be ready for clinical trial.

Methyl Inosine Monophosphate (MIMP)

Methyl inosine monophosphate (MIMP) is a derivative of IMP that is intended to replace isoprinosine. In preclinical studies and in *in vitro* studies using human peripheral blood leukocytes (PBL), it appears to have advantages over its predecessors. In mice infected with a murine leukemia virus, MIMP administered orally over a dose range of 1–50 mg/kg/day significantly increased survival as compared with placebo-treated controls (J. W. Hadden, *unpublished data*). Human PBL treated *in vitro* with MIMP showed increased blastogenic stimulation in response to phytohemagglutinin (J. W. Hadden, *unpublished data*). Importantly, PBL from AIDS patients also responded to mitogen in an improved manner in the presence of MIMP. Thus there is preliminary evidence to suggest that MIMP may be potentially beneficial as an AIDS therapy.

Diethyldithiocarbamate (Imuthiol)

Another orally active thymomimetic drug that has been examined as an AIDS therapeutic is diethyldithiocarbamate (DTC). This drug is more active and less toxic than its predecessor, levamisole (19,57). The drug was first shown to be promising in a murine retroviral infection model (58). Subsequently, clinical trials using DTC (10 mg/kg orally) in HIV-infected patients indicated that the drug could decrease the frequency of ARC symptoms and of conversion from ARC to AIDS (4.5% versus 13% in untreated controls) and could increase CD4+ lymphocyte counts (59,60). In a randomized trial of 25 patients with CD4+ cell counts greater than 200/mm^3, the group receiving DTC at a dose of 800 mg/M^2 administered iv twice weekly had a reduction in lymphadenopathy (61).

These studies were followed by a large multicenter trial of 389 patients (62), in which a significant (approximately 50%) reduction in opportunistic infections was observed in both the ARC and AIDS patients randomized to receive 400 mg/M^2 of DTC orally once per week. No significant increase in CD4+ cells was noted as compared to controls. Treatment of asymptomatic HIV-infected individuals with DTC is presently underway in Europe in a study involving 1600 patients. Preliminary results suggest that DTC can produce a reduction in symptomatology, lymphadenopathy, opportunistic infections, and progression of disease, while increasing CD4+ cell counts. Thus it appears that DTC and per-

haps other thymomimetic drugs may be an important adjunct to therapy for HIV-infected individuals.

Soluble CD4

Recombinant DNA technology has allowed the preparation of soluble CD4, the cellular receptor for HIV. Theoretically, this molecule will bind to HIV and thus prevent viral attachment to lymphocytes. Phase I/II testing indicates that, with frequent administration, serum CD4 levels of 10–100 ng/ml can be achieved without accompanying toxicity (63,64). These levels are sufficient to inhibit viral replication *in vitro*. Although there is no evidence to date of clinical benefit from soluble CD4 therapy, phase I/II trials are underway for HIV-seropositive, asymptomatic individuals with CD4+ cell counts between 200 and 500/mm^3 (65).

There are ongoing attempts to link bacterial toxins (e.g., *Pseudomonas aeruginosa* exotoxin) or other molecules to soluble CD4. The rational for this approach is based on the binding of soluble CD4 plus toxin to gp120 on the surface of HIV-infected cells, with internalization of toxin and death of the target cell selectively. Clinical trials are anticipated. A note of caution to this approach is that problems may be encountered with the antigenicity of the toxin.

AS 101

AS 101 is an ammonium salt of tellurium that can stimulate growth factor production by murine or human lymphocytes (CSF and IL-2) and can augment mitogen-induced lymphoblastogenesis. Phase I/II clinical trials are in progress in the United States, testing the efficacy of AS 101 alone or in combination with AZT (8).

SUMMARY OF CURRENT STATUS

Presently there is no evidence that an immunotherapeutic regimen is likely to provide a long-term cure for HIV infection. Nevertheless, several studies have provided enough favorable data to suggest that immunotherapy(ies) alone, or more likely as an adjunct to antiviral therapy, can benefit patients. Experience with the growth factor, erythropoietin, has indicated that adjunctive therapy with this compound can limit the degree of anemia caused by AZT. Interferon-α is unequivocally effective in the treatment of Kaposi's sarcoma in selected HIV-infected patients but has not benefited other HIV-infected patients without this neoplasm. A preliminary report suggesting that IFN-α given in low dose by the oral route is highly effective in limiting AIDS progression deserves further investigation but must be viewed

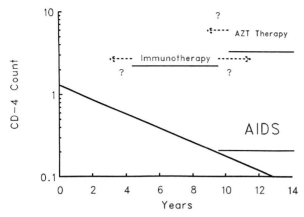

FIG. 1. Model for combined antiviral–immunostimulatory therapy for AIDS.

with limited enthusiasm until confirmed in more extensive trials.

Positive results have been attained with five other agents, IL-2, DTC, ImReg-1, thymopentin, and isoprinosine. The latter two agents have thymomimetic activity, suggesting that T lymphocyte upregulation may be a key to successful immune therapy. These five agents require further study both alone and in combination with antiviral agents. The data are not yet compelling enough to warrant adoption of any given protocol for general clinical use. Furthermore, at what point in the natural history of HIV infection immunostimulants should be administered either alone or with antiviral agents is unclear (Fig. 1). Thus investigators in this area are charged with refining their approach(es) (66) using the criteria discussed below.

PROSPECTS FOR FUTURE IMMUNOTHERAPY

Identifying the Defects to be Corrected

Our inability to understand fully the pathogenesis of HIV infection as it passes from clinical latency through the earliest symptoms to frank AIDS is the greatest impediment to developing effective immunotherapy. The central defect in the CD4+ cell population is quite obvious, but the cause for the defect must be clearly identified in order to identify measures necessary to correct the problem. Immune therapies that have boosted CD4+ cell counts have also been associated with certain clinical improvements in the short term, but as yet the long-term effects are unknown. Moreover, it is still uncertain as to what other defects in the immune system contribute to disease progression. Defects in NK cell activity, cytokine production, and others are noted in AIDS patients, but their significance remains ill defined. These gaps in our understanding of HIV infection increase the challenge of finding safe and effective immunotherapeutic approaches.

Goals for Immunotherapy

There are several approaches that can be taken to designing immunotherapy. Establishing immune therapy as the primary type of treatment for patients is somewhat different from using immune stimulants as an adjunct to antiviral (or antimicrobial) chemotherapy. Thus deciding whether trials will be one dimensional or combinational is critical to their design. In addition, determining whether therapy is intended to be immunoprophylactic or immunorestorative is necessary. Is the therapeutic approach intended to maintain "normal" immune function in asymptomatic HIV-infected persons or to restore function in patients already demonstrating depressed immune function? Another issue is whether therapy is intended to improve lymphocyte numbers and/or function or to reverse granulocyte or erythrocyte cytopenias. The most useful immunotherapeutic approach currently remains ill defined.

Definition of Timing of Administration

The optimal time to begin immune therapy is also unclear. Based on observations to date it seems likely that beginning therapy before CD4+ cell counts drop below 400–500/mm^3 would yield the greatest benefit. However, it is conceivable that introduction of immunotherapy at this stage will be problematic, since immune stimulation might either activate virus or lead to dysregulation of host immunity. Determination of the most beneficial time to initiate immunotherapy is likely to be a critical factor in the success of this approach.

Prospects for Combination Therapy

Studies of immunotherapy are more and more frequently examining combinations of an immunostimulant and AZT. Numerous problems and questions are raised by such combinations. For example, it is much more difficult to assess the benefits of each individual component when two or more agents are used together. Such studies will necessitate inclusion of larger numbers of patients randomized into several treatment arms, including an evaluation of either drug alone versus the combination. This type of study design should help to elucidate whether beneficial effects of drug combinations are based on additive or synergistic effects of the individual components.

Another key aspect of studies involving drug combinations is the timing and dosing of each component. For example, can antiviral drug levels that border on toxicity be reduced due to the added benefit of immunotherapy? Should the two components of therapy be administered simultaneously or sequentially, and if the latter approach is used, which should be administered first and for how long? How much time should elapse between administration of each component? Should combinations be tried involving three or more components? These are not readily answerable questions at present. They will require extensive study in preclinical and clinical trials.

A Role for Vaccines in Combination Treatment

Vaccine development against HIV has been deemed to be an important strategy for both disease management and prevention. Vaccines are currently being examined in both HIV-seropositive and -seronegative individuals. The concept of a postexposure vaccine for a virus that has already established latent infection in its target organs is unprecedented. In order to generate an immune response that is protective, it is possible that newer adjuvants, for example, muramyl dipeptides (67), may be necessary for administration with vaccines. An alternative to vaccines is passive immunotherapy using antibodies to HIV epitopes that can lead to virus neutralization. Reports that technology is emerging for the production of human–human hybridomas to generate anti-HIV monoclonal antibodies have surfaced recently. It will be interesting to see if immunostimulatory therapy might be used to boost anti-HIV immunity generated by either a vaccine or serotherapy.

CONCLUSIONS

The application of immunotherapy for AIDS has yet to realize the hope that is held for this approach. Despite the absence of great success with this approach, we have outlined herein some fruitful and encouraging beginnings. Immunotherapy combined with antiviral therapy has provided indications that such approaches may be of greater benefit than either component used alone. Agents such as interferon-α, growth factors, thymic hormones, and thymomimetic agents have contributed to the slowing of disease progression, increased CD4+ cell counts and clinical improvement. These results have tended to be more evident when therapy is applied before the onset of frank AIDS and when CD4+ lymphocyte counts are greater than 400/mm^3.

While the total elimination of virus in the infected host does not seem to be a reality at present, the use of combinations of immunotherapeutic agents and antiviral chemotherapy offers improved prospects for maintaining subclinical infection, continued health of the HIV-infected host, and a higher quality of life.

REFERENCES

1. Barré-Sinoussi F, Chermann JC, Rey F, et al. Isolation of a T-lymphotropic retrovirus from a patient at risk for acquired immune deficiency syndrome (AIDS). *Science* 1983;220:868–71.

2. Popovic M, Sarngadharan MG, Read E, Gallo RC. Detection, isolation, and continuous production of cytopathic retroviruses (HTLV-III) from patients with AIDS and pre-AIDS. *Science* 1984;224:840–2.

3. Ongradi J, Ceccherini-Nelli L, Soldaini E, Bendinelli M, Conaldi PG, Specter S, Friedman H. Endotoxin suppresses indirect activation of HIV-1 by human herpesvirus 6. In: Nowotny A, Spitzer JJ, Ziegler EJ, eds. *Cellular and molecular aspects of endotoxin reactions.* Amsterdam: Elsevier; 1990:387–94.

4. Wright K. Mycoplasma in the AIDS spotlight. *Science* 1990;248:682–3.

5. Lo S-C, Tsai S, Benish JR, Shih W-K, Wear DJ, Wong DM. Enhancement of HIV-1 cytocidal effects in CD4+ lymphocytes by the AIDS-associated mycoplasma. *Science* 1991;251:1074–6.

6. Watson RR. *Co-factors in HIV-1 infection and AIDS.* Boca Raton, FL: CRC Press; 1990.

7. Koenig S, Fauci AS. Immunology of AIDS and HIV infection. In: Gallo RC, Wong-Staal F, eds. *Retrovirus biology and human disease.* New York: Marcel Dekker; 1990:285–316.

8. Abrams D, Grieco M, Gottlieb M, Speer M (eds.). *AIDS/HIV experimental treatment,* AMFAR Directory Vol 3, No. 1. AMFAR;1989.

9. Sandstrom E. Antiviral therapy in human immunodeficiency virus infection. *Drugs* 1989;38(3):417–50.

10. de Clercq E. Targets and strategies for the antiviral chemotherapy of AIDS. *Trends Pharmacol* 1990;11:198–205.

11. Volberding PA, Lagakos SW, Kock MA, et al., AIDS Clinical Trials Group National Institute of Allergies and Infectious Diseases. Zidovudine in asymptomatic human immunodeficiency virus infection. *N Engl J Med* 1990;322:941–9.

12. Zagury D, Leonard R, Fouchard M, et al. Immunization against AIDS in humans. *Nature* 1987;326:249–50.

13. Ada G. Prospects for a vaccine against HIV. *Nature* 1989;339:331–2.

14. Bolognesi DP. Progress in vaccines against AIDS. *Science* 1989;246:1233–4.

15. Girard M. Prospects for an AIDS vaccine. *Cancer Detect Prev* 1990;14:411–3.

16. Koff W. Abstracts of the International Conference on Advances in AIDS Vaccine Development, US Public Health Service, 1990.

17. Pahwa S, Pahwa R, Saxinger C, Gallo RC, Good RA. Influence of the human T-lymphotropic virus/lymphadenopathy-associated virus on functions of human lymphocytes: evidence for immunosuppressive effects and polyclonal B-cell activation by banded viral preparations. *Proc Natl Acad Sci USA* 1985;82:8198–202.

18. Plata F. HIV-specific cytotoxic T lymphocytes. *Res Immunol* 1989;140:89–124.

19. Hadden JW. Current status of the immunotherapy of AIDS and the AIDS-related complex. In: Wormser GP, Stahl RE, Bottone EJ, eds. *AIDS and other manifestations of HIV Infection.* Park Ridge, NJ: Noyes Publications; 1987:992.

20. Lane HC, Masur H, Gelmann EP, Fauci AS. Therapeutic approaches to patients with AIDS. *Cancer Res* 1985;45:4674s–6.

21. Gupta S, Gottlieb MS. Treatment of the acquired immune deficiency syndrome. *J Clin Immunol* 1986;6:183–93.

22. Lane HC, Davey RT Jr, Sherwin SA, et al. A phase I trial of recombinant human interferon-γ in patients with Kaposi's sarcoma and acquired immunodeficiency syndrome (AIDS). *J Clin Immunol* 1989;9:351–61.

23. Hadden JW. Current immunotherapeutic efforts and future prospects in human HIV disease. In: Hadden JW, Spreafico F, Yamamura Y, Austen KF, Dukor P, Masek K, eds. *Advances in immunopharmacology 4.* New York: Pergamon Press; 1989:19.

24. Johnson VA, Hirsch MS. New developments in antiretroviral drug therapy for human immunodeficiency virus infections. In: Volberding P, Jacobson MA, eds. *AIDS clinical review 1990.* New York: Marcel Dekker; 1990:235–72.

25. Jackson GG, Perkins JT, Rubenis M, Paul DA, Knigge M, Despotas JC, Spencer P. Passive immunoneutralization of HIV p24 antigenemia in patients with advanced AIDS by infusion of human plasma. IV Int Conf AIDS 96:35-37 and *Lancet* 2(8612):647–52.

26. Karpas A, Hill F, Youle M, et al. Effects of passive immunization in patients with the acquired immunodeficiency syndrome-related complex and acquired immunodeficiency syndrome. *Proc Natl Acad Sci USA* 1988;85:9234–7.

27. NIH Consensus Conference. Intravenous immunoglobulin: prevention and treatment of disease. *JAMA* 1990;264:3189–93.

28. DeSimone C, Antonaci S, Chirigos S, et al. Report of the symposium on the use of intravenous gamma globulin (IVIG) in adults infected with HIV. *J Clin Lab Anal* 1990;4:313–7.

29. Holland HK, Saral R, Rossi JJ, et al. Allogenic bone marrow transplantation, zidovudine and human immunodeficiency virus type I (HIV-I) infection. *Ann Intern Med* 1989;111:973–81.

30. Brook MG, Gor D, Forster S, Harris JRW, Jeffries DJ, Thomas HC. Anti-HIV effects of α-interferon. *Lancet* 1989;1:42.

31. Davey V, Johnson RP, Lane HC. A placebo-controlled trial of interferon α-2b in asymptomatic HIV infection. 5th International Conference on AIDS, Montreal, Canada, June 1989.

32. Koech DK, Obel AO. Efficacy of Kemron (low dose oral interferon alpha) in the management of HIV-1 infection and acquired immunodeficiency syndrome (AIDS). *East Afr Med J* 1991; 67:S64–70.

33. Carter WA, Brodsky I, Pellegrino MG, et al. Clinical, immunological and virological effects of ampligen, a mismatched double-stranded RNA in patients with AIDS or AIDS-related complex. *Lancet* 1987;6:1286–92.

34. Strayer DR. Ampligen therapy in ARC/pre-ARC: immune/virological effects and clinical improvement. 4th International Conference on AIDS, Stockholm, Sweden, June 1988.

35. Lane HC. The role of immunomodulators in the treatment of patients with AIDS. *AIDS* 1989;3(suppl 1):181s–5.

36. Murphy PM, Lane HC, Gallin JI, Fauci AS. Marked disparity in incidence of bacterial infections in patients with the acquired immunodeficiency syndrome receiving interleukin-2 or interferon-γ. *Ann Intern Med* 1988;108:35–41.

37. Schwartz DH, Skowron G, Merigan TC. Safety and effects of interleukin-2 plus zidovudine in asymptomatic individuals infected with human immunodeficiency virus. Summary of Infectious Diseases and AIDS Meeting, San Francisco, 1990.

38. Groopman JE, Mitsuyasu RT, DeLeo MJ, Oette D, Golde DW. Effect of recombinant human granulocyte-macrophage colony-stimulating factor on myelopoiesis in the acquired immunodeficiency syndrome. *N Engl J Med* 1987;317:593–8.

39. Baldwin GC, Gasson JC, Quan SG, et al. Granulocyte-macrophage colony-stimulating factor enhances neutrophil function in acquired immunodeficiency syndrome patients. *Proc Natl Acad Sci USA* 1988; 85:2763–6.

40. Kimura S, Matsuda J, Ikematsu S, et al. Efficacy of recombinant human granulocyte colony-stimulating factor on neutropenia in patients with AIDS. *AIDS* 1990;12:1251–5.

41. Fischl M, Galpin JE, Levine JD, et al. Recombinant human erythropoietin for patients with AIDS treated with zidovudine. *N Engl J Med* 1990;322:1488–93.

42. Shepp D, Agins BD, Farber BF. Letter to the Editor. *N Engl J Med* 1990;323:1069–70.

43. Barcellini W, Meroni PL, Frasca D, et al. Effect of subcutaneous thymopentin treatment in drug addicts with persistent generalized lymphadenopathy. *Clin Exp Immunol* 1987;67:537–43.

44. Silvestris F, Gernone A, Frassanito M, Dammacco F. Immunologic effects of long-term thymopentin treatment in patients with HIV-induced lymphadenopathy syndrome. *J Lab Clin Med* 1989;113:139–44.

45. Conant MA, Goldstein G, Hirsch RL, Meyerson LA, Kremer AB. The effect of thymopentin treatment on progression of disease and surrogate markers in HIV-infected patients without AIDS. (UCLA Symposia on Molecular and Cell Biology, San Francisco AIDS Meeting Abstract #L411.) *J Cell Biochem [Suppl]* 1990;14D:148.

46. Handzel ZT, Galili-Weisstraub E, Burstein R, et al. Immune derangements in asymptomatic male homosexuals in Israel: a pre-AIDS condition? *Ann NY Acad Sci* 1984;437:549–53.

47. Carey JT, Lederman MM, Tossii Z, et al. Augmentation of skin test reactivity and lymphocyte blastogenesis in patients with AIDS treated with transfer factor. *JAMA* 1987;257:651–5.

48. Gottlieb AA, Trial Investigators. A phase 3 controlled trial of ImReg-1 in AIDS/ARC patients. 4th International Conference on AIDS, Stockholm, Sweden, June 1988.

49. Sinha SK, Sizemore RC, Gottlieb AA. Immunomodulatory components present in ImReg-1, an experimental immunosupportive biologic. *Biotechnology* 1988;6:810–5.

50. Glasky AJ, Gordon J. Inosiplex treatment of acquired immunodeficiencies: a clinical model for effective immunomodulation. *Methods Fund Exp Clin Pharmacol* 1986;8:35–40.

51. Bekesi JG, Tsang PH, Wallace JI, Roboz JP. Immunorestorative properties of isoprinosine in the treatment of patients at high risk of developing ARC or AIDS. *J Clin Lab Immunol* 1987;24: 155–61.

52. Hoehler F, Robins DS. Incidence of acquired immune deficiency syndrome in patients with persistent generalized lymphadenopathy: immunologic risk factors and effects of short-term immunotherapy with inosine pranobex. *Curr Ther Res* 1988;43:688–700.

53. Jurgensen HJ, Scandinavian Isoprinosine Study Group. Influence on development of AIDS in patients with human immunodeficiency virus (HIV) infection; efficacy and safety of isoprinosine (inosine pranobex, methisoprinol): a randomized, double blind, placebo-controlled, multicenter study in Denmark and Sweden. *EOS J Immunol Immunopharmacol* 1989;9:185–6.

54. Pedersen C, Sandstrom E, Petersen CS, et al. Scandinavian Isoprinosine Study Group. The efficacy of inosine pranobex in preventing the acquired immunodeficiency syndrome in patients with human immunodeficiency virus infection. *N Engl J Med* 1990;322:1757–63.

55. DeSimone C, Albertini F, Almaviva M, et al. Clinical and immunological assessment in HIV⁺ subjects receiving inosine-pranobex: a randomized, multicentric study. *Med Oncol Tumor Pharmacother* 1988;10:299–303.

56. DeSimone C, Albertini F, Almaviva M, et al. The place of methisoprinol (inosine pranobex, isoprinosine) for the therapy of HIV infected subjects. *EOS J Immunol Immunopharmacol* 1989;9: 184–5.

57. Renoux G, Renoux M. Diethyldithiocarbamate (DTC): a biological augmenting agent specific for T cells. In: Fenichel RL, Chirigos MA, eds. *Immune modulation agents and their mechanisms.* New York: Marcel Dekker; 1984:7.

58. Hersh EM, Funk CY, Peterson EA, Mosier DE. Biological activity of diethyldithiocarbamate (Ditiocarb, Imuthiol) in an animal model of retrovirus-induced immunodeficiency disease and in clinical trials in patients with HIV infection. The Ditiocarb Study Group. *Dev Biol Stand* 1990;72:355–63.

59. Lang J. Long term administration of dithiocarbamate in HIV-seropositive subjects. 5th International Conference on AIDS, Montreal, Canada, June 1989.

60. Reisinger EC, Kern P, Ernst M, Bock P, Flao HD, Dietrich M, German DTC Study Group. Inhibition of HIV progression by dithiocarb. *Lancet* 1990;335:679–82.

61. Kaplan CS, Peterson EA, Yocum D, Hersh EM. A randomized controlled dose response study of intravenous sodium diethyldithiocarbamate in patients with advanced human immunodeficiency virus infection. *Life Sci* 1989;45:iii–ix.

62. Hersh EM, Brewton G, Abrams D, et al. Ditiocarb sodium (diethyldithiocarbamate) in patients with symptomatic HIV infection and AIDS. A randomized, double-blind, placebo-controlled, multicenter study. *JAMA* 1991;265:1538–44.

63. Kahn JO, Allan JD, Hodges TL, et al. The safety and pharmacokinetics of recombinant soluble CD4 (rCD4) in subjects with the acquired immunodeficiency syndrome (AIDS) and AIDS-related complex. *Ann Intern Med* 1990;112:254–61.

64. Schooley RT, Merigan TC, Gaut P, et al. Recombinant soluble CD4 therapy in patients with the acquired immunodeficiency syndrome (AIDS) and AIDS-related complex. *Ann Intern Med* 1990;112:247–53.

65. Abrams D, Wong R, Grieco M, et al. Results of phase I/II placebo-controlled dose finding pilot study of lentinan in patients with HIV infection. Summary of Infectious Diseases and AIDS Meeting, San Francisco, 1990.

66. Hadden JW. Immunotherapy of human immunodeficiency virus infection. *TIPS Rev* 1991;12:107–11.

67. Audibert F, Jolivet-Reynaud C, Jolivet M, Lise D. Modulation of the immunogenic characters of the protective epitopes in synthetic vaccines. In: Hadden JW, Spreafico F, Yamamura Y, Austen KF, Kukor P, Masek K, eds. *Advances in immunopharmacology 4.* New York: Pergamon Press; 1989:133.

AIDS and Other Manifestations of HIV Infection,
Second Edition, Edited by Gary P. Wormser.
Raven Press, Ltd., New York © 1992.

CHAPTER 39

Progress in the Development and Testing of HIV Vaccines

G. L. Ada

It is some 8 years since the virus HIV, which infects humans and leads to the condition known as AIDS, was first discovered. Progress since that time in elucidating the structure of the virus, in defining the process of infection of a cell via the CD4 receptor, and in describing the immune response of the host and the events that lead to immunodeficiency and disease has been spectacular. By 1986–1987, there was considerable optimism that a vaccine would soon be forthcoming; after all, current viral vaccines for medical use were generally highly successful and there was an additional number close to registration for human use. However, the most effective of these prevented infection/disease by viruses that showed little or no antigenic variation, that induced acute infections, and that were not retroviruses. When these and other factors were realized, the potential difficulties of the task became more apparent (1,2). It seemed that an attenuated retroviral vaccine would be unacceptable, unless all else failed, and that there would be some concern even about a vaccine containing inactivated whole virus with its full complement of RNA (3). This meant that vaccine candidates would be developed using either peptide synthesis or application of recombinant DNA technology. To achieve this, the antigenic properties of the virus needed to be mapped in detail. Much of this has now been done.

G. L. Ada: Department of Immunology and Infectious Diseases, Johns Hopkins School of Hygiene and Public Health, Baltimore, Maryland 21205. Present address: Division of Cell Biology, John Curtin School of Medical Research, Australian National University, Canberra, ACT 2601, Australia.

ACHIEVEMENTS

Virus Structure

HIV-1 and HIV-2 have the most complex structure of any known retroviruses as far as the accessory or regulatory proteins are concerned (4). The HIV-1 proviral genome is 9.7 kb in length, which includes regulatory sequences at either end, long terminal repeats (LTRs), and genes coding viral proteins that have structural (env, gag) or enzymatic (pol) properties. The env protein consists of two segments linked non covalently: gp41, which has a transmembrane component, and gp120, which is entirely external to the viral membrane. The gag (group-specific) protein is translated as a polyprotein precursor molecule, p55, which is cleaved to form four products (p17, p24, p9, p7). The products of the *pol* gene have enzymatic activities, a reverse transcriptase, an endonuclease, a protease, and an integrase. There is an elaborate set of regulatory genes that determine whether or not virus is made and, if so, the level of production; they include *vpr, rev, vif, tat, vpu,* and *nef.* Their role in viral regulation will not be commented on further.

Process of Infection

There is general agreement that the CD4 molecule, which is expressed principally but not only on class II MHC-restricted T cells, is the major if not the only specific receptor for HIV (5). Complementary sites on this molecule and on gp120 have been mapped (6). HIV appears to use the second of the two known methods of viral entry into susceptible cells: pH-dependent fusion of virus particles with the membrane of endocytic vesicles, or pH-independent fusion with the plasma membrane. The CD4 molecule may be necessary both for viral attachment and for some subsequent step of entry into the cell. There is some evidence that another cell molecule in addition to CD4 may act as a receptor for HIV-2, as HIV-1 cannot superinfect HIV-2-infected cells, whereas HIV-2 can superinfect HIV-1-infected cells, though with delayed kinetics (7).

CD4 is expressed at low levels on a variety of other cells, including those of the myeloid line such as monocytes, macrophages, microglia, and dendritic and follicular dendritic cells. All these cells are susceptible to and become infected *in vivo* by HIV; the latter two strongly support viral replication (8). Other receptors (Fc and C) for aggregated immunoglobulins may with CD4 enhance entry of the virus into certain cells. A variety of other cells such as stromal fibroblasts and megakaryocytes in the bone marrow can be infected and may play a role in the suppression of hematopoiesis (9). Soluble CD4 can prevent infection of most cells by HIV (10) but is rather less effective if freshly isolated rather than cell-grown virus is used (11).

Antigens as Targets for Immune Attack

Vaccines especially for prophylaxis must stimulate the adaptive components of the immune response, that is, the lymphocyte that displays immunological memory. This next section describes the search for B and T cell epitopes on the various antigenic components of the virus.

B Cell Epitopes for Neutralization for ADCC, for Immune Enhancement, and for Autoimmunity

Neutralizing antibody is the major specific defense mechanism, preventing viral replication and possibly entry to the cell. The recent recognition that there is a principle neutralizing determinant (PND), the V3 loop in the gp120 molecule (12), is a very significant finding. This loop, formed by a disulfide bridge between two invariant cysteines at positions 303 and 338, is highly variable. The segment defined by residues 320–324 is relatively conserved, but the flanking regions are highly variable (Fig. 1). Sixty-five percent of 86 randomly chosen positive sera reacted with peptides containing the most common sequences. Though this is a linear determinant, there is now clear evidence that substitutions at residues downstream from this loop can affect the interaction of antibody with epitopes within the loop (13–15). Residue 582, which is external to the viral membrane in gp41, seems to be critical. It is thought that substitutions at this and at some of the other residues affects the conformation of the loop itself, so that anti-loop antibody, which otherwise neutralized viral infectivity, is now ineffective.

Other type-specific and some group-specific neutralization domains on both gp120 and gp41 have been identified; some are continuous and others discontinuous sequences (16,17). It has been proposed that they supplement rather than act independently of antibody to the V3 loop in preventing infection (18).

Antibody to viral proteins expressed at the surface of virus-infected cells may lyse those cells in one of two ways: by antibody-dependent cell-mediated cytotoxicity (ADCC) and by antibody- plus complement-mediated lysis. ADCC antibodies can be either isolate specific or group specific. In addition to the V3 loop, there are other epitopes distinct from neutralizing sites; one is the 46 amino acid sequence bridging the carboxy end of gp120 and the proximal NH_2 terminus of gp41 (19,20). ADCC can potentially have two roles in HIV infection. It may lyse HIV-infected cells and so be beneficial; if, however, free gp120 binds to uninfected cells via CD4, ADCC could conceivably destroy those cells and so accelerate progress to disease.

11	12	13	14	15	16	17	18	19	20	21	22	23	24	25	26	27
R 200	K 177	S 124	I 230	H 114	I 202	• 234	• 234	G 240	P 233	G 241	R 223	A 204	F 176	Y 196	• 243	T 137
K 20	R 57	G 69	L 5	T 27	M 17	Q 10	R 10	A 3	L 5	E 2	K 11	V 18	I 29	V 17	H 1	A 92
S 11	N 6	R 40	M 3	R 27	L 10	R 1	G 1	E 1	A 3	R 2	Q 4	N 5	V 14	H 13	T 1	• 5
I 6	Q 5	H 4	T 3	P 22	V 5			R 1	Q 2		• 3	T 5	L 10	L 8		V 4
E 3		K 4	V 2	N 16	T 3			S 2			S 2	R 4	Y 7	F 5		Q 3
P 1		A 3	E 1	S 16	R 2						M 1	K 4	W 6	R 3		Y 3
Q 1		• 1	F 1	Y 13	K 2						G 1	P 3	T 1	S 1		S 1
G 1				F 5	Y 2							S 1	S 1	M 1		
M 1				A 2	F 1							W 1	H 1	I 1		
T 1				G 1	S 1											
				V 1												
				K 1												

FIG. 1. Frequency of occurrence of amino acids at positions 11–27 of the consensus principle neutralizing determinant (PND). The 245 sequences were analyzed with a multiple-sequence alignment program to find the most frequently occurring amino acids and the extent of variability at positions in the central region of the PND. The amino acids occurring at positions 11–27 are shown with the number of times they occur at these positions. Periods indicate deletions. (From ref. 12, with permission.)

Antibody may have other unwanted effects. One is immune enhancement. If a virus replicates in cells expressing Fc and/or complement (C) receptors, uptake of virus–antibody (non-neutralizing) complexes may enhance viral infection within that cell and potentially hasten progression to disease. The classical example is dengue virus infections. Immune enhancement has been shown to occur in HIV-infected people and to correlate with disease, as judged by *in vitro* tests (21). Two separate enhancing domains, aa 579–613 and aa 644–663, both in gp41, have now been identified (22). It can be argued that these sequences should be deleted from future vaccines.

gp160 was also found to contain aa sequences that showed substantial homology with several normal host proteins, including class II MHC molecules (1). To date, there has been little evidence from either clinical trials or animal model systems to indicate that vaccination may cause significant autoimmunity and disease. As more potent adjuvants come to be used to enhance the immunogenicity of subunit and possibly polypeptide preparations, this possibility may need to be monitored.

T Cell Epitopes for Help, for Suppression, and for Cytotoxicity

T helper (Th) cells have been called the "leaders of the immunological orchestra" and as such they have a pivotal role in immune responses, aiding in the activation of both B cells and cytotoxic T (Tc) cells. Epitopes recognized by Th cells have been identified in the V3 loop and in conserved regions near the NH_2 terminus, in the CD4 binding area, in gp41, in gag, and in pol (23–27).

Suppressor cell activity in the peripheral blood lymphocytes (PBLs) of HIV-infected patients has also been reported (reviewed in ref. 6). Using synthetic peptides, a region (env aa sequence 581–597) within gp41, which specifically inhibits murine and human lymphoproliferation, has been identified (28). In HIV-seropositive individuals, antibody recognizing this peptide correlates with the absence of disease (29). However, whether a vaccine should aim to induce antibody to this region is not yet clear.

Many asymptomatic infected individuals maintain strong cytotoxic T cell (Tc) responses in their PBLs (without *in vitro* stimulation), sometimes for several years, and this has stimulated a search for epitopes recognized by these cells (30,31). To date, all the Tc cell responses to viral infections detected *in vivo* have been mediated by CD8+, class I MHC-restricted T cells; there is evidence from animal experiments using a range of viruses including influenza, Sendai, vaccinia, Kunjin, respiratory syncytial virus, and herpesviruses that such cells can clear viral infections (32). Although cultured or cloned CD4+ T cells have shown cytotoxic activity, such

a role for *primary* CD4+ cells *in vivo* remains to be proved (33). Based on our current understanding of the immune system, CD4+ cells, if cytotoxic, might lyse newly HIV antigen-activated B cells before antibody production occurred, hardly a desirable feature. Epitopes recognized by Tc cells have now been described in the env and/or gag antigens (34–36), p17 (37), reverse transcriptase (38,39), nef (40,41), and vif (42). Several aspects are worth emphasizing.

1. Of these proteins, nef and gag of HIV-1 seem to be important sources of Th and/or Tc epitopes.

2. The finding of continuing Tc lymphocyte activity in a viral infection is unusual and has been attributed to the continuing production of infectious virus from a source in the body that is not accessible/recognized by these cells (1).

3. The epitopes on the internal viral antigens are generally conserved sequences, for example, as in gag (43). This adds to the attraction of including at least some of these antigens in candidate vaccines in a form that would stimulate these responses.

4. Two properties of the epitopes in the gag and nef proteins have now been examined in some detail. By using synthetic peptides that may bind to cells expressing class I HLA molecules of different specificities, a number of peptides, occurring mainly in the midsection of the nef protein, have been identified. Sometimes, the same peptide binds to two (B17, B37) or three (A3, A11, B35) HLA molecules (44,45). Some peptides that bind to HLA molecules of different specificities, such as B18 and B7, overlap by about 50%.

5. By using a technique in which labeled HLA molecules can bind to immobilized synthetic peptides (46), many peptides have been found that mimic the results found using the above approach, but some have now been found that, so far, do not seem to be recognized by naturally occurring Tc cells.

6. As progression toward disease occurs, Tc cell activity declines. Several explanations for this have been proposed. One is the induction of escape mutants, as occurs with B cells; another is the progressive decrease in CD4+ cells; a third is the production of suppressor activity by CD8+ CD57+ cells, which are found particularly in the lung (47).

Though particular mixes of peptides might be a useful approach to vaccine development (see next section), inclusion of intact gag and nef as part of a subunit or live vector vaccine would have some advantage.

VACCINE CANDIDATES

Most attention to date has focused on the development of candidate HIV vaccines, using mainly five approaches. These are:

1. Inactivated whole virus. Attenuated strains of HIV are considered potentially too dangerous for human use.

2. Subunit preparations, based on part or all of some of the major antigens of HIV-1.

3. Live vectors containing DNA coding for one or more of the major antigens of the virus.

4. Complex oligopeptides, in which different viral epitopes and other sequences are linked together.

5. Anti-idiotypic preparations.

Each one of these approaches is being tried. Some preparations are in clinical trials and will be discussed further in the next section.

1. *Inactivated whole virus.* This is a traditional approach to vaccine development and several such preparations are effective vaccines, such as inactivated polio and Japanese encephalitis viruses. One HIV preparation (Immune Response Corporation), which has a depleted amount of the env gp120, is being used in clinical trials and this will be described in the next section. An alternative approach is to prepare pseudovirions, that is, whole virus particles that are noninfectious due to the deletion of key elements required for infectivity but not for virus assembly.

Much research is also being carried out with the related virus, simian immunodeficiency virus, particularly using whole inactivated virus.

2. *Subunit preparations.* Following the great success of the hepatitis B vaccine, which contains the surface antigen of the virus, this approach has become particularly favored. The env protein has been the major interest and several preparations have been made. One of the first candidates to become available is a preparation of HIV-1 gp160 made in baculovirus/insect cells (MicrogeneSyS). Recombinant vaccinia virus constructs have been used as a means of expressing very high titers of foreign proteins in mammalian cells; the protein may be secreted into the medium (48). A preparation of HIV-1 gp160 (Immuno-AG) has been made in this way and is under trial in chimpanzees. Preparations of gp120 and 160 (Genentech) have been made in transfected Chinese hamster ovary cells (49); the gp120 has protected chimpanzees and clinical trials are now in progress. A preparation of HIV-1 gp120 made in transfected yeast cells has been used in clinical trials in Switzerland.

There are two other subunit preparations. The gag protein is of interest because it is more conserved than the env protein and because high levels of antibodies to HIV gag proteins are said to be associated with stabilization of disease and improved clinical status (50). One group, British Biotechnology, has used a novel approach to make a subunit preparation (51). The *gag* gene was fused to a yeast transposon, Ty; this results in the formation of viruslike particles (VLPs), which may increase their immunogenicity. The other subunit preparation (Viral Technologies) is a synthetic analog of p17 (37,52).

Subunit preparations are almost invariably made using recombinant DNA technology and are likely to be relatively expensive to produce. They also require the use of an adjuvant. This is an area that has recently become very active.

3. *Live vector preparations.* Several viral and bacterial preparations, principally vaccinia, avipox, and adenoviruses, and the bacterial vaccine BCG, are being used as vectors of HIV-1 genes, principally the env, gag, and pol antigens. Viral vectors have the advantage that the protein, say, gp160, is synthesized, processed, and transported to the cell plasma membrane in a way that mimics that of the native protein following HIV infection (53). Most work has been with a chimeric vaccinia/gp160 construct, which has been administered to human volunteers and which will be described in the next section. A novel approach in this connection is the use of different avipox viruses, notably fowl and canary poxviruses. These viruses infect humans but only undergo an abortive replication cycle (54). Adenoviruses are now the center of much interest for two reasons: the current adenovirus vaccine administered to the U.S. armed forces has proved to be both safe and effective, and the vaccine is administered in an enteric coated pill, which is administered orally, thus inducing mucosal immunity. The gene coding for gp160 has been engineered into the virus and is expressed in infected mammalian cells (55).

BCG, a widely used vaccine given to babies shortly after birth, is under close investigation as a vector of genes coding for other antigens. Two recent publications (56,57) report the expression of gp120 in recombinant BCG. On administration to mice in initial experiments, both gave poor titers of anti-gp120 antibody but good T cell responses.

Live vectors have considerable potential advantages. Provided they are genetically stable, they should be relatively inexpensive to produce, should not require refrigeration, should be easy to administer, and should give long-lasting immunity after one or a few doses; these are properties that make them very attractive candidates for use in third world countries. The use of live vectors would be contraindicated for pregnant women and immunocompromised people, including those already infected with HIV.

4. *Peptide-based preparations.* Synthetic peptide preparations seek to include the epitopes necessary to induce both humoral and CMI responses, but to exclude the great majority of the protein, which can include sequences that, for example, mimic host proteins or are immunosuppressive. It is rare that a peptide by itself is immunogenic; it is usually conjugated to a carrier protein and the complex administered with an adjuvant. The examples in the case of HIV cover a spectrum. The

synthetic analog of p17, mentioned above, has been coupled to keyhole limpet hemocyanin (referred to as HGP30), is recognized by HIV-positive people, and has been administered to animals (37,58).

This approach seems to have been brought to its full potential by the conjugation of synthetic peptides, aligned in sequence and composed of an HIV-1 B cell epitope, a Th cell epitope, a Tc cell epitope, and a fusion peptide that allows entry of the complex into the cytoplasmic pathway of the cell. Immunization with this complex has resulted in the generation of neutralizing antibody, as well as Th and Tc responses, the latter being class I MHC restricted (59).

5. *Anti-idiotype antibodies.* Initially, there was considerable interest in the development of vaccines based on anti-idiotype antibodies. These would have the advantage that they could be made without knowing the details of viral structure. However, despite considerable work, no preparation has been made that shows sufficient promise of being effective to justify a greater effort.

PROTECTION STUDIES

Though the final test of any vaccine for medical use is its performance in humans, development of most vaccines is greatly facilitated if there is one or more appropriate animal models available. This has been a significant difficulty with HIV studies. The virus infects both the chimpanzee and the gibbon ape without causing disease; both of these animals are on the endangered list and are very expensive to use. Thus it has been stated that the cost of keeping a chimpanzee in captivity from birth to old age is approximately $250,000. Attempts to find other models have led to the use of SCID mice, which can be reconstituted with human cells and become susceptible to infection with HIV (60,61). A potentially promising use of this model is to reconstitute the mouse with PBLs and sera from immunized people (61) and to assess the ability of the reconstituted mice to withstand infection by HIV. It will be a significant step forward if this can be regularly achieved by defined preparations of cells and/or sera.

Protection Against HIV-1: Passive and Active Immunization Studies

There are numerous reports of monoclonal antibody (Mab) preparations against different regions of gp160 that neutralize HIV-1 infectivity *in vitro* and sometimes with a broad specificity (62). However, there are few reports where protection has been achieved following transfusion into the host before challenge. In an early study, protection had been achieved against the homologous virus by premixing the virus with the antibody (90

min) prior to injection into chimpanzees. More recently, the same group (63) reported that a chimpanzee transfused with 36 mg of a Mab specific for the V3 loop of the IIIB virus strain and challenged with 75 chimp infectious doses (CID_{50}) of the same virus 24 hr later was apparently protected against infection, as virus could not be recovered at any subsequent time from the host. This result clearly shows that antibody against this region in sufficient concentration and by itself can prevent infection by the homologous virus—a very significant finding.

There are three reports of protection of chimpanzees following immunization. In one report, chimpanzees were immunized (three injections) with gp120 (two animals) or gp160 (two animals) produced by transfected CHO cells. They were challenged with 10 CID_{50} of the homologous virus; the animals immunized with gp120 remained uninfected whereas those immunized with gp160 seroconverted more rapidly than a control, unimmunized animal. Protection correlated with high-titer neutralizing activity directed toward the intact V3 loop (50). The second example is rather more complex. Three chimpanzees were multiply immunized with a variety of HIV-1 preparations, including inactivated whole HIV or vaccinia/HIV protein constructs, but the final administration(s) was different V3 peptides; this resulted in high titers against this region. The dose of challenge virus was 40 CID_{50} and two of the animals have remained uninfected for well over 1 year; virus was recovered from the third animal about 7 months after challenge. In this experiment, there was no correlation between protection and neutralization titers (64). The third example is the Immuno-AG gp160 preparation, which exists as particles 20–30 nm in diameter. When administered twice with alum, only low levels of antibody resulted. Following three more injections using a lipid phase adjuvant, high titers of antibody resulted but only low levels of anti-V3 loop antibody; high T cell responses were generated. Following challenge with 100 $TCID_{50}$ of homologous virus, infection did not occur (65). In this trial, there was no apparent correlation between protection and anti-V3 loop antibody levels.

Protection Against SIV: Active Immunization

The lack of easily available, inexpensive animal models for HIV studies has prompted many more experiments with the closely related virus, simian immunodeficiency virus (SIV), which infects monkeys, some without causing disease but in others inducing a disease similar to AIDS. In contrast to HIV studies, the use of inactivated whole virus has been the most popular approach. Protection using formalin-inactivated SIV was first achieved in eight out of nine rhesus macaques challenged with about 10 MID_{50} (66) and this result has generally been repeatable. An alternative approach (67) was to immunize with SIV-infected cells after fixing the cells with glutaraldehyde and treating with B-propiolactone to destroy SIV infectivity. Initially, three to four injections were given but, recently, protection has been achieved after only two injections. An encouraging result has been the demonstration that immunization of monkeys with one SIV strain protected first against challenge with the same strain and later against challenge with a second strain that differed from the first by 10 to 16% in the outer envelope nucleotide and amino acid sequences (68). However, the amino acid sequences of the V3 loops differed by only two amino acid residues between the two strains. In contrast, cross-protection has not been achieved between SIV and HIV-2 in immunized monkeys; here, the amino acid sequences of the V3 loop differ by about 30% (68). With few exceptions, attempts to protect monkeys with subunit or recombinant live vector preparations of SIV have been unsuccessful (69), raising some concern whether studies with SIV will be as relevant to the attempts to develop HIV vaccines as was hoped. It is also worth noting that, as with the one HIV-chimpanzee experiment (64), immunization of monkeys with inactivated whole SIV has occasionally resulted in recovery of infectious virus 6–9 months after the challenge with live virus (68). This implies that it will be necessary to wait for a long period, of the order of 1 year, before it is certain that a given immunization schedule in the animal models has been successful in completely protecting against challenge with live virus.

STUDIES IN HUMANS

The main approach, the performance of clinical trials, is discussed later in this section. A complementary approach is to establish whether infected people respond to particular B and/or T cell epitopes; if so, it may be a reason to include those epitopes in the candidate vaccine. In addition to the work previously discussed (46), two other reports illustrate the usefulness of this approach. In one report (41), the fine specificity of a Tc cell epitope in HIV-1 nef was mapped, using target cells exposed to the peptides and PBLs from seropositive donors. Human cell transfectants expressing mutations of the HLA A3.1 molecule were used to define critical amino acids in the nef epitope. In the second report (70), fresh PBLs from seropositive donors were used to demonstrate that T cells from 19/25 seropositive donors recognized four synthetic peptides from different regions of gp160; furthermore, the same peptides could both stimulate Th cells and be recognized by Tc cells. Vaccine developers may increasingly adopt this approach to determine the extent to which different epitopes of antigens are recognized by infected people, findings that may be crucial

for the development of effective subunit and particularly peptide-based preparations.

Clinical Trials: Prophylaxis

A number of candidate vaccines are undergoing phase I clinical trials in several developed countries, including the United States. The baculovirus/insect cell produced rgp160 (MicroGeneSys) has been administered to more than 100 volunteers with no evidence of untoward effects after four injections using doses varying from 10 to 1280 μg (71,72). Volunteers receiving three doses of 40–80 μg almost invariably produced low levels of mainly IgG$_1$ antibody, which did not persist. A fourth dose of the antigen induced higher levels of antibody and some recipients showed low levels of neutralizing antibody activity (71). In subsequent studies, larger doses of antigen (up to 640 and 1280 μg) are being administered. The specific T cell proliferative responses that were generated occurred much earlier than initial Western blot reactivity and persisted for well over a year (72). Cloned CD4+ T cell clones have been generated from the PBLs of some recipients but the relevance of this finding is not clear.

A preparation of gp120 synthesized in transfected yeast in a nonglycosylated form and isolated as a denatured preparation has been administered in a multidose regimen with a novel adjuvant, muramyl tripeptide (MTP-PE). The preparation was well tolerated. Low antibody titers with no detectable neutralizing activity, but a significant specific T cell response, were induced in most recipients (73).

The first experimental immunization of humans against HIV-1 began in 1986, using a recombinant vaccinia virus construct expressing the env, gag, and pol antigens of the IIIB strain (74). The same group later changed their approach by switching to the injection of autologous cells infected by the vaccinia virus/bacteriophage T7 system (48) expressing the above HIV antigens of HIV (75). An anamnestic humoral and CMI response could be elicited more than a year later. Administration of an additional dose yielded high levels of neutralizing antibodies. Though this approach is unrealistic for vaccine development, it showed that a strong immune response could be generated to gp160.

More recently, extensive phase I trials of a recombinant vaccinia virus construct expressing the HIV-1 gp160 (HIVAC-1e) were begun in the United States. HIVAC-1e was administered to volunteers, most of whom had a history of smallpox vaccination (76). In the majority group, the preparation failed to induce antibody and the T cell responses were transient; in contrast, antibody and persisting T cell proliferative responses were generated in both of the two vaccinia naive individuals.

Several other candidate vaccines are under trial.

They include (a) the gp120 produced by transfected cells (50, Genentech); (b) the gp160 produced by the HIV-infected vaccinia virus/bacteriophage T7 system (48, Immuno-AG); (c) the Ty gag preparation (52, British Biotechnology); and (d) the p17 preparation (37, Viral Technologies).

Detailed information on the safety and immunogenicity in humans of these preparations is not yet available.

Clinical Trials: Therapy

Passive Immunization

To test the possible relationship between the presence of neutralizing antibodies and resistance to disease progression, sera from clinically healthy HIV-1 infected individuals, who were p24-antigen negative, had CD4+ counts above 400/mm^3, and had high anti-viral antibody titers, were transfused to two groups of recipients—some with ARC and some with advanced AIDS (77). A beneficial effect for the AIDS patients was short-lived; in contrast, there was complete p24 clearance in three ARC patients who showed evidence of immunological stability for at least 22 months (78). This result suggests that the presence of substantial levels of neutralizing antibody is beneficial.

Active Immunization

Vaccines are generally designed to be used as prophylactic reagents and rarely are deliberately used for immunotherapy. The classical exception is the administration of his rabies vaccine by Pasteur to subjects bitten by rabid dogs. However, it is likely that when a vaccine is used in an endemic third world country, some recipients may recently have been exposed to the infection.

Dr. J. Salk (79) first drew attention to the need to design a vaccine(s) that might be administered to asymptomatic, HIV-seropositive people in order to retard or prevent the progression toward disease. His preparation was an irradiated (^{60}Co) and β-propiolactone treated whole HIV, depleted of gp120. In initial studies, four groups (total, 86 patients) of seropositive, asymptomatic patients were given 100-μg doses (three to eight injections over 6–24 months) in Freund's incomplete adjuvant. About 60% of patients showed transient DTH reactivity at one or another time after immunization (80). A second double-blind study on 27 matched pairs was begun later and these recipients have shown enhanced DTH reactions. A second double-blind, placebo-controlled study involving 60 healthy, asymptomatic infected people with CD4+ levels greater than 550/mm^3 and HIV/DTH negative status has begun. It is also planned to initiate phase I studies on seronegative people (81).

Dr. D. Zagury and colleagues have extended their approach using homologous cells infected with a vaccinia/env:gag:pol construct and inactivated with paraformaldehyde. This preparation was infused every 12 weeks into one group of 14 HIV-infected people; a second group with the same initial CD4+ count acted as a control. Over a period of 1 year, seven opportunistic infections occurred in the control group and none in the immunized group. Similarly, immunization seemed to delay conversion to p24 antigenemia (82). There was no sign that this effect was caused by an enhanced specific immune response so consideration is being given to a possible role for nonadaptive immune responses. Promising as these results seem, three of the immunized group have since died from, it has been claimed, a vaccinia-like infection (83); Zagury is said to dispute this finding (84).

The gp160 (MicroGeneSys) preparation has recently been administered to 30 volunteer subjects in the early stages of HIV infection (85). Groups received three to six injections of 40–640 μg; 87% of those receiving six doses of antigen had increased antibody titers and T cell proliferation responses. Initially high (>600 CD4) cell counts and multiple, large doses of antigen correlated with these responses. Overall, 19/30 subjects showed humoral and T cell proliferation responses and, on the average, stable CD4 counts, whereas this latter count decreased 7.3% in the 11 nonresponders. These results are sufficiently favorable to warrant a larger trial to measure clinical efficacy.

CURRENT AND FUTURE TASKS

In addition to the above aspects, there are some general points to be investigated and some of these are addressed briefly in this section.

Antigen Presentation

The evidence to date suggests that individual proteins, such as the gp120/160 from this virus, and possibly the whole virus are poorly immunogenic. Multiple doses have been required to give reasonable antibody levels, and the generation of high neutralizing activity by any regimen has been relatively rare. There are three aspects:

1. *Physical form of the antigen.* Antigen as a particle is likely to be more immunogenic for several reasons. It would present a mosaic of repeating epitopes, preferably similar to that in the virion, to be recognized by the receptors on individual B cells; not infrequently, antibodies that neutralize viral infectivity recognize the tertiary or quaternary conformations formed by such mosaics. Particles are also more readily taken up by macrophages.

The long-lived presence of antibody after immunization depends on the persistence of antigen attached to follicular dendritic cells (86). Naturally occurring polymers of antigen are often found to be more resistant to proteolysis compared to monomeric preparations.

2. *The adjuvant.* Alum, which was first used more than 50 years ago, is still the only adjuvant licensed for general medical use. The most powerful adjuvant used in experimental animals, Freund's complete adjuvant, is not permissible for humans. An adjuvant has at least two properties—to activate the antigen-presenting cell (APC) so that appropriate interleukins are released and to act as a depot for the release over time of the antigen. The tubercle bacillus, the component in Freund's complete adjuvant that has the former activity, has been "chemically dissected" and two preparations have been isolated. A family of simple compounds, the muramyl dipeptides, is one active principle. Many different variants are available and some have been used in experimental human vaccines together with different oils and emulsifiers (87). More recently, a mixture consisting of squalane and the cell wall skeleton of mycobacteria has given enhanced antibody responses (88). Many other preparations have been tried (89); some like dextran sulfate have been found to affect the isotype of antibody formed (90), but none has greatly affected the quantity of the antibody response. The time when one or more interleukins will be used to generate particular responses is on the way but has not yet arrived.

3. *Formulations.* Three major approaches are being tried—liposomes, immunostimulating complexes (ISCOMS) (91), and biodegradable controlled release formulations, microcapsules or microspheres (92). Liposomes have given quite variable results in different hands. ISCOMS have generally given substantially enhanced antibody responses and have an additional advantage that they can induce the generation of class I MHC-restricted T cell responses (93,94). Microspheres/ capsules have been used with (92) and without (95) the incorporation of adjuvants and have been administered parenterally or orally. In one experimental model in which a peptide–diphtheria toxoid conjugate was administered I.M. as a single dose in such a preparation, the level of antibody at 70 weeks was approximately 40% of the maximal level (92, V. Stevens, *personal communication*).

Free Virus Versus Infected Cells

To date, almost all challenges with experimental model systems have been with infectious virus administered systemically. In practice, infection either by sexual transmission or intravenous injection involves infected cells as well as free virus. It is comparatively recently that attention has been directed to the nature of infected cells in semen (96). It remains to be established whether free virus or infected cells are the more usual mechanism of infection and, if the latter, which is the most effective immunological mechanism for their destruction.

A Need for Mucosal Immunity

Worldwide, the commonest route of infection is now heterosexual intercourse so that it is likely that in many, if not most, cases, infection occurs via a mucosal surface. To *prevent* infection, a vaccine would need to generate a strong secretory IgA response in the female reproductive tract (FRT). This may be difficult for two reasons: (a) in experimental work, immune responses following topical application of noninfectious preparations in the FRT are generally weak and short-lived; and (b) globally, this route of immunization may well be impracticable. Recently, there were two encouraging reports that immunization via the oral route could lead to immunity in the FRT; this approach needs to be pursued (97). The aim should be to generate both mucosal and systemic immunity to ensure the greatest chance of preventing and controlling an infection.

The two potentially most serious problems remain.

1. *How serious a problem is antigenic variation?* HIV displays more antigenic variation and undergoes more "antigenic drift" in individuals than any other known virus. On the one hand, it has been proposed that, as the chance of transmission by sexual intercourse is significantly below 1, infection via this route is by a single infectious unit (98). If this interpretation is correct, the strain present to highest titer may be the only infecting agent, but this is likely to vary between different people. In addition, this concept may not be valid if infected cells are the major transmitting agent. Currently, the intention is to use a cocktail of antigens; this approach has been only partially successful with influenza virus vaccines and such an HIV vaccine may initially protect only 70–80% of a population. The extent of success of this approach will only become apparent when efficacy trials are under way.

2. *Will the vaccine(s) be affordable?* In the past, the cost of vaccines in developed countries has not been a major public health concern. The opposite is the case in most developing countries. The World Health Organization's Expanded Programme of Immunization, which now has achieved about an 80% coverage of the world's children with vaccines against the six common childhood diseases, places an upper limit of $1 U.S. on the cost of a vaccine if it is to be incorporated into that program. It is estimated that by the year 2000, 30 million people worldwide will be infected by HIV. The incidence in developing countries will still be climbing so that very large amounts of vaccines at a very low cost will be required. Some candidate vaccines will potentially be con-

siderably less expensive than others. Continuing development of such preparations should be encouraged.

CONCLUDING REMARKS

The results obtained so far are sufficiently encouraging to suggest that it should be possible to develop a vaccine(s) to prevent HIV infection and to delay progression toward disease of those already infected. Not all scientists are convinced of this; Albert Sabin has drawn attention to several unresolved aspects (99).

Optimally, a prophylactic vaccine that depends on adaptive immune responses should generate three such responses: T helper cells for the generation of high-affinity antibody of different isotypes; cytotoxic T cells that may lyse infected cells or limit virus growth at an early stage after infection; and antibody that prevents infection or helps lyse infected cells expressing viral antigens. At the present time, the only marker that clearly can be identified with protection of chimpanzees following active or passive immunization is antibody to at least part of the V3 loop. Other responses, possibly T cell mediated, might also be protective but at present there are no clear indications of the type and specific target(s) of these responses. It is unclear why inactivated whole SIV preparations protect monkeys.

Until these questions can be answered more definitively, it is not possible to nominate top candidates in the current field of candidate vaccines. Clearly, a number of different approaches including whole virus, subunits, chimeric live vectors, and peptide-based preparations should continue to be studied. In the meantime, every attempt should be made to identify and prepare those sites where vaccine efficacy trials can be performed, so that when clear preferences for certain vaccine candidates can be made, they can be adequately tested without further delay.

REFERENCES

1. Ada GL. Prospects for HIV vaccines. *J AIDS* 1988;1:295–303.
2. Clements ML. AIDS vaccines. In: Mandel GL, Douglas RG Jr, Bennet JE, eds. *Principles and practice of infectious disease.* New York: Churchill Livingston; 1990:1112–21.
3. Ada GL. Commentry—prospects for a vaccine against HIV. *Nature* 1989;339:331–2.
4. Haseltine WA. Molecular biology of HIV-1. In: Dalgleish AG, Weiss RA, eds. *AIDS and the new viruses.* Orlando: Academic Press; 1990:11–40.
5. Sattentau QJ, Weiss RA. The CD4 antigen: physiological ligand and HIV receptor. *Cell* 1988;52:631–3.
6. Sattentau QJ. Molecular interactions between CD4 and the HIV envelope glycoproteins. In: Dalgleish AG, Weiss RA, eds. *AIDS and the new viruses.* Orlando: Academic Press; 1990:41–54.
7. Hart AR, Cloyd MW. Interference patterns of human immunodeficiency viruses, HIV-1 and HIV-2. *Virology* 1990;177:1–10.
8. Macatonia SE, Lau R, Patterson S, et al. Dendritic cell infection, depletion and dysfunction in HIV-infected individuals. *Immunology* 1990;71:38–45.
9. Groopman JE, Sakagichi M, Scadden DT. Pathogenesis of HIV mediated blood cell abnormalities. In: Girard M, Valette L, eds. *Fifth Colloquium of Cent Gardes; retroviruses of human AIDS and related animal diseases.* Paris: Pasteur-Merieux; 1990:5–8.
10. Smith DH, Byrn RA, Marsters SA, et al. Blocking of HIV-1 infectivity by a soluble secreted form of the CD4 antigen. *Science* 1987;238:1704–8.
11. Daar ES, Li XL, Moudgil T, Ho DD. High concentrations of recombinant soluble CD4 are required to neutralize primary human immunodeficiency virus type 1 isolates. *Proc Natl Acad Sci USA* 1990;87:6574–8.
12. LaRosa GJ, Davide JP, Weinhold K, et al. Conserved sequence and structural elements in the HIV-1 principal neutralizing determinant. *Science* 1990;249:932–5.
13. Reitz MS, Wilson C, Naugle C, et al. Generation of a neutralization-resistant variant of HIV-1 is due to selection for a point mutation in the envelope gene. *Cell* 1988;54:57–63.
14. Nara PL, Smit L, Dunlop N, et al. Emergence of viruses resistant to neutralization by V3 specific antibodies in experimental human immunodeficiency virus type 1 IIIB infection of chimpanzees. *J Virol* 1990;64:3779–91.
15. Wilson C, Reitz MS, Aldrich K, et al. The site of an immune-selected point mutation in the transmembrane protein of human immunodeficiency virus type 1 does not constitute the neutralization site. *J Virol* 1990;64:3240–8.
16. Veronese FDM, Rahman R, Kalyanaraman VS, et al. Monoclonal antibodies to HTLV-III451 gp41: delineation of an immunoreactive conserved epitope in the transmembrane region of divergent isolates of HIV-1. *AIDS Res Hum Retroviruses* 1989;5:479–86.
17. Profy AT, Salinas PA, Eckler LI, et al. Epitopes recognized by the neutralizing antibodies of an HIV-1-infected individual. *J Immunol* 1990;144:4641–7.
18. Broliden P-A, von Gegerfelt A, Clapham P, et al. Identification of human neutralizing regions of the human immunodeficiency virus type-1 envelope glycoproteins. *Proc Natl Acad Sci USA* 1992;89:461–5.
19. Tyler DS, Lyerly HK, Weinhold KJ. Mini-review: anti-HIV-1 ADCC. *AIDS Res Hum Retroviruses* 1989;5:557–63.
20. Evans LA, Thomson-Honnebier G, Steimer K, et al. Antibody-dependent cellular cytotoxicity is directed against both the gp120 and gp41 envelope proteins of HIV. *AIDS* 1989;3:273–6.
21. Homsy J, Meyer M, Levy JA. Serum enhancement of human immunodeficiency virus (HIV) infection correlates with disease in HIV-infected individuals. *J Virol* 1990;64:1437–40.
22. Zolla-Pazner S, Hersh E, Mitchell WM, Robinson WE. Antibody-dependent enhancement of HIV and SIV infection: domain mapping and vaccines. In: Girard M, Valette L, eds. *Fifth Colloquium of Cent Gardes: retroviruses of human AIDS and related animal diseases.* Paris: Pasteur-Merieux; 1990:161–7.
23. Cease KB, Margalit H, Cornette JL, et al. Helper T cell antigenic site identification in the acquired immunodeficiency syndrome virus gp120 envelope protein and induction of immunity in mice to the native protein using a 16 residue synthetic peptide. *Proc Natl Acad Sci USA* 1987;84:4249–53.
24. Palker TJ, Matthews TJ, Langlois A, et al. Polyvalent human immunodeficiency virus synthetic immunogen comprised of envelope gp120 T helper sites and B cell neutralization epitopes. *J Immunol* 1989;142:3612–9.
25. Ahearne PM, Matthews TJ, Lyerly HK, et al. Cellular immune responses to viral peptides in patients exposed to HIV. *AIDS Res Hum Retroviruses* 1988;4:259–67.
26. Berzofsky JA, Benussan A, Cease KB, et al. Antigenic peptides recognized by T lymphocytes from AIDS viral envelope-immune humans. *Nature* 1988;334:706–8.
27. Schrier RD, Gnann FW Jr, Landes R, et al. T cell recognition of HIV synthetic peptides in a natural infection. *J Immunol* 1989;142:1166–76.
28. Ruegg CL, Monell CR, Strand M. Inhibition of lymphocyte proliferation by a synthetic peptide with a sequence identity to gp41 of the human immunodeficiency virus type 1. *J Virol* 1989;63:3257–63.
29. Klasse RJ, Pipkorn R, Blomberg J. Presence of antibodies to a putatively immunosuppressive part of human immunodeficiency

virus (HIV) envelope glycoprotein gp41 is strongly associated with health among HIV-positive subjects. *Proc Natl Acad Sci USA* 1988;85:5225–9.

30. Walker BD, Chakrabarti S, Moss B, et al. HIV-specific cytotoxic T lymphocytes in seropositive individuals. *Nature* 1987;328:345–9.

31. Plata F, Autran B, Martins LP, et al. AIDS virus-specific cytotoxic T lymphocytes in lung disorders. *Nature* 1987;328:348–51.

32. Ada GL. The immunological principles of vaccine development. In: Webster RG, Granoff A, eds. *Encyclopedia of virology.* London: Saunders Scientific, 1992.

33. Shen L, Chen ZW, Miller MD, et al. Recombinant virus-induced SIV-specific CD8+ cytotoxic T lymphocytes. *Science* 1991;252: 440–3.

34. Takahashi H, Cohen J, Hosmalin A, et al. An immunodominant epitope of the human immunodeficiency virus envelope glycoprotein gp160 recognized by class I major histocompatibility complex molecule-restricted murine cytotoxic T lymphocytes. *Proc Natl Acad Sci USA* 1988;85:3105–9.

35. Nixon DF, Townsend ARM, Elvin JG, et al. HIV-1 gag-specific cytotoxic T lymphocytes defined with recombinant vaccinia virus and synthetic peptides. *Nature* 1988;336:484–7.

36. Riviere Y, Tanneau-Salvadori F, Regnault A, et al. Human immunodeficiency virus-specific cytotoxic responses of seropositive individuals; distinct type of effector cells mediate killing of targets expressing gag and env proteins. *J Virol* 1989;63:2270–7.

37. Achour A, Picard O, Zagury D, et al. HGP-30, a synthetic analogue of human immunodeficiency virus (HIV) p17, is a target for cytotoxic lymphocytes in HIV-infected individuals. *Proc Natl Acad Sci USA* 1990;87:7045–9.

38. Walker BD, Flexner C, Birch-Limberger K, et al. Long-term culture and fine specificity of human cytotoxic T-lymphocyte clones reactive with human immunodeficiency virus type 1. *Proc Natl Acad Sci USA* 1989;86:2344–8.

39. Hosmalin A, Clerici M, Houghten R, et al. An epitope of human immunodeficiency virus 1 reverse transcriptase recognized by both mouse and human cytotoxic T lymphocytes. *Proc Natl Acad Sci USA* 1990;87:2344–8.

40. Culmann B, Gomard E, Kieny M-P, et al. An antigenic peptide of the HIV-1 nef protein recognized by cytotoxic T lymphocytes of seropositive individuals in association with different HLA-B molecules. *Eur J Immunol* 1989;19:2383–6.

41. Koenig S, Fuerst TR, Wood LV, et al. Mapping the fine specificity of a cytolytic T cell response to HIV-1 nef protein. *J Immunol* 1990;145:127–35.

42. Chenciner N, Michel F, Dadaglio G, et al. Multiple sets of HIV-specific cytotoxic T lymphocytes in humans and in mice. *Eur J Immunol* 1989;19:1537–44.

43. Buseyne F, McChesney M, Porrot F, et al. Immune response against the gag protein of HIV-1. In: Girard M, Valette L, eds. *Fifth Colloquium of Cent Gardes: retroviruses of human AIDS and related animal diseases.* Paris: Pasteur-Merieux; 1990:153–5.

44. Gomard E, Choppin J, Culmann B, et al. Mapping of CTL reacting epitopes in the HIV-1 nef protein and possibility to predict such CTL epitopes in viral proteins. In: Girard M, Valette L, eds. *Fifth Colloquium of Cent Gardes: retroviruses of human AIDS and related animal diseases.* Paris: Pasteur-Merieux; 1990:147–52.

45. Frelinger JA, Gotch FM, Zweerink H, et al. Evidence of widespread binding of HLA class I molecules to peptides. *J Exp Med* 1990;172:827–8.

46. Bouillot M, Choppin J, Cornille F, et al. Physical association between MHC class I molecules and immunogenic peptides. *Nature* 1989;339:473–4.

47. Joly P, Guillon JM, Mayaud C, et al. Cell-mediated suppression of HIV-specific cytotoxic T lymphocytes. *J Immunol* 1989;143: 2193–201.

48. Fuerst TH, Moss B. Use of hybrid vaccinia virus/T7 RNA polymerase system for high level eukaryotic gene expression. In: Chanock RM, Lerner RA, Brown F, Ginsberg H, eds. *Vaccines 87.* Cold Spring Harbor, NY: Cold Spring Harbor Laboratory; 1987:356–9.

49. Berman PW, Gregory TJ, Riddle L, et al. Protection of chimpanzees from infection by HIV-1 after vaccination with recombinant glycoprotein gp120 but not gp160. *Nature* 1990;345:622–5.

50. Lange JMA, de Wolf F, Krone WJA, et al. Decline of antibody reactivity to outer viral core protein p17 is an earlier serological

51. Cherfas J. U.K. vaccine trial: stalking horse for the future. *Science* 1990;249:626.

52. Sarin PS, Sun D-K, Thornton AH, et al. Neutralization of HTLV-III/LAV replication by antiserum to thymosin-1. *Science* 1986; 232:1135–7.

53. Chakrabarti S, Mizukami T, Franchini G, Moss B. Synthesis, oligomerization, and biological activity of the human immunodeficiency virus type 2 envelope glycoprotein expressed by a recombinant vaccinia virus. *Virology* 1990;178:134–42.

54. Paoletti E. Poxviruses recombinant vaccines. *Ann NY Acad Sci* 1990;590:309–25.

55. Dewar RL, Natarajan V, Vasudevachari MB, Salzman NP. Synthesis and processing of human immunodeficiency virus type 1 envelope proteins encoded by a recombinant human adenovirus. *J Virol* 1989;63:129–36.

56. Stover CK, de la Cruz VF, Fuerst TR, et al. New use of BCG for recombinant vaccines. *Nature* 1991;351:456–9.

57. Aldovini A, Young RA. Humoral and cell-mediated immune responses to live recombinant BCG-HIV vaccines. *Nature* 1991;351:479–82.

58. Goldstein AL, Naylor PH, Gibbs CJ, Sarin PS. Progress in the development of an HIV-p17 based vaccine. *AIDS Res Hum Retroviruses* 1990;6:39–40.

59. Haynes BF, Hart MK, Palker TJ, et al. Design of HIV synthetic peptides containing T and B cell epitopes capable of inducing anti-HIV neutralizing antibody, T helper cell and CD8+ cytotoxic T cell responses *in vivo.* In: Girard M, Valette L, eds. *Fifth Colloquium of Cent Gardes: retroviruses of human AIDS and related animal diseases.* Paris: Pasteur-Merieux; 1990:185–8.

60. McCune JM. The SCID-hu mouse: application towards the development of antiviral compounds and vaccines against HIV-1. In: Girard M, Valette L, eds. *Fifth Colloquium of Cent Gardes: retroviruses of human AIDS and related animal diseases.* Paris: Pasteur-Merieux; 1990:105–10.

61. Mosier DE, Gulizia RJ, MacIsaac PD, et al. Evaluation of prototype vaccines in hu-PBL-SCID mice; nature of the protective response. In: Girard M, Valette L, eds. *Fifth Colloquium of Cent Gardes: retroviruses of human AIDS and related animal diseases.* Paris: Pasteur-Merieux; 1990:181–3.

62. Tilley SA, Honnen WJ, Racho ME, et al. Broadly neutralizing human monoclonal antibody against HIV gp120. In: Girard M, Valette L, eds. *Fifth Colloquium of Cent Gardes: retroviruses of human AIDS and related animal diseases.* Paris: Pasteur-Merieux; 1990:189–92.

63. Connelly A, Emini E. Report at the NIAID AIDS Vaccine Clinical Trials Network meeting, NIH, May 13, 1991.

64. Girard M, Kieny MP, Barré-Sinoussi F, et al. Immunization of chimpanzees confers protection against challenge with HIV. *Proc Natl Acad Sci USA* 1991;88:542–6.

65. Dorner F. Report at the NIAID AIDS Vaccine Clinical Trials Network meeting, NIH, May 13, 1991.

66. Murphey-Corb M, Martin LN, Davison-Fairburn B, et al. A formalin-inactivated whole SIV vaccine confers protection in macaques. *Science* 1989;246:1293–7.

67. Stott EJ, Chan WL, Mills KHG, et al. Preliminary report: protection of cynomolgus macaques against simian immunodeficiency virus by fixed-infected-cell vaccine. *Lancet* 1990;336:1538–41.

68. Gardner MB, Murphy-Corb M. Vaccine protection of rhesus monkeys against homologous and heterologous strains of SIV. In: Girard M, Valette L, eds. *Fifth Colloquium of Cent Gardes: retroviruses of human AIDS and related animal diseases.* Paris: Pasteur-Merieux; 1990:221–6.

69. Stott J. Report at the NIAID AIDS Vaccine Clinical Trials Network meeting, NIH, May 13, 1991.

70. Clerici M, Lucey DR, Zajac RA, et al. Detection of cytotoxic T lymphocytes specific for synthetic peptides of gp160 in HIV-seropositive individuals. *J Immunol* 1990;146:2214–9.

71. Dolin R, Graham BS, Greenberg SB, et al. The safety and immunogenicity of a human immunodeficiency virus type 1 (HIV-1) recombinant gp160 candidate vaccine in humans. *Ann Intern Med* 1991;114:119–27.

72. Keefer MC, Bonnez W, Roberts NJ, et al. Human immunodefi-

ciency virus (HIV-1) gp160-specific lymphocyte proliferative responses of mononuclear leukocytes from HIV-1 recombinant gp160 vaccine recipients. *J Infect Dis* 1991;163:448–53.

73. Wintsch J, Chaignat C-L, Braun DG, et al. Safety and immunogenicity of a genetically engineered human immunodeficiency virus vaccine. *J Infect Dis* 1991;163:219–25.

74. Zagury D, Leonard R, Fouchard M, et al. Immunization against AIDS in humans. *Nature* 1987;326:249–50.

75. Zagury D, Bernard J, Cheynier R, et al. A group specific anamnestic immune reaction against HIV-1 induced by a candidate vaccine against AIDS. *Nature* 1988;332:344–6.

76. Cooney EL, Collier AC, Greenberg PD, et al. Safety and immunological response to a recombinant vaccinia virus vaccine expressing HIV envelope glycoprotein. *Lancet* 1991;337:567–72.

77. Karpas A, Hill F, Youle M, et al. Effect of passive immunization in patients with acquired immunodeficiency syndrome-related complex and acquired immunodeficiency syndrome. *Proc Natl Acad Sci USA* 1988;85:9234–7.

78. Karpas A. Effects of passive immunization in patients with ARC and AIDS. In: Girard M, Valette L, eds. *Fifth Colloquium of Cent Gardes: retroviruses of human AIDS and related animal diseases.* Paris: Pasteur-Merieux; 1990:253–61.

79. Salk J. Prospects for the control of AIDS by immunizing seropositive individuals. *Nature* 1987;327:473–6.

80. Levine A, Henderson B, Groshen S, et al. Immunization of HIV-infected individuals with inactivated HIV immunogen. In: Girard M, Valette L, eds. *Fifth Colloquium of Cent Gardes: retroviruses of human AIDS and related animal diseases.* Paris: Pasteur-Merieux; 1990:247–52.

81. Slade H. Report at the NIAID AIDS Vaccine Clinical Trials Network meeting, NIH, May 13, 1991.

82. Picard O, Giral P, Defer MC, et al. AIDS vaccine therapy: phase I trial. *Lancet* 1990;336:179.

83. Guillaume JC, Salag P, Wechsler J, et al. Vaccinia from recombinant virus expressing HIV genes. *Lancet* 1991;337:1034–5.

84. Dorozynski A, Anderson A. Deaths in vaccine trials trigger French inquiry. *Science* 1991;252:501–2.

85. Redfield RR, Birx DL, Ketter N, et al. A phase I evaluation of the safety and immunogenicity of vaccination with recombinant gp160 in patients with early human immunodeficiency virus infection. *N Engl J Med* 1991;324:1677–84.

86. Ada GL. Vaccination and the immune response. *Curr Biol* 1991;1:221–3.

87. Jones WR, Bradley J, Judd SJ, et al. Phase I clinical trial of a World Health Organization birth control vaccine. *Lancet* 1988;1:1295–9.

88. Malcolm MS, Kan-Mitchell J, Kempf RA, et al. Active specific immunotherapy for melanoma: phase I trial of allogeneic lysates and a novel adjuvant. *Cancer Res* 1988;48:5883–93.

89. Ada GL. Vaccines. In: Paul WE, ed. *Fundamental immunology.* New York: Raven Press; 1988:985–1032.

90. Watson DL. Serological response of sheep to live and killed *Staphylococcus aureus* vaccines. *Vaccine* 1987;5:275–8.

91. Morein B, Fossum C, Lovgren K, Hoglund S. The Iscom—a modern approach to vaccines. *Semin Virol* 1990;1:49–56.

92. Stevens VC, Powell JE, Rickey M, et al. Studies of various delivery systems for a human choriogonadotrophin vaccine. In: Alexander NJ, Griffin D, Spieler JM, Waites GMH, eds. *Gamete interaction: prospects for immunocontraception.* New York: Wiley-Liss, 1990:549–63.

93. Jones PD, Tha Hla R, Morein B, Ada GL. Cellular immune responses in the murine lung to local immunization with influenza A virus glycoproteins in micelles and iscoms. *Scand J Immunol* 1988;27:645–52.

94. Takahashi H, Takeshita T, Morein B, et al. Induction of CD8+ cytotoxic T cells by immunization with purified HIV-1 envelope protein in ISCOMS. *Nature* 1989;342:561–4.

95. Eldridge JH, Gilley RM, Staas JK, et al. Biodegradable microspheres: vaccine delivery system for oral immunization. *Curr Top Microbiol Immunol* 1989;146:59–68.

96. Anderson DJ, Wolff H, Pudney J, et al. Presence of HIV in semen. In: Alexander NJ, Gabelnick HL, Spieler JM, eds. *Heterosexual transmission of AIDS.* New York: Wiley-Liss; 1990:167–79.

97. Ada GL. Prospects for vaccination at mucosal surfaces for the control of sexually transmitted diseases. In: Quinn TC, Gallin J, Fauci A, eds. *Advances in host defense mechanisms.* New York: Raven Press, in press.

98. Wigzell H. Prospects for an HIV vaccine. *FASEB J* (in press).

99. Sabin AB. Effectiveness of AIDS vaccines. *Science* 1991;251:1161.

AIDS and Other Manifestations of HIV Infection,
Second Edition, Edited by Gary P. Wormser.
Raven Press, Ltd., New York © 1992.

CHAPTER 40

AIDS Prevention Programs for Injecting Drug Users

Don C. Des Jarlais and Samuel R. Friedman

Approximately 30% of the recent cases of AIDS in the United States (1) and approximately 50% of such cases in Europe (2) have occurred in persons who inject illicit drugs (IDUs). Rapid spread of HIV has also occurred among IDUs in several developing countries, including Thailand (3), Brazil (4), Argentina (5), and India (6), so large numbers of AIDS cases can be anticipated in those countries. In areas where HIV becomes widespread among IDUs, they become a predominant source of both heterosexual and perinatal transmission of HIV. Of note, however, is that in all prevention programs for IDUs that have focused on both drug equipment sharing and sexual transmission, more subjects have reduced drug-related rather than sexual risks.

The first studies of AIDS risk reduction among injecting drug users were conducted in 1984 and 1985 in New York City (7–9). These studies found what was then a surprising amount of behavior change among IDUs to reduce the risk of AIDS. Since then a large and growing literature has developed, with consistent findings that large numbers of IDUs have changed their behavior because of concerns about AIDS. The behavior change observed in these studies should generally be considered risk reduction, not risk elimination, since the large majority of IDUs often still practice some level of risk behavior. Also, a worrisome minority of the subjects in most studies do not change their behavior at all because of AIDS.

AIDS risk reduction among IDUs has occurred in response to a variety of intervention programs and through a variety of mechanisms. Table 1 lists a compen-

dium of these studies through 1990. We have attempted to be as inclusive as possible in constructing this compendium but would not claim it to be fully comprehensive. We believe, however, that there is no systematic sampling bias with respect to published and presented studies that would affect our conclusions.

No scientific consensus has developed about a "best" way to prevent AIDS among IDUs. Indeed, there are many indications in the field that multiple simultaneous interventions are needed. Political considerations, however, have often led many localities to promulgate a preferred method of AIDS prevention for IDUs, sometimes to the exclusion of other methods. Ironically, syringe exchange programs and methadone maintenance programs—the methods for which there are the most data available indicating effectiveness in reducing AIDS risk —have been the most controversial types of AIDS prevention programs.

In this chapter, we review various types of AIDS prevention and behavior change programs for IDUs. For each type of program, one or more prototype program is described, major policy issues are discussed briefly, and data on the effectiveness of each type of program in preventing HIV infection—at both the individual and the community level—are assessed. We believe that it is important to distinguish between the individual and community levels when assessing the effectiveness of AIDS prevention programs for IDUs. At the individual level, we consider whether participation in the program has led individuals to change their behavior or has reduced their chances of becoming infected with HIV. At the community level, we consider whether the prevention program has led to large-scale behavior change in communities of IDUs and/or whether it has reduced the transmission of HIV within a group of IDUs.

It is quite possible that a given prevention program

D. C. Des Jarlais: Beth Israel Medical Center, New York, New York 10013.
S. R. Friedman: Narcotic and Drug Research, Inc., New York, New York 10013.

TABLE 1. *Recent studies of AIDS risk reduction among IV drug users, grouped by mechanism of change as reported by investigators*[a]

Counseling/testing
Raffi et al. (49)
Zerboni et al. (50)
Böttiger and Blaxhult (51)
Jones et al. (52)
Farley et al. (53)
Casadonte et al. (54)
Gibson et al. (55)
Cartter et al. (56)
McCoy et al. (57)
Inciardi (58)
Sorensen (59)
Friedman et al. (16)
Brown and Beschner (60)
Dow et al. (61)
Goldstein (62)
Howell and Niven (63)
Mersky (64)
Sorrell and Springer (65)
Wheat et al. (66)
Higgins et al. (67)
Methadone treatment
Rezza et al. (68)
Hartgers et al. (69)
Blix and Gronbladh (23)
Ball et al. (70)
Abdul-Quader et al. (21)
Hartel et al. (20)
Yancovitz et al. (71)
Keffelew et al. (72)
Arif (73)
Cartter et al. (56)
Nemoto et al. (74)
Torrens et al. (24)
Chaisson et al. (25)
Kolar et al. (75)
Magura et al. (76)
Harris et al. (77)
Zinberg (78)
Schoenbaum et al. (79)
Mersky (64)
Nathan and Karan (80)
Payte (81)
Sorensen et al. (82–84)
Outreach/bleach distribution
Wiebel et al. (85)
Thompson et al. (86)
Flynn et al. (87)
Watters et al. (88)
Friedman et al. (89)
Herb et al. (36)
Rivera-Beckman et al. (37)
Moss et al. (38)
Chitwood et al. (90)
Conviser and Rutledge (91)
Haverkos (92)

Syringe exchange
Lowe et al. (93)
Buning et al. (94)
Ljungberg et al. (28)
Hart et al. (95)
Stimson and Lart (96)
Harris et al. (97)
Des Jarlais et al. (98)
Jones (99)
Joseph (100)
Legal sale of syringes
Robertson et al. (32)
Espinoza et al. (33)
van den Hoek et al. (34)
Fuchs et al. (35)
Goldberg et al. (101)
McKeganey et al. (102)
Increased marketing of illicit syringes
Des Jarlais et al. (7)
Des Jarlais and Hopkins (103)
Media coverage/social support
Jason et al. (104)
Friedman et al. (8)
Battjes et al. (105)
Serrano (106)
Leukefeld (107)
Zich and Temoshok (108)
Weisse et al. (109)
Fisher and Misovich (110)
Outreach, increased treatment
Jackson and Rotkiewicz (10)
Neaigus et al. (111)
Thompson et al. (86)
Gagnon (112)
Cohen et al. (113)
Casriel et al. (114)
Guydish et al. (115)
Brown et al. (116)
Westermeyer et al. (117)
Education/information campaign
Getzenberg et al. (118)
Jackson and Baxter (119)
Graves (120)
Pott (121)
Bortolotti et al. (122)
Benedetti (123)
Carrillo et al. (124)
de la Loma et al. (13)
Mondanaro (125)
Jang et al. (126)
Longshore (127)
Maccoby (128)
Ostrow (129)
Multiple interventions
Battjes et al. (130)
Abdul-Quader et al. (47)
Robertson et al. (131)

[a] Several mechanisms may be involved in a single study.

could be effective at an individual level but could not be operated on a large enough scale to be effective at the community level. It is also possible that some interventions could be effective at the community level without differentially protecting their individual participants against HIV exposure. Special treatment programs for HIV-positive IDUs, or HIV counseling and testing, are examples of programs that could reduce HIV transmission *from* their participants, with possible community-level benefits—without, of course, being able to prevent HIV infection in those already infected.

When discussing either individual-level or community-level effectiveness, we focus the discussion on studies that used changes in HIV seroprevalence or frequency of seroconversion as the outcome measure. We do this fully aware of the limitations of these parameters as outcome measures. The great majority of studies, however, have used only behavioral change as the outcome measure and thus, although included in Table 1, are not discussed further. Evaluation of HIV seroprevalence or seroconversion usually requires a study with a large number of subjects, followed over a period of several years. Such studies are difficult and expensive. Even when sufficient resources (time, money, and scientific talent) are available, the causal linkages between behavior changes and rate of seroconversion, or changes in seroprevalence, are often unclear. Nevertheless, reducing HIV transmission is the ultimate goal of all AIDS prevention programs, and this must be assessed quantitatively in order to ascertain the extent to which prevention programs are succeeding.

AIDS EDUCATION

That "education is currently the only means for preventing AIDS" has frequently been repeated during the course of the HIV/AIDS epidemic. While there is general agreement on the importance of AIDS education for groups at risk of HIV infection, there are comparatively little data on the effectiveness of this modality, and even less conceptualization as to which of the various educational techniques should be used. The mass media, including news coverage, appear to have been relatively effective in conveying the basic information about how AIDS is transmitted to the U.S. population. Surveys of AIDS knowledge and attitudes conducted by the National Center for Health Statistics show that the general population understands the basic routes of transmission, although there continues to be some misinformation concerning the likelihood of casual-contact transmission. The first studies of AIDS risk reduction among IDUs in New York City found that almost 100% knew that AIDS was transmitted through sharing injection equipment (8,9) before any specific AIDS education programs were started for IDUs in the city. The IDUs had

learned about AIDS from the mass media and through oral communication networks within their own group.

The first AIDS education programs begun for IDUs were in New Jersey, San Francisco, Rotterdam, and New York. These involved outreach with trained ex-addicts, streetwise volunteers or staff, or members of drug users' organizations conducting AIDS education in high-drug-use neighborhoods. The outreach work was supplemented by printed media, including posters on buses and subways, as well as pamphlets and photo-novellas distributed by the outreach workers. These educational materials included not only the basics of AIDS transmission but also methods for disinfecting used injection equipment, such as boiling or soaking them in bleach or alcohol.

One particularly interesting finding from these outreach studies was that while the drug users contacted in the community were interested in learning how to disinfect injection equipment, many of them were also interested in coming into treatment for their drug problems. In response, the New Jersey program developed a "voucher" system in which the outreach workers handed out vouchers that could be redeemed for free entry into drug abuse treatment. Over 85% of the vouchers distributed were redeemed by drug users entering treatment programs (10).

Deliberate AIDS risk reduction clearly cannot occur among IDUs who do not know about AIDS. Insofar as is known, the instances where HIV has spread rapidly among IDUs have occurred in places where IDUs were not then aware of AIDS as a local threat, for example, New York (11), Italy (12), and Bangkok (3). Evaluations of AIDS education programs for IDUs, however, have tended to produce "disappointing" results (13). No study has shown that drug users with greater knowledge about AIDS are more likely to be HIV-seronegative. In part, this may be a ceiling effect of the relative simplicity of the knowledge needed to become concerned about AIDS—along with the power of the emotional and interpersonal factors that facilitate and/or retard AIDS risk reduction among IDUs. Cognitive education about AIDS and how the virus is transmitted may be one prerequisite for risk reduction, but the conjoined impact of several other factors will probably be required for that knowledge to be translated into lasting behavior changes.

DRUG ABUSE TREATMENT

Drug abuse treatment is not merely a method of preventing AIDS among IDUs but potentially offers very important additional benefits. Not only would successful treatment eliminate the risk of transmission of HIV through the sharing of drug injection equipment, it would also greatly reduce other health and social problems associated with illicit drug use. Even for persons who were already HIV-seropositive, successful treatment would eliminate the chance for them to transmit HIV to other IDUs through sharing injection equipment. It would also provide opportunities for counseling and life-style stabilization, both of which might reduce the possibility of sexual transmission of HIV. For this among other reasons, drug abuse treatment is usually the officially preferred method of preventing HIV transmission among IDUs. This official preference is particularly strong in Sweden and the United States, where opposition to "safer injection" programs has been the strongest (14).

No new forms of drug abuse treatment have been developed specific to preventing HIV infection among IDUs. The AIDS epidemic has, however, led many countries to consider expansion of their previous treatment systems, and some countries to adapt types of treatment that previously were ideologically unacceptable. The introduction of methadone maintenance in Germany is probably the most notable example of AIDS leading to implementation of a type of treatment that, prior to the epidemic, was considered unacceptable.

While no new forms of drug abuse treatment have been developed specific to the prevention of AIDS, the epidemic has led to many changes in previously existing programs in areas where there are large numbers of HIV-seropositive IDUs (15,16). Drug abuse treatment programs in such areas have had to (a) deal with concerns about casual contact and "body fluid" transmission within the program, (b) provide medical treatment for clients with HIV-related disease, (c) provide education and counseling to reduce transmission from seropositive clients to sexual partners, (d) provide education to reduce drug-related transmission by those for whom treatment does not succeed, and (e) work with seropositive clients who want to have additional children—even though they are aware of the possibility of perinatal transmission.

None of these responsibilities was traditionally part of staff training for drug abuse treatment programs, and none of them is easy, even after the staff have been trained. Most importantly, the AIDS epidemic has challenged the hope that drug abuse treatment programs had traditionally offered to their clients: if you stop using drugs, as difficult as that may be, you will also free yourself of the problems that drug use has created for you. AIDS may occur long after the person has stopped using drugs. The development of AIDS among seropositive clients who have stopped using drugs and the development of AIDS among program staff who are ex-users are thus particularly distressing to drug abuse treatment programs.

Prior to the emergence of AIDS, it was well established that drug abuse treatment produced dramatic reductions in drug injection for persons who enter and remain in the programs (17–19). Thus one would expect that these programs would also reduce the risk of HIV exposure for IDUs who entered and remained in the programs. Indeed, to date, drug abuse treatment is the only AIDS prevention technique with proven effectiveness at the individual level. There have been several studies of methadone maintenance treatment which show that IDUs who entered and stayed in such programs have lower HIV infection rates than those from the same community who did not enter or remain in methadone maintenance. Most of these studies are from New York City (20–22), where there are a large number of methadone programs, and HIV has been present among IDUs in the city for approximately 15 years. Another study, from Sweden, is particularly convincing because the comparison group was composed of persons who applied to the program but were not accepted because of the program's limited capacity (23).

On a methodological level, it is important to note that the observed differences in HIV seroprevalence between the IDUs who were in methadone maintenance, and those who were not, emerged only after years of treatment. Other studies that use HIV seroprevalence as an outcome measure may also require years of follow-up before statistically significant differences emerge. In the treatment studies, the IDUs who had entered methadone treatment did so prior to the periods of rapid transmission of HIV among IDUs in New York City and Sweden. A high rate of HIV transmission among the local community of IDUs may also be important in showing statistically significant differences between IDUs who enter and remain in methadone maintenance (or other) treatment, and those who do not participate in such treatment. On a final methodological note, the differences that were found in these studies developed when the communities were not yet aware of the local transmission of HIV among IDUs. Thus there were no "alternative" HIV prevention activities for the comparison subjects (nor supplementary prevention activities for those IDUs in methadone maintenance programs).

Protection against HIV exposure during methadone treatment is not absolute: some subjects in New York were exposed to HIV before entering such treatment, and some subjects in both New York and Sweden became exposed while participating in methadone maintenance treatment. The problem of cocaine injection has often been raised as a limitation to the effectiveness of methadone maintenance treatment against HIV exposure. Many IDUs in the United States inject both heroin and cocaine, and this pattern may be spreading to western Europe (24). Methadone as a medication relieves craving for narcotics and can provide a cross-tolerance "blockade" against the euphoric effects of injecting heroin but has no pharmacologic effect on cocaine use. Moreover, there is no reason to expect dramatic reductions in the frequency of cocaine injection among IDUs entering methadone maintenance, and a substantial number of those in treatment may even start injecting cocaine after they have entered treatment. Cocaine injection may put them at very high risk for exposure to HIV (25).

Concerns about cocaine injection as an HIV risk necessitate considering other forms of drug abuse treatment as a method of preventing HIV among IDUs. Pre-AIDS studies (17–19) show that long-term drug-free residential (therapeutic community) treatment is effective in reducing both heroin and cocaine use, so that this type of treatment should also be effective as a means for HIV prevention. To date, however, there have not been outcome studies of IDUs who entered long-term residential treatment that (a) had some form of comparison group and (b) used HIV exposure as an outcome measure. Even if such studies were to be performed, most of the methodological concerns noted above with respect to methadone maintenance studies would probably also apply.

In the pre-AIDS era, studies of short-term forms of treatment for IDUs, particularly of detoxification programs, showed little if any reduction in illicit drug use (17–19). Indeed, in the DARP study (17), short-term detoxification subjects did not differ in outcomes from subjects who had received no treatment. Rather than expecting short-term and detoxification-only treatment programs to provide protection against HIV for IDUs who enter these programs, it may be more realistic to consider short-term treatment as the basis for other opportunities: (a) AIDS education, (b) HIV counseling and testing; and (c) linkage to long-term modes of treatment.

While there is good evidence that long-term types of drug abuse treatment should provide effective protection against HIV exposure for IDUs who enter (and remain in) those programs, the extent to which such treatment can provide protection against HIV at the community level has yet to be determined. First, although the present state of the art for drug abuse treatment leads to substantial immediate reduction in individual illicit drug use, there is a very high likelihood (75% or greater) that the person will return to illicit drug use after leaving treatment (17,18). Thus indefinite treatment, or multiple episodes of treatment, may be required before an IDU is likely to cease using illicit drugs permanently. How to prevent HIV infection in the intervals between multiple episodes of treatment becomes a very difficult problem, and one that is not easily addressed while the person is currently in treatment.

Second, a major problem of utilizing drug abuse treatment for community-wide AIDS prevention is that only a modest proportion of IDUs are in treatment at any given time. Typically, this fraction is about one-sixth to one-fifth of the IDUs in developed countries and is considerably smaller in developing countries. Large-scale expansion of drug abuse treatment programming would

be relatively expensive, and it is not clear how many IDUs would actually enter treatment programs even if the treatment system were greatly expanded. Residential drug-free therapeutic communities, in particular, are attractive only to a relatively small percentage of IDUs. The development of new forms of treatment that are more attractive to IDUs, and more capable of successfully treating cocaine abuse, may be required. The difficulties in expanding a treatment system (and in enrolling enough IDUs into long-term programs) to protect an entire community of IDUs against an HIV epidemic are so vast that it is unlikely this method will even be tested in most locations.

Nonetheless, humanitarian concerns—along with the multiple benefits both to society and the individual of discontinuing illicit drug use—mean that some form of treatment system is likely to be one part of an overall comprehensive AIDS prevention programs for IDUs. As will be discussed below, complementary relationships often develop between "safer injection" programs and drug abuse treatment programs. In areas where the current HIV seroprevalence among IDUs is low, a strategy of inducing those who are HIV-infected into treatment (26) is becoming increasingly utilized. This requires a large-scale counseling and testing system (as discussed below) in order to identify such individuals. Drug abuse treatment should greatly reduce the extent to which HIV is transmitted to other IDUs, as well as provide easier access to better medical care.

SYRINGE EXCHANGE

The AIDS epidemic has led to the development of a variety of "safer injection" programs throughout the world. Since it is not illicit drug injection *per se* that transmits HIV, but rather the multiperson use of injection equipment, it should be possible to prevent HIV transmission even if illicit drug injection continues. Safer injection programs have focused on ways in which HIV transmission can be prevented without requiring IDUs to stop injecting.

Among the different types of safer injection programs, syringe exchange programs have received the most public attention. In a syringe exchange program, an IDU exchanges one or more used needles and syringes for new (sterile) ones, at no cost to the IDU. Such programs provide injection equipment that does not carry HIV and assures proper disposal of the used injection equipment, which may contain viable HIV. In addition, nearly all syringe exchange programs provide more services than the mere exchanging of injection equipment. Contact between IDUs and the health-care workers operating an exchange also provides opportunities for HIV counseling (particularly about sexual transmission), distribution of condoms, and, for those IDUs who need them, referral to drug abuse treatment and other medical and social services.

The syringe exchange system in Amsterdam has served as the model on which most other exchanges are based, and from which the various exchanges now operating in almost all developed countries evolved. The exchange program in Amsterdam actually was begun prior to the realization that HIV infection was a problem for IDUs in that city. Over-the-counter sale of needles and syringes to IDUs has always been permitted under Dutch law, but individual pharmacists have never been legally required to sell injection equipment to IDUs. In 1984, a pharmacy in Amsterdam that had been a major source of new injection equipment for injecting drug users decided to stop selling to injecting drug users. In response, the Amsterdam analog of a "junkiebond" (which included not only active IDUs, but ex-IDUs and interested health professionals) convinced the municipal health department to set up a syringe exchange program in the city. Concern about hepatitis B transmission was the rationale for the exchanges. (At this time, HIV antibody tests were not widely available, and it was not known that HIV infection was present among IDUs in Amsterdam.)

The exchange program was begun in the fall of 1984, and 100,000 sterile needles and syringes were distributed in Amsterdam by 1985, for a population of approximately 3000 IDUs. When HIV testing was begun in Amsterdam in 1985, the findings showed that approximately 30% of IDUs were already carrying the AIDS virus, so a massive expansion of the syringe exchange program was undertaken. Within several years, the number of needles and syringes distributed reached approximately 600,000 and has remained at that level for the same number (3000) of IDUs in the city. The Amsterdam syringe exchange operates out of a number of different sites, including some (but not all) drug treatment programs, as well as freestanding exchange sites.

Elsewhere, concern about HIV transmission among IDUs has led to syringe exchange programs in almost all developed countries. In addition to The Netherlands, national syringe exchange programs have been established in the United Kingdom, Australia, New Zealand, and Canada. Yet opposition to syringe exchanges has remained strong in the United States and Sweden. In the United States, the federal government has officially adopted a policy prohibiting any federal support for syringe exchanges. There is, however, growing local support for syringe exchanges and a number have been established through such efforts. But at present, there is no expectation of federal support, and opposition remains strong in most localities. In southern Sweden, syringe exchanges were established without official support. These were then evaluated by a national board, which recommended expansion of syringe exchanges. The Par-

liament, however, rejected this recommendation and limited syringe exchange to those programs that were already in operation.

There is considerable variation in the actual operation of syringe exchanges in terms of the number of syringes that may be exchanged at one time, whether syringes will be given or sold to an IDU who comes without a used syringe to exchange, hours of operation, and linkage to other services that IDUs may need. These operational factors are discussed below in relation to community effectiveness.

One additional factor relevant to syringe exchanges is that, in the United States, a number of syringe exchanges have an, at best, uncertain legal status. The current syringe exchanges in New York City and San Francisco (plus many others in the Northeast and in California) may be operating in violation of laws that (a) require prescriptions for the distribution of syringes and (b) prohibit the possession of drug paraphernalia. Persons operating syringe exchanges in several areas in the United States have been arrested and taken to trial. Yet, as of April 1991, only one trial has been completed, which ended with a not guilty verdict. Ironically, operating a syringe exchange in potential violation of the law may help one gain the trust of IDUs—but it also creates many limitations on the extent of services that can be provided.

At the individual level of effectiveness, there have been two studies of seroconversion rates among participants in syringe exchange programs, in London (27) and in Sweden (28). Both studies showed very low—almost zero—seroconversion rates among participants, although interpretation of the rates is somewhat difficult; for example, some of the seroconverters in the London sample may have been infected prior to beginning to use the exchange, while some of those with new infections in Sweden may have become infected in a different geographic area. Moreover, neither study had a comparison group, precluding definitive conclusions about the effectiveness of syringe exchanges in protecting individual IDUs from exposure to HIV. Also, in both areas, there were additional AIDS prevention activities operating concurrently with the syringe exchanges: not just AIDS education, but linkages from the exchange to drug abuse treatment in both areas, as well as over-the-counter sales of syringes in London, and large-scale HIV testing and counseling for IDUs in Sweden. Even in Amsterdam— where the expansion of the syringe exchange system has been associated with more IDUs using the system—studies have not yet demonstrated that syringe exchange is associated, at the individual level, with a reduced risk of HIV infection (29).

Studies of the potential community-level effectiveness of a syringe exchange program—can exchanges reduce HIV transmission among a group of IDUs?—have led to a better understanding of how syringe exchanges should operate and suggest that exchanges might be effective at the community level even without having an easily measurable effect at the individual level. To be effective at the community level, a syringe exchange needs to attract a large percentage of the IDUs in the community on a consistent basis. To do so, an exchange needs to be "user friendly" (27,30,31). A user-friendly exchange is (a) readily accessible to IDUs, (b) located preferably in or near areas where drugs are sold, and (c) open at the hours during which IDUs inject drugs—in short, it should be so convenient that IDUs would have to go out of their way to avoid the exchange. Staff of a user-friendly exchange take a nonjudgmental attitude toward the injection of illicit drugs. That is, they will not convey a condemnation of persons who continue to inject illicit drugs.

Many user-friendly exchanges also provide additional services to IDUs. Preventing sexual transmission of HIV, which includes condom distribution, is part of the mission of the exchange. Moreover, it may provide not only referrals to drug abuse treatment, medical treatment, and social services, but also assistance in negotiating the bureaucratic obstacles associated with trying to access those additional services. Finally, a user-friendly exchange will also make some provision for "satellite" exchange of sterile needles and syringes. Some users will be exchanging syringes not only for themselves as individuals, but for their friendship groups. They may bring in dozens, even hundreds, of used syringes at one time for exchange. A user-friendly exchange will take advantage of this opportunity to increase its coverage of the IDU community while maintaining an exchange—not simply a syringe distribution—operation, so that potentially contaminated used injection equipment is retrieved and properly disposed of.

A large-scale, user-friendly syringe exchange system may be effective at the community level without showing measurable effectiveness at the individual level, because such an exchange would attract both seronegative and (already) seropositive IDUs. Participation by seropositives would reduce HIV transmission from them to other IDUs, including those not using the exchange. This may already be occurring in Amsterdam, where HIV seroprevalence among IDUs has stabilized and the incidence of hepatitis B infection among IDUs has actually declined (29).

OVER-THE-COUNTER SALES

Selling sterile injection equipment without restrictions to IDUs at pharmacies or other commercial retail outlets has many potential advantages as a method of preventing HIV transmission. There is already a wide distribution system of pharmacies, including sites in or near high-drug-use areas. The cost of needles and syringes at pharmacies is quite low (in developed countries), and the marginal cost of expanding the sale of syringes to IDUs through pharmacies and vending machines would be quite low. Pharmacy staff can also be trained to provide some counseling and referral services for IDUs who purchase injection equipment. (In some places, such as New Zealand and parts of the United Kingdom, syringe exchanges are operated out of pharmacies. In these areas, it becomes quite difficult to distinguish between syringe exchange and over-the-counter sales as different methods of preventing HIV transmission among IDUs.)

In most developed countries, pharmacists had no legal restrictions on selling injection equipment to IDUs prior to the AIDS epidemic, although there was considerable variation in the extent to which pharmacists actually would sell to persons suspected of being IDUs. Indeed, the fact that pharmacists in Edinburgh, Scotland, were persuaded by law-enforcement officials to stop selling injection equipment to IDUs is believed to be an important factor in the rapid spread of HIV among IDUs in that city (32).

The French program for selling injection equipment to IDUs through pharmacies serves as a good example of how such programs can work. Prior to AIDS, French law required prescriptions for the sale of injection equipment and, of course, prescriptions were not permitted for the purpose of injecting illicit drugs. The law was changed because of the AIDS epidemic, and a national program for training pharmacy staff to work with IDUs on safer injection practices was established. Studies of IDUs entering the prison system in Paris showed that this change in the law, combined with the training program, led to a large increase in the percentage of IDUs who obtained sterile injection equipment from pharmacies (33).

Although a limited number of studies have shown that increasing the potential for IDUs to purchase injection equipment at pharmacies leads to an increase in the use of sterile injection equipment, it is not yet established whether this actually reduces the risk of exposure to HIV. Many IDUs who do not use syringe exchanges do purchase equipment at pharmacies, however, so that studies showing no difference in HIV seroprevalence between those who use exchanges and those who do not (34) may be seen as indirect evidence for the effectiveness of over-the-counter sales.

An over-the-counter sales policy appears to have led to a stabilization of HIV seroprevalence in Innsbruck, Austria (35). Prior to concern about AIDS, it was legally permissible for pharmacies to sell injection equipment to IDUs there, but the policy was to sell syringes only in lots of 100. This greatly limited the extent to which IDUs were able to purchase injection equipment. The threat of

AIDS in IDUs led health officials to convince the pharmacists to sell individual syringes to IDUs, and HIV seroprevalence has since stabilized in the city (though a strict cause-and-effect relationship has not been demonstrated).

The relative lack of studies showing the individual- or community-level effectiveness of over-the-counter sales of injection equipment should not be taken as an indication that this method of preventing HIV infection lacks support among AIDS prevention specialists. In most developed countries—with Sweden and the United States as notable exceptions—the need for over-the-counter sales is considered to be self-evident. (In developing countries, this strategy is limited because these countries often lack the financial resources to provide sterile injection equipment for medical injections, much less illicit drug injections.) Over-the-counter sales are considered to be a baseline against which to measure other, more expensive and labor-intensive, AIDS prevention strategies.

BLEACH DISTRIBUTION

Standard household bleach is a commonly used disinfectant in medical settings and, even at low concentrations, is capable of killing HIV. Bleach distribution programs were devised in the United States as a means for preventing HIV infection among IDUs despite the frequent legal restrictions on the distribution and possession of injection equipment. The Mid-City Consortium in San Francisco developed the specifics of the "small-bottles-of-bleach" program, based on their ethnographic studies of IDUs. Original recommendations for disinfection had been that equipment be soaked in a 1:10 solution of bleach and water for 10–15 min. But IDUs who have drugs to inject are usually in a hurry to do so, particularly if they are experiencing withdrawal symptoms. Locating bleach, mixing the proper solution, and waiting through the long soaking period are all quite impractical for IDUs when they are anxious to inject. In contrast, small bottles of bleach can be carried about and thus are likely to be on hand when IDUs want to inject. Also, rinsing twice in full-strength bleach, then twice in water, would take only 20–30 sec. There have not yet been any direct comparisons as to the viricidal effectiveness of the soaking (versus the rinsing) procedure, but full-strength bleach is quite effective in killing HIV. Thoroughness in rinsing out the needle and syringe may be the most important factor in proper bleach disinfection.

The small bottles of bleach have labels explaining the proper multiple-rinsing procedures (in both words and pictures) as well as the names and phone numbers of organizations that provide additional AIDS services for IDUs. The bottles are distributed by trained outreach workers in high-drug-use areas. These individuals also provide face-to-face AIDS education and referrals for other services, including drug abuse treatment. More recently, there has been an evolution from the distribution of bleach alone to more complete "AIDS prevention kits," including small bottles of clean water (for both rinsing the syringes and preparing the drug solution), a bottle cap to be used as a "cooker" (so that the IDUs do not need to share cookers), a ball of cotton (for use in filtering the drug solution—again, so that the IDUs do not need to share), alcohol swabs to prevent bacterial infection (36), several condoms, and literature with AIDS education and information about obtaining additional services. These are usually packaged in a small plastic bag. Outreach workers are often, but not always, ex-addicts themselves. It is not necessary to be an ex-addict in order to be successful at outreach/bleach-distribution work, provided the worker is knowledgeable in local street drug culture and is able to work with IDUs in a nonjudgmental way (37). Outreach workers usually work in pairs, both for mutual support and for mutual protection.

Through the National AIDS Demonstration Research (NADR) program sponsored by the National Institute on Drug Abuse, 63 outreach/bleach-distribution programs have been conducted in over 50 cities in the United States (although the extent to which a program emphasizes bleach distribution varies considerably across programs). Originally, some European health officials had considerable doubts about the use of bleach as a disinfectant, particularly whether virus contained within cells would be inactivated, and whether all the blood would be removed as a result of the rinsing procedures. Recently, however, some European syringe exchanges have reconsidered this position and begun distributing bleach for use by IDUs.

One difficulty that has been observed with the bleach-followed-by-water rinsing procedure is that full-strength bleach will degrade the ease with which the plunger moves in the barrel of the syringe—making it more difficult to operate and reducing the number of times a syringe can be used. Thus a successful bleach distribution strategy may also require at least a moderate degree of access to sterile injection equipment for IDUs, whether through licit or illicit channels.

Although there are several studies indicating that bleach disinfection is readily acceptable to IDUs, there are as yet no studies showing that bleach protects an IDU from infection with HIV. Seroconversion studies conducted in San Francisco (38) and Baltimore (D. Vlahov, *personal communication*, 1991), as well as our own study in New York, have not yet demonstrated that IDUs using bleach as a disinfectant are less likely to become infected with HIV. Nonetheless—given the inherent multiple difficulties in demonstrating that any type of AIDS prevention program works at the *individual* level—the results from these ongoing studies should not be construed to mean that bleach distribution is ineffective.

There is more evidence for the effectiveness of bleach distribution at the community level than at the individual level. HIV seroprevalence among IDUs in San Francisco had been increasing rapidly prior to the development of the bleach distribution program. Bleach was quickly adopted by a majority of IDUs in the city, and HIV seroprevalence then stabilized at approximately 15%, although a strict cause-and-effect relationship has not been demonstrated. In contrast, in other cities (such as New York and Bangkok) HIV seroprevalence among IDUs continued to rise to levels as high as 40–50%. It should be noted, however, that there were, at this time, other AIDS prevention services for IDUs in San Francisco (26), though none operated on the scale of the bleach program. In addition, bleach distribution was so linked with other prevention services that it is impossible to pinpoint precisely the role of the bleach program *per se* in the stabilization of HIV seroprevalence among IDUs in San Francisco.

The NIDA National AIDS Demonstration Research program should provide more definitive information within the next several years regarding the effectiveness of bleach distribution.

HIV COUNSELING AND TESTING

Identifying individual carriers of an infectious agent has been a central part of traditional public health strategies for control of infectious diseases. This tactic clearly works best in situations where screening is relatively cost-efficient, and there is some clear course of action to be taken that prevents further spread, which is perceived to be beneficial by the persons involved. HIV testing as a public health measure has been challenged on each of these grounds: it may be highly cost-ineffective in populations with low HIV seroprevalence, and, until recently, there was little action to be taken to assist an HIV-infected person, and the potential loss of confidentiality was a serious concern.

Based on a limited number of studies of the effect of HIV counseling and testing on IDUs, it may be concluded that voluntary testing (along with good counseling) does lead to reduced levels of AIDS risk/transmission behavior (38a). However, these studies have also demonstrated that even voluntary HIV counseling and testing should not be considered to have a simple, uniform effect on IDUs. An individual's expectations about the test results and the actual results are two obvious and important variables.

One interesting characteristic of HIV counseling and testing as an AIDS prevention tactic is that in those situations where it does not work, it might actually be counterproductive. There have been anecdotal reports of individual IDUs who increase their drug use (and other problem behavior) after learning that they are HIV-positive, although the frequency of this response is unclear. Concern has also been raised that perceived coerciveness in HIV testing, and loss of confidentiality of test results, may lead IDUs to avoid services they need, if HIV testing is connected to those services. (As indicated below, the development of early treatment for HIV infection is greatly changing the perception of HIV counseling and testing, including how it may act in prevention of further HIV transmission.)

It is disturbing to note how little research has been done on the impact of HIV testing, considering the amount of testing that goes on throughout the world. This applies not only to IDUs but to all other high-risk groups as well. One explanation is that such studies, particularly when they involve measuring HIV seroprevalence or seroconversion, are very difficult to conduct. In practical terms, it is hard to find appropriate controls for the group that did receive HIV counseling and testing. In addition, it would be ethically questionable to withhold HIV counseling and testing from members of a control group who wanted to be tested. There is a general consensus that an individual has the right to knowledge about his or her medical status, which would include HIV serostatus.

Sweden has attempted HIV testing for all IDUs, using multiple testing sites (including drug treatment programs and prisons) with the goal of regularly retesting those who are seronegative. Even the syringe exchange sites actively encourage IDUs to be tested for HIV. The scale of this program does permit some inferences about the potential effectiveness of HIV antibody testing and counseling on reducing spread of HIV among IDUs. Several reports indicate that HIV seroprevalence has stabilized among IDUs in Sweden (39,40), suggesting that the rate of new HIV infections has been reduced considerably. Olin (*personal communication*) has noted that a new social norm has arisen among IDUs in Sweden, which is indicative of the widespread acceptance of HIV testing; namely, when other IDUs ask to use their injection equipment, seropositive IDUs will tell the potential borrower of their positive serostatus.

There are, however, at least three reasons why it cannot be extrapolated that HIV testing *per se* would lead to stabilization of HIV seroprevalence among IDUs in areas other than Sweden. First, the HIV testing program in Sweden was accompanied by efforts to place all IDUs into drug abuse treatment. Second, concerns about confidentiality that may limit willingness to be tested for HIV, do not appear to be nearly as strong in Sweden as they are in most other developed countries. Finally, the majority of IDUs in Sweden inject amphetamines—and the dynamics of syringe sharing among amphetamine injectors may be different from syringe sharing among heroin or cocaine injectors. For reasons that are not yet understood, the HIV seroprevalence rate among amphetamine injectors in Sweden is less than 10%, while the seroprevalence among heroin injectors is approximately 50% (39).

As noted above, the development of treatments for preventing opportunistic infections among asymptomatic HIV-infected persons is changing the perception that HIV counseling and testing are only useful as a means of preventing HIV transmission. It now becomes ethically necessary to provide the greatest possible access to medical treatment for persons found to be infected in an HIV testing program. The effectiveness of HIV testing as a means of reducing HIV transmission was always linked to the quality of the counseling that accompanied it and, in the future, the effectiveness of HIV testing may also become closely linked to the quality of the medical treatment, drug abuse treatment, and social services that can be provided in conjunction with testing.

DRUG USERS' ORGANIZATIONS

Another method of preventing HIV transmission is by the organized efforts of the persons most at risk. The efforts of organized gay communities in a large number of cities seem to have led to declines in new HIV infections among gay men with ties to their gay subcultures (41). Some, but much less, self-organization has occurred among drug injectors. These organizations have (a) engaged in educational activities; (b) distributed syringes, bleach, and condoms; and (c) promulgated norms for how to minimize the risk of HIV transmission while engaging in drug-injecting and sexual practices.

In the early 1980s, there was an outburst of collective self-organization by drug users in The Netherlands who wanted acceptance and better treatment by their society. The *junkiebonden* that were formed also became involved in AIDS education and the distribution of syringes to drug injectors. These organizations, however, remained limited in size and have tended to vary over time in their effectiveness, with periods of high activity interspersed with periods in which little was done (42). In the last 2 years, there has been renewed self-organization, particularly in Germany, where at least 25 cities now have chapters of JES (Junkies, Ex-users, Substitutionists) and in Australia, where organizations exist in several cities which combine the efforts of current and former drug injectors. In New York, ADAPT (Association for Drug Abuse Prevention and Treatment)—an organization of ex-users, health professionals, and users—has tried since 1985 to prevent HIV transmission through outreach and other activities.

In the United States, efforts have been made to organize drug injectors against AIDS in Minneapolis–St.

Paul (43) and in the Williamsburg section of Brooklyn (by ADAPT, under subcontract to Narcotic and Drug Research, Inc.). The Williamsburg effort has met with only moderate success in establishing an organization, but a behavioral evaluation study found that considerable risk reduction has occurred among drug injectors in the neighborhood (44), including the regular use of condoms, reported by one-third of the study participants (45).

No individual level HIV seroconversion or seroprevalence data have been reported with which to evaluate the effectiveness of these organizations. Community-level data do show a leveling off of seroprevalence and decline in seroconversions in Amsterdam (46). Moreover, to the extent that this leveling off is the result of the syringe exchange, it should be noted that the exchange was itself initiated at the request of the MDHG, a mixed group of drug users and nonusers. In New York City, seroprevalence also seems to have leveled off, but at least in Manhattan this probably occurred prior to efforts by ADAPT —and certainly prior to the effort to organize drug injectors on a community basis in Williamsburg.

SUMMARY COMMENTS

Many studies have demonstrated that IDUs will change their behavior in response to the threat of AIDS, to the point where previous doubts as to the willingness or ability of IDUs to change their AIDS risk behaviors can now be dismissed. Unfortunately, it remains difficult to assess the epidemiologic importance of any specific behavior change. Only a limited number of studies have been able to use either HIV seroprevalence or seroincidence as an outcome variable, so that it is very difficult to compare the relative effectiveness of different types of AIDS prevention programs for IDUs.

Taken as a whole, the studies indicate that AIDS education alone is not sufficient. Prevention programs need to provide the practical means for behavior change, whether it is drug abuse treatment to reduce/eliminate drug injection itself, or a means for "safer injection" so that HIV transmission need not occur during illicit drug use.

Relatively little research has focused on the mechanisms through which AIDS risk reduction is initiated and maintained among IDUs. Basic knowledge of what AIDS is and how it is transmitted appears to be necessary for risk reduction, and several studies (8,47,48) suggest that social influence processes are important. The development of new norms among drug injectors that proscribe multiperson use of injection equipment would both extend the effects of an AIDS prevention program to IDUs not directly reached by the program, as well as maintain these effects over time if the prevention program ends.

Our present level of knowledge about AIDS risk reduction among IDUs does not permit identification of a single "best" type of program. The research data—as well as the practical experience of persons operating programs—suggest that multiple types of programs should operate simultaneously. A variety of methods of drug abuse treatment is needed, both because persons injecting at high frequencies cannot be expected always to practice safer injection, and because IDUs in contact with prevention programs often ask for treatment. Also, safer injection programs are needed, because not all IDUs want to enter treatment, and treatment is not uniformly successful with those who do enter.

Considering the difficulties in accurately measuring AIDS risk behavior among IDUs, and the inherent complexity of the problems, much has been learned in the last 7 years of research and practice. It is now clear that there are a variety of effective prevention strategies, and that the rate of new HIV infections among drug injectors can be greatly reduced—though no strategy or combination of strategies has yet succeeded in eliminating new infections. Questions arise with respect to the future of AIDS prevention for IDUs. Are there potential breakthroughs that have been missed so far? How will we learn more? No breakthroughs appear about to happen, but given the demonstrated creativity of people working on AIDS prevention for IDUs, the unexpected is certainly possible. One area in which a breakthrough is needed is the development of a treatment, on a public-health scale, for cocaine dependence. In terms of assessing AIDS prevention strategies for IDUs, it appears unlikely that traditional methods of evaluating experiments will be applicable to community-level prevention efforts. Such studies would be exceedingly expensive, and the community efforts are often a changing mixture of different programs. In order to assess changes in the prevalence and incidence of HIV infection, we need to develop better models of how HIV has and might spread among groups of drug injectors.

ACKNOWLEDGMENTS

The research in this chapter was supported by National Institute on Drug Abuse grant DA03574. The views expressed here do not necessarily reflect the positions of the granting agencies or of the institutions by which the authors are employed.

REFERENCES

1. *HIV/AIDS surveillance, year-end edition.* U.S. AIDS cases reported through December 1990. Atlanta GA: Centers for Disease Control; 1991.
2. *AIDS surveillance in Europe.* WHO-EC Collaborating Center on AIDS. Quarterly Report No. 27. Geneva: World Health Organization; September 30, 1990.
3. Vanichseni S, Sakuntanaga P. Results of three seroprevalence surveys for HIV in IVDU in Bangkok. 6th International Conference on AIDS, San Francisco, June, 1990.
4. Minister of Health. *AIDS Boletim Epidemiologico.* Rio de Janiero; Brazil, 1988.
5. Boxaca M, Libonatti O, Muzzio E, Segura E, Hosokawa R, Weissenbacher M. HIV-1 prevalence and the role of other infectious diseases in a group of drug users in Argentina. 6th International Conference on AIDS, San Francisco, June 1990.
6. Naik TN, Sarkar S, Singh SL, et al. Intravenous drug users—a new high-risk group for HIV infection in India. *AIDS* 1991;5(1):117–118.
7. Des Jarlais DC, Friedman SR, Hopkins W. Risk reduction for the acquired immunodeficiency syndrome among intravenous drug users. *Ann Intern Med* 1985;103:755–9.
8. Friedman SR, Des Jarlais DC, Sotheran JL. AIDS and self-organization among intravenous drug users. *Int J Addict* 1987;22(3):201–19.
9. Selwyn PA, Feiner C, Cox CP, Lipschutz C, Cohen R. Knowledge about AIDS and high-risk behavior among intravenous drug abusers in New York City. *AIDS* 1987;1(4):247–54.
10. Jackson J, Rotkiewicz L. A coupon program: AIDS education and drug treatment. 3rd International Conference on AIDS, Washington, DC, June 1987.
11. Des Jarlais DC, Friedman SR, Novick D, et al. HIV-1 infection among intravenous drug users in Manhattan. *JAMA* 1989; 261:1008–12.
12. Angarano G, Pastore G, Monno L, Santantonio F, Luchera N, Schiraldi O. Rapid spread of HTLV-III infection among drug addicts in Italy. *Lancet* 1985;2:1302.
13. de la Loma A, Garcia S, Ramos P, Neila MA. Poor lifestyle modification among IV drug users assisted at an STD clinic for HIV infection diagnosis. 4th International Conference on AIDS, Stockholm, Sweden, June 1988.
14. Des Jarlais DC, Friedman SR. AIDS and IV drug use. *Science* 1989;245:578.
15. Des Jarlais DC. Stages in the response of the drug abuse treatment system to the AIDS epidemic in New York City. *J Drug Issues* 1990;20(2):335–47.
16. Friedman SR, Des Jarlais DC, Goldsmith DS. An overview of AIDS prevention efforts aimed at intravenous drug users circa 1987. *J Drug Issues* 1989;19(1):93–112.
17. Simpson DD, Savage LJ, Sells SB. *Data book on drug treatment outcomes: follow-up study of 1969–1972 admissions to the Drug Abuse Reporting Program (DARP) 1978.* Report 78-10. Fort Worth, TX: Institute of Behavior Research, Texas Christian University; 1978.
18. Hubbard RL, Marsden ME, Rachal JV, Harwood HJ, Cavanaugh ER, Ginzburg HM. *Drug abuse treatment: a national study of effectiveness.* Chapel Hill: University of North Carolina Press; 1989.
19. Gerstein DR, Harwood HJ, eds. *Treating drug problems.* Washington, DC: National Academy Press; 1990.
20. Hartel D, Selwyn PA, Schoenbaum EE, Klein RS, Friedland GH. Methadone maintenance treatment (MMTP) and reduced risk of AIDS and AIDS-specific mortality in intravenous drug users (IVDUs). 4th International Conference on AIDS, Stockholm, Sweden, June 1988.
21. Abdul-Quader AS, Friedman SR, Des Jarlais DC, Marmor M, Maslansky R, Bartelme S. Methadone maintenance and behavior by intravenous drug users that can transmit HIV. *Contemp Drug Problems* 1987;14(3):425–34.
22. Novick DM, Kreek MJ, Des Jarlais DC, et al. Antibody to LAV, the putative agent of AIDS, in parenteral drug abusers and methadone-maintained patients: therapeutic, historical, and ethical aspects. In: Harris LJ, ed. *Problems of drug dependence 1985.* National Institute on Drug Abuse, Research Monograph 67. Rockville, MD: National Institute on Drug Abuse; 1986:318–20.
23. Blix O, Gronbladh L. AIDS and IV heroin addicts: the preventive effect of methadone maintenance in Sweden. 4th International Conference on AIDS, Stockholm, Sweden, June 1988.
24. Torrens M, San L, Peri J, Olle J. Cocaine abuse among heroin addicts in Spain. *Drug Alcohol Dependence* 1991;27:29–34.
25. Chaisson RE, Bacchetti P, Osmond D, Brodie B, Sande MA, Moss

AR. Cocaine use and HIV infection in intravenous drug users in San Francisco. *JAMA* 1989;261(4):561–5.

26. Moss AR, Chaisson RE. AIDS and intravenous drug use in San Francisco. *AIDS Public Policy J* 1988;3(2):37–41.

27. Hart GJ, Carvell ALM, Woodward N, Johnson AM, Williams P, Parry J. Evaluation of needle exchange in central London: behaviour change and anti-HIV status over one year. *AIDS* 1989;3(5):261–5.

28. Ljungberg B, Andersson B, Christensson B, Hugo-Persson M, Tunving K, Ursing B. Distribution of sterile equipment to IV drug abusers as part of an HIV prevention program. 4th International Conference on AIDS, Stockholm, June 1988.

29. Van Haastrecht HJA, van den Hoek JAR, Bardoux C, Leentvaar-Kuypers A, Coutinho RA. The course of the HIV epidemic among intravenous drug users in Amsterdam, The Netherlands. *AJPH* 1991;81(1):59–62.

30. Des Jarlais DC. Outcomes of HIV infection in intravenous drug users in New York City. NIDA National Conference on Drug Abuse Research and Practice, Washington, Jan 12–15, 1991.

31. Friedman SR. Syringe availability and AIDS. Read before the Minnesota Department of Human Services, St. Paul, Nov 4, 1988.

32. Robertson JR, Bucknall ABV, Welsby PD, et al. Epidemic of AIDS related virus (HTLV-III/LAV) infection among intravenous drug users. *Br Med J* 1986;292:527–9.

33. Espinoza P, Bouchard I, Ballian P, Polo Devoto J. Has the open sale of syringes modified the syringe exchanging habits of drug addicts? 4th International Conference on AIDS, Stockholm, Sweden, June 1988.

34. van den Hoek JAR, Coutinho A, van Haastrecht HJA, van Zadelhoff AW, Goudsmit J. Prevalence and risk factors of HIV infections among drug users and drug-using prostitutes in Amsterdam. *AIDS* 1988;2:55–60.

35. Fuchs D, Unterweger B, Hausen A, et al. Anti-HIV-1 antibodies, anti-HTLV-1 antibodies and neopterin levels in parenteral drug addicts in the Austrian Tyrol. *J AIDS* 1988;1(1):65–6.

36. Herb F, Watters JK, Case P, Pettiti D. Endocarditis, subcutaneous abscesses, and other bacterial infections in intravenous drug users and their association with skin-cleaning at drug injection sites. 5th International Conference on AIDS, Montreal, Canada, June 1989.

37. Rivera-Beckman J, Friedman SR, Clatts MC, Curtis R. "Inside"–"outside": social process in AIDS outreach. In: *Proceedings of the Second National AIDS Demonstration Research Conference.* Rockville, MD: National Institute on Drug Abuse; in press.

38. Moss AR, Bachetti P, Osmond D, Meakin R, Kefelew A, Gorter R. Seroconversion for HIV in intravenous drug users in San Francisco. 5th International Conference on AIDS, Montreal, Canada, June 1989.

38a. Rugg DL, MacGowan RJ. Assessing the effectiveness of HIV counseling and testing: a practical guide. Background paper for WHO Global Programme on AIDS, Geneva, November 13–16, 1990.

39. Kall K, Olin R. HIV status and changes in risk behavior among intravenous drug users in Stockholm 1987–88. *AIDS* 1990;4(2):153–7.

40. Böttiger M, Forsgren M, Grillner L, Biberfeld G, Eriksson G, Janzon R. Monitoring of HIV infection among IV drug users in Stockholm. 4th International Conference on AIDS, Stockholm, Sweden, June 1988.

41. Coutinho RA, van Griensven GJP, Moss A. Effects of preventive efforts among homosexual men. *AIDS* 1989;3(suppl 1):S53–6.

42. Friedman SR, de Jong WM, Des Jarlais DC. Problems and dynamics of organizing intravenous drug users for AIDS prevention. *Health Educ Res* 1988;3:49–57.

43. Carlson J, Needle R. Sponsoring addict self-organization (Addicts Against AIDS): a case study. First Annual National AIDS Demonstration Research Conference, Rockville, MD, 1989.

44. Friedman SR, Neaigus A, Jose B, et al. Behavioral outcomes of organizing drug injectors against AIDS. In: *Proceedings of the Second National AIDS Demonstration Research Conference.* Rockville, MD: National Institute on Drug Abuse; in press.

45. Jose B, Friedman SR, Neaigus A, Sufian M. Condom use among drug injectors in an organizing project neighborhood. In: *Proceed-*

ings of the Second National AIDS Demonstration Research Conference. Rockville, MD: National Institute on Drug Abuse; in press.

46. Van Haastrecht HJA, van den Hoek JAR, Coutinho RA. No trend in yearly HIV-seroprevalence rates among IVDU in Amsterdam: 1986–1988. 5th International Conference on AIDS, Montreal, Canada, June 1989.

47. Abdul-Quader AS, Tross S, Friedman SR, Kouzi AC, Des Jarlais DC. Street-recruited intravenous drug users and sexual risk reduction in New York City. *AIDS* 1990;4(11):1075–9.

48. Klee H, Faugier J, Hayes C, Boulton T, Morris J. Factors associated with risk behavior among injecting drug users. *AIDS Care* 1990;2:133–45.

49. Raffi F, Milpied B, Charonnat M-F. Free and anonymous HIV testing center of Nantes, France: 1989 experience. 6th International Conference on AIDS, San Francisco, June 1990; SC 646 (abst).

50. Zerboni R, D'Orso M, Cusini M, et al. HIV infection in the STD centre of Milan–Italy. 6th International Conference on AIDS, San Francisco, June 1990; FC 636 (abst).

51. Böttiger M, Blaxhult A. Evaluation of true number of HIV infected persons in Sweden. 6th International Conference on AIDS, San Francisco, June 1990; FC 646 (abst).

52. Jones ST, Moore M, Cahill K, Gardom JC, Poppe PO, Kirby CD, Bowen GS. HIV antibody counseling and testing (CT) for intravenous drug users and their sexual partners—United States, 1988–89. 6th International Conference on AIDS, San Francisco, June 1990; SC 659 (abst).

53. Farley T, Cartter M, Hadler J. HIV counseling and testing in methadone programs: effect on treatment compliance. 6th International Conference on AIDS, San Francisco, June 1990; SC 660 (abst).

54. Casadonte P, Des Jarlais DC, Friedman SR, Rotrosen J. Psychological and behavioral impact among intravenous drug users of learning H.I.V. test results. *Int J Addict* 1990;25(4):409–26.

55. Gibson DR, Guydish J, Case P et al. Using forensic techniques to corroborate IV drug users' self-reports of needle sharing. 6th International Conference on AIDS, San Francisco, June 1990; SC 741 (abst).

56. Cartter ML, Petersen LR, Savage RB, Donagher J. Providing HIV counseling and testing services in methadone maintenance programs. *AIDS* 1990;4(5):463–5.

57. McCoy CB, Chitwood DD, Khoury EL, Miles CE. The implementation of an experimental research design in the evaluation of an intervention to prevent AIDS among IV drug users. *J Drug Issues* 1990;20(2):215–22.

58. Inciardi JA. Federal efforts to control the spread of HIV and AIDS among IV drug users. *Am Behavioral Sci* 1990;33(4):408–18.

59. Sorensen JL. Preventing AIDS: prospects for change in white male intravenous drug users. National Institute on Drug Abuse, Research Monograph 93. Rockville, MD: National Institute on Drug Abuse; 1990:83–107.

60. Brown BS, Beschner GM. AIDS and HIV infection: implications for drug abuse treatment. *J Drug Issues* 1989;19(1):141–62.

61. Dow MG, Knox MD, Cotton DA. Administrative challenges to working with HIV-positive clients: experiences of mental health and substance abuse program directors in Florida. *J Ment Health Admin* 1989;16(2):80–90.

62. Goldstein DA. AIDS and drug use: breaking the link. *AIDS Educ Prevent* 1989;1(3):231–46.

63. Howell EF, Niven RG. The argument for HIV-antibody testing in chemical dependence treatment programs. *J Psychoactive Drugs* 1989;21(4):415–7.

64. Mersky SA. Testing for human immunodeficiency virus in chemical dependence treatment programs. *J Psychoactive Drugs* 1989;21(4):407–13.

65. Sorrell SJ, Springer ER. The argument against HIV-antibody testing in chemical dependence treatment programs. *J Psychoactive Drugs* 1989;21(4):419–21.

66. Wheat M, Devons C, Solomon S, Hyman R. HIV risk-factor counseling by medical housestaff. 6th International Conference on AIDS, San Francisco, June 1990.

67. Higgins DL, Galavotti C, Johnson R, O'Reilly KR, Rugg DL.

The effect of HIV antibody counseling and testing on risk behaviors: Are the studies consistent? 6th International Conference on AIDS, San Francisco, June 1990.

68. Rezza G, Oliva C, Sasse H. Preventing AIDS among Italian drug addicts: evaluation of treatment programs and informative strategies. 4th International Conference on AIDS, Stockholm, Sweden, June 1988; 8531 (abst).

69. Hartgers C, van den Hoek JAR, Krijnen P, Coutinho RA. Risk factors and heroin and cocaine use trends among injection drug users (IDU) in low threshold methadone programs, Amsterdam 1985–1989. 6th International Conference on AIDS, San Francisco, June 1990; FC 638 (abst).

70. Ball JC, Lange WR, Myers CP, Friedman SR. Reducing the risk of AIDS through methadone maintenance treatment. *J Health Soc Behav* 1988;29(3):214–26.

71. Yancovitz S, Des Jarlais DC, Peyser N, et al. Innovative AIDS risk reduction project: interim methadone clinic. 4th International Conference on AIDS, Stockholm, Sweden, June 1988; 8547 (abst).

72. Keffelew A, Clark G, Bacchetti P, Gorter R, Osmond D, Moss AR. Use of needle exchange program by San Francisco drug users in methadone treatment. 6th International Conference on AIDS, San Francisco, June 1990; FC 107 (abst).

73. Arif A, ed. *Methadone maintenance in the management of opioid dependence: an international review.* New York: Praeger Publishers; 1990.

74. Nemoto T, Brown LS, Foster K, Chu A. Behavioral risk factors of human immunodeficiency virus infection among intravenous drug users and implications for preventive interventions. *AIDS Educ Prevent* 1990;2(2):116–26.

75. Kolar AF, Brown BS, Weddington WW, Ball JC. A treatment crisis: cocaine use by clients in methadone maintenance programs. *J Substance Abuse Treatment* 1990;7(2):101–7.

76. Magura S, Shapiro JL, Grossman JI, Siddiqi Q. Reactions of methadone patients to HIV antibody testing. *Adv Alcohol Substance Abuse* 1990;8(3–4):97–111.

77. Harris RE, Langrod J, Hebert JR, Lowinson J. Changes in AIDS risk behavior among intravenous drug abusers in New York City. *NY State J Med* 1990;90(3):123–6.

78. Zinberg NE. Social policy: AIDS and intravenous drug use. *Daedalus* 1989;118(3):23–46.

79. Schoenbaum EE, Hartel D, Selwyn PA, et al. Risk factors for human immunodeficiency virus infection in intravenous drug users. *N Engl J Med* 1989;321(13):874–9.

80. Nathan JA, Karan LD. Substance abuse treatment modalities in the age of HIV spectrum disease. *J Psychoactive Drugs* 1989;21(4):423–9.

81. Payte JT. Combined treatment modalities: the need for innovative approaches. *J Psychoactive Drugs* 1989;21(4):431–4.

82. Sorensen JL, Batki SL, Good P, Wilkinson K. Methadone maintenance program for AIDS-affected opiate addicts. *J Substance Abuse Treatment* 1989;6:87–94.

83. Sorensen JL, Gibson DR, Heitzmann C, et al. Psychoeducational group approach to AIDS prevention with drug abusers in residential treatment: impact 6 months after intervention. 5th International Conference on AIDS, Montreal, Canada, June 1989.

84. Sorensen JL, Costantini MF, London JA. Coping with AIDS: strategies for patients and staff in drug abuse treatment programs. *J Psychoactive Drugs* 1989;21(4):435–40.

85. Wiebel W, Chene D, Johnson W. Adoption of bleach use in a cohort of street intravenous drug users in Chicago. 6th International Conference on AIDS, San Francisco, June 1990; SC 742 (abst).

86. Thompson PI, Jones TS, Cahill K, Medina V. Promoting HIV prevention outreach activities via community-based organizations. 6th International Conference on AIDS, San Francisco, June 1990; FD 797 (abst).

87. Flynn NM, Jain S, Harper S, et al. Sharing of paraphernalia in intravenous drug users (IVDU): knowledge of AIDS is incomplete and doesn't affect behavior. 3rd International Conference on AIDS, Washington, DC, June 1987; TP 184 (abst).

88. Watters JK, Case P, Huang K, Cheng Y-T, Lorvick J, Carlson J. HIV seroepidemiology and behavior change in intravenous drug users: progress report on the effectiveness of street-based preven-

tion. 4th International Conference on AIDS, Stockholm, Sweden, June 1988; 8523 (abst).

89. Friedman SR, Sterk C, Des Jarlais DC, Sufian M. Will bleach decontaminate needles during cocaine binges in shooting galleries? *JAMA* 1989;262(11):1467.

90. Chitwood DD, McCoy CB, Comerford M. Risk behaviors of intravenous cocaine users: implications for intervention. National Institute on Drug Abuse, Research Monograph 93. Rockville, MD: National Institute on Drug Abuse; 1990:120–33.

91. Conviser R, Rutledge JH. Can public policies limit the spread of HIV among IV drug users? *J Drug Issues* 1989;19(1):113–28.

92. Haverkos HW. AIDS update: prevalence, prevention, and medical management. *J Psychoactive Drugs* 1989;21(4):365–70.

93. Lowe D, Milechman B, Cotton R, Vumbaca G, McDermott R, Ward S. Maximizing return rates and safe disposal of injection equipment in Australian needle & syringe exchange programs. 6th International Conference on AIDS, San Francisco, June 1990; SC 746 (abst).

94. Buning EC, Hartgers C, Verster AD, van Santen GW, Coutinho RA. The evaluation of the needle/syringe exchange in Amsterdam. 4th International Conference on AIDS, Stockholm, Sweden, June 1988; 8513 (abst).

95. Hart GJ, Woodward NJ, Johnson AM, Querubin G, Connell J, Adler MW. Risk behaviour and HIV infection in clients of needle-exchange in central London. 6th International Conference on AIDS, San Francisco, June 1990; SC 745 (abst).

96. Stimson G, Lart R. National survey of syringe-exchanges in England. 6th International Conference on AIDS, San Francisco, June 1990; 3079 (abst).

97. Harris E, Fullilove R, Gross S, Fullilove M, Dasher T. Feasibility of needle exchange program in San Francisco: a survey of street-based addicts. 6th International Conference on AIDS, San Francisco, June 1990; SC 744 (abst).

98. Des Jarlais DC, Hagan H, Purchase D, Reid T, Friedman SR. Safer injection among participants in the first North American syringe exchange program. 5th International Conference on AIDS, Montreal, Canada, June 1989; TAO20 (abst).

99. Jones LD. Working with drug users to prevent the spread of HIV: the application of an analytical framework to a range of programmes. *Health Educ Res* 1990;5(1):5–16.

100. Joseph SC. Current challenges of AIDS in New York City. *NY State J Med* 1989;89(9):517–9.

101. Goldberg D, Watson H, Stuart F, Miller M, Gruer L, Follett E. Pharmacy supply of needles and syringes—the effect on spread of HIV intravenous drug misusers. 4th International Conference on AIDS, Stockholm, Sweden, June 1988; 8521 (abst).

102. McKeganey N, Barnard M, Watson H. HIV-related risk behavior among a non-clinic sample of injecting drug users. *Br J Addict* 1989;84(12):1481–90.

103. Des Jarlais DC, Hopkins W. "Free" needles for intravenous drug users at risk for AIDS: current developments in New York City. *N Engl J Med* 1985;313(23):1476.

104. Jason J, Vlahov D, Solomon L, Smith M. Potential media channels for intravenous drug users' (IVDUs) AIDS prevention messages. 6th International Conference on AIDS, San Francisco, June 1990; FD 852 (abst).

105. Battjes RJ, Leukefeld CG, Amsel Z. Community prevention efforts to reduce the spread of AIDS associated with intravenous drug abuse. National Institute on Drug Abuse, Research Monograph 93. Rockville, MD: National Institute on Drug Abuse; 1990:288–90.

106. Serrano Y. The Puerto Rican intravenous drug user. National Institute on Drug Abuse, Research Monograph 93. Rockville, MD: National Institute on Drug Abuse; 1990:24–34.

107. Leukefeld CG, ed. *AIDS and intravenous drug use: future directions for community-based prevention research.* National Institute on Drug Abuse, Research Monograph 93. Rockville, MD: National Institute on Drug Abuse; 1990.

108. Zich J, Temoshok L. Perceptions of social support, distress and hopelessness in men with AIDS and ARC: clinical implications. In: Temoshok L, Baum A, eds. *Psychosocial perspectives on AIDS: etiology, prevention, and treatment.* Hillsdale, NJ: Lawrence Erlbaum Associates; 1990:201–27.

109. Weisse CS, Nesselhof-Kendall SEA, Fleck-Kandath C, Baum A.

Psychosocial aspects of AIDS prevention among heterosexuals. In: Edwards J, Tindale RS, Heath L, eds. *Social influence processes and prevention.* New York: Plenum Press; 1990:15–38.

110. Fisher JD, Misovich SJ. Social influences and AIDS-preventive behavior. In: Edwards J, Tindale RS, Heath L, eds. *Social influence processes and prevention.* New York: Plenum Press; 1990:39–70.

111. Neaigus A, Sufian M, Friedman SR, et al. Effects of outreach intervention on risk reduction among intravenous drug users. *AIDS Educ Behav* 1990;2:253–71.

112. Gagnon JH. Disease and desire. *Daedalus* 1989;118(3):47–77.

113. Cohen JB, Hauer LB, Wofsy CB. Women and IV drugs: parenteral and heterosexual transmission of human immunodeficiency virus. *J Drug Issues* 1989;19(1):39–56.

114. Casriel C, Des Jarlais DC, Rodriguez R, Friedman SR. Working with heroin sniffers: clinical issues in preventing drug injection. *J Substance Abuse Treatment* 1990;7(1):1–10.

115. Guydish J, Temoshok L, Dilley J, Rinaldi J. Evaluation of a hospital-based abuse intervention and referral service for HIV-affected patients. *Gen Hosp Psychiatry* 1990;12(1):1–7.

116. Brown BS, Hickey JE, Chung AE, Craig RD. The functioning of individuals on a drug abuse treatment waiting list. *Am J Drug Alcohol Abuse* 1989;15(3):261–74.

117. Westermeyer J, Seppala M, Gasow S, Carlson G. AIDS-related illness and AIDS risk in male homo/bisexual substance abusers: case reports and clinical issues. *Am J Drug Alcohol Abuse* 1989;15(4):443–61.

118. Getzenberg J, Lenihan P, Salem E. You *can* get there from here: a city's strategic response to AIDS. 6th International Conference on AIDS, San Francisco, June 1990; FD 776 (abst).

119. Jackson J, Baxter R. Inner-city mobile units: AIDS education and prevention. 4th International Conference on AIDS, Stockholm, Sweden, June 1988; 9024 (abst).

120. Graves G. Peer participation in poster production. 6th International Conference on AIDS, San Francisco, June 1990; FD 785 (abst).

121. Pott E. AIDS prevention and health education in the Federal Republic of Germany. 6th International Conference on AIDS, San Francisco, June 1990; FD 887 (abst).

122. Bortolotti F, Stivanello A, Carraro L, et al. Effect of AIDS prevention campaign on the behavior of drug abusers in Italy. 4th International Conference on AIDS, Stockholm, Sweden, June 1988; 8525 (abst).

123. Benedetti P. Phone counselling to persons at risk for HIV: the Italian experience. 6th International Conference on AIDS, San Francisco, June 1990; FD 903 (abst).

124. Carrillo ME, Tovar SM, Cipriano PB, et al. AIDS hotline in a developing country. 6th International Conference on AIDS, San Francisco, June 1990; FD 902 (abst).

125. Mondanaro J. Community-based AIDS prevention interventions: special issues of women intravenous drug users. National Institute on Drug Abuse, Research Monograph 93. Rockville, MD: National Institute on Drug Abuse; 1990:68–82.

126. Jang M, Forst M, Moore M, Gandelman A. AIDS education and prevention programs for intravenous drug users: the California experience. *J Drug Educ* 1990;20(1):1–13.

127. Longshore D. AIDS education for three high-risk populations. *Evaluation Program Planning* 1990;13(1):67–72.

128. Maccoby N. Communication and health education research: potential sources for education for prevention of drug use. National Institute on Drug Abuse, Research Monograph 93. Rockville, MD: National Institute on Drug Abuse; 1990:1–23.

129. Ostrow DG. AIDS prevention through effective education. *Daedalus* 1989;118(3):229–54.

130. Battjes RJ, Pickens R, Amsel Z. Trends in HIV infection and AIDS risk behaviors among intravenous drug abusers in selected US cities. 6th International Conference on AIDS, San Francisco, June 1990; FC 552 (abst).

131. Robertson JR, Skidmore CA, Roberts JJK. HIV infection in intravenous drug users: a follow-up study indicating changes in risk-taking behaviour. *Br J Addict* 1988;83:387–91.

AIDS and Other Manifestations of HIV Infection,
Second Edition, Edited by Gary P. Wormser.
Raven Press, Ltd., New York © 1992.

CHAPTER 41

Public Health Strategies for Prevention of HIV Infection

Donald P. Francis

PREVENTION

It is probable that HIV-1 (for simplicity referred to as HIV) first infected humans centuries ago and has moved from person to person ever since. Through transmission routes limited to the exchange of blood or plasma, the exchange of vaginal or seminal fluid, or from mother to unborn fetus or newborn, HIV has successfully propagated and spread worldwide.

Because of its extreme virulence (Table 1), HIV poses a unique public health problem. No other human virus has a mortality rate like HIV. In the past, when there were local outbreaks of severe infectious diseases, major campaigns were launched to control them. Yet for HIV, no "launching" has been seen. There has been no "AIDS Sunday," no national mobilization for HIV prevention. Political and public health leaders have often tried to stay clear of HIV rather than launch prevention campaigns. Why has there seemingly been so little concern for HIV? A major factor has been the long incubation period from infection to disease and death. This long "disease-free" period has confused individuals, communities, and societies and allowed them to deny the extent and importance of the epidemic. In reality, however, the long incubation period with continued viral excretion should have *increased* our public health concern rather than decreased it. Another factor has been the absence of a "magic bullet" for HIV. Without a vaccine or therapeutic agent, programs have had to rely on the "vaccine" of behavior change. Although quite effective and obviously essential for survival, implementing educational programs that must deal with people's sexual and intravenous drug-using behaviors has not been easy, at least in

the American political climate. Can we expect such inappropriate responses in the future? Possibly not. The climate seems to be slowly changing. As our knowledge has increased, individuals, communities, and society as a whole are beginning to understand HIV and make appropriate choices to minimize its future damage. Hopefully, the second decade of HIV will see better choices made than did the first.

The damage caused by HIV can be prevented either primarily, by interrupting transmission, or secondarily, by preventing progression to disease. This chapter stresses primary prevention—the process of preventing HIV from moving from an infected person to a susceptible one (Fig. 1).

TRANSMISSION

As with other infectious agents, the transmission of HIV appears to be a function of the amount of virus excreted in the transmitting fluid and the site of inoculation of that fluid. Since the amount of virus excreted by HIV-infected persons is relatively small, its modes of transmission are rather limited and the rate of transmission per exposure is rather low. For example, when heterosexual contacts of HIV-infected men are tested for antibodies, commonly 10–25% of them are found to be infected (1,2). This relatively low rate of transmission occurs despite multiple unprotected sexual exposures over a period of several years in many cases (1).

Why are some infected and others not? It appears that, at least early in the natural history of HIV infection, infectiousness varies widely among infected persons. Some transmit rather efficiently and others not (1,3,4). Given that 10–25% of sexual partners are infected, we can conclude that most infected persons appear to be rather poor transmitters. However, occasionally one ap-

D. Francis: Department of Health Service, Berkeley, California 94704.

TABLE 1. *Mortality from viral infections of humans*

Infection	Mortality (%)
Rabies	99
HIV-1	>75
Ebola/Marburg	25–80
Smallpox	
Major	30
Intermediate	3–11
Minor	1
Hepatitis B (acute and chronic)	5
Lassa	3–5
Polio	<0.1

pears to be quite contagious (3,4). These high transmitters, presumably carrying and excreting high titers of virus, are probably important contributors to the continuing transmission of HIV. In addition to variations in viral titers among individuals, there may also be variations in each individual over time. It appears that viral titers may be greater very early and very late in the course of infection (5,6). Moreover, open lesions on either the infected or susceptible person's genitals or skin facilitate transmission (7).

The association of transmissibility with inoculum of virus is most strikingly demonstrated in blood-borne infections. For small inocula, as occurs with a needlestick, the risk of infection is rather low, approximately 3/1000 (8). On the other extreme, the recipient of a large volume, for example, the 500 ml in a unit of blood, is almost guaranteed to be infected (9). For heterosexual vaginal intercourse, one might logically presume, merely from the volume of inoculum left in a woman compared to that left in a man, that male-to-female transmission would be greater than female-to-male transmission. Such probably is the case (10–12); however, the available data on the subject are conflicting (13).

Regarding the site of inoculation, for heterosexual intercourse, anal intercourse appears to be more likely to transmit infection than vaginal intercourse (1). Similarly, for homosexual intercourse between men, it is clear that the partner receiving the ejaculate rectally is at far greater risk than either the recipient of ejaculate

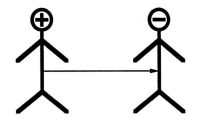

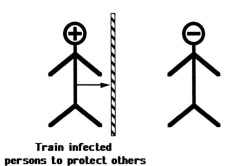

Train infected
persons to protect others

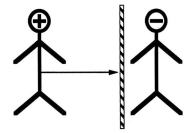

Train susceptible persons
to protect themselves

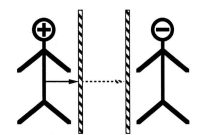

FIG. 1. Prevention of HIV from moving from an infected person to a susceptible person.

orally or the donor of ejaculate in either situation (14,15). Furthermore, when studied in the chimpanzee, inoculation vaginally readily infected while inoculation orally did not (16).

Thus, to summarize all data, the risk of HIV infection depends on the amount of virus in the transmitting fluid and the site of inoculation of that fluid. There are some fluid–site combinations likely to result in infection and others that are unlikely to result in infection. Blood given intravenously must be the combination with the highest probability of infection. For sexual intercourse, semen placed on the rectal mucosa, followed by semen placed on vaginal/cervical mucosa, followed by vaginal fluid placed (presumably) on the male urethral mucosa are all quite likely to result in infection. Rectal fluid placed (presumably) on the male urethral mucosa is less likely to result in infection. Finally, semen placed on the oral mucosa appears very unlikely to transmit infection.

What about skin exposure? In blood-borne transmission the infectious inoculum transgresses the skin through a needle and can establish infection. On the other hand, normal unbroken skin appears to be an effective barrier to HIV since massive exposure, for example, that which occurred among clinical laboratory workers prior to the discovery of HIV and the institution of universal precautions, is not known to have resulted in transmission (17). Yet, from a few anecdotal reports (8), if introduced onto broken skin, HIV will clearly infect.

Perinatal transmission is common where the prevalence of infection among child-bearing women is high. Approximately, one-third or less of infected women will transmit infection to their unborn fetus or their infant before or during delivery (18–20). Higher rates may be found when infants are born to women with more advanced disease (20). Infection has also been documented to have been transmitted after delivery through breast milk by women who were infected at the time of delivery via transfusion (21).

Other modes of transmission appear extremely rare (22).

Given HIV's relative inefficiency of transmission, one would not predict sudden outbreaks. Indeed, HIV in rural, traditional African villages appears to stabilize at a low prevalence [0.8% in 1976 and 0.8% in 1986 (23)]. Moreover, introductions of HIV into urban areas of the United States (24) and Europe (25) in past decades did not spread.

But more recent introductions into groups of people linked together through frequent sexual or blood-sharing exposures have resulted in a massive pandemic (26). When sex with multiple partners, sharing of drug injection equipment, or the therapeutic use of HIV-infected blood or blood products is common, HIV can spread rapidly. This has been especially true in urban areas of much of the world (26,27). From being a relatively rare

infection in the early 1970s, HIV is now estimated to infect 8–12 million persons worldwide.

MODALITIES FOR PREVENTION

To interrupt further transmission, we must design and implement effective public health intervention programs (28). Such programs have been fielded for other infectious diseases. For example, syphilis, gonorrhea, and tuberculosis control programs have been launched that target infected persons and, by using antimicrobial agents, render them noncontagious. For other diseases, like measles, polio, or smallpox, control programs have been launched that use immunizing agents to protect susceptible persons from infection. But no highly effective treatment or immunization is available for HIV. Without such options, we must turn to more basic prevention modalities.

PUBLIC HEALTH RESPONSIBILITY

Public health's responsibility is to protect the public's health. Its prime role therefore for HIV is to prevent transmission between an infected person and a susceptible one. If, for example, HIV were transmitted through respiratory aerosols, public health would clearly screen entire populations, identify all infectious persons, and keep their air separate from the air breathed by susceptible persons. Breathing air is not optional; thus keeping it safe is clearly a public health responsibility.

With such a virulent agent one could suggest that quarantine, more properly "mandatory isolation," would be a logical option to follow for HIV. Indeed, at least one country, Cuba, has followed such an approach (29). Yet mandatory isolation, to be effective, is quite complex and expensive. Its purpose, after all, is to establish a net through which no infected person or infectious material crosses. Consider the ramifications of placing such a net on today's highly mobile society.

If, as hypothesized above, HIV were transmitted by aerosol or other "nonconsensual" means, such expense and inconvenience may be justifiable. But HIV transmission is rather unique in that it transmits almost exclusively through consensual acts. With sexual intercourse and self-injection of drugs being the main routes of HIV transmission, both parties involved have a choice regarding the risk they are willing to take. Thus with the consensual nature of HIV transmission, public health need not institute mandatory isolation as other, less disruptive and less costly options exist. Commonly, public health has, through information, motivation, and skill building, attempted to provide the public with information, motivation, and skills so that individuals can take responsibility to protect themselves. Since success with such an "educational" approach requires a close and trusting relationship with at-risk persons, it can be very difficult to combine such an approach with the more coercive actions required for mandatory isolation procedures. Indeed, there is ample evidence to suggest that even the perception of adverse consequences of, for example, mandatory testing can drive people away from prevention programs (30).

Yet some mandatory components exist for most HIV prevention programs. For example, in the United States mandatory testing is required of blood donors, military applicants, Job Corps applicants, some prisoners, and, in Nevada, licensed prostitutes.

In the end, the overall effectiveness of HIV prevention programs will depend on a balance of approaches that, on the one hand, encourage individual responsibility through voluntary programs that change social norms, while, on the other hand, require certain actions through mandated programs. The balance of the different modalities will be essential for success.

PROGRAM PLANNING AND DESIGN

Random application of any disease control modality is not effective. Instead, an organized approach is required that reviews the tools (modalities) available, plans how to apply the modalities, identifies the resources necessary to apply them, develops a structure through which to deliver them, delivers them, and then evaluates their effect.

First, let us review the prevention modalities available for HIV. These can be grouped according to when during the process of transmission, exposure, infection, or disease they are applied. For example, those modalities that operate at the earliest time in the transmission process are those that will decrease the risk of *exposure* to an HIV-infected person. The next group are those modalities that, given a fixed risk of exposure, will decrease the chance that the exposure will cause *infection.* The last group are those modalities that, given exposure and infection, will prevent progression to *disease.* Other chapters discuss therapeutically preventing or delaying disease progression in those already infected. This chapter focuses on ways to decrease the risk of exposure and ways to decrease the probability of infection once exposure occurs.

Changing Behavior

All HIV prevention modalities involve modification of behavior or of practices that place people at risk of infection. Changing human behavior, especially when it involves sexual and drug-using practices, can be challenging. Yet, for HIV, considerable success has been achieved and examination of the reasons for this success can teach us some lessons that, if applied, can increase our chances for future success.

These lessons can be summarized into guiding principles (31). First, information is essential, but not sufficient, to induce behavior change. In other words, it is relatively easy to instill knowledge, but it takes more to change behavior. Second, strong motivation to change one's behavior is essential for success. Motivation for HIV prevention is accentuated if the targeted person carries a clear image of the clinical picture of AIDS as it would affect him or her. In other words, the person him/herself must feel personally threatened. Third, in addition to information and motivation, the actual skills necessary to avoid infection must be taught. These include both motor skills, for example, how to put on a condom or how to clean injection equipment, and interpersonal skills, for example, how to negotiate safe sex or safe injection with a potential partner. Fourth, the message is most effective when delivered by peers who are respected by the target audience and who are sensitive to the ethnic, cultural, and educational backgrounds of the audience. Fifth, the delivery must include activities that help give the person being educated the self-confidence (empowerment) that he or she can actually do what is prescribed. Sixth, repeat counseling is the rule for success. In other words, training will often not be successful if given only in a single session. Seventh, behavior change is most dramatic and long-lasting when community-wide programs coexist that endeavor to change the standards (norms) of the community in which the target person/group interacts. And last, people generically adjust to change better if they are given choices rather than absolute rules.

Before moving on to specific program design and application, we should discuss general issues of target audiences and specific HIV-prevention messages. In relation to HIV, all populations can be divided into three general groups (see Fig. 2): one group with little or no risk of HIV infection, another with substantial risk of infection but still uninfected, and a group already infected. The messages to be delivered to the three groups are different.

The first group, those at minimal risk, need to be taught how HIV is not transmitted so that they do not harbor unnecessary fears regarding the conduct of their daily lives. The second, those at substantial risk but not infected, need to be taught how to protect themselves from becoming infected. The last, those already infected, need to be taught how to protect others from infection (and how to gain access to medical care and other services).

General Population

The means by which to reach the various groups differ substantially. Using the mass media has been the most common approach to reach the general population. This has been shown to be quite effective in giving informa-

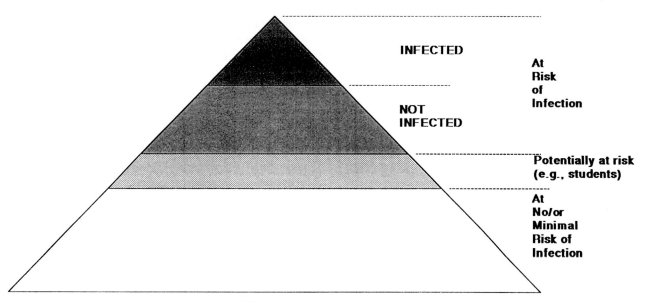

FIG. 2. Target populations.

tion. Moreover, some intense mass media programs, for example, the condom campaign in Switzerland, have had considerable effect in positively changing normative behavior (32).

Schools

School-based programs are another common avenue used to reach youth in the general population. School and youth-directed campaigns are essential for HIV prevention. In the future, these programs should form the bulwark of HIV prevention, supplying graduates who are educated and trained with information on how to keep themselves uninfected. Effective general education and school programs have, however, been difficult to launch in many areas because of concerns that teaching safer sexual and drug-using practices will actually accelerate the initiation and frequency of these behaviors. Although substantial data exist to refute such concerns (32), resistance to aggressive school-based programs continues to jeopardize HIV prevention. Such resistance has been highlighted recently by attempts by the New York City school system to follow their initial school education campaign with the provision of condoms within the school. This confrontation has revealed the essence of the school program debate: Are we going to ignore reality and pretend that adolescents do not have sex or are we going to face reality and improve the chance of youngsters to have healthy lives?

Targeted Programs

Targeted programs can be subdivided into those that target individuals and those that target whole communities. These two subdivisions, although overlapping, attempt to accomplish two different objectives. On the one hand, individual programs provide persons known to be at increased risk with information, motivation, and the skills necessary to prevent themselves from becoming infected or infecting others. On the other hand, community norm-changing programs change the foundation of normative behavior of an entire targeted community that support the new, safer practices honed by individual counseling programs. Both programs have been found to be necessary for successful behavior change to occur and to be maintained (31).

Targeted programs focus on similar groups around the world, although varied emphasis is placed in different geographic areas. Some programs are "active" with workers venturing into localities where drug use, prostitution, or other at-risk activities are prevalent. For example, paraphernalia exchange and/or bleach provision has proved remarkably effective in reaching intravenous drug users (33–36) and prostitute outreach has been useful for contacting street prostitutes (37,38). Such programs have most commonly used outreach workers who know and understand the target audience well and are familiar with the local customs and geography. Other programs are "passive." These programs are geographically fixed and at-risk persons come to them. Some take advantage of the fact that HIV risk-prone behaviors often cause other events that bring risk-taking people to health care or law enforcement facilities. For example, counseling and HIV testing services have frequently been provided at clinics for sexually transmitted diseases, injection drug users, or prostitutes (38). Also, counseling and testing services have been established in jails and prisons. Others take advantage of locations where people at-risk for HIV seek out services, for example, HIV test sites (see below).

Individual Counseling Programs

Individual counseling, provided through a variety of avenues, is an essential part of HIV prevention. Counseling can be provided through private physicians, specialized counseling programs, programs associated with serologic testing, or targeted programs associated with sexually transmitted disease clinics or drug treatment clinics. In addition, telephone hot lines are a unique and important way for people to seek advice conveniently. (The advice to be given to people is discussed below.)

Community-Based Norm Changing

In localized areas having a high prevalence of transmission-prone behavior, special programs have been designed to change the behavioral norms of the population. Such programs have had remarkable success with prostitutes (37,38), gay men (39–41), and intravenous drug users (33–36,42).

Difficult-to-Influence Persons

As the influence of general population, targeted population, and community-based norm-change programs grows, increasing numbers of people adopt safer behaviors. Indeed, many in the behavioral field have been impressed with the extent of change that HIV prevention programs have instilled. Yet in all communities some people continue to take risks. In the future, no doubt, we will find that a high proportion of HIV transmission is occurring among this small proportion of the at-risk population. This small group will have to be a major target of future prevention activities. Current programs must look ahead so that today's program designs will be flexible enough to accommodate tomorrow's clients. Many of these clients will be a real challenge for program staffs. They will often be people with multiple problems including low income, poor mental health, and substance abuse. If we are to be successful in stopping HIV, we must be prepared to assist them with these problems along with their HIV risk.

Serologic Testing

Extremely sensitive and specific HIV antibody tests are available for detecting HIV infection (43). The role of testing in prevention programs has been debated in the past. However, the beneficial effect of antiviral (44,45) and anti-*Pneumocystis* (46,47) therapies given prior to the development of clinically apparent disease has made such discussions moot. In areas of the world that have the resources and facilities for serologic testing and subsequent clinical monitoring, many persons at risk have

sought out such services and are being followed. This passive approach to testing has been relatively successful for self-identified gay men in major cities, for example, in San Francisco and Los Angeles, where the majority have been tested. Programs such as prenatal testing have made it clear, however, that depending on individuals to assess their own risk and determine the need for testing is, in some cases, not very reliable (48,49). Thus a trend is approaching where, in areas with a substantial prevalence of infection (perhaps greater than 1 per 1000), routine voluntary testing will be offered and recommended at every contact with the health-care or law enforcement systems.

Early Intervention

As HIV prevention programs become more sophisticated, many are offering specific prevention services to HIV-infected persons and their contacts in conjunction with ongoing clinical follow-up. Such services, known collectively as early intervention, may be of considerable benefit to both the infected person (50) and their susceptible contacts (51). In such a program, a commitment is made to provide life-long medical management, together with behavioral and psychosocial support and case management services to HIV-infected persons and their at-risk contacts. These services are designed to minimize the risk of further transmission and maximize the healthy and productive lives of those already infected. Although just in the formative stages, it has been suggested that these programs are an essential part of all testing programs (50), and that testing without early intervention services may be unethical (52). Ethical considerations aside, it seems illogical from a medical and public health standpoint not to provide these services to all HIV-infected persons in a well designed and structured manner that maximizes effect and minimizes cost.

Couple Counseling and Partner Notification

The issue of contacts is an important one for prevention of person-to-person infection. As the importance of early medical intervention increases, the need to inform people of their exposure to HIV assumes greater importance and the controversy that in the past has surrounded partner notification loses much of its basis. The frequency of infection in exposed contacts is significant. For example, for heterosexual contacts, infection rates are commonly over 10%. All staff that provide counseling services to HIV-infected persons must assume some role in dealing with the issues of contacts. First in importance are those persons having ongoing sexual or drug injection contact with HIV-infected persons. They, together with the infected partner, need to be informed of their risk and offered serologic testing. If one partner remains uninfected, careful, long-term counseling is required of both partners to ensure that no further transmission occurs (see below).

Contacts who are not in an ongoing relationship with the infected index case should be notified to inform them of their exposure and the need for serologic testing. This is especially true for partners who may not self-identify with at-risk groups and therefore not suspect exposure to HIV. This aspect of partner notification has often been a lightning rod sparking more controversy than is justified. Hopefully, as the logic of the program in light of early intervention becomes better understood, as the satisfaction of clients who have participated becomes well known (51), and as the ability of health departments to maintain confidentiality becomes evident, opposition to this important program component will lessen.

Ideally, partner notification should be performed by the patient him/herself. However, if the patient is unable or uncomfortable performing such notification, public health staff, well trained in this delicate endeavor, should perform this service. Such services should follow standard practice, keeping the index patient's name strictly confidential and never revealing the name to the notified contact.

Counseling Advice

What advice can one give to people regarding HIV risk? Regarding sexual encounters, the advice depends on the prevalence of HIV infection among partners of the person being counseled, frequency of changing partners, and the specific risk-taking activities in which the person engages. Decreasing the number of partners with whom risk-taking activity is shared is an obvious recommendation that makes clear sense. The effect of such advice will vary, however, depending on the prevalence of infection among the person's contacts. Where prevalence is high, for example, among gay men in the United States and Europe, the effect will be less than where prevalence is low.

The most extreme recommendation for decreasing the number of partners is to have none or only one. This has often been stated in terms of making abstinence or monogamy the primary call of HIV prevention programs. Much fruitless debate has often followed such calls. As mentioned earlier, one of the principal keys to the success of behavior change is to give people choices. Abstinence or monogamy are very reasonable choices to offer. But it is equally important to provide people who continue to have multiple partners the means by which to protect themselves and others.

For sexual intercourse, condoms are an extremely effective barrier to HIV transmission. Most studies examining condom use have reported high rates of protection (53,54). Condoms introduce a physical barrier between two persons that cannot be crossed by even something as small as a virus (55,56). Of course failures occur, even with pregnancy prevention, and clearly sperm are far larger than viruses. More often than not, however, the reason for failure is presumably human error. For example, some people fail to put condoms on during foreplay, allowing for mucous to mucous membrane contact. Others use condoms with mineral oil-containing lubricants that dissolve latex.

Condom use during sexual activity should become the social norm. Regardless of the prevalence of HIV infection, it is wise to recommend condom use during all sexual relations prior to the establishment of a long-term monogamous relationship or the decision to have children. This recommendation is made not only to prevent HIV infection but also to prevent all the other miserable yet preventable infections that are transmitted through sexual intercourse. With the frequency of chronic, often untreatable, genital infections, such as herpes, papillomavirus, and pelvic inflammatory disease, it seems wise to strictly limit the number of persons with whom one has unprotected sexual intercourse.

After condom recommendations are made for vaginal and anal sex, the next question is often about oral sex. Although the rates must be extremely low, transmission by fellatio has been reported (15,54). Thus, in counseling at-risk persons, these data should be discussed. Although the risk appears extremely low, it does exist. The risk from cunnilingus with an HIV-infected woman must be present, but also must be very low. The risk for both would approach zero if condoms or latex dams were used appropriately.

The next sexually related issue deals with hand to genital contact (mutual masturbation). Here, except for persons with chronic dermatitis or open skin lesions (8), the risk approaches zero.

Couples

Advice regarding HIV infection is most frequently given as a statistical probability of transmission within a certain setting. As mentioned before, enough data are available to say that anal and vaginal intercourse have a high risk of transmission, anal being higher, and that oral intercourse carries a low risk and that hand to genital contact carries a negligible risk. And that condoms, used properly, offer good protection from all risk. It should be stressed, however, that most advice is given when discussing an untested, hypothetical partner. Advice becomes far more difficult when counseling couples where one partner is known to be HIV infected and the other is known to be susceptible ("discordant"). Here, since every sexual act involves at-risk contact between an infected person and a susceptible one, even activities with extremely low risks of transmission per encounter become significant. In this situation counseling must be extremely conservative. Given the gravity of infection, many may choose not to have insertive sexual activity. Others may choose to use condoms compulsively at each encounter. Although safe sexual activity appears to be possible (N. Padian, *personal communication,* 1991), further evaluation is clearly indicated before solid assurances can be made. To ensure safety in this potentially dangerous situation, counselors should err on the side of conservatism.

Advice for intravenous drug users is quite straightforward. First, if the user wants to get off drugs, he/she should be given assistance in obtaining appropriate treatment. Because of the frequency of continued injection of people in treatment, however, all users, whether or not in treatment, must be taught how to inject safely. Clearly, the best advice for needle users is to *never* share injection equipment. In areas where exchange programs have been established and users have ready access to sterile injection paraphernalia, sharing decreases dramatically (33,34,36). Aside from community concerns, most public health experts have become convinced that exchange programs should be an integral part of AIDS and drug prevention and care. Despite this consensus, most communities do not have needle and syringe exchange programs and users do not always have access to their own equipment. In the absence of having their own "works," injectors need to be taught disinfection. HIV is very sensitive to a variety of disinfectants (57), but the most common one used is household bleach. Flushing a syringe and needle with water, followed by bleach and water again, should be very effective in eliminating HIV as well as most other infectious agents.

Reaching injection drug users is a challenge. Many programs have now recruited street-knowledgeable staff who know where and how to contact users in the street. Perhaps the best contact means for existing users has been paraphernalia exchange programs where users seek out exchange personnel who, if staffing is sufficient, can deal with other needs including education and access to drug treatment if desired. Another access point for users is the corrections system. Drug users are frequently arrested. Thus jail/prison counseling and testing programs, if maintained with high clinical standards in a caring environment, could be quite successful.

Advising women of child-bearing age is complex. For an HIV-infected woman, the decision whether to become pregnant is one that she must decide herself. She must be given all the information and, if possible, provided access to other infected women who have made their decisions. The risk of infection to an infant born to an HIV-infected mother is 30% or less (18,19,58). The prognosis for the infant once infected is poor. In addition, it is not uncommon for the mother to begin to get sick at the same time as the child. If this is compounded with the husband and other children being ill, the situation becomes extremely difficult to manage.

Even when the infant is not infected, caring for an infant and child as an ill parent is not an easy task. This decision is an important one and should not be taken lightly.

PROGRAM ORGANIZATION

As this discussion has progressed, multiple program components like counseling and testing, school and community education and norm-changing programs, and early intervention have been discussed. These components are each designed to fill a specific niche in the overall AIDS prevention scheme. But not all components are usually supplied by a single provider. Who provides each component service will vary in different locales. Some can best be provided through the private or nonprofit sectors. Others can best be provided through government agencies. Indeed, diversity of persons at risk usually requires a diversity in service providers. Yet without some cohesion, the maximal effect of the programs cannot be realized. In an organizational sense, that cohesion and leadership should be provided by local public health authorities.

However individual locales organize their HIV prevention and care programs, the design should be flexible enough to accommodate future changes. The likelihood of new therapies or preventive modalities coming in the future is very high and program design must anticipate and be able to rapidly integrate such changes.

At the distal end of organization, HIV prevention (and care) programs must concentrate around the infected person. If transmission chains are to be interrupted, an intense prevention effort must be accorded the infected person and his/her at-risk contacts. Furthermore, for secondary and tertiary prevention, specific services to prevent disease progression and unnecessary hospitalization must be provided for infected persons. As more and more infected persons volunteer for testing and are found positive, medical and public health responses can be more effectively directed because community and patient needs will become more easily quantifiable. Some link is required, however, through which these services are provided and through which data are collected to plan for future needs.

Reporting and the Counselor-Advisor Link

A link between every HIV-infected person and the health and public health systems is key to manage HIV prevention and care programs effectively. Often this need is expressed in terms of "reporting" infected persons. Such expression misses the point since it is not a computerized list of names that is the overall objective. The true objective is to provide services that improve both medical and preventive care. Instead of mandatory reporting in the absence of preventive services, we have suggested that a counselor-advisor be linked to every person identified as being positive to ensure that all available medical, mental health, and public health services are provided to that person. And, if all services are not available, the counselor-advisor assures that unmet needs are reported to a planning council so that future resources can be directed to fill those unmet needs.

Considering the number of infected and ill persons and the variety of services required to meet their needs, all sectors of society will have to contribute their part. Yet, as with other national disasters, government will have to shoulder a large share. It is not necessarily government's responsibility to provide all these services, but rather it should be the government's role to ensure that all HIV-infected persons have access to the essential services. If the person does not have the resources to obtain essential services, then it is logical for the government to supply them.

HEALTH-CARE WORKERS

There are some prevention issues that are specific to those providing health care. These issues involve both risk of infection for the susceptible health-care worker (HCW) from the infected patient and the risk of infection of the susceptible patient from the infected HCW.

Any HCW working with potentially infectious body fluids, especially blood, is at risk for HIV infection. The discovery of HIV has led to much concern regarding HCW's risk of blood-borne infections, yet such concern among infection control personnel long preceded HIV (59). The concern is a real one, not just for HIV but for other known and unknown infections that can be transmitted via blood or other body fluids. Thus blood contact with mucous membranes and abraded skin should be avoided. The application of recent recommendations, often referred to as "universal precautions" (60), should add significantly to the safety of HCWs. The implementation of universal precautions, however, will not eliminate all risk. Although small, some risk will remain. That risk is primarily due to accidents involving sharp instruments. Some "accidents" are inevitable, especially those associated with emergency procedures where speed can make a difference to the life of a patient. Others, however, are clearly preventable (16).

Although the greatest health-care-associated HIV risk is from patient to HCW, there is at least some risk from HCW to patient (61). Our understanding of hepatitis B virus (HBV) infection documented that the vast majority of HBV infections transmitted from HCW to patient have been due to some significant violation of accepted surgical technique, for example, sticking of a gloved finger to determine if the needle has pierced a tissue pedicle (62).

For HIV to be transmitted from a HCW to a patient, infected material, most likely blood, would have to exit from the HCW and *remain in the patient.* If standard surgical practice, which requires removing needles or scalpels that have injured a HCW and regloving after an injury, is followed, such incidents should be extremely rare.

BLOOD AND BLOOD PRODUCTS

In most places in the world, HIV testing of therapeutic blood products, estimated to be highly effective (32), has become standard practice. In addition, obtaining histories for infection-prone behavior of donors has been added in many areas. To decrease transfusion-associated infection further, attempts have been made to ensure that transfusion is used only where clearly indicated.

SURVEILLANCE AND EVALUATION

Surveillance, classically defined as collecting and analyzing data on disease occurrence, is complex for HIV because of the long incubation period from infection to disease. For data to be valuable for program evaluation, they should reflect what is currently happening. AIDS case data reflect infection that occurred as long as a decade or more before the data were collected and therefore are not very useful for program evaluation. Continually monitoring the source of infection for AIDS cases is useful, however, to ensure that modes of transmission are not changing (22).

An ideal evaluation program would monitor the incidence of HIV infection rather than end-stage HIV disease (AIDS). But monitoring incidence of infection, even in high-incidence groups like cohorts of gay men, is very expensive as large numbers of susceptible persons must be contacted and serologically tested and interviewed at regular intervals.

Various less expensive approaches have been used as alternatives to cohort studies. The most common has been cross-sectional serologic surveys. Such surveys, for example, among prostitutes, young gay men, and intravenous drug users, have been useful to show that infection is occurring in these populations and therefore preventive intervention is required. However, because of sampling biases, projecting incidence from multiple prevalence surveys is not easy. The most successful approach has been the testing of infant blood specimens obtained on filter paper for genetic disease screening. This approach is inexpensive and valuable in that true population-based data can be obtained (63).

With the need for serologic data over and above clinical AIDS case data, there has been a continuing move in many countries to require reporting of positive HIV test results rather than just AIDS. Such a requirement is clearly logical and would parallel requirements for other infectious diseases such as syphilis. Many states in the

United States now require reporting. But states with the highest prevalences of infection have been reluctant to mandate HIV test result reporting for fear of driving HIV-infected people away from prevention and care programs. There are data to support such fears (30); however, it is clear from our work in California that if services are provided to care for HIV-infected persons in trusting and caring environments, the fear of "being reported" disappears. Thus the issue to report or not to report HIV infection status needs to be reformatted. If you are willing to care for people comprehensively, they will come to receive service and reporting becomes a moot issue. On the contrary, if programs are not willing to provide service, then what is the point of requiring reporting?

Short of serologic testing, other surrogate measurements have been used that can indirectly reflect HIV incidence. One is the incidence of sexually transmitted diseases (STD). An early observation from San Francisco showed that rectal gonorrhea rates among men declined in parallel with HIV incidence rates (64). Using STD incidence as an indicator of safer sexual practices is valid as long as the method of STD surveillance has remained constant over time. If laboratory tests used to determine a case have changed or if laboratory screening of asymptomatic persons were instituted or discontinued during the period in question, then changes over time are more difficult to interpret.

A straightforward approach to assessing risk-taking behavior has been to survey sexual and needle-sharing behaviors. Remarkable data have been obtained from targeted populations or general population surveys undertaken in schools or through random digit dialing telephone surveys. There has been a remarkable correlation of self-reported behavior and HIV incidence in areas having both data sets (41).

In addition to evaluation of specific infection or behavioral outcomes, process evaluation data are important to guide HIV prevention programs. Documentation of smaller waiting lists, number of drug treatment slots filled, number of visits to an early intervention program, percentage of nonsuspecting contacts notified and tested, and so on are very useful for program planning and evaluation.

TRAINING

The HIV epidemic is new and evolving. To field all the essential program components, trained staff will be required. Although many of the principles of HIV prevention and care follow other diseases, specific HIV training of all staff will be necessary. Such training needs should be planned for in advance to avoid unnecessary delays and confusion.

REFERENCES

1. Padian N, Marquis L, Francis DP, Anderson RE, Rutherford GW, O'Malley PM, Winkelstein W Jr. Male-to-female transmission of human immunodeficiency virus. *JAMA* 1987;258:788–90.
2. Toomey KE, Cates W Jr. Partner notification for the prevention of HIV infection. *AIDS* 1989;3:S57–62.
3. Taylor AF, Johnson S, Wyant SR, Dassey DE. Heterosexual and perinatal transmission of human immunodeficiency virus in a low prevalence community. *West J Med* 1989;148:171–5.
4. Clumeck N, Taelman H, Hermans P, et al. A cluster of HIV infection among heterosexual people without apparent risk factors. *N Engl J Med* 1989;321:1460–2.
5. Ho DD, Moudgil T, Alam M. Quantitation of the human immunodeficiency virus type 1 in the blood of infected persons. *N Engl J Med* 1989;321:1621–5.
6. Daar ES, Moudgil T, Meyer RD, Ho DD. Transient high levels of viremia in patients with primary human immunodeficiency virus type 1 infection. *N Engl J Med* 1991;324:961–4.
7. Piot P, Laga M. Genital ulcers, other sexually transmitted diseases, and the sexual transmission of HIV. *Br Med J* 1989;298:623–4.
8. Centers for Disease Control. Update. Human immunodeficiency virus in health-care workers exposed to blood of infected patients. *MMWR* 1987;36:285–9.
9. Busch MP, Young MJ, Samson SM, Mosley JW, Ward JW, Perkins HA. Risk of human immunodeficiency virus (HIV) transmission by blood transfusion before the implementation of HIV-1 antibody screening. The transfusion safety study group. *Transfusion* 1991;31:4–11.
10. Padian NS. Heterosexual transmission of acquired immunodeficiency syndrome: international perspectives and national projections. *Rev Infect Dis* 1987;9:947–60.
11. Padian NS. Sexual histories of heterosexual couples with one HIV-infected partner. *Am J Public Health* 1990;80:990–1.
12. European Study Group. Risk factors for male to female transmission of HIV. *Br Med J* 1989;298:411–5.
13. Fischl MA, Dickinson GM, Scott GB, Klimas N, Fletcher MA, Parks W. Evaluation of heterosexual partners, children, and household contacts of adults with AIDS. *JAMA* 1987;257:640–4.
14. Winkelstein W Jr, Lyman DM, Padian NS, et al. Sexual practices and risk of infection by the human immunodeficiency virus. The San Francisco men's health study. *JAMA* 1987;257:321–5.
15. Lifson AR, O'Malley PM, Hessol NA, Buchbinder SP, Cannon L, Rutherford GW. HIV seroconversion in two homosexual men after receptive oral intercourse with ejaculation: implications for counseling concerning safe sexual practices. *Am J Public Health* 1990;80:1509–11.
16. Fultz PA, McClure HM, Daugharty H, et al. Vaginal transmission of human immunodeficiency virus (HIV) to a chimpanzee. *J Infect Dis* 1986;154:896–900.
17. Gerberding JL, Bryant-LeBlanc CE, Nelson KN, et al. Risk of transmitting the human immunodeficiency virus, cytomegalovirus, and hepatitis B virus to health care workers exposed to patients with AIDS and AIDS-related conditions (ARC). *J Infect Dis* 1987;156:1–8.
18. Rogers MF, Ou CY, Rayfield M, et al. Use of polymerase chain reaction for early detection of the proviral sequences of human immunodeficiency virus in infants born to seropositive mothers. New York City collaborative study of maternal HIV transmission and Montefiore Medical Center HIV perinatal transmission study group. *N Engl J Med* 1989;320:1649–54.
19. European Collaborative Study. Children born to women with HIV-infection: natural history and risk transmission. *Lancet* 1991;1:253–60.
20. Hira SK, Kamanga J, Bhat GJ, Mwale C, Tembo G, Luo N, Perine PL. Perinatal transmission of HIV-I in Zambia. *Br Med J* 1989;299:1250–2.
21. Ziegler JB, Johnson RO, Cooper DA, et al. Postnatal transmission of AIDS-associated retrovirus from mother to infant. *Lancet* 1985;1:896–97.
22. Lifson AR. Do alternate modes for transmission of human immunodeficiency virus exist? A review. *JAMA* 1988;259:1353–6.
23. Nzilambi N, DeCock KM, Forthal DN, et al. The prevalence of

infection with human immunodeficiency virus over a 10-year period in rural Zaire. *N Engl J Med* 1988;318:276–9.

24. Huminer D, Rosenfeld JB, Pitlik SD. HIV infection in 1968. *JAMA* 1989;261:2198–9.

25. Bygbjerg IC. AIDS in a Danish surgeon (Zaire 1976). *Lancet* 1983;1:925.

26. Chin J, Mann J. Global surveillance and forecasting of AIDS. *Bull WHO* 1989;67:1–7.

27. Brundage JF, Burke DS, Gardner LI, et al. Tracking the spread of the HIV infection epidemic among young adults in the United States: results of the first four years of screening among civilian applicants for U.S. military service. *J AIDS* 1990;3:1168–80.

28. Francis DP, Kaslow RA. Prevention: general considerations. In: Kaslow RA, Francis DP, eds. *The epidemiology of AIDS.* New York: Oxford University Press; 1989:253–65.

29. Bayer R, Healton C. Controlling AIDS in Cuba. The logic of quarantine. *N Engl J Med* 1989;320:1022–4.

30. Kegeles SM, Catania JA, Coates TJ, Pollack LM, Lo B. Many people who seek anonymous HIV-antibody testing would avoid it under other circumstances. *AIDS* 1990;4:585–8.

31. Stall R, Coates TJ, Mandel JS, Morales ES, Sorensen JL. Behavioral factors and intervention. In: Kaslow RA, Francis DP, eds. *The epidemiology of AIDS.* New York: Oxford University Press; 1989:266–81.

32. Hauser D. Prevention strategies and assessment: the Swiss experience presented at "Assessing AIDS Prevention," Montreux, Switzerland, Oct 29–Nov 1, 1990.

33. Watters JK, Downing M, Case P, Lorvick J, Cheng YT, Fergusson B. AIDS prevention for intravenous drug users in the community: street-based education and risk behavior. *Am J Community Psychol* 1990;18:587–96.

34. Coutinho RA. Epidemiology and prevention of AIDS among intravenous drug users. *J AIDS* 1990;3:413–6.

35. Nicolosi A, Musicco M, Saracco A, Molinari S, Ziliani N, Lazzarin A. Incidence and risk factors of HIV infection: a prospective study of seronegative drug users from Milan and northern Italy. *Epidemiology* 1990;1:453–9.

36. Brickner PW, Torres RA, Barnes M, et al. Recommendations for control and prevention of human immunodeficiency virus (HIV) infection in intravenous drug users. *Ann Intern Med* 1989;110:833–7.

37. Ngugi EN, Simonsen JN, Bosire M, et al. Prevention of transmission of human immunodeficiency virus in Africa: effectiveness of condom promotion and health education among prostitutes. *Lancet* 1988;2:887–90.

38. Papaevangelou G, Roumeliotou A, Kallinikos G, Papoutsakis G, Trichopoulou E, Stefanou T. Education in preventing HIV infection in Greek registered prostitutes. *J AIDS* 1988;1:386–9.

39. Kelly JA, St Lawrence JS, Diaz YE, et al. HIV risk behavior reduction following intervention with key opinion leaders of population: an experimental analysis. *Am J Public Health* 1991;81:168–71.

40. Stall RD, Coates TJ, Hoff C. Behavioral risk reduction for HIV infection among gay and bisexual men, a review of results from the United States. *Am Psychol* 1988;43:878–85.

41. Communication Technologies. Designing an effective AIDS risk reduction program for San Francisco: results from the first probability sample of multiple/high-risk partner heterosexual adults. June 30, 1986. Prepared by the San Francisco AIDS Foundation.

42. Des Jarlais DC, Friedman SR, Stoneburner RL. HIV infection and intravenous drug use: critical issues in transmission dynamics, infection outcomes, and prevention. *Rev Infect Dis* 1988;10:151–8.

43. Hausler WJ Jr. Report of the third consensus conference of HIV testing sponsored by the association of state and territorial public health laboratories. *Infect Control Hosp Epidemiol* 1988;9:345–9.

44. Fischl MA, Parker CB, Pettinelli C, et al. A randomized controlled trial of a reduced daily dose of zidovudine in patients with the acquired immunodeficiency syndrome. *N Engl J Med* 1990;323:1009–14.

45. Volberding PA, Lagakos SW, Koch MA, et al. Zidovudine in asymptomatic human immunodeficiency virus infection, a controlled trial in persons with fewer than 500 CD-4 positive cells per cubic millimeter. *N Engl J Med* 1990;322:941–49.

46. Montgomery AB. Prophylaxis of *Pneumocystis carinii* pneumonia in patients infected with the human immunodeficiency virus type 1. *Semin Respir Infect* 1989;4:311–7.

47. Kemper CA, Tucker RM, Lang OS, et al. Low-dose dapsone prophylaxis of *Pneumocystis carinii* pneumonia in AIDS and AIDS-related complex. *AIDS* 1990;11:1145–8.

48. Landesman S, Minkoff H, Holman S, McCalla S, Siijin O. Serosurvey of human immunodeficiency virus infection in parturients: implications for human immunodeficiency virus testing programs of pregnant women. *JAMA* 1987;258:2701–3.

49. Krasinski K, Borkowshy W, Bebenroth B, Moor T. Failure of voluntary testing for human immunodeficiency virus to identify infected parturient women in a high-risk population. *N Engl J Med* 1988;318:185.

50. Francis DP, Anderson RE, Gorman ME, et al. Targeting AIDS prevention treatment toward HIV-1-infected persons. The concept of early intervention. *JAMA* 1989;262:2572–6.

51. Wykoff RF, Heath CW Jr, Hollis SL, et al. Contact tracing to identify human immunodeficiency virus infection in a rural community. *JAMA* 1988;259:3563–6.

52. Levine C, Bayer R. The ethics of screening for early intervention in HIV disease. *Am J Public Health* 1989;79:1661–7.

53. Mann JM, Nzilambi N, Piot P. HIV infection and associated risk factors in female prostitutes in Kinshasa, Zaire. *AIDS* 1988;2:249–54.

54. Deteis R, English P, Visscher BR, et al. Seroconversion, sexual activity and condom use among 2915 HIV seronegative men followed for up to 2 years. *J AIDS* 1989;2:77–83.

55. Conant MC, Hardy D, Sernatinger J, et al. Condoms prevent transmission of AIDS-associated retrovirus. *JAMA* 1986;255:1706.

56. Rietmeijer CAM, Krebs JW, Feorino PM, Judson FN. Condoms as physical and chemical barriers against human immunodeficiency virus. *JAMA* 1988;259:1851–3.

57. Guidelines on sterilization and high-level disinfection methods effective against human immunodeficiency virus (HIV). *Bull Int Union Against Tuberc Lung Dis* 1988;63:7–11.

58. Ryder RW, Nsa W, Hassig SE, et al. Perinatal transmission of the human immunodeficiency virus type 1 to infants of seropositive women in Zaire. *N Engl J Med* 1989;320:1637–42.

59. Maynard JE. Nosocomial viral hepatitis. *Am J Med* 1981;70:439–44.

60. Centers for Disease Control. Recommendations for prevention of HIV transmission in health-care settings. *MMWR* 1987;36:S1–S18.

61. Centers for Disease Control. Possible transmission of human immunodeficiency virus to a patient during an invasive dental procedure. *MMWR* 1990;39:489–93.

62. Carl M, Blakey D, Francis D, et al. Interruption of hepatitis B transmission by modification of a gynaecologist's surgical technique. *Lancet* 1982;1:731–3.

63. Gwinn M, Pappaioanou M, George JR, et al. Prevalence of HIV infection in childbearing women in the United States. *JAMA* 1991;265:1704–8.

64. City and County of San Francisco. Sexually transmitted diseases in San Francisco: changes in incidence, 1984–1988. *San Francisco Epidemiol Bull* Apr 1989.

AIDS and Other Manifestations of HIV Infection,
Second Edition, Edited by Gary P. Wormser.
Raven Press, Ltd., New York © 1992.

CHAPTER 42

Immunizations, Vaccine-Preventable Diseases, and HIV Infection

Ida M. Onorato and Lauri E. Markowitz

In the decade since acquired immunodeficiency syndrome (AIDS) was first reported, advances in therapy of the disease and elucidation of the pathophysiology have been achieved. Studies in San Francisco show improved median survival time for AIDS patients diagnosed in 1986 and 1987 compared to those diagnosed in the first 5 years of the epidemic (1). Zidovudine improves survival of patients with AIDS and prolongs the time from HIV infection to progression to AIDS in patients with CD4 counts below 500 cells/mm³ (2,3). The use of prophylactic aerosolized pentamidine and other agents can prevent the development of *Pneumocystis carinii* pneumonia, an AIDS-defining disease (4). Other antiviral and chemoprophylactic agents for prevention of clinical HIV disease and opportunistic infections now being developed will also increase life expectancy. As AIDS takes on more of the characteristics of a chronic disease, other causes of morbidity and mortality become more important. Although opportunistic infections will account for much of the morbidity in HIV-infected persons, other infectious diseases are potentially preventable by immunizations.

The first recommendations for immunization of HIV-infected children and young adults were published in 1986 (5). Data concerning immunization of children have recently been reviewed (6) and current recommendations are presented in Table 1 (7). This chapter focuses on recommendations for adults. In 1990, the American College of Physicians included recommendations for immunization of HIV-infected adults in the *Guide for Adult Immunization* (8). In spite of the substantial mor-

bidity and mortality of hepatitis B, influenza, and pneumococcal disease in older age groups, immunization levels of recommended vaccines for healthy adults have been low (9). The increase in numbers of HIV-infected adults in the United States and increases in their life expectancy necessitate an understanding of the epidemiology of vaccine-preventable diseases and immunizations and a renewed priority on immunization of adults.

CONCERNS ABOUT IMMUNIZATION OF HIV-INFECTED PERSONS

Two types of concerns about the safety of immunizing HIV-infected persons have been raised: (a) the safety of the vaccines themselves and (b) potential adverse effects on the progression of HIV infection. HIV infection is associated with profound defects in cell-mediated and humoral immunity, resulting in increased susceptibility to a variety of infectious agents. Historically, live virus [e.g., oral poliovaccine (OPV); measles, mumps, and rubella (MMR) vaccine] and bacterial [i.e., bacille Calmette-Guérin (BCG)] vaccines have not been recommended for immunocompromised persons because replication of live, attenuated agents may be enhanced, while inactivated bacterial and viral vaccines [e.g., diphtheria and tetanus toxoids and pertussis vaccine (DTP), influenza vaccine, pneumococcal vaccine, *Haemophilus influenzae* type b conjugate vaccine (HbCV), inactivated poliovaccine (IPV)] are recommended. In the 1960s a child with leukemia immunized with a less attenuated strain of measles vaccine than is used in the United States today developed measles pneumonia (10). Vaccine-associated poliomyelitis, like infection with wild poliovirus, is more frequent and severe in persons with immunologic abnormalities (11). BCG has been reported to produce disseminated BCG disease in persons with T-cell deficiency (12).

I. M. Onorato: Division of HIV/AIDS, Center for Infectious Diseases, Centers for Disease Control, Atlanta, Georgia 30333.
L. E. Markowitz: Division of Immunizations, Center for Prevention Services, Centers for Disease Control, Atlanta, Georgia 30333.

TABLE 1. *Recommendations for routine immunization of HIV-infected children: United States*

Vaccine	Known HIV infection	
	Asymptomatic	Symptomatic
DTP[a]	Yes	Yes
OPV[b]	No	No
IPV[c]	Yes	Yes
MMR[d]	Yes	Yes[e]
HbCV[f]	Yes	Yes
Pneumococcal	Yes	Yes
Influenza	No[g]	Yes

[a] DTP, diphtheria and tetanus toxoids and pertusis vaccine, adsorbed. DTP may be used up to the seventh birthday.
[b] OPV, poliovirus vaccine live oral, trivalent: contains poliovirus types 1, 2, and 3.
[c] IPV, poliovirus vaccine inactivated: contains poliovirus types 1, 2, and 3.
[d] MMR, measles, mumps, and rubella virus vaccine.
[e] Should be considered.
[f] HbCV, vaccine composed of *Haemophilus influenzae b* polysaccharide antigen conjugated to a protein carrier.
[g] Not contraindicated.

A corollary concern is the risk of vaccine-associated poliomyelitis in HIV-infected household contacts of recently immunized children. Because most HIV-infected children acquire HIV perinatally, their parents are infected as well. OPV viruses are excreted by healthy vaccinees for up to 8 weeks and excretion may be prolonged in HIV-infected children. In contrast, extensive experience has shown that the attenuated viruses in MMR are not transmissible to close contacts.

SAFETY OF IMMUNIZATION OF HIV-INFECTED PERSONS

The safety of immunization in HIV infection has been studied mostly in children. The New York City Department of Health conducted a retrospective survey of 221 HIV-infected children with valid immunization records to evaluate the frequency of vaccine-associated adverse events (13). No adverse reactions were noted after receipt of a total of 468 doses of OPV and 70 doses of MMR or measles vaccine, some of which were given after the onset of AIDS. Prospective studies of cohorts of children born to HIV-infected mothers in Africa, the United States, and other countries provide further evidence of the safety of vaccines in HIV-infected children (6). For example, in the best studied cohorts in Zaire and Rwanda, 362 children with HIV infection and 586 non-infected children were vaccinated with BCG, DTP, OPV, and measles vaccine and observed for adverse events (6,14). Rates of common adverse reactions, specifically fever and rash, were similar in both groups of children and no serious reactions were noted. National surveillance for adverse reactions to immunization conducted by the Centers for Disease Control (CDC) has noted no increase in serious adverse events due to measles vaccine and no cases of vaccine-associated poliomyelitis in HIV-infected persons (CDC, *unpublished data*). Onorato et al. (6) estimated the maximal theoretical risk (upper boundary 95% confidence interval) of serious adverse events occurring after OPV and measles immunization to be 0.8% and 1.4%, respectively. Adults have been immunized with influenza and pneumococcal vaccines in a small number of prospective studies. No unusual or more frequent adverse reactions have been observed in the immediate postvaccination period (15,16).

The only adverse effects from vaccination that have been reported have occurred in HIV-infected adults receiving vaccines not recommended for general use in the United States. An asymptomatic HIV-infected military recruit developed generalized vaccinia and was diagnosed with AIDS after receiving smallpox vaccine during basic training (17). Disseminated disease and regional lymphadenitis have occurred in adults with symptomatic HIV infection who received BCG (18,19). However, no cases of disseminated BCG infection have been documented among HIV-infected children receiving routine BCG vaccination (6).

Recent data suggest that there may be an unexpected consequence of hepatitis B vaccine in HIV-infected adults. In one study, HIV-infected men who received vaccine at the time they developed new hepatitis B infection were at increased risk of developing chronic hepatitis B surface antigen (HBsAg) carriage compared to exposed unvaccinated HIV-infected men (20). Eighty percent of those who received their first dose and 56% of those who received a second dose at the time of hepatitis infection became carriers compared with 21% of exposed unvaccinated men. This suggests that hepatitis B vaccine may temporarily impair the immune response to hepatitis B virus infection in HIV-infected men.

Concern has been expressed that simultaneous administration of multiple antigens (even inactivated vaccines) may accelerate the progression of HIV disease by increasing HIV replication and activating CD4 cells (17). Clinical and laboratory data refute this possibility. Retrospective review of clinical disease in a group of HIV-infected children who had received routine immunizations did not reveal any correlation between the number of vaccines received and subsequent progression to AIDS (13). Prospective follow-up of HIV-infected men immunized with influenza and pneumococcal vaccines in immunogenicity studies have showed no clinical deterioration, although the observation period was short (4–6 weeks) for the majority of vaccinees (15,21,22). One of 21 asymptomatic HIV-infected drug users and their partners who received pneumococcal vaccine developed generalized lymphadenopathy at 7 months follow-up, as did one HIV-infected unvaccinated control (16). During the longest prospective observation period reported (36–57 weeks), none of 13 asymptomatic pneumococcal vaccine recipients developed AIDS (22). A cohort of 489 homosexual men enrolled in hepatitis B vaccine trials in 1978–1980 were retrospectively studied to determine progression to AIDS following hepatitis B infection or vaccination after seroconversion to HIV. When controlling for duration of HIV infection, there were no significant differences between 30 HBsAg carriers and noncarriers, 22 hepatitis B-infected and noninfected men or 56 hepatitis B vaccine recipients versus unvaccinated men in rates of progression to AIDS (23).

Laboratory indicators of increased HIV replication or adverse effect on immune function following vaccination have been studied by several investigators. In two studies, no reduction in T4 cells was observed in vaccinated HIV-infected adults compared to unvaccinated or HIV-negative controls (15,16). Among 102 HIV-infected adult influenza vaccine recipients and six children who received measles vaccine, a significant increase in p24 antigen postvaccination was noted in only one man (21,24,25). In a small study of MR vaccination of HIV-infected adults (most of whom had prevaccination measles antibody), no decline in CD4 cells and no increase in number of vaccinees who were p24 antigenemic were detected postvaccination (26). Currently, data from several sources support the safety of immunization of HIV-infected children and adults.

VACCINE-PREVENTABLE DISEASES IN HIV-INFECTED ADULTS

Pneumococcus and *Haemophilus influenzae*

Polyclonal activation of B cells caused by HIV and the resulting decreases in specific antibody responses and opsonization render HIV-infected persons susceptible to infection with the encapsulated bacteria, *Streptococcus pneumoniae* and *Haemophilus influenzae*. The increased incidence and severity of these infections in HIV-infected adults have been documented by examining mortality reports and pneumonia and influenza (P&I) surveillance data. U.S. death rates for pneumonia and influenza (excluding *Pneumocystis carinii* pneumonia) in men 25–44 years had been declining for two decades until 1981. Since 1981, rates have increased each year with a 176% increase in P&I-attributable deaths in cities with the highest AIDS incidence (27). The increased mortality was greatest in cities with a comparatively high proportion of AIDS cases occurring in intravenous drug users. In New York City, a retrospective medical record review of 192 persons dying from pneumonia in 1986 showed that 80% belonged to groups at increased risk for AIDS (82% were intravenous drug users) and 40% had a diagnosis of thrush or an AIDS-defining condition (28).

Pneumococcal and *H. influenzae* pneumonias were reported in homosexual men and intravenous drug users with AIDS early in the epidemic (29–31). The first case report, in 1984, also raised a question about the efficacy of pneumococcal vaccine in AIDS patients since one of the five cases had recently been immunized (29). Estimates of the annual incidence of community-acquired pneumococcal pneumonia in patients with symptomatic HIV infection were 17.9/1000, 45.5/1000, and 95/1000 in hospital-based clinical case series (29,32,33). These rates are several-fold higher than those in the general population or in non-AIDS patients admitted to the same hospitals (29,33,34). AIDS patients in San Francisco also had a higher rate of pneumococcal bacteremia (9.4/1000 person-years) than splenectomized patients (0.92–2.1/1000), adults with sickle-cell disease (0.86/1000), or community-based rates reported before the AIDS epidemic (7.5–16.4/100,000)(35). Finally, among a cohort of methadone maintenance clients followed prospectively for 1 year, asymptomatic HIV-infected clients were five times as likely to be hospitalized with pneumococcal or *H. influenzae* pneumonia than seronegative drug users (36). Clinical complications, including bacteremia and recurrent pneumonias, are also more frequent in HIV-infected persons, suggesting that effective prevention (if possible) of pneumococcal and *H. influenzae* infections would substantially decrease morbidity and mortality (29–33).

Pertussis, Influenza

Although *Bordetella pertussis* is increasingly recognized as a cause of respiratory illness in adults, and immunocompromised persons are known to be at risk of complications of influenza, these pathogens have rarely been reported in HIV-infected patients (37,38). Several case reports document the isolation of influenza viruses and *B. pertussis* from patients initially suspected of having *P. carinii* pneumonia, indicating that influenza pneumonia or pertussis may incorrectly be attributed to other respiratory agents (39–42). The increases in mortality in P&I surveillance data noted above occurred in the winter, concurrent with influenza activity, but the relative contributions of influenza and bacterial pneumonia are not known (28).

Measles

Measles is known to be severe in immunocompromised persons with defects in cell-mediated immunity, including HIV-infected children both in the United States and in developing countries (43–45). In the United States, severe measles and measles-associated deaths in HIV-infected adults have been reported to CDC (CDC, *unpublished data*). Because of the current epidemiology of measles in the United States, characterized by recurrent outbreaks of measles in inner city areas, HIV-infected persons may be at increased risk of exposure to measles. Except for the 1990 measles epidemic when most measles cases occurred in preschool-age children, during the past decade, the majority of measles cases have occurred in persons over 10 years of age (46). Outbreaks have been reported among adults in colleges or universities. In 1989, 93 colleges reported measles (47).

Hepatitis B

Behaviors such as intravenous drug use and homosexual relations that place individuals at risk for HIV infection also increase their risk for hepatitis B. In addition, HIV-infected persons are at increased risk of becoming chronic HBsAg carriers once exposed. Hadler et al. (20) reported that among exposed HIV-uninfected men, 7% became carriers compared with 21% of 14 exposed HIV-infected men. Bodsworth et al. (48) found a similar increased risk of HBsAg carriage in HIV-infected men.

Similar findings were reported by Taylor et al. (49): 20% of HIV-infected men became carriers compared with 6% of those without HIV infection. HIV-infected persons also have higher levels of viremia (50–52). These data indicate that the current epidemiology of HIV will have a major impact on the risk of hepatitis B carriage. In contrast to the early years of the AIDS epidemic, many high-risk persons will now be exposed to hepatitis B after they are infected with HIV, resulting in higher carriage rates and facilitating transmission.

Varicella Zoster

Since over 90% of adults in the United States have serologic evidence of previous varicella zoster virus exposure, reactivation (herpes zoster) is a frequent manifestation of immune compromise in HIV-infected adults. However, recently, primary varicella infection, documented by seroconversion, was reported in nine HIV-infected adults with no history of varicella (53). One fatality occurred in spite of acyclovir therapy. Although four of the nine patients reported household contact with a child with chickenpox and two were infected by other hospitalized patients, postexposure prophylaxis with varicella immune globulin was not given in any of these cases.

Other Vaccine-Preventable Diseases

There have been no reports of mumps, rubella, poliomyelitis, diphtheria, or tetanus in HIV-infected persons. Although often considered childhood illnesses, all these diseases except polio have been reported increasingly in adults in recent years and the more serious complications occur in older persons or their fetuses. The age distribution for mumps and rubella cases has shifted from the under-10 year old age group in the prevaccination era to adolescents and young adults, a group that is relatively underimmunized (54,55). Recent outbreaks of mumps and rubella on college campuses and in the workplace have led to recommendations for vaccination of susceptible adolescents on college entry and childbearing women postpartum (54,55). In 1985–1989, 92% of tetanus and 64% of diphtheria patients were adults who were inadequately immunized (9).

IMMUNOGENICITY OF RECOMMENDED VACCINES IN HIV-INFECTED PERSONS

A number of studies have compared immunogenicity (i.e., the serologic response postvaccination) in HIV-infected persons with that in seronegative controls (Table 2). Difficulties comparing studies include different classifications of HIV disease, different vaccines used, and different serologic measures of immunity reported. In general, these studies have shown that responses are impaired as HIV-induced immunosuppression progresses and that even in responders, antibody levels achieved may be lower than in healthy persons. Responses to immunization attempted after the onset of HIV infection appear to be lower than secondary responses to antigens encountered prior to HIV infection. Vaccine-induced antibody may also decline over time to a nonprotective level as other immunologic functions deteriorate. As HIV-infected patients survive for longer periods, more follow-up studies are needed.

Polysaccharide Vaccines

One of the earliest indications of the B-cell dysfunction characteristic of AIDS was the poor response of AIDS patients to immunization with T-cell-independent antigens, such as pneumococcal polysaccharides. Evaluating responses to pneumococcal vaccine is complex since there are 23 serotypes in the present vaccine, laboratory tests are not standardized [radioimmunoassay (RIA) and enzyme-linked immunoassay (EIA) are used most often], and there is no agreement on the level of antibody or increase in titer that correlates with protection. RIA measures total antibody while the ELISA can also measure immunoglobulin class-specific antibody; results of RIA and EIA do not always agree.

Immunogenicity studies in different groups of HIV-infected people have shown that fewer HIV-infected persons respond to vaccination than seronegative controls (Table 2). A vaccine failure in an AIDS patient has been reported (29). Response rates are higher in asymptom-

TABLE 2. *Immunogenicity of recommended vaccines in HIV-infected patients compared to seronegative adults*

Vaccine	Reference	Stage of HIV infection	HIV-infected patients		Controls	
			Number tested	Response[a]	Number tested	Response[a]
Pneumococcal	83	AIDS	18	51%	20	99%
	84	PGL	25	36%	10	100%
	59	AIDS/ARC	13	15%	23	100%
		Asymptomatic	11	18%		
	15	PGL	25	10/12 types[b]	39	
		Asymptomatic	15	11/12 types	53	
	22	AIDS	21	61%	53	88%
		Asymptomatic	27	63%		
	16	Asymptomatic	21	7/12 types[b]	23	
Hib	57	Asymptomatic	7	3.1 ± 1[c]	14	42 ± 19[c]
Influenza	59	AIDS/ARC	13	1.5[d]	23	2.8
		Asymptomatic	11	2.1		
	15	PGL	25	72–96%	19	58–95%
		Asymptomatic	10	60–100%		
	21	AIDS	15	13–40%	38	71–100%
		AIDS, on AZT	10	17–50%		
		ARC	14	15–54%		
		Asymptomatic/PGL	27	32–89%		
	24	AIDS	7	13–37%	31	25–100%
		AIDS, on AZT	30	0–43%		
		ARC	9	11–78%		
		Asymptomatic/PGL	32	22–84%		
Diphtheria	85	Asymptomatic	21	57%	21	45%
	86	Asymptomatic	8	3[d]	6	8
Tetanus	85	Asymptomatic	21	48%	21	43%
	84	PGL	25	5.25[d]	12	5.85
	62	Asymptomatic	5	1.7[d]	9	8.6
	86	Asymptomatic	8	6.5[d]	6	10
IPV	62	Asymptomatic	5	$9–10 \pm 3$[c]	8	$11–12 \pm 3$[c]
	87	AIDS/ARC/PGL	5	63–102[c]	3	5955–9410[c]
		Asymptomatic	12	5250–6277[c]		
HBV-plasma	68	Asymptomatic/PGL	17	53%	18	94%
	67	NA	16	56%	68	91%
	69	Asymptomatic	4	50%	69	93%
	70	NA/hemophiliacs	12	50%	29	93%
HBV-recomb	71	NA	10	40%	19	91%
	72	Asymptomatic	14	43%	37	86%
	69	Asymptomatic	9	22%	72	81%

AIDS, acquired immunodeficiency syndrome; AIDS, on AZT, AIDS patients receiving zidovudine (AZT); ARC, AIDS-related complex; PGL, persistent generalized lymphadenopathy; Hib, *Haemophilus infuenzae* type b polysaccharide and conjugate vaccines; IPV, inactivated poliovirus vaccine; HBV-plasma, plasma-derived vaccine; HBV-recomb, hepatitis B recombinant vaccine; NA, not available.

[a] Definition of response varied by study and type of serologic test performed. Percent indicates proportion attaining specified antibody level or significant titer rise. When a range is given, the percent varied by serotype.

[b] Geometric mean titer (GMT) in HIV-infected persons equal to controls for specified number of capsular types.

[c] Mean titer of antibody postvaccination in μg/ml or reciprocal log dilutions. When a range is given, titers varied by serotype.

[d] Ratio of postvaccination to prevaccination titers.

atic HIV-infected persons but mean antibody levels in all immunoglobulin classes were lower in responders than in controls (15,22). In spite of the generally poorer response of HIV-infected persons, there are indications that vaccination may be useful. Klein et al. (16) noted that 87% of all HIV-infected intravenous drug users and persons infected via heterosexual transmission had a rise

in antibody to greater than 400 ng AbN/ml to one or more vaccine types. Overall, protective levels were achieved in intravenous drug users and infected sex partners to 35% and 54% of the capsular types, respectively. At 1 year follow-up, in another study there were no significant differences in the proportions of asymptomatic HIV-infected homosexual men and of seronegative homosexual men, who retained antibody although the level of antibody was lower in HIV-infected men (22). Other data indicate that AIDS patients who were treated with zidovudine for 13 weeks prior to vaccination had a significantly increased response compared to untreated AIDS patients (aggregate GMT 942.9 versus 763.8)(56). Thus it may be expected that zidovudine prophylaxis should have a greater effect on responses of asymptomatic HIV-infected patients.

Although asymptomatic HIV-infected men immunized with *H. influenzae b* polysaccharide vaccine had lower levels of antibody postvaccination than seronegative controls, levels in both groups were protective (≥1.0 μg/ml)(57). As has been shown in normal children and adults, HIV-infected men respond with higher antibody levels to polyribosylribitol phosphate (PRP) conjugated with diphtheria toxoid than to PRP vaccine alone (58). Among AIDS patients, 3/3 developed protective antibody levels to conjugated vaccine compared to 1/6 given PRP.

Influenza Vaccine

The influence of stage of HIV disease on the ability to respond to immunization is clearly demonstrated in prospective studies of influenza vaccination of HIV-infected patients with a spectrum of clinical manifestations (Table 2). Interestingly, at all stages of HIV disease, responses to influenza A hemagglutinins H1 and H3 were higher than responses to influenza B antigen (21,24). The proportion of symptomatic HIV-infected patients who respond to monovalent influenza A and trivalent influenza A and B vaccines was much lower than for seronegative controls (21,24,59). The number of CD4 cells present at vaccination was related to antibody titers achieved postvaccination (21). AIDS patients receiving zidovudine had similar CD4 numbers as ARC patients and their responses to immunization were intermediate between those of untreated AIDS patients and ARC patients. The proportions of asymptomatic patients and those with persistent generalized lymphadenopathy who acquired protective levels of antibody were equal to controls for all three vaccine antigens in two studies (15,24) and for one or two antigens in the other two reported studies (21,59). Thus influenza vaccination, if given early in the course of HIV infection, should provide a measure of protection.

In an attempt to improve vaccine responses, Miotti et al. (24) studied the effect of a booster dose of vaccine given 1 month after the first dose. Only a few HIV-infected persons who did not respond to the first vaccine dose seroconverted after the booster dose. The booster dose increased antibody to protective levels (≥1:64) in only one asymptomatic HIV-infected person and had no effect on levels in ARC patients. Of 30 AIDS patients on zidovudine therapy, the proportion who reached a protective level of antibody increased from 30% to 33% for

H1 antibody, from 37% to 47% for H3 antibody, and from 13% to 17% for antibody to influenza B after the booster dose.

Diphtheria and Tetanus Toxoids

After primary immunization with diphtheria and tetanus toxoids in childhood, almost all HIV-infected adults maintain protective levels of antibody (≥0.01 μg/ml) after the onset of HIV infection. Similar experiences have been reported from Africa and Haiti, where HIV-infected women were found to have the same levels of tetanus antibody after two doses of vaccine given during pregnancy as seronegative women (60,61). In all but one study, the increases in antibody levels after booster doses of diphtheria and/or tetanus toxoid vaccine were the same in asymptomatic HIV-infected persons and in controls (62). The decreased response in HIV-infected men in this study correlated with the lack of proliferative responses of peripheral blood mononuclear cells postvaccination when exposed to tetanus toxoid *in vitro* (62). However, when tetanus toxoid was coupled to agarose beads creating a T-cell-independent antigen, *in vitro* responses did occur.

Measles, Mumps, and Rubella Vaccine

Most data on the response to measles vaccine are from children in developing countries (45,63,64). There are few data for rubella vaccine and none for mumps. In one study in Zaire, seroconversion rates after measles immunization at 9 months of age were related to severity of HIV infection. Among HIV-uninfected, asymptomatic HIV-infected, and symptomatic HIV-infected children 89%, 77%, and 36% responded to vaccine, respectively (45). In a small retrospective study in the United States, only 3 (12.5%) of 24 vaccinated HIV-infected children had antibody to measles virus. However, a larger number of children had antibody when tested by a more sensitive assay. Among children studied prospectively, only two (25%) of eight responded to measles vaccination (25).

Most HIV-infected adults will either have received MMR vaccine during childhood or have had natural disease. Two studies have found that almost all HIV-infected adults have protective levels of measles antibody (65,66). Thus there are no data to suggest that after primary immunization or disease in childhood, HIV-infected adults lose protective measles antibody. Only one study has evaluated the response of MR vaccination of HIV-infected adults. In this study only 3 of 39 HIV-seropositive and 2 of 17 healthy vaccinees were measles seronegative at the time of vaccination. None of the HIV-infected and one of the healthy adults seroconverted (26). Four HIV-infected and three healthy vaccinees were rubella seronegative at the time of vaccination; three and two, respectively, responded to vaccination.

Hepatitis B

Several studies have demonstrated an impaired response to hepatitis B vaccine in HIV-infected adults. Three studies in homosexual HIV-infected men, using plasma-derived vaccine, found that 50–56% of HIV-infected adults seroconverted compared with over 80% of uninfected controls (67–69). Similar results have been reported in studies of HIV-infected hemophiliacs (70). Studies of recombinant vaccine in homosexual men have found similarly low immunogenicity in those HIV-infected (69,71,72). Revaccination of HIV-infected persons who do not respond to the three-dose primary series produces poor results. In a small study, one of six HIV-infected nonresponders seroconverted after a second series compared with 50% of uninfected adults (73). Among those who responded to vaccine, no difference in geometric mean titers between HIV-infected and uninfected vaccinees was reported by Carne et al. (68); however, lower levels were found in other studies (67,71). In addition to low seroconversion rates in HIV-infected persons, accelerated loss of hepatitis B surface antibody in responders has been reported (74). Thirty-six percent of 75 men without HIV infection lost protective levels of antibody within 5 years of vaccination compared with 63–86% of 21 men who acquired HIV infection before or during the hepatitis B vaccination series. However, good persistence was reported in another study (75). Among HIV-infected persons who respond to vaccine, protec-tion against serious illness appears to be good: among 17 HIV-infected responders who were infected with hepatitis B virus, none had severe illness or became chronic carriers (20).

Poliovirus Vaccines

In two small studies, all but one of 22 HIV-infected patients had antibody to all three poliovirus types prior to vaccination with inactivated poliovaccine (IPV) (Table 2). The patients had all been vaccinated with poliovirus vaccine in childhood or were exposed to wild polioviruses. Following vaccination, asymptomatic HIV-infected men all responded similarly as uninfected men with substantial increases in antibody. However, none of the symptomatic HIV-infected men had a booster response to IPV.

RECOMMENDATIONS FOR IMMUNIZATION AND PROPHYLAXIS OF HIV-INFECTED ADULTS

Pneumococcal and *H. influenzae* Vaccines

The use of inactivated vaccines poses no risk of adverse events and may be beneficial for HIV-infected persons. Although the response to immunization may be less than optimal in HIV-infected persons, the Immunizations Practices Advisory Committee (ACIP) and the American College of Physicians (ACP) recommend that all HIV-infected persons be immunized with pneumococcal vaccine regardless of disease status (Table 3)(8,34). As yet there are no data on which to base a

TABLE 3. *Recommendations for immunization and prophylaxis of asymptomatic and symptomatic HIV-infected adults*

	Vaccine		Prophylaxis	
Disease	Asymptomatic status	Symptomatic status	Asymptomatic status	Symptomatic status
Diphtheria[a]	Td	Td		
Tetanus[a]	Td[b]	Td[b]	TIG[b]	TIG[b]
Pneumococcal	Pneumococcal	Pneumococcal		
Haemophilus influenzae	HbCV	HbCV		
Influenza	Influenza	Influenza	Amantadine	Amantadine
Poliomyelitis[a]	IPV	IPV		
Measles[a]	MMR	MMR[c]		IG[d]
Mumps[a]	MMR	MMR[c]		
Rubella[a]	MMR	MMR[c]		
Hepatitis B	HBV	HBV	HBIG	HBIG
Varicella			VZIG	VZIG

Td, diphtheria and tetanus toxoids formulated for adults; TIG, tetanus immune globulin; HbCV, *Haemophilus influenzae b* conjugate vaccine; HBV, hepatitis B vaccine; VZIG, varicella zoster immune globulin; HBIG, hepatitis B immune globulin; MMR, measles, mumps, rubella vaccine.

[a] Primary immunization usually completed during childhood. Booster doses are recommended as for immunocompetent adults.

[b] Irrespective of immunization history or wound severity, a booster dose of Td should be administered as part of wound management. A prophylactic dose of TIG should also be given when the wound is other than clean and minor.

[c] Should be considered. MMR is recommended for all persons born after 1956 who lack adequate evidence of immunity.

[d] Irrespective of immunization history.

recommendation for revaccination with pneumococcal vaccine. *H. influenzae b* vaccine should also be considered in view of the known immunologic deficiencies in humoral immunity in HIV-infected persons. Chemoprophylaxis with oral penicillin or other drugs for patients with recurrent episodes of pneumococcal or *H. influenzae* pneumonia may be used, although efficacy data are lacking. The greatest benefit from immunization will occur when HIV-infected patients are immunized before the onset of immunocompromise. Thus persons possibly at risk for HIV infection because of their life-styles or exposures must be encouraged to seek voluntary HIV counseling and testing.

Influenza Vaccine

Influenza vaccine should be given annually, because the prevalent virus strains and thus vaccine composition changes each year (76). In addition, medical personnel and household members who may expose HIV-infected persons should be vaccinated to prevent transmission of influenza virus. Because vaccine efficacy cannot be assured, chemoprophylaxis should be considered for certain situations. Amantadine should be considered for HIV-infected patients with AIDS or low CD4 cells who may be expected to have a poor response to immunization (76). During nosocomial outbreaks, amantadine should be given to all institutionalized patients regardless of previous influenza vaccination. Amantadine may also be given during the 2-week period after influenza vaccination and before the development of antibodies if an influenza outbreak has begun in the community. Finally, during periods of influenza A activity, amantadine may be given to unvaccinated institutionalized HIV-infected persons and to those who will be exposed in the community. There are almost no data on the safety of amantadine in HIV-infected persons (37). Patients should be carefully observed for adverse drug reactions, especially when neurologic conditions or renal insufficiency is present. During influenza outbreaks, unvaccinated hospital and clinic personnel and household caregivers should also receive prophylaxis to prevent transmission of virus to HIV-infected persons.

Diphtheria and Tetanus Toxoids, Inactivated Poliovaccine

Other inactivated vaccines (i.e., diphtheria and tetanus toxoids and inactivated poliovaccines) may be used for immunization of unvaccinated or inadequately vaccinated HIV-infected adults or for boosters as recommended for immunocompetent adults. In addition, children residing in households or having close contact with known HIV-infected adults should receive IPV for primary immunization. A history of immunization with tetanus and diphtheria toxoids (which is often not known for adults) may not indicate present immunity. Prophylaxis with tetanus immune globulin (TIG) and a tetanus booster are recommended for HIV-infected adults who sustain a significant wound exposure.

Measles Vaccine, MMR

All adults born in or after 1957 should have evidence of immunity to measles: either documentation of receipt of measles vaccine after the first birthday; laboratory evidence of immunity; or history of physician documented measles disease. Adults born before 1957 can generally be considered to be immune from natural disease. The ACIP recommends that asymptomatic HIV-infected adults without evidence of immunity to measles receive MMR vaccine. Vaccination should also be considered for symptomatic HIV-infected adults. In 1989, a routine two-dose MMR schedule was implemented in the United States (77). Both doses are recommended in childhood; however, documentation of two doses of vaccine has also been recommended for young adults who are attending college or other post-high-school educational institutions, who are working in situations at high risk of measles transmission (such as health-care facilities) or in the setting of a measles outbreak. These same recommendations apply to HIV-infected adults. Because of the reduced immunogenicity of measles vaccine in HIV-infected persons, previously vaccinated persons, as well as those with no history of vaccination or disease, should receive intramuscular immune globulin within 6 days of measles exposure.

Hepatitis B Vaccine

A routine three-dose schedule (with an interval of 1 month between the first and second doses and 6 months between the second and third doses) is recommended for all HIV-infected persons who lack evidence of prior immunity [antibody to hepatitis B surface or core antigens [anti-Hbs or anti-Hbc)]. A larger than normal vaccine dose, 40 μg, which is recommended for some immunocompromised persons, may be considered but has not been studied in HIV-infected adults. Postvaccination serologic testing is recommended for all HIV-infected persons between 1 and 6 months after completion of the vaccination series. Revaccination with one or more doses should be considered if the anti-Hbs is below 10 MIU/ml. Postexposure recommendations for HIV-infected persons are similar to those for uninfected persons (78). Hepatitis B immune globulin and initiation of the hepatitis B vaccination series is recommended for all nonimmune HIV-infected persons who have accidental percutaneous or mucous membrane exposure to blood containing hepatitis B surface antigen or who have sexual exposure.

Varicella Zoster Postexposure Prophylaxis

All HIV-infected patients who are exposed to varicella should be given prophylaxis with varicella immune globulin (VZIG) within 96 hr of exposure, as recommended for other immunocompromised persons (79). Most adults with a history of chickenpox will be immune; however, a past history of varicella, a previous positive serologic test for varicella antibody, or recent administration of VZIG does not guarantee immunity (8). Varicella vaccine may be licensed for use in the United States in the near future, but initial indications will not include the use of vaccine in HIV-infected persons. Susceptible medical personnel and household members should be immunized to decrease the risk of nosocomial transmission to HIV-infected patients.

HIV-Infected Travelers

HIV-infected persons who wish to travel to developing countries pose a special problem. They should be made aware of the risks of travel to areas in which many diseases are endemic and that lack supportive medical care. There are no data concerning adverse reactions, immunogenicity, or efficacy of vaccines usually recommended only for travel outside the United States. The live attenuated virus vaccines for prevention of yellow fever and typhoid are contraindicated for symptomatic HIV-infected persons (80,81). For necessary travel to countries requiring proof of vaccination, a waiver letter should be provided by the traveler's physician. For asymptomatic persons with adequate numbers of CD4 cells who cannot avoid possible exposure to yellow fever, the physician should inform the patient of the risks and benefits of immunization and offer the choice of vaccination. Prior to travel, determination of an adequate antibody response to vaccination is desirable. All HIV-infected persons should be advised to avoid exposure to mosquitoes by using barrier methods of protection. An inactivated typhoid vaccine is available and theoretically may be a safe alternative for symptomatic and asymptomatic HIV-infected persons (80). Inactivated cholera vaccine has been shown to be only about 50% effective in preventing illness. Nevertheless, many countries continue to require evidence of cholera vaccination for entry; a physician's waiver seems appropriate for HIV-infected persons. Travelers should be advised that careful selection of food and drink remains the best prevention for *S. typhi* and *V. cholerae* infections.

For HIV-infected travelers planning longer sojourns in developing countries, passive immunization with immune globulin is safe and protective against clinical hepatitis A disease. Other vaccine-preventable diseases, including rabies, Japanese encephalitis, meningococcal infection, and plague, are rare in American travelers. The vaccines are inactivated and could be considered in the unusual circumstance when exposure cannot be avoided.

CONCLUSION

As the number of HIV-infected persons continues to increase, as more patients are identified earlier in their disease, and as survival is increased, there will be more opportunity for acquisition of vaccine-preventable diseases. Current vaccines are most likely to be effective when HIV-infected persons are immunized before the onset of immune compromise. Past experiences with adult immunizations indicate that provision of recommended vaccines and immuno- and chemoprophylaxis to HIV-infected persons needs to be much more aggressive. Additional techniques to improve responses to immunization are necessary. Research should include modifications of vaccination schedules including booster or multiple dose schedules, vaccination concurrent with anti-HIV therapy, and development of more immunogenic vaccines. Recent studies of the use of immunoadjuvants to increase the efficacy of existing vaccines are a very promising step in this direction (82).

REFERENCES

1. Lemp GF, Payne SF, Rutherford GW, et al. Projections of AIDS morbidity and mortality in San Francisco. *JAMA* 1990; 263:1497–501.
2. Fischl MA, Richman DD, Grieco MH, et al. The efficacy of azidothymidine (AZT) in the treatment of patients with AIDS and AIDS-related complex. *N Engl J Med* 1987;317:185–91.
3. Volberding PA, Lagakos SW, Koch MA, et al. Zidovudine in asymptomatic human immunodeficiency virus infection. *N Engl J Med* 1990;322:941–9.
4. Centers for Disease Control. Guidelines for prophylaxis against *Pneumocystis carinii* pneumonia for persons infected with human immunodeficiency virus. *MMWR* 1989;38(S-5):1–9.
5. Immunization Practices Advisory Committee. Immunization of children infected with HTLVIII/LAV lymphadenopathy associated-virus. *MMWR* 1986;35:595–606.
6. Onorato IM, Markowitz LE, Oxtoby MJ. Childhood immunization, vaccine-preventable diseases and infection with human immunodeficiency virus. *Pediatr Infect Dis* 1988;6:588–95.
7. Immunization Practices Advisory Committee. General recommendations on immunization. *MMWR* 1989;38:205–216,219–27.
8. American College of Physicians. *Guide for adult immunization*, 2nd ed. Philadelphia: American College of Physicians;1990.
9. Centers for Disease Control. Public health burden of vaccine-preventable diseases among adults: standards for adult immunization practices. *MMWR* 1990;39:725–9.
10. Mitus A, Holloway A, Evans AE, et al. Attenuated measles vaccine in children with acute leukemia. *Am J Dis Child* 1962;103:243–8.
11. Nkowane BM, Wassilak SGF, Orenstein WA, et al. Vaccine-associated paralytic poliomyelitis. *JAMA* 1987;257:1335–40.
12. Lotte A, Wasz-Hockert O, Poisson N, et al. BCG complications. *Adv Tuberc Res* 1984;21:107–93.
13. McLaughlin M, Thomas P, Onorato I, et al. Use of live virus vaccines in HIV-infected children: a retrospective survey. *Pediatrics* 1988;82:229–33.

14. Dabis F, Msellati P, Lepage P, Bazubagira A, Hitimana DG, Van de Perre P. HIV and adverse reactions following routine childhood immunization in Africa: a cohort study in Kigali, Rwanda. 6th International AIDS Conference, San Francisco, June 1990.

15. Huang KL, Ruben FL, Rinaldo CR, Kingsley L, Lyter DW, Ho M. Antibody responses after influenza and pneumococcal immunization in HIV-infected homosexual men. *JAMA* 1987;257:2047–50.

16. Klein RS, Selwyn PA, Maude D, Pollard C, Freeman K, Schiffman G. Response to pneumococcal vaccine among asymptomatic heterosexual partners of persons with AIDS and intravenous drug users infected with human immunodeficiency virus. *J Infect Dis* 1989;160:826–31.

17. Redfield RR, Wright DC, James WD, et al. Disseminated vaccinia in a military recruit with human immunodeficiency virus disease. *N Engl J Med* 1987;316:673–6.

18. Armbruster C, Junker W, Vetter N, Jaksch G. Disseminated bacille Calmette-Guérin infection in an AIDS patient 30 years after BCG vaccination. *J Infect Dis* 1990;162:1216.

19. Centers for Disease Control. Disseminated *Mycobacterium bovis* infection from BCG vaccination of a patient with acquired immunodeficiency syndrome. *MMWR* 1985;34:227–8.

20. Hadler SC, Judson FN, O'Malley PM, et al. Outcome of hepatitis B virus infection in homosexual men and its relation to prior human immunodeficiency virus infection. *J Infect Dis* 1991; 163:454–9.

21. Nelson KE, Clements ML, Miotti P, Cohn S, Polk BF. The influence of human immunodeficiency virus infection on antibody responses to influenza vaccines. *Ann Intern Med* 1988;109:383–8.

22. Janoff EN, Douglas JM, Gabriel M, et al. Class-specific antibody response to pneumococcal capsular polysaccharides in men infected with human immunodeficiency virus type 1. *J Infect Dis* 1988;158:983–90.

23. Buchbinder S, Hessol N, Lifson A, et al. Does infection with hepatitis B virus or vaccination with plasma-derived hepatitis B vaccine accelerate progression to AIDS? 6th International Conference on AIDS, San Francisco, June 1990.

24. Miotti PG, Nelson KE, Dallabetta GA, Farzadegan H, Margolick J, Clements ML. The influence of HIV infection on antibody responses to a two-dose regimen of influenza vaccine. *JAMA* 1989;262:779–83.

25. Krasinski K, Borkowsky W. Measles and measles immunity in children infected with human immunodeficiency virus. *JAMA* 1989;261:2512–6.

26. Sprauer MA, Markowitz LE, Dales L, et al. Evaluation of measles and rubella vaccination among HIV-infected adults. 6th International Conference on AIDS, San Francisco, June 1990.

27. Beuhler JB, Devine OJ, Berkelman RL, Chevarley FM. Impact of human immunodeficiency virus epidemic on mortality trends in young men, United States. *Am J Public Health* 1990;80:1080–6.

28. Centers for Disease Control. Increase in pneumonia mortality among young adults and the HIV epidemic—New York City, United States. *MMWR* 1988;37:593–6.

29. Simberkoff MS, El Sadr W, Schiffman G, Rahal JJ. *Streptococcus pneumoniae* infections and bacteremia in patients with acquired immune deficiency syndrome, with report of a vaccine failure. *Am Rev Respir Dis* 1984;130:1174–6.

30. Murata GH, Ault MJ, Meyer RD. Community-acquired bacterial pneumonias in homosexual men: presumptive evidence for a defect in host resistance. *AIDS Res* 1984/5;1:379–93.

31. Schlamm HT, Yancovitz SR. *Haemophilus influenzae* pneumonia in young adults with AIDS, ARC, or risk of AIDS. *Am J Med* 1989;86:11–4.

32. Polsky B, Gold JWM, Whimbey E, et al. Bacterial pneumonia in patients with acquired immunodeficiency syndrome. *Ann Intern Med* 1986;104:38–41.

33. Witt DJ, Craven DE, McCabe WR. Bacterial infections in adult patients with the acquired immune deficiency syndrome (AIDS) and AIDS-related complex. *Am J Med* 1987;82:900–6.

34. Immunization Practices Advisory Committee. Pneumococcal polysaccharide vaccine. *MMWR* 1989;38:64–76.

35. Redd SC, Rutherford GW, Sande MA, et al. The role of human immunodeficiency virus infection in pneumococcal bacteremia in San Francisco residents. *J Infect Dis* 1990;162:1012–7.

36. Selwyn PA, Feingold AR, Hartel D, et al. Increased risk of bacterial pneumonia in HIV-infected intravenous drug users without AIDS. *AIDS* 1988;2:267–72.

37. Cohen JP, Macauley C. Susceptibility to influenza A in HIV-positive patients. *JAMA* 1989;261:245.

38. Centers for Disease Control. Pertussis surveillance—United States —1986–1988. *MMWR* 1990;39:57–58,63–6.

39. Thurn JR, Henry K. Influenza A pneumonitis in a patient infected with the human immunodeficiency virus. *Chest* 1989;95:807–10.

40. Safrin S, Rush JD, Mills J. Influenza in patients with human immunodeficiency virus infection. *Chest* 1990;98:33–7.

41. Ng V, York M, Hadley WK. Unexpected isolation of *Bordetella pertussis* from patients with the acquired immunodeficiency syndrome. *J Clin Microbiol* 1989;27:337–8.

42. Doebbeling BN, Feilmeier ML, Herwalt LA. Pertussis in an adult man infected with the human immunodeficiency virus. *J Infect Dis* 1990;161:1296–8.

43. CDC. Measles in HIV-infected children in the United States. *MMWR* 1988;37:183–6.

44. Sension MG, Markowitz LE, Linnan MJ, et al. Measles in hospitalized African children with human immunodeficiency virus. *Am J Dis Child* 1988;142:1271–2.

45. Oxtoby MS, Mvula M, Ryder R, Baende E, Nsa W, Onorato IM. Measles and measles immunity in African children with HIV. Twenty-eighth Interscience Conference on Antimicrobial Agents and Chemotherapy, Los Angeles, Oct 23–26, 1988.

46. CDC. Measles—United States, 1988. *MMWR* 1989;38:601–5.

47. Hersh BS, Markowitz LE, Hoffman RE, et al. A measles outbreak at a college with a prematriculation immunization requirement. *Am J Public Health* 1991;81:360–4.

48. Bodsworth NJ, Cooper DA, Conovan B. The influence of human immunodeficiency virus type 1 infection on the development of the hepatitis B virus carrier state. *J Infect Dis* 1991;163:1138–40.

49. Taylor PE, Stevens CE, Rodriquez de Cordoba S, Rubenstein P. Hepatitis B virus and human immunodeficiency virus: possible interactions. In: Zuckerman AH, ed. *Viral hepatitis and liver disease.* New York: Alan R Liss; 1988:198–200.

50. Perrillo RP, Regenstein FG, Roodman ST. Chronic hepatitis B in asymptomatic homosexual man with antibody to the human immunodeficiency virus. *Ann Intern Med* 1986;105:382–3.

51. Bodsworth N, Donovan B, Nightingale BN. The effect of concurrent human immunodeficiency virus infection on chronic hepatitis B: a study of 150 homosexual men. *J Infect Dis* 1989; 160:577–82.

52. Krogsgaard K, Lindhardt BO, Nielson JO, et al. The influence of HTLV-III infection on the natural history of hepatitis B virus infection in male homosexual HBsAg carriers. *Hepatology* 1987;7:37–41.

53. Perronne C, Lazanas M, Leport C, et al. Varicella in patients infected with human immunodeficiency virus. *Arch Dermatol* 1990;126:1033–6.

54. Centers for Disease Control. Mumps—United States, 1985–1988. *MMWR* 1989;38:101–5.

55. Centers for Disease Control. Rubella and congenital rubella syndrome—United States, 1985–1988. *MMWR* 1989;38:173–8.

56. Glaser JB, Volpe S, Schiffman G. AZT's effect on responses to pneumococcal vaccine. 5th International Conference on AIDS, Montreal, Canada, June 1989.

57. Janoff EN, Worel S, Douglas JM. Natural immunity and response to conjugate vaccine for *Haemophilus influenzae* type B in men with HIV. Thirtieth Interscience Conference on Antimicrobial Agents and Chemotherapy, Atlanta, Oct 21–24, 1990.

58. Auerbach BS, Steinhoff M, Nelson K, et al. Protein conjugation enhances immunogenicity of *H. influenzae* type b polysaccharide vaccine in HIV-infected adults. 6th International Conference on AIDS, San Francisco, June 1990.

59. Ragni MV, Ruben FL, Winkelstein A, Spero JA, Bontempo FA, Lewis JH. Antibody responses to immunization of patients with hemophilia with and without evidence of human immunodeficiency virus infection. *J Lab Clin Med* 1987;109:545–9.

60. Halsey NA, Boulos R, Donnenberg AD, et al. Anti-tetanus antibody in umbilical cord blood from HIV-seropositive Haitian women. 4th International Conference on AIDS, Stockholm, Sweden, June 1988.

61. Baende E, Ryder R, Halsey N, Donnenberg A, Quinn T. Equally

poor response to tetanus vaccine in HIV seropositive and seronegative mothers in Zaire. 5th International AIDS Conference, Montreal, Canada, June 1989.

62. Teeuwsen VJP, Logtenberg T, Siebelink KHJ, et al. Analysis of the antigen- and mitogen-induced differentiation of B lymphocytes from asymptomatic human immunodeficiency virus-seropositive male homosexuals. *J Immunol* 1987;139:2929-35.

63. Halsey NA, Boulos R, Robert-Guroff M, et al. Measles vaccination of infants born to LAV/HTLVIII infected mothers. 2nd International Conference on AIDS Paris, France, 1986.

64. Ndikuyeze A, Taylor E, Faradegan H, et al. Measles immunization in children with human immunodeficiency virus infection. *Vaccine* 1987;5:168.

65. Kovamees J, Sheshberadaran H, Chiodi F, et al. Accentuated antibody response to paramyxoviruses in individuals infected with human immunodeficiency virus. *J Med Virol* 1988;26:41-8.

66. Kemper C, Zolopa A, Bhatia G, et al. Measles immunity in HIV infection. 7th International Conference on AIDS, Florence, Italy, June 1991.

67. Collier AC, Corey L, Murphy VL, Handsfield HH. Antibody to human immunodeficiency virus and suboptimal response to hepatitis B vaccination. *Ann Intern Med* 1988;109:101-5.

68. Carne CA, Weller IVD, Waite J, et al. Impaired responsiveness of homosexual men with HIV antibodies to plasma derived hepatitis B vaccine. *Br Med J* 1987;294:866-8.

69. Odaka N, Elred L, Cohn S, et al. Comparative immunogenicity of plasma and recombinant hepatitis B vaccines in homosexual men. *JAMA* 1988;260:3635-7.

70. Drake JH, Parmley RT, Britton HA. Loss of hepatitis B antibody in human immunodeficiency virus-positive hemophilia patients. *Pediatr Infect Dis* 1987;6:1051-4.

71. Geseman M, Scheiemann N, Brockmeyer N, et al. Clinical evaluation of a recombinant hepatitis B vaccine in HIV-infected vs. uninfected persons. In: Zuckerman AJ, ed. *Viral hepatitis and liver disease.* New York: Alan R Liss; 1988:1076-8.

72. Loke RHT, Anderson MG, Tsiquaye KN, et al. Reduced immunogenicity of recombinant yeast-derived hepatitis B vaccine in HIV antibody positive male homosexuals. In: Zuckerman AJ, ed. *Viral hepatitis and liver disease.* New York: Alan R Liss; 1988:1074-5.

73. Hadler SC, Judson F, Echenberg D, et al. Effect of prior human immunodeficiency virus infection on the outcome of hepatitis B virus infection. *J Med Virol* 1987;21:87A.

74. Hadler SC, Judson FN, O'Malley PM, et al. Studies of hepatitis B vaccine in homosexual men. In: Coursaget P, Tong MJ, eds. *Progress in hepatitis B immunization.* London: John Libbey Eurotext;1990:165-75.

75. Taylor PE, Stevens CE. Persistence of antibody to hepatitis B surface antigen after vaccination with hepatitis B vaccine. In: Zuckerman AJ, ed. *Viral hepatitis and liver disease.* New York: Alan R Liss;1988:995-7.

76. Immunization Practices Advisory Committee. Prevention and control of influenza. *MMWR* 1990;39(RR-7):1-15.

77. Immunization Practices Advisory Committee. Measles prevention: recommendations of the Immunization Practices Advisory Committee (ACIP). *MMWR* 1989;38(S-9):1-18.

78. Immunization Practices Advisory Committee. Protection against viral hepatitis: recommendations of the Immunization Practices Advisory Committee (ACIP). *MMWR* 1990;39(RR-2):1-26.

79. Immunization Practices Advisory Committee. Varicella-zoster immune globulin for the prevention of chickenpox. *MMWR* 1984;33:84-90,95-100.

80. Immunization Practices Advisory Committee. Typhoid immunization. *MMWR* 1990;39(RR-10):1-5.

81. Immunization Practices Advisory Committee. Yellow fever vaccine. *MMWR* 1990;39(RR-6):1-6.

82. Hibberd PL, Rubin RH. Immunization strategies for the immunocompromised host. *Ann Intern Med* 1989;110:955-6.

83. Ammann AJ, Schiffman G, Abrams D, Volberding P, Ziegler J, Conant M. B-cell immunodeficiency in acquired immune deficiency syndrome. *JAMA* 1984;251:1447-9.

84. Ballet JJ, Sulcebe G, Couderc LJ, et al. Impaired anti-pneumococcal antibody response in patients with AIDS-related persistent generalized lymphadenopathy. *Clin Exp Immunol* 1987;68:479-87.

85. Rhoads JL, Birx DL, Wright DC, Brundage J, Redfield RR, Burke DS. Response to vaccination in HIV seropositive subjects. 3rd International Conference on AIDS, Washington, DC, June 1987.

86. Janoff EN, Hardy WD, Smith PD, Chafey S, Fall H, Wahl SM. Humoral immune responses to recall antigens are intact in persons with HIV infection. Twenty-ninth Interscience Conference on Antimicrobial Agents and Chemotherapy, Houston, TX, Sept 17-20, 1989.

87. Varidinon N, Handsher R, Burke M, Zacut V, Yust I. Poliovirus vaccination responses in HIV-infected patients: correlation with T4 cell counts. *J Infect Dis* 1990;162:238-41.

*AIDS and Other Manifestations of HIV Infection,
Second Edition,* Edited by Gary P. Wormser.
Raven Press, Ltd., New York © 1992.

CHAPTER **43**

Nursing Perspectives in the Care of Patients with AIDS

Carol Joline

The AIDS epidemic is now in its 11th year in the United States, still without a cure or vaccine for prevention, and with a 100% mortality rate. Every day hundreds of individuals are newly diagnosed as seropositive for the human immunodeficiency virus (HIV) antibody, which indicates infection with HIV. Unlike most infectious diseases in the 20th century, AIDS, along with its multiple array of symptoms and debilitating infections, carries with it fear, prejudice, social stigma, and a tangle of political and ethical issues.

FEAR OF CONTAGION

The fear of contagion surrounding AIDS, especially during the first years of the epidemic, might be compared to that described by Garrison, writing about the bubonic plague epidemic in 15th century Europe (1). He states that there were many state and city ordinances against the plague, and in France, plague-stricken homes were burned to the ground while many patients were tortured and put to death. He states that "the physicians delegated to treat the plague wore a strange prophylactic garb, consisting of a long red or black gown of smooth material (often Morocco or Cordovan leather) with leather gauntlets, leather masks having glass-covered openings for the eyes, and a long beak or snout, filled with fumigants for the nose. In his hand the pest-doctor carried a wand to feel the pulse. In spite of the comic opera makeup, he was a highly esteemed functionary, often drawing a large salary."

This same fear of the unknown and fear of contagion have been observed in many nurses and other health-care workers caring for AIDS patients, especially those in

that role for the first time. While morally and legally bound to deliver quality health care to all patients, many nurses still struggle to overcome their anxiety when assigned to care for an AIDS patient. They must examine their commitment to nursing, as well as their own individual values.

There have always been certain risks in caring for patients with communicable diseases. In the past, nurses have accepted personal risks in caring for patients with such diseases as hepatitis B and tuberculosis. AIDS should be no different. Nursing is a chosen profession. The nurse accepts the moral and legal obligation to care for all sick people and is charged by the ethics of his/her profession to treat patients with all forms of sickness and disease (including AIDS)(2).

KNOWLEDGE AND ATTITUDES

We must recognize that the AIDS epidemic has created an arduous and difficult atmosphere for nurses. Although the stress is constant, there can also be rewards and great satisfaction in providing care for these patients.

Pasacreta and Jacobson (3) have classified nurses into two groups. The first group are nurses with limited or no AIDS experience, and the second, nurses specializing in AIDS care. They stated that nurses with little or no experience in caring for AIDS patients react in the ways most health-care workers did in the early 1980s when there was a paucity of knowledge about the disease. This group has great fear of contagion, will devote minimal time to the care of the AIDS patient, with minimal physical contact, and is likely to request a transfer. This group of nurses needs extensive in-service education. They stated that "ongoing professional education promotes learning about AIDS and affects attitudes in a positive direction, thus improving patient care and staff well-being."

C. Joline: AIDS Management Program, Westchester County Medical Center, Valhalla, New York 10595.

For the second group, nurses *specializing* in AIDS care, fear of contagion is no longer a primary issue. (However, it may resurface if a nurse becomes pregnant or sustains an accidental exposure such as a needlestick.) The experienced AIDS nurses are more concerned with burnout and professional isolation. Burnout is a term used for emotional and physical exhaustion causing occupational stress (3–5). Factors contributing to burnout are low staffing, lack of emotional support, and a feeling of helplessness as patients deteriorate toward eventual death.

Gignac and Oermann (6) report similar findings in studying student nurses. They found that there was a significant relationship between knowledge about AIDS and attitudes toward AIDS patients. They stated that in the few studies that have been done on the willingness of student nurses to care for AIDS patients, senior nursing students were more knowledgeable and willing to provide care than students in the first 2 years of school. The authors cited a study by Carwein and Bowles (1988) who reviewed AIDS policies and guidelines in 242 baccalaureate nursing programs. They stated that 86% had no guidelines for dealing with AIDS issues, and 49% had no plans to develop such policies. Gignac and Oermann also cited a study by Lawrence and Lawrence (1989), which found that factual information presented both in lecture format and small group discussion was most effective in increasing knowledge about AIDS as well as changing attitudes toward persons with AIDS. They also noted that van Servellen et al. (1988) have stated that educational programs are needed that are guided by principles of attitudinal change and that explore any biases student nurses may have about homosexuals and intravenous drug users. AIDS education should be ongoing, with frequent in-service programs and discussion groups, including reinforcement of universal precautions and other infection control issues (3,6).

EMOTIONAL ISOLATION OF THE PATIENT

Nurses and other health-care workers may contribute to an AIDS patient's sense of isolation and abandonment by practicing unnecessary or exaggerated isolation precautions and by avoiding all but the most essential interactions with the patient. These emotional and physical barriers may add to the patient's loneliness, depression, and anger. Brock (7) writes about visiting a patient who told him "you've got to wear a space suit to come in this room. Didn't they tell you?" The *patient* was being isolated instead of his disease. The patient went on to reveal that this visit by a health-care worker *not* in a space suit was the first time he had touched another person in 12 days. (Most AIDS patients will express how important it is for them to be touched and hugged.)

Lack of knowledge by health-care providers early in the AIDS epidemic elicited some strange actions and be-

havior. A family member reported that he was told by a health-care worker to burn everything at home that the patient had touched (8). AIDS hysteria fosters use of excessive barrier precautions and occasionally a nurse's or physician's flat refusal to care for patients with AIDS (4,9). In addition to their fear of AIDS, many are biased against persons with socially unaccepted life-styles such as homosexuality and illicit drug use.

NURTURING AND COMPASSION

Nurses possibly represent the largest group of health-care professionals caring for AIDS patients. As stated by Chow (9): "The physician gives the patient the diagnosis, but it is the nurse who picks the patient up after the diagnosis. It is the nurse who listens to the patient's fears and doubts. It is the nurse who talks with the patient's family about the obstacles that must be overcome and the adjustments that need to be made." As is the case for any hospitalized patient, patient satisfaction is due in large part to nursing. In addition, primary care nursing allows the nurse to provide all the care for his/her patients and fosters greater trust and communication. This is a key factor in caring for the AIDS patient.

NOSOCOMIAL TRANSMISSION

AIDS presents a significant conflict for nurses—caring for patients for whom there is no cure and from whom they may accidentally contract the disease themselves. Although AIDS is not transmitted by casual contact, there have been at least 11 documented nosocomial infections with HIV seroconversion among health-care workers in the United States, from needlesticks or mucous membrane splashes of blood or body fluids from HIV infected patients (10). Brown (11) stated that nurses are forced to review their commitment to nursing and their individual values and beliefs. Moral and ethical decisions must be made. Values need to be reexamined. Brown also stated that nurses caring for AIDS patients need two dominant characteristics—courage and impartiality. "Courage is needed to confront risks, particularly in facing an illness that poses a threat. Impartiality is needed to temper prejudice" (11). Although it is well known that AIDS may infect any person and is not limited to homosexual men and intravenous drug users, many people still associate it with these groups. Nurses must be knowledgeable about the mechanisms of transmission of HIV and the necessary actions to follow (universal precautions) to prevent transmission.

ACCIDENTAL OCCUPATIONAL EXPOSURE

An occupational exposure is defined as one in which an individual sustains a percutaneous injury (such as a needlestick or a cut with a sharp instrument), or a splash onto a mucous membrane or nonintact skin, with blood, tissues, or certain body fluids from an HIV-infected person (12). If such an exposure should occur, the individual should wash his/her hands and other sites of exposure immediately (preferably with an antimicrobial soap) and report the incident without delay. Studies have shown that the risk of HIV infection after a percutaneous exposure is small (0.4%) (13). However, there is risk nonetheless. At present there is no established prophylaxis against HIV infection after an exposure, although zidovudine (AZT) is often used for this purpose (12). The best line of defense is prevention of exposure.

PSYCHOSOCIAL ISSUES

In caring for AIDS patients, nurses must not only address the medical aspects of the illness but must be concerned with the psychosocial impact of the illness and the diagnosis upon the patient. Upon learning of the diagnosis, AIDS patients will experience various emotions, including anxiety, fear, denial, anger, and guilt. They will have an overwhelming sense of powerlessness, grieving, depression, and social isolation (14). Nurses and other professionals should support AIDS patients in confronting and accepting death at an early age. AIDS patients must develop coping skills to make their remaining years or months meaningful to them. Since AIDS usually affects a younger population than most chronic and fatal illnesses, these individuals lack the experience to cope with death and dying. In addition, a patient's anger against him/herself, his/her disease, or the manner in which he/she became infected may often be targeted against his/her nurses and others. This should be recognized for what it is. We must try to help the patient direct this anger toward positive action.

FAMILIES AND FRIENDS

Today, AIDS remains a socially unacceptable disease to a large portion of society. While the families of some AIDS patients may be caring and supportive, many may have rejected their family members even prior to their diagnoses because of dislike of their life-styles (homosexuality and/or intravenous drug use). Many parents will further reject their children upon learning of the diagnosis of AIDS. Families may not wish to be associated with the disease because of fear of stigmatization and/or the fear of contagion. Making it even more difficult for families is that they must watch their previously healthy, relatively young loved ones progress toward total debilitation and unavoidable death. Often, the only available "family" are friends and/or a significant other. For many patients, health-care professionals will become part of their family.

THE DEDICATED AIDS UNIT

Factors to consider when deciding whether to care for AIDS/HIV patients on a dedicated unit or in scatter-site beds include the projected average daily census of eligible patients and the availability of staff and support services. For those institutions treating fewer than 10 patients a day, the scatter-site model can be effective. However, for those with an inpatient census of 10–20 or more, the establishment of a dedicated unit would be ideal (15–17). Advantages of a dedicated AIDS care unit are many, as the AIDS and HIV patients require comprehensive multidisciplinary care and case management services. Nursing care of the adult AIDS patient differs from that of other patients admitted with a serious illness, in that the prognosis is always poor, there is often multisystem failure, and there are many psychosocial needs to be met (18,19). The nursing staff assigned to a unit are there because they wish to care for AIDS patients. This ensures both the quality and quantity of care delivered to these patients. The dedicated unit concept also facilitates communication among the various staff members and disciplines involved.

The multidisciplinary case management model includes nursing, medicine, social work, nutritional care, psychiatry, psychology, and occupational and physical therapy. Closely related in a consultative capacity are the dental, ophthalmology, gynecology, and pharmacy departments. This model facilitates better continuity of care as well as a closer relationship between patients and care givers (16). Weekly case management rounds are held as well as more informal nursing rounds on a daily basis. Advantages extend to the patients' psychosocial needs as well. Case managers can provide individual therapeutic care, as well as act as facilitators in group therapy. Patients are able to receive support from team members as well as from other patients. Many patients develop positive relationships with each other that may continue after discharge. AIDS patients may be subjected to periods of acute illness interspersed with periods of wellness eventually leading to the need for terminal care; continued support is essential (20). In New York State the guidelines for a dedicated AIDS/HIV inpatient care unit recommend between 7.2 and 10.3 nursing hours per patient over a 24-hr period (a regular medical–surgical patient would require about 4.5 hr) (M. Carraher, *personal communication, 1991*). AIDS patients require more nursing hours due to the complexity of illness in which a patient may have multiple disease processes simultaneously. As a result of their immunocompromised state, HIV-infected patients are prone to numerous opportunistic infections and certain malignancies. Upon admission to the unit, the patient's nursing needs are assessed, including the following categories: respiratory status, cardiovascular status, general nutrition and diet regimen, functions of elimination (bladder and bowel), neurological and sensory orientation, skin and mucous membrane integrity, pain management, sleep patterns, ability to perform the activities of daily living, current status of sexual activity, social support systems, educational needs (including the ability to learn and to understand), and the patient's medication history (18,21,22). Discharge planning also starts at this time. This should involve the patient's family and/or significant other, as well as members of the AIDS care team. This facilitates the patient's discharge to home or transfer to alternate care at the end of hospitalization. Comprehensive case management also includes follow-up care as an outpatient. Services in this area include periodic checkups, monitoring of laboratory values, and outpatient treatments for preventive therapy. The physical nursing care as well as the emotional support received on the dedicated AIDS unit will assist the patient in coming to terms with the illness and accepting the prognosis (18).

A POSITIVE APPROACH

A positive approach by nursing and other health-care workers is essential and ideally should transfer to the patient. Patients should be assisted in developing a clear understanding of the disease and a positive attitude toward their care and general state of health, in other words, not to give up hope.

It is also important for the patient to develop positive feelings about death and dying. This includes completing unfinished business and making peace with one's self. If the health-care worker is not in touch with his/her own feelings about death and dying, he/she will not be able to provide comprehensive care to the AIDS patient.

In addition, the health-care worker must be comfortable in caring for AIDS patients without fear of contagion. Only then will it be possible to develop a meaningful relationship with the patient. Most AIDS patients, after years of rejection, isolation, and painful loneliness, have developed a keen sense of awareness in perceiving other's feelings and fears in relation to their disease. Nurses and other health-care workers must be able to achieve a nonjudgmental, caring, touching approach to their patients (who are first individuals and secondly happen to have a fatal illness, AIDS). Touching is necessary and important. Farrell et al. (23) state "a good nurse should know when to lead, when to follow, when to be side by side and when just to be there."

SUPPORT SYSTEMS FOR THE HEALTH-CARE PROVIDERS

The emotional well-being of the health-care providers is necessary in order to promote optimal care of AIDS patients (3). The question often asked is: While the health-care provider is providing care to patients, who is

providing care to the health-care provider? Bolle (24) states that "AIDS . . . has brought a new dimension to stress and burnout in terminal care." Weekly support groups for care providers can help individuals learn how to maintain a positive attitude.

CONCLUSION

AIDS patients should be helped to view themselves as *living* with their disease, not dying from it. It is most important that we help the patient accomplish the very highest quality of life possible and maintain a positive approach toward the future, whatever it may hold.

ACKNOWLEDGMENTS

I am grateful to Margaret Carraher, Patricia Ames, and Alida Pereira for their help and suggestions in preparing this chapter.

REFERENCES

1. Garrison FH. *An introduction to the history of medicine.* Philadelphia: Saunders, 1929.
2. Health and Public Policy Committee, American College of Physicians; Infectious Diseases Society of America. The acquired immunodeficiency virus (HIV). *Ann Intern Med* 1988;108:460–9.
3. Pasacreta JV, Jacobson PB. Addressing the need for staff support among nurses caring for the AIDS population. *Oncol Nurs Forum* 1989;16:653–9.
4. Lovejoy NC. Family and care giver responses to HIV infection. In: Gee G, Moran TA, eds. *AIDS: concepts in nursing practice.* Baltimore: Williams & Wilkins; 1988:379–401.
5. Christ GH, Siegal K, Moynihan RT. Psychosocial issues: prevention and treatment. In: De Vita V, Hellman S, Rosenberg S, eds. *AIDS: etiology, diagnosis, treatment, and prevention.* Philadelphia: Lippincott; 1988:321–37.
6. Gignac D, Oermann MH. Willingness of nursing students and faculty to care for patients with AIDS. *Am J Infect Control* 1991;19:191–7.
7. Brock R. Beyond fear: the next step in nursing the patient with AIDS. *Nurs Manage* 1988;19:46–7.
8. Cecchi R. Living with AIDS: when the system fails. *Am J Nurs* 1986;86:45–7.
9. Chow M. Nursing's response to the challenge of AIDS. *Nurs Outlook* 1989;37:82–3.
10. CDC. Update: acquired immunodeficiency syndrome and human immunodeficiency virus infection among health care workers. *MMWR* 1988;37:229–39.
11. Brown ML. AIDS and ethics: concerns and considerations. In: Gee G, Moran TA, eds. *AIDS: concepts in nursing practice.* Baltimore: Williams & Wilkins; 1988:351–60.
12. CDC. Public Health Service statement on management of occupational exposure to human immunodeficiency virus, including considerations regarding zidovudine postexposure use. *MMWR* 1990;39(RR-1):1–14.
13. Marcus R, CDC Cooperative Needlestick Study Group. Surveillance of health-care workers exposed to blood from patients infected with the human immunodeficiency virus. *N Engl J Med* 1988;319:1118–23.
14. Gee G. Individual psychosocial responses to HIV infection. In: Gee G, Moran TA, eds. *AIDS: concepts in nursing practice.* Baltimore: Williams & Wilkins; 1988:361–78.
15. Morrison C. Nursing perspectives in the care of patients with AIDS. In: Wormser GP, Stall R, Bottone E, eds. *AIDS—acquired*

immune deficiency syndrome—and other manifestations of HIV infection. Park Ridge, NJ: Noyes Publications; 1987:1082–95.

16. Pellegrino V, Spicehandler D. Dedicated AIDS units: pros and cons. *AIDS Patient Care* 1988;2(4):8–11.

17. Oberlink M. The AIDS cluster. *AIDS Patient Care* 1988; 2(2):26–9.

18. Rosenthal Y, Haneiwich S. Nursing management of adults in the hospital. *Nurs Clin of North Am* 1988;23(4):707–18.

19. New York State Office of Mental Health. *Nursing management of the patient with AIDS.* New York: NYS Office of Mental Health; 1991.

20. Grady C. Acquired immunodeficiency syndrome, the impact on professional nursing practice. *Cancer Nurs* 1989;12(1):1–9.

21. Ungvarski PJ. Nursing management of the adult client. In: Flaskerund JH, ed. *AIDS/HIV infection, a reference guide for nursing professionals.* Philadelphia: Saunders; 1989:74–110.

22. Reno CL, Walker AP. Providing direct nursing care in the adult inpatient setting. In: Lewis A, ed. *Nursing care of the patients with AIDS/ARC.* Rockville, MD: Aspen Publishers; 1988:73–89.

23. Farrell M, Wells R, Nygaard OM. Janforum: AIDS—an interview with Ole Morten Nygaard who is HIV positive. *J Adv Nurs* 1990;15:859–64.

24. Bolle JL. Supporting the deliverers of care: strategies to support nurses and prevent burnout. *Nurs Clin North Am* 1988; 23(4):843–50.

AIDS and Other Manifestations of HIV Infection,
Second Edition, Edited by Gary P. Wormser.
Raven Press, Ltd., New York © 1992.

CHAPTER 44

AIDS and the Ethics of Prevention, Research, and Care

Ronald Bayer

AIDS, the first serious epidemic disease to strike advanced industrial nations in more than a generation, has posed an extraordinary array of ethical challenges. As a lethal illness, spread in the context of the most intimate relationships, it has forced us to confront many difficult questions, including what constitutes the appropriate public health role of the state. As a disease of the socially vulnerable, those who have been subject to irrational reactions stemming from fears associated with HIV infection, AIDS has compelled Americans to face issues involving the need to employ the power of the state to protect the weak at moments of social stress. As a disease that has affected large numbers of poor individuals without adequate health insurance, AIDS has required us once again to consider what justice demands in terms of the protection of all against the costs associated with illness. Thus the roles of government in advancing the public health, defending the weak, and assuring access to health care have all been called upon by the AIDS epidemic.

In this chapter, three broad topics are considered: the ethics of prevention and protection, the ethics of research, and the ethics of care.

THE ETHICS OF PREVENTION AND PROTECTION

In the United States as well as in other nations bounded by the liberal tradition, ethical considerations and pragmatic concerns have both contributed to the adoption of public health strategies to control the spread of HIV infection that may be broadly defined as voluntaristic—stressing mass education, counseling, and re-

R. Bayer: Columbia University School of Public Health, New York, New York 10032.

spect for privacy (1). This general consensus has affected policies on testing for HIV infection, the protection of confidentiality, and the use of the coercive powers of the state to restrict those whose behaviors are thought to pose a risk of HIV transmission.

Testing and Voluntarism

From the outset, the test developed to detect antibody to HIV—first used on a broad scale in blood banking—was mired in controversy. Uncertainty about the significance of the test's findings and about the quality and accuracy provided the technical substrate of disputes that inevitably took on a political and ethical character, since issues of privacy, communal health, social and economic discrimination, coercion, and liberty were always involved. How would the test be used outside the context of blood banking? Would groups at increased risk for AIDS be encouraged to take the test? How forceful would such encouragement be? How would those who agreed to be tested be counseled about the test's significance for themselves and others? Would, and could, the results be kept confidential? Would voluntary testing be a prelude to compulsory screening? What would be the consequence of testing for the right to work? To go to school? To obtain insurance? To bear children? To remain free? Each of these questions would force a confrontation over the fundamental matter of the relationship between the defense of privacy and the protection of the public health; over the roles of voluntarism and coercion in the social response to the threat of AIDS.

Out of the controversies that whirled about the antibody test, there emerged a broad voluntarist consensus. Except for clearly circumscribed circumstances, testing was to be done under conditions of voluntary, informed consent only after counseling that outlined both the benefits and risks of testing, and the results were to be protected by stringent confidentiality safeguards. In the United States, to underscore the importance of protecting the privacy of tested individuals, the option of anonymous testing was made broadly available. The voluntarist consensus was supported by gay leaders (2), civil libertarians (3), bioethicists (4), public health officials (5), and professional organizations representing clinicians (6). But as broad as the consensus was, it was also fragile, because it was based on differing interests and commitments. It was a consensus shaped by the relative impotence of medicine in the epidemic's first years.

Remarkable advances in therapeutics and a wide range of clinical trials for which the infected may be eligible have changed the outlook for patients with HIV infection. Under these new circumstances, the potential benefits of testing have become apparent (7). Persons who formerly urged those at risk for infection to exercise great caution before seeking to know their antibody status now encourage voluntary confidential or anonymous testing. Under such circumstances, a growing number of clinicians want to loosen the requirements for specific informed consent before HIV-antibody testing occurs. In short, clinicians have begun to assert that the time has come to "return AIDS to the medical mainstream."

Given the traditions of medicine, such impatience is not surprising. But ethicists have continued to argue for the centrality of consent (8). A number of arguments have been put forward in this regard. First, as much as the clinical picture has begun to change, there is no definitive therapeutic course for HIV-infected, but otherwise asymptomatic, individuals. At the same time, the prospects of stigma and discrimination have remained a threat to the social well-being of HIV-infected persons. Under these conditions, the arguments for specific informed consent have been viewed as important as ever. But ethicists have gone further, arguing that even were the clinical picture to improve dramatically, the moral basis for insisting on informed consent before HIV testing would not change. Their conclusions are derived from the well-established principle of medical ethics that competent adults have the right to determine whether or not to undergo treatment or to terminate treatments already begun. The principle that limits the paternalistic authority of the physician to order therapies in the interest of the patient, it has been argued, extends to the authority to order those tests that would serve as the basis for commencing treatment.

But if those concerned with respect for the autonomy of the patient have continued to assert that physicians should exercise restraint, they have also begun to claim that the physician's ethical responsibility to provide appropriate care, the principle of beneficence, now requires physicians to offer HIV-antibody testing routinely to those patients whose social histories suggest some in-

creased possibility of infection. Only by being offered such tests can patients have the opportunity to learn whether or not they are infected. Only then can they exercise their right to choose whether or not to begin therapy or enter available clinical trials. The process of reaching the informed consent of patients for such testing, however, must clearly define the social risks associated with being identified as infected as well as the clinical benefits that may be associated with treatment.

More complex is the question of whether the current situation justifies the routine or mandatory screening of infants born to mothers at risk for HIV infection (9). Some pediatricians have asserted that the early identification of infected newborns provides an opportunity to initiate aggressive intervention, including the prophylactic administration of zidovudine (AZT), or the early commencement of *Pneumocystis carinii* pneumonia prophylaxis. Others have been more skeptical of what can be done for asymptomatic infants. Furthermore, current testing technology does not permit the routine identification of babies infected with HIV. The enzyme-linked immunosorbent assay test merely reveals the presence of maternal antibody. Since 70–80% of those born to infected mothers are uninfected, the antibody test is inadequate for identifying newborns who could hypothetically benefit from therapeutic or prophylactic intervention. The polymerase chain reaction (PCR) technique, though experimental now, may make early identification possible in the future. What current testing can do is identify the existence of an infected mother. Thus the mandatory testing of newborns is, in fact, the mandatory testing of women who have given birth. From an ethical perspective, before such identification can be permitted, without consent, it will be necessary to demonstrate more than a hypothetical benefit to the infant.

The debate over newborn testing takes place against a background of widely accepted mandatory or routine testing of newborns to permit the identification of those in need of special treatment (10). Screening in these instances is held to represent a legitimate exercise of the state's power to protect the vulnerable. Screening for phenylketonuria (PKU) is a good example of such testing. Early identification of newborns with PKU is critical so that a special dietary regime can be initiated. The failure to undertake such a therapeutic intervention can be catastrophic for the child. A definitive diagnostic test, a definitive therapeutic intervention, and an imperative to act quickly are the conditions that provide the empirical and moral grounds for the routine screening of newborns without first seeking parental consent.

None of these conditions now prevails in the case of HIV. Thus there is, from an ethical perspective, no basis for mandatory newborn screening. Were a diagnostic procedure for identifying infection in the newborn developed, and were a therapy for such infants available, the clinical and ethical bases for making a claim on behalf of the vulnerable child would exist. Such developments might well be sufficient to establish the grounds for testing without prior parental consent.

Screening for Safety

Because AIDS represented the first major infectious threat with which advanced industrial societies had to contend in almost a generation, and because the causative agent was not identified until 3 years after the first case reports, it is not surprising that it provoked considerable social anxiety. How was it spread? Who posed a risk? Who was endangered? That AIDS was a disease of socially marginal, and not infrequently despised, individuals only intensified the urge toward discrimination. Employers, landlords, school personnel, and even the staff of some health-care institutions evidenced a willingness to exclude those with the new disease. With the discovery of HIV, and the development of a test that could detect antibody to the virus, the potential scope for discriminatory activity increased, despite the epidemiological evidence about how infection was spread.

In the United States, the Centers for Disease Control moved swiftly to contain the irrational impulse toward exclusion. At the end of 1985, guidelines to prevent the spread of HIV infection in schools (11) and the workplace (12) were issued. Early in 1986, detailed guidelines for health-care workers on preventing the spread of infection while engaged in invasive procedures were published (13). In each instance, the goal was to convey information, to provide protection, and to prevent panic. The message was clear: HIV could not be casually transmitted, and so there were no grounds for exclusion of infected individuals, who otherwise were capable of performing their expected functions, from school and workplace. There were thus no grounds for mandatory testing for HIV. In the context of the health-care setting, universal blood and body fluid precautions would protect workers not only from HIV but from the far more infectious hepatitis B. Screening could only provide illusory protections.

Five years of careful surveillance have revealed the fundamental wisdom of the CDC's recommendations on schools and workplaces (14). No cases of casual transmission have been recorded. Although there are still shameful occurrences of efforts to exclude or isolate school children with AIDS or HIV infection, and although cases of discrimination by employers continue to occur, they are almost universally deplored as irrational, unscientific, and retrograde. There are some notable exceptions: the U.S. government screens all applicants for the armed forces, the foreign service, and the Job Corps, an employment program for poor youth (1). In the case of the military and foreign service, it is clear that exclusionary efforts are motivated both by political concerns

over relations between the United States and other governments, and by a long-standing official antihomosexual bias; in the case of the Job Corps, by concerns about sexual relations between those who would reside in special camps. Such policies, whatever their justification, have little bearing on the more general recognition that screening in the workplace is unnecessary for the protection and safety of workers.

The situation in health care has not been so clear-cut. The relatively few cases of transmission that have occurred as a result of needlesticks, and the even smaller number of transmissions linked to blood splashes (15), have provoked distress among health-care workers, especially among surgeons, obstetricians, nurses, and emergency room personnel. Those whose work regularly brings them into contact with their patients' blood have felt vulnerable. On rare occasions they have asserted the right to refuse to care for the infected (16)—rejecting fundamental principles of medical ethics (17). Far more frequently, such clinicians have publicly challenged the adequacy of the recommendations for universal blood and body fluid precautions. Instead, they have demanded the right to know whether or not their patients are infected, and the right to screen on a routine or mandatory basis for HIV infection. The level of vigilance demanded by the threat of a lethal infection cannot, they have argued, be maintained at all times. Protection requires knowledge of infection. The conflict between public health officials who have declared that universal precautions are adequate, and clinicians who have asserted that they are not, has not abated; indeed, it has intensified. A deep fissure has thus emerged, rupturing the broad alliance that had existed within the medical profession. This is not a situation that can long endure.

Paralleling this debate has been a revived interest in the question of the appropriate measures to protect patients from HIV-infected clinicians. Some have argued that although professionals have a moral duty to assume some risks—especially those that are quite small—in caring for their patients, patients do not have an equivalent duty to expose themselves to even small risks when being cared for (18). Dismissing as irrational those who would deny all infected health-care workers, whatever their functions, the right to engage in clinical work, many have asserted that physicians whose invasive work can place their patients at some risk ought not to engage in those procedures. Both the American Dental Association and the American Medical Association have asserted that infected clinicians have a duty to either inform their patients or to desist from invasive procedures. But if those who know themselves to be infected with HIV have such professional duties, are there correlative institutional obligations to identify the infected, to exclude them from certain functions? Are they obligated to screen health-care workers, and if so, at what frequency? Might concern about protecting patients provide the basis for mandatory screening and surveillance after so much effort to forestall such programs? And if screening and surveillance were to be adopted, what would be the impact on an anxious social climate? These matters have taken on a new urgency with the first report by the CDC that a dentist with AIDS may have transmitted HIV to several of his patients.

Finally, it is necessary to comment on the trend toward the screening and segregation of infected individuals who reside in "total institutions," not because of irrational fears of casual transmission or because of the uncertainties that surround transmission in health-care settings, but because of the possibility of sexual transmission. Prisons in the United States with large numbers of inmates with histories of intravenous drug use—especially on the East Coast—and where homosexual relations, including rape, occur more frequently than officials would like to acknowledge are paradigmatic.

In general, the support for HIV screening and segregation has been stronger in locales with few cases, where the administrative consequences of separating the infected would not be too burdensome. In New York, by contrast, such a strategy might well require the creation of a parallel prison system. Prisoners' rights advocates have almost universally opposed such measures, viewing them as repressive, an extension of the practice of administrative segregation that always represents an intensification of the punitive regime. Instead, they have advocated education, the provision of condoms (what an acknowledgement of prison homosexuality that would require!), and the segregation of only those who are sexually assaultive. Prisoners are, after all, despite their crimes, capable of making crucial decisions about matters involving sexual expression and the assumption of risks if only they were to be given the information and paraphernalia associated with "safer sex."

It is more difficult to define the appropriate course in psychiatric hospitals or residential facilities for the mentally retarded. There, too, there is sexual activity. But those for whom responsibility has been assumed are by definition limited in their capacities. They are vulnerable and, in a fundamental sense, require protection. Should they be screened and, if infected, separated or kept under very careful watch? How far does the obligation to protect the health of the uninfected extend? And what burden or restriction on the infected is tolerable? Who will benefit? Who will lose? These are matters of profound clinical and ethical importance in those areas where HIV represents a threat. They are questions in need of urgent and nuanced attention rather than formulaic responses.

In years to come, new controversies over screening will surely arise. In each of these conflicts, those who confront each other will predictably seek to appropriate the mantle of value-free decision making and will charge that those with whom they disagree have deserted the

standards of science. On some occasions, the risk posed by the infected will be understood to be so small and the implications of screening and exclusion so burdensome that even the most cautious will find it hard to justify compulsory testing and the imposition of restrictions; on other occasions, the choices will not be clear-cut. But in each case, more than "science" will be involved. Decisions about screening policy will reflect the balance of moral commitments to privacy, reason, and communal well-being.

Confidentiality and Its Limits

There is perhaps no ethical issue involving AIDS that has received more attention than that of confidentiality. That gay men and those who have spoken on their behalf have placed such great stress on confidentiality should come as no surprise. A history of oppression and the existence of antisodomy laws have made the protection of privacy a critical feature of the struggle for social survival. But the call for the protection of confidentiality has come as well from the Surgeon General (19), the Centers for Disease Control (20), the Institute of Medicine and the National Academy of Sciences (21), the Presidential Commission on the HIV Epidemic (22), and public health officials across the nation (23).

The issue of confidentiality had surfaced even before the discovery of HIV. When little was known about the etiology of AIDS, broad-scale epidemiological research was necessary to begin the process of unraveling the mysteries of the new disease. Such studies required careful investigations of the sexual behavior of those who had become sick—recent emigrants from Haiti, gay men, and intravenous drug users. Socially vulnerable, none could be expected to speak with candor or to cooperate with investigators unless ironclad assurances could be given that what they revealed about themselves would be kept in confidence—that none of the information would be shared with law enforcement officials, immigration authorities, employers, or insurers (24).

When the role of HIV as the etiological agent responsible for AIDS was discovered and an antibody test was developed to reveal infection, the importance of confidentiality became all the more important. If individuals were to come forward for testing and counseling, it was imperative for them to believe that in doing so they would not be placing themselves at social risk. Thus at the same time as public health officials began to press aggressively for wide-scale voluntary testing, they were also impelled to insist that the results of testing be carefully shielded. The protection of the public health and the protection of privacy were intimately linked.

And so in those states that were so profoundly affected by AIDS, public health officials pressed for the enactment of especially stringent legislative and administrative safeguards. The centrality of confidentiality to the pursuit of public health objectives provided an explanation for the unique decision in states with relatively high AIDS case counts not to require reporting of the names of individuals with HIV infection to public health registries, despite the fact that AIDS itself has been a reportable condition in all states since 1983 (1). Although the late 1980s witnessed a gradual shift on this policy matter, respect for the privacy of those who are infected with HIV has continued to influence policymakers in many states.

But what of the role of confidentiality in the clinical setting? The importance of confidentiality in the clinical encounter derives from two quite distinct sources. On moral grounds, respect for the dignity and autonomy of the patient is held to require that those communications made with an expectation that they will be shielded from others will be treated as inviolable. From a pragmatic perspective, confidentiality is held to be critical to candor on the part of the patient; without assurances of confidentiality patients might be inhibited from revealing clinically relevant information. Without confidentiality the very possibility of establishing a therapeutic relationship might thus be subverted.

But despite the importance of confidentiality to the practice of medicine, physicians on their own, under pressure from colleagues, and most frequently as a result of state requirements, have at times revealed their patients' secrets when some threat to the safety or well-being of others was involved (25). The moral and pragmatic underpinnings of confidentiality have thus yielded to supervening moral and societal claims.

Many courts in the United States have acknowledged the moral imperative of protecting third parties in immediate danger (26). The course of judicial opinion has, however, been fraught with controversy. The most celebrated case is *Tarasoff* v. *Regents of the State of California* (27). The Supreme Court of California held that if a psychotherapist reasonably believes that a patient poses a direct physical threat to a third party, he or she must warn the endangered person. The *Tarasoff* decision produced an avalanche of concern about the extent to which patients would be discouraged from confiding their dangerous thoughts to their therapists.

Those who have considered the ethical, as contrasted with the legal, dimensions of the conflict between the claims of confidentiality and the duty to warn have, in general, asserted that there are circumstances under which the sanctity of the clinical encounter may be breached (28). When a physician is uniquely positioned to warn an identifiable individual about an intended grave harm, the principles of medical ethics cannot, according to most interpretations, be held to prevent clinicians from warning potential victims in a timely and effective manner. There is less agreement on the extent to which breaches of confidentiality under such circumstances should be morally obligatory or left to the physician's discretion.

It is against this backdrop that clinicians, public health officials, and politicians have struggled with the question of how to act when an HIV-infected patient refuses to inform identifiable, unsuspecting past or current partners about the dangers of infection. In the case of past partners, concern has centered on the possibility that an unknowingly infected individual might act as unwitting agent of transmission to yet others. In the case of current partners, the focus has been on the possibility of preventing the transmission of HIV to an as yet uninfected individual. As these issues were considered, it became clear that the process of warning past sexual partners did not require the identification of the source of potential infection. No public health goal would be served by breaching the cloak of anonymity of the index case. Where an infected individual refused to warn a current partner, the situation posed graver difficulties. Without revealing the source of potential infection, it was possible that no effective protective warning could be made.

Informing the dispute about how it might be best to proceed has been a deep concern about the consequences that could well follow were it to be widely believed that physicians would routinely breach confidentiality when presented with a patient who refused to warn past or current partners about the risk of HIV infection. Would the consequence be a reduction in clinical candor? Would patients be discouraged from seeking to know their HIV status? Would they be less accessible to the efforts of clinicians to convince them of the importance of warning those who might be at risk? In sum, would breaching confidentiality to warn unsuspecting individuals result in a net loss from the perspective of public health? Here a troubling irony became clear. Conventionally, the ethics of the diadic clinical encounter has been thought to involve the greatest commitment to privacy and confidentiality; the ethics of public health to place less weight on such values. Yet under these circumstances the ethics of the clinical encounter—overriding confidentiality to warn another—appeared to dictate a course that from the perspective of public health might well be counterproductive. The ethics of public health, concerned with the well-being of the community, might require a greater commitment to confidentiality than the ethics of the clinical encounter!

Beginning in the latter part of 1987, a number of efforts were made in the United States to resolve the issues associated with the warning of unsuspecting third parties. Each reflected an effort to define appropriate professional roles and to chart a prudential course that would achieve the greatest overall protection of the public health without too grave a sacrifice of the principled and pragmatic defense of confidentiality.

At the end of 1987, the American Medical Association

issued a broad set of statements on the ethical issues posed by the AIDS epidemic (29). In that document the AMA addressed the issue of warning in a forthright manner. Physicians were to try to convince patients of their obligation to warn the unsuspecting. If they failed in that task, they were to seek the intervention of public health officials. Only if public health officials refused or were unwilling to take on the responsibility of warning was it the obligation of the physician to act directly.

When the Presidential Commission on the HIV Epidemic addressed this issue in mid-1988, it too endorsed the notion that physicians should have the right to breach confidentiality in order to warn the unsuspecting, despite the centrality of confidentiality to its overall strategy (30). Reflecting, however, a commitment to professional autonomy, the Commission held that the decision about whether to breach confidentiality was to remain with the physician and was not to be imposed as a matter of law.

That too was the stance of a wide spectrum of public health officials, including the Association of State and Territorial Health Officials (31), who chose to speak of a "privilege to disclose" rather than a duty to warn. Concerned about the potential public health impact of such efforts, the mid-1988 publication, *Guide to Public Health Practice: HIV Partner Notification Strategies,* urged that the identity of the index case only be revealed in the "rare case" of ongoing exposure by an individual who would under no conditions be suspected as a potential source of harm. Under such circumstances, it was public health officials, rather than clinicians, who were to be responsible for making the critical determinations and interventions. More than 20 state legislatures have adopted the privilege to disclose doctrine, while only two have imposed such a duty.

Coercive Controls

The question of how to respond to individuals whose behavior represented a threat to unknowing partners inevitably provoked discussion of the public health tradition of imposing restrictions on liberty in the name of communal welfare. The specter of quarantine has haunted all such discussions, not because there was any serious consideration in the United States of the Cuban approach to AIDS—which mandates the isolation of all persons infected with HIV (32)—but because of fears that even a more limited recognition of the authority to quarantine would lead to egregious intrusions upon privacy and invidiously imposed deprivations of freedom.

Although fierce opposition has surfaced to all efforts to bring AIDS within the scope of state quarantine statutes, more than a dozen states had done so between 1987 and 1990, typically using the occasion to modernize their disease control laws to reflect contemporary constitutional standards, which detail procedural guarantees, and to require that restrictions on freedom represent the "least restrictive alternative" available to achieve a "compelling state interest" (33).

Soon after he resigned as Commissioner of Health in New York City at the end of 1989, Stephen Joseph bluntly made the case for the careful exercise of the power of quarantine (34). He noted that among his last formal acts had been the signing of a detention order for a woman with infectious tuberculosis because of her repeated unwillingness to take the medication that would render her noninfectious. "It is virtually certain that at some point, a New York City Health Commissioner will be faced with an analogous situation concerning the transmission of the AIDS virus. When all lesser remedies have failed, can anyone doubt what would be the proper course of action for the Commissioner to take, faced with . . . an infected individual who knowingly and repeatedly sold his blood for transfusion?" When and if a treatment became available that would render HIV-infected persons less infectious, "would there not then be a clear obligation to take all reasonable measures to ensure that the infected take their medication, thus protecting others?"

With the exception of the few notable cases that have received press attention, there is no well-documented review of the extent to which newly revised quarantine statutes have been applied to the AIDS epidemic. There are, however, data to suggest that the power vested in public health officials by such laws has been used more often to warn those whose behavior has posed a risk of HIV transmission than to incarcerate. But in any case the numbers have been small.

The enactment of statutes criminalizing behaviors linked to the spread of AIDS has paralleled the political receptivity to laws extending the authority of public health officials to control individuals whose behavior posed a risk of HIV transmission. Such use of the criminal law, broadly endorsed by the Presidential Commission on the HIV Epidemic, called upon a tradition of state enactments that made the knowing transmission of venereal disease a crime (30). Though they almost never were enforced, the existence of these older laws served as a rationale for new legislative initiatives. Between 1987 and 1989, 20 states enacted such statutes, the vast majority of which defined the proscribed acts as felonies despite the fact that older statutes typically treated knowing transmission as a misdemeanor (33). As important, aggressive prosecutors have relied on laws defining assaultive behavior and attempted murder to bring indictments even in the absence of AIDS-specific legislation.

Any effort to determine the extent to which prosecutions for HIV-related acts have occurred must confront the difficulty of monitoring the activity of local courts when there is neither a guilty verdict nor an appeal to a higher state tribunal. One survey, relying on newspaper accounts as well as official court reports, estimated that between 50 and 100 prosecutions had been initiated involving acts as diverse as spitting, biting, blood splattering, blood donation, and sexual intercourse with an unsuspecting partner (35). Though small in number, these cases have drawn great attention. In the vast majority, there was either an acquittal or the prosecution was dropped. In the small number of cases that produced guilty verdicts, there have been some unusually harsh sentences. In Nevada, where prostitution is both legal and regulated, a woman was sentenced to 20 years imprisonment in 1989 under a statute that made solicitation by those who tested positive for HIV a felony. In the same year, an Indiana appeals court upheld a conviction for attempted murder against an individual who had splattered blood on emergency workers seeking to prevent him from committing suicide (36).

Whatever the allure of such measures and of the rediscovery of traditional public health approaches in the effort to combat the spread of HIV infection, it has remained clear that the future course of the AIDS epidemic will be determined by the creation of a social and institutional milieu within which radical voluntary changes in behavior can occur and be sustained. Educational campaigns and counseling programs, most effectively undertaken by groups linked to the populations at risk, have remained the centerpiece of that preventive effort.

THE ETHICS OF RESEARCH

In the absence of effective therapies for those with AIDS and HIV-related disease in the epidemic's first years, research on potentially effective treatments for opportunistic infections and on antiviral agents took on enormous significance. The desperation of those who were diagnosed with what was almost uniformly viewed as an ultimately fatal condition generated demands for a reconsideration not only of how research was funded, about the level of federal support for such efforts, but of the premises of the ethical regime that governed such work.

The contemporary history of human experimentation is haunted by the specter of abuse. The work of the Nazi doctors exposed at Nuremberg, the Tuskegee syphilis study that exploited poor black men in the American South, the catalog of misdeeds made public by Henry Knowles Beecher in the *New England Journal of Medicine* (37), all provided the backdrop to the effort to formulate ethical standards to guide the conduct of investigators dependent on the collaboration of women, men, and children as they sought to advance the scientific understanding of disease and its cures.

In the mid-1970s the National Commission for the Protection of Human Subjects of Biomedical and Behav-

ioral Research examined these issues and in its Belmont Report (38) codified a set of ethical principles to guide the work of researchers. Those norms provided the foundations for regulations subsequently enacted by the Department of Health and Human Services (39) and the Food and Drug Administration (40). At the core of those guidelines was the radical distinction between research designed to produce socially necessary, generalizable knowledge, and therapy designed to benefit individuals. Against the former, individuals—but especially those who were socially vulnerable—needed protection against conscription.

AIDS has forced a reconsideration of this formulation. There had been challenges to federal protections in the past, for example, when prisoners at Jackson State Prison in Michigan demanded that they be permitted to serve as research subjects because participation provided them with *social* advantages (41). But the HIV epidemic has provided the circumstances for the emergence of a broad and potent political movement that has sought to reshape radically the conditions under which research is undertaken. The role of the randomized clinical trial, the importance of placebo controls, the centrality of academic research institutions, the dominance of scientists over subjects, the sharp distinction between research and therapy, and the protectionist ethos of the Belmont Report have all been brought into question.

Although scholars concerned with the methodological demands of sound research and ethicists committed to the protection of research subjects have played a crucial role in the ensuing discussions, both as defenders of the received wisdom and as critics, the debate has been driven by the articulate demands of those most threatened by AIDS. Most prominent have been groups such as the People With AIDS Coalition and ACT-UP, organizations made up primarily of white gay men. But advocates of women's, children's, and prisoners' rights have also made their voices heard. What has been so stunning, disconcerting to some, and exciting to others has been the rhythm of challenge and response. Rather than the careful exchange of academic arguments, we have been witness to the mobilization of disruptive and effective political protest.

The threat of death has hovered over the process. As Carol Levine has noted in her essay "Has AIDS Changed the Ethics of Human Subjects Research?" (42), "the shortage of proven therapeutic alternatives for AIDS and the belief that trials are, in and of themselves, beneficial have led to the claim that people have a right to be research subjects. This is the exact opposite of the tradition starting with Nuremberg—that people have a right *not* to be research subjects." It is that striking reversal that has resulted in a rejection of the model of research conducted at remote academic centers, with restrictive (protective) standards of access, and strict adherence to the "gold standard" of the randomized clinical trial. Blurring the distinction between research and treatment—"A Drug Trial is Health Care Too"—those insistent on radical reform have sought to open wide the points of entry to new "therapeutic" agents both within and outside clinical trials, have demanded that the paternalistic ethical warrant for the protection of the vulnerable from research be replaced by an ethical regime informed by respect for the autonomous choice of potential subjects who could weigh, for themselves, the potential risks and benefits of new treatments for HIV infection. Thus demands have been made that women be enrolled in trials in greater numbers; that prisoners and drug users be granted access; that children be included in trials at a much (earlier) point than had been considered acceptable. Moreover, the revisionists have demanded a basic reconceptualization of the relationship between researchers and subjects. In place of protocols imposed from above, they have proposed a more egalitarian and democratic model in which negotiation would replace scientific authority.

The reformulation of the ethics of research that has begun under the impact of AIDS has implications that go far beyond the epidemic of HIV disease, since the emerging new conceptions and standards could govern the conduct of the entire research enterprise. Furthermore, the role of the carefully controlled clinical trial, as providing protection against the wide-scale use of drugs whose safety and efficacy have not yet been proved, no longer commands unquestioned support. At this moment, protagonists who have been locked in often acrimonious debate foretell very different consequences of the changing social standards of research. Proponents of the new ethos hold out the prospect of a new regime that is both respectful of individual rights and the requirements of good science. Martin Delaney of Project Inform in San Francisco, for example, has stated that "regulatory practices contribute to the failure of science, demean the public good, and tread heavily on our civil liberties. . . . Science and patient alike would be better served by a system that permits life-threatened patients some form of access to the most promising experimental therapies, peacefully coexisting alongside a program of unencumbered clinical research" (43). Those who are less sanguine have spoken in a different voice. George Annas has warned that the blurring of the distinction between research and treatment can only harm the desperate. "It is not compassionate to hold out false hope to terminally ill patients so that they spend their last dollars on unproven 'remedies' that they might live longer" (44). Jerome Groopman of New England Deaconess Hospital in Boston has gone further and sees the contemporary liberalization as a threat to the research enterprise itself. "If the philosophy is that anyone can decide at any point what drugs he or she wants to take, then you will not be able to do a clinical trial" (45). Whether such dire predictions will prove prescient or utterly mistaken, it is still too soon to tell. What is possible now is to understand how the debate thus far has shaped the process of reform.

THE ETHICS OF CARE

For almost four decades, health-care workers in the United States, as well as in other advanced industrial societies, were largely shielded from what had been the routine experience of those who had in prior eras worked with the sick: the acquisition of their patients' infections and sometimes lethal diseases (46). Though never as total as many had come to believe, this invincibility was psychologically ruptured by the intrusion of AIDS, beginning in 1981. AIDS forced physicians and health-care workers to consider the possibility that theirs was indeed a "dangerous trade."

Early in the history of this epidemic, broad-scale uncertainty about what accounted for the collapse of the immune systems of those who had fallen ill contributed to considerable anxiety in the general population, but especially among those who came into physical contact with AIDS patients or with materials that they had touched. Morticians, garbage collectors, correctional officials, and health-care workers expressed alarm and sought to distance themselves from those they feared as a source of contamination (47). Anecdotal reports began to surface about hospital aides leaving food trays at the doors of those who were sick, and of nurses, physicians, and dentists refusing to treat patients with the new disease. With greater epidemiologic experience it became clear that there was nothing to fear from what was termed "casual transmission." With the isolation of the viral agent responsible for AIDS and the rapid development of a better understanding of how the virus behaved, it became even clearer that those who came into contact with infected patients had little to fear if appropriate precautions were taken with body fluids, and especially with blood.

As noted earlier in this chapter, the Centers for Disease Control contributed to the containment of the anxiety by the publication in late 1985 and 1986 of a series of reports in *Morbidity and Mortality Weekly Report* that sought to provide guidance for sound infection control practice and rational social policy. The special context of health-care facilities with the possibility of exposure to blood and other body fluids was subjected to careful attention. For purposes of establishing a margin of safety, the CDC asserted that the risk of hepatitis B provided a worst case scenario. Infection control precautions adequate to the prevention of the transmission of hepatitis B would be more than adequate to the protection of health-care workers from HIV (13).

Since those initial recommendations were issued, epidemiologic studies of health-care workers have repeatedly demonstrated how very low are the risks of acquiring HIV. Even among those exposed to needlesticks involving blood from AIDS patients, the rate of infection has been very low. Perhaps 0.5% to 3/1000 have seroconverted (14).

But to say that the risks of HIV transmission among health-care workers are extremely low does not mean that the risk is zero. Rare events, though of low frequency, do occur. The relatively few cases of HIV transmission that have occurred in the context of the health-care setting led to a number of well-publicized instances of physicians refusing to treat infected patients. At times such refusals were justified explicitly in terms of the right of the physician to self-protection.

Confronted with the challenge represented by the voice of narrow self-interest and the threat of patient abandonment, those committed to staunching the emerging trend turned to history (17) in hopes that an unambiguous lesson on responsibility of physicians would emerge. Physicians had, after all, been called to respond when epidemics were more common, when morbidity was awesome. For those who had hoped to discover a univocal message from the chronicles of the past, history proved a disappointment. Although some physicians had stayed behind to care for their patients, many had fled. At times they did so in order that they might attend to their fleeing patrons, sometimes simply to protect themselves. Perhaps most significant as a reflection of the extent to which many physicians refused to remain with those afflicted in earlier plagues was the need to make arrangements for the care of the sick through the special institution of the "plague doctor." Employed by local merchants and the political elites, these physicians took up where others had failed (48).

If history failed to provide clear guidance, what of the codes of ethics that have expressed the aspirations of the guilds and associations of medical practitioners? What of the statements of those who have sought to provide a moral standard against which to measure physician conduct? Remarkably, such statements and codes had been silent on the duty of physicians to treat in the time of epidemics (17). In this regard, the AMA code of 1847 (49) was unique in its forthright assertion of such a responsibility. "And when pestilence prevails, it is their duty to face the danger and to continue their labors for the alleviation of suffering, even at the jeopardy of their own lives." This provision remained in the code until 1957, when a revised and shortened statement eliminated the stipulation that must certainly have seemed an anachronism. After all, the era of epidemics had come to an end in the advanced industrial world.

But remaining in the code was a provision—first incorporated into the AMA's statement of professional responsibility of 1912—that, in the absence of a strong assertion of a duty to care, was to be a source of great confusion when AIDS confronted American medicine. "A physician shall," stated Section VI of the AMA's code, "in the provision of appropriate patient care, except in emergencies, be free to choose whom to serve" (50). A statement of unbounded professional discretion—and of opposition to state interference in the medical entrepreneur's freedom—Section VI was ultimately incompatible with any notion of moral responsibility on the part of physicians. Amending the blunt articulation of an unencumbered professional freedom, the AMA's Judicial Council has ruled that refusals to treat on the basis of race, religion, or creed were unethical (51). In November 1987, in the seventh year of the AIDS epidemic, the Council ruled that "a physician may not ethically refuse to treat a patient whose condition is within the physician's current realm of competence solely because the patient is seropositive" (52).

As philosophers have attempted to struggle with this issue, they, at times, have stressed the importance of a *social* responsibility to guarantee each HIV-infected individual with access to health care, the responsibility of the health-care *professions* (46) as collective entities to provide appropriate care to those in need, rather than the responsibility of each individual health-care worker to treat. In short, some argued, if somewhat reluctantly, that as long as the needs of the HIV infected were met, there might be no sound ethical grounds for insisting that each health-care worker share in the responsibility.

Others have argued for a more universal obligation (53). Acknowledging the right of individuals to opt out of the duty to treat could well subvert the ultimate capacity of the system as a whole to meet the responsibility to treat in a humane, respectful, and efficient manner. Permitting large numbers of individuals to opt out could create serious burdens for those who agreed to treat, making them bear an unfair share of social responsibility, thus contributing to the problem of "burnout." Recognizing the right of health-care professionals to opt out would represent one more step in the erosion of the special role and status of medicine. It was Edmund Pellegrino, the physician–philosopher, who warned that "to refuse to care for AIDS patients, even if the danger were greater than it is, is to abnegate what is essential to being a physician" (54). Since house staff, nurses, and other hospital personnel do not generally enjoy the same discretion as private physicians, permitting individuals to opt out would create a bifurcated system within which those "employed" as health-care workers would be held to one standard, while "free professionals" would be held to another. Finally, permitting physicians to opt out of the duty to care because of *their* fears of HIV transmission could foster an atmosphere of irrational fear in other social realms. Rather than physicians serving as a moral yardstick against which to judge the actions of laypeople (e.g., employers and school administrators), they would give succor to those whose fears—no matter how exaggerated—drove them to the wholesale exclusion from social life of all HIV-infected individuals.

For many who stressed a universal obligation to treat, it is clear that the relatively low risk of infection has been central. Were the risks of HIV transmission very much greater, it would have required an ethics of heroism to insist that each health-care worker bear the responsibility of assuring adequate and appropriate health care for the infected. Given the level of risk entailed in the face of HIV infection, even among surgeons and obstetricians, those who stressed the obligation to treat argued that it was not heroism but more straightforward duty that was involved.

The issue of access to care is not, however, primarily raised by the specter of physician abandonment. Rather, it centers on the problem of the structure of the American health-care system. Despite the extraordinary increase in expenditures for health care over the past three decades and the rise in government financing through Medicare and Medicaid, significant and growing inequities continue to plague the health-care system. Millions of Americans either have no health insurance at all or are inadequately protected by limited and intermittent coverage (55). With growing concern about the rise in health-care costs, public attention has shifted from the social goal of securing equitable access for the unprotected to the issue of "cost containment." The reformist drive of the 1960s, which sought to create an equitable health-care system, is nearly exhausted.

For those concerned with the ethics of health care, the creation of a just and adequate health-care system capable of responding to persons with HIV infection, as well as to those with other diseases, requires the elimination of the prevailing economic barriers to medical services. A central feature of any such program of reform, they have held, must be the creation of a system of universal health insurance protection. But we are far from such a system. And it is the current pattern of inequality that has set the stage for a uniquely American question: How will we assure access to care on the part of those not only with AIDS but of those with asymptomatic HIV infection who will need early clinical intervention?

The striking contrast between important clinical advances in the care of those with HIV infection and the social organization of American medicine led the National Commission on Acquired Immune Deficiency Syndrome to warn in a December 1989 report to the President (56) that medical breakthroughs would "mean little unless the health care system can incorporate them and make them accessible to people in need." The existence of a medically disenfranchised class meant that, for many, access to care was almost solely through the "emergency room door of one of the few hospitals in the country that treats people with HIV infection and AIDS."

The looming crisis in health care for those with HIV disease set the stage for congressional action in mid-1990 that could scarcely have been imagined a short time earlier. Such action represented the fruit of dogged efforts on the part of AIDS activists, their allies, and some political leaders from the cities and states that had borne the disproportionate share of AIDS cases. In the winter of 1990, Senator Edward Kennedy, the exemplar of Democratic party liberalism, and Senator Orin Hatch, a Republican whose stance on abortion often cast him in the role of a conservative, jointly sponsored legislation—the Comprehensive AIDS Resource Emergency Act of 1990 —that would have provided a major infusion of federal assistance to those localities most severely burdened by AIDS. As the government had responded to natural disasters, the Kennedy–Hatch Bill asked it to respond to the medical disaster of AIDS. "The human immunodeficiency virus constitutes a crisis as devastating as an earthquake, flood or drought. Indeed, the death toll of the unfolding AIDS tragedy is already a hundredfold greater than any natural disaster to strike our nation in this century" (57).

As remarkable as the joint sponsorship of this legislation, which promised to provide $2.9 billion over 5 years in a complex political formula to the cities and states most severely struck by AIDS, was the overwhelming support the legislation received in the Senate, where the vote in favor was 95–4 (58). When similar legislation, with even greater resource commitments, was voted on by the House of Representatives, the vote was 408–14 (59).

However late in coming, this legislation represented on both symbolic and practical levels an important act of national solidarity. But the hopes of early summer were dashed by the fall as the Congress, confronted with a severe budgetary crisis, slashed funds for the now renamed Ryan White Act. What allocations will be made in successive years cannot be foretold. It is certain, however, that such an emergency act cannot be a substitute for the fundamental change in the organization and financing of health care in the United States that will be required by the chronic management of the medical and social needs of all HIV-infected persons at a moment when so many other medical needs of the nation's poor remain unmet.

In the meantime, those with HIV disease will require ongoing, often expensive, medical care. Their needs will force an answer to the question: Can a fundamentally unjust health-care system respond equitably to the challenges posed by AIDS?

Typically, efforts directed at preventing disease and those that seek to provide clinical care are viewed as conceptually distinct. In the day-to-day world of competition for limited resources, funds made available to one often mean funds not available to the other. That is true in the case of AIDS as well. But from another perspective these efforts can be seen as intimately linked. Attempts to slow the spread of HIV infection among gay men have been strikingly effective. Success has been more illusive among those whose risk of infection is linked to intravenous drug use and among those who are the sexual partners of drug users, the vast majority of whom are poor, black, and Hispanic.

The possibility of reaching such individuals with life-prolonging clinical services provides an unparalleled opportunity—as would the provision of drug abuse services—to council repeatedly about the necessity of behavioral change. Thus the failure to provide care will not only mean needlessly foreshortened lives and needless misery but a lost opportunity to reinforce the message of prevention and in so doing to affect the future trajectory of the epidemic itself.

The AIDS epidemic has posed a series of pressing ethical challenges to American society. Although the disease is relatively new, the issues posed are, at the most fundamental level, not at all new. They go to the heart of the complex task of policymaking in a liberal society, one that proclaims respect for individual rights and social justice. By compelling us to confront these issues in the context of a lethal epidemic, AIDS has revealed not only the strength of those values but the extent to which they remain aspirations rather than realities. More troubling is the realization that those values may at times serve to mask a profound unwillingness to transform the shape of the health-care system. AIDS thus provides a mirror on American life in the last decade of the 20th century.

REFERENCES

1. Bayer R. *Private acts, social consequences: AIDS and the politics of public health,* 2nd ed. New Brunswick: Rutgers University Press; 1991.
2. American Association of Physicians for Human Rights. Nov 12, 1985, unpublished.
3. Northern California Branch, American Civil Liberties Union. *AIDS and civil liberties.* San Francisco: Northern California Branch, ACLU, Mar 1986.
4. Bayer R, Levine C, Wolf SM. HIV antibody screening: an ethical framework for evaluating proposed programs. *JAMA* 1986;256: 1768–74.
5. Association of State Territorial Health Officials. *ASTHO guide to public health practice: HTLV III antibody testing and community approaches.* Washington, DC: Public Health Foundation; 1985.
6. American Medical Association. *Report of the Council on Ethical and Judicial Affairs: ethical issues involved in the growing AIDS crisis.* Chicago: American Medical Association; 1987.
7. US Public Health Service. Guidelines for prophylaxis against *Pneumocystis carinii* pneumonia for persons infected with human immunodeficiency virus disease. *MMWR* 1989;38(suppl 5):1–9.
8. Levine C, Bayer R. The ethics of screening for early intervention in HIV disease. *Am J Public Health* 1989;79(12):1661–7.
9. Bayer R. Should newborns be routinely tested for HIV? *Med Ethics* 1990;5(1):18.
10. Faden R, Holtzman N, Chwalow A. Parental rights, child welfare, and public health: the case of PKU screening. *Am J Public Health* 1982;72:1396–400.
11. Centers for Disease Control. Education and foster care for children infected with human T-lymphotropic virus type III/lymphadenopathy-associated virus. *MMWR* 1985;34:517–21.
12. Centers for Disease Control. Recommendations for preventing transmission of infection with human T-lymphotropic virus type III/lymphadenopathy-associated virus in the workplace. *MMWR* 1985;34:681–6,691–5.
13. Centers for Disease Control. Recommendations for preventing transmission of infection with human T-lymphotropic virus type III/lymphadenopathy-associated virus during invasive procedures. *MMWR* 1986;35:221–3.
14. Friedland GH, Klein RS. Transmission of the human immunodeficiency virus. *N Engl J Med* 1987;317:1125–35.
15. Centers for Disease Control. Update: acquired immunodeficiency syndrome and human immunodeficiency virus infection among health-care workers. *MMWR* 1988;37:229–39.
16. *New York Times,* Nov 9, 1987.
17. Zuger A, Miles SH. Physicians, AIDS and occupational risk: historic traditions and ethical obligations. *JAMA* 1987;258:1924–28.
18. Gostin L. HIV-infected physicians and the practice of seriously invasive procedures. *Hastings Center Report* 1989;19:32–9.
19. *Surgeon General's Report on acquired immune deficiency syndrome.* Washington, DC: US Government Printing Office; 1986.
20. Centers for Disease Control. Recommendations for assisting in the prevention of perinatal transmission of human T-lymphotropic virus type III/lymphadenopathy-associated virus and acquired immunodeficiency syndrome. *MMWR* 1985;34:721–6,731–2.
21. Institute of Medicine and National Academy of Sciences. *Confronting AIDS.* Washington, DC: National Academy Press; 1986:96.
22. Presidential Commission on the Human Immuno Deficiency Virus Epidemic. *Final Report,* 1986.
23. Association of State and Territorial Health Officials. *ASTHO guide to public health practice: HTLV III antibody testing and community approaches.* Washington, DC: Public Health Foundation; 1985:16.
24. Bayer R, Levine C, Murray TH. Guidelines for confidentiality in research on AIDS. *IRB: Rev Hum Subjects Res* 1984;6(6):1–7.
25. Hermann DHJ. AIDS malpractice and transmission liability. *Univ Colorado Law Rev* 1986–1987;58:63–107.
26. Bayer R, Gostin L. Legal and ethical issues in AIDS. In: Gottlieb MS, et al., eds. *Current Topics in AIDS,* vol 2. New York: Wiley; 1989:1–29.
27. *Tarasoff* v. *Regents of the State of California,* 17 Cal. 3d 425,551p. 2d334,131 *Cal Rptr* 14(Cal) 1976.
28. Dickens BM. Legal limits of AIDS confidentiality. *JAMA* 1988;259:3449–51.
29. American Medical Association. Prevention and control of acquired immunodeficiency syndrome. *JAMA* 1987;258:2097–103.
30. Report of the Presidential Commission on the Human Immunodeficiency Virus Epidemic. Washington, DC, 1988.
31. Association of State and Territorial Health Officials. *Guide to public health practice: HIV partner notification strategies.* Washington, DC: Public Health Foundation; 1988.
32. Bayer R, Healton C. Controlling AIDS in Cuba. *N Engl J Med* 1989;320:1022–4.
33. Based on a review of all AIDS-related legislation in the files of the Intergovernmental Health Policy Project, Washington, DC. See Field M, Sullivan K. AIDS and the criminal law. *Law Med Health Care* 1987;Summer:46–60.
34. *New York Times,* Feb 10, 1990:25.
35. Gostin LO. The AIDS Litigation Project: a national review of court and Human Rights Commission decisions, part I: the social impact of AIDS. *JAMA* 1990;263:1963.
36. Gostin LO. The politics of AIDS: compulsory state powers, public health, civil liberties. *Ohio State Law J* 1989:1041.
37. Beecher HN, Ethics in clinical research. *N Engl J Med* 1966;274:1354–60.
38. National Commission for the Protection of Human Subjects of Biomedical and Behavioral Research. *The Belmont report: ethical principles and guidelines for the protection of human subjects of research.* Washington, DC: Department of Health, Education and Welfare; 1978.

39. Department of Health and Human Services. Rules and regulations. 1983; 45 CFR 46.

40. Food and Drug Administration. Protection of human subjects: prisoners as the subjects of research. 1980; 45 CFR 36.

41. Dubler NW, Sidel VW. On research on HIV infection and AIDS in correctional facilities. *Milbank Q* 1989;67:171–207.

42. Levine C. Has AIDS changed the ethics of human subjects research? *Law Med Health Care* 1988;16:167–73.

43. Delaney M. The case for patient access to experimental therapy. *J Infect Dis* 1989;159:416–9.

44. Annas G. Faith (healing), hope and charity at the FDA: the politics of AIDS drug trials. *Villanova Law Rev* 1989;34:771–97.

45. CDC. *AIDS Weekly* Dec 1989;11:3.

46. Arras J. The fragile web of professional responsibility: AIDS and the duty to treat. *Hastings Center Report,* Special Suppl April/May 1988.

47. Bayer R. AIDS and the gay community: between the promise and the spectre of medicine. *Social Res* 1985;52(3):581–606.

48. Fox D. The politics of physicians' responsibility in epidemics: a note on history. *Hastings Center Report,* Special Suppl April/May 1988.

49. Council on Ethical and Judicial Affairs. American Medical Association: ethical issues involved in the growing AIDS crisis. Report A(1-87);1.

50. American Medical Association. *Principles of medical ethics.* Chicago: American Medical Association; 1980.

51. Current Opinions of the Council on Ethical and Judicial Affairs. American Medical Association: ethical issues, sections 9,11. 1986.

52. Current Opinions of the Council on Ethical and Judicial Affairs. American Medical Association: ethical issues. Nov 1987.

53. Bayer R. AIDS and the duty to treat: risk, responsibility, and health care workers. *Bull NY Acad Med* 1988;64(6):498–505.

54. Pellegrino E. Altruism, self interest and medical ethics. *JAMA* 1987;258(14):1939–40.

55. Davis K, Rowland D. Uninsured and undeserved: inequities in health care in the US. *Milbank Memorial Fund Q* 1987;61(2):149.

56. National Commission on AIDS. Report Nov 1, 1989.

57. Senator Edward Kennedy. Letter. Feb 1990, unpublished.

58. *New York Times,* May 17, 1990:B-10.

59. *New York Times,* June 14, 1990:B-9.

Subject Index

A

Acquired immunodeficiency syndrome, (AIDS) *see also* HIV infection
  in Africa, 25, 28–30, 88–89, 532–533
  age and, 4–5, 6, 7, 202, 209
  animal models for, 117–123
  antibodies in, 146–147, 634
  in Asia, 25, 31–32
  B-cell function in, 157–158, 207–208, 269
  case reporting, 2
  CD4+ T cells in, 63–64, 79–81, 145–146, 149, 221
  in children, 208–210, 323–324, 375, 527–530
  clinical progression of, 77–78, 89–90
  CMV infection in, 249, 251, 252, 253–259, 261–262, 565
  confidentiality of, 363–364
  cryptococcus infections and, 331, 360, 393–396, 397–401, 507, 563–564
  definition of, 2, 26–27, 217–218, 499
  diagnosis, 2, 104, 173, 209
  earliest cases, 2
  epidemiology, 1–14, 25–32, 279–283, 596–600
  ethical concerns in, 363–364, 689–699
  in Europe, 31
  in health care workers, 7, 8, 599–604
  HIV-2 and, 25, 29–30, 89–91, 102
  immunosuppression and, 145, 146, 253–254, 594
  incubation period of, 77
  infection control, 585–595, 645–655
  mortality, 7, 9, 28, 32, 259
  neoplasms in, 1, 28, 50–51, 259, 337–338, 419, 425–426, 443–452
  neurological complications in, 256–257, 315–340, 374–375, 543–551, 575–578
  nutritional status and, 427–428
  PC and, 1, 27, 66, 132, 225, 226, 239–240,
  progression, 77–78, 90, 146, 209
  protozoan infections in, 383–390, 423–424, 433–439
  prevention programs, 645–655
  reporting completeness, 3
  risk reduction, 645–655
  stigma of, 349–350
  suicide and, 353–354
  surveillance, 2–6, 10, 13–14, 27, 217–218
  survival rate, 611

  toxoplasmosis and, 384–385, 387, 389, 558–563
  tuberculosis and, 278–297
  viral cofactors, 77, 78–82
  in United States, 3–8, 30, 280–283
Acyclovir
  in HSV treatment, 333
  in ocular herpes infection, 484
Adolescent HIV infection
  age and, 202
  classification of, 219
  heterosexual transmission in, 202
  HIV diagnosis in, 203–205
  in United States, 18, 202
  by year of reporting, 18
Adrenal gland
  in AIDS, 258
  in CMV infection, 258
  pathology, 258
Africa
  AIDS incidence in, 25, 28
  AIDS mortality in, 29
  AIDS pathology in, 532–533
  HIV-1 in 25, 28, 88–89, 91
  HIV-2 in, 88–89, 91
  HIV epidemiology in, 25, 26, 28–30, 88–89
  HIV transmission in, 28, 29
  immunization of HIV infected in, 672
  tuberculosis in, 28, 533
Age
  AIDS cases by, 4–5, 6, 7, 29, 202
  AIDS mortality and, 7
  of AIDS diagnosis, 19
  CD4+ cell counts and, 204
  of HIV infection 202, 203–204
  HIV transmission and, 29, 90
  MAC infection and, 300
  TB cases by, 282
AIDS cases
  by age, 4–5, 6, 8, 90
  annual incidence, 7, 8
  definition of, 26–27
  by exposure category, 4–5, 8
  in Europe, 31
  in females, 4–5, 6, 8
  geographic distribution, 9–10
  in health-care workers, 7, 8, 600, 603, 604
  heterosexually infected, 4, 6, 8
  in homosexuals, 3–4, 6, 8, 9–10
  in IV drug users, 4–5, 6, 8, 9

  in males, 3, 4–5, 6, 8
  by minority populations, 7, 8
  in no identified risk group, 6–7, 8, 201
  pediatric, 5, 8, 17–21, 89, 201–202
  by racial/ethnic populations, 6, 7
  in United States, 1–14, 17–18, 25, 201–202
  in world, 25
AIDS-dementia complex, (ADC)
  Alzheimer's disease and, 377
  cerebral cortex in, 551
  in children, 323–324, 375
  classification of, 543
  clinical features, 322–324, 374–375, 378
  CMV and, 543
  CSF analysis in, 322–323, 375, 376, 377
  CT in, 323–324, 375, 544, 545, 548
  dementia and, 549, 550, 551
  demyelination in, 324
  depression and, 375
  development of, 322–323, 374
  diagnosis, 375–377, 543
  EEG findings in, 320
  epidemiology, 377
  focal microglial infiltration in, 544–546
  gp 120 protein and, 553–554
  herpes infection and, 320
  histopathology in, 544–545, 547, 549, 550–551, 555
  HIV infection and, 315, 320, 322–324, 543, 544, 552
  immune system in, 379
  incidence, 543
  JC virus and, 543, 547
  leukoencephalopathy in, 546, 547–548, 549–550
  MNCs in, 543, 544–546, 549, 550, 551
  motor function in, 374, 375
  MS findings in, 547–548
  myelopathy in, 324–325, 545
  neuroimaging in, 323, 375–376, 377
  neuronal density in, 551
  pathogenic model for, 553
  pathophysiology, 324, 373, 378, 380, 543–551
  prevention, 380
  progression of, 377
  psychological testing in, 375
  relation to HIV-1 infection, 378, 379
  terminology in, 373–374, 543–544